CLINICAL HANDBOOK OF PSYCHOLOGICAL DISORDERS

CLINICAL HANDBOOK OF
PSYCHOLOGICAL
DISORDERS

A Step-by-Step Treatment Manual

FOURTH EDITION

EDITED BY
DAVID H. BARLOW

THE GUILFORD PRESS
New York   London

To Beverly
For love, loyalty, and dedication

© 2008 The Guilford Press
A Division of Guilford Publications, Inc.
72 Spring Street, New York, NY 10012
www.guilford.com

Printed in the United States of America

This book is printed on acid-free paper.

Last digit is print number: 9 8 7 6 5 4

The authors have checked with sources believed to be reliable in their efforts to provide
information that is complete and generally in accord with the standards of practice that are
accepted at the time of publication. However, in view of the possibility of human error or
changes in medical sciences, neither the authors, nor the editor and publisher, nor any other
party who has been involved in the preparation or publication of this work warrants that
the information contained herein is in every respect accurate or complete, and they are not
responsible for any errors or omissions or the results obtained from the use of such
information. Readers are encouraged to confirm the information contained in this book with
other sources.

Library of Congress Cataloging-in-Publication Data

Clinical handbook of psychological disorders : a step-by-step treatment manual / edited by
David H. Barlow.—4th ed.
    p. ; cm.
  Includes bibliographical references and index.
  ISBN-13: 978-1-59385-572-7 (hardcover : alk. paper)
  ISBN-10: 1-59385-572-9 (hardcover : alk. paper)
  1. Behavior therapy—Handbooks, manuals, etc. 2. Medical protocols—Handbooks,
manuals, etc. I. Barlow, David H.
  [DNLM: 1. Mental Disorders—therapy. 2. Psychotherapy—methods. WM 420 C6415
2008]
  RC489.B4C584 2008
  616.89′1—dc22
                                                              2007015429

About the Editor

David H. Barlow, PhD, is Professor of Psychology and Psychiatry and Founder and Director Emeritus of the Center for Anxiety and Related Disorders at Boston University. He has published over 500 articles and chapters and close to 50 books and clinical manuals—some translated in over 20 languages, including Arabic, Chinese, and Russian—mostly in the area of emotional disorders and clinical research methodology. Dr. Barlow has been the recipient of numerous awards throughout his career, most recently the American Board of Professional Psychology's Distinguished Service Award to the Profession of Psychology in 2006. He is past president of the Society of Clinical Psychology (Division 12) of the American Psychological Association and the Association for Advancement of Behavior Therapy (now the Associaton for Behavioral and Cognitive Therapies) and past editor of the journals *Behavior Therapy*, the *Journal of Applied Behavior Analysis*, and *Clinical Psychology: Science and Practice*. Dr. Barlow was chair of the American Psychological Association Task Force on Psychological Intervention Guidelines, a member of the DSM-IV Task Force of the American Psychiatric Association, and a cochair of the DSM-IV work group for revising the anxiety disorder categories. He is a Diplomate in Clinical Psychology of the American Board of Professional Psychology and maintains a private practice.

Contributors

Michael E. Addis, PhD, Department of Psychology, Clark University, Worcester, Massachusetts

Laura B. Allen, PhD, Center for Anxiety and Related Disorders and Department of Psychology, Boston University, Boston, Massachusetts

Amy K. Bach, PhD, Department of Psychiatry and Human Behavior, Brown University, Providence, Rhode Island

David H. Barlow, PhD, Center for Anxiety and Related Disorders and Department of Psychology, Boston University, Boston, Massachusetts

Aaron T. Beck, MD, Department of Psychiatry, School of Medicine, University of Pennsylvania, Philadelphia, Pennsylvania, and Beck Institute for Cognitive Therapy and Research, Bala Cynwyd, Pennsylvania

Kathryn L. Bleiberg, PhD, Department of Psychiatry, Weill Cornell Medical College, Cornell University, New York, New York

Andrew Christensen, PhD, Department of Psychology, University of California, Los Angeles, California

Zafra Cooper, DPhil, Department of Psychiatry, University of Oxford, Oxford, United Kingdom

Michelle G. Craske, PhD, Department of Psychology, University of California, Los Angeles, California

Elizabeth T. Dexter-Mazza, PsyD, Department of Psychology, University of Washington, Seattle, Washington

Sona Dimidjian, PhD, Department of Psychology, University of Colorado, Boulder, Colorado

Christopher G. Fairburn, MD, Department of Psychiatry, Oxford University, Oxford, United Kingdom

Edna B. Foa, PhD, Department of Psychiatry and Center for the Treatment and Study of Anxiety, University of Pennsylvania, Philadelphia, Pennsylvania

Martin E. Franklin, PhD, Department of Psychiatry and Center for the Treatment and Study of Anxiety, University of Pennsylvania, Philadelphia, Pennsylvania

Sarah H. Heil, PhD, Departments of Psychiatry and Psychology, University of Vermont, Burlington, Vermont

Richard G. Heimberg, PhD, Adult Anxiety Clinic and Department of Psychology, Temple University, Philadelphia, Pennsylvania

Ruth Herman-Dunn, PhD, private practice, Seattle, Washington

Stephen T. Higgins, PhD, Departments of Psychiatry and Psychology, University of Vermont, Burlington, Vermont

Neil S. Jacobson, PhD (deceased), Department of Psychology, University of Washington, Seattle, Washington

Marsha M. Linehan, PhD, Departments of Psychology and Psychiatry and Behavioral Sciences, University of Washington, Seattle, Washington

Leanne Magee, MA, Adult Anxiety Clinic and Department of Psychology, Temple University, Philadelphia, Pennsylvania

John C. Markowitz, MD, Department of Psychiatry, New York State Psychiatric Institute, New York, New York

Christopher R. Martell, PhD, private practice, Seattle, Washington, and Department of Psychiatry and Behavioral Sciences, University of Washington, Seattle, Washington

Barbara S. McCrady, PhD, Center on Alcoholism, Substance Abuse, and Addictions, and Department of Psychology, University of New Mexico, Albuquerque, New Mexico

R. Kathryn McHugh, MA, Center for Anxiety and Related Disorders and Department of Psychology, Boston University, Boston, Massachusetts

David J. Miklowitz, PhD, Department of Psychology, University of Colorado, Boulder, Colorado

Candice M. Monson, PhD, National Center for PTSD, VA Boston Healthcare System, Boston, Massachusetts

Patricia A. Resick, PhD, National Center for PTSD, VA Boston Healthcare System, Boston, Massachusetts

Shireen L. Rizvi, PhD, Department of Psychology, New School for Social Research, New York, New York

Jayne L. Rygh, PhD, Cognitive Therapy Center of New York, New York, New York

Roz Shafran, PhD, School of Psychology and Clinical Language Science, Reading University, Reading, United Kingdom

Stacey C. Sigmon, PhD, Departments of Psychiatry and Psychology, University of Vermont, Burlington, Vermont

Nicholas Tarrier, PhD, Division of Clinical Psychology, School of Psychological Sciences, University of Manchester, Manchester, United Kingdom

Cynthia L. Turk, PhD, Anxiety Clinic and Department of Psychology, Washburn University, Topeka, Kansas

Arthur D. Weinberger, PhD, Cognitive Therapy Center of New York, New York, New York

Jennifer G. Wheeler, PhD, private practice, Seattle, Washington

G. Terence Wilson, PhD, Graduate School of Applied and Professional Psychology, Rutgers, The State University of New Jersey, Piscataway, New Jersey

John P. Wincze, PhD, Department of Psychiatry and Human Behavior and Department of Psychology, Brown University, Providence, Rhode Island

Jeffrey E. Young, PhD, Department of Psychiatry, Columbia University, and Cognitive Therapy Center of New York, New York, New York

Preface

Evidence-based practice (EBP) is one of those ideas that comes along occasionally and takes the world by storm. Although some of the tenets of EBP have been around for decades (as has this *Handbook*), it is only in the past 10 years that EBP has been formally identified as a systematic method of delivering clinical care (Institute of Medicine, 2001; Sackett, Strauss, Richardson, Rosenberg, & Haynes, 2000).

Since that time the "tipping point" (Gladwell, 2000) for EBP has clearly occurred, and health care policymakers and governments as well as professional societies around the world have collectively decided that the delivery of health care, including behavioral health care, should be based on evidence (APA Task Force on Evidence-Based Practice, 2006). Fulfilling this mandate comprises the goals of EBP, and has also been the goal of this book since the first edition was published in 1985.

The fourth edition of this book continues to represent a distinct departure from any number of similar books reviewing advances in the treatment of psychological disorders from the perspective of EBP. Over the past two decades we have developed a technology of behavior change that necessarily differs from disorder to disorder.

This technology consists of a variety of techniques or procedures with more or less proven effectiveness for a given disorder (and increasingly for classes of disorders). Naturally, we have more evidence of the effectiveness of these treatments for some disorders than for others. It also has become more apparent since the earlier editions that considerable clinical skill is required to apply this technology most effectively. Therefore, this book, in its fourth edition, is *not* another review of therapeutic procedures for a given problem with recommendations for further research. Rather, it is a detailed description of actual treatment protocols in which experienced clinicians implement the technology of behavior change in the context of the most frequently encountered disorders.

In this edition, the originators of some of the best-known psychological treatment protocols have revised and updated the descriptions of their interventions to reflect the latest developments in an increasingly powerful array of psychological treatments. Among these revisions to existing chapters, several deserve comment. Patricia A. Resick, Candice M. Monson, and Shireen L. Rizvi have updated their chapter on posttraumatic stress disorder with a new and tragic case fresh from the battlefields of Iraq. Their successful treatment of this individual suffering from the unspeakable (and intolerable) trauma of war is one consequence of today's headlines that seldom makes it into print. Drug abuse continues as a scourge that ruins individual lives, the functioning of families, and the very fabric of society. Stephen T. Higgins, Stacey C. Sigmon, and Sarah H. Heil have expanded their chapter from a more narrow focus on cocaine to a broader focus on all serious drugs of abuse. The body of evidence supporting interpersonal psychotherapy (IPT) has continued to grow in recent years, and for the first time in this edition two of the leading clinicians and teachers of IPT, Kathryn L. Bleiberg and John C. Markowitz, illustrate their fascinating approach to the treatment of depression in the context of an illuminating case.

In addition, there is much that appears for the first time in this edition, reflecting major developments in the past several years. Four original treatment protocols make their appearance—two that focus on specific disorders and two that cut across disorders. Chapter 8, by Sona Dimidjian, Christopher R. Martell, Michael E. Addis, and Ruth Herman-Dunn, describes the application of behavioral activation to depression. A variety of new evidence suggests that this approach is one of the more exciting innovations in recent years, but because it is so new, few are aware of the intricacies of its application to depressed patients. Chapter 11, by Nicholas Tarrier, presents the latest developments on psychological approaches to schizophrenia directed mostly at the "positive" symptoms of hallucinations and delusions. Much of this work has been innovated in the United Kingdom, and is unfamiliar to many in North America despite the robust nature of evidence for efficacy.

Finally, there is growing consensus that the future of EBP will be to distill principles of effective change that cut across diagnostic conditions, making them more generally applicable. Two of these "unified" or "transdiagnostic" protocols are presented for the first time in this edition. Chapter 5 presents our own unified approach to emotional disorders, and Chapter 14 describes a transdiagnostic approach to eating disorders by the originators, Christopher G. Fairburn, Zafra Cooper, Roz Shafran, and G. Terence Wilson. As with all chapters, the nuts and bolts of clinical application are emphasized.

As with the previous editions, this book was motivated by countless clinical psychology graduate students, psychiatric residents, and other mental health professionals, either in training or in practice, asking, "But how do I do it?" Realizing that there is no single source in which to find step-by-step treatment protocols for use as a guide to practice, this book attempts to fill the void. To accomplish this purpose, a number of specific topics are common to most chapters. Each chapter begins with a brief review of our knowledge of the specific disorder (or class of disorders), followed by a description of the particular model or mini-theory that guides the technology utilized with the disorder in question. This model, or mini-theory, typically answers the question, What particular facets of the disorder should be assessed and treated? While clinical application always dilutes theoretical models, clinicians will recognize behavioral and systems approaches with some psychodynamic contributions as the predominant theoretical context.

This model is followed by a description of the typical setting in which the treatment is carried out. The setting varies from disorder to disorder, ranging from the more usual office setting to the home environment of the patient. Similar detailed descriptions of the social context of treatment (e.g., the importance of the involvement of family or friends) as well as therapist and client variables that are important within the context of the particular problem are discussed. For example, therapist variables that may be important in implementing techniques for treatment of agoraphobia or couple distress are described. In addition, the implications for treatment of client variables such as dependency and unassertiveness in individuals with panic disorder with agoraphobia are discussed.

A detailed description of the actual step-by-step process of assessment and treatment follows, liberally sprinkled in many chapters with transcripts of therapy sessions. Important components of this process are the specifics of the rationale given to the patient before treatment, as well as typical problems that arise during the implementation of the technology. Where data exist, information on clinical predictors of success or failure is provided.

In accomplishing the rather ambitious goals described above, I was very fortunate in this edition of the book, as in previous editions, to have leading clinicians and researchers document in some detail how they actually treat their patients. Once again, these authorities reported that the number of details they had to include in order to convey how they actually applied their treatment programs went far beyond their expectations. My hope is that practicing clinicians and clinical students everywhere will benefit from acquaintance with these details.

In closing, I would like to express my deep appreciation to Mara Fleischer, my research and administrative assistant during the editing of this book. She worked with me and the authors every step of the way. I am sure this information will come in handy as she is now pursuing her own doctorate in clinical psychology.

DAVID H. BARLOW, PhD

REFERENCES

APA Task Force on Evidence-Based Practice. (2006). Evidence-based practice in psychology. *American Psychologist, 61,* 271–285.

Gladwell, M. (2000). *The tipping point: How little things can make a big difference.* Boston: Little, Brown.

Institute of Medicine. (2001). *Crossing the quality chasm: A new health system for the 21st century.* Washington, DC: National Academies Press.

Sackett, D. L., Strauss. S. E., Richardson, W. S., Rosenberg, W., & Haynes, R. B. (2000). *Evidence-based medicine: How to practice and teach EBM* (2nd ed.). London: Churchill Livingstone.

Contents

Panic Disorder and Agoraphobia

MICHELLE G. CRASKE
DAVID H. BARLOW

The treatment protocol described in this chapter represents one of the success stories in the development of empirically supported psychological treatments. Results from numerous studies indicate that this approach provides substantial advantages over placebo medication or alternative psychosocial approaches containing "common" factors, such as positive expectancies and helpful therapeutic alliances. In addition, this treatment forms an important part of every clinical practice guideline in either public health or other sources from countries around the world, describing effective treatments for panic disorder and agoraphobia. Results from numerous studies evaluating this treatment protocol, both individually and in combination with leading pharmacological approaches, suggest that this approach is equally effective as the best pharmacological approaches in the short term and more durable over the long term. But this treatment protocol has not stood still. For example, we have learned a great deal in the past 5 years about neurobiological mechanisms of action in fear reduction, and the best psychological methods for effecting these changes. In this chapter we present the latest version of this protocol, incorporating these changes and additions as illustrated in a comprehensive account of the treatment of "Julie."—D. H. B.

Advances continue in the development of biopsychosocial models and cognitive-behavioral treatments for panic disorder and agoraphobia. The conceptualization of panic disorder as an acquired fear of certain bodily sensations, and agoraphobia as a behavioral response to the anticipation of such bodily sensations or their crescendo into a full-blown panic attack, continues to be supported by experimental, clinical, and longitudinal research. Furthermore, the efficacy of cognitive-behavioral treatments that target fear of bodily sensations and associated agoraphobic situations is well established. In addition to presenting an up-to-date review of treatment outcome data, this chapter covers recent theoretical and empirical developments in reference to etiological factors, the role of comorbid diagnoses in treatment, ways of optimizing learning during exposure therapy, and the effect of medication on cognitive-behavioral treatments. The chapter concludes with a detailed, session-by-session outline of cognitive-behavioral treatment for panic disorder with agoraphobia (PDA). This protocol has been developed in our clinics; the full protocol is detailed in available treatment manuals (Barlow & Craske, 2006; Craske & Barlow, 2006).

NATURE OF PANIC
AND AGORAPHOBIA

Panic Attacks

"Panic attacks" are discrete episodes of intense dread or fear, accompanied by physical and cognitive symptoms, as listed in the DSM-IV-TR panic attack checklist (American Psychiatric Association, 2000). Panic attacks are discrete by virtue of their sudden or abrupt onset and brief duration, as opposed to gradually building anxious arousal. Panic attacks in panic disorder often have an unexpected quality, meaning that from the patient's perspective, they appear to happen without an obvious trigger or at unexpected times. Indeed, the diagnosis of panic disorder is given in the case of recurrent "unexpected" panic attacks, followed by at least 1 month of persistent concern about their recurrence and their consequences, or by a significant change in behavior consequent to the attacks (American Psychiatric Association, 1994).

As with all basic emotions (Izard, 1992), panic attacks are associated with strong action tendencies; Most often, these are urges to escape, and less often, urges to fight. These fight and flight tendencies usually involve elevated autonomic nervous system arousal needed to support such fight–flight reactivity. Furthermore, perceptions of imminent threat or danger, such as death, loss of control, or social ridicule, often accompany such fight–flight reactivity. However, the features of urgency to escape, autonomic arousal, and perception of threat are not present in every self-reported occurrence of panic. For example, despite evidence for elevated heart rate or other indices of sympathetic nervous system activation during panic attacks on average (e.g., Wilkinson et al., 1998), Margraf, Taylor, Ehlers, Roth, and Agras (1987) found that 40% of self-reported panic attacks were not associated with accelerated heart rate. Moreover, in general, patients with panic disorder are more likely than non-anxious controls to report arrhythmic heart rate in the absence of actual arrhythmias (Barsky, Clearly, Sarnie, & Ruskin, 1994). Heightened anxiety about signs of autonomic arousal may lead patients to perceive cardiac events when none exist (Barlow, Brown, & Craske, 1994; Craske & Tsao, 1999). We believe that self-reported panic in the absence of heart rate acceleration or other indices of auto-nomic activation reflects anticipatory anxiety rather than true panic (Barlow et al., 1994), especially because more severe panics are more consistently associated with accelerated heart rate (Margraf et al., 1987). Another example of discordance occurs when perceptions of threat or danger are refuted despite the report of intense fear. This has been termed "noncognitive" panic (Rachman, Lopatka, & Levitt, 1988). Finally, the urgency to escape is sometimes weakened by situational demands for continued approach and endurance, such as performance expectations or job demands, thus creating discordance between behavioral responses on the one hand, and verbal or physiological responses on the other.

A subset of individuals with panic disorder experience nocturnal panic attacks. "Nocturnal panic" refers to waking from sleep in a state of panic with symptoms that are very similar to panic attacks during wakeful states (Craske & Barlow, 1989; Uhde, 1994). Nocturnal panic does *not* refer to waking from sleep and panicking after a lapse of waking time, or nighttime arousals induced by nightmares or environmental stimuli (e.g., unexpected noises). Instead, nocturnal panic is an abrupt waking from sleep in a state of panic, without an obvious trigger. Nocturnal panic attacks reportedly most often occur between 1 and 3 hours after sleep onset, and only occasionally more than once per night (Craske & Barlow, 1989). Surveys of select clinical groups suggest that nocturnal panic is relatively common among individuals with panic disorder: 44–71% report having experienced nocturnal panic at least once, and 30–45% report repeated nocturnal panics (Craske & Barlow, 1989; Krystal, Woods, Hill, & Charney, 1991; Mellman & Uhde, 1989; Roy-Byrne, Mellman, & Uhde, 1988; Uhde, 1994). Individuals who suffer frequent nocturnal panic often become fearful of sleep and attempt to delay sleep onset. Avoidance of sleep may result in chronic sleep deprivation, which in turn precipitates more nocturnal panics (Uhde, 1994).

"Nonclinical" panic attacks occur occasionally in approximately 3–5% of people in the general population who do not otherwise meet criteria for panic disorder (Norton, Cox, & Malan, 1992). Also, panic attacks occur across a variety of anxiety and mood disorders (Barlow et al., 1985), and are not limited to panic disorder. As stated earlier, the defining feature of panic disorder is not the presence of panic attacks per se, but involves additional anxiety about the recurrence of panic or its consequences, or a significant behavioral change because of the panic attacks. It is the additional anxiety about panic combined with catastrophic cognitions in the face of panic that differentiate between the person with panic disorder and the occasional nonclinical panicker (e.g., Telch, Lucas, & Nelson, 1989) or the person with other anxiety disorders who also happens to panic. The following scenario exemplifies the latter point.

PATIENT: Sometimes I lay awake at night thinking about a million different things. I think about what is going to happen to my daughter if I get sick. Who will look after her, or what would happen if my husband died and we didn't have enough money to give my daughter a good education? Then I think about where we would live and how we would cope. Sometimes I can work myself up so much that my heart starts to race, my hands get sweaty, and I feel dizzy and scared. So I have to stop myself from thinking about all those things. I usually get out of bed and turn on the TV—anything to get my mind off the worries.

THERAPIST: Do you worry about the feelings of a racing heart, sweating, and dizziness happening again?

PATIENT: No. They're unpleasant, but they are the least of my concerns. I am more worried about my daughter and our future.

This scenario illustrates the experience of panic that is *not* the central focus of the person's anxiety. More likely, this woman has generalized anxiety disorder, and her uncontrollable worry leads her to panic on occasion. The next example is of someone with social phobia, who becomes very concerned about panicking in social situations, because the possibility of a panic attack increases her concerns about being judged negatively by others.

PATIENT: I am terrified of having a panic attack in meetings at work. I dread the thought of others noticing how anxious I am. They must be able to see my hands shaking, the sweat on my forehead, and worst of all, my face turning red.

THERAPIST: What worries you most about others noticing your physical symptoms?

PATIENT: That they will think that I am weird or strange.

THERAPIST: Would you be anxious in the meetings if the panic attacks were fully preventable?

PATIENT: I would still be worried about doing or saying the wrong thing. It is not just the panic attacks that worry me.

THERAPIST: Are you worried about panic attacks in any other situations?

PATIENT: Formal social events and sometimes when I meet someone for the first time.

In this case, even though the patient experiences panic attacks, the real concern is about being judged negatively by others consequent to panic attacks, and the panic attacks do not occur in situations other than social ones. Hence, this presentation is most aptly described as social phobia.

Agoraphobia

"Agoraphobia" refers to avoidance or endurance with dread of situations from which escape might be difficult or help unavailable in the event of a panic attack, or in the event of developing symptoms that could be incapacitating and embarrassing, such as loss of bowel control or vomiting. Typical agoraphobic situations include shopping malls, waiting in line, movie theaters, traveling by car or bus, crowded restaurants, and being alone. "Mild" agoraphobia is exemplified by the person who hesitates about driving long distances alone but manages to drive to and from work, prefers to sit on the aisle at movie theaters but still goes to movies, and avoids crowded places. "Moderate" agoraphobia is exemplified by the person whose driving is limited to a 10-mile radius from home and only if accompanied, who shops at off-peak times and avoids large supermarkets, and who avoids flying or traveling by train. "Severe" agoraphobia refers to very limited mobility, sometimes even to the point of becoming housebound.

Not all persons who panic develop agoraphobia, and the extent of agoraphobia that emerges is highly variable (Craske & Barlow, 1988). Various factors have been investigated as potential predictors of agoraphobia. Although agoraphobia tends to increase as history of panic lengthens, a significant proportion of individuals panic for many years without developing agoraphobic limitations. Nor is agoraphobia related to age of onset or frequency of panic (Cox, Endler, & Swinson, 1995; Craske & Barlow, 1988; Kikuchi et al., 2005; Rapee & Murrell, 1988). Some studies report more intense physical symptoms during panic attacks when there is more agoraphobia (e.g., de Jong & Bouman, 1995; Goisman et al., 1994; Noyes, Clancy, Garvey, & Anderson, 1987; Telch, Brouillard, Telch, Agras, & Taylor, 1989). Others fail to find such differences (e.g., Cox et al., 1995; Craske, Miller, Rotunda, & Barlow, 1990). On the one hand, fears of dying, going crazy, or losing control do not relate to level of agoraphobia (Cox et al., 1995; Craske, Rapee, & Barlow, 1988). On the other hand, concerns about social consequences of panicking may be stronger when there is more agoraphobia (Amering et al., 1997; de Jong & Bouman, 1995; Rapee & Murrell, 1988; Telch, Brouilard, et al., 1989). In addition, in a recent investigation, Kikuchi and colleagues (2005) found that individuals who developed agoraphobia within 6 months of the onset of panic disorder had a higher prevalence of generalized anxiety disorder but not major depression. However, whether the social evaluation concerns or comorbidity are precursors or are secondary to agoraphobia remains to be determined. Occupational status also predicts agoraphobia, accounting for 18% of the variance in one study (de Jong & Bouman, 1995). Perhaps the strongest predictor of agoraphobia is sex; the ratio of males to females shifts dramatically in the direction of female predominance as level of agoraphobia worsens (e.g., Thyer, Himle, Curtis, Cameron, & Nesse, 1985).

PRESENTING FEATURES

From the latest epidemiological study, the National Comorbidity Survey Replication (NCS-R; Kessler, Berglund, Demler, Jin, & Walters, 2005; Kessler, Chiu, Demler, & Walters, 2005) prevalence estimates for panic disorder with or without agoraphobia (PD/PDA) are 2.7% (12 month) and 4.7% (lifetime). These rates are higher than those reported in the original NCS (Kessler et al., 1994) and the older Epide-miologic Catchment Area (ECA; Myers et al., 1984) study.

Individuals with agoraphobia *who seek treatment* almost always report that a history of panic preceded their development of avoidance (Goisman et al., 1994; Wittchen, Reed, & Kessler, 1998). In contrast, epidemiological data indicate that a subset of the population experiences agoraphobia without a history of panic disorder: 0.8% in the last 12 months (Kessler, Chiu, et al., 2005) and 1.4% lifetime prevalence (Kessler, Berglund, et al., 2005). The discrepancy between clinical and epidemiological data has been attributed to misdiagnosis of generalized anxiety, specific and social phobias, and reasonable cautiousness about certain situations (e.g., walking alone in unsafe neighborhoods) as agoraphobia in epidemiological samples (Horwath, Lish, Johnson, Hornig, & Weissman, 1993), and to the fact that individuals who panic are more likely to seek help (Boyd, 1986).

Rarely does the diagnosis of PD/PDA occur in isolation. Commonly co-occurring Axis I conditions include specific phobias, social phobia, dysthymia, generalized anxiety disorder, major depressive disorder, and substance abuse (e.g., Brown, Campbell, Lehman, Grishman, & Mancill, 2001; Goisman, Goldenberg, Vasile, & Keller, 1995; Kessler, Chiu, et al., 2005). Also, 25–60% of persons with panic disorder also meet criteria for a personality disorder, mostly avoidant and dependent personality disorders (e.g., Chambless & Renneberg, 1988). However, the nature of the relationship between PD/PDA and personality disorders remains unclear. For example, comorbidity rates are highly dependent on the method used to establish Axis II diagnosis, as well as the co-occurrence of depressed mood (Alneas & Torgersen, 1990; Chambless & Renneberg, 1988). Moreover, the fact that abnormal personality traits improve and some "personality disorders" even remit after successful treatment of PD/PDA (Black, Monahan, Wesner, Gabel, & Bowers, 1996; Mavissakalian & Hamman, 1987; Noyes, Reich, Suelzer, & Christiansen, 1991) raises questions about the validity of Axis II diagnoses. The issue of comorbidity with personality disorders and its effect on treatment for PD/PDA is described in more detail in a later section.

The modal age of onset is late teenage years and early adulthood (Kessler, Berglund, et al., 2005). In fact, a substantial proportion of adolescents report panic attacks (e.g., Hayward et al., 1992), and panic disorder in children and adolescents tends to be chronic and comorbid with other anxiety, mood, and disruptive disorders (Biederman, Faraone, Marrs, & Moore, 1997). Treatment is usually sought at a much later age, around 34 years (e.g., Noyes et al., 1986). The overall ratio of females to males is approximately 2:1 (Kessler et al., 2006), and, as mentioned already, the ratio shifts dramatically in the direction of female predominance as level of agoraphobia worsens (e.g., Thyer et al., 1985).

Most (approximately 72%) (Craske et al., 1990) report identifiable stressors around the time of their first panic attack, including interpersonal stressors and stressors related to physical well-being, such as negative drug experiences, disease, or death in the family. However, the number of stressors does not differ from the number experienced prior to the onset of other types of anxiety disorders (Pollard, Pollard, & Corn, 1989; Rapee, Litwin, & Barlow, 1990; Roy-Byrne, Geraci, & Uhde, 1986). Approximately one-half report having experienced panicky feelings at some time before their first panic, suggesting that onset may be either insidious or acute (Craske et al., 1990).

Finally, PD/PDA tend to be chronic conditions, with severe financial and interpersonal costs; that is, only a minority of untreated individuals remit without subsequent relapse within a few years (30%), although a similar number experience notable improvement, albeit with a waxing and waning course (35%) (Katschnig & Amering, 1998; Roy-Byrne & Cowley, 1995). Also, individuals with panic disorder overutilize medical resources compared to the general public and individuals with other "psychiatric" disorders (e.g., Katon et al., 1990; Roy-Byrne et al., 1999).

HISTORY OF PSYCHOLOGICAL TREATMENT FOR PANIC DISORDER AND AGORAPHOBIA

It was not until the publication of DSM-III (American Psychiatric Association, 1980) that PD/PDA was recognized as a distinct anxiety problem. Until that time, panic attacks were viewed primarily as a form of free-floating anxiety. Consequently, psychological treatment approaches were relatively nonspecific. They included relaxation and cognitive restructuring

for stressful life events in general (e.g., Barlow et al., 1984). Many presumed that pharmacotherapy was necessary for the control of panic. In contrast, the treatment of agoraphobia was quite specific from the 1970s onward, with primarily exposure-based approaches to target fear and avoidance of specific situations. However, relatively little consideration was given to panic attacks in either the conceptualization or treatment of agoraphobia. The development of specific panic control treatments in the middle to late 1980s shifted interest away from agoraphobia. Interest in agoraphobia was subsequently renewed, specifically in terms of whether panic control treatments are sufficient for the management of agoraphobia, and whether their combination with treatments that directly target agoraphobia is superior overall. We address these questions in more detail after describing the conceptualization that underlies cognitive-behavioral approaches to the treatment of panic and agoraphobia.

CONCEPTUALIZATION OF ETIOLOGICAL AND MAINTAINING FACTORS FOR PANIC DISORDER AND AGORAPHOBIA

Several independent lines of research (Barlow, 1988; Clark, 1986; Ehlers & Margraf, 1989) converged in the 1980s on the same basic conceptualization of panic disorder as an acquired fear of bodily sensations, particularly sensations associated with autonomic arousal. Psychological and biological predispositions are believed to enhance the vulnerability to acquire such fear. These interacting vulnerabilities have been organized into an etiological conception of anxiety disorders in general, referred to as "triple vulnerability theory" (Barlow, 1988, 2002; Suárez, Bennett, Goldstein, & Barlow, in press). First, genetic contributions to the development of anxiety and negative affect constitute a generalized (heritable) biological vulnerability. Second, evidence also supports a generalized psychological vulnerability to experience anxiety and related negative affective states, characterized by a diminished sense of control arising from early developmental experiences. Although the unfortunate co-occurrence of generalized biological and psychological vulnerabilities may be sufficient to produce anxiety and related states, particularly generalized anxiety disorder and depression, a third vulnerability seems necessary to account for the development of at least some specific anxiety disorders, including panic disorder; that is, early learning experiences in some instances seem to focus anxiety on particular areas of concern. In panic disorder, the experience of certain somatic sensations becomes associated with a heightened sense of threat and danger. This specific psychological vulnerability, when coordinated with the generalized biological and psychological vulnerabilities mentioned earlier, seems to contribute to the development of panic disorder. Fear conditioning, avoidant responding, and information-processing biases are believed to perpetuate such fear. It is the perpetuating factors that are targeted in the cognitive-behavioral treatment approach. What follows is a very brief review of some contributory factors with practical relevance for panic disorder.

Three Vulnerability Factors

Genetics and Temperament

The temperament most associated with anxiety disorders, including panic disorder, is neuroticism (Eysenck, 1967; Gray, 1982), or proneness to experience negative emotions in response to stressors. A closely linked construct, "negative affectivity," is the tendency to experience a variety of negative emotions across a variety of situations, even in the absence of objective stressors (Watson & Clark, 1984). Structural analyses confirm that negative affect is a higher-order factor that distinguishes individuals with each anxiety disorder (and depression) from controls with no mental disorder: Lower-order factors discriminate among anxiety disorders, with "fear of fear" being the factor that discriminates panic disorder from other anxiety disorders (Brown, Chorpita, & Barlow, 1998; Zinbarg & Barlow, 1996). The anxiety disorders load differentially on negative affectivity, with more pervasive anxiety disorders, such as generalized anxiety disorder, loading more heavily, panic disorder loading at an intermediate level, and social anxiety disorder loading the least (Brown et al., 1998).[1] However, these findings derive from cross-sectional data sets.

Longitudinal prospective evidence for the role of neuroticism in predicting the onset of panic disorder is relatively limited. Specifically, neuroticism predicted the onset of panic at-

tacks in adolescents (Hayward, Killen, Kraemer, & Taylor, 2000; Schmidt, Lerew, & Jackson, 1997, 1999), and "emotional reactivity" at age 3 was a significant variable in the classification of panic disorder in 18- to 21-year-old males (Craske, Poulton, Tsao, & Plotkin, 2001). Ongoing studies, such as the Northwestern/UCLA Youth Emotion Project, are comprehensively evaluating the role of neuroticism in the prediction of subsequent panic disorder.

Numerous multivariate genetic analyses of human twin samples consistently attribute approximately 30–50% of variance in neuroticism to additive genetic factors (Eley, 2001; Lake, Eaves, Maes, Heath, & Martin, 2000). In addition, anxiety and depression appear to be variable expressions of the heritable tendency toward neuroticism (Kendler, Heath, Martin, & Eaves, 1987). Symptoms of panic (i.e., breathlessness, heart pounding) may be additionally explained by a unique source of genetic variance that is differentiated from symptoms of depression and anxiety (Kendler et al., 1987) and neuroticism (Martin, Jardine, Andrews, & Heath, 1988).

Analyses of specific genetic markers remain preliminary and inconsistent. For example, panic disorder has been linked to a locus on chromosome 13 (Hamilton et al., 2003; Schumacher et al., 2005) and chromosome 9 (Thorgeirsson et al., 2003), but the exact genes remain unknown. Findings regarding markers for the cholecystokinin-B receptor gene have been inconsistent (cf. Hamilton et al. [2001] and van Megen, Westenberg, Den Boer, & Kahn [1996]). Also, association and linkage studies implicate the adenosine receptor gene in panic disorder (Deckert et al., 1998; Hamilton et al., 2004). But studies of genes involved in neurotransmitter systems associated with fear and anxiety have produced inconsistent results (see Roy-Byrne, Craske, & Stein, 2006). Thus, there is no evidence at this point for a specific link between genetic markers and temperament, on the one hand, and panic disorder on the other. Rather, neurobiological factors seem to comprise a nonspecific biological vulnerability.

Anxiety Sensitivity

As described earlier, neuroticism is viewed as a higher-order factor characteristic of all anxiety disorders, with "fear of fear" being more unique to panic disorder. The construct "fear of fear" overlaps with the construct anxiety sensitivity, or the belief that anxiety and its associated symptoms may cause deleterious physical, social, and psychological consequences that extend beyond any immediate physical discomfort during an episode of anxiety or panic (Reiss, 1980). Anxiety sensitivity is elevated across most anxiety disorders, but it is particularly elevated in panic disorder (e.g., Taylor, Koch, & McNally, 1992; Zinbarg & Barlow, 1996), especially the Physical Concerns subscale of the Anxiety Sensitivity Index (Zinbarg & Barlow, 1996; Zinbarg, Barlow, & Brown, 1997). Therefore, beliefs that physical symptoms of anxiety are harmful seem to be particularly relevant to panic disorder and may comprise a specific psychological vulnerability.

Anxiety sensitivity is presumed to confer a risk factor for panic disorder, because it primes fear reactivity to bodily sensations. In support, anxiety sensitivity predicts subjective distress and reported symptomatology in response to procedures that induce strong physical sensations, such as CO_2 inhalation (Forsyth, Palav, & Duff, 1999), balloon inflation (Messenger & Shean, 1998), and hyperventilation (Sturges, Goetsch, Ridley, & Whittal, 1998) in nonclinical samples, even after researchers control for the effects of trait anxiety (Rapee & Medoro, 1994). In addition, several longitudinal studies indicate that high scores on the Anxiety Sensitivity Index predict the onset of panic attacks over 1- to 4-year intervals in adolescents (Hayward et al., 2000), college students (Maller & Reiss, 1992), and community samples with specific phobias or no anxiety disorders (Ehlers, 1995). The predictive relationship remains after controlling for prior depression (Hayward et al., 2000). In addition, Anxiety Sensitivity Index scores predicted spontaneous panic attacks and worry about panic (and anxiety more generally), during an acute military stressor (i.e., 5 weeks of basic training), even after controlling for history of panic attacks and trait anxiety (Schmidt et al., 1997, 1999). Finally, panic attacks themselves elevate anxiety sensitivity over a 5-week period in adults (Schmidt et al., 1999), and over a 1-year period in adolescents, albeit to a lesser extent (Weems, Hayward, Killen, & Taylor, 2002).

However, we (Bouton, Mineka, & Barlow, 2001) have noted that the relationship between anxiety sensitivity and panic attacks in these studies is relatively small, not exclusive to panic, and is weaker than the relationship between panic and neuroticism. Furthermore, these studies have evaluated panic attacks and worry about panic, but not the prediction of diagnosed panic disorder. Thus, the causal significance of anxiety sensitivity for panic disorder remains to be fully understood.

History of Medical Illness and Abuse

Other studies highlight the role of medical illnesses as contributing to a specific psychological vulnerability for panic disorder. For example, using the Dunedin Multidisciplinary Study database, we found that experience with personal respiratory disturbance (and parental poor health) as a youth predicted panic disorder at age 18 or 21 (Craske et al., 2001). This finding is consistent with reports of more respiratory disturbance in the history of patients with panic disorder compared to other patients with anxiety disorders (Verburg, Griez, Meijer, & Pols, 1995). Furthermore, in a recent study, first-degree relatives of patients with panic disorder had a significantly higher prevalence of chronic obstructive respiratory disease, and asthma in particular, than first-degree relatives of patients with other anxiety disorders (van Beek, Schruers, & Friez, 2005).

Childhood experiences of sexual and physical abuse may also prime panic disorder. Retrospective reports of such childhood abuse were associated with panic disorder onset at ages 16–21 years in a recent longitudinal analysis of New Zealanders from birth to age 21 (Goodwin, Fergusson, & Horwood, 2005). This finding is consistent with multiple cross-sectional studies in both clinical and community samples (e.g., Bandelow et al., 2002; Kendler et al., 2000; Kessler, Davis, & Kendler, 1997; Moisan & Engels, 1995; Stein et al., 1996). The association with childhood abuse is stronger for panic disorder than for other anxiety disorders, such as social phobia (Safren, Gershuny, Marzol, Otto, & Pollack, 2002; Stein et al., 1996) and obsessive–compulsive disorder (Stein et al., 1996). In addition, some studies reported an association between panic disorder and exposure to violence between other family members, generally interparental violence (e.g., Bandelow et al., 2002; Moisan & Engels, 1995), whereas the most recent study did not (Goodwin et al., 2005). Retrospective reporting of childhood abuse and familial violence in all of these studies, however, limits the findings.

Interoceptive Awareness

Patients with panic disorder, as well as non-clinical panickers, appear to have heightened awareness of, or ability to detect, bodily sensations of arousal (e.g., Ehlers & Breuer, 1992, 1996; Ehlers, Breuer, Dohn, & Feigenbaum, 1995; Zoellner & Craske, 1999). Discrepant findings (e.g., Antony et al., 1995; Rapee, 1994) exist but have been attributed to methodological artifact (Ehlers & Breuer, 1996). Ability to perceive heartbeat, in particular, appears to be a relatively stable individual-difference variable given that it does not differ between untreated and treated patients with panic disorder (Ehlers & Breuer, 1992), or from before to after successful treatment (Antony, Meadows, Brown, & Barlow, 1994; Ehlers et al., 1995). Thus, interoceptive accuracy may be a predisposing trait for panic disorder. Ehlers and Breuer (1996) suggested that "although good interoception is considered neither a necessary nor a sufficient condition for panic disorder, it may enhance the probability of panic by increasing the probability of perceiving sensations that may trigger an attack if perceived as dangerous" (p. 174). Whether interoceptive awareness is learned, and represents another specific psychological vulnerability, or is more dispositional remains to be determined.

Separate from interoception is the issue of propensity for intense autonomic activation. As noted earlier, some evidence points to a unique genetic influence on the reported experience of breathlessness, heart pounding, and a sense of terror (Kendler et al., 1987). Conceivably, cardiovascular reactivity presents a unique physiological predisposition for panic disorder. In support of this, cardiac symptoms and shortness of breath predict later development of panic attacks and panic disorder (Keyl & Eaton, 1990). Unfortunately, these data derive from *report* of symptoms, which is not a good index of actual autonomic state (Pennebaker & Roberts, 1992) and may instead reflect interoception.

Initial Panic Attacks

From an evolutionary standpoint, fear is a natural and adaptive response to threatening stimuli. However, the fear experienced during the first unexpected panic attack is often unjustified due to the lack of an identifiable trigger or antecedent; hence, it represents a "false alarm" (Barlow, 1988, 2002). The large majority of initial panic attacks are recalled as occurring outside of the home, while driving, walking, at work, or at school (Craske et al., 1990), generally in public (Lelliott, Marks, McNamee, & Tobena, 1989), and on a bus, plane, subway, or in social-evaluative situations (Shulman, Cox, Swinson, Kuch, & Reichman, 1994). We (Barlow, 1988; Craske & Rowe, 1997b) believe situations that set the scene for initial panic attacks are ones in which bodily sensations are perceived as posing the most threat, because of impairment of functioning (e.g., driving), entrapment (e.g., air travel, elevators), negative social evaluation (e.g., job, formal social events), or distance from safety (e.g., unfamiliar locales). Entrapment concerns may be particularly salient for subsequent development of agoraphobia (Faravelli, Pallanti, Biondi, Paterniti, & Scarpato, 1992).

Maintenance Factors

Acute "fear of fear" (or, more accurately, anxiety focused on somatic sensations) that develops after initial panic attacks in *vulnerable individuals* refers to anxiety about certain bodily sensations associated with panic attacks (e.g., racing heart, dizziness, paresthesias) (Barlow, 1988; Goldstein & Chambless, 1978), and is attributed to two factors. The first is interoceptive conditioning, or conditioned fear of internal cues, such as elevated heart rate, because of their association with intense fear, pain, or distress (Razran, 1961). Specifically, interoceptive conditioning refers to low-level somatic sensations of arousal or anxiety becoming conditioned stimuli, so that early somatic components of the anxiety response come to elicit significant bursts of anxiety or panic (Bouton et al., 2001). An extensive body of experimental literature attests to the robustness of interoceptive conditioning (e.g., Dworkin & Dworkin, 1999), particularly with regard to early interoceptive drug-onset cues becoming conditioned stimuli for larger drug effects (e.g., Sokolowska, Siegel, & Kim, 2002). In addition, interoceptive conditioned responses are not dependent on conscious awareness of triggering cues (Razran, 1961); thus, they have been observed in patients under anesthesia (e.g., Block, Ghoneim, Fowles, Kumar, & Pathak, 1987). Within this model, then, slight changes in relevant bodily functions that are not consciously recognized may elicit conditioned anxiety or fear and panic due to previous pairings with panic (Barlow, 1988; Bouton et al., 2001).

The second factor, offered by Clark (1986) to explain acute fear of panic-related body sensations, is catastrophic misappraisals of bodily sensations (misinterpretation of sensations as signs of imminent death, loss of control, etc.). Debate continues as to the significance of catastrophic misappraisals of bodily sensations versus conditioned (emotional, non-cognitively-mediated) fear responding. We have taken issue with the purely cognitive model of panic disorder by stating that it cannot account for panic attacks devoid of conscious cognitive appraisal without turning to constructs such as "automatic appraisals," which prove to be untestable (Bouton et al., 2001). Catastrophic misappraisals may accompany panic attacks because they are a natural part of the constellation of responses that go with panic, or because they have been encouraged and reinforced much like sick role behaviors during childhood. In addition, such thoughts may become conditioned stimuli that trigger anxiety and panic, as demonstrated via panic induction through presentation of pairs of words involving sensations and catastrophic outcomes (Clark et al., 1988). In this case, catastrophic cognitions may well be sufficient to elicit conditioned panic attacks, but not necessary.

Whether cognitively or noncognitively based, excessive anxiety over panic-related bodily sensations in panic disorder is well supported. Persons with panic disorder endorse strong beliefs that bodily sensations associated with panic attacks cause physical or mental harm (e.g., Chambless, Caputo, Bright, & Gallagher, 1984; McNally & Lorenz, 1987). They are more likely to interpret bodily sensations in a catastrophic fashion (Clark et al., 1988), and to allocate more attentional resources to words that represent physical threat, such as "disease" and "fatality" (e.g., Ehlers, Margraf, Davies, & Roth, 1988; Hope, Rapee, Heimberg, & Dombeck, 1990); catastrophe words, such as "death" and "insane" (e.g., Maidenberg, Chen, Craske, Bohn, & Bystritsky, 1996; McNally, Riemann, Louro, Lukach, & Kim, 1992); and heartbeat stimuli (Kroeze & van den Hout, 2000). Also, individuals with panic disorder show enhanced brain potentials in response to panic-related words (Pauli, Amrhein, Muhlberger, Dengler, &

Wiedemann, 2005). In addition, they are more likely to become anxious in procedures that elicit bodily sensations similar to the ones experienced during panic attacks, including benign cardiovascular, respiratory, and audiovestibular exercises (Antony, Ledley, Liss, & Swinson, 2006; Jacob, Furman, Clark, & Durrant, 1992), as well as more invasive procedures, such as CO_2 inhalations, compared to patients with other anxiety disorders (e.g., Perna, Bertani, Arancio, Ronchi, & Bellodi, 1995; Rapee, 1986; Rapee, Brown, Antony, & Barlow, 1992) or healthy controls (e.g., Gorman et al., 1994). The findings are not fully consistent, however, because patients with panic disorder did not differ from patients with social phobia in response to an epinephrine challenge (Veltman, van Zijderveld, Tilders, & van Dyck, 1996). Nonetheless, individuals with panic disorder also fear signals that ostensibly reflect heightened arousal and false physiological feedback (Craske & Freed, 1995; Craske, Lang, et al., 2002; Ehlers, Margraf, Roth, Taylor, & Birnbaumer, 1988).

Distress over bodily sensations is likely to generate ongoing distress for a number of reasons. First, in the immediate sense, autonomic arousal generated by fear in turn intensifies the feared sensations, thus creating a reciprocating cycle of fear and sensations that is sustained until autonomic arousal abates or the individual perceives safety. Second, because bodily sensations that trigger panic attacks are not always immediately obvious, they may generate the perception of unexpected or "out of the blue" panic attacks (Barlow, 1988) that causes even further distress (Craske, Glover, & DeCola, 1995). Third, the perceived uncontrollability, or inability to escape or terminate bodily sensations, again, is likely to generate heightened anxiety (e.g., Maier, Laudenslager, & Ryan, 1985; Mineka et al., 1984). Unpredictability and uncontrollability, then, are seen as enhancing general levels of anxiety about "When is it going to happen again?" and "What do I do when it happens?", thereby contributing to high levels of chronic anxious apprehension (Barlow, 1988, 2002). In turn, anxious apprehension increases the likelihood of panic by directly increasing the availability of sensations that have become conditioned cues for panic and/or attentional vigilance for these bodily cues. Thus, a maintaining cycle of panic and anxious apprehension develops. Also, subtle avoidance behaviors are believed to maintain negative beliefs about feared bodily sensations (Clark & Ehlers, 1993). Examples include holding onto objects or persons for fear of fainting, sitting and remaining still for fear of a heart attack, and moving slowly or searching for an escape route because one fears acting foolish (Salkovskis, Clark, & Gelder, 1996). Finally, anxiety may develop over specific contexts in which the occurrence of panic would be particularly troubling (i.e., situations associated with impairment, entrapment, negative social evaluation, and distance from safety). These anxieties may contribute to agoraphobia, which in turn maintains distress by preventing disconfirmation of catastrophic misappraisals and extinction of conditioned responding.

TREATMENT VARIABLES

Setting

There are several different settings for conducting cognitive-behavioral therapy for panic disorder and agoraphobia. The first, the outpatient clinic–office setting, is suited to psychoeducation, cognitive restructuring, assignment and feedback regarding homework assignments, and role-play rehearsals. In addition, certain exposures can be conducted in the office setting, such as interoceptive exposure to feared bodily sensations described later. Recently, outpatient settings have extended from mental health settings to primary care suites (e.g., Craske, Roy-Byrne, et al., 2002; Roy-Byrne et al., 2005; Sharp, Power, Simpson, Swanson, & Anstee, 1997). This extension is particularly important because of the higher prevalence of panic disorder in primary care settings (e.g., Shear & Schulberg, 1995; Tiemens, Ormel, & Simon, 1996). However, whether a mental health or a primary care office is being used, the built-in safety signals of such an office may limit the generalizability of learning that takes place in that setting. For example, learning to be less afraid in the presence of the therapist, or in an office located near a medical center, may not necessarily generalize to conditions in which the therapist is not present, or the perceived safety of a medical center is not close by. For this reason, homework assignments to practice cognitive-behavioral skills in a variety of different settings are particularly important.

In the second setting, the natural environment, cognitive restructuring and other anxiety management skills are put into practice, and the patient faces feared situations. The latter is called *in vivo* exposure and can be conducted with the aid of the therapist or alone. Therapist-directed exposure is particularly useful for patients who lack a social network to support *in vivo* exposure assignments, and more valuable than self-directed exposure for patients with more severe agoraphobia (Holden, O'Brien, Barlow, Stetson, & Infantino, 1983). Therapist-directed exposure is essential to guided mastery exposure, in which the therapist gives corrective feedback about the way the patient faces feared situations to minimize unnecessary defensive behaviors. For example, patients are taught to drive in a relaxed position at the wheel and to walk across a bridge without holding the rail. On the one hand, guided mastery exposure has been shown to be more effective than "stimulus exposure" when patients attempt simply to endure the situation alone until fear subsides, without the benefit of ongoing therapist feedback (Williams & Zane, 1989). On the other hand, self-directed exposure is very valuable also, especially to the degree that it encourages independence and generalization of the skills learned in treatment to conditions in which the therapist is not present. Thus, the most beneficial approach in the natural environment is to proceed from therapist-directed to self-directed exposure.

In an interesting variation that combines the office and the natural environment, telephone-guided treatment, therapists direct patients with agoraphobia by phone to conduct *in vivo* exposure to feared situations (NcNamee, O'Sullivan, Lelliot, & Marks, 1989; Swinson, Fergus, Cox, & Wickwire, 1995) or provide instruction in panic control skills (Cote, Gauthier, Laberge, Cormier, & Plamondon, 1994). In addition, one small study showed that cognitive-behavioral therapy was as effective when delivered by videoconference as in person (Bouchard et al., 2004).

Self-directed treatments, with minimal direct therapist contact, take place in the natural environment, and are beneficial for highly motivated and educated patients (e.g., Ghosh & Marks, 1987; Gould & Clum, 1995; Gould, Clum, & Shapiro, 1993; Lidren et al., 1994; Schneider, Mataix-Cols, Marks, & Bachofen, 2005). On the other hand, self-directed treatments are less effective for more severely affected patients (Holden et al., 1983), or those with more comorbidity (Hecker, Losee, Roberson-Nay, & Maki, 2004), less motivation, and less education; or for patients who are referred as opposed to recruited through advertisement (Hecker, Losee, Fritzler, & Fink, 1996). Self-directed treatments have expanded beyond workbooks and manuals to computerized and Internet versions (e.g., Carlbring, Ekselius, & Andersson, 2003; Richards, Klein, & Austen, 2006; Richards, Klein, & Carlbring, 2003). In general, these treatments yield positive results, although not quite as positive as fully therapist-delivered treatments. Specifically, a four-session computer-assisted cognitive-behavioral therapy for panic disorder was less effective than 12 sessions of therapist-delivered cognitive-behavioral therapy at posttreatment, although the groups did not differ at follow-up (Newman, Kenardy, Herman, & Taylor, 1997). More recently, 12 sessions of therapist-delivered cognitive-behavioral therapy was more effective than six sessions of either therapist-delivered or computer-augmented therapy (Kenardy et al., 2003). Also, findings from computerized programs for emotional disorders in general indicate that such treatments are more acceptable and successful when combined with therapist involvement (e.g., Carlbring et al., 2003).

The third setting, the inpatient facility, is most appropriate when conducting very intensive cognitive-behavioral therapy (e.g., daily therapist contact), or treating severely disabled persons who can no longer function at home. In addition, certain medical or drug complications may warrant inpatient treatment. The greatest drawback to the inpatient setting is poor generalization to the home environment. Transition sessions and follow-up booster sessions in an outpatient clinic–office or in the patient's own home facilitate generalization.

Format

Cognitive-behavioral therapy for panic disorder and agoraphobia may be conducted in individual or group formats. Several clinical outcome studies have used group treatments (e.g., Craske, DeCola, Sachs, & Pontillo, 2003; Evans, Holt, & Oei, 1991; Feigenbaum, 1988; Hoffart, 1995; Telch et al., 1993). The fact that their outcomes are generally consistent with the summary statistics obtained from individu-

ally formatted treatment suggests that group treatment is as effective as individual therapy. Also, Lidren and colleagues (1994) found that group therapy is as effective as individual bibliotherapy, although they did not include a comparison with individualized cognitive-behavioral therapy. In direct comparisons, a slight advantage is shown for individual formats. Specifically, Neron, Lacroix, and Chaput (1995) compared 12–14 weekly sessions of individual or group cognitive-behavioral therapy ($N = 20$), although the group condition received two additional 1-hour individual sessions. The two conditions were equally effective for measures of panic and agoraphobia at posttreatment and 6-month follow-up. However, the individual format was more successful in terms of generalized anxiety and depressive symptoms by the follow-up point. In addition, individual treatments resulted in more clinically significant outcomes than group formats in primary care (Sharp, Power, & Swanson, 2004). Furthermore, 95% of individuals assigned to the waiting-list condition in the latter study stated a clear preference for individual treatment when given the choice at the end of the waiting list.

Most studies of cognitive-behavioral therapy for panic and agoraphobia involve 10–20 weekly treatment sessions. Several studies show that briefer treatments may be effective as well. Evans and colleagues (1991) compared a 2-day group cognitive-behavioral treatment to a waiting-list condition, although without random assignment. The 2-day program comprised lectures (3 hours); teaching skills, such as breathing, relaxation, and cognitive challenging (3 hours); *in vivo* exposure (9 hours); and group discussion plus a 2-hour support group for significant others. Eighty-five percent of treated patients were reported to be either symptom-free or symptomatically improved, and these results were maintained 1 year later. In contrast, the waiting-list group did not demonstrate significant changes. A recent pilot study similarly indicated effectiveness with intensive cognitive-behavioral therapy over 2 days (Deacon & Abramowitz, 2006). Other studies have evaluated the effectiveness of cognitive-behavioral therapy when delivered over a fewer number of sessions. In a randomized study, patients with PDA who awaited pharmacotherapy treatment were assigned to four weekly sessions of either cognitive-behavioral therapy or supportive nondirective therapy (Craske, Maidenberg, & Bystritsky, 1995). Cognitive-behavioral therapy was more effective than supportive therapy, particularly with less severely affected patients, although the results were not as positive as those typically seen with more sessions. Also, we found that up to six sessions (average of three sessions) of cognitive-behavioral therapy combined with medication recommendations yielded significantly greater improvements on an array of measures, including quality of life, compared to treatment as usual for individuals with panic disorder in primary care settings (Roy-Byrne et al., 2005). Notably, however, the treatment effects substantially increased as the number of cognitive-behavioral therapy sessions (up to six) and follow-up booster phone call sessions (up to six) increased (Craske et al., 2006). Finally, in a direct comparison, results were equally effective whether cognitive-behavioral therapy was delivered across the standard 12 sessions or across approximately 6 sessions (Clark et al., 1999).

Interpersonal Context

Interpersonal context variables have been researched in terms of the development, maintenance, and treatment of agoraphobia. The reason for this research interest is apparent from the following vignettes:

"My husband really doesn't understand. He thinks it's all in my head. He gets angry at me for not being able to cope. He says I'm weak and irresponsible. He resents having to drive me around, and doing things for the kids that I used to do. We argue a lot, because he comes home tired and frustrated from work only to be frustrated more by the problems I'm having. But I can't do anything without him. I'm so afraid that I'll collapse into a helpless wreck without him, or that I'll be alone for the rest of my life. As cruel as he can be, I feel safe around him because he always has everything under control. He always knows what to do."

This vignette illustrates dependency on the significant other for a sense of safety despite a nonsympathetic response that may only serve to increase background stress for the patient. The second vignette illustrates inadvertent reinforcement of fear and avoidance through attention from the significant other.

"My boyfriend really tries hard to help me. He's always cautious of my feelings and doesn't push me to do things that I can't do. He phones me from work to check on me. He stays with me and holds my hand when I feel really scared. He never hesitates to leave work and take me home if I'm having a bad time. Only last week we visited some of his friends, and we had to leave. I feel guilty because we don't do the things we used to enjoy doing together. We don't go to the movies anymore. We used to love going to ball games, but now its too much for me. I am so thankful for him. I don't know what I would do without him."

Perhaps some forms of agoraphobia represent a conflict between desire for autonomy and dependency in interpersonal relationships (Fry, 1962; Goldstein & Chambless, 1978). In other words, the "preagoraphobic" is trapped in a domineering relationship without the skills needed to activate change. However, the concept of a distinct marital system that predisposes toward agoraphobia lacks empirical evidence. That is not to say that marital or interpersonal systems are unimportant to agoraphobia. For example, interpersonal discord/dissatisfaction may represent one of several possible stressors that precipitate panic attacks. Also, interpersonal relations may be negatively impacted by the development of agoraphobia (Buglass, Clarke, Henderson, & Presley, 1977), and in turn contribute to its maintenance. Not unlike one of the earlier vignettes, consider the woman who has developed agoraphobia and now relies on her husband to do the shopping and other errands. These new demands upon the husband lead to resentment and marital discord. The marital distress adds to background stress, making progress and recovery even more difficult for the patient.

Aside from whether interpersonal dysregulation contributes to the onset or maintenance of PD/PDA, some studies suggest that poor marital relations adversely impact exposure-based treatments (Bland & Hallam, 1981; Dewey & Hunsley, 1989; Milton & Hafner, 1979). However, other studies show no relationship between marital distress and outcome from cognitive-behavioral therapy (Arrindell & Emmelkamp, 1987; Emmelkamp, 1980; Himadi, Cerny, Barlow, Cohen, & O'Brien, 1986). Another line of research suggests that involving significant others in every aspect of treatment may override potential negative impacts of poor marital relations on phobic improvement (Barlow, O'Brien, & Last, 1984; Cerny, Barlow, Craske, & Himadi, 1987). Furthermore, involvement of significant others resulted in better long-term outcomes from cognitive-behavioral therapy for agoraphobia (Cerny et al., 1987). Similarly, communications training with significant others, compared to relaxation training, after 4 weeks of *in vivo* exposure therapy, resulted in significantly greater reductions on measures of agoraphobia by posttreatment (Arnow, Taylor, Agras, & Telch, 1985), an effect that was maintained over an 8-month follow-up. Together, these studies suggest the value of including significant others in the treatment for agoraphobia.

Yet another question is the degree to which treatment for panic disorder and agoraphobia influences marital/interpersonal relations. Some have noted that successful treatment can have deleterious effects (Hafner, 1984; Hand & Lamontagne, 1976). Others note that it has no effect or a positive effect on marital functioning (Barlow et al., 1983; Himadi et al., 1986). We (Barlow et al., 1983) suggested that when negative effects do occur, it may be because exposure therapy is conducted intensively, without the significant other's involvement, which causes major role changes that the significant other perceives as being beyond his or her control. This again speaks to the value of involving significant others in the treatment process.

Therapist Variables

Only a few studies have evaluated therapist variables in relation to cognitive-behavioral treatments for anxiety disorders. Williams and Chambless (1990) found that patients with agoraphobia who rated their therapists as caring/involved, and as modeling self-confidence, achieved better outcomes on behavioral approach tests. However, an important confound in this study was that patient ratings of therapist qualities may have depended on patient responses to treatment. Keijsers, Schaap, Hoogduin, and Lammers (1995) reviewed findings regarding therapist relationship factors and behavioral outcome. They concluded that empathy, warmth, positive regard, and genuineness assessed early in treatment predict positive outcome; patients who view their therapists as understanding and respectful improve the most; and patient perceptions of therapist

expertness, self-confidence, and directiveness relate positively to outcome, although not consistently. In their own study of junior therapists who provided cognitive-behavioral treatment for PD/PDA, Keijsers and colleagues (1995) found that more empathic statements and questioning occurred in Session 1 than in later sessions. In Session 3, therapists became more active and offered more instructions and explanations. In Session 10, therapists employed more interpretations and confrontations than previously. Most importantly, directive statements and explanations in Session 1 predicted poorer outcome. Empathic listening in Session 1 related to better behavioral outcome, whereas empathic listening in Session 3 related to poorer behavioral outcome. Thus, they demonstrated the advantages of different interactional styles at different points in therapy.

Most clinicians assume that therapist training and experience improve the chances of successful outcome. Some believe this to be the case particularly with respect to the cognitive aspects of cognitive-behavioral therapy (e.g., Michelson et al., 1990), and some indirect evidence for this supposition exists. Specifically, cognitive-behavioral therapy conducted by "novice" therapists in a medical setting (Welkowitz et al., 1991) was somewhat less effective in comparison to the same therapy conducted by inexperienced but highly trained therapists in a psychological setting (Barlow, Craske, Czerny, & Klosko, 1989), or by experienced and highly trained therapists in a community mental health setting (Wade, Treat, & Stuart, 1998). Huppert and colleagues (2001), who directly evaluated the role of therapist experience, found that, in general, therapist experience positively related to outcome, seemingly because these therapists were more flexible in administering the treatment and better able to adapt it to the individual being treated. Obviously, there is a need for more evaluation of the role of therapist experience and training in cognitive-behavioral therapy.

Equally, if not more important is the need to evaluate how much training of either novice or experienced therapists is necessary to attain therapeutic competency in cognitive-behavioral therapy. This is critically important in the current environment of dissemination of cognitive-behavioral treatments for anxiety disorders to real-world settings, in which training procedures must be adequate but not so costly that they are prohibitive and therefore not disseminable. Ongoing research in our settings is addressing exactly these issues. Others are investigating the benefits of training general practitioners in cognitive-behavioral therapy for panic disorder (Heatley, Ricketts, & Forrest, 2005).

Patient Variables

There has been a recent interest in the effect of comorbidity upon the outcomes of cognitive-behavioral therapy for PD/PDA. Brown, Antony, and Barlow (1995) found that comorbidity with other anxiety disorders did not predict response to cognitive-behavioral therapy overall, although social phobia was unexpectedly associated with superior outcome for PD/PDA. In contrast, we (Tsao, Lewin, & Craske, 1998) found a trend for comorbidity that comprised mostly other anxiety disorders to be associated with slightly lower rates of overall success. In a subsequent study, however, we replicated the finding by Brown et al. (1995) of no relationship between baseline comorbidity comprising mostly other anxiety disorders, and either immediate or 6-month outcome for PD/PDA (Tsao, Mystkowski, Zucker, & Craske, 2002).

Depressive disorders are highly comorbid with PD/PDA (e.g., Goisman et al., 1994). In contrast to expectations and to pharmacology trials, the available evidence does not consistently demonstrate detrimental effects of initial depression upon outcome from cognitive-behavioral therapy for PD/PDA. On the one hand, several studies found no relationship with outcome, regardless of whether depression was the principal diagnosis or secondary to PD/PDA (Brown et al., 1995; Laberge, Gauthier, Cote, Plamondon, & Cormier, 1993; McLean, Woody, Taylor, & Koch, 1998). On the other hand, Mennin and Heimberg's (2000) review led them to conclude a mixed pattern of results given evidence that patients without major depression showed greater reductions in fears of bodily sensations (Laberge et al., 1993), that patients with primary, but not secondary, depression had worse outcomes than those without depression (Maddock & Blacker, 1991), and that treatment completers were less likely than noncompleters to have comorbid depression (Wade et al., 1998). Some propose that depression impedes engagement in cognitive-behavioral therapy homework exercises. However, McLean and colleagues (1998) reported no relationship between depression

and compliance with cognitive-behavioral therapy homework. Similarly, Murphy, Michelson, Marchione, Marchione, and Testa (1998) found that depressed persons with PD/PDA engaged in as many self-directed exposures as nondepressed persons, although the depressed group reported more subjective anxiety during exposures.

A relatively high co-occurrence exists between PD/PDA and avoidant, dependent, and histrionic personality disorders (e.g., Reich et al., 1994). Questions of diagnostic reliability and validity aside, comorbid personality disorders are sometimes associated with poorer response than usual to cognitive-behavioral therapy for PD/PDA (e.g., Hoffart & Hedley, 1997; Marchand, Goyer, Dupuis, & Mainguy, 1998). However, closer examination reveals that although individuals with comorbid personality disorders have greater severity of PD/PDA at pre- and post–cognitive-behavioral therapy, the rate of decrease in PD/PDA symptoms usually is not affected by the comorbid personality disorder. Thus, Dreessen, Arntz, Luttels, and Sallaerts (1994) and van den Hout, Brouwers, and Oomen (2006) found that comorbid personality disorders did not affect response to cognitive-behavioral therapy for PD/PDA. Moreover, Hofmann and colleagues (1998) found that scores on questionnaire subscales reflecting Axis II personality disorders did not predict panic disorder treatment response to either cognitive-behavioral therapy or to medication. In fact, some personality traits may associate positively with outcome, as was reported by Rathus, Sanderson, Miller, and Wetzler (1995) with respect to compulsive personality features.

Substance-related disorders also commonly co-occur with PD/PDA. On the one hand, in a series of single cases ($N = 3$), Lehman, Brown, and Barlow (1998) demonstrated successful control of panic attacks in individuals who were abusing alcohol. On the other hand, the addition of anxiety treatment to a relapse prevention program for abstinent individuals with a primary diagnosis of alcohol dependence and a comorbid diagnosis of PDA or social phobia decreased anxiety symptoms relative to a relapse prevention program alone (Schade et al., 2005). However, adding the anxiety treatment did not affect rates of alcohol relapse in that study.

Another source of comorbidity is medical conditions, such as cardiac arrhythmias or asthma, that may slow improvement rates given the additional complications involved in discriminating between anxiety and disease symptomatology, increases in actual medical risk, and the stress of physical diseases. Although the effect of medical comorbidity on outcome has not been assessed to date, cognitive-behavioral therapy for panic disorder has been shown to alleviate self-reported physical health symptoms (Schmidt et al., 2003).

Other patient variables include socioeconomic status and general living conditions. We evaluated perceived barriers to receiving mental health treatment in our primary care study of panic disorder (Craske, Golinelli, et al., 2005). Commonly reported barriers included inability to find out where to go for help (43%), worry about cost (40%), lack of coverage by one's health plan (35%), and inability to get an appointment soon enough (35%). Also, in our multicenter trial, attrition from cognitive-behavioral and/or medication treatment for panic disorder with minimal agoraphobia was predicted by lower education, which in turn was dependent on lower income (Grilo et al., 1998). Similarly, level of education and motivation were associated with dropout rates in another sample, although the effects were small (Keijsers, Kampman, & Hoogduin, 2001). Low education–income may reflect less discretionary time to engage in activities such as weekly treatment. Consider the woman who is a mother of two, a full-time clerk, whose husband is on disability due to back injury, or the full-time student who works an extra 25 hours a week to pay his way through school. Under these conditions, treatment assignments of daily *in vivo* exposure exercises are much less likely to be completed. Frustration with lack of treatment progress is likely to result. Therapeutic success requires either a change in lifestyle that allows the cognitive-behavioral treatment to become a priority or termination of therapy until a later time, when life circumstances are less demanding. In fact, these kinds of life-circumstance issues may explain the trend for African Americans to show less treatment benefit in terms of mobility, anxiety, and panic attacks, than European Americans (Friedman & Paradis, 1991; Williams & Chambless, 1994). Although, in contrast to these two studies, Friedman, Paradis, and Hatch (1994) found equivalent outcomes across the two racial groups, and the results from another study yielded outcomes from a female African American sample that were judged to be comparable to those of European Americans (Carter, Sbrocco, Gore, Marin, & Lewis, 2003). The influence of ethnic and cultural differences on treatment outcome and delivery clearly needs more evaluation.

Finally, patients' understanding of the nature of their problem may be important to the success of cognitive-behavioral treatments. Given the somatic nature of panic disorder, many patients seek medical help first. Beyond that, however, differences in the way the problem is conceptualized could lead to the perception that pharmacological or analytical treatment approaches are more credible than cognitive-behavioral treatment approaches. For example, individuals who strongly believe their condition is due to "a neurochemical imbalance" may be more likely to seek medication and to refute psychological treatments. Similarly, individuals who attribute their condition to "something about my past—it must be unconscious influences" may resist cognitive-behavioral interpretations. Also, Grilo and colleagues (1998) found that patients with PD/PDA who attributed their disorder to specific stressors in their lives were more likely to drop out of cognitive-behavioral or medication treatment, perhaps because they saw the offered treatment as irrelevant.

Concurrent Pharmacological Treatment

Many more patients receive medications than cognitive-behavioral therapy for panic disorder and agoraphobia, partly because primary care physicians are usually the first line of treatment. Thus, one-half or more of patients with panic disorder who attend psychology research clinics already are taking anxiolytic medications. The obvious questions, therefore, are the extent to which cognitive-behavioral therapy and medications have a synergistic effect, and how medications impact cognitive-behavioral therapy.

Results from large clinical trials, including our own multisite trial (Barlow, Gorman, Shear, & Woods, 2000), suggest no advantage during or immediately after the conclusion of treatment combining cognitive-behavioral and pharmacological approaches. Specifically, both individual cognitive-behavioral and drug treatment and a combination treatment were immediately effective following treatment. Furthermore, following medication discontinuation, the combination of medication and cognitive-behavioral therapy fared worse than cognitive-behavioral therapy alone, suggesting the possibility that state- (or context-) dependent learning in the presence of medication may have attenuated the new learning that occurs during cognitive-behavioral therapy. On the other hand, in the primary care setting, we found that the addition of even just one component of cognitive-behavioral therapy to medications for PD/PDA resulted in statistically and clinically significant improvements at posttreatment and 12 months later (Craske, Golinelli, et al., 2005).

More recently, our multisite collaborative team has been investigating long-term strategies in the treatment of panic disorder. We examined sequential combination strategies to determine whether this approach was more advantageous than simultaneously combining treatments. In this study, currently in preparation for publication, 256 patients with panic disorder with all levels of agoraphobia completed 3 months of initial treatment with cognitive-behavioral therapy. Fifty-eight of those patients did not reach an optimal level of functioning (high end-state functioning) and entered a trial in which they received either continued cognitive-behavioral therapy or paroxetine. Paroxetine was administered for up to 1 year, whereas cognitive-behavioral therapy was delivered twice a month for 3 months. At the end of the 1-year period, there was a strong suggestion, represented as a statistical trend, that more of the patients receiving paroxetine achieved responder status compared to those receiving continued cognitive-behavioral treatment. Specifically, 60% of the nonresponders receiving paroxetine became responders, compared to 35% receiving continued cognitive-behavioral therapy ($p \leq .083$). Further evaluation of effect sizes will help us to evaluate the importance of this difference. This study also evaluated long-term strategies for maintaining gains in those patients who responded to cognitive-behavioral therapy, as described below.

In another study with similar results, patients who did not respond to cognitive-behavioral therapy also benefited more from the addition of a serotonergic drug (paroxetine) to continued cognitive-behavioral therapy than from the addition of a drug placebo, with substantially different effect sizes (Kampman, Keijsers, Hoogduin, & Hendriks, 2002). Con-

versely, individuals who are resistant to pharmacotherapy may respond positively to cognitive-behavioral therapy, although these findings were part of an open trial without randomization (Heldt et al., 2006).

Findings from the combination of fast-acting anxiolytics and, specifically, the high-potency benzodiazepines with behavioral treatments for agoraphobia are contradictory (e.g., Marks et al., 1993; Wardle et al., 1994). Nevertheless, several studies have reliably demonstrated the detrimental effects of chronic use of high-potency benzodiazepines on short-term and long-term outcome in cognitive-behavioral treatments for panic or agoraphobia (e.g., Otto, Pollack, & Sabatino, 1996; van Balkom, de Beurs, Koele, Lange, & van Dyck, 1996; Wardle et al., 1994). Specifically, there is evidence for more attrition, poorer outcome, and more relapse with chronic use of high-potency benzodiazepines. In addition, use of benzodiazepines as needed was associated with poorer outcome than regular use or no use in one small naturalistic study (Westra, Stewart, & Conrad, 2002).

Finally, the cost-effectiveness of cognitive-behavioral and medication treatments alone versus in combination requires further evaluation; currently, cognitive-behavioral therapy is considered to be more cost-effective (e.g., disability costs, work days missed, health care use) than pharmacotherapy (Heuzenroeder et al., 2004).

Understanding the ways in which psychotropic medications influence cognitive-behavioral therapy may prove useful for developing methods that optimize the combination of these two approaches to treatment. First, medications, particularly fast-acting, potent medications that cause a *noticeable* shift in state and are used on an as-needed basis (e.g., benzodiazepines, beta-blockers), may contribute to relapse, because therapeutic success is attributed to them rather than to cognitive-behavioral therapy. Patients' resultant lack of perceived self-control may increase relapse potential when medication is withdrawn or contribute to maintenance of a medication regimen under the assumption that it is necessary to functioning. In support, attribution of therapeutic gains to alprazolam, and lack of confidence in coping without alprazolam, even when given in conjunction with behavioral therapy, predicted relapse (Basoglu, Marks, Kilic, Brewin, & Swinson, 1994). Second, medications may assume the role of safety signals, or objects to which persons erroneously attribute their safety from painful, aversive outcomes. Safety signals contribute to maintenance of fear and avoidance in the long term (Hermans, Craske, Mineka, & Lovibond, 2006) and may interfere with corrections of misappraisals of bodily symptoms. Third, medications may block the capacity to experience fear, which, at least initially in exposure therapy, is a positive predictor of overall outcome (for a review, see Craske & Mystkowski, 2006). Fourth, medications may reduce the motivation to engage in practices of cognitive-behavioral skills, especially ones that effectively reduce panic and anxiety. Finally, learning that takes place under the influence of medications may not necessarily generalize to the time when medications are removed, thus contributing to relapse (Bouton & Swartzentruber, 1991). Some of these points are illustrated in the following vignettes:

"I had been through a program of cognitive-behavioral therapy, but it was really the Paxil that helped. Because I was feeling so much better, I considered tapering off the medication. At first I was very concerned about the idea. I had heard horror stories about what people go through when withdrawing. However, I thought it would be OK as long as I tapered slowly. So, I gradually weaned myself off. It really wasn't that bad. Well, I had been completely off the medication for about a month when the problem started all over again. I remember sitting in a restaurant, feeling really good because I was thinking about how much of a problem restaurants used to be for me before, and how easy it seemed now. Then, whammo. I became very dizzy and I immediately thought, 'Oh no, here it comes.' I had a really bad panic attack. All I could think of was why didn't I stay on the medication."

"I started to lower my dose of Xanax. I was OK for the first couple of days. . . . I felt really good. Then, when I woke up on Friday morning, I felt strange. My head felt really tight and I worried about having the same old feelings all over again. The last thing I want to do is to go through that again. So I took my usual dose of Xanax and, within a few minutes, I felt pretty good again. I need the medication. I can't manage without it right now."

Continuation of exposure after medication is withdrawn may offset relapse, because it enhances attributions of personal mastery and reduces the safety signal function of medications. In addition, opportunities to practice exposure and cognitive and behavioral strategies without the aid of medication overcome state dependency and enhance generalization of therapeutic gains once treatment is over.

CASE STUDY

Julie, a 33-year-old European American, mother of two, lives with Larry, her husband of 8 years. For the past 3 years she has been chronically anxious and panic stricken. She describes her panic attacks as unbearable and increasing in frequency. The first time she felt panicky was just over 3 years ago, when she was rushing to be by her grandmother's side in the last moments before she died. Julie was driving alone on the freeway. She remembers feeling as if everything were moving in slow motion, as if the cars were standing still, and things around her seemed unreal. She recalled feeling short of breath and detached. However, it was so important to reach her destination that she did not dwell on how she felt until later. After the day was over, she reflected upon how lucky she was not to have had an accident. A few weeks later, the same type of feeling happened again when driving on the freeway. This time it occurred without the pressure of getting to her dying grandmother. It scared Julie because she was unable to explain the feelings. She pulled off to the side of the road and called her husband, who came to meet her. She followed him home, feeling anxious all the way.

Now, Julie has these feelings in many situations. She describes her panic attacks as feelings of unreality, detachment, shortness of breath, a racing heart, and a general fear of the unknown. It is the unreality that scares her the most. Consequently, Julie is sensitive to anything that produces "unreal" types of feelings, such as the semiconsciousness that occurs just before falling asleep, the period when daylight changes to night, bright lights, concentrating on the same thing for long periods of time, alcohol or drugs, and being anxious in general. Even though she has a prescription for

Klonopin (a high-potency benzodiazepine), she rarely, if ever, uses it because of her general fear of being under the influence of a drug, or of feeling an altered state of consciousness. She wants to be as alert as possible at all times, but she keeps the Klonopin with her in the event that she has no other way of managing her panic. She does not leave home without the Klonopin. Julie is very sensitive to her body in general; she becomes scared of anything that feels a little different than usual. Even coffee, which she used to enjoy, is distressing to her now because of its agitating and racy effects. She was never a big exerciser, but to think of exerting herself now is also scary. Julie reports that she is constantly waiting for the next panic attack to occur. She avoids freeways, driving on familiar surface streets only. She limits herself to a 10-mile radius from home. She avoids crowds and large groups as well, partly because of the feeling of too much stimulation and partly because she is afraid to panic in front of others. In general, she prefers to be with her husband or her mother. However, she can do most things as long as she is within her "safety" region.

Julie describes how she differs from the way she used to be: how weak and scared she is now. The only other incident similar to her current panic attacks occurred in her early 20s, when she had a negative reaction to smoking marijuana. Julie became very scared of the feeling of losing control and feared that she would never return to reality. She has not taken drugs since then. Otherwise, there is no history of serious medical conditions, or any previous psychological treatment. Julie had some separation anxiety and was shy as a young child and throughout her teens. However, her social anxiety improved throughout her 20s to the point that until the onset of her panic attacks, she was mostly very comfortable around people. Since the onset of her panic attacks, Julie has become concerned that others will notice that she appears anxious. However, her social anxiety is limited to panic attacks and does not reflect a broader social phobia.

In general, Julie's appetite is good, but her sleep is restless. At least once a week she wakes abruptly in the middle of the night, feeling short of breath and scared, and has great difficulty going to sleep when her husband travels. In addition to worrying about her panic attacks, Julie worries about her husband and her children, although these latter worries are sec-

ondary to her worry about panicking and are not excessive. She has some difficulty concentrating but is generally able to function at home and at work, because of the familiarity of her environment and the safety she feels in the presence of her husband. Julie works part-time as the manager of a business that she and her husband own. She sometimes becomes depressed about her panic and the limitations on how far she can travel. Occasionally she feels hopeless about the future, doubting whether she will ever be able to escape the anxiety. Although the feelings of hopelessness and the teariness never last than more than a few days, Julie has generally had a low-grade depressed mood since her life became restricted by the panic attacks.

Julie's mother and her uncle both had panic attacks when they were younger. Julie is now worried that her oldest child is showing signs of being overly anxious, because he is hesitant about trying new things or spending time away from home.

ASSESSMENT

A functional behavioral analysis depends on several different modes of assessment, which we describe next.

Interviews

An in-depth interview is the first step in establishing diagnostic features and the profile of symptomatic and behavioral responses. Several semistructured and fully structured interviews exist. The Anxiety Disorders Interview Schedule—Fourth Edition (ADIS-IV; Di Nardo, Brown, & Barlow, 1994) primarily assesses anxiety disorders, as well as mood and somatoform disorders. Psychotic and drug conditions are screened by this instrument also. The ADIS-IV facilitates gathering the necessary information to make a differential diagnosis among anxiety disorders and offers a means to distinguish between clinical and subclinical presentations of a disorder. Data on the frequency, intensity, and duration of panic attacks, as well as details on avoidance behavior, are embedded within the ADIS-IV; this information is necessary for tailoring treatment to each individual's presentation. The value of structured interviews is in their contribution to a differential diagnosis and interrater reliability. Interrater agreement ranges from satisfactory to excellent for the various anxiety disorders using the ADIS-IV (Brown, Di Nardo, Lehman, & Campbell, 2001).

Similarly, the Schizophrenia and Affective Disorders Schedule—Lifetime Version (modified for the study of anxiety) produces reliable diagnoses for most of the anxiety disorders (generalized anxiety disorder and simple phobia are the exceptions) (Manuzza, Fyer, Liebowitz, & Klein, 1990), as does the Structured Clinical Interview for DSM-IV (SCID), which covers all of the mental disorders (First, Spitzer, Gibbon, & Williams, 1994).

Differential diagnosis is sometimes difficult because, as described earlier, panic is a ubiquitous phenomenon (Barlow, 1988) that occurs across a wide variety of emotional disorders. It is not uncommon for persons with specific phobias, social phobia, generalized anxiety disorder, obsessive–compulsive disorder, and posttraumatic stress disorder to report panic attacks. For Julie, there was a differential diagnostic question regarding social phobia and PDA. Shown in Figure 1.1 are the ADIS-IV questions that addressed this differentiation (Julie's answers are in italics).

As demonstrated in Figure 1.1, Julie experiences panic attacks in social situations and is concerned about being negatively evaluated by others if her anxiety becomes visibly apparent. However, despite her history of shyness, Julie's current social discomfort is based primarily on the possibility of panicking. Because of this, and because she meets the other criteria for PDA (i.e., uncued/nonsocial panic attacks and pervasive apprehension about future panic attacks), the social distress is best subsumed under the domain of PDA. If Julie reported that she experiences panic attacks in social situations only, or that she worries about panic attacks in social situations only, then a diagnosis of social phobia would be more probable. A report of uncued panic attacks, as well as self-consciousness about things that she might do or say in social situations regardless of the occurrence of panic, would be consistent with a dual diagnosis of PDA and social phobia. In general, individuals with PDA may continue to feel anxious even when playing a passive role in a social setting, whereas a patient with social phobia is more likely to feel relaxed when he or she is not the center of attention and does not anticipate being evaluated or judged (Dattilio & Salas-Auvert, 2000).

The same types of diagnostic questioning are useful for distinguishing between PDA and claustrophobia. Other differential diagnostic issues can arise with respect to somatoform disorders, real medical conditions, and avoidant or dependent personality disorders.

Medical Evaluation

A medical evaluation is generally recommended, because several medical conditions should be ruled out before assigning the diagnosis of PD/PDA. These include thyroid conditions, caffeine or amphetamine intoxication, drug withdrawal, or pheochromocytoma (a rare adrenal gland tumor). Furthermore, certain medical conditions can exacerbate PD/PDA, although it is likely to continue even when the symptoms are under medical control. Mitral valve prolapse, asthma, allergies, and hypoglycemia fall into this latter category. According to the model described earlier, these medical conditions exacerbate PD/PDA to the extent that they elicit the feared physical sensations. For example, mitral valve prolapse sometimes produces the sensation of a heart flutter, asthma produces shortness of breath, and hypoglycemia produces dizziness and weakness, all of which overlap with symptoms of panic and may therefore become conditioned cues for panic.

Self-Monitoring

Self-monitoring is a very important part of assessment and treatment for panic disorder–agoraphobia. Retrospective recall of past episodes of panic and anxiety, especially when made under anxious conditions, may inflate estimates of panic frequency and intensity (Margraf et al., 1987; Rapee, Craske, & Barlow, 1990). Moreover, such inflation may contribute to apprehension about future panic. In contrast, ongoing self-monitoring generally yields more accurate, less inflated estimates (for a comprehensive review of self-monitoring for panic and anxiety, see Craske & Tsao, 1999). Also, ongoing self-monitoring is believed to contribute to an objective self-awareness. Objective self-monitoring replaces negative affect-laden self-statements such as "I feel horrible. This is the worst its ever been—my whole body is out of control" with "My anxiety level is 6. My symptoms include tremulousness, dizziness, unreal feelings, and short-

Parts of ADIS-IV Panic Disorder Section

Do you currently have times when you feel a sudden rush of intense fear or discomfort? *Yes.*

In what kinds of situations do you have those feelings? *Driving, especially on freeways . . . alone at home . . . at parties or in crowds of people.*

Did you ever have those feelings come "from out of the blue," for no apparent reason, or in situations where you did not expect them to occur? *Yes.*

How long does it usually take for the rush of fear/discomfort to reach its peak level? *It varies, sometimes a couple of seconds and at other times it seems to build more slowly.*

How long does the fear/discomfort usually last at its peak level? *Depends on where I am at the time. If it happens when I'm alone, sometimes it is over within a few minutes or even seconds. If I'm in a crowd, then it seems to last until I leave.*

In the last month, how much have you been worried about, or how fearful have you been about having another panic attack?

0	1	2	3	4	5	6	7	8
No worry no fear		Rarely worried/mild fear		Occasionally worried/moderate fear		Frequently worried/ severe fear		Constantly worried/ extreme fear

Parts of ADIS-IV Social Phobia Section

In social situations, where you might be observed or evaluated by others, or when meeting new people, do you feel fearful, anxious, or nervous? *Yes.*

Are you overly concerned that you might do and/or say something that might embarrass or humiliate yourself in front of others, or that others may think badly of you? *Yes.*

What are you concerned will happen in these situations? *That others will notice that I am anxious. My face turns white and my eyes look strange when I panic. I am worried that I'll flip out in front of them, and they won't know what to do.*

Are you anxious about these situations because you are afraid that you will have an unexpected panic attack? *Yes (either a panic or that I'll feel unreal).*

Other than when you are exposed to these situations, have you experienced an unexpected rush of fear/anxiety? *Yes.*

FIGURE 1.1. Julie's responses to ADIS-IV questions.

ness of breath—and this episode lasted 10 minutes." Objective self-awareness usually reduces negative affect. Finally, self-monitoring provides feedback for judging progress and useful material for in-session discussions.

Panic attacks are recorded in the Panic Attack Record, a version of which is shown in Figure 1.2. This record is to be completed as soon as possible after a panic attack occurs; therefore, it is carried on-person (wallet size). Daily levels of anxiety, depression, and worry

about panic are monitored with the Daily Mood Record shown in Figure 1.3. This record is completed at the end of each day. Finally, activities may be recorded by logging daily excursions in a diary, or by checking off activities completed from an agoraphobia checklist.

A common problem with self-monitoring is noncompliance. Sometimes noncompliance is due to misunderstanding or lack of perceived credibility in self-monitoring. Most often, however, noncompliance is due to anticipation of

Date 2/16/06   Time began 5:20 P.M.

Triggers Home alone and shortness of breath

Expected x   Unexpected

Maximum Fear   0——1——2——3——4——5——6——7——8——9——10
                None   Mild   Moderate   Strong   Extreme

Check all symptoms present to at least a mild degree:

Chest pain or discomfort	_____	Sweating	x_____
Heart racing/palpitations/pounding	x_____	Nausea/upset stomach	_____
Short of breath	x_____	Dizzy/unsteady/lightheaded/faint	_____
Shaking/trembling	x_____	Chills/hot flushes	_____
Numbness/tingling	_____	Feelings of unreality	x_____
Feelings of choking	_____	Fear of dying	_____
Fear of losing control/going crazy	x_____		

Thoughts: I am going crazy, I will lose control
Behaviors: Called my mother

FIGURE 1.2. Julie's Panic Attack Record.

more anxiety as a result of monitoring. This is particularly true for individuals whose preferred style of coping is to distract themselves as much as possible, and to avoid "quiet" times, when thoughts of panic might become overwhelming: "Why should I make myself worse by asking myself how bad I feel?" In Julie's case, the self-monitoring task was particularly difficult, because explicit reminders of her anxiety elicited strong concerns about losing touch with reality. Prompting, reassurance that anxiety about self-monitoring would subside with perseverance at self-monitoring, and emphasis on objective versus subjective self-monitoring were helpful for Julie. In addition, cognitive restructuring in the first few sessions helped Julie to be less afraid of the feelings of unreality; therefore, she was less afraid to be reminded of those feelings by self-monitoring. Finally, therapist attention to the self-monitored information and corrective feedback about the method of self-monitoring at the start of each

0——1——2——3——4——5——6——7——8——9——10
None   Mild   Moderate   Strong   Extreme

Date	Average anxiety	Average depression	Average worry about panic
2/16	7	5	7
2/17	5	4	5
2/18	4	4	5
2/19	4	3	4
2/20	4	4	5
2/21	2	1	1
2/22	2	2	2

FIGURE 1.3. Julie's Daily Mood Record.

treatment session reinforced Julie's self-monitoring.

Standardized Inventories

Several standardized self-report inventories provide useful information for treatment planning and are sensitive markers of therapeutic change. The Anxiety Sensitivity Index (Reiss, Peterson, Gursky, & McNally, 1986) has received wide acceptance as a trait measure of threatening beliefs about bodily sensations. It has good psychometric properties and tends to discriminate between panic disorder–agoraphobia and other types of anxiety disorders (e.g., Taylor et al., 1992; Telch, Sherman, & Lucas, 1989), especially the Physical Concerns subscale (Zinbarg et al., 1997). More specific information about which particular bodily sensations are feared the most and what specific misappraisals occur most often may be obtained from the Body Sensations and Agoraphobia Cognitions Questionnaire (Chambless et al., 1984). The Mobility Inventory (Chambless, Caputo, Gracely, Jasin, & Williams, 1985) lists agoraphobic situations rated in terms of degree avoidance when alone and when accompanied. This instrument is very useful for establishing *in vivo* exposure hierarchies. Measures of trait anxiety include the State–Trait Anxiety Inventory (Speilberger, Gorsuch, Lushene, Vagg, & Jacobs, 1983) and the Beck Anxiety Inventory (Beck, Epstein, Brown, & Steer, 1988).

In addition, we have developed two standardized self-report inventories that are useful for panic disorder and agoraphobia. The first, the Albany Panic and Phobia Questionnaire (Rapee, Craske, & Barlow, 1995), is a 32-item questionnaire designed to assess fear and avoidance of activities that produce feared bodily sensations, as well as more typical agoraphobia and social situations. Factor analyses confirmed three distinct factors labeled Agoraphobia, Social Phobia, and Interoceptive Fears. The questionnaire has adequate psychometric properties and is useful in profiling agoraphobic versus interoceptive avoidance. The second, the Anxiety Control Questionnaire, is a 30-item scale that assesses perceived lack of control over anxiety-related events and occurrences, such as internal emotional reactions or externally threatening cues (Rapee, Craske, Brown, & Barlow, 1996). This scale is designed to assess locus of control, but in a more specific and targeted manner relevant to anxiety and anxiety disorders compared to more general locus-of-control scales. A revised 15-item version yields three factors, Emotion Control, Threat Control, and Stress Control, with a higher-order dimension of perceived control (Brown, White, Forsyth, & Barlow, 2004). Changes in this scale from pre to posttreatment predicted reductions in comorbidity at follow-up in one study (Craske et al., 2007). Finally, measures of interpersonal context include the Dyadic Adjustment Scale (Spanier, 1976), and the Marital Happiness Scale (Azrin, Naster, & Jones, 1973).

Behavioral Tests

The behavioral test is a useful measure of degree of avoidance of specific interoceptive cues and external situations. Behavioral approach tests can be standardized or individually tailored. The standardized behavioral test for agoraphobic avoidance usually involves walking or driving a particular route, such as a 1-mile loop around the clinic setting. Standardized behavioral tests for anxiety about physical sensations involve exercises that induce panic-like symptoms, such as spinning in a circle, running in place, hyperventilating, and breathing through a straw (Barlow & Craske, 2006). Anxiety levels are rated at regular intervals throughout the behavioral tests, and actual distance or length of time is measured. The disadvantage of standardized behavioral tests is that the specific task may not be relevant to all patients (e.g., a 1-mile walk or running in place may be only mildly anxiety provoking); hence, the value of individually tailored tasks. In the case of agoraphobia, this usually entails attempts at three to five individualized situations that the patient has identified as ranging from *Somewhat difficult* to *Extremely difficult*, such as driving two exits on freeway, waiting in a bank line, or shopping in a local supermarket for 15 minutes. For anxiety about physical sensations, individually tailored behavioral tests entail exercises designed specifically to induce the sensations feared most by a given patient, and may include a tongue depressor to induce sensations of gagging, smells to induce sensations of nausea, or nose plugs to induce sensations of difficulty breathing. As with standardized tests, ongoing levels of anxiety and degree of approach behavior are measured in relation to individually tailored behavioral tests.

Individually tailored behavioral tests are more informative for clinical practice, although they confound between-subject comparisons for research purposes. On the one hand, standardized and individually tailored behavioral tests are susceptible to demand biases for both fear and avoidance prior to treatment, and improvement after treatment (Borkovec, Weerts, & Bernstein, 1977). On the other hand, behavioral tests are an important supplement to self-report of agoraphobic avoidance, because patients tend to underestimate what they can actually achieve (Craske et al., 1988). In addition, behavioral tests often reveal important information for treatment planning of which the individual is not yet fully aware. For example, the tendency to remain close to supports, such as railings or walls, may not be apparent until one observes the patient walk through a shopping mall. In Julie's case, the importance of changes from daylight to night was not apparent until she was asked to drive on a section of road as a behavioral test. Her response was that it was too late in the day to drive, because dusk made her feel as if things were unreal. Similarly, it was not until Julie completed a behavioral test that we recognized the importance of air-conditioning when Julie was driving. Julie believed that the cool air blowing on her face helped her to remain "in touch with reality." Finally, we noticed that her physical posture while driving was a factor that contributed to anxiety: Julie's shoulders were hunched, she leaned toward the wheel, and she held the wheel very tightly. All of these were targeted in the treatment: driving at dusk was included in her hierarchy; air-conditioning was regarded as a safety signal from which she should be weaned; and driving in a more relaxed position was part of mastery exposure.

Psychophysiology

Ongoing physiological measures are not very practical tools for clinicians, but they can provide important information. In particular, the discrepancy described earlier between reports of symptoms and actual physiological arousal (i.e., report of heart rate acceleration in absence of actual heart rate acceleration) may serve as a therapeutic demonstration of the role of attention and cognition in symptom production. Similarly, actual recordings provide data to disconfirm misappraisals such as "My heart feels like its going so fast that it will explode" or "I'm sure my blood pressure is so high that I could have a stroke at any minute." Finally, baseline levels of physiological functioning, which are sometimes dysregulated in anxious individuals, may be sensitive measures of treatment outcome (e.g., Craske, Golinelli, et al., 2005).

Functional Analysis

The various methods of assessment provide the material for a full functional analysis for Julie. Specifically, the topography of her panic attack is as follows: most common symptoms include a feeling of unreality, shortness of breath, and racing heart; average frequency is three per week; each panic attack on average lasts from a few seconds to 5 minutes, if Julie is not in a crowd; in terms of apprehension, Julie worries about panic 75% of the day; and she has mostly expected panic attacks but some unexpected ones as well. Julie has both situational and internal antecedents to her panic attacks. The situational antecedents include driving on freeways; crowds of people; being alone, especially at night; restaurants; dusk; reading and concentrating for long periods of time; and aerobic activity. The internal antecedents include heart rate fluctuations, lightheaded feelings, hunger feelings, weakness due to lack of food, thoughts of the "big one" happening, thoughts of not being able to cope with this for much longer, and anger. Her misappraisals about panic attack symptoms include beliefs that she will never return to normality, that she will go crazy or lose control, and that others will think she is weird. Her behavioral reactions to panic attacks include escape behaviors such as pulling off to the side of the road, leaving restaurants and other crowded places, calling her husband or mother, and checking for her Klonopin. Her behavioral reactions to the anticipation of panic attacks include avoidance of driving long distances alone, driving on unfamiliar roads and freeways or at dusk, crowded areas, exercise, quiet time with nothing to do, and doing one thing for a long period of time. In addition, she tries not to think about anxiety or feelings of unreality. Her safety signals and safety-seeking behaviors include having her Klonopin on hand at all times, always knowing the location of husband, and having the air-conditioning on. The consequences of her PDA affect her family: Julie's husband is concerned and supportive, but her mother thinks she should pull herself together because "it's all in her head." In addition, Julie works but has cut back the number of hours, and she travels and socializes much less. Her general mood includes some difficulty concentrating and sleeping, restlessness, headaches, and muscular pains and aches. In addition, she is occasionally tearful, sad, and hopeless, and generally feels down.

COMPONENTS OF COGNITIVE-BEHAVIORAL THERAPY

The components of the cognitive-behavioral treatment described in this section are integrated into a session-by-session treatment program in the next section.

Education

The treatment begins with education about the nature of panic disorder, the causes of panic and anxiety, and the ways panic and anxiety are perpetuated by feedback loops among physical, cognitive, and behavioral response systems. In addition, specific descriptions of the psychophysiology of the fight–flight response are provided, as well as an explanation of the adaptive value of the various physiological changes that occur during panic and anxiety. The purpose of this education is to correct the common myths and misconceptions about panic symptoms (i.e., beliefs about going crazy, dying, or losing control) that contribute to panic and anxiety. The survival value of alarm reactions (panic attacks) is emphasized throughout.

Education also distinguishes between the state of anxiety and the emotion of fear/panic, both conceptually and in terms of its three response modes (subjective, physiological, and behavioral). This distinction is central to the model of panic disorder and to the remainder of the treatment. Anxiety is viewed as a state of preparation for future threat, whereas panic is the fight–flight emotion elicited by imminent threat. Panic/fear is characterized by (1) perception or awareness of imminent threat, (2) sudden autonomic discharge, and (3) fight–flight behavior. Anxiety is characterized by (1) perception or awareness of future threat, (2) chronic tension, and (3) cautiousness, avoidance, and disruption of performance.

Self-Monitoring

Self-monitoring is considered essential to the personal scientist model of cognitive-behavioral therapy. Self-monitoring is introduced as a way to enhance objective self-awareness and increase accuracy in self-observation. As noted earlier, patients are asked to keep at least two types of records. The first, a Panic Attack Record, is completed as soon after each panic attack as possible; this record provides a description of cues, maximal distress, symptoms, thoughts, and behaviors. The second, a Daily Mood Record, is completed at the end of each day to record overall or average levels of anxiety, depression, and whatever else is considered important to record. Additionally, patients may keep a daily record of activities or situations completed or avoided.

Breathing Retraining

Breathing retraining is a central component early on in the development of panic-control treatments, because many panic patients describe symptoms of hyperventilation as being very similar to their panic attack symptoms. It is noteworthy, however, that hyperventilation symptom report does not always accurately represent hyperventilation physiology: only 50% or fewer patients show actual reductions in end-tidal carbon dioxide values during panic attacks (Hibbert & Pilsbury, 1989; Holt & Andrews, 1989; Hornsveld, Garssen, Fiedelij Dop, & van Spiegel, 1990).

In early conceptualizations, panic attacks were related to stress-induced respiratory changes that either provoke fear because they are perceived as threatening or augment fear already elicited by other phobic stimuli (Clark, Salkovskis, & Chalkley, 1985). Several studies illustrated a positive effect of breathing retraining. Kraft and Hoogduin (1984) found that six biweekly sessions of breathing retraining and progressive relaxation reduced panic attacks from 10 to 4 per week, but were no more effective than either repeated hyperventilation plus control of symptoms by breathing into a bag or identification of life stressors and problem solving. Other studies were uncontrolled reports that combined breathing retraining and cognitive restructuring, sometimes with *in vivo* exposure (Clark et al., 1985; Rapee, 1985; Salkovskis, Warwick, Clark, & Wessels, 1986).

More recently, the value of breathing retraining has been questioned. For example, it is unclear whether breathing retraining alone is therapeutic for agoraphobia, and several studies suggest that the addition of breathing retraining alone does not improve upon *in vivo* exposure (e.g., de Beurs, van Balkom, Lange, Koele, & van Dyck, 1995). We found breathing retraining to be slightly less effective than interoceptive exposure when each was added to cognitive restructuring and *in vivo* exposure (Craske, Rowe, Lewin, & Noriega-Dimitri, 1997), and in another study, the inclusion of breathing retraining resulted in poorer outcomes than cognitive-behavioral therapy without breathing retraining, although the findings were not robust (Schmidt et al., 2000). From their review of efficacy and mechanisms of action, Garssen, de Ruiter, and van Dyck (1992) concluded that breathing retraining probably effects change not through breathing per se, but through distraction and/or a sense of control. Given the recent recognition that tolerance of fear and anxiety may be a more critical learning experience than the elimination of fear (see Eifert & Forsyth, 2005), breathing retraining has been deemphasized, because it may become a method of avoidance of physical symptoms or a safety behavior, and thereby be antitherapeutic. When it is included in the treatment, it is essential that patients not rely upon breathing retraining as a method of avoidance or safety seeking.

Applied Relaxation

A form of relaxation known as applied relaxation has shown good results as a treatment for panic attacks. Applied relaxation entails training patients in progressive muscle relaxation (PMR) until they are skilled in cue control relaxation, at which point relaxation is used as a coping skill for practicing exposure to items from a hierarchy of anxiety-provoking tasks. A theoretical basis for relaxation as a treatment for panic attacks has not been elaborated beyond the provision of a somatic counter-response to the muscular tension that is likely to occur during anxiety and panic. However, evidence does not lend support to this notion (Rupert, Dobbins, & Mathew, 1981). An alternative suggestion is that, as with breathing retraining, fear and anxiety are reduced to the extent that relaxation provides a sense of control or mastery (Bandura, 1977; Rice & Blanchard, 1982). The procedures and mechanisms accountable for therapeutic gains are further clouded in the case of applied forms of relaxation given the involvement of exposure-based procedures as anxiety-provoking situations are faced.

Ost (1988) reported very favorable results with applied PMR: 100% of an applied PMR group ($N = 8$) were panic-free after 14 sessions in comparison to 71.7% of a nonapplied PMR group ($N = 8$). Furthermore, the results of the first group were maintained at follow-up (approximately 19 months after treatment completion): All members of the applied PMR group were classified as high end state (i.e., nonsymptomatic) at follow-up, compared to 25% of the nonapplied PMR group. Michelson and colleagues (1990) combined applied PMR with breathing retraining and cognitive training for 10 panickers. By treatment completion, all subjects were free of "spontaneous" panics, all but one were free of panic attacks altogether, and all met criteria for high end-state functioning. However, the specific contribution of applied PMR to these results is not known. Two subsequent studies by Ost (Ost & Westling, 1995; Ost, Westling, & Hellstrom, 1993) indicate that applied relaxation was as effective as *in vivo* exposure and cognitive therapy. In contrast, we (Barlow et al., 1989) found that applied PMR was relatively ineffective for panic attacks, although we excluded all forms of interoceptive exposure from the hierarchy of tasks to which PMR was applied, which was not necessarily the case in the studies by Ost. Clark and colleagues (1994) found that cognitive therapy was superior to applied PMR when conducted with equal amounts of *in vivo* exposure, whereas Beck, Stanley, Baldwin, Deagle, and Averill (1994) found very few differences between cognitive therapy and PMR when each was administered without exposure procedures.

Cognitive Restructuring

Initially, cognitive therapy for panic disorder and agoraphobia did not directly target misappraisals of bodily sensations, but instead fostered coping self-statements in anxiety-provoking situations. Michelson, Mavissakalian, and Marchione (1985) published the first of their series of investigations comparing different behavioral treatments to various coping-oriented cognitive treatments for agoraphobia. They compared paradoxical intention, graduated exposure, and progressive deep muscle relaxation, although all participants conducted self-directed *in vivo* exposure between sessions. At posttreatment and 3 months later, paradoxical intention demonstrated equivalent rates of improvement, but significantly more participants remained symptomatic compared to those treated with graduated exposure and relaxation. Michelson, Mavissakalian, and Marchione (1988) replicated this design with almost twice as many participants. Contrary to the first study, few significant differences were detected between treatments. Lack of differences was replicated in a third study (Michelson et al., 1990). Thus, coping-oriented cognitive treatments appeared to be as effective as behaviorally oriented treatments, although the cognitive treatments were all heavily contaminated by behavioral self-directed exposure. In a slightly different design, Murphy, Michelson, Marchione, Marchione, and Testa (1998) compared cognitive therapy combined with therapist- and self-directed exposure, relaxation combined with therapist- and self-directed exposure, and just therapist and self-directed exposure. Again, overall there were few significant differences, although the condition that included cognitive therapy yielded the most potent and stable changes. Without the self-directed exposure component, Emmelkamp and colleagues found that coping-oriented cognitive therapy (rational–emotive therapy and self-instruction training) was significantly less effective than prolonged *in vivo* exposure for agoraphobia on an array of behavioral and self-report measures of anxiety and avoidance (Emmelkamp, Brilman, Kuiper, & Mersch, 1986; Emmelkamp, Kuipers, & Eggeraat, 1978; Emmelkamp & Mersch, 1982).

Cognitive therapy that targets misappraisals of bodily sensations is clearly effective with samples with mild to moderate levels of agoraphobia, producing results that are either as effective as or superior to applied relaxation (Arntz & van den Hout, 1996; Beck et al., 1994; Clark et al., 1994; Ost & Westling, 1995; Stanley et al., 1996). Results with more severe levels of agoraphobia are mixed. One study indicated that cognitive therapy targeting misappraisals of bodily sensations is as effective as guided mastery exposure delivered intensively over 6 weeks for individuals with moderate to severe agoraphobia (Hoffart, 1995), and other studies showed that cognitive restructuring combined with breathing retraining and/or interoceptive exposure is as effective as self-directed *in vivo* exposure (Craske et al., 2003; de Ruiter, Garssen, Rijken, & Kraaimaat, 1989; Rijken, Kraaimaat, de Ruiter, & Garssen, 1992) for individuals with varying levels of agoraphobia. Other studies found that cognitive therapy is slightly less effective than guided mastery and *in vivo* exposure for agoraphobia (Bouchard et al., 1996; Williams & Falbo, 1996). Furthermore, several studies found no added benefit when cognitive therapy that targeted misappraisals of bodily sensations was added to *in vivo* exposure (Ost, Thulin, & Ramnero, 2004; van den Hout, Arntz, & Hoekstra, 1994).

Behavioral exposure-based strategies are usually included in cognitive therapy as vehicles for obtaining data that disconfirm misappraisals. The importance of exposure-based strategies to the effectiveness of cognitive therapy is not known, although 2 weeks of focused cognitive therapy with antiexposure instructions reduced panic attacks in all but one of a series of seven cases in a single-case, multiple baseline design (Salkovskis, Clark, & Hackmann, 1991).

In terms of implementation, cognitive therapy begins to provide a treatment rationale with discussion of the role of thoughts in generating emotions. Next, thoughts are recognized as hypotheses rather than fact, and are therefore open to questioning and challenge. Detailed self-monitoring of emotions and associated cognitions is instituted to identify specific beliefs, appraisals, and assumptions. Once relevant cognitions are identified, they are categorized into types of typical errors that occur during heightened emotion, such as overestimations of risk of negative events or catastrophizing of meaning of events. The process of categorization, or labeling of thoughts, is consistent with a personal scientist model and facilitates an objective perspective by which the validity of the thoughts can be evaluated. Thus, in labeling the type of cognitive distortion, the patient is encouraged to use an empirical approach to examine the validity of his or her thoughts by considering all of the available evidence. Therapists use Socratic questioning to help patients make guided discoveries and question their anxious thoughts. Next, more evidence-based alternative hypotheses are generated. In addition to surface-level appraisals (e.g., "That person is frowning at me because I look foolish"), core-level beliefs or schemas (e.g., "I am not strong enough to withstand further distress" or "I am unlikable") are questioned in the same way. Importantly, cognitive restructuring is not intended as a direct means of minimizing fear, anxiety, or unpleasant symptoms. Instead, cognitive restructuring is intended to correct distorted thinking; eventually fear and anxiety are expected to subside, but their diminution is not the first goal of cognitive therapy.

Exposure

Exposure is a critical phase of treatment and once begun, is a major focus of treatment sessions as well as between treatment session homework, since limited exposure practice is of small benefit and may even be detrimental. The exposure is designed to disconfirm misappraisals and extinguish conditioned emotional responses to external situations and contexts, through *in vivo* exposure, as well as to bodily sensations, through interoceptive exposure.

In Vivo Exposure

In vivo exposure refers to repeated and systematic real-life exposure, in this case, to agoraphobic situations. As indicated from the studies reviewed earlier, a long history of research has established the efficacy of *in vivo* exposure for agoraphobia.

Most often, *in vivo* exposure is conducted in a graduated manner, proceeding from the least to the most anxiety-provoking situations on an avoidance hierarchy. However, there is some evidence to suggest that intensive or ungraduated exposure may be effective. In a study by Feigenbaum (1988), treatment sessions were conducted in a massed format over the course of 6–10 consecutive days. One group received ungraded exposure ($N = 25$), beginning with the most feared items from avoidance hierarchies. Another group received graded exposure ($N = 23$), beginning with the least feared hierarchy items. Approximately one-third of this severely agoraphobic sample was housebound at initial assessment. At posttreatment and 8 months later, the conditions proved to be equally effective (although, intriguingly, the graded group reported the treatment to be more distressing). However, ungraded exposure was clearly superior at the 5-year follow-

up assessment: 76% of the intensive group versus 35% of the graded group reported themselves to be completely free of symptoms. When 104 subjects were added to the intensive exposure format, the same results were obtained. Of 129 subjects, 78% were reportedly completely symptom-free 5 years later. This dramatic set of results suggests that an intensive approach, which is likely to produce higher levels of arousal than a graduated approach, can be very beneficial (at least when conducted in a massed format). Unfortunately, the validity of the outcome measures in this study is somewhat questionable, and replication by independent investigators has yet to be reported.

Critical to *in vivo* exposure is the removal of safety signals and safety behaviors. Examples of safety signals include other people, water, money (to call for help), empty or full medication bottles, exit signs, and familiar landmarks when traveling. Safety behaviors similarly provide a sense of safety, and include seeking reassurance or checking for exits. Reliance on safety signals and safety behaviors attenuate distress in the short term but maintain excessive anxiety in the long term. With the therapist's guidance, the patient identifies and finds ways gradually to eliminate his or her own safety signals and behaviors. In addition, *in vivo* exposure is eventually combined with interoceptive exposure, by deliberately inducing feared sensations in feared situations.

The amount of time devoted to *in vivo* exposure is very dependent on the patient's agoraphobia profile. Obviously, more time is needed for patients with more severe agoraphobia. Also, as reviewed earlier, evidence indicates that inclusion of significant others in the treatment process can improve treatment outcomes (e.g., Cerny et al., 1987). The benefit obtained from involving significant others may depend on the pervasiveness of agoraphobia and the extent to which family roles and interactions have been affected by or contribute to the agoraphobic pattern.

Interoceptive Exposure

In interoceptive exposure, the goal is to deliberately induce feared physical sensations a sufficient number of times, and long enough each time so that misappraisals about the sensations are disconfirmed and conditioned anxiety responses are extinguished. A series of studies have reported on the effects of interoceptive exposure independent of other therapeutic strategies. Early on, Bonn, Harrison, and Rees (1971) and Haslam (1974) observed successful reduction in reactivity with repeated infusions of sodium lactate (a drug that produces panic-type bodily sensations). However, panic was not monitored in these investigations. Griez and van den Hout (1986) compared six sessions of graduated CO_2 inhalations to a treatment regimen of propranolol (a beta-blocker chosen because it suppresses symptoms induced by CO_2 inhalations), both conducted over the course of 2 weeks. CO_2 inhalation treatment resulted in a mean reduction from 12 to 4 panic attacks, which was superior to the results from propranolol. In addition, inhalation treatment resulted in significantly greater reductions in reported fear of sensations. A 6-month follow-up assessment suggested maintenance of treatment gains, although panic frequency was not reported. Beck and Shipherd (1997) similarly found positive effects from repeated CO_2 inhalations, although it had little effect on agoraphobia (Beck, Shipherd, & Zebb, 1997). Broocks and colleagues (1998) tested the effects of exercise (with once-weekly supportive contact from a therapist) in comparison to clomipramine or drug placebo over 10 weeks. The exercise group was trained to run 4 miles, three times per week. Despite high attrition from exercise (31%), exercise was more effective than the drug placebo condition. However, clomipramine was superior to exercise.

In the first comparison to other cognitive and behavioral treatments, we (Barlow et al., 1989) compared applied PMR, interoceptive exposure plus breathing retraining and cognitive restructuring, their combination with applied PMR, and a waiting-list control, in a sample with panic disorder with limited agoraphobia. The two conditions involving interoceptive exposure, breathing retraining and cognitive restructuring, were significantly superior to applied PMR and waiting-list conditions. The results were maintained 24 months following treatment completion for the group receiving interoceptive exposure, breathing retraining, and cognitive restructuring without PMR, whereas the combined group tended to deteriorate over follow-up (Craske, Brown, & Barlow, 1991). As already mentioned, we compared interoceptive exposure, cognitive therapy, and *in vivo* exposure to

breathing retraining, cognitive therapy, and *in vivo* exposure for individuals with varying levels of agoraphobia. The condition that included interoceptive exposure was slightly superior to breathing retraining at posttreatment and 6 months later (Craske et al., 1997). Similarly, Ito, Noshirvani, Basoglu, and Marks (1996) found a trend for those who added interoceptive exposure to their self-directed *in vivo* exposure and breathing retraining to be more likely to achieve at least a 50% improvement in phobic fear and avoidance. Recently, an intensive, 8-day treatment with a sensation-focused approach was developed for individuals with moderate to severe agoraphobia, and initial results are promising (Morisette, Spiegel, & Heinrichs, 2005). But breathing education, breathing retraining, and repeated interoceptive exposure to hyperventilation did not increase the effectiveness of *in vivo* exposure for agoraphobia (de Beurs, Lang, van Dyck, & Koele, 1995).

Interoceptive exposure is now a standard component of cognitive-behavioral therapy for panic disorder (e.g., Barlow et al., 2000; Craske, Lang, et al., 2005), although different groups give different emphases to interoceptive exposure, with some emphasizing it as a means for extinguishing fear responses (Barlow & Craske, 2006) and others, as a vehicle for disconfirming misappraisals (Clark, 1996).

In terms of implementation, a standard list of exercises, such as hyperventilating and spinning, are used to establish a hierarchy of interoceptive exposures. With a graduated approach, exposure begins with the less distressing physical exercises and continues with the more distressing exercises. It is essential that the patient endure the sensations beyond the point at which they are first noticed, for at least 30 seconds to 1 minute, because early termination of the task may eliminate the opportunity to learn that the sensations are not harmful and that the anxiety can be tolerated. The coping skills of cognitive restructuring and slow diaphragmatic breathing are used after each exercise, followed by a discussion of what the patient learned during the exercise about bodily sensations, fear, and avoidance. These interoceptive exercises are practiced daily outside of the therapy session to consolidate the process of learning. Interoceptive exposure extends to naturalistic activities that inherently induce somatic sensations (e.g., caffeine consumption, exercise).

Optimizing Learning during Exposure

The ways in which learning during exposure therapy is optimized are open to continuing investigation. In this section, we highlight the latest developments in the research.

LENGTH OF AN EXPOSURE PRACTICE

Expectancies regarding the likelihood of aversive events are central to human fear conditioning. For example, contingency awareness (i.e., knowledge that a specific conditional stimulus [CS] predicts a specific unconditioned stimulus [US]), although of debatable *necessity* for conditioned responding (cf. Lovibond & Shanks [2002] and Ohman & Mineka [2001]) is a strong correlate of conditioned responding. Differential autonomic conditioning in particular is strongly associated with verbal measures of contingency knowledge (e.g., Purkis & Lipp, 2001). Expectancies also are important for extinction; extinction is posited to follow from a mismatch between the expectancy of an aversive event and the absence of its occurrence (Rescorla & Wagner, 1972), or from the perception of a negative change in the rate at which aversive events are associated with the CS (Gallistel & Gibbon, 2000); that is, expectancies for the US are violated during extinction. Thus, exposure tasks designed to violate expectancies for negative outcomes are hypothesized to be the most effective form of exposure (Craske & Mystkowski, 2006). Indirect evidence derived from several studies of phobic samples indicates that a single, massed exposure is more effective than a series of short exposures of the same total duration, such as one 60-minute duration versus three 20-minute durations of exposure (e.g., Chaplin & Levine, 1981; Marshall, 1985). Conceivably, the lengthier (massed) exposure is more effective, because it provides sufficient time to learn that aversive outcomes do not occur (i.e., to disconfirm negative outcome expectancies) (Craske & Mystkowski, 2006). However, no study to date has directly evaluated outcome expectancies or manipulated exposure duration in relation to outcome expectancies.

Related, however, is the body of work on the role of distraction during exposure, because distraction in essence represents disrupted (i.e., unmassed) exposure. We (Craske, Street, & Barlow, 1989) administered therapist- and self-directed exposure to patients with agoraphobia in small groups for 11 sessions. In one condition (N = 16), patients were instructed to monitor bodily sensations and thoughts objectively throughout *in vivo* exposures, and to use thought stopping and focusing self-statements to interrupt distraction. In a second condition (N = 14), they were taught to use specific distraction tasks during *in vivo* exposures (word rhymes, spelling, etc.), and to use thought stopping and distracting self-statements to interrupt the focus of attention upon feared bodily sensations and images. The treatment groups did not differ at posttreatment or at follow-up assessment, but, consistent with previous findings with obsessive–compulsive disorder (Grayson, Foa, & Steketee, 1982), the focused exposure group improved significantly from posttreatment to follow-up, in contrast to a slight deterioration in the distracted exposure group. However, the degree to which participants were actually distracted versus focused was not ascertainable. Also, other results regarding the detrimental effects of distraction during exposure therapy have been contradictory (e.g., Kamphuis & Telch, 2000; Oliver & Page, 2003; Rodriguez & Craske, 1995; Rose & McGlynn, 1997). The equivocal nature of the findings may derive from lack of an operational definition of "distraction," from confounds with the affective quality of the distractor, and from the unknown amount of distraction that actually takes place.

Nonetheless, given the recent advances in research, showing that neither physiological habituation nor the amount of fear reduction *within an exposure trial* is predictive of overall outcome (see Craske & Mystkowski, 2006), and given that self-efficacy through performance accomplishment is predictive of overall phobia reductions (e.g., Williams, 1992), and that toleration of fear and anxiety may be a more critical learning experience than the elimination of fear and anxiety (see Eifert & Forsyth, 2005), the focus now is on staying in the phobic situation until the specified time, when patients learn that what they are most worried about never or rarely happens, and/or that they can cope with the phobic stimulus and tolerate the anxiety. Thus, the length of a given exposure trial is based not on fear reduction but on the conditions necessary for new learning, in which fear and anxiety eventually subside across trials of exposure. Essentially, the level of fear or fear reduction within a given trial of exposure is no longer considered an index of learning, but a reflection of performance; learning is best measured by the level of anxiety experienced the next time the patient encounters the phobic situation or at some later time. Therefore, we have moved away from the model of "Stay in the situation until fear has declined" to "Stay in the situation until you have learned what you need to learn, and sometimes that means learning that you can tolerate fear." Exposure tasks, therefore, are to be defined clearly in advance, independent of level of fear reduction in a given day of practice. For example, patients are encouraged to practice inducing sensations of shortness of breath for a predetermined amount of time, and driving on the freeway for a predetermined distance to gain experience that disconfirms what they fear most. If patients are most worried about their fear remaining elevated throughout the entire exposure, then the goal of exposure is reframed as learning to be able to tolerate a sustained level of fear. Nevertheless, there may be occasions when the therapist judges that the most effective learning comes from enduring an exposure task until fear has declined, such as would be the case for patients who maintain that their fear will decrease only when they exit from the situation.

SCHEDULE OF EXPOSURE PRACTICES

A second way of potentially optimizing exposure is through the scheduling of exposure sessions. Spacing *between* exposure days (as opposed to the duration of a given exposure practice) pertains to consolidation of learning. Unfortunately, research in human samples has failed simultaneously to address both massing within exposure trials and spacing between exposure trials; that is, studies of spacing *between* exposure days have been conducted without ensuring necessarily that exposure is sufficiently lengthy *within* each exposure day to violate negative expectancies effectively; hence, the results have been mixed. Foa, Jameson, Turner, and Payne (1980) found greater decrements in anxiety and avoidance behavior in those receiving massed rather than spaced exposure sessions for agoraphobia, whereas Ramsay, Barends, Brueker, and Kruseman (1966) found spaced schedules to be superior to massed schedules for desensitization for specific phobias. Chambless (1990) found no differences between weekly versus daily sessions of graduated *in vivo* exposure and training in

respiratory control, distraction techniques, and paradoxical intention. However, some subjects were unwilling to accept massed exposure, creating a sample selection bias. In addition, Chambless pointed out that her results may lack generalization, because spaced exposure is usually interspersed with homework assignments, which may increase outcome efficacy. Nevertheless, she concluded by suggesting that the choice for massed versus spaced exposure is the decision of the therapist and patient. Some of the contradiction arises from inconsistent operationalization of massed and spaced scheduling across studies. Studies have compared arbitrarily chosen fixed durations and schedules of exposure, and sometimes what is labeled as "massed" in one study is labeled as "spaced" in another.

Nonetheless, given the strength of the experimental data on spacing of learning trials for nonemotional learning (Bjork & Bjork, 1992), the evidence for superior outcomes from a schedule of progressively increasing durations between exposure trials in circumscribed phobias (e.g., Rowe & Craske, 1998), and the evidence for substantially improved outcomes with monthly follow-up phone calls after weekly cognitive-behavioral therapy for panic disorder in primary care settings (Craske et al., 2006), a schedule of weekly sessions followed by progressively longer intervals between sessions may be advisable.

LEVEL OF AROUSAL WITHIN AN EXPOSURE PRACTICE

Clinically, on the one hand, there is wide subscription to the theory that corrective learning is maximal when physiological arousal is initially activated, then allowed to subside within and between exposure sessions (i.e., emotional processing theory) (Foa & McNally, 1996). However, recent post hoc analyses indicate that the degree to which physiological responding declines from the beginning to the end of an exposure trial is not predictive of overall outcome (see Craske & Mystkowski, 2006). In addition, empirical and theoretical developments suggest that a certain level of sustained excitation during extinction training may yield even more effective results upon retesting. Specifically, Cain, Blouin, and Barad (2004) have found that anxiogenic drugs such as yohimbine facilitate extinction in mice, and in general suggest that drugs or conditions that enhance adrenergic transmission overcome a natural inhibitory constraint upon extinction. However, extant data in humans are limited to post hoc observations of a positive relationship between sustained excitation (i.e., heart rate) during exposure and overall outcome with circumscribed phobias (e.g., Rowe & Craske, 1998).

On the other hand, there is evidence for detrimental effects of safety signals and safety behaviors, which presumably lower anxiety and arousal during exposures. As mentioned earlier, common safety signals for patients with panic disorder are the presence of another person, therapists, medications, and food or drink (Barlow, 1988). Although they alleviate distress in the short term, safety signals are assumed to sustain anxiety in the long term (Siddle & Bond, 1988). These effects have been explained by associative and attributional mechanisms. The associative model assumes that the negative associative strength of the inhibitory stimulus cancels out the positive associative strength of the excitatory stimulus, so that there is no change from what is predicted by all cues (Lovibond, Davis, & O'Flaherty, 2000). The attributional model implies that if subjects attribute the absence of an expected outcome to the inhibitory stimulus, then there is no reason to change the causal status of the excitatory stimulus (Lovibond et al., 2000).

In terms of treatment, Sloan and Telch (2002) reported that claustrophobic participants who received an exposure treatment in which they were encouraged to use safety signals, reported more fear at posttest and follow-up than those encouraged to focus on their fear during exposure. In a subsequent study, Powers, Smits, and Telch (2004) found that the perception of safety (i.e., availability of safety behaviors regardless of whether they were used) rather than use of safety was detrimental to treatment outcome, because level of fear reduction was unaffected by actual use of safety behaviors. However, in both studies, the effects of safety signal encouragement may have been attributable to distraction, and the results were limited to circumscribed phobias. In another study, Salkovskis (1991) showed that "within-situation safety behaviours" interfered with the benefits of exposure therapy for panic and anxiety, and that teaching anxious patients to refrain from these behaviors leads to greater fear reduction after an exposure session. Clearly much more direct investigation is needed on the effects of safety signals and avoidance responses during exposure therapy, especially given the very direct implications for clinical practice.

Such research may be directed at medications that can become safety signals, because their availability reassures patients that the dangers of extreme fear are controllable. Attribution of safety to medications impedes correction of misperceived danger (e.g., "It is safe for me to drive on the freeway even when unmedicated"), and attribution of therapeutic gains to a medication (alprazolam) in patients with panic disorder and agoraphobia predicted subsequent withdrawal symptoms and relapse (Basoglu et al., 1994). Thus, the greater relapse following exposure combined with anxiolytics (especially high-potency, short-acting drugs) compared to exposure alone (e.g., Marks et al., 1993) may be attributable to medications functioning as safety signals.

THE EFFECT OF CONTEXT ON RETURN OF FEAR

A fourth consideration to optimize learning during exposure therapy derives from conditioning models in which extinction involves learning new, inhibitory CS–no US associations as opposed to unlearning original CS–US associations. Thus, Bouton (1993) proposed that the original excitatory *meaning* of the CS is not erased during extinction; rather, an additional inhibitory *meaning* is learned. The resulting dual meaning of the CS creates an ambiguity that is resolved only by the current context of the CS. Bouton uses the analogy of an ambiguous word; that is, reaction to the word "fire" depends largely on the context in which it occurs; "fire" may elicit a panic reaction in a crowded theater and elicit very little reaction in a carnival shooting gallery. Thus, the context determines which meaning is expressed at any given time. In terms of anxiety treatments, bodily sensations may mean "sudden death" when experienced in a context that reminds the person of intense panic attacks before treatment, whereas the same sensations may mean "unpleasant but harmless" when experienced in a context that reminds a person of his or her success with treatment. The effects of context shifts have been tested in circumscribed phobias, and indeed, return of fear is greater when participants are subsequently assessed in a context distinctly different rather than the same as that in which they were treated (for reviews, see Craske & Mystkowski, 2006; Hermans et al., 2006). Hence, what is learned in the context of exposure therapy may not be retrieved at reencounters with the previously feared phobic object or situation after therapy is over.

Conceivably, conducting exposure therapy in multiple contexts minimizes the context renewal effect after therapy is over. Unfortunately, extant research with humans is limited to one study of circumscribed phobias (Vansteenwegen et al., 2007). Because it is not always feasible to conduct exposures in original fear-acquisition or multiple contexts, we (Mystkowski, Craske, Echiverri, & Labus, 2006) sought to investigate whether a contextually based return of fear could be counteracted via mental rehearsal. Phobic participants who were instructed to recall the exposure learning environment just prior to being retested with a spider in a novel context showed less return of fear than those who were instructed to recall unrelated events. Although these findings were based on circumscribed phobias, they raise the possibility that simply reminding patients to recall their treatment experiences may offset return of fear when they reencounter their previously feared situations after treatment is over.

OVERALL EFFICACY OF COGNITIVE-BEHAVIORAL THERAPY

Cognitive-behavioral therapy, involving most or all of the components just listed, yields panic-free rates in the range of 70–80% and high end-state rates (i.e., within normative ranges of functioning) in the range of 50–70%, for panic disorder with minimal agoraphobia (e.g., Barlow et al., 1989; Clark et al., 1994). Two meta-analyses reported very large effect sizes of 1.55 and 0.90 for cognitive-behavioral therapy for panic disorder (Mitte, 2005; Westen & Morrison, 2001). Also, results generally maintain over follow-up intervals for as long as 2 years (Craske et al., 1991). One analysis of individual profiles over time suggested a less optimistic picture in that one-third of patients who were panic-free 24 months after cognitive-behavioral therapy had experienced a panic attack in the preceding year, and 27% had received additional treatment for panic over that same interval of time (Brown & Barlow, 1995). Nevertheless, this approach to analysis did not take into account the general trend toward continuing improvement over

time. Thus, rates of eventual therapeutic success may be underestimated when success is defined by continuous panic-free status since the end of active treatment.

The effectiveness extends to patients who experience nocturnal panic attacks (Craske, Lang, Aikins, & Mystkowski, 2005). Also, cognitive-behavioral therapy is effective even when there is comorbidity, and some studies indicate that comorbidity does not reduce the effectiveness of cognitive-behavioral therapy for panic disorder (e.g., Allen & Barlow, 2006; Brown, Antony, & Barlow, 1995; McLean et al., 1998). Furthermore, cognitive-behavioral therapy results in improvements in comorbid anxiety and mood disorders (Brown et al., 1995; Tsao et al., 1998; Tsao, Mystkowski, Zucker, & Craske, 2002, 2005), although results in one study indicated that the benefits for comorbid conditions may lessen over time, when assessed 2 years later (Brown et al., 1995). Nonetheless, the general finding of improvement in comorbidity is significant given that it suggests the value of remaining focused on the treatment for panic disorder even when comorbidity is present, because the comorbidity will be benefited as well, at least up to 1 year. Finally, applications of cognitive-behavioral therapy have proven very helpful in lowering relapse rates upon discontinuation of high-potency benzodiazepines (e.g., Otto et al., 1993; Spiegel, Bruce, Gregg, & Nuzzarello, 1994).

Results in samples with moderate to severe agoraphobia are generally slightly less positive than those in samples with no or mild agoraphobia (e.g., Williams & Falbo, 1996). However, data typically show patterns of continuing improvement over time. Furthermore, Fava, Zielezny, Savron, and Grandi (1995) found that only 18.5% of their panic-free patients relapsed over a period of 5–7 years after exposure-based treatment for agoraphobia. As mentioned, some research suggests that the trend for improvement after acute treatment is facilitated by involvement of significant others in every aspect of treatment for agoraphobia (e.g., Cerny et al., 1987).

As noted earlier, recently, our multicenter group evaluated strategies for maintaining response in those who are considerably improved after cognitive-behavioral treatment. Specifically, 157 patients who had responded well to initial treatment were randomized to receive either no further cognitive-behavioral treatment or one maintenance session a month for 9 months. At that point all treatment was discontinued for 1 year. At the end of that year, 97.3% of the patients receiving the booster sessions continued to maintain their response, whereas 81.9% maintained their response without the booster sessions; that is, 18.1% showed some loss of response compared to only 2.7% of those receiving the booster sessions, a significant difference. In this large study, the value of occasional continued booster sessions was demonstrated.

Most of the outcome studies to date are conducted in university or research settings, with select samples (although fewer exclusionary criteria are used in more recent studies). Consequently, of major concern is the degree to which these treatment methods and outcomes are transportable to nonresearch settings, with more severe or otherwise different populations, and with less experienced or trained clinicians—a topic that is just now receiving attention. Wade and colleagues (1998) used a benchmarking strategy to compare their results from a community mental health center with results from research sites. One hundred ten individuals underwent cognitive-behavioral therapy for PD/PDA, concomitant with psychopharmocotherapy where appropriate. Therapists were trained extensively. As in prior studies, treatment completion correlated positively with years of education. Overall, the percent of panic-free individuals and the percent achieving normative levels of functioning on a variety of measures were comparable to percents obtained from research sites. As mentioned, we are now evaluating the degree to which these treatment results can be obtained in other settings (e.g., primary care) and with less-well-trained therapists. In our first study of panic disorder in primary care, we found that offering a treatment combination of cognitive-behavioral therapy (up to six sessions) and pharmacotherapy yielded highly significant outcomes relative to treatment as usual (TAU) in primary care settings, with relatively novice therapists (Roy-Byrne et al., 2005).

TREATMENT DESCRIPTION: PROTOCOL

What follows is a description of a 12-session cognitive-behavioral therapy for PDA tailored to Julie's presentation. Of course, the degree to which the various components of treatment are emphasized vary by the functional assessment conducted for each patient.

Overview

The basic aim of the treatment protocol is to influence directly the catastrophic misappraisals and avoidance of bodily sensations and agoraphobic situations. This is done first through the provision of accurate information as to the nature of the fight–flight response. By provision of such information, patients are taught that they experience "sensations" and not "panics," and that these sensations are normal and harmless. Second, treatment aims to teach a set of skills for developing evidence-based appraisals regarding bodily sensations and agoraphobic situations. At the same time, specific information concerning the effects of hyperventilation and its role in panic attacks is provided, with extensive practice of breathing retraining. Then, the crux of the treatment involves repeated exposure to feared internal cues and agoraphobic situations.

Session 1

The goals of Session 1 are to describe fear and anxiety; to help patients understand the cyclical influences among behavioral, physiological, and cognitive responses; to understand that panic attack symptoms are not harmful; and to begin self-monitoring, if it was not already begun with the initial assessment. Therapy begins with identifying anxiety patterns and the situations in which anxiety and panic attacks are likely to occur. Many patients have difficulty identifying specific antecedents, reporting that panic can occur at almost any time. Therapists help patients to identify internal triggers, specifically, negative verbal cognitions, catastrophic imagery, and physical sensations. The following interchange took place for Julie:

THERAPIST: In what situations are you most likely to panic?

JULIE: Crowded restaurants and when I'm driving on the freeway. But sometimes I am driving along, feeling OK, when all of a sudden it hits. And other times I can be sitting at home feeling quite relaxed and it just hits. That's when I really get scared, because I can't explain it.

THERAPIST: So, when you are driving on the freeway, what is the very first thing you notice that tells you you're about to panic?

JULIE: Well, the other cars on the road look as if they are moving really slowly.

THERAPIST: And what is the first thing you notice when you're at home?

JULIE: An unreal feeling, like I'm floating.

THERAPIST: So, it sounds like the panic attacks that seem to occur for no reason are actually tied in with the sensations of unreality or when things look as if they are moving in slow motion.

JULIE: I guess so. I always thought the physical feelings were the panic attack, but maybe they start the panic attack.

Next, the three-response system model for describing and understanding anxiety and panic is introduced. This model contributes to an objective self-awareness—to becoming a personal scientist—and provides the groundwork for an alternative conceptual framework for explaining panic and anxiety that replaces the patient's own misassumptions. Patients are asked to describe cognitive, physiological, and behavioral aspects to their responding: to identify the things that they *feel*, *think*, and *do* when they are anxious and panicky. As described earlier, differences between the response profiles of anxiety and panic are highlighted. After grasping the notion of three responses that are partially independent, interactions among the response systems are described. The patient is asked to describe the three-response system components in a recent panic attack and to identify ways in which they interacted to produce heightened distress. For example,

THERAPIST: How would you describe the three parts to the panic attack you had at home last week?

JULIE: Well, physically, my head felt really light, and my hands were clammy. I thought that I would either pass out or that I would somehow dissolve into nothingness. My behavior was to lie down and call my husband, who was at work.

THERAPIST: What was the very first thing you noticed?

JULIE: When I stood up, my head started to feel really weird, as if it was spinning inside.

THERAPIST: What was your very next reaction to that feeling?

JULIE: I held onto the chair. I thought something was wrong. I thought it could get worse and that I'd collapse.

THERAPIST: So it began with a physical sensation, and then you had some very specific thoughts about those sensations. What happened next?

JULIE: I felt very anxious.

THERAPIST: And what happened next?

JULIE: Well, the dizziness seemed to be getting worse and worse. I became really concerned that it was different from any other experience I had ever had. I was convinced that this was "it."

THERAPIST: So, as you became more anxious, the physical feelings and the thoughts that something bad was going to happen intensified. What did you do next?

JULIE: I called my husband and lay on the bed until he came home. It was horrible.

THERAPIST: Can you see how one thing fed off another, creating a cycle? That it began with a sensation, then some anxious thoughts, then feeling anxious, then more sensations and more thoughts, and more fear, and so on?

Reasons why panic attacks first began are addressed briefly. Patients are informed that it is not necessary to understand the reasons why they began to panic to benefit from the treatment, because factors involved in onset are not necessarily the same as the factors involved in the maintenance of a problem. Nevertheless, the initial panic attack is described as a manifestation of anxiety/stress. The stressors surrounding the time of the first panic attack are explored with the patient, particularly in terms of how stressors may have increased levels of physical arousal and primed certain danger-laden cognitive schemas.

Next, the therapist briefly describes the physiology underlying anxiety and panic, and the myths about what the physical sensations might mean. The main concepts covered in this educational phase are (1) the survival value or protective function of anxiety and panic; (2) the physiological basis to the various sensations experienced during panic and anxiety, and the survival function of the underlying physiology; and (3) the role of specific learned and cognitively mediated fears of certain bodily sensations. The model of panic we described earlier in this chapter is explained. In particular, the concepts of misappraisals and interoceptive conditioning are explained as accounting for panic attacks that seem to occur from out of the blue—that are triggered by very subtle internal cues or physical sensations that may occur at any time. Not only does this information reduce anxiety by decreasing uncertainty about panic attacks but it also enhances the credibility of the subsequent treatment procedures. This information is detailed in a handout given to the patient to read over the next week (for the handout, see Barlow & Craske, 2006).

This information was very important for Julie, because the inability to explain her panic attacks was a major source of distress. Here are some of the questions she asked in her attempt to understand more fully:

JULIE: So, if I understand you correctly, you're saying that my panic attacks are the same as the fear I experienced the time we found a burglar in our house. It doesn't feel the same at all.

THERAPIST: Yes, those two emotional states—an unexpected panic attack and fear when confronted with a burglar—are essentially the same. However, in the case of the burglar, where were you focusing your attention—on the burglar or on the way you were feeling?

JULIE: The burglar, of course, although I did notice my heart was going a mile a minute.

THERAPIST: And when you have a panic attack, where are you focusing your attention—on the people around you or on the way you are feeling?

JULIE: Well, mostly on the way I'm feeling, although it depends on where I am at the time.

THERAPIST: Being most concerned about what's going on inside can lead to a very different type of experience than being concerned about the burglar, even though basically the same physiological response is occurring. For example, remember our description of the way fear of sensations can intensify the sensations.

JULIE: But what about the feelings of unreality? How can they be protective or how can feeling unreal help me deal with a danger situation?

THERAPIST: OK, remember that it's the physiological events that are protective—not the sensations. The sensations are just the end result of those events. Now, feelings of unreality can be caused by changes in your blood flow to your brain (although not dangerously so), or from overbreathing, or from concentrating too intensely on what's going on inside you. So the unreality sensation may not be protective, but the changes in blood flow and overbreathing are.

JULIE: I understand how I can create a panic attack by being afraid of my physical feelings, like my heart racing or feeling unreal. But sometimes it happens so quickly that I don't have time to think.

THERAPIST: Yes, these reactions can occur very quickly, at times automatically. But remember, we are tuned to react instantaneously to things (including our own bodies) that we think mean danger. Imagine yourself walking through a dark alley, and you have reason to believe that somewhere in the darkness lurks a killer. Under those conditions, you would be extremely attentive to any sign, any sound, or any sight of another person. If you were walking through the same alley and were sure there were no killers, you might not hear or detect the same signals you picked up on in the first case. Now let's translate this to panic; the killer in the dark alley is the panic attack, and the signs, sounds, and smells are the physical sensations you think signal the possibility of a panic attack. Given the acute degree of sensitivity to physical symptoms that signal a panic attack, it is likely that you are noticing normal "noises" in your body that you would otherwise not notice, and on occasion, immediately become fearful because of those "noises." In other words, the sensations are often noticeable because you attend to them.

Next, the method of self-monitoring was described and demonstrated with in-session practice of completing a Panic Attack Record. Julie was concerned that self-monitoring would only elevate her distress, by reminding of the very thing she was afraid of (panic and unreality). The therapist clarified the difference between objective and subjective self-monitoring, and explained that distress would subside as Julie persevered with self-monitoring.

The homework for this session was to self-monitor panic attacks, daily anxiety, and mood and to read the handout. In fact, we encourage patients to reread the handout several times, and to actively engage in the material by circling or marking the most personally relevant sections or areas in need of clarification, because effort enhances long-term retention of the material learned. Of course, for some patients, reading the material draws their attention to things they fear (just as with self-monitoring). In this case, therapists can discuss the role of avoidance versus that of exposure, and how, with repeated readings, distress levels will most likely subside.

At the end of the session, Julie suddenly became highly anxious. She felt unable to tolerate either the treatment procedures or her anticipation of them. She became very agitated in the office and reported feelings of unreality. She opened the office door to find her husband, who was waiting outside. The therapist helped Julie understand how the cycle of panic had emerged in the current situation: (1) The trigger was the treatment description—having to eventually face feared sensations and situations; (2) this was anxiety producing, because Julie believed that she could not cope with the treatment demands, that the treatment would cause her so much anxiety that she would "flip out" and lose touch with reality permanently, or that she would never improve because she could not tolerate the treatment; (3) the current anxiety in the office elicited sensations of unreality and a racing heart; (4) Julie began to worry that she might panic and lose touch with reality permanently within the next few minutes; (5) the more anxious Julie felt, and the stronger her attempts to escape and find safety, the stronger the physical sensations became; and (6) she felt some relief upon finding her husband, because his presence reassured her that she would be safe. Julie was reassured that treatment would progress at a pace with which she was comfortable, but at the same time she was helped to understand that her acute distress about the feeling of unreality would be the precise target of this type of treatment, therefore attesting to the relevance of this treatment for her. She was also calmed by preliminary cognitive restructuring of the probability of permanently losing touch with reality. After a lengthy discussion, Julie became more receptive to treatment. A team approach to treatment planning and progress was agreed upon, so that Julie did not feel that she would be forced to do things she did not think she could do.

Session 2

The goals of this session are to begin the development of a hierarchy of agoraphobic situations and coping skills of breathing retraining and cognitive restructuring. The individualized hierarchy comprises situations that range from mild to moderate anxiety, all the way up to extreme anxiety. These situations become the basis of graduated *in vivo* exposure. Although *in vivo* exposure exercises are not scheduled to take place until Session 4, the hierarchy is introduced now, so that cognitive restructuring skills can be practiced in relation to each situation on the hierarchy before *in vivo* exposure begins. Moreover, the hierarchy will be refined as a result of the cognitive restructuring practice, because the latter highlights specific features of agoraphobic situations that are most anxiety provoking.

Julie was asked to develop a hierarchy over the following week. She expressed some doubt that she would ever be able to accomplish any, let alone all, of the items on her hierarchy. The therapist helped Julie by asking her to think of any situation in her lifetime that used to be difficult but became easier with practice. Julie remembered how anxious she used to be when she first started working with customers at her husband's office—and how that discomfort subsided over time. This was used to help Julie realize that the same might happen with the situations listed on her hierarchy. Julie's final hierarchy comprised the following situations: driving home from work alone; sitting in a crowded movie theater; spending 2 hours alone at home during the day; alone at home as day turned to night; driving on surface streets to her brother's house (10 miles) alone; driving two exits on freeway 444, with her husband following in the car behind; driving two exits on freeway 444, alone; driving four exits on freeway 444; and driving on the freeway to her brother's house alone. Then, Julie was to repeat all of these tasks without taking Klonopin, and without knowing the location of her husband.

Breathing retraining also is begun in this session. Patients are asked to hyperventilate voluntarily by standing and breathing fast and deep, as if blowing up a balloon, for 1½ minutes. With prompting and encouragement from the therapist, patients can often complete the full 1½ minutes, after which time they are asked to sit, close their eyes, and breathe very slowly, pausing at the end of each breath, until the symptoms have abated. The experience is then discussed in terms of the degree to which it produced symptoms similar to those that occur naturally during anxiety or panic. Approximately 50–60% of patients report close similarity of the symptoms. Often, however, similarity of the symptoms is confused with similarity of the anxiety. Because the exercise is conducted in a safe environment and the symptoms have an obvious cause, most patients rate the experience as less anxiety provoking than if the same symptoms had occurred naturally. This distinction is important to make, because it demonstrates the significance of perceived safety for the degree of anxiety experienced. Julie rated the hyperventilation exercise as very anxiety provoking (8 on a 0- to 10-point scale), and rated the symptoms as being quite similar to her panic symptoms (6 on a 0- to 10-point scale). She terminated the task after approximately 40 seconds, in anticipation of experiencing a full-blown panic attack. The therapist and Julie discussed this experience in terms of the three response systems, and the role of misappraisals and interoceptive conditioning described during the previous session.

Then, Julie was briefly educated about the physiological basis to hyperventilation (see Barlow & Craske, 2006). As before, the goal of the didactic presentation was to allay misinterpretations of the dangers of overbreathing, and to provide a factual information base on which to draw when actively challenging misinterpretations. The educational content is tailored to the patient's own educational level and covered only to the degree that it is relevant to the patient.

In the next step, the therapist teaches breathing retraining, which begins by teaching patients to rely more on the diaphragm (abdomen) than chest muscles. In addition, patients are instructed to concentrate on their breathing, by counting on their inhalations, and thinking the word "relax" on exhalations. (Slow breathing is introduced in Session 3.) Therapists model the suggested breathing patterns, then provide corrective feedback to patients while they practice in the office setting.

Initial reactions to the breathing exercise may be negative for patients who are afraid of respiratory sensations, because the exercise directs their attention to breathing. It also can be difficult for patients who are chronic overbreathers, and patients for whom any interruption of habitual breathing patterns initially increases respiratory symptomatology. In both cases, continued practice is advisable, with reassurance that sensations such as shortness of breath are not harmful. The goal is to use breathing skills training to encourage continued approach toward anxiety and anxiety-producing situations. On occasion, patients mistakenly view breathing retraining as a way of relieving themselves of terrifying symptoms, thus falling into the trap of fearing dire consequences should they not succeed in correcting their breathing. This is what happened for Julie:

JULIE: So, all I have to do is to slow down my breathing, then everything will be OK.

THERAPIST: Certainly, slowing down your breathing will help to decrease the physical symptoms that you feel, but I am not sure what you mean when you ask whether everything will be OK.

JULIE: That proper breathing will prevent me from losing touch with reality—that I won't disappear.

THERAPIST: Remember, whether you breathe slowly or quickly, from your chest or from your abdomen, you will not disappear. In other words, it is a misinterpretation to think that the sense of unreality means that you are permanently losing touch with reality or that you will disappear. Breathing retraining will help you to feel more relaxed and, therefore, less likely to feel the sense of unreality, but the sense of unreality is not a sign of actual loss of touch with reality and disappearance.

The homework is to practice diaphragmatic breathing for at least 10 minutes, two times a day in relaxing environments.

Therapists introduce in this session cognitive restructuring by explaining that errors in thinking occur for everyone when anxious, thus helping the patient to expect his or her thinking to be distorted. Patients are informed that these distortions have an adaptive function: Chances of survival are greater if we perceive danger as probable and worthy of attention than if we minimize danger. Therefore, anxiety leads us to judge threatening events as being more likely and more threatening than they really are. However, the cognitive distortions are unnecessary, because there is no real threat in the case of panic disorder.

Then, patients are taught to treat their thoughts as hypotheses or guesses rather than as facts. The notions of automatic thinking and discrete predictions are also explained, to emphasize the need of becoming an astute observer of one's own habitual self-statements in each situation. This leads to a "downward arrow technique" to identify specific predictions made at any given moment, as shown with Julie.

THERAPIST: What is it that scared you about feeling detached in the movie theater last night?

JULIE: It is just such a horrible feeling.

THERAPIST: What makes it so horrible?

JULIE: I can't tolerate it.

THERAPIST: What makes you think you cannot tolerate it? What is the feeling of detachment going to do to you that makes you think it is horrible and intolerable?

JULIE: It might get to be so intense that it overwhelms me.

THERAPIST: And if it overwhelms you, what would happen?

JULIE: I could become so distressed that I lose touch with reality.

THERAPIST: What would it mean if you lost touch with reality?

JULIE: That I would be in a different mind state forever—I would never come back to reality. That I would be so crazy that I would have to be carted out of the movie theater to a mental hospital and locked away forever.

Overly general self-statements, such as "I feel terrible—something bad could happen," are insufficient, nontherapeutic, and may serve to intensify anxiety by virtue of their global and nondirective nature. Instead, detail in thought content, such as "I am afraid that if I get too anxious while driving, then I'll lose control of the wheel and drive off the side of the road and die," permits subsequent cognitive restructuring.

Analysis of anxious thought content yields two broad factors that are labeled as "risk"

and "valence." These two main types of cognitive errors are described to patients. Risk translates to overestimation, or jumping to conclusions by viewing negative events as being probable events, when in fact they are unlikely to occur. The patient is asked to identify overestimations from the anxiety and panic incidents over the past couple of weeks: "Can you think of events that you felt sure were going to happen when you panicked, only to find out in the end that they did not happen at all?" Usually, patients can identify such events easily, but with protestations. For example,

JULIE: Well, several times I thought that I really was going to lose it this time . . . that I would flip out and never return to reality. It never actually happened, *but* it could still happen.

THERAPIST: Why do you think "it" could still happen?

JULIE: Part of me feels like I've always managed to escape it just in time, by either removing myself from the situation or by having my husband help me, or by holding on long enough for the feeling to pass. But what if next time I can't hold on?

THERAPIST: Knowing what we know about our thoughts when we are anxious, can you classify any of the ideas you just expressed, of "just holding on" or "just escaping in time," as overestimations?

JULIE: I suppose you're saying that I can hold on or I can always escape in time.

THERAPIST: More that you feel the need to hold on and the need to escape, because you are overestimating the likelihood of flipping out and never returning to reality.

JULIE: But it really feels like I will.

THERAPIST: The confusion between what you think will happen and what actually happens is the very problem that we are addressing in this session.

The reasons why overestimations persist despite repeated disconfirmation are explored. Typically, patients misattribute the absence of danger to external safety signals or safety behaviors (e.g., "I only made it because I managed to find help in time," "If I had not taken Xanax last week when I panicked in the store, I'm sure I would have passed out" or "I wouldn't have made it if I hadn't pulled off the road in time"), or to "luck," instead of realizing the inaccuracy of the original prediction. Similarly, patients may assume that the only reason they are still alive, sane, and safe, is because the "big one" has not happened. In this case, patients err by assuming that intensity of panic attacks increases the risk of catastrophic outcomes.

The method for countering overestimation errors is to question the evidence for probability judgments. The general format is to treat thoughts as hypotheses or guesses rather than as facts and to examine the evidence and generate alternative, more realistic predictions. This is best done by the therapist using a Socratic style, so that patients learn the skill of examining the content of their statements and arrive at alternative statements or predictions after they have considered all of the evidence. Questioning of the logic (e.g., "How does a racing heart lead to heart attack?"), or the bases from which judgments are made (e.g., misinformation from others, unusual sensations) is useful in this regard. Continuing with the previous example from Julie, the questioning took the following course:

THERAPIST: One of the specific thoughts you have identified is that you will flip out and never return to reality. What specifically leads you to think that that is likely to happen?

JULIE: Well, I guess it really feels like that.

THERAPIST: Describe the feelings?

JULIE: Well, I feel spacey and unreal, like things around me are different and that I'm not connected.

THERAPIST: And why do you think those feelings mean that you have actually lost touch with reality?

JULIE: I don't know—it feels as if I have.

THERAPIST: So, let's examine that assumption. What is your behavior like when you feel unreal? For example, do you respond if someone asks you a question during those episodes?

JULIE: Well, I respond to you even though I feel that way sometimes in here.

THERAPIST: OK, and can you walk or write or drive when you feel that way?

JULIE: Yes, but it feels different.

THERAPIST: But you do perform those functions despite feeling detached. So, what does that tell you?

JULIE: Well, maybe I haven't lost complete touch with reality. But what if I do?

THERAPIST: How many times have you felt detached?

JULIE: Hundreds and hundreds of times.

THERAPIST: And how many times have you lost touch with reality permanently?

JULIE: Never. But what if the feelings don't go away? Maybe I'll lose it then?

THERAPIST: So what else tells you that this is a possibility?

JULIE: Well, what about my second cousin? He lost it when he was about 25, and now he's just a mess. He can hardly function at all, and he is constantly in and out of psychiatric hospitals. They have him on a bunch of heavy-duty drugs. I'll never forget the time I saw him totally out of it. He was talking to himself in jibberish.

THERAPIST: So, do you make a connection between him and yourself?

JULIE: Yes.

THERAPIST: What are the similarities between the two of you?

JULIE: There are none really. It's just that he *is* what I think I will become.

THERAPIST: Did he ever feel the way you feel now?

JULIE: I don't know.

THERAPIST: And if another one of your cousins had severe back problems, would you be concerned that you would end up with severe back problems?

JULIE: No.

THERAPIST: Why not?

JULIE: Because it never crosses my mind. It is not something that I worry about.

THERAPIST: So, it sounds like you think you will end up like your cousin because you are afraid of ending up like him.

JULIE: I suppose so.

THERAPIST: So, let's look at all of the evidence and consider some alternatives. You have felt unreal hundreds of times, and you've never lost touch with reality, because you've continued to function in the midst of those feelings, and they have never lasted. You are afraid of becoming like your cousin, but there are no data to show that you and he have the same problem. In fact, the data suggest otherwise, because you function and he does not. So what is the realistic probability that you will lose touch with reality permanently? Use a scale of 0 to 100, where 0 = *No chance at all* and 100 = *Definitely will happen.*

JULIE: Well, maybe it is lower than I thought. Maybe 20%.

THERAPIST: So that would mean that you have actually lost touch with reality in a permanent way once every five times you have felt unreal.

JULIE: When it's put like that, I guess not. Maybe it's a very small possibility.

THERAPIST: Yes, so what is an alternative explanation?

JULIE: Perhaps the feelings of unreality are caused by feeling anxious or overbreathing, and having those feelings does not mean that I am actually losing touch with reality, and that I am not like my cousin at all.

For homework, in addition to continuation of self-monitoring and practice of diaphragmatic breathing, Julie was asked to identify her anxious thoughts in relation to every item on her agoraphobia hierarchy, and to use the in-session steps of examining the evidence and generating alternative evidence based interpretations for errors of overestimating the risk. She was to do the same for every panic attack that occurred over the next week.

Session 3

The goals of this session are to develop breathing retraining and to continue active cognitive restructuring. The therapist reviews the patient's week of diaphragmatic breathing practice. Julie was disappointed with her attempts to practice.

JULIE: I just didn't seem to be able to do it the right way. Sometimes I would start off OK and then the more I tried, the more it felt like I was running out of air, and I'd have to take a big gulp between breaths. At other times, I felt dizzy and the unreal feelings would start, at which point I would stop and do "busy work" to keep my mind occupied.

THERAPIST: It sounds like quite a few things were going on. First of all, remember that this is a skill, just like learning to ride a bike, and you cannot expect it to be easy from the get-go. Second, it sounds like you experienced some uncomfortable physical symptoms that worried you. You said it felt like you were running out of air. Based on what we talked about last week, what do you think might have caused that feeling?

JULIE: Well, maybe I wasn't getting enough air into my lungs, because it's really hard for me to use my diaphragm muscle. I felt like I was suffocating myself.

THERAPIST: Possibly it's just a matter of learning to use the diaphragm muscle, but were you really suffocating or was it an interpretation that you might be suffocating?

JULIE: I don't know. I've had the feeling of suffocating before, especially when I'm trapped in a crowded room.

THERAPIST: So, how do you know you were suffocating?

JULIE: I don't know. It just felt that way.

THERAPIST: So, let's put the evidence together. You've had the feelings before and never suffocated. As we discussed last time, anxiety can sometimes create a sensation of shortness of breath even though you are getting plenty of air. Can you think of an alternative explanation?

JULIE: Well, maybe I wasn't suffocating. Maybe it just felt like that.

Julie's complaints represent typical concerns that should be addressed. The next step is to slow the rate of breathing until the patient can comfortably span a full inhalation and exhalation cycle of 6 seconds. Again, the therapist models slowed breathing, then provides corrective feedback on practice in the session. The patient is instructed to continue to practice slow breathing in "safe" or relaxing environments, and is discouraged from applying slow breathing when anxious or panicking, until fully skilled in its application.

Also, cognitive restructuring is continued by addressing the second cognitive error, which involves viewing an event as "dangerous," "insufferable," or "catastrophic," when in actuality it is not. Typical examples of catastrophic errors are "If I faint, people will think that I'm weak and that would be unbearable" or "Panic attacks are the worst thing I can imagine," and "The whole evening is ruined if I start to feel anxious." "Decatastrophizing" means to face the worst, to realize that the occurrences are not as "catastrophic" as stated, and to think about actual ways to cope with negative events rather than how "bad" they are. A key principle underlying decatastrophizing is that events can be endured even though they are uncomfortable. Recognition of the time-limited nature of discomfort contributes to the development of a sense of being able to cope. The critical distinction here is that although patients might prefer that these events not occur, they can tolerate the discomfort, if necessary. Thus, for the person who states that negative judgments from others are unbearable, it is important to discuss what he or she would do to cope should someone else make a direct negative judgment. Similarly, for the person who states that the physical symptoms of panic are intolerably embarrassing, the following type of questioning is helpful:

JULIE: I am really worried that I might lose control and do something crazy, like yell and scream.

THERAPIST: Aside from the low likelihood of that happening (as we discussed before), lets face the worst and find out what is so bad about it. What would be so horrible about yelling and screaming?

JULIE: I could never live it down.

THERAPIST: Well, lets think it through. What are the various things you could do in the situation? You have just yelled and screamed—now what?

JULIE: Well, I guess the yelling and screaming would eventually stop.

THERAPIST: That's right—at the very least you would eventually exhaust yourself. What else?

JULIE: Well, maybe I would explain to the people around me that I was having a really bad day but that I would be OK. In other words, reassure them.

THERAPIST: Good. What else?

JULIE: Maybe I would just get away—find someplace to calm down and reassure myself that the worst is over.

THERAPIST: Good.

JULIE: But what if the police came and took me away, locked me up in a mental ward?

THERAPIST: Again, lets face the worst. What if the police did come when you were yelling and screaming, and what if the police did take you away? As scary as that may sound to you, lets consider what actually would happen.

JULIE: I have this image of myself not being able to tell them what is really going on—that I am so out of it I don't have the ability to let them know I am just anxious.

THERAPIST: If you were so distraught that you could not clearly communicate, how long would that last?

JULIE: You're right. I would eventually exhaust myself and then I could speak more clearly. But what if they didn't believe me?

THERAPIST: What if they did not believe you at first? How long would it take before they would realize that you were not crazy?

JULIE: I guess that after a while they would see that I was OK, and maybe I could call a friend or my doctor to explain what was going on.

THERAPIST: That's right. Now remember, all of this is about events that are unlikely to happen. At the same time, it is helpful to face worst-case scenarios (even though unlikely) and realize that they are not as bad as you first thought.

The homework for this session, in addition to continued self-monitoring, is to practice slow and diaphragmatic breathing in relaxing environments, and to identify errors of catastrophizing in relation to each item on the agoraphobia hierarchy, followed by practice of decatastrophizing and generation of ways to cope. In addition, Julie was to use the skill of decatastrophizing for panic attacks that occurred over the following week.

Session 4

The main goal of this session is to use breathing retraining skills as a coping tool, to review cognitive restructuring skills, and to begin *in vivo* exposure to the first item on the agoraphobia hierarchy.

Now that patients have practiced slow and diaphragmatic breathing sufficiently in relaxing environments, they are ready to use these methods in distracting environments and in anxious situations. Patients are encouraged to use breathing skills as a coping technique as they face fear, anxiety, and anxiety-provoking situations. Some patients use breathing skills as a safety signal or a safety behavior; in other words, they believe that they will be at risk for some mental, physical, or social calamity if they do not breathe correctly. This issue came up with Julie, as shown below.

JULIE: When I panicked during the week, I tried to use the breathing. It didn't work. It made me feel worse.

THERAPIST: It sounds as if you might have attempted to use the breathing exercise as a desperate attempt to control the feelings you were experiencing.

JULIE: Yes, that's right.

THERAPIST: What did you think would have happened if you had not been able to control the feelings?

JULIE: I was really worried that I might not be able to handle the feelings.

THERAPIST: And if you weren't able to handle the feelings, what would happen?

JULIE: It just feels like I will lose it, permanently.

THERAPIST: So this is one of those thoughts that we were talking about last time. What does your evidence tell you about the likelihood of losing touch with reality permanently?

JULIE: So you mean even if I don't control my breathing, then I will be OK?

THERAPIST: Well, you had not lost touch with reality permanently before you learned the breathing exercise, so what does that tell you?

JULIE: OK, I get it.

THERAPIST: The breathing exercise is best thought of as a tool to help you face whatever is provoking anxiety. So, as you face situations and your anxiety increases, use the breathing exercise first, then use your cognitive skills, so that you can continue to face rather than run away from anxiety.

Patients who consistently use the breathing skills as a safety behavior might be discouraged from using the breathing skills, so that they learn that what they are most worried about either does not happen or it can be managed without using the breathing skills.

In terms of the cognitive restructuring, therapists give corrective feedback to patients on the methods of questioning the evidence to generate realistic probabilities, facing the worst, and generating ways of coping with each item on the agoraphobia hierarchy and any panic attacks that occurred over the past week. Particular "corrective" feedback is given when patients lack specificity in their cognitive restructuring (e.g., patients who record that they are most worried about panicking should be encouraged to detail what it is about panicking that worries them) or rely on blanket reassurance (e.g., patients who record that "Everything will be OK" as their evidence and/or ways of coping should be encouraged to list the evidence and/or generate actual coping steps).

Next, attention is given to how to practice the first item on the agoraphobia hierarchy. If appropriate, reasons why previous attempts at *in vivo* exposure may have failed are reviewed. Typical reasons for patients' past failures at *in vivo* exposure include attempts that are too haphazard and/or brief, or spaced too far apart, and attempts conducted without a sense of mastery, or while maintaining beliefs that catastrophe is very possible. Julie had tried to face agoraphobic situations in the past, but each time she had escaped, feeling overwhelmed by panic and terrified of losing touch with reality permanently. The therapist helped Julie realize how to approach the agoraphobic situations differently to benefit from the exposure. Julie's typical safety signals were the presence of her husband, or at least knowing his whereabouts, and Klonopin (which she carried but rarely used). The therapist discussed the importance of eventual weaning from those safety signals.

As mentioned earlier, the goal of exposure therapy is not immediate reduction in fear and anxiety; rather the goal is for the patient to learn something new as a result of exposure. Clarification of what patients are most worried about as they face their feared situations and the conditions that best help patients to learn that what they are most worried about never or rarely happens, and/or that they can cope with the situation and tolerate anxiety is essential for effective exposure. If a patient is most worried that fear and anxiety will remain elevated for the entire duration of the practice, then corrective learning involves toleration of sustained anxiety. For Julie, the first situation on her hierarchy was to drive home from work, alone. She stated that what most worried her in that situation was that she would panic and lose touch with reality, therefore losing control of the car and dying in an accident. She also stated that to drive at dusk was the condition under which she was most convinced of these eventualities. Thus, the task that the therapist considered most effective in teaching Julie that she would not lose touch with reality and have an accident, or that she could cope with the sensations of unreality and panic, was to drive home from work at dusk.

Delineation of the exposure task as concretely as possible, so that patients clearly understand exactly what the practice entails (e.g., "Walk around inside of mall for 10 minutes by myself"), reduces uncertainty about whether the practice was conducted correctly. Without such concrete details, patients might decide that they "failed." Importantly, the practice should not be ended because of anxiety (e.g., "Continue driving on the freeway until I feel anxious") because the exposure practice would then reinforce avoidance of anxiety.

Julie was reminded to use her coping skills should she panic as she practiced the task; that is, in moments of fear, patients are encouraged to use their breathing and thinking skills to complete the assigned task; the coping skills are not intended as means to reduce fear and anxiety, but to tolerate it.

Patients are encouraged to maintain a regular schedule of repeated *in vivo* exposure practices at least three times per week, and to conduct these practices regardless of internal (e.g., having a "bad day," feeling ill) or external (e.g., inclement weather, busy schedules) factors that may prompt postponement of practices. Julie expressed some concerns about being able to practice at least three times over the following week:

JULIE: I don't know if I can practice three times, because more days than not I feel pretty worn down; maybe I can practice on just Monday and Tuesday, because they are the days I typically feel better.

THERAPIST: What is it you are worried about happening if you practice on a day when you already feel worn down?

JULIE: I feel more fragile on those days.

THERAPIST: And if you feel more fragile, what might happen?

JULIE: I just don't think I could do it. It would be too hard. I might really freak out and lose touch with reality for ever.

THERAPIST: OK, so let's think about that thought. What does your experience tell you? How many times have you permanently lost touch with reality, including days when you were worn down?

JULIE: Well, never.

THERAPIST: So, what does that tell you?

JULIE: OK, but it still feels difficult to drive on those days.

THERAPIST: How about you start with Monday or Tuesday, but quickly move to the other days of the week when you are feeling worn down, so that you get a really good opportunity to learn whether you permanently lose touch with reality or not?

The homework for this session involves continued self-monitoring, continued use of cognitive restructuring and breathing retraining in the event of elevated anxiety or panic, and practicing the first item on the agoraphobia hierarchy at least three times, with at least one of those times being without her husband Larry.

Session 5

The goals of this session are to review the practice of *in vivo* exposure, to design another exposure task to be practiced over the next week, and to begin interoceptive exposure. Note that *in vivo* and interoceptive exposure can be done simultaneously or sequentially. For Julie, *in vivo* exposure was begun in Session 4, whereas interoceptive exposure was begun in this session, but they could easily have been done in the opposite order.

It is essential to review the week's practice of *in vivo* exposure. An objective evaluation of performance is considered necessary to offset subjective and damaging self-evaluations. As demonstrated in experimental literature on learning and conditioning, appraisals of aversive events after they have occurred can influence anxiety about future encounters with the same types of aversive events. Any practice that is terminated prematurely is to be reviewed carefully for contributing factors, which can then be incorporated into subsequent trials of *in vivo* exposure. Recognition of the precipitant to escape is very important, because the urge to escape is usually based on the prediction that continued endurance would result in some kind of danger. For example, patients may predict that the sensations will become intense and lead to an out-of-control reaction. This prediction can be discussed in terms of jumping to conclusions and blowing things out of proportion. At the same time, escape itself need not be viewed catastrophically (i.e., as embarrassing, or as a sign of failure). In addition, therapists reinforce the use of breathing and cognitive skills to help patients remain in the situation until the specified duration or task has been completed, despite uncomfortable sensations.

Again, it is important for patients to recognize that the goal is to repeatedly face situations despite anxiety, not to achieve a total absence of anxiety. Toleration of fear rather than immediate fear reduction is the goal for each exposure practice; this approach leads to an eventual fear reduction. Anxiety that does not decline over repeated days of *in vivo* exposure may result from too much emphasis on immediate fear and anxiety reduction; that is, trying too hard or wishing too much for anxiety to decline typically maintains anxiety.

Julie had success with her first *in vivo* exposure practice; she managed to drive home from work at dusk, alone, four different times. She noted that the first time was easier than she had expected; the second was harder, and the one time she pulled off to the side of the road. The therapist helped Julie identify the thoughts and sensations that led her to "escape" from the situation: the sensations of unreality and fears of losing touch with reality. Julie had waited for a few minutes, then continued driving home—an action that was highly reinforced by the therapist. The third and fourth times were easier.

Julie's husband Larry attended Session 5, so that he could learn how to help Julie overcome her PDA. He was supportive and eager to help in any way possible, expressing frustration at having had no idea how to help in the past.

The general principles for involvement of significant others in treatment are as follows. First, a treatment conceptualization is provided to the significant other to reduce his or her frustration and/or negative attributions about the patient's emotional functioning (e.g., "Oh, she's just making it up. There's nothing really wrong with her" or "He has been like this since before we were married, and he'll never

change"). The way in which the agoraphobic problem has disrupted daily routines and distribution of home responsibilities is explored and discussed also. Examples might include social activities, leisure activities, and household chores. The therapist explains that family activities may be structured around the agoraphobic fear and avoidance to help the patient function without intense anxiety. At the same time, reassignment of the patient's tasks to the significant other may actually reinforce the agoraphobic pattern of behavior. Consequently, the importance of complying with *in vivo* exposure homework instructions, even though the patient may experience some distress initially, is emphasized.

The significant other is encouraged to become an active participant by providing his or her perception of the patient's behavior and fearfulness, and the impact on the home environment. Sometimes significant others have provided information of which the patient was not fully aware, or did not report, particularly in relation to how the patient's behavior affects the significant other's own daily functioning. Larry, for example, described how he felt restricted at home in the evenings; whereas, before, he occasionally played basketball with his friends at the local gym, he now stays at home, because he feels guilty if he leaves Julie alone.

The next step is to describe the role of the significant other regarding *in vivo* exposure tasks. The significant other is viewed as a coach, and the couple is encouraged to approach the tasks as a problem-solving team. This includes deciding exactly where and when to practice *in vivo* exposure. In preparation for practices, the patient identifies his or her misappraisals about the task and generates cognitive alternatives. The significant other is encouraged to help the patient question his or her own "anxious" thoughts. Role plays of this type of questioning of the patient by the significant other may be conducted in the session, so that the therapist can provide corrective feedback to each partner. Throughout *in vivo* exposure, the significant other reminds the patient to apply cognitive challenges and/or breathing skills. Because the significant other is usually a safety signal, tasks are less anxiety provoking. However, the patient must be weaned from the safety signal eventually. Therefore, initial attempts at facing agoraphobic situations are conducted with the significant other, and later trials are conducted alone. Weaning from the significant other may be graduated, as in the case of (1) Julie driving first with Larry in the car, (2) with him in a car behind, (3) meeting the significant other at a destination point, and (4) driving alone.

Very important to the success of this collaboration is style of communication. On the one hand, significant others are discouraged from magnifying the experience of panic and are encouraged to help the patient apply coping statements when anxious. On the other hand, significant others are encouraged to be patient given the fact that progress for the patient may be erratic. The patient and significant other are instructed to use a 0- to 10-point rating scale to communicate with each other about the patient's current level of anxiety or distress, as a way of diminishing the awkwardness associated with discussion of anxiety, especially in public situations. The patient is warned about the potential motivation to avoid discussing his or her feelings with the significant other, due to embarrassment or an attempt to avoid the anxiety for fear that such discussion and concentration on anxiety may intensify his or her distress level. Avoidance of feelings is discouraged, because distraction is viewed as less beneficial in the long term than is objectively facing whatever is distressing and learning that predicted catastrophes do not occur. The patient is reassured that the initial discomfort and embarrassment will most likely diminish as the couple becomes more familiar with discussing anxiety levels and their management. Furthermore, the patient's concerns about the significant other being insensitive or too pushy are addressed. For example, a significant other may presume to know the patient's level of anxiety and anxious thoughts without confirmation from the patient, or the significant other may become angry toward the patient for avoiding or escaping from situations, or being fearful. All of these issues are described as relatively common and understandable patterns of communication that are nevertheless in need of correction. In-session role-playing of more adaptive communication styles during episodes of heightened anxiety is a useful learning technique. On occasion, more specific communications training may be beneficial, especially if the partners frequently argue in their attempts to generate items or methods for conducting *in vivo* exposure.

The next *in vivo* exposure task for Julie was to sit in a crowded movie theater, gradually moving away from the aisle, toward the middle of the row, because that was the condition in which she was most concerned that she would lose control and draw attention to herself. Julie and Larry rehearsed their approach to the *in vivo* exposure task in session, while the therapist provided corrective feedback using the principles of communication and coping described earlier. They were instructed to practice this task at least three times over the next week. On at least one occasion, Julie was to practice the task alone.

Next, interoceptive exposure was introduced. As with *in vivo* exposure, through repeated exposures to feared sensations, patients learn that they are not harmed by the sensations, and they achieve increased confidence in their ability to tolerate symptoms of anxiety. The procedure begins with assessment of the patient's response to a series of standardized exercises. The therapist models each exercise first. Then, after the patient has completed the exercise, the therapist records the sensations, anxiety level (0 to 10), sensation intensity (0 to 10), and similarity to naturally occurring panic sensations (0 to 10). The exercises include shaking the head from side to side for 30 seconds; placing the head between the legs for 30 seconds and lifting the head to an upright position quickly; running in place or using steps for 1 minute; holding one's breath for as long as possible; complete body muscle tension for 1 minute or holding a push-up position for as long as possible; spinning in a swivel chair for 1 minute; hyperventilating for 1 minute; breathing through a narrow straw (with closed nasal passages) or breathing as slowly as possible for 2 minutes; and staring at a spot on the wall or at one's mirror image for 90 seconds. If none of these exercises produce sensations at least moderately similar to those that occur naturally, other, individually tailored exercises are generated. For example, tightness around the chest may be induced by a deep breath before hyperventilating; heat may be induced by wearing heavy clothing in a heated room; choking sensations may be induced by a tongue depressor, high-collared sweater, or a necktie; and startle may be induced by an abrupt, loud noise in the midst of relaxation. For Julie, the sensations produces by hyperventilating, spinning, and staring at a spot on the wall were most anxiety provoking.

Patients who report little or no fear because they feel safe in the presence of the therapist are asked to attempt each exercise alone, either with the therapist out of the office or at home. At the same time, discussing the influence of perceived safety as a moderating factor in the amount of fear experienced reinforces the value of cognitive restructuring. For a minority of patients, the known cause and course of the sensations override the fear response; that is, because the sensations are predictably related to a clear cause (the interoceptive exercise), and because the sensations can be relatively easily controlled by simply terminating the interoceptive exercise, fear is minimal. Under these conditions, discussion can productively center on the misassumptions that render naturally occurring sensations more frightening than the ones produced by the interoceptive exercises. Typically, these misassumptions are that naturally occurring sensations are unpredictable, that unpredictable sensations are more harmful, and that if naturally occurring sensations are not controlled, then they pose a potential threat. The majority of patients fear at least several of the interoceptive exercises despite knowing the cause of the sensations and their controllability.

Interoceptive exercises rated as producing at least somewhat similar sensations to naturally occurring panic (at least 3 on the 0- to 10-point scale) are selected for repeated exposure. A graduated approach is used for interoceptive exposure, beginning with the lowest item on the hierarchy established in Session 4. For each trial of exposure, the patient is asked to begin the induction, to indicate when the sensations are first experienced (e.g., by raising a hand), and to continue the induction for at least 30 seconds longer to permit corrective learning. After terminating the induction, anxiety is rated, and the patient is given time to apply cognitive and breathing coping skills. Finally, the therapist reviews the induction experience and the application of management strategies with the patient. During this review, the therapist emphasizes the importance of experiencing the sensations fully during the induction, of concentrating objectively on the sensations versus distracting from them, and the importance of identifying specific cognitions and challenging them by considering all of the evidence. In addition, the therapist asks key questions to help the patient realize his or her safety (e.g., "What would have happened if you had continued spinning for another 60 seconds?"), and to generalize to naturally occurring experiences

(e.g., "How is this different from when you feel dizzy at work?"). In other words, cognitive restructuring extends the cognitive reprocessing already taking place implicitly as a result of repeated interoceptive exposure.

Specific, previously unrecognized cognitions sometimes become apparent during repeated exposure. For example, when Julie began to conduct repeated exposures to hyperventilation and spinning, she became more aware of her implicit assumption that sensations of spaciness or lightheadedness would lead her to lose control of her limbs. This related to her concern about causing an accident when driving. During repeated hyperventilation exercises, and with prompting of "what ifs" from the therapist, Julie discovered her fear of not being able to move her arms or legs. The therapist then behaviorally challenged this assumption by having Julie overbreathe for longer periods of time, followed immediately by walking, picking up objects, and so on.

Homework practice is very important, because safety signals present in the clinic setting or that derive from the therapist per se may, again, prevent generalizability to the natural setting. Patients are instructed to practice the interoceptive items conducted in session on a daily basis, three times each day. Julie was to practice hyperventilation over the following week. She expressed some concern at doing the exercises alone, so the therapist helped Julie to use her cognitive restructuring skills in relation to being alone. In addition, more graduation of homework was suggested, so that Julie would practice hyperventilating when her husband was at home the first couple of days, then when he was not at home the rest of the time.

Sessions 6 and 7

The primary goal of these sessions is to review the past week of *in vivo* exposure practices, design new exposures, review between-session practices of interoceptive exposure, conduct repeated interoceptive exposure in session, and assign those as homework for the next week.

The *in vivo* exposure is reviewed, as in the previous session. In this case, Julie and Larry had done well with the movie theater practice. Julie even practiced going to the movies on her own. On that occasion she reported higher anxiety than when she was with Larry for fear of having to get up and leave the theater and worries about bothering others in the audience.

The therapist helped Julie to identify what worry led her to think about leaving in the first place; in other words, what did she think might happen if she could not leave? Julie indicated that she had thoughts of losing control and causing a scene, to which she was then prompted to apply her cognitive restructuring skills of evidence-based analyses and decatastrophizing. She was ready to move to the next items on her hierarchy: to spend 2 hours alone at home during the day and to stay alone at home as day turned to night. As with every *in vivo* exposure task, Julie identified what she most feared happening in those situations, and the best conditions under which to practice to learn that either those eventualities would not happen and/or that she could cope with the worst.

The past week of interoceptive exposure practice is reviewed in session with a mind toward avoidance: either overt failure to practice, or covert avoidance by minimizing the intensity or duration of the sensations induced, or limiting practice to the presence of a safety signal (e.g., a significant other) or times when background anxiety is minimal. Reasons for avoidance may include continued misinterpretation of the dangers of bodily sensations (i.e., "I don't want to hyperventilate, because I'm afraid that I won't be able to stop overbreathing and no one will be there to help me") or the belief that anxiety will not reduce with repetition of the task.

For the first week, Julie practiced interoceptive exposure exercises about half of the days between sessions. The therapist used a "downward arrow" method to explore Julie's reasons for not practicing every day.

JULIE: I tried hyperventilating on my own. However, I wasn't very successful, because I felt too scared and I stopped it as soon as I noticed the strange feelings.

THERAPIST: What did you think would happen if the sensations became more intense?

JULIE: I thought the feelings would get worse and worse and worse, and just overwhelm me. I didn't want to have that feeling of panic again.

THERAPIST: If you did become overwhelmed, then what would happen to you?

JULIE: Then I'd feel really terrible.

THERAPIST: And if you felt really terrible?

JULIE: Well, nothing. I'd just feel terrible.

THERAPIST: The word "terrible" carries a lot of meaning. Let's see if we can pin down your anxious thoughts that make the feelings so terrible.

JULIE: I just can't tolerate the feeling.

THERAPIST: What tells you that you cannot tolerate it? How do you know you can't tolerate it?

And the discussion continued, so that Julie realized what was most important for her to learn by the repeated hyperventilation: She could tolerate the sensations and anxiety.

However, after the subsequent week of repeated practice, Julie remained cautious for fear that the exercises would cause her to revert to her state of several weeks earlier; that is, she was concerned that the inductions would leave her in a persistent symptomatic state. Furthermore, she was particularly reluctant to practice interoceptive exposure at the end of the day, when she was more likely to feel unreal, or on a day when an important social event was scheduled. Again, these avoidance patterns were related to fears that the symptoms would become too intense or result in some type of mental or social catastrophe. These types of avoidance patterns are addressed in the following vignette:

THERAPIST: When did you practice deliberately spinning and hyperventilating?

JULIE: Usually in the mornings. One day I left it until the end of the day, and that turned out to be a bad idea. I felt terrible.

THERAPIST: Let's think about that a bit more. What made it terrible when you practiced at the end of the day?

JULIE: Well, I was already feeling pretty unreal—I usually do around that time of the day. So I was much more anxious about the symptoms.

THERAPIST: Being more anxious implies that you thought the symptoms were more harmful. Is that what happened on the day that you practiced interoceptive exposure when you were already feeling unreal?

JULIE: Yes, I felt that because I was already feeling unreal, I was on the edge, and that I might push myself over the edge if I tried to increase the feelings of unreality.

THERAPIST: What do you mean by "push myself over the edge"?

JULIE: That I would make the feelings so intense that I really would lose it—go crazy.

THERAPIST: So there is one of those hypotheses: to feel more intense unreality means to be closer to going crazy. Let's examine the evidence. Is it necessarily the case that more intense unreality means you are closer to craziness?

In sessions, the therapist continued practice of interoceptive exposure with the next item on Julie's hierarchy, which was to stare at a spot on the wall and to spin around.

The homework from this session is to continue self-monitoring, *in vivo* exposure to an item from the agoraphobia hierarchy at least three times, and daily practice of interoceptive exposure.

Sessions 8 and 9

The primary goals of these sessions are to continue *in vivo* exposure, as described in the prior sessions, and to extend interoceptive exposure to natural activities. Julie had practiced staying at home for 2 hours alone during the day and as daylight turned to dusk, with good results. In particular, she experienced a couple of panic attacks during these *in vivo* exposure practices but continued with the assigned practice regardless. This was critical for Julie, as it allowed her to learn that she could survive the feeling of panic; it was the first time she had remained in a situation despite panicking.

In reviewing the week's practice of interoceptive exposure, it became apparent that Julie was separating the practices from real-life experiences of bodily sensations in a way that would limit generalization. This was addressed as follows:

JULIE: After spinning and hyperventilating several times, I really do feel much less anxious. I was terrified at the start, but now I am only mildly anxious, if at all. But this is different than what happens to me when I'm on the freeway or at home.

THERAPIST: How is it different?

JULIE: I don't know when the feelings of dizziness and unreality are going to hit.

THERAPIST: From our previous discussions, let's think of potential reasons why you might feel dizzy or unreal at a particular time?

JULIE: I know. I have to keep remembering that it could be my breathing, or just feeling anxious, or tired, or a bunch of different things.

THERAPIST: OK. And why is it so important to know when those feelings will occur?

JULIE: Because I don't want them to be there at all.

THERAPIST: And why not . . . what are you afraid of?

JULIE: I guess it's the same old thing . . . that I'll lose it somehow?

THERAPIST: So let's go back to the cognitive restructuring that you have been doing. What specifically are you afraid of? How likely is it to happen? What are the alternatives?

JULIE: I understand.

THERAPIST: So, now you see that whether the sensations of dizziness or unreality are produced by anxiety, overbreathing, diet, or the exercises we do here, they're all the same—they are just uncomfortable physical sensations. The only reason they perturb you more when you are driving or at home is because of the meaning you still give to them in those situations.

"Naturalistic" interoceptive exposure refers to exposure to daily tasks or activities that have been avoided or endured with dread because of the associated sensations. Typical examples include aerobic exercise or vigorous physical activity, running up flights of stairs, eating foods that create a sensation of fullness or are associated with sensations of choking, saunas or steamy showers, driving with the windows rolled up and the heater on, caffeine consumption, and so on. (Of course, these exercises may be modified in the event of actual medical complications, such as asthma or high blood pressure.) From a list of typically feared activities and generation of items specific to the individual's own experience, a hierarchy is established. Each item is ranked in terms of anxiety ratings (0–10). Julie's hierarchy was as follows: looking out through venetian blinds (anxiety = 3); watching *One Flew over the Cuckoo's Nest* (anxiety = 4); playing tennis (anxiety = 4); scanning labels on a supermarket shelf (anxiety =

5); concentrating on needlework for an hour (anxiety = 6); driving with windows closed and heater on (anxiety = 7); a nightclub with strobe lights (anxiety = 8); and rides at Disneyland (anxiety = 10).

Like the symptom exercises, the activity exercises are designed to be systematically graduated and repetitive. Patients may apply the breathing and cognitive skills while the activity is ongoing. This is in contrast to the symptom induction exercises, in which coping skills are used only after completion of the symptom exercise, because the activities often are considerably longer than the symptom induction exercises. Nevertheless, patients are encouraged to focus on the sensations and experience them fully throughout the activity, and not use the coping skills to prevent or remove the sensations.

Patients are instructed to identify maladaptive cognitions and rehearse cognitive restructuring before beginning each activity. In-session rehearsal of the cognitive preparation allows therapists to provide corrective feedback. Julie did this with her therapist for her first two naturalistic activities, which were to look at venetian blinds and to watch *One Flew over the Cuckoo's Nest*. Julie realized that she was most worried about sensations of unreality and fears of going crazy, although, as a result of her various exposure exercises up to this point, she quickly was able to recognize that such sensations were harmless and that she could tolerate them, and that such fears were unrealistic based on the evidence.

As with all exposures, it is important to identify and remove (gradually, if necessary) safety signals or protective behaviors, such as portable phones, lucky charms, walking slowly, standing slowly, and staying in close proximity to medical facilities. These safety signals and behaviors reinforce catastrophic misappraisals about bodily sensations. Julie's safety behaviors were identified as checking the time on the clock (as a reassurance that she was in touch with reality) and pinching herself (again, to feel reality). She was asked to practice the two naturalistic interoceptive exposures at least three times each before the next treatment session, without the safety behaviors.

Sessions 10 and 11

The primary goals of these sessions are to review the *in vivo* and naturalistic exposure exercises over the past week, and to combine exposure to feared and avoided agoraphobic situations with deliberate induction of feared sensations into those situations. As with earlier interoceptive exposure homework assignments, it is important to evaluate and correct tendencies to avoid naturalistic interoceptive exposure tasks, mainly by considering the underlying misassumptions that are leading to avoidance. Remember also that a form of avoidance is to rely on safety signals or safety behaviors, so careful questioning of the way in which the naturalistic exposure was conducted, and under what conditions, may help to identify inadvertent reliance on these unnecessary precautions. Julie reported that she was successful in looking at the venetian blinds, even though she experienced sensations of unreality. She had more difficulty watching *One Flew over the Cuckoo's Nest*, because it tapped directly into her worst fears of losing touch with reality permanently; she tried but terminated the film early. The second time she watched it with Larry, who prompted Julie to remember her cognitive and breathing skills, and she was able to watch the entire film. She watched the film one more time on her own. Two new naturalistic exposure items were selected for the coming week, with special attention to weaning or removing safety signals and safety behaviors, and rehearsal of cognitive restructuring in session. For Julie, these were playing tennis (something she had avoided for years) and scanning items on supermarket shelves.

The notion of deliberately inducing feared bodily symptoms within the context of feared agoraphobic situations derives from the evidence that compound relationships between external and internal cues can be the most potent anxiogenic agent; that is, it is neither just the situation nor just the bodily sensation that triggers distress, but the combination of the bodily sensation and the situation that is most distressing. Thus, effective exposure targets both types of cues. Otherwise, patients run the risk of later return of fear. For example, repeated practice walking through a shopping mall without feeling dizzy does not adequately prepare patients for occasions on which they feel dizzy walking through a shopping mall, and without such preparation, patients may be likely to panic and escape should they feel dizzy in this or similar situations in the future. Wearing heavy clothing in a restaurant helps patients to learn to be less afraid of not only the restaurant but also of feeling hot in a restaurant. Other examples include drinking coffee before any of the agoraphobic tasks, turning off the air-conditioning or turning on the heater while driving, breathing very slowly in a crowded area, and so on.

Patients choose an item from their hierarchy of agoraphobia situations, either one already completed or a new item, and also choose which symptom to induce and ways of inducing that symptom in that situation. Julie's task was to drink coffee as she went to a movie. She expressed the following concerns:

JULIE: Do you really think I am ready to drink coffee and go to the movie?

THERAPIST: What worries you about the combination of coffee and the movie theater?

JULIE: Well, I've practiced in the movie theaters a lot, so that feels pretty good, but the coffee is going to make me feel very anxious.

THERAPIST: And if you feel very anxious in the movie theater, then what?

JULIE: Then, I don't know what. Maybe I will get those old feelings again, like I have to get out.

THERAPIST: Based on everything you have learned, how can you manage those feelings?

JULIE: Well, I guess my number one rule is never to leave a situation because I am feeling anxious. I will stick it out, no matter what.

THERAPIST: That sounds great. It means you are accepting the anxiety and taking the opportunity to learn that you can tolerate it. What else?

JULIE: I can ask myself what is the worst that can happen. I know I am not going to die or go crazy. I will probably feel my heart rate going pretty fast because of the coffee.

THERAPIST: And if your heart rate goes fast, what does that mean?

JULIE: I guess it just means that my heart rate will go fast.

THERAPIST: This will be a really good way for you to learn that you can tolerate the anxiety and the symptoms of a racing heart.

The homework for this session is to continue self-monitoring, to practice *in vivo* exposure combined with interoceptive exposure, and to continue naturalistic interoceptive exposure.

Session 12

The last treatment session reviews the principles and skills learned and provides the patient with a template of coping techniques for potential, high-risk situations in the future. Julie finished the program after 12 sessions, by which time she had not panicked in 8 weeks, rarely experienced dizziness or feelings of unreality, and was driving further distances. There were some situations still in need of exposure practices (e.g., driving very long distances away from home and on the freeway at dusk). However, Julie and Larry agreed to continue *in vivo* exposure practices over the next few months to consolidate her learning and to continue her improvement.

CONCLUSION

As noted earlier in this chapter, cognitive-behavioral treatments for panic disorder and agoraphobia are highly effective and represent one of the success stories of psychotherapy. Between 80 and 100% of patients undergoing these treatments will be panic free at the end of treatment and maintain these gains for up to 2 years. These results reflect substantially more durability than medication treatments. Furthermore, between 50 and 80% of these patients reach a point of "high end state," meaning within normative realms of symptoms and functioning, and many of the remainder have only residual symptomatology. Nevertheless, major difficulties remain.

First, these treatments are not foolproof. As many as 50% of patients retain substantial symptomatology despite improvement from baseline, and this is particularly likely for those with more severe agoraphobia. Further research must determine how treatments can be improved or better individualized to alleviate continued suffering. For example, one of us (D. H. B.) saw a patient several years ago who had completed an initial course of treatment but required continued periodic visits for over 4 years. This patient was essentially improved for approximately 9 months but found himself relapsing during a particularly stressful time at work. A few booster sessions restored his functioning, but he was back in the office 6 months later with reemerging symptomatology. This pattern essentially continued for 4 years and was characterized by symptom-free periods followed by (seemingly) stress-related relapses. Furthermore, the reemerging panic disorder would sometimes last from 3 to 6 months before disappearing again, perhaps with the help of a booster session.

Although this case was somewhat unusual in our experience, there was no easy explanation for this pattern of relapses and remissions. The patient, who has a graduate degree, understood and accepted the treatment model and fully implemented the treatment program. There was also no question that he fully comprehended the nature of anxiety and panic, and the intricacies of the therapeutic strategies. While in the office, he could recite chapter and verse on the nature of these emotional states, as well as the detailed process of his own reaction while in these states. Nevertheless, away from the office, the patient found himself repeatedly hoping that he would not "go over the brink" during a panic, despite verbalizing very clearly the irrationality of this concept while in the office. In addition, he continued to attempt to reduce minor physiological symptoms associated with anxiety and panic, despite a full rational understanding of the nature of these symptoms (including the fact that they are the same symptoms that he experienced during a state of excitement, which he enjoyed). His limited tolerance of these physical sensations was also puzzling in view of his tremendous capacity to endure pain.

Any number of factors might account for what seemed to be "overvalued ideation" or very strongly held irrational ideas during periods of anxiety, including the fact that the patient has several relatives who have repeatedly been hospitalized for emotional disorders (seemingly mood disorders or schizoaffective disorder). Nevertheless, the fact remains that we do not know why this patient did not respond as quickly as most people. Eventually he made a full recovery, received several promotions at work, and considered treatment to be the turning point in his life. But it took 5 years.

Other patients, as noted earlier, seem uninterested in engaging in treatment, preferring to conceptualize their problems as chemical imbalances. Still others have difficulty grasping some of the cognitive strategies, and further attempts are necessary to make these treatments more "user-friendly."

It also may seem that this structured, protocol-driven treatment is applied in a very standard fashion across individuals. Nothing could be further from the truth. The clinical art involved in this, and in all treatments described in this book, requires a careful adaptation to these treatment strategies to the individual case. Many of Julie's symptoms revolved around feelings of unreality (derealization and depersonalization). Emphasizing rational explanations for the production of such feelings, as well as adapting cognitive and exposure exercises to maximize these sensations, is an important part of this treatment program. Although standard interoceptive provocation exercises seemed sufficient to produce relevant symptomatology in Julie's case, we have had to develop new procedures to deal with people with more idiosyncratic symptoms and fears, particularly those involving feelings of unreality or dissociation. Other innovations in both cognitive and behavioral procedures will be required by individual therapists as they apply these procedures.

Although these new treatments seem highly successful when applied by trained therapists, treatment is not readily available to individuals with these disorders. In fact, these treatments, although brief and structured, are far more difficult to deliver than, for example, pharmacological treatments (which are also often misapplied). Furthermore, few people are currently skilled in the application of these treatments. What seems to be needed for these and other successful psychosocial treatments is a new method of disseminating them, so that they reach the maximum number of patients. Modification of these treatment protocols into more user-friendly formats, as well as brief periods of training for qualified therapists to a point of certification, would be important steps in successfully delivering these treatments. This may be difficult to accomplish.

NOTE

1. Specific phobias were not assessed, but by being most circumscribed, they would be hypothesized to load the least on negative affectivity.

REFERENCES

Allen, L. B., & Barlow, D. H. (2006). The treatment of panic disorder: Outcomes and basic processes. In B. O. Rothbaum (Ed.), *Pathological anxiety: Emotional processing in etiology and treatment* (pp. 166–180). New York: Guilford Press.

Alneas, R., & Torgersen, S. (1990). DSM-III personality disorders among patients with major depression, anxiety disorders, and mixed conditions. *Journal of Nervous and Mental Disease, 178,* 693–698.

American Psychiatric Association. (1980). *Diagnostic and statistical manual of mental disorders* (3rd ed.). Washington, DC: Author.

American Psychiatric Association. (1994). *Diagnostic and statistical manual of mental disorders* (4th ed.). Washington, DC: Author.

American Psychiatric Association. (2000). *Diagnostic and statistical manual of mental disorders* (4th ed., text rev.). Washington, DC: Author.

Amering, M., Katschnig, H., Berger, P., Windhaber, J., Baischer, W., & Dantendorfer, K. (1997). Embarrassment about the first panic attack predicts agoraphobia in disorder patients. *Behaviour Research and Therapy, 35,* 517–521.

Antony, M. M., Brown, T. A., Craske, M. G., Barlow, D. H., Mitchell, W. B., & Meadows, E. A. (1995). Accuracy of heartbeat perception in panic disorder, social phobia, and nonanxious subjects. *Journal of Anxiety Disorders, 9,* 355–371.

Antony, M. M., Ledley, D. B., Liss, A., & Swinson, R. P. (2006). Responses to symptom induction exercises in panic disorder. *Behaviour Research and Therapy, 44,* 85–98.

Antony, M. M., Meadows, E. A., Brown, T. A., & Barlow, D. H. (1994). Cardiac awareness before and after cognitive-behavioral treatment for panic disorder. *Journal of Anxiety Disorders, 8,* 341–350.

Arnow, B. A., Taylor, C. B., Agras, W. S., & Telch, M. J. (1985). Enhancing agoraphobia treatment outcome by changing couple communication patterns. *Behavior Therapy, 16,* 452–467.

Arntz, A., & van den Hout, M. (1996). Psychological treatments of panic disorder without agoraphobia: Cognitive therapy versus applied relaxation. *Behaviour Research and Therapy, 34,* 113–121.

Arrindell, W., & Emmelkamp, P. (1987). Psychological states and traits in female agoraphobics: A controlled study. *Journal of Psychopathology and Behavioral Assessment, 9,* 237–253.

Azrin, N., Naster, B., & Jones, R. (1973). Reciprocity counselling: A rapid learning-based procedure for marital counselling. *Behaviour Research and Therapy, 11,* 365–382.

Bandelow, B., Spath, C., Tichaner, G. A., Brooks, A., Hajak, G., & Ruther, E. (2002). Early traumatic life events, parental attitudes, family history, and birth risk factors in patients with panic disorder. *Comprehensive Psychiatry, 43,* 269–278.

Bandura, A. (1977). Self-efficacy: Toward a unifying theory of behavioral change. *Psychological Review, 84,* 191–215.

Barlow, D. H. (1988). *Anxiety and its disorders: The nature and treatment of anxiety and panic.* New York: Guilford Press.

Barlow, D. H. (2002). *Anxiety and its disorders: The nature and treatment of anxiety and panic* (2nd ed.). New York: Guilford Press.

Barlow, D. H., Brown, T. A., & Craske, M. G. (1994). Definitions of panic attacks and panic disorder in the DSM-IV: Implications for research. *Journal of Abnormal Psychology, 103,* 553–564.

Barlow, D. H., Cohen, A., Waddell, M., Vermilyea, J., Klosko, J., Blanchard, E., et al. (1984). Panic and generalized anxiety disorders: Nature and treatment. *Behavior Therapy, 15,* 431–449.

Barlow, D. H., & Craske, M. G. (2006). *Mastery of your anxiety and panic: Patient workbook* (4th ed.). New York: Oxford University Press.

Barlow, D. H., Craske, M. G., Cerny, J. A., & Klosko, J. S. (1989). Behavioral treatment of panic disorder. *Behavior Therapy, 20,* 261–282.

Barlow, D. H., Gorman, J. M., Shear, M. K., & Woods, S. W. (2000). Cognitive-behavioral therapy, imipramine, or their combination for panic disorder: A randomized controlled trial. *Journal of the American Medical Association, 283*(19), 2529–2536.

Barlow, D. H., O'Brien, G. T., & Last, C. G. (1984). Couples treatment of agoraphobia. *Behavior Therapy, 15*(1), 41–58.

Barlow, D. H., O'Brien, G. T., Last, C. G., & Holden, A. E. (1983). Couples treatment of agoraphobia. In K. D. Craig & R. J. McMahon (Eds.), *Advances in clinical behavior therapy* (pp. 99–127). New York: Brunner/Mazel.

Barlow, D. H., Vermilyea, J., Blanchard, E., Vermilyea, B., Di Nardo, P., & Cerny, J. (1985). Phenomenon of panic. *Journal of Abnormal Psychology, 94,* 320–328.

Barsky, A. J., Cleary, P. D., Sarnie, M. K., & Ruskin, J. N. (1994). Panic disorder, palpitations, and the awareness of cardiac activity. *Journal of Nervous and Mental Disease, 182,* 63–71.

Basoglu, M., Marks, I. M., Kilic, C., Brewin, C. R., & Swinson, R. P. (1994). Alprazolam and exposure for panic disorder with agoraphobia: Attribution of improvement to medication predicts subsequent relapse. *British Journal of Psychiatry, 164,* 652–659.

Beck, A. T., Epstein, N., Brown, G., & Steer, R. A. (1988). An inventory for measuring clinical anxiety: Psychometric properties. *Journal of Consulting and Clinical Psychology, 56,* 893–897.

Beck, J. G., & Shipherd, J. C. (1997). Repeated exposure to interoceptive cues: Does habituation of fear occur in panic disorder patients?: A preliminary report. *Behaviour Research and Therapy, 35,* 551–557.

Beck, J. G., Shipherd, J. C., & Zebb, B. J. (1997). How does interoceptive exposure for panic disorder work?: An uncontrolled case study. *Journal of Anxiety Disorders, 11,* 541–556.

Beck, J. G., Stanley, M. A., Baldwin, L. E., Deagle, E. A., & Averill, P. M. (1994). Comparison of cognitive therapy and relaxation training for panic disorder. *Journal of Consulting and Clinical Psychology, 62,* 818–826.

Biederman, J., Faraone, S. V., Marrs, A., & Moore, P. (1997). Panic disorder and agoraphobia in consecutively referred children and adolescents. *Journal of the American Academy of Child and Adolescent Psychiatry, 36*(12), 214–223.

Bjork, R. A., & Bjork, E. L. (1992). A new theory of disuse and an old theory of stimulus fluctuation. In A. Healy, S. Kosslyn, & R. Shiffrin (Eds.), *From learning processes to cognitive processes: Essays in honor of William K. Estes* (Vol. 2, pp. 35–67). Hillsdale, NJ: Erlbaum.

Black, D. W., Monahan, P., Wesner, R., Gabel, J., & Bowers, W. (1996). The effect of fluvoxamine, cognitive therapy, and placebo on abnormal personality traits in 44 patients with panic disorder. *Journal of Personality Disorders, 10*, 185–194.

Bland, K., & Hallam, R. (1981). Relationship between response to graded exposure and marital satisfaction in agoraphobics. *Behaviour Research and Therapy, 19*, 335–338.

Bonn, J. A., Harrison, J., & Rees, W. (1971). Lactate-induced anxiety: Therapeutic application. *British Journal of Psychiatry, 119*, 468–470.

Borkovec, T., Weerts, T., & Bernstein, D. (1977). Assessment of anxiety. In A. Ciminero, K. Calhoun, & H. Adams (Eds.), *Handbook of behavioral assessment* (pp. 367–428). New York: Wiley.

Bouchard, S., Gauthier, J., Laberge, B., French, D., Pelletier, M., & Godbout, D. (1996). Exposure versus cognitive restructuring in the treatment of panic disorder with agoraphobia. *Behaviour Research and Therapy, 34*, 213–224.

Bouchard, S., Paquin, B., Payeur, R., Allard, M., Rivard, V., Gournier, T., et al. (2004). Delivering cognitive-behavior therapy for panic disorder with agoraphobia in videoconference [Special issue: Telemedicine in Canada]. *Telemedicine Journal and E-Health, 10*(1), 13–24.

Bouton, M. E. (1993). Context, time and memory retrieval in the interference paradigms of Pavlovian learning. *Psychological Bulletin, 114*, 90–99.

Bouton, M. E., Mineka, S., & Barlow, D. H. (2001). A modern learning-theory perspective on the etiology of panic disorder. *Psychological Review, 108*(1), 4–32.

Bouton, M. E., & Swartzentruber, D. (1991). Sources of relapse after extinction in Pavlovian conditioning and instrumental conditioning. *Behavioral Neuroscience, 104*, 44–55.

Boyd, J. H. (1986). Use of mental health services for the treatment of panic disorder. *American Journal of Psychiatry, 143*, 1569–1574.

Broocks, A., Bandelow, B., Pekrun, G., George, A., Meyer, T., Bartmann, U., et al. (1998). Comparison of aerobic exercise, clomipramine, and placebo in the treatment of panic disorder. *American Journal of Psychiatry, 155*, 603–609.

Brown, T. A., Antony, M. M., & Barlow, D. H. (1995). Diagnostic comorbidity in panic disorder: Effect on treatment outcome and course of comorbid diagnoses following treatment. *Journal of Consulting and Clinical Psychology, 63*, 408–418.

Brown, T. A., & Barlow, D. H. (1995). Long-term outcome in cognitive-behavioral treatment of panic disorder: Clinical predictors and alternative strategies for assessment. *Journal of Consulting and Clinical Psychology, 63*, 754–765.

Brown, T. A., Campbell, L. A., Lehman, C. L., Grisham, J. R., & Mancill, R. B. (2001). Current and lifetime comorbidity of the DSM-IV anxiety and mood disorders in a large clinical sample. *Journal of Abnormal Psychology, 110*(4), 585–599.

Brown, T. A., Chorpita, B. F., & Barlow, D. H. (1998). Structural relationships among dimensions of the DSM-IV anxiety and mood disorders and dimensions of negative affect, positive affect, and autonomic arousal. *Journal of Abnormal Psychology, 107*(2), 179–192.

Brown, T. A., Di Nardo, P. A., Lehman, C. L., & Campbell, L. A. (2001). Reliability of DSM-IV anxiety and mood disorders: Implications for the classification of emotional disorders. *Journal of Abnormal Psychology, 110*(1), 49–58.

Brown, T. A., White, K. S., Forsyth, J. P., & Barlow, D. II. (2004). The structure of perceived emotional control: Psychometric properties of a revised Anxiety Control Questionnaire. *Behavior Therapy, 35*(1), 75–99.

Buglass, P., Clarke, J., Henderson, A., & Presley, A. (1977). A study of agoraphobic housewives. *Psychological Medicine, 7*, 73–86.

Cain, C. K., Blouin, A. M., & Barad, M. (2004). Adrenergic transmission facilitates extinction of conditional fear in mice. *Learning and Memory, 11*(2), 179–187.

Carlbring, P., Ekselius, L., & Andersson, G. (2003). Treatment of panic disorder via the Internet: A randomized trial of CBT vs. applied relaxation. *Journal of Behavior Therapy and Experimental Psychiatry, 34*, 129–140.

Carter, M. M., Sbrocco, T., Gore, K. L., Marin, N. W., & Lewis, E. L. (2003). Cognitive-behavioral group therapy versus a wait-list control in the treatment of African American women with panic disorder. *Cognitive Therapy and Research, 27*(5), 505–518.

Cerny, J. A., Barlow, D. H., Craske, M. G., & Himadi, W. G. (1987). Couples treatment of agoraphobia: A two-year follow-up. *Behavior Therapy, 18*, 401–415.

Chambless, D. L. (1990). Spacing of exposure sessions in treatment of agoraphobia and simple phobia. *Behavior Therapy, 21*, 217–229.

Chambless, D. L., Caputo, G., Bright, P., & Gallagher, R. (1984). Assessment of fear in agoraphobics: The Body Sensations Questionnaire and the Agoraphobic Cognitions Questionnaire. *Journal of Consulting and Clinical Psychology, 52*, 1090–1097.

Chambless, D. L., Caputo, G., Gracely, S., Jasin, E., & Williams, C. (1985). The Mobility Inventory for Agoraphobia. *Behaviour Research and Therapy, 23,* 35–44.

Chambless, D. L., & Renneberg, B. (1988, September). *Personality disorders of agoraphobics.* Paper presented at World Congress of Behavior Therapy, Edinburgh, Scotland.

Chaplin, E. W., & Levine, B. A. (1981). The effects of total exposure duration and interrupted versus continuous exposure in flooding therapy. *Behavior Therapy, 12*(3), 360–368.

Clark D. A. (1996). Panic disorder: From theory to therapy. In P. M. Salkovskis (Ed.), *From frontiers of cognitive therapy: The state of the art and beyond* (pp. 318–344). New York: Guilford Press.

Clark, D. M. (1986). A cognitive approach to panic. *Behaviour Research and Therapy, 24,* 461–470.

Clark, D. M., & Ehlers, A. (1993). An overview of the cognitive theory and treatment of panic disorder. *Applied and Preventive Psychology, 2,* 131–139.

Clark, D. M., Salkovskis, P., & Chalkley, A. (1985). Respiratory control as a treatment for panic attacks. *Journal of Behavior Therapy and Experimental Psychiatry, 16,* 23–30.

Clark, D. M., Salkovskis, P., Gelder, M., Koehler, C., Martin, M., Anastasiades, P., et al. (1988). Tests of a cognitive theory of panic. In I. Hand & H. Wittchen (Eds.), *Panic and phobias II* (pp. 71–90). Berlin: Springer-Verlag.

Clark, D. M., Salkovskis, P. M., Hackmann, A., Middleton, H., Anastasiades, P., & Gelder, M. (1994). A comparison of cognitive therapy, applied relaxation and imipramine in the treatment of panic disorder. *British Journal of Psychiatry, 164,* 759–769.

Clark, D. M., Salkovskis, P. M., Hackmann, A., Wells, A., Ludgate, J., & Gelder, M. (1999). Brief cognitive therapy for panic disorder: A randomized controlled trial. *Journal of Consulting and Clinical Psychology, 67,* 583–589.

Cote, G., Gauthier, J. G., Laberge, B., Cormier, H. J., & Plamondon, J. (1994). Reduced therapist contact in the cognitive behavioral treatment of panic disorder. *Behavior Therapy, 25,* 123–145.

Cox, B. J., Endler, N. S., & Swinson, R. P. (1995). An examination of levels of agoraphobic severity in panic disorder. *Behaviour Research and Therapy, 33,* 57–62.

Craske, M. G., & Barlow, D. H. (1988). A review of the relationship between panic and avoidance. *Clinical Psychology Review, 8,* 667–685.

Craske, M. G., & Barlow, D. H. (1989). Nocturnal panic. *Journal of Nervous and Mental Disease, 177*(3), 160–167.

Craske, M. G., & Barlow, D. H. (2006). *Mastery of your anxiety and panic: Therapist guide* (3rd ed.). New York: Oxford University Press.

Craske, M. G., Brown, T. A., & Barlow, D. H. (1991). Behavioral treatment of panic disorder: A two-year follow-up. *Behavior Therapy, 22,* 289–304.

Craske, M. G., DeCola, J. P., Sachs, A. D., & Pontillo, D. C. (2003). Panic control treatment of agoraphobia. *Journal of Anxiety Disorders, 17*(3), 321–333.

Craske, M. G., Farchione, T., Allen, L., Barrios, V., Stoyanova, M., & Rose, D. (2007). Cognitive behavioral therapy for panic disorder and comorbidity: More of the same or less of more. *Behaviour Research and Therapy, 45*(6), 1095–1109.

Craske, M. G., & Freed, S. (1995). Expectations about arousal and nocturnal panic. *Journal of Abnormal Psychology, 104,* 567–575.

Craske, M. G., Glover, D., & DeCola, J. (1995). Predicted versus unpredicted panic attacks: Acute versus general distress. *Journal of Abnormal Psychology, 104,* 214–223.

Craske, M. G., Golinelli, D., Stein, M. B., Roy-Byrne, P., Bystritsky, A., & Sherbourne, C. (2005). Does the addition of cognitive behavioral therapy improve panic disorder treatment outcome relative to medication alone in the primary-care setting? *Psychological Medicine, 35*(11), 1645–1654.

Craske, M. G., Lang, A. J., Aikins, D., & Mystkowski, J. L. (2005). Cognitive behavioral therapy for nocturnal panic. *Behavior Therapy, 36,* 43–54.

Craske, M. G., Lang, A. J., Rowe, M., DeCola, J. P., Simmons, J., Mann, C., et al. (2002). Presleep attributions about arousal during sleep: Nocturnal panic. *Journal of Abnormal Psychology, 111,* 53–62.

Craske, M. G., Maidenberg, E., & Bystritsky, A. (1995). Brief cognitive-behavioral versus non directive therapy for panic disorder. *Journal of Behavior Therapy and Experimental Psychiatry, 26,* 113–120.

Craske, M. G., Miller, P. P., Rotunda, R., & Barlow, D. H. (1990). A descriptive report of features of initial unexpected panic attacks in minimal and extensive avoiders. *Behaviour Research and Therapy, 28,* 395–400.

Craske, M. G., & Mystkowski, J. L. (2006). Exposure therapy and extinction: Clinical studies. In M. G. Craske, D. Hermans, & D. Vansteenwegen (Eds.), *Fear and learning: From basic processes to clinical implications* (pp. 217–233). Washington, DC: American Psychological Association.

Craske, M. G., Poulton, R., Tsao, J. C. I., & Plotkin, D. (2001). Paths to panic–agoraphobia: An exploratory analysis from age 3 to 21 in an unselected birth cohort. *American Journal of Child and Adolescent Psychiatry, 40,* 556–563.

Craske, M. G., Rapee, R. M., & Barlow, D. H. (1988). The significance of panic–expectancy for individual patterns of avoidance. *Behavior Therapy, 19,* 577–592.

Craske, M. G., & Rowe, M. K. (1997a). A comparison of behavioral and cognitive treatments of phobias. In G. C. L. Davey (Ed.), *Phobias—a handbook of theory, research and treatment* (pp. 247–280). West Sussex, UK: Wiley.

Craske, M. G., & Rowe, M. K. (1997b). Nocturnal panic. *Clinical Psychology: Science and Practice, 4,* 153–174.

Craske, M. G., Rowe, M., Lewin, M., & Noriega-Dimitri, R. (1997). Interoceptive exposure versus breathing retraining within cognitive-behavioural therapy for panic disorder with agoraphobia. *British Journal of Clinical Psychology, 36*, 85–99.

Craske, M. G., Roy-Byrne, P., Stein, M. B., Donald-Sherbourne, C., Bystritsky, A., Katon, W., et al. (2002). Treating panic disorder in primary care: A collaborative care intervention. *General Hospital Psychiatry, 24*(3), 148–155.

Craske, M. G., Roy-Byrne, P., Stein, M. B., Sullivan, G., Hazlett-Stevens, H., Bystritsky, A., et al. (2006). CBT intensity and outcome for panic disorder in a primary care setting. *Behavior Therapy, 37*, 112–119.

Craske, M. G., Street, L., & Barlow, D. H. (1989). Instructions to focus upon or distract from internal cues during exposure treatment for agoraphobic avoidance. *Behaviour Research and Therapy, 27*, 663–672.

Craske, M. G., & Tsao, J. I. C. (1999). Self-monitoring with panic and anxiety disorders. *Psychological Assessment, 11*, 466–479.

Dattilio, F. M., & Salas-Auvert, J. A. (2000). *Panic disorder: Assessment and treatment through a wide-angle lens.* Phoenix, AZ: Zeig, Tucker.

Deacon, B., & Abramowitz, J. (2006). A pilot study of two-day cognitive-behavioral therapy for panic disorder. *Behaviour Research and Therapy, 44*, 807–817.

de Beurs, E., Lange, A., van Dyck, R., & Koele, P. (1995). Respiratory training prior to exposure *in vivo* in the treatment of panic disorder with agoraphobia: Efficacy and predictors of outcome. *Australian and New Zealand Journal of Psychiatry, 29*, 104–113.

de Beurs, E., van Balkom, A. J., Lange, A., Koele, P., & van Dyck, R. (1995). Treatment of panic disorder with agoraphobia: Comparison of fluvoxamine, placebo, and psychological panic management combined with exposure and of exposure *in vivo* alone. *American Journal of Psychiatry, 152*, 683–691.

Deckert, J., Nothen, M. M., Franke, P., Delmo, C., Fritze, J., Knapp, M., et al. (1998). Systematic mutation screening and association study of the A1 and A2a adenosine receptor genes in panic disorder suggest a contribution of the A2a gene to the development of disease. *Molecular Psychiatry, 3*, 81–85.

de Jong, M. G., & Bouman, T. K. (1995). Panic disorder: A baseline period: Predictability of agoraphobic avoidance behavior. *Journal of Anxiety Disorders, 9*, 185–199.

De Ruiter, C., Garssen, B., Rijken, H., & Kraaimaat, F. (1989). The hyperventilation syndrome in panic disorder, agoraphobia, and generalized anxiety disorder. *Behaviour Research and Therapy, 27*(4), 447–452.

Dewey, D., & Hunsley, J. (1990). The effects of marital adjustment and spouse involvement on the behavioral treatment of agoraphobia: A meta-analytic review. *Anxiety Research, 2*(2), 69–83.

Di Nardo, P., Brown, T. A., & Barlow, D. H. (1994). *Anxiety Disorders Interview Schedule—Fourth Edition (ADIS-IV).* New York: Oxford University Press.

Dreessen, L., Arntz, A., Luttels, C., & Sallaerts, S. (1994). Personality disorders do not influence the results of cognitive behavior therapies for anxiety disorders. *Comprehensive Psychiatry, 35*(4), 265–274.

Dworkin, B. R., & Dworkin, S. (1999). Heterotopic and homotopic classical conditioning of the baroreflex. *Integrative Physiological and Behavioral Science, 34*(3), 158–176.

Ehlers, A. (1995). A 1-year prospective study of panic attacks: Clinical course and factors associated with maintenance. *Journal of Abnormal Psychology, 104*, 164–172.

Ehlers, A., & Breuer, P. (1992). Increased cardiac awareness in panic disorder. *Journal of Abnormal Psychology, 101*, 371–382.

Ehlers, A., & Breuer, P. (1996). How good are patients with panic disorder at perceiving their heartbeats? *Biological Psychology, 42*, 165–182.

Ehlers, A., Breuer, P., Dohn, D., & Fiegenbaum, W. (1995). Heartbeat perception and panic disorder: Possible explanations for discrepant findings. *Behaviour Research and Therapy, 33*, 69–76.

Ehlers, A., & Margraf, J. (1989). The psychophysiological model of panic attacks. In P. M. G. Emmelkamp (Ed.), *Anxiety disorders: Annual series of European research in behavior therapy* (Vol. 4, pp. 1–29). Amsterdam: Swets.

Ehlers, A., Margraf, J., Davies, S., & Roth, W. T. (1988). Selective processing of threat cues in subjects with panic attacks. *Cognition and Emotion, 2*, 201–219.

Ehlers, A., Margraf, J., Roth, W. T., Taylor, C. B., & Birbaumer, N. (1988). Anxiety induced by false heart rate feedback in patients with panic disorder. *Behaviour Research and Therapy, 26*(1), 1–11.

Eifert, G. H., & Forsyth, J. P. (2005). *Acceptance and commitment therapy for anxiety disorders: A practitioner's treatment guide to using mindfulness, acceptance, and value-based behavior change strategies.* Oakland, CA: New Harbinger.

Eley, T. C. (2001). Contributions of behavioral genetics research: Quantifying genetic, shared environmental and nonshared environmental influences. In M. W. Vasey & M. R. Dadds (Eds.), *The developmental psychopathology of anxiety* (pp. 45–59). New York: Oxford University Press.

Emmelkamp, P. (1980). Agoraphobic's interpersonal problems. *Archives of General Psychiatry, 37*, 1303–1306.

Emmelkamp, P. M., Brilman, E., Kuiper, H., & Mersch, P. (1986). The treatment of agoraphobia: A comparison of self-instructional training, rational emotive therapy, and exposure *in vivo. Behavior Modification, 10*, 37–53.

Emmelkamp, P. M., Kuipers, A. C., & Eggeraat, J. B. (1978). Cognitive modification versus prolonged exposure *in vivo*: A comparison with agoraphobics as subjects. *Behaviour Research and Therapy, 16,* 33–41.

Emmelkamp, P. M., & Mersch, P. P. (1982). Cognition and exposure *in vivo* in the treatment of agoraphobia: Short-term and delayed effects. *Cognitive Therapy and Research, 6,* 77–90.

Evans, L., Holt, C., & Oei, T. P. S. (1991). Long term follow-up of agoraphobics treated by brief intensive group cognitive behaviour therapy. *Australian and New Zealand Journal of Psychiatry, 25,* 343–349.

Eysenck, H. J. (1967). *The biological basis of personality.* Springfield, IL: Charles C. Thomas.

Faravelli, C., Pallanti, S., Biondi, F., Paterniti, S., & Scarpato, M. A. (1992). Onset of panic disorder. *American Journal of Psychiatry, 149,* 827–828.

Fava, G. A., Zielezny, M., Savron, G., & Grandi, S. (1995). Long-term effects of behavioural treatment for panic disorder with agoraphobia. *British Journal of Psychiatry, 166,* 87–92.

Feigenbaum, W. (1988). Long-term efficacy of ungraded versus graded massed exposure in agoraphobics. In I. Hand & H. Wittchen (Eds.), *Panic and phobias: Treatments and variables affecting course and outcome.* Berlin: Springer-Verlag.

First, M. B., Spitzer, R. L., Gibbon, M., & Williams, J. B. W. (1994). *Structured Clinical Interview for Axis I DSM-IV Disorders.* New York: Biometric Research Department, New York State Psychiatric Institute.

Foa, E. B., Jameson, J. S., Turner, R. M., & Payne, L. L. (1980). Massed vs. spaced exposure sessions in the treatment of agoraphobia. *Behaviour Research and Therapy, 18,* 333–338.

Foa, E. B., & McNally, R. J. (1996). Mechanisms of change in exposure therapy. In R. M. Rapee (Ed.), *Current controversies in the anxiety disorders* (pp. 329–343). New York: Guilford Press.

Forsyth, J. P., Palav, A., & Duff, K. (1999). The absence of relation between anxiety sensitivity and fear conditioning using 20% versus 13% CO_2-enriched air as unconditioned stimuli. *Behaviour Research and Therapy, 37*(2), 143–153.

Friedman, S., & Paradis, C. (1991). African-American patients with panic disorder and agoraphobia. *Journal of Anxiety Disorders, 5,* 35–41.

Friedman, S., Paradis, C. M., & Hatch, M. (1994). Characteristics of African-American and white patients with panic disorder and agoraphobia. *Hospital ande Community Psychiatry, 45,* 798–803.

Fry, W. (1962). The marital context of an anxiety syndrome. *Family Process, 1,* 245–252.

Gallistel, C. R., & Gibbon, J. (2000). Time, rate, and conditioning. *Psychological Review, 107*(2), 289–344.

Garssen, B., de Ruiter, C., & van Dyck, R. (1992). Breathing retraining: A rational placebo? *Clinical Psychology Review, 12,* 141–153.

Ghosh, A., & Marks, I. M. (1987). Self-treatment of agoraphobia by exposure. *Behavior Therapy, 18,* 3–16.

Goisman, R. M., Goldenberg, I., Vasile, R. G., & Keller, M. B. (1995). Comorbidity of anxiety disorders in a multicenter anxiety study. *Comprehensive Psychiatry, 36,* 303–311.

Goisman, R. M., Warshaw, M. G., Peterson, L. G., Rogers, M. P., Cuneo, P., Hunt, M. F., et al. (1994). Panic, agoraphobia, and panic disorder with agoraphobia: Data from a multicenter anxiety disorders study. *Journal of Nervous and Mental Disease, 182,* 72–79.

Goldstein, A. J., & Chambless, D. L. (1978). A reanalysis of agoraphobia. *Behavior Therapy, 9,* 47–59.

Goodwin, R. D., Fergusson, D. M., & Horwood, L. J. (2005). Childhood abuse and familial violence and the risk of panic attacks and panic disorder in young adulthood. *Psychological Medicine, 35,* 881–890.

Gorman, J. M., Papp, L. A., Coplan, J. D., Martinez, J. M., Lennon, S., Goetz, R. R., et al. (1994). Anxiogenic effects of CO_2 and hyperventilation in patients with panic disorder. *American Journal of Psychiatry, 151*(4), 547–553.

Gould, R. A., & Clum, G. A. (1995). Self-help plus minimal therapist contact in the treatment of panic disorder: A replication and extension. *Behavior Therapy, 26,* 533–546.

Gould, R. A., Clum, G. A., & Shapiro, D. (1993). The use of bibliotherapy in the treatment of panic: A preliminary investigation. *Behavior Therapy, 24,* 241–252.

Gray, J. A. (1982). *The neuropsychology of anxiety: An enquiry into the functions of the septo-hippocampal system.* New York: Oxford University Press.

Grayson, J. B., Foa, E. B., & Steketee, G. (1982). Habituation during exposure treatment: Distraction versus attention-focusing. *Behaviour Research and Therapy, 20,* 323–328.

Griez, E., & van den Hout, M. A. (1986). CO_2 inhalation in the treatment of panic attacks. *Behaviour Research and Therapy, 24,* 145–150.

Grilo, C. M., Money, R., Barlow, D. H., Goddard, A. W., Gorman, J. M., Hofmann, S. G., et al. (1998). Pretreatment patient factors predicting attrition from a multicenter randomized controlled treatment study for panic disorder. *Comprehensive Psychiatry, 39,* 323–332.

Hafner, R. J. (1984). Predicting the effects on husbands of behavior therapy for agoraphobia. *Behaviour Research and Therapy, 22,* 217–226.

Hamilton, S. P., Fyer, A. J., Durner, M., Heiman, G. A., Baisre de Leon, A., Hodge, S. E., et al. (2003). Further genetic evidence for a panic disorder syndrome mapping to chromosome 13q. *Proceedings of National Academy of Science USA, 100,* 2550–2555.

Hamilton, S. P., Slager, S. L., De Leon, A. B., Heiman, G. A., Klein, D. F., Hodge, S. E., et al. (2004). Evidence for genetic linkage between a polymorphism in the adenosine 2A receptor and panic disorder. *Neuropsychopharmacology, 29,* 558–65.

Hamilton, S. P., Slager, S. L., Helleby, L., Heiman, G. A., Klein, D. F., Hodge, S. E., et al. (2001). No association or linkage between polymorphisms in the genes encoding cholecystokinin and the cholecystokinin B receptor and panic disorder. *Molecular Psychiatry, 6,* 59–65.

Hand, I., & Lamontagne, Y. (1976). The exacerbation of interpersonal problems after rapid phobia removal. *Psychotherapy: Theory, Research and Practice, 13,* 405–411.

Haslam, M. T. (1974). The relationship between the effect of lactate infusion on anxiety states and their amelioration by carbon dioxide inhalation. *British Journal of Psychiatry, 125,* 88–90.

Hayward, C., Killen, J. D., Hammer, L. D., Litt, I. F., Wilson, D. M., Simmonds, B., et al. (1992). Pubertal stage and panic attack history in sixth- and seventh-grade girls. *American Journal of Psychiatry, 149,* 1239–1243.

Hayward, C., Killen, J. D., Kraemer, H. C., & Taylor, C. B. (2000). Predictors of panic attacks in adolescents. *Journal of the American Academy of Child and Adolescent Psychiatry, 39*(2), 1–8.

Heatley, C., Ricketts, T., & Forrest, J. (2005). Training general practitioners in cognitive behavioural therapy for panic disorder: Randomized-controlled trial. *Journal of Mental Health, 14*(1), 73–82.

Hecker, J. E., Losee, M. C., Fritzler, B. K., & Fink, C. M. (1996). Self-directed versus therapist-directed cognitive behavioral treatment for panic disorder. *Journal of Anxiety Disorders, 10,* 253–265.

Hecker, J. E., Losee, M. C., Roberson-Nay, R., & Maki, K. (2004). Mastery of your anxiety and panic and brief therapist contact in the treatment of panic disorder. *Journal of Anxiety Disorders, 18*(2), 111–126.

Heldt, E., Manfro, G. G., Kipper, L., Blaya, C., Isolan, L., & Otto, M. W. (2006). One-year follow-up of pharmacotherapy-resistant patients with panic disorder treated with cognitive-behavior therapy: Outcome and predictors of remission. *Behaviour Research and Therapy, 44*(5), 657–665.

Hermans, D., Craske, M. G., Mineka, S., & Lovibond, P. F. (2006). Extinction in human fear conditioning. *Biological Psychiatry, 60,* 361–368.

Heuzenroeder, L., Donnelly, M., Haby, M. M., Mihalopoulos, C., Rossell, R., Carter, R., et al. (2004). Cost-effectiveness of psychological and pharmacological interventions for generalized anxiety disorder and panic disorder. *Australian and New Zealand Journal of Psychiatry, 38*(8), 602–612.

Hibbert, G., & Pilsbury, D. (1989). Hyperventilation: Is it a cause of panic attacks? *British Journal of Psychiatry, 155,* 805–809.

Himadi, W., Cerny, J., Barlow, D., Cohen, S., & O'Brien, G. (1986). The relationship of marital adjustment to agoraphobia treatment outcome. *Behaviour Research and Therapy, 24,* 107–115.

Hoffart, A. (1995). A comparison of cognitive and guided mastery therapy of agoraphobia. *Behaviour Research and Therapy, 33,* 423–434.

Hoffart, A., & Hedley, L. M. (1997). Personality traits among panic disorder with agoraphobia patients before and after symptom-focused treatment. *Journal of Anxiety Disorders, 11,* 77–87.

Hofmann, S. G., Shear, M. K., Barlow, D. H., Gorman, J. M., Hershberger, D., Patterson, M., et al. (1988). Effects of panic disorder treatments on personality disorder characteristics. *Depression and Anxiety, 8*(1), 14–20.

Holden, A. E. O., O'Brien, G. T., Barlow, D. H., Stetson, D., & Infantino, A. (1983). Self-help manual for agoraphobia: A preliminary report of effectiveness. *Behavior Therapy, 14,* 545–556.

Holt, P., & Andrews, G. (1989). Hyperventilation and anxiety in panic disorder, agoraphobia, and generalized anxiety disorder. *Behaviour Research and Therapy, 27,* 453–460.

Hope, D. A., Rapee, R. M., Heimberg, R. G., & Dombeck, M. J. (1990). Representations of the self in social phobia: Vulnerability to social threat. *Cognitive Therapy and Research, 14,* 177–189.

Hornsveld, H., Garssen, B., Fiedeldij Dop, M., & van Spiegel, P. (1990). Symptom reporting during voluntary hyperventilation and mental load: Implications for diagnosing hyperventilation syndrome. *Journal of Psychosomatic Research, 34,* 687–697.

Horwath, E., Lish, J. D., Johnson, J., Hornig, C. D., & Weissman, M. M. (1993). Agoraphobia without panic: Clinical reappraisal of an epidemiologic finding. *American Journal of Psychiatry, 150,* 1496–1501.

Huppert, J. D., Bufka, L. F., Barlow, D. H., Gorman, J. M., Shear, M. K., & Woods, S. W. (2001). Therapist, therapist variables, and cognitive-behavioral therapy outcome in a multicenter trial for panic disorder. *Journal of Consulting and Clinical Psychology, 69*(5), 747–755.

Ito, L. M., Noshirvani, H., Basoglu, M., & Marks, I. M. (1996). Does exposure to internal cues enhance exposure to external exposure to external cues in agoraphobia with panic. *Psychotherapy and Psychosomatics, 65,* 24–28.

Izard, C. E. (1992). Basic emotions, relations among emotions, and emotion cognition relations. *Psychological Review, 99,* 561–565.

Jacob, R. G., Furman, J. M., Clark, D. B., & Durrant, J. D. (1992). Vestibular symptoms, panic, and phobia: Overlap and possible relationships. *Annals of Clinical Psychiatry, 4*(3), 163–174.

Kamphuis, J. H., & Telch, M. J. (2000). Effects of distraction and guided threat reappraisal on fear reduction during exposure-based treatments for specific fears. *Behaviour Research and Therapy, 38*(12), 1163–1181.

Kampman, M., Keijsers, G. P. J., Hoogduin, C. A. L., & Hendriks, G.-J. (2002). A randomized, double-blind, placebo-controlled study of the effects of adjunctive paroxetine in panic disorder patients unsuccessfully treated with cognitive-behavioral therapy alone. *Journal of Clinical Psychiatry, 63*(9), 772–777.

Katon, W., Von Korff, M., Lin, E., Lipscomb, P., Russo, J., Wagner, E., et al. (1990). Distressed high utilizers of medical care: DSM-III-R diagnoses and treatment needs. *General Hospital Psychiatry, 12*(6), 355–362.

Katschnig, H., & Amering, M. (1998). The long-term course of panic disorder and its predictors. *Journal of Clinical Psychopharmacology, 18*(6, Suppl. 2), 6S–11S.

Keijsers, G. P., Kampman, M., & Hoogduin, C. A. (2001). Dropout prediction in cognitive behavior therapy for panic disorder. *Behavior Therapy, 32*(4), 739–749.

Keijsers, G. P., Schaap, C. P., Hoogduin, C. A., & Lammers, M. W. (1995). Patient–therapist interaction in the behavioral treatment of panic disorder with agoraphobia. *Behavior Modification, 19*, 491–517.

Kenardy, J. A., Dow, M. G., Johnston, D. W., Newman, M. G., Thomson, A., & Taylor, C. B. (2003). A comparison of delivery methods of cognitive-behavioral therapy for panic disorder: An international multicenter trial. *Journal of Consulting and Clinical Psychology, 71*(6), 1068–1075.

Kendler, K. S., Bulik, C. M., Silberg, J., Hettema, J. M., Myers, J., & Prescott, C. A. (2000). Childhood sexual abuse and adult psychiatric and substance use disorders in women: An epidemiological and co-twin analysis. *Archives of General Psychiatry, 57*, 953–959.

Kendler, K. S., Heath, A. C., Martin, N. G., & Eaves, L. J. (1987). Symptoms of anxiety and symptoms of depression: Same genes, different environments? *Archives of General Psychiatry, 44*, 451–457.

Kessler, R. C., Berglund, P., Demler, O., Jin, R., & Walters, E. E. (2005). Lifetime prevalence and age-of-onset distributions of DSM-IV disorders in the National Comorbidity Survey Replication. *Archives of General Psychiatry, 62*, 593–602.

Kessler, R. C., Chiu, W. T., Demler, O., & Walters, E. E. (2005). Lifetime prevalence and age-of-onset distributions of DSM-IV disorders in the National Comorbidity Survey Replication. *Archives of General Psychiatry, 62*(6), 593–602.

Kessler, R. C., Chiu, W. T., Jin, R., Ruscio, A. M., Shear, K., & Walters, E. E. (2006). The epidemiology of panic attacks, panic disorder, and agoraphobia in the National Comorbidity Survey Replication. *Archives of General Psychiatry, 63*, 415–424.

Kessler, R. C., Davis, C. G., & Kendler, K. S. (1997). Childhood adversity and adult psychiatric disorder in the U.S. National Comorbidity Survey. *Psychological Medicine, 27*, 1101–1119.

Kessler, R. C., McGonagle, K. A., Zhao, S., Nelson, C. B., Hughes, M., Eshkeman, S., et al. (1994). Lifetime and 12 month prevalence of DSM-III-R psychiatric disorders in the United States: Results from the National Comorbidity Study. *Archives of General Psychiatry, 51*, 8–19.

Keyl, P. M., & Eaton, W. W. (1990). Risk factors for the onset of panic disorder and other panic attacks in a prospective, population-based study. *American Journal of Epidemiology, 131*, 301–311.

Kikuchi, M., Komuro, R., Hiroshi, O., Kidani, T., Hanaoka, A., & Koshino, Y. (2005). Panic disorder with and without agoraphobia: Comorbidity within a half-year of the onset of panic disorder. *Psychiatry and Clinical Neurosciences, 58*, 639–643.

Kraft, A. R., & Hoogduin, C. A. (1984). The hyperventilation syndrome: A pilot study of the effectiveness of treatment. *British Journal of Psychiatry, 145*, 538–542.

Kroeze, S., & van den Hout, M. A. (2000). Selective attention for cardiac information in panic patients. *Behaviour Research and Therapy, 38*, 63–72.

Krystal, J. H., Woods, S. W., Hill, C. L., & Charney, D. S. (1991). Characteristics of panic attack subtypes: Assessment of spontaneous panic, situational panic, sleep panic, and limited symptom attacks. *Comprehensive Psychiatry, 32*(6), 474–480.

Laberge, B., Gauthier, J. G., Cote, G., Plamondon, J., & Cormier, H. J. (1993). Cognitive-behavioral therapy of panic disorder with secondary major depression: A preliminary investigation. *Journal of Consulting and Clinical Psychology, 61*, 1028–1037.

Lake, R. I., Eaves, L. J., Maes, H. H., Heath, A. C., & Martin, N. G. (2000). Further evidence against the environmental transmission of individual differences in neuroticism from a collaborative study of 45,850 twins and relatives of two continents. *Behavior Genetics, 30*(3), 223–233.

Lehman, C. L., Brown, T. A., & Barlow, D. H. (1998). Effects of cognitive-behavioral treatment for panic disorder with agoraphobia on concurrent alcohol abuse. *Behavior Therapy, 29*, 423–433.

Lelliott, P., Marks, I., McNamee, G., & Tobena, A. (1989). Onset of panic disorder with agoraphobia: Toward an integrated model. *Archives of General Psychiatry, 46*, 1000–1004.

Lidren, D. M., Watkins, P., Gould, R. A., Clum, G. A., Asterino, M., & Tulloch, H. L. (1994). A comparison of bibliotherapy and group therapy in the treatment of panic disorder. *Journal of Consulting and Clinical Psychology, 62*, 865–869.

Lovibond, P. F., Davis, N. R., & O'Flaherty, A. S. (2000). Protection from extinction in human fear conditioning. *Behaviour Research and Therapy, 38*, 967–983.

Lovibond, P. F., & Shanks, D. R. (2002). The role of awareness in Pavlovian conditioning: Empirical evidence and theoretical implications. *Journal of Experimental Psychology: Animal Behavior Processes, 28*, 3–26.

Maddock, R. J., & Blacker, K. H. (1991). Response to treatment in panic disorder with associated depression. *Psychopathology, 24*(1), 1–6.

Maidenberg, E., Chen, E., Craske, M., Bohn, P., & Bystritsky, A. (1996). Specificity of attentional bias in panic disorder and social phobia. *Journal of Anxiety Disorders, 10,* 529–541.

Maier, S. F., Laudenslager, M. L., & Ryan, S. M. (1985). Stressor controllability, immune function and endogenous opiates. In F. R. Brush & J. B. Overmeier (Eds.), *Affect, conditioning and cognition: Essays on the determinants of behavior* (pp. 183–201). Hillsdale, NJ: Erlbaum.

Maller, R. G., & Reiss, S. (1992). Anxiety sensitivity in 1984 and panic attacks in 1987. *Journal of Anxiety Disorders, 6(3),* 241–247.

Mannuzza, S., Fyer, A. J., Liebowitz, M. R., & Klein, D. F. (1990). Delineating the boundaries of social phobia: Its relationship to panic disorder and agoraphobia. *Journal of Anxiety Disorders, 4(1),* 41–59.

Marchand, A., Goyer, L. R., Dupuis, G., & Mainguy, N. (1998). Personality disorders and the outcome of cognitive-behavioural treatment of panic disorder with agoraphobia. *Canadian Journal of Behavioural Science, 30(1),* 14–23.

Margraf, J., Taylor, C. B., Ehlers, A., Roth, W. T., & Agras, W. S. (1987). Panic attacks in the natural environment. *Journal of Nervous and Mental Disease, 175,* 558–565.

Marks, I. M., Swinson, R. P., Basoglu, M., Kuck, K., Noshirvani, H., O'Sullivan, G., et al. (1993). Alprazolam and exposure alone and combined in panic disorder with agoraphobia: A controlled study in London and Toronto. *British Journal of Psychiatry, 162,* 776–787.

Marshall, W. L. (1985). The effects of variable exposure in flooding therapy. *Behavior Therapy, 16,* 117–135.

Martin, N. G., Jardine, R., Andrews, G., & Heath, A. C. (1988). Anxiety disorders and neuroticism: Are there genetic factors specific to panic? *Acta Psychiatrica Scandinavica, 77,* 698–706.

Mavissakalian, M., & Hamman, M. (1987). DSM-III personality disorder in agoraphobia: II. Changes with treatment. *Comprehensive Psychiatry, 28,* 356–361.

McLean, P. D., Woody, S., Taylor, S., & Koch, W. J. (1998). Comorbid panic disorder and major depression: Implications for cognitive-behavioral therapy. *Journal of Consulting and Clinical Psychology, 66,* 240–247.

McNally, R. J., & Lorenz, M. (1987). Anxiety sensitivity in agoraphobics. *Journal of Behavior Therapy and Experimental Psychiatry, 18(1),* 3–11.

McNally, R. J., Riemann, B. C., Louro, C. E., Lukach, B. M., & Kim, E. (1992). Cognitive processing of emotional information in panic disorder. *Behaviour Research and Therapy, 30,* 143–149.

McNamee, G., O'Sullivan, G., Lelliott, P., & Marks, I. M. (1989). Telephone-guided treatment for housebound agoraphobics with panic disorder: Exposure vs. relaxation. *Behavior Therapy, 20,* 491–497.

Mellman, T. A., & Uhde, T. W. (1989). Sleep panic attacks: New clinical findings and theoretical implications. *American Journal of Psychiatry, 146,* 1204–1207.

Mennin, D. S., & Heimberg, R. G. (2000). The impact of comorbid mood and personality disorders in the cognitive-behavioral treatment of panic disorder. *Clinical Psychology Review, 20(3),* 339–357.

Messenger, C., & Shean, G. (1998). The effects of anxiety sensitivity and history of panic on reactions to stressors in a non-clinical sample. *Journal of Behavior Therapy, 29,* 279–288.

Michelson, L., Mavissakalian, M., & Marchione, K. (1985). Cognitive and behavioral treatments of agoraphobia: Clinical, behavioral, and psychophysiological outcomes. *Journal of Consulting and Clinical Psychology, 53,* 913–925.

Michelson, L., Mavissakalian, M., & Marchione, K. (1988). Cognitive, behavioral, and psychophysiological treatments of agoraphobia: A comparative outcome investigation. *Behavior Therapy, 19,* 97–120.

Michelson, L., Mavissakalian, M., Marchione, K., Ulrich, R., Marchione, N., & Testa, S. (1990). Psychophysiological outcome of cognitive, behavioral, and psychophysiologically-based treatments of agoraphobia. *Behaviour Research and Therapy, 28,* 127–139.

Milton, F., & Hafner, J. (1979). The outcome of behavior therapy for agoraphobia in relation to marital adjustment. *Archives of General Psychiatry, 36,* 807–811.

Mineka, S., Cook, M., & Miller, S. (1984). Fear conditioned with escapable and inescapable shock: The effects of a feedback stimulus. *Journal of Experimental Psychology: Animal Behavior Processes, 10,* 307–323.

Mitte, K. A. (2005). Meta-analysis of the efficacy of psycho- and pharmacotherapy in panic disorder with and without agoraphobia. *Journal of Affective Disorders, 88,* 27–45.

Moisan, D., & Engels, M. L. (1995). Childhood trauma and personality disorder in 43 women with panic disorder. *Psychological Reports, 76,* 1133–1134.

Morisette, S. B., Spiegel, D. A., & Heinrichs, N. (2005). Sensation-focused intensive treatment for panic disorder with moderate to severe agoraphobia. *Cognitive and Behavioral Practice, 12(1),* 17–29.

Murphy, M. T., Michelson, L. K., Marchione, K., Marchione, N., & Testa, S. (1998). The role of self-directed *in vivo* exposure in combination with cognitive therapy, relaxation training, or therapist-assisted exposure in the treatment of panic disorder with agoraphobia. *Behaviour Research and Therapy, 12,* 117–138.

Myers, J., Weissman, M., Tischler, C., Holzer, C., Orvaschel, H., Anthony, J., et al. (1984). Six-month prevalence of psychiatric disorders in three communities. *Archives of General Psychiatry, 41,* 959–967.

Mystkowski, J. L., Craske, M. G., Echiverri, A. M., & Labus, J. S. (2006). Mental reinstatement of context and return of fear in spider-fearful participants. *Behavior Therapy, 37*(1), 49–60.

Neron, S., Lacroix, D., & Chaput, Y. (1995). Group vs individual cognitive behaviour therapy in panic disorder: An open clinical trial with a six month follow-up. *Canadian Journal of Behavioural Science, 27,* 379–392.

Newman, M. G., Kenardy, J., Herman, S., & Taylor, C. B. (1997). Comparison of palmtop-computer-assisted brief cognitive-behavioral treatment to cognitive-behavioral treatment for panic disorder. *Journal of Consulting and Clinical Psychology, 65,* 178–183.

Norton, G. R., Cox, B. J., & Malan, J. (1992). Nonclinical panickers: A critical review. *Clinical Psychology Review, 12,* 121–139.

Noyes, R., Clancy, J., Garvey, M. J., & Anderson, D. J. (1987). Is agoraphobia a variant of panic disorder or a separate illness? *Journal of Anxiety Disorders, 1,* 3–13.

Noyes, R., Crowe, R. R., Harris, E. L., Hamra, B. J., McChesney, C.M., & Chaudhry, D. R. (1986). Relationship between panic disorder and agoraphobia: A family study. *Archives of General Psychiatry, 43,* 227–232.

Noyes, R., Reich, J., Suelzer, M., & Christiansen, J. (1991). Personality traits associated with panic disorder: Change associated with treatment. *Comprehensive Psychiatry, 32,* 282–294.

Ohman, A., & Mineka, S. (2001). Fears, phobias, and preparedness: Toward an evolved module of fear and fear learning. *Psychological Review, 108,* 483–522.

Oliver, N. S., & Page, A. C. (2003). Fear reduction during *in vivo* exposure to blood–injection stimuli: Distraction vs. attentional focus. *British Journal of Clinical Psychology, 42*(1), 13–25.

Ost, L.-G. (1988). Applied relaxation vs. progressive relaxation in the treatment of panic disorder. *Behaviour Research and Therapy, 26,* 13–22.

Ost, L.-G., Thulin, U., & Ramnero, J. (2004). Cognitive behavior therapy vs exposure *in vivo* in the treatment of panic disorder with agoraphobia. *Behaviour Research and Therapy, 42*(1), 1105–1127.

Ost, L. G., & Westling, B. E. (1995). Applied relaxation vs cognitive behavior therapy in the treatment of panic disorder. *Behaviour Research and Therapy, 33,* 145–158.

Ost, L. G., Westling, B. E., & Hellstrom, K. (1993). Applied relaxation, exposure *in vivo,* and cognitive methods in the treatment of panic disorder with agoraphobia. *Behaviour Research and Therapy, 31,* 383–394.

Otto, M. W., Pollack, M. H., & Sabatino, S. A. (1996). Maintenance of remission following cognitive behavior therapy for panic disorder: Possible deleterious effects of concurrent medication treatment. *Behavior Therapy, 27,* 473–482.

Otto, M. W., Pollack, M. H., Sachs, G. S., Reiter, S. R., Meltzer-Brody, S., & Rosenbaum, J. F. (1993). Discontinuation of benzodiazepine treatment: Efficacy of cognitive-behavioral therapy for patients with panic disorder. *American Journal of Psychiatry, 150*(10), 1485–1490.

Pauli, P., Amrhein, C., Muhlberger, A., Dengler, W., & Wiedemann, G. (2005). Electrocortical evidence for an early abnormal processing of panic-related words in panic disorder patients. *International Journal of Psychophysiology, 57,* 33–41.

Pennebaker, J. W., & Roberts, T. (1992). Toward a his and hers theory of emotion: Gender differences in visceral perception. *Journal of Social and Clinical Psychology, 11*(30), 199–212.

Perna, G., Bertani, A., Arancio, C., Ronchi, P., & Bellodi, L. (1995). Laboratory response of patients with panic and obsessive–compulsive disorders to 35% CO_2 challenges. *American Journal of Psychiatry, 152,* 85–89.

Pollard, C. A., Pollard, H. J., & Corn, K. J. (1989). Panic onset and major events in the lives of agoraphobics: A test of contiguity. *Journal of Abnormal Psychology, 98,* 318–321.

Powers, M. B., Smits, J. A. J., & Telch, M. J. (2004). Disentangling the effects of safety behavior utilization and safety-behavior availability during exposure based treatments: A placebo- controlled trial. *Journal of Consulting and Clinical Psychology, 72,* 448–454.

Purkis, H. M., & Lipp, O. V. (2001). Does affective learning exist in the absence of contingency awareness? *Learning and Motivation, 32,* 840–899.

Rachman, S., Lopatka, C., & Levitt, K. (1988). Experimental analyses of panic: II. Panic patients. *Behaviour Research and Therapy, 26,* 33–40.

Ramsay, R. W., Barends, J., Breuker, J., & Kruseman, A. (1966). Massed versus spaced desensitization of fear. *Behaviour Research and Therapy, 4*(3), 205–207.

Rapee, R. (1986). Differential response to hyperventilation in panic disorder and generalized anxiety disorder. *Journal of Abnormal Psychology, 95,* 24–28.

Rapee, R. M. (1985). A case of panic disorder treated with breathing retraining. *Behavior Therapy and Experimental Psychiatry, 16,* 63–65.

Rapee, R. M. (1994). Detection of somatic sensations in panic disorder. *Behaviour Research and Therapy, 32,* 825–831.

Rapee, R. M., Brown, T. A., Antony, M. M., & Barlow, D. H. (1992). Response to hyperventilation and inhalation of 5.5% carbon dioxide-enriched air across the DSM-III-R anxiety disorders. *Journal of Abnormal Psychology, 101,* 538–552.

Rapee, R. M., Craske, M. G., & Barlow, D. H. (1990). Subject described features of panic attacks using a new self-monitoring form. *Journal of Anxiety Disorders, 4,* 171–181.

Rapee, R. M., Craske, M. G., & Barlow, D. H. (1995). Assessment instrument for panic disorder that includes fear of sensation-producing activities: The Albany Panic and Phobia Questionnaire. *Anxiety, 1,* 114–122.

Rapee, R. M., Craske, M. G., Brown, T. A., & Barlow, D. H. (1996). Measurement of perceived control over anxiety-related events. *Behavior Therapy, 27*(2), 279–293.

Rapee, R. M., Litwin, E. M., & Barlow, D. H. (1990). Impact of life events on subjects with panic disorder and on comparison subjects. *American Journal of Psychiatry, 147,* 640–644.

Rapee, R. M., & Medoro, L. (1994). Fear of physical sensations and trait anxiety as mediators of the response to hyperventilation in nonclinical subjects. *Journal of Abnormal Psychology, 103*(4), 693–699.

Rapee, R. M., & Murrell, E. (1988). Predictors of agoraphobic avoidance. *Journal of Anxiety Disorders, 2,* 203–217.

Rathus, J. H., Sanderson, W. C., Miller, A. L., & Wetzler, S. (1995). Impact of personality functioning on cognitive behavioral treatment of panic disorder: A preliminary report. *Journal of Personality Disorders, 9,* 160–168.

Razran, G. (1961). The observable unconscious and the inferable conscious in current soviet psychophysiology: Interoceptive conditioning, semantic conditioning, and the orienting reflex. *Psychological Review, 68,* 81–147.

Reich, J., Perry, J. C., Shera, D., Dyck, I., Vasile, R., Goisman, R. M., et al. (1994). Comparison of personality disorders in different anxiety disorder diagnoses: Panic, agoraphobia, generalized anxiety, and social phobia. *Annals of Clinical Psychiatry, 6*(2), 125–134.

Reiss, S. (1980). Pavlovian conditioning and human fear: An expectancy model. *Behavior Therapy, 11,* 380–396.

Reiss, S., Peterson, R., Gursky, D., & McNally, R. (1986). Anxiety sensitivity, anxiety frequency, and the prediction of fearfulness. *Behaviour Research and Therapy, 24,* 1–8.

Rescorla, R. A., & Wagner, A. R. (1972). A theory of Pavlovian conditioning: Variations in the effectiveness of reinforcement and nonreinforcement. In A. H. Black & W. F. Prokasy (Eds.), *Classical conditioning II: Current research and theory* (pp. 64–99). New York: Appleton-Century-Crofts.

Rice, K. M., & Blanchard, E. B. (1982). Biofeedback in the treatment of anxiety disorders. *Clinical Psychology Review, 2,* 557–577.

Richards, J., Klein, B., & Carlbring, P. (2003). Internet-based treatment for panic disorder. *Cognitive Behaviour Therapy, 32,* 125–135.

Richards, J. C., Klein, B., & Austin, D. W. (2006). Internet cognitive behavioural therapy for panic disorder: Does the inclusion of stress management information improve end-state functioning? *Clinical Psychologist, 10*(1), 2–15.

Rijken, H., Kraaimaat, F., de Ruiter, C., & Garssen, B.

(1992). A follow-up study on short-term treatment of agoraphobia. *Behaviour Research and Therapy, 30,* 63–66.

Rodriguez, B. I., & Craske, M. G. (1995). Does distraction interfere with fear reduction during exposure? A test among animal-fearful subjects [Special issue: Experimental pain as a model for the study of clinical pain]. *Behavior Therapy, 26*(2), 337–349.

Rose, M. P., & McGlynn, F. D. (1997). Toward a standard experiment for studying post-treatment return of fear. *Journal of Anxiety Disorders, 11*(3), 263–277.

Rowe, M. K., & Craske, M. G. (1998). Effects of an expanding-spaced vs massed exposure schedule on fear reduction and return of fear. *Behaviour Research and Therapy, 36,* 701–717.

Roy-Byrne, P., Craske, M. G., Stein, M. B., Sullivan, G., Bystritsky, A., Katon, W., et al. (2005). A randomized effectiveness trial of cognitive-behavioral therapy and medication for primary care panic disorder. *Archives of General Psychiatry, 62,* 290–298.

Roy-Byrne, P. P., & Cowley, D. S. (1995). Course and outcome in panic disorder: A review of recent follow-up studies. *Anxiety, 1,* 151–160.

Roy-Byrne, P. P., Craske, M. G., & Stein, M. B. (2006). Panic disorder. *Lancet, 368,* 1023–1032.

Roy-Byrne, P. P., Geraci, M., & Uhde, T. W. (1986). Life events and the onset of panic disorder. *American Journal of Psychiatry, 143,* 1424–1427.

Roy-Byrne, P. P., Mellman, T. A., & Uhde, T. W. (1988). Biologic findings in panic disorder: Neuroendocrine and sleep-related abnormalities [Special issue: Perspectives on panic-related disorders]. *Journal of Anxiety Disorders, 2,* 17–29.

Roy-Byrne, P. P., Stein, M. B., Russo, J., Mercier, E., Thomas, R., McQuaid, J., et al. (1999). Panic disorder in the primary care setting: Comorbidity, disability, service utilization, and treatment. *Journal of Clinical Psychiatry, 60*(7), 492–499.

Rupert, P. A., Dobbins, K., & Mathew, R. J. (1981). EMG biofeedback and relaxation instructions in the treatment of chronic anxiety. *American Journal of Clinical Biofeedback, 4,* 52–61.

Safren, S. A., Gershuny, B. S., Marzol, P., Otto, M. W., & Pollack, M. H. (2002). History of childhood abuse in panic disorder, social phobia, and generalized anxiety disorder. *Journal of Nervous and Mental Disease, 190*(7), 453–456.

Salkovskis, P., Clark, D., & Hackmann, A. (1991). Treatment of panic attacks using cognitive therapy without exposure or breathing retraining. *Behaviour Research and Therapy, 29,* 161–166.

Salkovskis, P., Warwick, H., Clark, D., & Wessels, D. (1986). A demonstration of acute hyperventilation during naturally occurring panic attacks. *Behaviour Research and Therapy, 24,* 91–94.

Salkovskis, P. M. (1991). The importance of behaviour in the maintenance of anxiety and panic: A cognitive account [Special issue: The changing face of behavioural psychotherapy]. *Behavioural Psychotherapy*, 19(1), 6–19.

Salkovskis, P. M., Clark, D. M., & Gelder, M. G. (1996). Cognition–behaviour links in the persistence of panic. *Behaviour Research and Therapy*, 34, 453–458.

Schade, A., Marquenie, L. A., van Balkom, A. J., Koeter, M. W., de Beurs, E., van den Brink, W., et al. (2005). The effectiveness of anxiety treatment on alcohol-dependent patients with a comorbid phobic disorder: A randomized controlled trial. *Alcoholism: Clinical and Experimental Research*, 29(5), 794–800.

Schmidt, N. B., Lerew, D. R., & Jackson, R. J. (1997). The role of anxiety sensitivity in the pathogenesis of panic: Prospective evaluation of spontaneous panic attacks during acute stress. *Journal of Abnormal Psychology*, 106, 355–364.

Schmidt, N. B., Lerew, D. R., & Jackson, R. J. (1999). Prospective evaluation of anxiety sensitivity in the pathogenesis of panic: Replication and extension. *Journal of Abnormal Psychology*, 108, 532–537.

Schmidt, N. B., McCreary, B. T., Trakowski, J. J., Santiago, H. T., Woolaway-Bickel, K., & Ialong, N. (2003). Effects of cognitive behavioral treatment on physical health status in patients with panic disorder. *Behavior Therapy*, 34(1), 49–63.

Schmidt, N. B., Woolaway-Bickel, K., Trakowski, J., Santiago, H., Storey, J., Koselka, M., et al. (2000). Dismantling cognitive-behavioral treatment for panic disorder: Questioning the utility of breathing retraining. *Journal of Consulting and Clinical Psychology*, 68(3), 417–424.

Schneider, A. J., Mataix-Cois, D., Marks, I. M., & Bachofen, M. (2005). Internet-guided self-help with or without exposure therapy for phobic and panic disorders. *Psychotherapy and Psychosomatics*, 74(3), 154–164.

Schumacher, J., Jamra, R. A., Becker, T., Klopp, N., Franke, P., Jacob, C., et al. (2005). Investigation of the DAOA/G30 locus in panic disorder. *Molecular Psychiatry*, 10, 428–429.

Sharp, D. M., Power, K. G., Simpson, R. J., Swanson, V., & Anstee, J. A. (1997). Global measures of outcome in a controlled comparison of pharmacological and psychological treatment of panic disorder and agoraphobia in primary care. *British Journal of General Practice*, 47, 150–155.

Sharp, D. M., Power, K. G., & Swanson, V. (2004). A comparison of the efficacy and acceptability of group versus individual cognitive behaviour therapy in the treatment of panic disorder and agoraphobia in primary care. *Clinical Psychology and Psychotherapy*, 11(2), 73–82.

Shear, M. K., & Schulberg, H. C. (1995). Anxiety disorders in primary care. *Bulletin of the Menninger Clinic*, 59(2, Suppl. A), A73–A85.

Shulman, I. D., Cox, B. J., Swinson, R. P., Kuch, K., & Reichman, J. T. (1994). Precipitating events, locations and reactions associated with initial unexpected panic attacks. *Behaviour Research and Therapy*, 32, 17–20.

Siddle, D. A., & Bond, N. W. (1988). Avoidance learning, Pavlovian conditioning, and the development of phobias. *Biological Psychology*, 27, 167–183.

Sloan, T., & Telch, M. J. (2002). The effects of safety-seeking behavior and guided threat reappraisal on fear reduction during exposure: An experimental investigation. *Behaviour Research and Therapy*, 40(3), 235–251.

Sokolowska, M., Siegel, S., & Kim, J. A. (2002). Intraadministration associations: Conditional hyperalgesia elicited by morphine onset cues. *Journal of Experimental Psychology: Animal Behavior Processes*, 28(3), 309–320.

Spanier, G. (1976). Measuring dyadic adjustment: New scales for assessing the quality of marriage and similar dyads. *Journal of Marriage and the Family*, 38, 15–38.

Spiegel, D. A., Bruce, T. J., Gregg, S. F., & Nuzzarello, A. (1994). Does cognitive behavior therapy assist slow-taper alprazolam discontinuation in panic disorder? *American Journal of Psychiatry*, 151(6), 876–881.

Spielberger, C. D., Gorsuch, R. L., Lushene, R., Vagg, P. R., & Jacobs, G. A. (1983). *Manual for the State–Trait Anxiety Inventory (STAI, Form Y)*. Palo Alto, CA: Consulting Psychologists Press.

Stanley, M. A., Beck, J. G., Averill, P. M., Baldwin, L. E., Deagle, E. A., & Stadler, J. G. (1996). Patterns of change during cognitive behavioral treatment for panic disorder. *Journal of Nervous and Mental Disease*, 184, 567–572.

Stein, M. B., Walker, J. R., Anderson, G., Hazen, A. L., Ross, C. A., Eldridge, G., et al. (1996). Childhood physical and sexual abuse in patients with anxiety disorders and a community sample. *American Journal of Psychiatry*, 153, 275–277.

Sturges, L. V., Goetsch, V. L., Ridley, J., & Whittal, M. (1998). Anxiety sensitivity and response to hyperventilation challenge: Physiologic arousal, interoceptive acuity, and subjective distress. *Journal of Anxiety Disorders*, 12(2), 103–115.

Suárez, L., Bennett, S., Goldstein, C., & Barlow, D. H. (in press). Understanding anxiety disorders from a "triple vulnerabilities" framework. In M. M. Anthony & M. B. Stein (Eds.). *Oxford handbook of anxiety and related disorders*. New York: Oxford University Press.

Swinson, R. P., Fergus, K. D., Cox, B. J., & Wickwire, K. (1995). Efficacy of telephone-administered behavioral therapy for panic disorder with agoraphobia. *Behaviour Research and Therapy*, 33, 465–469.

Taylor, S., Koch, W. J., & McNally, R. J. (1992). How does anxiety sensitivity vary across the anxiety disorders? *Journal of Anxiety Disorders*, 6, 249–259.

Telch, M. J., Brouillard, M., Telch, C. F., Agras, W. S., & Taylor, C. B. (1989). Role of cognitive appraisal in panic-related avoidance. *Behaviour Research and Therapy, 27,* 373–383.

Telch, M. J., Lucas, J. A., & Nelson, P. (1989). Nonclinical panic in college students: An investigation of prevalence and symptomatology. *Journal of Abnormal Psychology, 98,* 300–306.

Telch, M. J., Lucas, J. A., Schmidt, N. B., Hanna, H. H., LaNae, Jaimez, T., et al. (1993). Group cognitive-behavioral treatment of panic disorder. *Behaviour Research and Therapy, 31,* 279–287.

Telch, M. J., Sherman, M., & Lucas, J. (1989). Anxiety sensitivity: Unitary personality trait or domain specific appraisals? *Journal of Anxiety Disorders, 3,* 25–32.

Thorgeirsson, T. E., Oskarsson, H., Desnica, N., Kostic, J. P., Stefansson, J. G., Kolbeinsson, H., et al. (2003). Anxiety with panic disorder linked to chromosome 9q in Iceland. *American Journal of Human Genetics, 72,* 1221–1230.

Thyer, B. A., Himle, J., Curtis, G. C., Cameron, O. G., & Nesse, R. M. (1985). A comparison of panic disorder and agoraphobia with panic attacks. *Comprehensive Psychiatry, 26,* 208–214.

Tiemens, B. G., Ormel, J., & Simon, G. E. (1996). Occurrence, recognition, and outcome of psychological disorders in primary care. *American Journal of Psychiatry, 153,* 636–644.

Tsao, J. C. I., Lewin, M. R., & Craske, M. G. (1998). The effects of cognitive-behavior therapy for panic disorder on comorbid conditions. *Journal of Anxiety Disorders, 12,* 357–371.

Tsao, J. C. I., Mystkowski, J. L., Zucker, B. G., & Craske, M. G. (2002). Effects of cognitive-behavioral therapy for panic disorder on comorbid conditions: replication and extension. *Behavior Therapy, 33,* 493–509.

Tsao, J. C. I., Mystkowski, J. L., Zucker, B. G., & Craske, M. G. (2005). Impact of cognitive-behavioral therapy for panic disorder on comorbidity: A controlled investigation. *Behaviour Research and Therapy, 43,* 959–970.

Uhde, T. W. (1994). The anxiety disorders: Phenomenology and treatment of core symptoms and associated sleep disturbance. In M. Kryger, T. Roth, & W. Dement (Eds.), *Principles and practice of sleep medicine* (pp. 871–898). Philadelphia: Saunders.

van Balkom, A. J., de Beurs, E., Koele, P., Lange, A., & van Dyck, R. (1996). Long-term benzodiazepine use is associated with smaller treatment gain in panic disorder with agoraphobia. *Journal of Nervous and Mental Disease, 184,* 133–135.

van Beek, N., Schruers, K. R. J., & Friez, E. J. L. (2005). Prevalence of respiratory disorders in first-degree relatives of panic disorder patients. *Journal of Affective Disorders, 87,* 337–340.

van den Hout, M., Arntz, A., & Hoekstra, R. (1994). Exposure reduced agoraphobia but not panic, and cognitive therapy reduced panic but not agoraphobia. *Behaviour Research and Therapy, 32,* 447–451.

van den Hout, M., Brouwers, C., & Oomen, J. (2006). Clinically diagnosed Axis II co-morbidity and the short term outcome of CBT for Axis I disorders. *Clinical Psychology and Psychotherapy, 13*(1), 56–63.

van Megen, H. J., Westenberg, H. G., Den Boer, J. A., & Kahn, R. S. (1996). The panic-inducing properties of the cholecystokinin tetrapeptide CCK4 in patients with panic disorder. *European Neuropsychopharmacology, 6,* 187–94.

Vansteenwegen, D., Vervliet, B., Iberico, C., Baeyens, F., van den Bergh, O., & Hermans, D. (2007). The repeated confrontation with videotapes of spiders in multiple contexts attenuates renewal of fear in spider-anxious students. *Behavior Research and Therapy, 45*(6), 1169–1179.

Veltman, D. J., van Zijderveld, G., Tilders, F. J., & van Dyck, R. (1996). Epinephrine and fear of bodily sensations in panic disorder and social phobia. *Journal of Psychopharmacology, 10*(4), 259–265.

Verburg, K., Griez, E., Meijer, J., & Pols, H. (1995). Respiratory disorders as a possible predisposing factor for panic disorder. *Journal of Affective Disorders, 33,* 129–134.

Wade, W. A., Treat, T. A., & Stuart, G. L. (1998). Transporting an empirically supported treatment for panic disorder to a service clinic setting: A benchmarking strategy. *Journal of Consulting and Clinical Psychology, 66,* 231–239.

Wardle, J., Hayward, P., Higgitt, A., Stabl, M., Blizard, R., & Gray, J. (1994). Effects of concurrent diazepam treatment on the outcome of exposure therapy in agoraphobia. *Behaviour Research and Therapy, 32,* 203–215.

Watson, D., & Clark, L. A. (1984). Negative affectivity: The disposition to experience aversive emotional states. *Psychological Bulletin, 96*(3), 465–490.

Weems, C. F., Hayward, C., Killen, J., & Taylor, C. B. (2002). A longitudinal investigation of anxiety sensitivity in adolescence. *Journal of Abnormal Psychology, 111*(3), 471–477.

Welkowitz, L., Papp, L., Cloitre, M., Liebowitz, M., Martin, L., & Gorman, J. (1991). Cognitive-behavior therapy for panic disorder delivered by psychopharmacologically oriented clinicians. *Journal of Nervous and Mental Disease, 179,* 473–477.

Westen, D., & Morrison, K. (2001). A multidimensional meta-analysis of treatments for depression, panic, and generalized anxiety disorder: An empirical examination of the status of empirically supported therapies. *Journal of Consulting and Clinical Psychology, 69*(6), 875–899.

Westra, H. A., Stewart, S. H., & Conrad, B. E. (2002). Naturalistic manner of benzodiazepine use and cognitive behavioral therapy outcome in panic disorder and agoraphobia. *Journal of Anxiety Disorders, 16*(3), 223–246.

Wilkinson, D. J., Thompson, J. M., Lambert, G. W., Jennings, G. L., Schwarz, R. G., Jefferys, D., et al.

(1998). Sympathetic activity in patients with panic disorder at rest, under laboratory mental stress, and during panic attacks. *Archives of General Psychiatry, 55*(6), 511–520.

Williams, K. E., & Chambless, D. (1990). The relationship between therapist characteristics and outcome of *in vivo* exposure treatment for agoraphobia. *Behavior Therapy, 21,* 111–116.

Williams, K. E., & Chambless, D. L. (1994). The results of exposure-based treatment in agoraphobia. In S. Friedman (Ed.), *Anxiety disorders in African Americans* (pp. 149–165). New York: Springer.

Williams, S. L. (1992). Perceived self-efficacy and phobic disability. In R. Schwarzer (Ed.), *Self-efficacy: Thought control of action* (pp. 149–176). Washington, DC: Hemisphere.

Williams, S. L., & Falbo, J. (1996). Cognitive and performance-based treatments for panic attacks in people with varying degrees of agoraphobic disability. *Behaviour Research and Therapy, 34,* 253–264.

Williams, S. L., & Zane, G. (1989). Guided mastery and stimulus exposure treatments for severe performance anxiety in agoraphobics. *Behaviour Research and Therapy, 27,* 237–245.

Wittchen, H.-U., Reed, V., & Kessler, R. C. (1998). The relationship of agoraphobia and panic in a community sample of adolescents and young adults. *Archives of General Psychiatry, 55*(11), 1017–1024.

Zinbarg, R. E., & Barlow, D. H. (1996). Structure of anxiety and the anxiety disorders: A hierarchical model. *Journal of Abnormal Psychology, 105*(2), 184–193.

Zinbarg, R. E., Barlow, D. H., & Brown, T. A. (1997). Hierarchical structure and general factor saturation of the Anxiety Sensitivity Index: Evidence and implication. *Psychological Assessment, 9,* 277–284.

Zoellner, L. A., & Craske, M. G. (1999). Interoceptive accuracy and panic. *Behaviour Research and Therapy, 37,* 1141–1158.

CHAPTER 2

Posttraumatic Stress Disorder

PATRICIA A. RESICK
CANDICE M. MONSON
SHIREEN L. RIZVI

Severe, unexpected trauma may occur in less than a minute but have lifelong consequences. The tragedy that is post traumatic stress disorder (PTSD) is brought into stark relief when the origins of the trauma occur in the context of man's inhumanity to man. In this chapter, the case of "Tom" illustrates the psychopathology associated with PTSD in all its nuances and provides a very personal account of its impact. In one of any number of events summarized dryly every day in the middle pages of the newspaper, Tom, in the fog of war in Iraq, shoots and kills a pregnant woman and her young child in the presence of the husband and father. The impact of this event devastates him. The sensitive and skilled therapeutic intervention described in this chapter is a model for new therapists, and belies the notion that, in these severe cases, manualized therapy can be rote and automated. In addition, the next generation of treatment for PTSD, termed "cognitive processing therapy" by the authors, is sufficiently detailed to allow knowledgeable practitioners to incorporate this treatment program into their practice. This comprehensive treatment program takes advantage of the latest developments in our knowledge of the psychopathology of trauma impact by incorporating treatment strategies specifically tailored to overcome trauma-related psychopathology.—D. H. B.

DIAGNOSIS

Unlike most other psychiatric diagnoses, posttraumatic stress disorder (PTSD) requires a specific type of event to occur from which the person affected does not recover. First, to qualify for a diagnosis of PTSD according to the *Diagnostic and Statistical Manual of Mental Disorders*, fourth edition (DSM-IV; American Psychiatric Association, 1994), the individual must have experienced, witnessed, or otherwise been confronted with an event that involved actual or threatened death, serious injury, or threat to physical integrity. Second, the individual's response to the event must include intense fear, helplessness, or horror. Thus, an event is defined as traumatic when it has involved death or serious injury, or the threat of death or injury, and the individual experiences strong negative affect in response to the event (criterion A). Symptom criteria fall into three broad categories: reexperiencing symptoms (criterion B), avoidance and numbing symptoms (criterion C), and physiological hyperarousal (criterion D). According to criterion B, the reexperiencing symptoms must be experienced in one of the following ways: Memories of the trauma may intrude into consciousness repetitively, without warning, seemingly "out of the blue," without triggers or reminders to elicit them. The person with PTSD may experience intensely vivid reenactment experiences, or flashbacks. Intrusive memories may also occur during the sleeping state in the form of thematically related nightmares. Additionally, when faced with cues associated with the traumatic event, whether actual or symbolic, the individual may exhibit intense psychological reactions (e.g., terror, disgust, depression) and/or physiological responses (e.g., increased heart rate, perspiration, and rapid breathing).

These reexperiencing symptoms are generally experienced as distressing and intrusive, because the individual has no control over when or how they occur, and they elicit strong negative emotions associated with the initial trauma (Janoff-Bulman, 1992; Resick & Schnicke, 1992). Fear stimuli (cues) are sometimes obvious, such as the combat veteran who ducks in fear when a car backfires because it sounds like gunfire. However, sometimes the relationship between the trauma and the cue is not immediately clear. For example, one survivor of rape was fearful of taking showers, even though the rape had occurred away from her home. However, as she began to deal with the rape in treatment, she realized that every time she took a shower, she felt very vulnerable because she was alone, naked, had no escape routes, and had diminished vision and hearing—all stimuli that reminded her of the rape.

Avoidance and numbing symptoms (criterion C) reflect the individual's attempt to gain psychological and emotional distance from the trauma. Some have suggested that avoidance symptoms are a response to reexperiencing symptoms (Creamer, Burgess, & Pattison, 1992), although some factor-analytic studies of PTSD symptoms suggest that effortful avoidance is more strongly associated with reexperiencing symptoms, whereas numbing is associated with high arousal symptoms (Buckley, Blanchard, & Hickling, 1998; Taylor, Kuch, Koch, Crockett, & Passey, 1998). As traumatic memories intrude into consciousness, so do the painful negative emotions associated with the original trauma. Thus, the individual may avoid thoughts and feelings about the trauma, avoid situations and events reminiscent of the trauma, or may actually forget significant aspects of the trauma. Avoidance of the trauma memory leads to a temporary decrease in pain-

ful emotions, which increases avoidance behavior. Similarly, detachment or numbing symptoms are an attempt to cut off the aversive feelings associated with intrusive memories (Astin, Layne, Camilleri, & Foy, 1994; Resick & Schnicke, 1992). This detachment may then generalize to all emotions, both positive and negative. Trauma survivors commonly state that they no longer have any strong feelings, or that they feel numb a great deal of the time. This sort of pervasive detachment may interfere profoundly with the individual's ability to relate to others, enjoy daily life, remain productive, and plan for the future. Trauma survivors have frequently reported highly constricted lifestyles after the traumatic experience due to the need to avoid reminders of the traumatic memory and associated emotions. At least three types of avoidance behavior are required before diagnosis can be made.

The trauma survivor may also experience symptoms of increased physiological arousal (criterion D). This suggests that the individual is in a constant state of "fight or flight," which is similar to how the individual's body responded during the actual traumatic event. In this state of alert, the individual is primed to react to new threats of danger, even in relatively "safe" situations. During a crisis, this is adaptive because it facilitates survival. However, as a steady state, hyperarousal interferes with daily functioning and leads to exhaustion. In this state, the individual spends a great deal of energy scanning the environment for danger cues (hypervigilance). The individual is likely to experience sleep disturbance, decreased concentration, irritability, and an overreactivity to stimuli (exaggerated startle response). There is evidence to suggest that this constant state of tension has deleterious effects on overall physical health (e.g., Kulka et al., 1990). At least two of the criterion D behaviors must be present for a diagnosis of PTSD.

The previously described symptom criteria must be met concurrently for at least 1 month to receive a diagnosis of PTSD, and the symptoms must be perceived as distressing or cause functional impairment. A substantial proportion of trauma survivors exhibit symptoms consistent with a PTSD diagnosis immediately after the traumatic event. However, these rates drop almost in half within 3 months posttrauma, then tend to stabilize. For example, rape trauma survivors assessed at 2 weeks, 1 month, 3 months, 6 months, and 9 months exhibited

PTSD diagnostic rates of 94, 65, 47, 42, and 42%, respectively (Rothbaum & Foa, 1993). Thus, after 3 months, PTSD rates did not drop substantially. Another study that assessed survivors of rape trauma at approximately 2-weeks and at 3-months postcrime found very similar rates of PTSD (Gutner, Rizvi, Monson, & Resick, 2006). At the first time point, 81% of the rape trauma survivors met symptom criteria for PTSD (minus the time criterion), and at 3-months postrape, 53% continued to meet the criteria. Other, more heterogeneous events (greater variability in the severity of the event), such as combat, disasters, or assaults, are associated with lower rates of PTSD than rape (Kessler, Sonnega, Bromet, Hughes, & Nelson, 1995). Delayed onset of PTSD is rare and may reflect earlier subthreshold symptoms (perhaps due to dissociation, amnesia, or extensive avoidance) or a change in the meaning of the event at a later time (the perpetrator kills a later victim, thereby changing the meaning of the event for the survivor).

In the dozen years that have passed since these criteria were last reviewed, an expanding body of research has questioned this diagnostic structure, as well as specific items included in the current nosology. For example, at least seven factor-analytic studies have been conducted (e.g., Amdur & Liberzon, 2001; Asmundson et al., 2000; Buckley et al., 1998; King, Leskin, King, & Weathers, 1998; Simms, Watson, & Doebbeling, 2002; Smith, Redd, DuHamel, Vicksberg, & Ricketts, 1999; Taylor et al., 1998), and none have found the three-factor structure that comprises the current diagnosis. Most typically, researchers have found either four or two factors. The four-factor solution separates effortful avoidance from numbing. The two-factor solutions pair numbing with arousal and intrusions with avoidance. At the item level, intrusions have been found to be largely sensory, particularly visual images, and distinct from cognitions (Ehlers et al., 2002). The merger of images and thoughts into one symptom item is probably a misrepresentation of both the clinical phenomenology, and brain structure and functioning (Shin, Rauch, & Pitman, 2005). An increasing body of literature has implicated guilt and shame in the development and maintenance of PTSD (Andrews, Brewin, Rose, & Kirk, 2000; Beckham, Feldman, & Kirby, 1998; Glover, Pelesky, Bruno, & Sette, 1990; Henning & Frueh, 1997; Kubany et al., 1995; Kubany, Haynes, Abueg, & Manke, 1996; Leskela, Dieperink, & Thuras, 2002; Wong & Cook, 1992), yet the diagnostic criteria do not include anything about guilt or shame.

PREVALENCE

Epidemiological studies have demonstrated high rates of trauma exposure and PTSD in the population (Kessler et al., 1995; Kilpatrick, Saunders, Veronen, Best, & Von, 1987; Kulka et al., 1990). In a national (U.S.) random probability sample of 4,008 women, Resnick, Kilpatrick, Dansky, Saunders, and Best (1993) found a very high rate of trauma experiences (69%). When they extrapolated their results to the U.S. population based on census statistics for 1989, they estimated that 66 million women in the U.S. had experienced at least one major traumatic event. Of those who had experienced a criterion A stressor, Resnick and colleagues found the following lifetime PTSD rates: completed rape, 32%; other sexual assault, 31%; physical assault, 39%; homicide of family or friend, 22%; any crime victimization, 26%; noncrime trauma (e.g., natural and man-made disasters, accidents, injuries), 9%.

In the first large national civilian prevalence study of the psychological effects of trauma, Kessler and colleagues (1995) surveyed a representative U.S. national sample of 5,877 persons (2,812 men and 3,065 women). This study, which included both men and women, assessed 12 categories of traumatic stressors. They found that a majority of people had experienced at least one major traumatic event. They found that, whereas 20.4% women and 8.2% of men were likely to develop PTSD following exposure to trauma, the rates for specific traumas were often much higher. For example, rape was identified as the trauma most likely to lead to PTSD among men, as well as women, and 65% of men and 46% of women who identified rape as their worst trauma developed PTSD. Among men who identified other worst traumas, the probability of developing PTSD was 39% of those with combat exposure, 24% with childhood neglect, and 22% who had experienced childhood physical abuse. Among women, aside from rape PTSD was likely to be associated with physical abuse in childhood (49%), threat with a weapon (33%), sexual molestation (27%), and physical attack (21%). As with the Resnick and colleagues (1993) study, accidents and natural disasters were much less likely to precipitate PTSD among men and women. On the other hand, Norris (1992) has pointed out although motor vehicle accidents (MVAs) are less frequent than some traumas (e.g., tragic death or robbery), and less traumatic than some events (sexual and physical assault), when both frequency and impact are considered together, MVAs may be the single most significant event. The lifetime frequency of MVAs is 23%, and the PTSD rate is 12%, which results in a rate of 28 seriously distressed people for every 1,000 adults in the United States, just from one type of event.

More recently, Kessler and his colleagues (Kessler, Berglund, et al., 2005; Kessler, Chiu, et al., 2005), reported on another large National Comorbidity Survey with over 9,200 respondents. The overall prevalence of PTSD was 6.8% in this study that included people who had not experienced trauma. This compares to 7.8% population prevalence reported in the 1995 study (Kessler et al., 1995).

The largest study of combat veterans, the National Vietnam Veterans Readjustment Study (NVVRS; Kulka et al., 1990), was mandated by the U.S. Congress in 1983 to assess PTSD and other psychological problems following the Vietnam war. During the years of the war, over 8 million people served in the U.S. military. Of those, 3.1 million served in Vietnam (theater veterans) and the remainder served in other areas abroad or in the United States (era veterans). Women comprised 7,200 of those serving in Vietnam, and over 255,000 of those serving elsewhere during the Vietnam era. The NVVRS conducted in-depth interviews and assessments with three groups: 1,632 Vietnam theater veterans, 716 Vietnam era veterans, and 668 nonveterans/civilian counterparts, for a total of 3,016 participants.

The results of the NVVRS indicated that the majority of Vietnam theater veterans made a successful readjustment to civilian life and did not suffer from PTSD or other problems. However, the researchers also found that 31% of male and 27% of female veterans had a full diagnosis of PTSD at some time during their lives. Furthermore, 15% of male and 9% of female veterans had PTSD at the time of the study, over a decade after the end of the war. These rates translated to 479,000 Vietnam veterans with current PTSD. In addition, 11% of male and 8% of female veterans were found to have significant symptoms and distress but did

not meet the full criteria for PTSD. This translated to an additional 350,000 men and women in the United States alone who were still suffering in the aftermath of the Vietnam war.

Recently the data from the NVVRS were reevaluated using very strict criteria that only included those incidents that could be verified through historical records. Dohrenwend and colleagues (2006) found very little falsification of events and a strong relationship between the amount of trauma exposure and rates of PTSD (i.e., the dose–response relationship). They did, however, find lower rates of PTSD after controlling for people who developed PTSD before or after their deployment to Vietnam and eliminating those people with unverifiable events. Using these stricter criteria, they found that 18.7% of the veterans met the criteria for war-related PTSD at some point, and 9.1% still had PTSD when assessed 11–12 years later. These rates should be considered minimum likelihood rates given that people can be traumatized by events that may not be verifiable (e.g., rape, accidents) in historical accounts of the war.

Also recent, with the wars in Iraq and Afghanistan, are the first attempts to assess PTSD *during* a war (Hoge et al., 2004; Hoge, Auchterlonie, & Milliken, 2006). In the first study, Hoge and his colleagues (2004) studied 2,530 Army soldiers and Marines before and 3,671 after deployment to Iraq or Afghanistan. They found that mental heath problems were significantly greater among those who had returned from deployment than those who had not yet deployed, and that mental health problems were greater in those who deployed to Iraq compared with Afghanistan. Prior to deployment, 9% of the service personnel exceeded the cutoff used for likely PTSD, whereas 11.5% of those deployed to Afghanistan and 18–20% of those deployed to Iraq exceeded the cutoff. There was a linear relationship between the number of firefights reported and the severity of PTSD. Being wounded or otherwise physically injured was also associated with greater PTSD symptomatology.

Because the military began screening all military personnel for PTSD following deployment, the second study was actually a population-based study for a 1-year period (May 2003 to April 2004) of 303,905 Army soldiers and Marines who deployed to Afghanistan, Iraq, or other locations (Hoge et al., 2006). As with the previous report, service men and women were more likely to report mental health problems (19.1%) after serving in Iraq than in Afghanistan (11.3%) or other locations (8.5%). In this study 32,500 women were also assessed, comprising 10.7% of the total sample. There was an overall gender difference in mental health concerns, with 23.6% of women reporting a mental health concern compared with 18.6% of men. However, this gender comparison did not take into account preexisting traumas or PTSD, exposure to combat traumas or sexual assault, or other variables that might be used to explain these differences. Also, the PTSD screen was a four-item questionnaire for which two yes answers indicated possible PTSD. On this screen 9.8% of those who had served in Iraq indicated possible PTSD, and there was again an association between the amount of combat exposure and PTSD.

THEORETICAL MODELS OF PTSD

As researchers and behavioral therapists began to study and treat survivors of rape trauma and Vietnam veterans in the 1970s, they began to draw upon learning theory as an explanation for the symptoms they were observing. Mowrer's two-factor theory (1947) of classical and operant conditioning was first proposed to account for posttrauma symptoms (Becker, Skinner, Abel, Axelrod, & Cichon, 1984; Holmes & St. Lawrence, 1983; Keane, Zimering, & Caddell, 1985; Kilpatrick, Veronen, & Best, 1985; Kilpatrick, Veronen, & Resick, 1982). Classical conditioning was used to explain the high levels of distress and fear that were observed in trauma victims in reaction to trauma-related stimuli. Operant conditioning explained the development of PTSD avoidance symptoms and maintenance of fear over time, despite the fact that the unconditioned stimulus, the traumatic stressor, does not recur. Because the trauma memory and other cues (conditioned stimuli) elicit fear and anxiety (conditioned emotional responses), these cues are avoided (or escaped from), and the result is a reduction in fear and anxiety. In this manner, avoidance of the conditioned stimuli is negatively reinforced, which prevents extinction of the link between the trauma cues and anxiety, which would normally be expected without repetition of the trauma itself. Although learning theory accounts for much of the development and maintenance of the

fear and avoidance in PTSD, it does not fully explain intrusion symptoms (i.e., the repetitive memories of the trauma that intrude into the survivors' thoughts in both conscious and unconscious states such as nightmares). Based on Lang's (1977) information processing theory of anxiety development, Foa, Steketee, and Rothbaum (1989) suggested that PTSD emerges due to the development of a fear network in memory that elicits escape and avoidance behavior. Mental fear structures include stimuli, response, and meaning elements. Anything associated with the trauma may elicit the fear structure or schema and subsequent avoidance behavior. The fear network in people with PTSD is thought to be stable and broadly generalized, so that it is easily accessed. Chemtob, Roitblat, Hamada, Carlson, and Twentyman (1988) proposed that these structures are always at least weakly activated in individuals with PTSD and guide their interpretation of events as potentially dangerous. When the fear network is activated by reminders of the trauma, the information in the network enters consciousness (intrusive symptoms). Attempts to avoid this activation result in the avoidance symptoms of PTSD. According to information processing theory, repetitive exposure to the traumatic memory in a safe environment results in habituation of the fear and subsequent change in the fear structure. As emotion decreases, clients with PTSD begin to modify their meaning elements spontaneously, and change their self-statements and reduce their generalization.

Social-cognitive theories are also concerned with information processing, but they focus on the impact of trauma on a person's belief system and the adjustments that are necessary to reconcile a traumatic event with prior beliefs and expectations. The first and most influential social-cognitive theorist was Horowitz, who moved from a more psychodynamic to a cognitive processing theory. Horowitz (1986) proposed that processing is driven by a "completion tendency," the psychological need for new, incompatible information to be integrated with existing beliefs. The completion tendency keeps the trauma information in active memory until the processing is complete and the event is resolved. Horowitz also theorized that there is a basic conflict between the need to resolve and reconcile the event into the person's history, and the desire to avoid emotional pain. When the images of the event (flashbacks, nightmares, intrusive recollections), thoughts about the meanings of the trauma, and emotions associated with the trauma become overwhelming, psychological defense mechanisms take over, and the person exhibits numbing or avoidance. Horowitz suggested that a person with PTSD oscillates between phases of intrusion and avoidance, and that if successfully processed, the oscillations become less frequent and less intense. Chronic PTSD would mean that the event stays in active memory without becoming fully integrated; therefore, it is still able to stimulate intrusive and avoidant reactions.

Several other social-cognitive researchers and theorists have focused more on the actual content of the cognitions in PTSD, and propose that basic assumptions about the world and oneself are "shattered." Constructivist theories are based on the idea that people actively create their own internal representations of the world (and themselves). New experiences are assigned meaning based on a person's model of the world (Janoff-Bulman, 1985, 1992; Mahoney & Lyddon, 1988; McCann & Pearlman, 1990). The task for recovery is to reconstruct fundamental beliefs and establish equilibrium. Janoff-Bulman (1985) suggested that this process is accomplished by reinterpreting the event to reduce the distance between the prior beliefs and the new beliefs. Other theorists have proposed that if one's preexisting beliefs are particularly positive or particularly negative, then more severe PTSD symptoms result (Foa, 1996; McCann & Pearlman, 1990; Resick & Schnicke, 1992). Foa (1996) focused particularly on beliefs regarding the predictability and controllability of the trauma, whereas McCann and Pearlman (1990) proposed that several areas of cognition might be either disrupted or seemingly confirmed, that is, beliefs regarding safety, trust, control/power, esteem, and intimacy.

Resick and Schnicke (1992, 1993) have argued that posttrauma affect is not limited to fear, and that individuals with PTSD may be just as likely to experience a range of other strong emotions, such as shame, anger, or sadness. Emotions such as fear, anger, or sadness may emanate directly from the trauma (primary emotions), because the event is interpreted as dangerous and/or abusive, and results in losses. It is possible that secondary, or manufactured, emotions can also result from faulty interpretations made by the trauma survivor.

For example, if someone is intentionally attacked by another person, the danger of the situation would lead to a fight–flight response, and the attending emotions might be anger or fear (primary). However, if in the aftermath, a person blamed him- or herself for the attack, that person might experience shame or embarrassment. These manufactured emotions would have resulted from thoughts and interpretations about the event rather than from the event itself.

In a social-cognitive model, affective expression is needed, not for habituation, but for the trauma memory to be processed fully. It is assumed that the natural affect, once accessed, dissipates rather quickly, and that the work of accommodating the memory with beliefs can begin. Once faulty beliefs regarding the event (self-blame, guilt) and overgeneralized beliefs about oneself and the world (e.g., safety, trust, control, esteem, intimacy) are challenged, then the secondary emotions also vanish, along with the intrusive reminders. The fact that both stress inoculation training without trauma exposure exercises (Foa, Rothbaum, Riggs, & Murdock, 1991; Foa et al., 1999) and cognitive therapy (e.g., Ehlers et al., 2003; Tarrier et al., 1999) are effective treatments for PTSD undermines the assumption that habituation or extinction is the sole mechanism of change.

Ehlers and Clark (2000) proposed a cognitive model of PTSD that focuses on threat and memory. Although the event has occurred in the past, Ehlers and Clark propose that the people with PTSD are unable to see the event as time-limited and assume that it has larger implications for the future. Individuals with PTSD appraise the event such that they believe themselves to be currently at risk. There are several ways in which this misappraisal happens. One is to overgeneralize based on the event and begin to assume that normal activities are more dangerous than they actually are. They may overestimate the probability that the event will recur. After the trauma happens, people may misconstrue the meaning of their PTSD symptoms such that they perceive themselves to be in greater danger (false alarms are assumed to be true alarms) or interpret their symptoms to mean that they cannot cope with events in the future.

Ehlers and Clark's (2000) cognitive theory also considers the apparent memory disturbance that occurs with PTSD such that persons with PTSD may have trouble intentionally accessing their memory of the event but have involuntary intrusions of parts of the event. They propose that because memory encoded at the time of the trauma is poorly elaborated and integrated with other memories with regard to details, context of time, sequence, and so forth, this might explain why people with PTSD may have poor autobiographical memory, yet may be triggered to have memory fragments that have a here-and-now quality (no time context) or lack appropriate posttrauma appraisals (e.g., "I did not die"). Like the emotional processing models, Ehlers and Clark also propose that strong associative learning is paired with fear responses and may become generalized. In response to the perceptions of threat, people with PTSD adopt various maladaptive coping strategies, depending on their appraisals. For example, people who believe they will go crazy if they think about the traumatic event try to avoid thoughts about the trauma and keep their minds occupied all of the time. Someone who believes that he or she must figure out why the traumatic event happened to keep it from happening again will ruminate about how it could have been prevented. Those who think that they were being punished for their actions may become immobilized and unable to make decisions. These maladaptive strategies, most often avoidance behaviors, may (1) increase symptoms, (2) prevent change in negative appraisals, or (3) prevent change in the trauma memory.

In an attempt to reconcile the theories of PTSD, Brewin, Dalgleish, and Joseph (1996) proposed a dual-representation theory that incorporates both information processing and social-cognitive theories, and introduces research and theory from cognitive science with regard to memory. Brewin and colleagues have suggested that the concept of a single emotional memory is too narrow to describe the full range of memory that has been evident in research and clinical observations. Based on prior research, they proposed that sensory input is subject to both conscious and nonconscious processing. The memories that are conscious can be deliberately retrieved and are termed "verbally accessible memories" (VAMs). VAMs contain some sensory information, information about emotional and physical reactions, and the personal meaning of the event. Although VAMs might be reasonably detailed, they may also be very selective, because attention is narrowed under conditions of stress, and short-term memory capacity may be decreased.

The other type of memory is theorized to be nonconsious and are termed "situationally accessed memories" (SAMs). This type of information, which is probably much more extensive than the autobiographical memories of the event, cannot be accessed deliberately and is not as easily altered or edited as the more explicitly accessed VAMs. SAMs comprise sensory (e.g., auditory, visual, tactile), physiological, and motoric information that may be accessed automatically when a person is exposed to a stimulus situation similar in some fashion to the trauma, or when that person consciously thinks about the trauma. The SAM is then experienced as an intrusive sensory image or flashback accompanied by physiological arousal.

Dual representation theory posits two types of emotional reactions: One is conditioned during the event (e.g., fear, anger), recorded in the SAMs, and activated along with reexperienced sensory and physiological information. The other type, secondary emotions, result from the consequences and implications (meaning) of the trauma. These secondary emotions may include not only fear and anger but also guilt, shame, and sadness.

Brewin and colleagues (1996) proposed that emotional processing of the trauma has two elements. One element of the processing is the activation of SAMS (as suggested by information processing theories), the purpose of which is to aid in cognitive readjustment by supplying the detailed sensory and physiological information concerning the trauma. The activation of SAMs may eventually diminish in frequency when they are blocked by the creation of new SAMs, or when they are altered by the incorporation of new information. When the SAMs are brought into consciousness, they can be altered by being paired with different bodily states (e.g., relaxation or habituation) or different conscious thoughts. Eventually, if the SAMs are replaced or altered sufficiently, there is a reduction in negative emotions and a subsequent reduction in attentional bias and accessibility of the memory.

The second element (as proposed by the social-cognitive theorists) is the conscious attempt to search for meaning, to ascribe cause or blame, and to resolve conflicts between the event and prior expectations and beliefs. The goal of this process is to reduce the negative emotions and to restore a sense of relative safety and control in one's environment. To obtain this second goal, the traumatized person may have to edit his or her autobiographical memory (VAMs) to reconcile conflicts between the event and the person's belief system. The traumatized person may either alter the memory of the event in some way to reestablish the preexisting belief system or alter preexisting beliefs and expectations to accommodate this new information.

Brewin and colleagues (1996) suggested that for cases in which the emotions are primary and driven by SAMs, exposure therapy may be all that is needed. However, when secondary emotions are present, when clients are reporting self-blame, guilt, or shame and consequent depression, cognitive therapy may be needed. Although both exposure and cognitive therapies have been found to be effective in treating PTSD, no research thus far has matched types of therapy to client profiles.

Another multirepresentational cognitive model called SPAARS (Dalgleish, 2004) was originally proposed to explain everyday emotional experience and was then applied to PTSD. This model also endeavors to encompass the previous theories. The model proposes four types or levels of mental representation systems: the Schematic, Propositional, Analogue, and Associative Representational Systems. The schematic level represents abstract generic information, or schemas. Propositional-level information is verbally accessible meanings, similar to VAMs, whereas information at the analogue level is stored as "images" across all types of sensory systems, similar to SAMs. Associative representations are similar to the fear structures hypothesized in emotional processing theory as representing the connections between other types of representations. In the SPAARS model, emotions are generated through two routes. One, similar to the Ehlers and Clark (2000) cognitive model, is through appraisals at the schematic level, in which events are compared against important goals. A person appraises an event to be threatening if it blocks an important goal, then experiences fear. Because traumatic events are threats to survival, they are appraised as threatening and elicit fear. The second route to emotion is through associative learning, which is automatic and similar to the fear activation described by Foa and her colleagues (1989).

Within this SPAARS model, a traumatic event triggers intense appraisal-driven fear, helplessness, or horror, as well as a range of other emotions. Information about the traumatic event is encoded in the schematic, propositional, and analogue levels simultaneously. Because the memory of the traumatic event represents an ongoing threat to goals, the person is left with low-level fear activation, cognitive bias to attend to threat appraisals, and intrusive sensory images and appraisals. The trauma memory exists across different levels of mental representation but is unincorporated into the person's larger mental representations; the memory may be elicited as flashbacks or nightmares. Such strong memory and emotional intrusions result in efforts to cope through avoidance.

ASSESSMENT

Any comprehensive assessment of PTSD must capture whether or not a life event meets the seriousness and subjective response requirements of a traumatic stressor (criterion A), as well as the presence and severity of 17 associated symptoms (criteria B–D). Although interview-based measures are considered the "gold standard" for assessing PTSD, a number of self-report measures have been developed in recent years to provide a quicker, less resource-heavy method for assessing PTSD.

Assessment of Traumatic Events

The first essential step in the assessment of PTSD is to identify major traumas in the patient's history. Often this is difficult to achieve, because many trauma survivors, especially rape and child sexual abuse trauma survivors, do not spontaneously disclose their trauma history. This is consistent with general patterns of avoidance of trauma-related reminders and may reflect shame, embarrassment, and self-blame regarding the incidents. Even when seeking treatment for mental health problems, trauma survivors often fail to recognize that their psychological difficulties may be associated with their trauma history. Kilpatrick (1983) suggested several other reasons survivors might not be forthcoming with this information, including fear of a negative reaction to disclosure, especially if previous disclosure has resulted in disbelief or blame. Additionally, many trauma survivors do not recognize or label their experience as "trauma," "rape," or "abuse," especially if the assailant was an acquaintance or a relative, or if the trauma was experienced by many people, as in combat. Finally, in the absence of a strong alliance with the therapist, many people choose not to disclose such deeply personal information. It is therefore important for the clinician to forge a positive alliance as early as possible and be forthcoming about the purpose of the questioning, any limits of confidentiality, and how the obtained information may be used (i.e., diagnosis, treatment planning, research purposes).

In terms of questions regarding the presence of traumatic experiences, a behavioral, descriptive prompt such as "Has anyone ever made you have unwanted sexual contact by physical force or threat of force?" is more detailed and is preferable to asking, "Have you ever been raped?" In the latter case, someone who is married (or dating) and who has been sexually assaulted may say "no" because "rape" might not be a term that is associated with forced sex by one's partner. The same problem may exist with child abuse. A patient may indicate that he was not abused as a child but readily admits, when asked, that a parent whipped him with a belt until he had welts. In general, it is recommended that the clinician always begin with broad questions about experiences, then move to more specific behaviorally-anchored questions.

In recent years, some structured interviews have been developed with the primary purpose of assessing traumas in more detail. The Potential Stressful Events Interview (Kilpatrick, Resnick, & Freedy, 1991) has behaviorally anchored questions that are particularly good for assessing interpersonal victimizations, as well as a range of other traumatic stressors. The DSM-IV version of the Clinician-Administered PTSD Scale (CAPS; Blake et al., 1995) (reviewed in more detail later), includes a self-report screening scale (Life Events Checklist), followed by interviewer prompts to establish whether a trauma meets criterion A.

Many clinicians may choose to circumvent some of these extensive questions by using self-report measures, such as checklists, to acquire some initial information. Although clinicians should not rely on them exclusively, a number of checklists can be used as a springboard for further inquiry. In addition to the Life Events Checklist, the Traumatic Stress Schedule

(Norris, 1990), the Trauma History Questionnaire (THQ; Green, 1996), the Traumatic Life Events Questionnaire (TLEQ; Kubany, Haynes, et al., 2000), and the Traumatic Events Scale (Vrana & Lauterbach, 1994) all assess a number of different types of trauma, including accidents, natural disaster, sexual assault, and threats of, or actual, physical harm. The Posttraumatic Stress Diagnostic Scale (PDS; Foa, 1995) has two sections prior to assessment of symptoms. The first section assesses 13 potentially traumatic events, whereas the second has questions to determine whether an event meets the definition of criterion A. With regard to combat in particular, the Combat Exposure Scale (Keane, Fairbank, Caddell, & Zimering, 1989) has been used widely to assess the degree of combat exposure.

Structured Diagnostic Interviews

The CAPS, developed by Blake and others (1995), has become, perhaps, the "gold standard" assessment of PTSD and is now the most widely used diagnostic interview (Weathers, Keane, & Davidson, 2001; Weathers, Ruscio, & Keane, 1999). The CAPS has several attractive features. In addition to a detailed assessment of individual trauma experiences, it assesses both severity and frequency of symptoms, using specific criteria. Furthermore, the CAPS includes questions on associated features of PTSD, including dissociation, survivor guilt, and social and occupational impairment. Additionally, it gives clear guidelines for assessing changes in behavior following exposure to trauma. The CAPS, the best and most thorough assessment of PTSD, has a large body of research demonstrating its reliability and validity across a wide variety of trauma populations. One disadvantage is its length of administration, which is, on average, about 1 hour, and the need for administration by a mental health clinician. The length of administration may be decreased slighted by assessing only the 17 core symptoms.

The Structured Clinical Interview for DSM-IV (SCID; First, Spitzer, Williams, & Gibbon, 1995) is one of the most widely used diagnostic scales. The SCID includes assessment of PTSD symptomatology and was developed for use by experienced clinicians. Although it assesses all of the symptoms of PTSD and can provide information about whether an individual meets criteria for the diagnosis, it is important to note that the interview does not assess for frequency or severity of individual symptoms. Furthermore, by using the SCID, one can only determine a count of the number of positive symptoms, thereby limiting its utility in research or clinical settings in which a continuous measure of severity may be desirable. Resnick, Kilpatrick, and Lipovsky (1991) recommended certain modifications of the SCID for use with rape victims, including more sensitive screening questions for history of rape and other major traumatic events.

Another structured interview, the Diagnostic Interview Schedule (DIS; Robins, Helzer, Croughan, & Ratcliff, 1981), is highly structured and has the advantage of requiring less training and experience to administer than the CAPS and SCID. Like the SCID, the DIS results in diagnosis but does not have continuous severity scores. One potential problem is that the PTSD section assesses exposure to civilian trauma, including sexual assault, but uses the term "rape" without any further specification. Thus, the modifications suggested by Resnick and colleagues (1991) relative to rape may be appropriate for this instrument, as well as when assessing interpersonal traumas. Kessler and colleagues (1995) also have modified the DIS for better diagnosis of PTSD in large studies with lay interviewers.

The PTSD Symptom Scale—Interview (PSS-I; Foa, Riggs, Dancu, & Rothbaum, 1993) has a particular advantage in its ease of administration and brevity, with 17 items and prompts matching the 17-symptom PTSD criteria. The PSS-I can result in continuous scores reflecting frequency of symptoms, or to determine PTSD diagnosis. Another advantage is its companion self-report measure (PSS-SR), to which scores on the interview can be compared. Thus, after conducting an initial interview, one could administer the PSS-SR on a more regular basis (e.g., biweekly) to monitor symptom change, without having to readminister the interview frequently. A disadvantage of the interview is that symptoms are assessed only over a current, 2-week period instead of 1 month, so it is possible that some diagnoses may be incorrect. The time frame should be modified if careful diagnosis is required.

Self-Report Instruments

There are now a number of self-report scales of PTSD that have good psychometric properties.

Among them are the PSS-SR (Falsetti, Resnick, Resick, & Kilpatrick, 1993; Foa et al., 1993), the Purdue PTSD Scale—Revised (Lauterbach & Vrana, 1996), the PTSD Checklist (PCL; Weathers, Litz, Herman, Huska, & Keane, 1993), the Distressing Event Questionnaire (DEQ; Kubany, Leisen, Kaplan, & Kelly, 2000), the Mississippi Scale for Combat-Related PTSD (Keane, Caddell, & Taylor, 1988), and the Posttraumatic Stress Diagnostic Scale (PDS; Foa, 1995). Most of these scales were developed with specific populations, such as rape trauma survivors (e.g., PSS) or combat veterans (e.g., Mississippi Scale, PCL), and research on their validity with other populations in some cases is minimal. Thus, it is important for clinicians to think about their target population before adopting a measure. Moreover, as with any self-report measure, there are limitations to relying exclusively on questionnaires for diagnosis or symptom severity. Used in conjunction with structured interviews, however, they can be useful for screening purposes or for demonstrating changes over time as a result of a particular intervention.

The Impact of Event Scale (IES; Horowitz, Wilner, & Alvarez, 1979; Weiss & Marmar, 1997) and the Mississippi Scale (Keane et al., 1988, 1989) are two of the oldest self-report measures. The IES is useful for measuring trauma impact and was revised from its original version, which included only intrusion and avoidance symptoms, to include arousal symptoms as well; thus, it maps onto the DSM-IV criteria (IES-R; Weiss & Marmar, 1997). The original 35-item Mississippi Scale, which assesses both diagnostic criteria and associated features of PTSD in combat veterans, a newer version has been created for use with civilians. The PDS (Foa, 1995), a 49-item scale designed to assess all five PTSD criteria, has strong psychometrics. Griffin, Uhlmansiek, Resick, and Mechanic (2004) found a strong correlation between the PDS and the CAPS.

Two measures of PTSD have been empirically derived from other scales. The Keane PTSD Scale (PK) of the Minnesota Multiphasic Personality Inventory (MMPI) and MMPI-2 has been used successfully to discriminate between Vietnam combat veterans with and without PTSD (Keane, Malloy, & Fairbank, 1984; Weathers & Keane, 1999). The Symptom Checklist 90—Revised (SCL-90-R; Derogatis, 1983) has also been examined by Saunders, Arata, and Kilpatrick (1990) and by Weathers and colleagues (1999), who developed PTSD subscales derived from different sets of items for female crime victims and combat veterans, respectively.

The PCL is widely used in Department of Veterans Affairs (VA) and military settings with a version (PCL-M) that specifically refers to military-related traumas. The civilian version of the scale (PCL-C) assesses civilian traumas, and the PCL-S allows the assessor to identify the specific trauma of reference. Like the PDS, the PCL reflects DSM-IV symptoms of PTSD.

In response to a need to screen large numbers of people for PTSD after combat or disasters, or in medical settings when time is limited, a brief PTSD screen has been developed for use in primary care settings or for large-group administrations, such as those with military personnel following deployment (Prins et al., 2004). The Primary Care PTSD Screen (PC-PTSD) was developed for such a purpose and is now being used routinely in the United States with anyone returning from military deployment or receiving any kind of treatment in the VA medical system (Hoge et al., 2006). This scale has four yes–no items that represent the four major symptom clusters found in most PTSD factor-analytic studies that separate effortful avoidance from numbing. These four items were found to be highly associated with PTSD as measured by the CAPS. In fact, the PC-PTSD outperformed the PCL with regard to sensitivity and specificity, as well as efficiency. A cutoff of 3 was recommended as an optimally efficient score for both men and women, and a cutoff of 2 was recommended for maximum sensitivity.

Finally, it should be noted that only one trauma-related scale, the Trauma Symptom Inventory (TSI; Briere, 1995), includes scales to assess response bias. For forensic purposes, in which response bias may be of particular concern, the assessor may wish to include the TSI or administer the MMPI-2, which contains both the PK scale and validity subscales. In addition to clinical scales, the TSI also includes subscales assessing tendencies to overendorse unusual or bizarre symptoms, to respond in an inconsistent or random manner, and to deny symptoms that others commonly endorse. In addition to PTSD-related subscales, such as Intrusive Experiences, Defensive Avoidance, and Anxious Arousal, it also includes subscales that measure frequently observed problems: Depression, Anger, Dissociation, Tension-Reduction Behaviors, and Disruptions in Self-Perception and Sexual Functioning.

Psychophysiological Assessment

The ideal assessment includes measurement in multiple response channels, including physiological responses. This is especially true in PTSD assessment, because physiological reactivity to trauma cues is one of the criteria of the disorder. However, a psychophysiological test might not be feasible in clinical settings, because the required technology and expertise are not always available. Despite this limitation, it is important to be aware of the research in this area and to be alert to obvious physiological symptoms in patients when talking about their trauma experiences (e.g., signs of agitation, sweating, flushing). Research has demonstrated consistent group differences in physiological reactivity between individuals with and without PTSD when exposed to trauma-related stimuli, such as through the use of individualized trauma scripts (for a systematic review of this body of research, see Orr, Metzger, Miller, & Kaloupek, 2004). Vietnam veterans with PTSD have been found to be consistently more reactive to combat imagery than combat veterans without PTSD, even when the comparison samples had other anxiety disorders or other psychological problems (Keane, Kolb, et al., 1998; Pitman, Orr, Forgue, & Altman, 1990; Pitman, Orr, Forgue, de Jong, & Claiborn, 1987). Similar results have been found in people with PTSD as a result of MVAs and child sexual abuse (Blanchard, Hickling, Buckley, & Taylor, 1996; Orr et al., 1998).

The largest investigation of physiological reactivity was a multisite study of over 1,300 veterans (Keane, Kaloupek, & Kolb, 1998). Using four psychophysiological measures, Keane and colleagues were able to classify correctly two-thirds of those who had PTSD. This indicates that whereas psychophysiological reactivity can help to distinguish between many members of PTSD and non-PTSD groups, it should not be used as a sole measure of diagnostic assessment. In fact, a number of factors may affect physiological reactivity, and these must be taken into account when assessing the validity of psychophysiological findings. For example, the presence of psychotropic drugs (i.e., benzodiazepines, beta-adrenergic blockers) can affect an individual's response. Furthermore, it has been demonstrated that antisocial characteristics can suppress levels of psychophysiological responding (Miller, Kaloupek, & Keane, 1999). In addition to people who do not respond physiologically, some people appear to have an alternative response to arousal.

Griffin, Resick, and Mechanic (1997) studied psychophysiological reactivity in recent rape trauma survivors using a methodology that differed in two significant ways from prior studies. First, rather than listening to generated scripts, participants were asked to talk for 5 minutes on both a neutral recall topic and their rapes. These neutral and trauma phases were interspersed with baseline conditions. Second, instead of looking at the PTSD group as a whole, the researchers examined physiological reactivity by degree of "peritraumatic dissociation" (PD), which refers to the extent to which someone dissociated during the traumatic event. Griffin and colleagues found that a small group of women with high PD responded in a very different manner than other women with PTSD. Whereas skin conductance and heart rate of women with low PD scores increased as expected while they were talking about the rape, those with high PD scores showed a decrease in the physiological measures. When the participants' subjective distress during each of the phases was examined, the high-PD group reported the same level of distress as the low-PD group. Therefore, despite experiencing distress, the physiological responses of the high-PD group were suppressed. Griffin and colleagues speculated that there may be a dissociative subtype of subjects with PTSD who physiologically respond quite differently than those with the more phobic type of PTSD.

In general, there are two major aims in assessment in clinical practice: diagnosis and treatment planning. Whether the primary purpose of assessment is diagnosis or treatment planning, a multidimensional, multiaxial approach is desirable. Because a cross-sectional view taken at a single point in time may fail to capture the full range and pattern of symptoms, a longitudinal approach to assessment has been advocated by Denny, Robinowitz, and Penk (1987) and Sutker, Uddo-Crane, and Allain (1991). Certainly for purposes of treatment, ongoing assessment of symptom patterns and treatment effectiveness is essential. Even when measuring PTSD cross-sectionally, it has been suggested that multiple measures and methods be used, depending on the purpose of the assessment (Keane, Brief, Pratt, & Miller, 2007; Weathers & Keane, 1999).

Some final notes regarding assessment are in order. First, given the empirical evidence linking PTSD with increased risk of suicide, suicide risk should always be carefully assessed and monitored. The National Women's Study (Kilpatrick, Edmunds, & Seymour, 1992) found that 13% of rape trauma survivors had made a suicide attempt compared to 1% of nonvictims. Additionally, 33% of the rape trauma survivors compared to 8% of nonvictims stated that they had seriously considered suicide at some point. Furthermore, the presence of comorbid PTSD has been associated with a greater number of suicide attempts among individuals with major depressive disorder (Oquendo et al., 2003). These data highlight the need for careful monitoring of suicidal ideation and behavior among individuals being assessed or treated for PTSD.

Second, a growing body of research suggests that individuals with PTSD are at increased risk of perpetrating physical aggression against others. McFall, Fontana, Raskind, and Rosenheck (1999) found that male Vietnam veteran inpatients with PTSD were more likely than inpatients without PTSD or a community sample of Vietnam veterans to perpetrate acts of violence toward objects or others. Results from the NVVRS indicated that 33% of Vietnam veterans with PTSD had assaulted their partner within the previous year (Jordan et al., 1992). Unfortunately, risk of violence does not appear to be limited to Vietnam veterans. There is evidence of increased risk of violence in other traumatized populations, including women (e.g., Miller, Kaloupek, Dillon, & Keane, 2004). Given also that an outburst of anger is one of the DSM-IV symptoms of PTSD, it is important that history of aggressive acts, as well as current impulses toward aggression, are carefully assessed and addressed.

TREATMENT

Types of Therapy for PTSD

There have been four predominant forms of therapy for PTSD: coping, skills-focused treatments; exposure-based treatments; cognitive therapy; and combination treatments and eye movement desensitization and reprocessing (EMDR) (which may be a combination treatment). Before reviewing the research on treatment outcome for PTSD, we describe some of the treatment protocols.

Stress Inoculation Training

The earliest comprehensive approach described specifically for use with rape trauma survivors was stress inoculation training (SIT; Kilpatrick & Amick, 1985; Kilpatrick et al., 1982). Based on Meichenbaum's (1985) approach to anxiety, its aim is to give clients a sense of mastery over their fears by teaching a variety of coping skills. The approach is tailored to the individual problems and needs of each client, so it is flexible and can be used in individual or group settings. SIT is approached in phases. The first phase, preparation for treatment, includes an educational element to provide an explanatory or conceptual framework from which the client can understand the nature and origin of her or his fear and anxiety and make sense of the trauma and its aftermath. In SIT, a social learning theory explanation is used. Along with this, fear and anxiety reactions are explained as occurring along three channels (Lang, 1968): (1) the physical or autonomic channel, (2) the behavioral or motoric channel, and (3) the cognitive channel. Specific examples are given for each, and the patient identifies her or his own reactions within each channel. Interrelationships among the three channels are explained and discussed. The second phase of SIT is the training of coping skills directed at each of these channels of response. It includes, in sequence, a definition of the coping skill, a rationale, an explanation of the mechanism by which the skill works, a demonstration of the skill, application by the client of the skill to a problem area unrelated to the target behaviors, a review of how well the skill worked, and, finally, application and practice of the skill with one of the target fears. Skills taught most often for coping with fear in the physical channel are muscle relaxation and breathing control.

For the behavioral channel, covert modeling and role playing are the coping skills usually taught. The client is taught to visualize a fear or anxiety-provoking situation and to imagine her- or himself confronting it successfully. For the cognitive channel, the client is taught guided self-dialogue. The client is taught to focus on her or his internal dialogue and trained to label negative, irrational, and maladaptive self-statements. She or he is then taught to substitute more adaptive self-verbalizations. Self-dialogue is taught in four categories: preparation, confrontation and management, coping with feelings of being overwhelmed, and reinforcement. For each of these categories, a series of questions and/or statements is generated that encourage the client to assess the actual probability that the negative event will occur, to manage the overwhelming fear and avoidance behavior, to control self-criticism and self-devaluation, to engage in the feared behavior, and finally to reinforce her- or himself for making the attempt and following the steps.

Exposure Techniques

Beginning in the early 1980s, forms of exposure therapy were investigated as a treatment for PTSD. Although systematic desensitization (SD) has been demonstrated to be effective for treating PTSD in a number of case study reports and controlled studies, it has not been widely adopted as a preferred treatment (Bowen & Lambert, 1986; Brom, Kleber, & Defares, 1989; Frank et al., 1988; Frank & Stewart, 1983, 1984; Schindler, 1980; Shalev, Orr, & Pitman, 1992; Turner, 1979). Because people with PTSD may fear and avoid a wide range of trauma-related stimuli, SD may require a number of hierarchies that can be quite inefficient.

Extended exposure to feared cues or to the trauma memory itself is a more efficient treatment and has been employed more widely. Known variously as direct therapeutic exposure (DTE), flooding, or prolonged exposure, these exposure techniques require clients to confront feared situations *in vivo*, to imagine themselves in a fear-producing situation, or to recall their particular trauma for extended periods of time. Rothbaum (1998) experimented with the use of virtual reality for treating Vietnam veterans. The veteran with PTSD can take a virtual helicopter trip in Vietnam, complete with gunfire and other stimuli that may evoke memories of traumatic events.

Foa and colleagues (1991; Rothbaum & Foa, 1992) were the first to focus extensively on the specific trauma memory rather than fear-producing stimuli. Prolonged exposure (PE) is conducted individually in 9–12 weekly or biweekly 90-minute sessions. The first two sessions are for information gathering, treatment planning, and explanation of the treatment rationale. Clients are also taught breathing retraining. A hierarchical list is generated of major stimuli that are feared and avoided. Clients are instructed to confront feared cues for at least 45 minutes a day, starting with a moderately anxiety-provoking stimulus on the hierarchy. Beginning with Session 3, the trauma scene is relived in imagination, and the client is asked to describe it aloud in the present tense. The level of detail is left to the client for the first two exposures, but thereafter she or he is encouraged to include more and more detail about external cues and internal cues, such as thoughts, physiological responses, and feared consequences. Descriptions are repeated several times each session (for 60 minutes) and tape-recorded. Clients are assigned homework, to listen to the tape and to engage in *in vivo* tasks. Care is taken in sessions to ensure that the client's anxiety decreases before the session is terminated, aided by the therapist, if necessary (Foa & Rothbaum, 1998).

Marks, Lovell, Noshirvani, Livanou, and Thrasher (1998) have conducted exposure therapy somewhat differently. Their version of the therapy includes five sessions of imaginal exposure, then five sessions of live exposure. During the imaginal exposure, clients are asked to relive the experience aloud in the first person, present tense about the details of their experience, and then to imagine and describe critical aspects of the event (rewind and hold). Clients listen to their therapy tapes daily between sessions. During the live exposure portion of therapy, clients (most often therapist-accompanied) progress through a hierarchy of feared, avoided, and disabling trauma-related stimuli. They are asked to practice the live exposure for an hour a day between sessions.

Cognitive Therapy/Cognitive Restructuring

Cognitive therapy for PTSD has generally taken two forms. One form is more present-focused and typically uses daily diaries or monitoring forms to elicit thoughts that the client has recorded during the week. These homework sheets form the basis of the cognitive restructuring training that occurs during treatment through the use of teaching and Socratic questioning. Clients are taught to identify and to dispute their unrealistic or exaggerated thoughts about themselves, the world, and their futures with more probabilistic reasoning

and evidence-based argument. Examples of studies that have used this model of cognitive restructuring are Blanchard and colleagues (2003) and Foa and colleagues (2005).

The other form of cognitive therapy is more trauma-focused and constructivist, focusing on the particular meanings that the event has for the client and how those interpretations of the event contradict or seemingly confirm previously held beliefs about self and others. These distorted assumptions about the event (e.g., "I should have been able to stop the event, so it is my fault that it happened") may maintain a belief in a just world or a sense of controllability, but typically at the cost of reduced self-esteem, shame, or guilt. The focus of treatment is on how clients may have distorted the event itself to maintain prior beliefs about justice or the role of others (assimilation), or conversely, how they may have changed their beliefs about themselves and the world too much (over-accommodation) in an attempt to regain a sense of control or safety in the present or the future ("I cannot trust other people at all any more"). Treatment includes Socratic questioning and teaching clients to challenge their thinking about their traumatic events and the implications they have constructed through the use of progressive worksheets. Examples of trauma-focused cognitive therapy are studies by Resick, Nishith, Weaver, Astin, and Feuer (2002) or Tarrier and colleagues (1999).

Combination Treatments/Additive Studies

Some studies that we review below refer to their protocols as cognitive-behavioral therapy (CBT; e.g., Blanchard et al., 2003; Bryant, Harvey, Dang, Sackville, & Basten, 1998). These therapy packages are typically combinations of various forms of exposure (imaginal, *in vivo*, written) and cognitive restructuring or cognitive therapy, but they may also include relaxation or other coping skills. These protocols may have been developed as a combination treatment to begin with, or may reflect additive studies in which a new component is added to an existing treatment to determine whether the extra component adds value to the existing therapy. An important distinction between these two types of protocols is that the combination treatments were designed to be a specific length to accommodate the components of the treatment. In other words, the therapy package was designed to achieve the optimal goals of the exposure or cognitive components. Additive studies must accommodate to the original protocol length; therefore, they may not be designed with the optimal amount of therapy needed to achieve the goals of the components. In additive studies, the amount of exposure, stress management, or cognitive therapy in combination is shortened to maintain the length of the original protocol being compared.

STAIR/MPE

Cloitre, Koenen, Cohen, and Han (2002) proposed that survivors of child sexual abuse trauma have problems of affect regulation and interpersonal effectiveness, in addition to their PTSD, that compromise their ability to profit from trauma-focused interventions. Thus, they developed a protocol called STAIR (i.e., skills training in affective and interpersonal regulation) that included treatment for these problems prior to implementing a modification of prolonged exposure (MPE). This combination treatment first trained patients in emotion management and interpersonal skills for 8 weeks, followed by a second phase of treatment with imaginal exposure. The imaginal exposure phase also included postexposure emotional management and cognitive therapy.

COGNITIVE PROCESSING THERAPY

Unlike the additive studies, cognitive processing therapy (CPT) was initially developed specifically as a combination treatment to treat the specific symptoms of PTSD in sexual assault trauma survivors (Resick & Schnicke, 1992, 1993), but it has since been tested with other populations. CPT, which can be delivered in either individual or group formats, is a 12-session, structured therapy program that includes a written form of exposure to the traumatic memory but is predominantly a cognitive therapy. After an introduction to PTSD symptoms and the therapy, clients are asked to write an impact statement, a statement of how their worst traumatic event has affected them. Clients are asked to focus on any self-blame they have regarding the trauma and the effects of the event on their beliefs about self and others. This statement is used to understand how they may have distorted the cause of the event or overgeneralized its meaning, such that their functioning has been compromised. For exam-

ple, if someone thought that she or he should have been able to stop the event, then the individual might feel guilt afterward. If a client decided that the event means that no one is to be trusted, then she or he will behave as though that were true.

Before examining the trauma in depth, the client is taught to label emotions and recognize the connection among events, thoughts, and feelings, then is asked to write a detailed account of the worst traumatic event and read it to her- or himself every day. In sessions she or he reads it to the therapist and is encouraged to feel whatever emotions emerge. The therapist begins to challenge faulty thinking about the traumatic event with Socratic questioning. After writing and reading the account for a second time, the therapist focuses on teaching the client to learn the skill of challenging thoughts and assumptions with Socratic questions for her- or himself through a series of worksheets. The client is first taught to question a single thought, then look for patterns of problematic thinking, and, finally, to generate alternative, more balanced thoughts about the event itself and then overgeneralized assumptions about self and world. In the last five sessions, clients are provided modules to assist them in thinking about specific themes that are commonly disrupted following traumatic events: safety, trust, power and control, esteem, and intimacy.

Eye Movement Desensitization and Reprocessing (EMDR)

Eye movement desensitization and reprocessing therapy (EMDR) is a controversial therapy that evolved not from theory or application of effective techniques for other disorders, but from a personal observation. As originally developed by Shapiro (1989, 1995), EMDR was based on a chance observation that troubling thoughts were resolved when her eyes followed the waving of leaves during a walk in the park. Shapiro developed EMDR on the basis of this observation and argued that lateral eye movements facilitate cognitive processing of the trauma. Subsequently, EMDR was conceptualized as a cognitive-behavioral treatment aimed at facilitating information processing of traumatic events and cognitive restructuring of negative, trauma-related cognitions. In the early presentations of EMDR, it was touted as a one-session cure for a range of disorders. However, more recent studies are typically of trauma-related symptoms, with a course more similar to the other trauma therapies. EMDR is now described as an eight-phase treatment that includes history taking, client preparation, target assessment, desensitization, installation, body scan, closure, and reevaluation of treatment effects. EMDR includes exposure and cognitive components, as well as the lateral eye movements.

In the basic EMDR protocol, clients are asked to identify and focus on a traumatic image or memory (target assessment phase). Next, the therapist elicits negative cognitions or belief statements about the memory. Clients are asked to assign a rating to the memory and negative cognitions on an 11-point scale of distress and to identify the physical location of the anxiety. The therapist helps clients generate positive cognitions that would be preferable to associate with the memory. These are rated on a 7-point scale of how much the clients believe the statement. Once the therapist has instructed a client in the basic EMDR procedure, she or he is asked to do four things simultaneously (desensitization phase): (1) Visualize the memory; (2) rehearse the negative cognitions; (3) concentrate on the physical sensations of the anxiety; and (4) visually track the therapist's index finger. While the client does this, the therapist rapidly moves his or her index finger back and forth from right to left, 30 to 35 cm from the client's face, with two back-and-forth movements per second. These are repeated 24 times. Then the client is asked to blank out the memory and take a deep breath. Subsequently, she or he brings back the memory and cognitions and rates the level of distress. Sets of eye movements (saccades) are repeated until the distress rating equals 0 or 1. At this point, the client is asked about how she or he feels about the positive cognition and gives a rating for it (installation phase).

Evidence for Treatment Efficacy

Because so many of the studies have compared more than one type of treatment or combinations of components, this section is presented generally in chronological order. Only controlled trials are presented here. Foa and colleagues (1991) compared a modified SIT to PE, supportive counseling, and a waiting-list control group, seeing clients individually. Because they did not want overlapping techniques in their comparison, Foa and colleagues eliminated the *in vivo* exposure component, confronting feared cues from SIT. In this study, SIT was most effective immediately posttreatment in reducing PTSD symptoms, anxiety, and depression. However, at 3.5-month follow-up, there was a trend for the exposure approach to show the greatest efficacy.

Marks and colleagues (1998) compared four groups: exposure therapy, cognitive restructuring, exposure combined with cognitive restructuring, and relaxation training. The participants were 87 men and women who had PTSD from a range of traumatic stressors. Seventy-seven participants completed treatment and 52 completed the 36-week follow-up. The authors found that overall, the cognitive, exposure, and combined treatments were more effective than relaxation, but there were no major differences among any of the three treatments. The treatment gains were maintained through the 6-month follow-up. Marks and colleagues, in responding to these findings, modified the theory. They suggested that emotions may be viewed as response syndromes that comprise loosely linked reactions of many physiological, behavioral, and cognitive components. The intensity of an emotion may be reduced by acting on any of several components. A change in one component may affect the others. Several components can be acted on at the same time by certain treatment combinations.

In an additive study, Foa and colleagues (1999) compared modified SIT, PE, and a combination of SIT and PE. They found that the combination did not improve the results over SIT or PE alone. However, as discussed earlier, it should be pointed out that because of the nature of the research, the participants only received half as much SIT or PE as the other participants, because they had the same length of sessions but half SIT and half PE at each session. It should also be pointed out that neither of the Foa and colleagues studies were powered to detect anything but large treatment differences. The small sample sizes may not have been able to detect differences that might have emerged with samples large enough to find small to medium effect sizes.

Tarrier and colleagues (1999) compared imaginal exposure and cognitive therapy. At posttreatment and follow-up, the investigators did not find a difference between the two therapies. However at a 5-year follow-up with 52% of the original sample, no patients who received cognitive therapy were diagnosed with

PTSD compared to 29% of those receiving exposure treatment (Tarrier & Sommerfield, 2004). Those receiving exposure treatment reported significantly more PTSD and depressive symptoms than the cognitive therapy group.

Beginning in the early to mid-1990s, a series of studies compared EMDR to other treatments and examined the necessity of the eye movements for the treatment. In a sample of 61 combat veterans, all of whom met diagnostic criteria for PTSD, Boudewyns, Hyer, Peralme, Touze, and Kiel (1995) found EMDR to be equally as effective as PE in reducing symptoms of PTSD, depression, anxiety, and accelerated heart rate. In this study, subjects were randomly assigned to one of three groups. All three groups received the standard treatment at their facility, which comprised eight group therapy sessions and a few spontaneous individual sessions. One group received only this form of treatment; the second and third groups also received either five to eight sessions of EMDR or five to eight sessions of PE. All three groups improved significantly on symptoms of PTSD. The therapy-only group did not improve on depression and showed increases in anxiety and heart rate, whereas the two other groups improved on all measures.

Two studies had mixed or negative results for EMDR. The Pitman and colleagues (1993) study of 17 combat veterans compared 12 sessions of EMDR to an eyes-fixed procedure in which the therapist alternately tapped each leg of the subject. The EMDR group reported significantly greater improvement on measures of subjective distress, self-report measures of PTSD intrusion and avoidance, and psychiatric symptoms. No effects were observed, however, on other standardized self-report and structured interviews of PTSD. Jensen (1994) compared two sessions of EMDR with no treatment in 25 combat veterans and found no improvements in either group on standardized measures of PTSD.

Devilly and Spence (1999) found a statistical and effect size advantage (Cohen's $d = 0.67$) for a CBT intervention including exposure and cognitive elements compared to EMDR. These results were maintained at 3-month follow-up assessment. Taylor and colleagues (2003) also found that exposure therapy was statistically superior to EMDR, which was not significantly different from relaxation therapy in a mixed sample. The proportion of individuals achieving clinically significant reductions in their PTSD symptoms

(i.e., improvement greater than two standard deviations on clinician assessment of PTSD) was greater in the exposure group.

Several studies have compared EMDR to various combinations of CBT. Three of these studies report effect size advantages for EMDR in those who complete treatment. Ironson, Freund, Strauss, and Williams (2002) compared EMDR to PE in a relatively small mixed sample and found no statistical differences between the two treatments. However, there was an effect size advantage of 0.65 for EMDR compared to prolonged exposure in completer analyses. Lee, Gavriel, Drummond, Richards, and Greenwald (2002) compared EMDR to a combination of SIT and PE in another small sample and found no statistical differences between the treatments, with exception of a statistical advantage of EMDR in intrusive symptoms and an overall effect size advantage ($d = 0.62$) in completer analyses. In a large mixed-trauma sample, Power and colleagues (2002) compared EMDR to a combination of exposure therapy and cognitive restructuring, and found no significant differences. They reported effect size advantages for EMDR in the frequency and intensity of PTSD symptoms clusters.

Most recently, Rothbaum, Astin, and Marsteller (2005), compared EMDR, PE, and a waiting-list control group in a very well-controlled study of 74 women with rape-related PTSD. They found no differences between the two active conditions on PTSD at posttreatment or 6-month follow-up; both groups improved substantially. They only found differences among the subsample with multiple comorbidities, in which the EMDR sample with multiple comorbidities did not fare as well as the PE sample participants with such comorbidity.

While Shapiro has maintained that lateral eye movements are an essential therapeutic component of EMDR, studies that have examined this have had mixed results. Renfrey and Spates (1994) treated a sample of 23 heterogeneous trauma survivors with standard EMDR, a variant in which lateral eye movements were engendered via a light-tracking task, or another variant in which no lateral eye movements were induced and subjects were instructed to fix their visual attention. All three groups improved significantly on measures of PTSD, depression, anxiety, heart rate, and subjective units of distress (SUDs) scores at posttreatment and at 1- to 3-month follow-up. No differences were found among treatments. In contrast, in 18 heterogeneous trauma survivors, Wilson, Silver, Covi, and Foster (1996) found significant improvements in subjects who received EMDR, but not in subjects who were instructed to fix their visual attention, or in subjects who alternated tapping their right and left thumbs to a metronome. Physiological measures and SUDs, but no standardized distress measures, were used to measure outcome. Pitman and colleagues (1993), as noted earlier, found mixed results.

Given these results, it is not clear whether lateral eye movements are an essential component of EMDR. EMDR forces clients to think about the trauma, to identify the negative cognitions associated with the trauma, and to work toward positive cognitions as they process the traumatic memory. Without the lateral eye movements, EMDR is quite similar to a form of CPT that facilitates the processing of the traumatic memory. Therefore, any efficacy demonstrated by EMDR may be more attributable to engagement of the traumatic memory and the facilitation of cognitive reassessment than to eye movements. Nevertheless, EMDR appears to be as effective as other exposure and combination CBT packages in these relatively small studies.

In a comparison of exposure and a combination protocol, Paunovic and Öst (2001) compared a package of cognitive-behavioral interventions, including exposure therapy, cognitive restructuring, and controlled breathing, to exposure therapy only in a relatively small sample of refugees. No statistical differences were found between the two conditions, but there was a small effect size advantage (0.13) for the combination of interventions.

Cloitre and colleagues (2002) compared the STAIR/MPE protocol for adults who had been sexually abused as children and a waiting-list control group. Compared to the waiting-list condition, this combination of treatments was found to be efficacious, with an effect size of d = 1.3 at posttreatment. The treatment had significant effects on affect regulation and interpersonal measures, as well as PTSD. Only 23% of the treated group still met criteria for PTSD after treatment. Cloitre and colleagues also found that the participants continued to improve from posttreatment to 3-month follow-up and then again at 9-month follow-up. In a further analysis of the study, Cloitre, Stovall-

McClough, Miranda, and Chemtob (2004) examined the effect of therapeutic alliance and affect regulation (Phase 1) on the outcome of Phase 2 exposure treatment. They found that therapeutic alliance led to greater affect regulation in Phase 1, which then resulted in better treatment outcome following the modified PE.

Resick and her colleagues (2002) conducted a large randomized controlled trial comparing individually delivered CPT, PE, and minimal attention waiting-list conditions with survivors of completed rape. Participants in both CPT and PE conditions showed large decreases in PTSD symptoms (75% decrease on average) compared to the waiting-list control condition, which did not change over the same period. A small effect size difference favored CPT over PE. Eighty percent of participants in both treatment groups remitted from their PTSD diagnosis. CPT was more effective with specific guilt cognitions than PE, although both conditions improved significantly. In addition to PTSD, there were similar decreases in depression, anger, dissociation, and other indicators of complex PTSD (Resick, Nishith, & Griffin, 2003).

Several studies compared active treatments to nonspecific treatments rather than a waiting-list control. These designs control for nonspecific effects of treatment and are not expected to produce the large differences typically found with comparisons to waiting-list control groups. For example, Blanchard and colleagues (2003) compared CBT to supportive counseling and a waiting list in a sample of MVA survivors. They found that CBT (relaxation, written exposure, *in vivo* exposure, cognitive restructuring, and behavioral activation) was significantly better than supportive counseling, which was significantly better than waiting list. There was a 0.63 effect size advantage for CBT compared to supportive counseling in those who completed the treatment. Neuner, Schauer, Klaschik, Karunakara, and Elbert (2004) also used supportive counseling, as well as a psychoeducation intervention for control groups, and compared them to their narrative exposure therapy. In this form of therapy, clients are asked to construct their entire autobiography verbally, including all of the traumatic events they experienced. In a sample of Sudanese refugees, there were no differences among the three conditions at posttreatment. However, narrative exposure therapy was significantly better than both conditions, which were equal to one another in effectiveness, at 1-year follow-up.

In one of the largest studies published to date, a multisite trial of group CBT treatment was compared to a present-centered problem-solving group treatment (Schnurr et al., 2003). Three hundred sixty male veterans were randomly assigned to one of the two conditions and provided weekly therapy for 7 months. The CBT treatment included education and self-management of symptoms, autobiographies, war-zone scene identification, imaginal exposures, cognitive restructuring, and relapse prevention. Using intention-to-treat (ITT) analyses with the entire randomized sample, about 38% of each group exhibited clinically significant improvements after treatment and 44% of each group 1 year after the beginning of treatment, but there were no differences between the two treatment conditions on any measure. When examining only those clients who received an "adequate dose" of 24 sessions, there were some significant differences in PTSD symptoms between conditions, and it appeared that the differences were larger in the latter cohorts of the study than in the first cohort, perhaps a practice effect by therapists. In considering the modest findings and lack of differences between the CBT and control condition, the investigators questioned whether the number of exposures in the group setting was adequate, whether more experienced CBT therapists might have made a difference, or whether veterans, with their multiple comorbid conditions, might be a more difficult population to treat.

Ehlers and colleagues (2003) conducted a randomized control trial comparing cognitive therapy, a self-help booklet, and repeated assessments with victims of MVA survivors after a period of self-monitoring. They found that a small percentage of patients (12%) improved by self-monitoring alone. The remaining patients with PTSD were randomized into one of the three conditions approximately 3 months after the MVA. Although the 64-page booklet included cognitive-behavioral principles and education about PTSD, it was found to be less effective (as were repeated assessments only) compared to cognitive therapy. The cognitive therapy was highly effective and had no dropouts. In contrast, the educational self-help approach did not differ from repeated assessment, although both groups did improve. It should be pointed out, though, that this sample of patients with PTSD could still have been in

the natural recovery stage, so the important finding is the clear superiority of the cognitive therapy.

Bryant, Moulds, Guthrie, Dang, and Nixon (2003) compared imaginal exposure, a combination of imaginal exposure and cognitive restructuring, and a supportive counseling therapy with 58 civilian survivors of mixed traumas. The participants received eight 90-minute sessions. In the combined condition, therapists began with the cognitive therapy focusing on catastrophic beliefs about the trauma and skills training to challenge participants' beliefs. They spent 25 minutes of each session on the cognitive component. Bryant and colleagues found that the combination resulted in lower PTSD scores and better end-state functioning than the imaginal exposure condition only, which performed better than the supportive psychotherapy. They concluded that the addition of cognitive therapy enhanced treatment effectiveness.

In contrast, a recent study compared PE and PE plus present-focused cognitive restructuring (Foa et al., 2005). This study examined treatment in a sample of female sexual or physical assault survivors treated in either a community rape crisis center or an academic treatment center. Foa and her colleagues found no differences between PE and PE plus cognitive restructuring, although both showed marked improvement compared to the waiting-list control. They also found no differences in the effects of treatment based on the setting in which the treatment was provided. In a second study that examined a larger range of Axis II disorders, Hembree, Cahill, and Foa (2004) examined data from the Foa and colleagues (2005) study. A second purpose of the study was to compare the effectiveness of expert research therapists and community counselors on these comorbid conditions. They found that 39% of the 75 participants met criteria for at least one personality disorder, that there were no significant differences in PTSD outcome at posttreatment, that those without personality disorders tended to have better end-state functioning, but that community counselors tended to have better results than the research therapists with comorbid clients. The main results of this study contrast those of Bryant and colleagues (2003) in which the cognitive intervention enhanced the results of exposure alone. However, it is possible that the cognitive intervention in Bryant and colleagues was more trauma-focused than the present-oriented cognitive restructuring of the Foa and colleagues study, and that the different type of cognitive intervention may make a difference.

Chard (2005) expanded CPT to work with the range of problems observed in adults who were sexually abused as children (CPT-SA). In addition to the core CPT protocol, Chard provided the treatment in a combination of group and individual therapy in a 17-week protocol. The group supports the cognitive therapy and compliance with homework, whereas the detailed written exposure and cognitive challenging occurred in the individual therapy. This protocol also added modules for examining preexisting family "rules" and developmental abilities, communication skills, and social support. Compared with the waiting-list control group, which did not change, the CPT-SA was very successful. Sixty percent of the ITT and 93% of the treatment completer samples remitted from their PTSD by posttreatment, and their treatment gains were maintained through the 1-year follow-up.

Monson and colleagues (2006) conducted a waiting-list controlled study of CPT in male and female veterans with chronic, military-related PTSD. CPT was superior to waiting-list in reducing PTSD and comorbid symptoms; 40% of the ITT sample receiving CPT no longer met criteria for a PTSD diagnosis at the end of treatment. Monson and colleagues also found that PTSD-related disability status was not associated with the outcomes. This trial provides some of the most encouraging results to date in the treatment of veterans with military-related PTSD.

Finally, another multisite study conducted within the VA with women veterans compared PE to a present-centered therapy (PCT) control condition (Schnurr et al., 2007). The PCT condition was an active treatment that provided nonspecific control for attending therapy and having a relationship with a therapist but did not have a specific intervention beyond focusing on present life circumstances. Unlike the first multisite VA study (Schnurr et al., 2003), which used an untested CBT group treatment, this study implemented treatment individually with PE, which had been established to be efficacious. Similar to the Monson and colleagues (2006) study, 41% of the female veterans remitted from their PTSD diagnosis as a result of treatment. Schnurr and colleagues (2003) also found that neither having a service-connected

disability as a result of PTSD nor being a survivor of military sexual trauma specifically affected the outcomes of treatment. The PE and PCT conditions differed at posttreatment and at 3-month follow-up but not at 6-month follow-up on overall PTSD symptoms. This lack of statistical difference at 6-month follow-up was not because the PE group worsened; rather, the PCT group continued to improve. These findings speak to the power of the nonspecific elements of good psychotherapy. Future studies will need to focus on parsing out the active intervention components of the therapeutic relationship and other nonspecific factors, such as repeated assessments.

Therapist, Client, and Setting Variables

Gender and Ethnicity

According to the recent National Comorbidity Survey Replication study (Kessler, Berglund, et al., 2005) lifetime prevalence rates of PTSD are nearly three times higher in women (9.7%) compared with men (3.6%). The recent Tolin and Foa (2006) meta-analysis of sex differences in risk for potentially traumatic events and PTSD indicated that females were more likely than males to meet criteria for PTSD but less likely to have experienced potentially traumatic events. Females were more likely than males to experience sexual assault and child sexual abuse but less likely to experience accidents, nonsexual assaults, witnessing death and injury, disaster or fire, and war-related trauma. Within specific types of traumatic events, females still exhibited greater PTSD, suggesting that risk of exposure to particular types of trauma only partially explains the differential PTSD risk in males and females.

Because sexual assault is predominantly perpetrated by men, and is a highly personal and intimate crime, survivors of sexual assault often distrust men. Consequently, the issue of therapist gender can be relevant. Frequently, clients prefer or insist on a female therapist. The effectiveness of male therapists has not been studied specifically, but they may be quite effective, if well trained (Resick, Jordan, Girelli, Hutter, & Marhoeder-Dvorak, 1988). Issues for male therapists, discussed by Silverman (1977) and Koss and Harvey (1991), include the tendency for men to view rape more as a sexual crime than as a crime of violence (Burt, 1980), therefore focusing too much on sexual aspects of the experience and its aftermath.

In treating survivors of sexual assault, regardless of therapist gender, it is essential that the therapist be knowledgeable about rape and PTSD. This includes the literature on reactions to rape, rape myths, and attitudes about rape. Therapists bring their culturally learned perceptions with them, as do clients, and these can interfere with their effectiveness if they adhere to any of the common misperceptions about rape (e.g., rape is primarily about sex, most rapists are strangers, it is not rape unless the woman actively resists). Sexual assault survivors are extremely sensitive to insinuations that they might have been to blame, for example, and many drop out of treatment if they sense that the therapist might harbor victim-blaming attributions.

Similarly, combat veterans are often hesitant to start treatment with novice therapists who may not know particular war details or relevant history. It is important for therapists to acknowledge their level of familiarity and work with clients to understand more fully their trauma experiences and the context surrounding them.

The role of ethnicity in CBT for PTSD has received little attention in outcome research. This limitation, unfortunately, is not restricted to PTSD treatment research; the minority-focused supplement of the Surgeon General's report on mental health (U.S. Department of Health and Human Services, 2001) made clear that there is a paucity of empirical research on treatment for depression and anxiety in minorities. The few studies of prevalence rates among ethnic groups have shown mixed results that, in part, may reflect differential rates of trauma exposure (Breslau, Davis, & Andreski, 1995; Norris, 1992).

Two program evaluation studies compared African American and European American male veterans with PTSD. Rosenheck, Fontana, and Cottrol (1995) found less improvement among African American veterans on some measures. However, Rosenheck and Fontana (1996) did not support this finding. Only one study to date has examined the efficacy of CBT with African American women with PTSD. Zoellner, Feeny, Fitzgibbons, and Foa (1999) compared African American and European American women who were survivors of either sexual or nonsexual assault. Treatment comprised PE, SIT, or a combination of the two. There were no ethnic group differences in treatment efficacy. These results were achieved in spite of an inability to match clients and therapists on ethnicity. Although these results are encouraging, continued attention to ethnic and cultural issues in treatment is important (see McNair & Neville, 1996).

Vicarious Traumatization

Working with trauma victims can have negative effects on therapists that are similar to problems experienced by their clients. This has been labeled "secondary" or "vicarious" traumatization. McCann and Pearlman (1990) discussed this impact as disruption of the therapist's own cognitive schemas about self and the world. Hearing clients' traumatic experiences may be shocking and lead to lasting alterations in assumptions and expectations, which in turn affect therapists' feelings, behaviors, and relationships. Working with trauma victims may challenge therapists' assumptions about personal invulnerability and safety, as well as beliefs that the world is a meaningful, orderly place filled with trustworthy people. According to McCann and Pearlman's model, an individual therapist's reaction depends on the degree of discrepancy between the survivor's trauma and the therapist's cognitive schemas. For example, if the therapist's own complex experiences have led to the development of safety assumptions (schemas) as central to his or her well-being, working with trauma survivors may be distressing due to a heightened sense of vulnerability. In addition, the therapist's memory system may be altered to incorporate traumatic imagery that can become intrusive.

To counteract the effects of vicarious traumatization, therapists should be prepared to recognize and acknowledge these effects and take steps to deal with them. McCann and Pearlman (1990) recommend the use of one's professional network as a source of support and to prevent isolation. Talking to other professionals who work with trauma survivors is especially useful, because they can help the therapist to recognize the effects of vicarious traumatization and to normalize these reactions. Other coping strategies suggested by McCann and Pearlman include balancing one's caseload with trauma and nontrauma cases, engaging in other professional and personal activities, recognizing one's own limitations, working for social change, and focusing on the positive personal impact of work with trauma survivors and ways it can enrich one's life.

"Resistance"

Clients with PTSD can be notoriously difficult due to their ambivalence about therapy. They want help, but they fear confronting their memories and have difficulty trusting others, including therapists. They may also have strong feelings of shame about the traumatic event that interfere with their willingness to disclose information that they feel may lead to rejection by others. Of course, it is important to remember that avoidance behaviors, including avoiding thoughts about the trauma, are part of the criteria for PTSD. Therefore, it is to be expected that avoidance will also occur in the context of treatment. No-shows are common, and both subtle and obvious avoidance behaviors are seen throughout the beginning stages of therapy. If possible, therapists should consider treatment as starting on the telephone prior to the first session. The no-show rate is likely to decrease if the therapist expresses understanding of the client's hesitance to come in and encourages attendance. Early in therapy, the therapist should describe avoidance as a symptom of PTSD and an ineffective, though understandable, means of coping. Labeling this as "resistance" likely only increases judgmentalness toward the client and hinders therapist effectiveness. This and other challenges in working with rape trauma survivors are discussed by Koss and Harvey (1991) and Kilpatrick and Veronen (1983). Shay and Munroe (1999) discuss the challenges of working with combat veterans with complex PTSD.

Multiply Traumatized Victims

The treatment approaches presented here have been shown to produce significant improvement in civilian trauma victims within a brief time. Moreover, in a secondary analysis of Resick and colleagues' (2002) trial, Resick and colleagues (2003) showed that patients with childhood sexual abuse experiences in addition to their adult index trauma had significant improvements in their PTSD. In recent years, there has been a surge in evidence of treatment success in individuals with more chronic or repeated trauma histories, such as domestic violence (Kubany et al., 2004), combat (Monson et al., 2006), and long-standing childhood sex-

ual abuse (Chard, 2005; Cloitre et al., 2004). This research points to the utility of evidence-based treatment for complex cases and debunks the myth that cognitive-behavioral treatments only work for "simple" cases of a single trauma. That said, therapists should be aware of attending to special issues in working with these cases. For example, some research suggests that PTSD in sexual assault trauma survivors may play a role in repeat traumatization (e.g., Kilpatrick et al., 1987), although this relationship appears to be complex (Wilson, Calhoun, & Bernat, 1999). Survivors of child sexual abuse may present additional challenges (Cloitre, 1998), because their traumatization may have interfered with processes of normal development. Given that the abuse often involves a relative or trusted adult, it represents a serious betrayal by someone on whom the child depended for basic safety and protection. They may need more help with skills development as well, especially interpersonal and emotion regulation skills. In some cases, sexual dysfunctions must be addressed. This can be added to an individual treatment program or the client may be referred to a sex therapy specialist, but only after the treatment for other trauma-related problems is complete. Veterans may present with issues specific to committing acts of violence or killing others, distrust of the government and authority figures, ethnic/racial stereotyping, and protracted grief reactions (Monson, Price, & Ranslow, 2005).

Group Treatment

The decision whether to use a group or an individual format for treatment is usually made on the basis of clinical judgment and practicality. There is scant research comparing the two procedures. Most interventions that have been used with trauma victims are adaptable for use in either format. Recent research has shown that standardized group treatments may be successful for combat veterans and child sexual abuse trauma survivors (Chard, 2005; Creamer, Morris, Biddle, & Elliott, 1999).

Group treatment has several advantages that make it popular among both trauma survivors and professionals. Koss and Harvey (1991) discussed a number of these. Group treatment reduces the sense of isolation felt by most survivors, who withdraw from interactions and believe that others cannot understand their feelings. It provides social support that is unambiguous and nonblaming. It helps to validate and to normalize feelings and reactions to the trauma. Group treatment confirms the reality of the traumatic experience and allows sharing of coping strategies. It counteracts self-blame and promotes self-esteem. Because it is more egalitarian than individual therapy, group treatment can promote reempowerment and decrease dependency. It provides a safe environment for developing attachment and intimacy with others and an opportunity for sharing grief and loss. Finally, group treatment can help trauma survivors assign meaning to the event, promoting cognitive processing.

Group approaches have drawbacks as well, and care should be taken to screen clients to assess their readiness for joining a group. McCann and Pearlman (1990) suggest that clients with severe PTSD should be in individual therapy simultaneously with group treatment, because groups may elicit strong affect and memories that can overwhelm an unprepared client. For similar reasons, Resick and Markaway (1991) warn against having group members share their rape experiences during the first few sessions. Although important for recovery, the sharing of "war stories" should be done later in the group process or in individual sessions, to avoid frightening other group members or sensitizing them to other vulnerable situations. Poor candidates for group treatment, as suggested by Koss and Harvey (1991) and McCann and Pearlman (1990), are suicidal clients, those with heavy substance abuse problems, self-mutilating or substance-abusing clients with a borderline personality disorder diagnosis, clients with very unstable, disorganized lives, and clients who have never before spoken about the trauma or whose memory of it is incomplete.

CASE STUDY

"Tom" is a 23-year-old single, white male who presented for treatment approximately 1 year after a traumatic event that occurred during his military service in Iraq. Tom received CPT while on active duty in the Army.

Background

Tom was born the third of four children to his parents. He described his father as an alcoholic who was frequently absent from the home due to work travel prior to his parents' divorce. Tom indicated that his father was always emotionally distant from the family, and especially after the divorce. Tom had close relationships with his mother and siblings. He denied having any significant mental health or physical health problems in his childhood. However, he described two significant traumatic events in his adolescence. Specifically, he described witnessing his best friend commit suicide by gunshot to the head. Tom indicated that this event severely affected him, as well as his entire Midwestern community. He went on to report that he still felt responsible for not preventing his friend's suicide. The second traumatic event was the death of Tom's brother in an automobile accident when Tom was 17 years old. Tom did not receive any mental health treatment during his childhood or after these traumatic events, though he indicated that he began using alcohol and illicit substances after these traumatic events in his youth. He admitted to using cannabis nearly daily during high school, as well as daily use of alcohol, drinking as much as a 24-pack of beer per day until he passed out. Tom reported that he decreased his alcohol consumption and ceased using cannabis after his enlistment.

Tom served in the Infantry. He went to Basic Training and then attended an advanced training school prior to being deployed directly to Iraq. While in Iraq, Tom witnessed and experienced a number of traumatic incidents. He spoke about fellow soldiers who were killed and injured in service, as well as convoys that he witnessed being hit by improvised explosive devices (IEDs). However, the traumatic event that he identified as most distressing and anxiety-provoking was shooting a pregnant woman and child.

Tom described this event as follows: There had been suicide bombers who detonated several bombs in the area where Tom served, and a control point had been set up to contain the area. During the last few days of his deployment, Tom was on patrol at this control point. It was dark outside. A car began approaching the checkpoint, and officers on the ground signaled for the car to stop. The car did not stop in spite of these warnings. It continued to approach the control point, entering the area where the next level of Infantrymen were guarding the entrance. Per protocol, Tom fired a warning shot into the air to stop the approaching car, but the car continued toward the control point. About 25 yards from the control point gate, Tom and at least one other soldier fired upon the car several times.

After a brief period of disorientation, a crying man with clothes soaked with blood emerged from the car with his hands in the air. The man quickly fell to his knees, with his hands and head resting on the road. Tom could hear the man sobbing. According to Tom, the sobs were guttural and full of despair. Tom looked over to find in the pedestrian seat a dead woman who was apparently pregnant. A small child in the backseat was also dead. Tom never confirmed this, but he and his fellow soldiers believed that the man crying on the road was the husband of the woman and the father of the child and fetus.

Tom was immediately upset by the event, and a Combat Stress Control unit in the field eventually had him air-lifted from the field because of his increasing reexperiencing and hypervigilance symptoms that were beginning to have a paranoid quality. Tom was brought to a major Army hospital and received individual CPT within this setting.

Tom was administered the CAPS at pretreatment; his score was in the severe range, and he met diagnostic criteria for PTSD. He also completed the Beck Depression Inventory (BDI) and the State–Trait Anxiety Inventory (STAI). His depression and anxiety symptoms at pretreatment were in the severe range. Tom was provided feedback about his assessment results in a session focused on an overview of his psychological assessment results and on obtaining his informed consent for a course of CPT. After providing feedback about his assessment, the therapist gave Tom an overview of CPT, with an emphasis on its trauma-focused nature, expectation of homework compliance, and the client's active role in getting well. Tom signed a "CPT Treatment Contract" detailing this information, and was provided a copy of the contract for his records. The CPT protocol began in the next session.

Session 1

Tom arrived 15 minutes prior to his first scheduled appointment of CPT. He sat down in the chair that the therapist gestured that he sit in, but he was immediately restless and repositioned frequently. Tom quickly asked to move to a different chair in the room, so that his back was not facing the exterior door and his gaze

could monitor both the door and the window. He asked the therapist how long his session would take and whether he would have to "feel anything." The therapist responded that this session would last 50–60 minutes, and that, compared to other future sessions, she would be doing most of the talking. She added that, as discussed during the treatment contracting session, the focus would be on Tom's feelings in reaction to the traumatic event, but that the current session would focus less on this. The therapist also explained that she would have the treatment manual in her lap, and would refer to it throughout to make sure that she delivered the psychotherapy as it was prescribed. The therapist also encouraged Tom to ask any questions he might have as the session unfolded.

The therapist explained that at the beginning of each session, they would develop an agenda for the session. The purposes of the first therapy session were to (1) describe the symptoms of PTSD; (2) give Tom a framework for understanding why these symptoms had not remitted; (3) present an overview of treatment to help Tom understand why homework completion and therapy attendance were important, to elicit cooperation, and to explain the progressive nature of the therapy; (4) build rapport between the client and therapist; and (5) give the client an opportunity to talk briefly about Tom's worst traumatic event or other issues.

The therapist then proceeded to give didactic information about the symptoms of PTSD. She asked Tom to provide examples of the various clusters of PTSD symptoms that he was experiencing, emphasizing how reexperiencing symptoms are related to hyperarousal symptoms, and how hyperarousal symptoms elicit a desire to avoid or become numb. The paradoxical effect of avoidance in maintaining, or even increasing, PTSD symptoms was also discussed. Tom indicated that this was the first time someone had specifically explained the symptoms of PTSD to him, and put them "in motion" by describing how they interact with one another.

The therapist transitioned to describe trauma aftereffects within an information processing framework. She described how traumas may be schema-discrepant events; traumatic events often do not fit with prior beliefs about oneself, others, or the world. To incorporate this event into one's memory, the person may alter one's perception of the event (assimilate the event into an existing belief system). Examples of assimilation include looking back on the event and believing that some other course of action should have been taken ("undoing" the event) or blaming oneself because it occurred. The therapist went on to explain that Tom could have also attempted to radically change his prior belief system to overaccommodate for the event. "Overaccommodation" was described as changing beliefs too much as a result of the traumatic event (e.g., "I can't trust myself about anything"). She explained that several areas of beliefs are often affected by trauma, including safety, trust, power/control, esteem, and intimacy. The therapist described how people have beliefs in these areas regarding themselves and others, and that beliefs in both areas could be affected. The therapist also pointed out that if Tom had negative beliefs prior to the traumatic event relative to any of these topics, the event could serve to strengthen these preexisting negative beliefs.

At this point, Tom described his childhood and adolescent experiences, and how they had contributed to his premilitary trauma beliefs. The therapist noted that Tom tended to blame himself and to internalize the bad things that had happened in his family, and the suicide of his friend. She also noted his comment, "I wonder if my father drank to cope with me and my siblings." In Tom's case, it seemed likely that the traumatic experience served to confirm further his preexisting beliefs that he had caused or contributed to bad things happening around and to him.

Tom then spent some time describing how drastically things had changed after his military traumas. Prior to his military experiences and, specifically, the shooting of the woman and child, Tom described himself as "proud of being a soldier" and for "pulling his life together." He indicated that the military structure had been very good for him in developing self-discipline and improving his self-esteem. He indicated that he felt good about "the mission to end terrorism" and was proud to serve his country. He felt camaraderie with his fellow soldiers and considered a career in the military. He denied any authority problems and in fact believed that his commanding officers had been role models of the type of leader he wished to be. Prior to his deployment to Iraq, Tom met and married his wife, and they appeared to have a stable, intimate relationship. After his return from Iraq, Tom indicated that he did not trust anyone, especially anyone associated with the U.S. Federal government. Tom expressed his disillusionment with the war effort and distrust of the individuals who commanded his unit. He also articulated distrust of himself: "I always make bad decisions when the chips are down." He stated that he felt completely unsafe in his environment. At times in his immediate postdeployment, Tom had believed snipers on the base grounds had placed him in their crosshairs to kill him. He indicated that he minimally tolerated being close to his wife, including sexual contact between the two of them.

The therapist introduced the notion of "stuck points," or ways of making sense of the trauma or of thinking about himself, others, and the world, getting in the way of Tom's recovery from the traumatic events. The therapist noted that a large number of individuals are exposed to trauma. In fact, military personnel are among the most trauma-exposed individuals. However, most people recover from their trauma exposure. Thus, a primary goal of the therapy was to figure out what had prevented Tom from recovering (i.e., how his thinking had got him "stuck," leading to the maintenance of his PTSD symptoms).

The therapist then asked Tom to provide a 5-minute account of his worst traumatic event. Tom immediately responded, "There were so many bad things over there. How could I pick one?" The therapist asked, "Which of those events do you have the most thoughts or images about? Which of those events do you dislike thinking about the most?" The therapist indicated that Tom did not need to provide a fine-grained description of the event, but rather a brief overview of what happened. Tom provided a quick account of the shooting of the woman and child. The therapist praised Tom for sharing the account with her and asked about his feelings as a result of sharing the information. Tom said that he felt anxious and wanted the session to be over. The therapist used this as an opportunity to describe the differences between "natural" and "manufactured" emotions.

The therapist first described "natural" emotions as those feelings that occur in response to events that are normal or that occur naturally. For example, if we perceive that someone has wronged us, it is natural to feel anger. If we encounter a threatening situation, it is natural to feel fear. Natural emotions have a self-limited and diminishing course. If we allow ourselves to feel these natural emotions, they will naturally dissipate. The therapist used the analogy of the energy contained in a bottle of carbonated soda to illustrate this concept. If the top of the bottle is removed, the pressure initially comes out with some force, but that force subsides and eventually has no energy forthcoming. On the other hand, there are "manufactured" emotions, or emotions that a person has a role in making. Our thoughts contribute to the nature and course of these emotions. The more that we "fuel" these emotions with our self-statements, the more we can increase the "pressure" of these emotions. For example, if a person tells himself over and over that he is a stupid person and reminds himself of more and more situations in which he perceived that he made mistakes, then he is more likely to have more and more anger toward himself. The therapist reiterated that the goals of the therapy were (1) to allow Tom to feel the natural emotions that he has "stuffed," which keep him from recovering from his trauma; and (2) to figure out how Tom was manufacturing emotions that were not helpful to him.

The therapist summarized for Tom the three major goals of the therapy: (1) to remember and to accept what happened to him by not avoiding those memories and associated emotions; (2) to allow himself to feel his natural emotions and let them run their course, so the memory could be put away without such strong feelings still attached, and (3) to balance beliefs that had been disrupted or reinforced so that Tom did not manufacture unhelpful emotions.

The therapist made a strong pitch for the importance of homework compliance before assigning Tom the first practice assignment. The therapist told Tom that there appeared to be no better predictor of response to the treatment than how much effort a patient puts into it. She pointed out that of the 168 hours in a week, Tom would be spending 1–2 hours of that week in psychotherapy sessions (*Note.* We have found it helpful to do twice-weekly sessions, at least in the initial portion of the therapy, to facilitate rapport building, to overcome avoidance, and to capitalize on early gains in the therapy.) If Tom only spent the time during psychotherapy sessions focused on these issues, he would be spending less than 1% of his week focused on his recovery. To get better, the therapist used daily worksheets or other writing assignments to promote needed skills into Tom's

daily life and decrease his avoidance. The therapist also pointed out that at the beginning of each session they would review the homework Tom has completed. The therapist asked Tom if this made sense, and he responded, "Sure. It makes sense that you get out of it what you put into it."

Tom's first assignment was to write an Impact Statement about the meaning of the event to determine how he had made sense of the traumatic event, and to help him begin to determine what assimilation, accommodation, and overaccommodation had occurred since the event. Stuck points that get in the way of recovery are identified with this first assignment. Tom was instructed to start writing the assignment later that day to address directly any avoidance about completing the assignment. He was specifically reminded that this was *not* a trauma account (that would come later) and that this assignment was specifically designed to get at the meaning of the event in his life, and how it had impacted his belief systems.

The specific assignment was as follows:

Please write at least one page on what it means to you that you that this traumatic experience happened. Please consider the effects that the event has had on your beliefs about yourself, your beliefs about others, and your beliefs about the world. Also consider the following topics while writing your answer: safety, trust, power/competence, esteem, and intimacy. Bring this with you to the next session.

Session 2

The purposes of the second session are (1) to discuss the meaning of the event and (2) to help Tom begin to recognize thoughts, label emotions, and see the connection between what he says to himself and how he feels. Tom arrived with obvious anger and appeared defensive throughout most of the session. He stated that he had been feeling quite angry all week, and that he was "disgusted" with society and particularly politicians, who were "all self-interested or pandering to those with money." He expressed a great deal of anger over the reports of alleged torture at Abu Ghraib prison, which was a major news item during his therapy. The therapist was interested in the thinking behind Tom's anger about the events at Abu Ghraib. However, she first reviewed Tom's practice assignment, writing the first Impact Statement, to reinforce the completion of homework and to maintain the session structure she had outlined in the first session.

The therapist asked Tom to read his Impact Statement aloud. Clients in individual CPT are always asked to read their homework assignments aloud. Should the therapist read them, the client could dissociate or otherwise avoid his or her own reactions to their material. Tom had written:

The reason that this traumatic event happened is because I was friggin' stupid and made a bad decision. I killed an innocent family, without thinking. I murdered a man's wife and child. I can't believe that I did it. I took that man's wife and child, and oh, yeah, his unborn child, too. I feel like I don't deserve to live, let alone have a wife and child on the way. Why should I be happy when that man was riddled with despair, and that innocent woman, child, and unborn child died? Now, I feel like I'm totally unsafe. I don't feel safe even here on the hospital grounds, let alone in the city or back home with my family. I feel like someone is watching me and is going to snipe at me and my family because the terrorists had information about the situation and passed it on. I also don't feel that people are safe around me. I might go off and hurt someone, and God forbid it be my own family. With my wife pregnant, I am really concerned that I might hurt her. I don't trust anyone around me, and especially the government. I don't even trust the military treating me. I also don't trust myself. If I made a bad decision at that time, who is to say that I won't make a bad decision again? About power and control, I feel completely out of control of myself, and like the military and my commanding officer have complete control over me. My self-esteem is in the toilet. Why wouldn't it be given the crappy things that I have done? I don't think there are many positive things that I've done with my life, and when the chips are down, I always fail and let others down. I'm not sure what other-esteem is, but I do like my wife. In fact, I don't think she deserves to have to deal with me, and I think they would be better without me around. I don't want to be close to my wife, or anyone else for that matter. It makes me want to crawl out of my skin when my wife touches me. I feel like I'll never get over this. It wasn't supposed to be like this.

The therapist asked Tom what it was like to write and then read the Impact Statement aloud. Tom responded that it had been very difficult, and that he had avoided the assignment until the evening before his psychotherapy session. The therapist immediately reinforced Tom for his hard work in completing the assignment. She also used the opportunity to gently address the role of avoidance in maintaining PTSD symptoms. She asked specific Socratic questions aimed at elucidating the distress associated with anticipatory anxiety, and wondered aloud with Tom about what it would have been like to have completed the homework earlier in the week. She also asked Socratic questions aimed at highlighting the fact that Tom felt better, not worse, after completing the assignment.

Tom's first Impact Statement and the information he shared in the first session made evident the stuck points that would have to be challenged. In CPT, areas of assimilation are prioritized as the first targets of treatment. Assimilation is targeted first, because changes in the interpretation of the event itself are integrally related to the other, more generalized beliefs involved in overaccommodation. In Tom's case, he was assimilating the event by blaming himself. He used the term "murderer" to describe his role in the event, disregarding important contextual factors that surrounded the event. These beliefs would be the first priority for challenging. Tom's overaccommodation is evident in his general distrust of society and authority figures, and in his belief that he made bad decisions in difficult situations. His overaccommodation is also evident in his sense of threat in his environment (e.g., snipers), difficulty being emotionally and physically intimate with his wife, and low esteem for others and himself.

The therapist returned to Tom's anger about Abu Ghraib to get a better sense of possible stuck points, and also to experiment with Tom's level of cognitive rigidity or openness to cognitive restructuring. The following exchange ensued between Tom and the therapist:

THERAPIST: Earlier you mentioned that you were feeling angry about the reports from Abu Ghraib. Can you tell me what makes you angry?

TOM: I can't believe that they would do that to those prisoners.

THERAPIST: What specifically upsets you about Abu Ghraib?

TOM: Haven't you heard the reports? I can't believe that they would humiliate and hurt them like that. Once again, the U.S. military's use of force is unacceptable.

THERAPIST: Do you think your use of force as a member of the U.S. military was unacceptable?

TOM: Yes. I murdered innocent civilians. I am no different than those military people at Abu Ghraib. In fact, I'm worse, because I murdered them.

THERAPIST: "Murder." That's a strong word.

TOM: Yeah?

THERAPIST: From what you've told me, it seems like you killed some people who may or may not have been "innocent." Your shooting occurred in a very specific place and time, and under certain circumstances.

TOM: Yes, they died at my hands.

THERAPIST: Yes, they died, and it seems, at least in part, because of your shooting. Does that make you a murderer?

TOM: Innocent people died and I pulled the trigger. I murdered them. That's worse than what happened at Abu Ghraib.

THERAPIST: (Quietly) Really, you think it is worse?

TOM: Yes. In one case, people died, and in another they didn't. Both are bad, and both were caused by soldiers, but I killed people and they didn't.

THERAPIST: The outcomes are different. I'm curious whether how it happened matters.

TOM: Huh?

THERAPIST: Does it matter what the soldiers' intentions were in those situations, never mind the outcome?

TOM: No. The bottom line is killing versus no killing.

THERAPIST: (Realizing that there was minimal flexibility at this point) I agree that there is no changing the fact that the woman and child died, and that your shooting had something to do with that. However, I think we might disagree on the use of the term "mur-

der." It is clear that their deaths have been a very difficult thing for you to accept, and that you are trying to make sense of that. The sense that you appear to have made of their deaths is that you are a "murderer." I think this is a good example of one of those stuck points that has prevented you from recovering from this traumatic event. We'll definitely be spending more time together on understanding your role in their deaths. I'm not sure "murder" is the right word to describe what happened.

In addition to testing Tom's cognitive flexibility, the therapist also wanted to plant the seeds of a different interpretation of the event. She was careful not to push too far and retreated when it was clear that Tom was not amenable to an alternative interpretation. He was already defensive and somewhat angry, and she did not want exacerbate his defensiveness or possibly contribute to dropout from the therapy.

From there, the therapist described how important it was to be able to label emotions and to begin to identify what Tom was saying to himself. The therapist and Tom discussed how different interpretations of events can lead to very different emotional reactions. They generated several examples of how changes in thoughts result in different feelings. The therapist also reminded Tom that some interpretations and reactions follow naturally from situations and do not need to be altered. For example, Tom indicated that he was saddened by the death of the family; the therapist did not challenge that statement. She encouraged Tom to feel his sadness and to let it run its course. He recognized that he had lost something, and it was perfectly natural to feel sad as a result. At this point Tom responded, "I don't like to feel sad. In fact, I don't like to feel at all. I'm afraid I'll go crazy." The therapist gently challenged this belief. "Have you ever allowed yourself to feel sad?" Tom responded that he worked very hard to avoid any and all feelings. The therapist encouraged Tom. "Well, given that you don't have much experience with feeling your feelings, we don't know that you're going to go crazy if you feel your feelings, right?" She also asked him whether he had noticed anyone in his life who had felt sad, and had not gone crazy. He laughed. The therapist added, "Not feeling your feelings hasn't been working for you so far. This is your opportunity to experiment with feeling these very natural feelings about the traumatic event to see whether it can help you recover now from what has happened."

Tom was given a number of A-B-C Sheets as homework to begin to identify what he was telling himself and his resulting emotions. In the first column under A, "Something happens," Tom was instructed to write down an event. Under the middle column, B, "I tell myself something," he was asked to record his thoughts about the event. Under column C, "I feel and/or do something," Tom was asked to write down his behavioral and emotional responses to the event. The therapist pointed out that if Tom says something to himself a lot, it becomes automatic. After a while, he does not need to think the thought consciously, he can go straight to the feeling. It is important to stop and recognize automatic thoughts to decide whether they either make sense or should be challenged and changed.

Session 3

Tom handed the therapist his homework as soon as he arrived. The therapist went over the individual A-B-C Sheets that Tom had completed and emphasized that he had done a good job in identifying his feelings and recognizing his thoughts. Some of the homework is shown in Figure 2.1.

The purpose of reviewing this homework at this point in the therapy is to identify thoughts and feelings, not to heavily challenge the content of those thoughts. The therapist did a minor correction of Tom's identification of the thought "I feel like I'm a bad person" (bolded in Figure 2.1) as a feeling. She commented that feelings are almost always one word and what you feel in your "gut," and that adding the stem "I feel . . . " does not necessarily make it a feeling. The therapist noticed the pattern of thoughts that Tom tended to record (i.e., internalizing and self-blaming), as well as the characteristic emotions he reported.

The therapist noted the themes of assimilation that again emerged (i.e., self-blame) and chose to focus on mildly challenging these related thoughts. She specifically chose to focus on Tom's thoughts and feelings related to his wife's pregnancy, which ultimately seemed to be related to his assimilation of the traumatic event.

THERAPIST: You don't think you deserve to have a family? Why is that?

TOM: Why should I get to have a family when I took someone else's away?

THERAPIST: OK, so it sounds like this relates to the first thought that you wrote down on the A-B-C Sheet about being a murderer. When you say to yourself, "I took someone else's family away," how do you feel?

TOM: I feel bad.

THERAPIST: Let's see if we can be a bit more precise. What brand of bad do you feel? Remember how we talked about the primary colors of emotion? Which of those might you feel?

TOM: I feel so angry at myself for doing what I did.

THERAPIST: OK. Let's write that down—anger at self. So, I'm curious, Tom, do the other people that you've told about this situation, or who were there at the time, think what you did was wrong?

TOM: No, but they weren't the ones who did it, and they don't care about the Iraqi people like I do.

THERAPIST: Hmm . . . that makes me think about something, Tom. I'm curious, in the combat zone in which you were involved in Iraq, how easy was it to determine who you were fighting?

TOM: Not always particularly easy. There were lots of insurgents who looked like everyday people.

THERAPIST: Like civilians? *Innocent* civilians? (*pause*)

TOM: I see where you are going. I feel like it is still wrong because they died.

THERAPIST: I believe you when you say that it *feels* that way. However, feeling a certain way doesn't necessarily mean that it is based on the facts or the truth. We're going to work together on seeing whether that feeling of guilt or wrongdoing makes sense when we look at the situation very carefully in our work together.

Because the goal is for Tom to challenge and dismantle his own beliefs, the therapist probed and planted seeds for alternative interpretations of the traumatic event but did not pursue

ACTIVATING EVENT A "Something happens"	BELIEF B "I tell myself something"	CONSEQUENCE C "I feel something"
I killed an innocent family.	"I am a murderer."	**I feel like I'm a bad person.** Avoid talking about it.
My wife is pregnant.	"I don't deserve to have a family."	Guilty
Abu Ghraib	"The government sucks."	Angry
Going to therapy	"I'm weak. I shouldn't have PTSD. PTSD is only for the weak."	Angry

Are my thoughts in B *realistic*?

Yes.

What can you tell yourself on such occasions in the future?

?

FIGURE 2.1. A-B-C Sheet.

the matter too far. Although Tom did move some from his extreme stance within the session, the therapist was not expecting any dramatic changes. She focused mostly on being supportive, building rapport, and helping Tom get the connections among thoughts, feelings, and behaviors.

The therapist praised Tom for his ability to recognize and label thoughts and feelings, and said that she wanted Tom to attend to both during the next assignment, which was writing about the traumatic event. Tom was asked to write as homework a detailed account of the event, and to include as many sensory details as possible. He was asked to include his thoughts and feelings during the event. He was instructed to start as soon as possible on the assignment, preferably that day, and to pick a time and place where he would have privacy and could allow himself to experience his natural emotions. Wherever he had to stop writing his account of the event, he was asked to draw a line. (The place where the client stops is often the location of a stuck point in the event, where the client gave up fighting, where something particularly heinous occurred, etc.) Tom was also instructed to read the account to himself every day until his next session. The therapist predicted that Tom would want to avoid writing the account, and procrastinate until as late as possible. She asked him why it would be important for him to do the assignment, and do it as soon as possible. This was a technique to determine how much Tom was able to recount the rationale for the therapy, and to strengthen his resolve to overcome avoidance. Tom responded that he needed to stop avoiding, or he would remain scared of his memory. The therapist added that the assignment was to help Tom get his full memory back, to feel his emotions about it, and for the therapist and client to begin to look for stuck points. She also reassured Tom that although doing so could be difficult for a relatively brief period of time, it would not continue to be so intense, and he would soon be over the hardest part of the therapy.

Session 4

During the settling-in portion of the session, Tom indicated that he had written the account of the event the evening before, although he had thought about and dreaded it every day prior to that. He admitted that he had been avoidant due to his anxiety. The therapist asked Tom to read his account aloud to her. Before starting, Tom asked why it was important to read it in the session. The therapist reminded Tom of what they had talked about the previous session, and added that the act of reading aloud would help him to access the whole memory and his feelings about it. Tom read what he wrote quickly, like a police report, and without much feeling:

There were several of us who were assigned to guard a checkpoint south of Baghdad. We were there because insurgents were beginning to take over the particular area, and we were there to contain the area. I was placed on top of the checkpoint, about 10 feet in the air. It was dusk. It had been a fairly routine day, with people coming through the checkpoint like they were going through a toll booth. Off in the distance I noticed a small, dark car that was going faster than most cars. I could tell it was going faster, because there was more sand smoke kicking up behind it. Men out in front of the checkpoint were motioning for the car to slow down, but it didn't seem to be slowing down. Someone shot into the air to warn them, but they kept on coming. I could see two heads in the car coming toward us. We had been told to shoot at any vehicle that came within 25 yards of the gate to protect those around the gate, and the area beyond the gate. The car kept coming. I shot a bunch of rounds at the car.

At least one other person shot, too. There was so much chaos after that. I remember feeling my gun in my hand as I stood there. After a few moments, I also remember my legs carrying me down to the car. I don't really remember how I got there, but I did. Several men had surrounded the car, and a man got out of it. The man was crying. No, sobbing. He was speaking fast while he cried. He turned toward the car, resisting the men who attempted to remove him from the scene. I turned to see what the man was looking at and saw them for the first time. I saw the woman first.

There was blood everywhere, and her face had been shot. Then I saw the little girl in the backseat slumped over, holding a doll. There was blood all over her too. I saw the gunshots through the car. I looked back at the woman, but avoided looking at her face. I saw a bump under her dress. She was pregnant.

I don't remember much else after that. I know I went back to camp and basically fell apart. They took me off duty for a couple of days, but eventually they sent me back home because I was such a mess.

After reading the account, Tom quickly placed it in his binder of materials and closed the binder as if to indicate that he was ready to move onto something else. The therapist asked Tom what he was feeling, and he indicated that he was feeling "nothing" The therapist followed up, saying, "Nothing at all?" Tom reluctantly admitted that he was feeling anxious. The therapist then asked him to read the account again, but this time to slow down his reading rate, and allow himself to experience the emotions he had felt at the time of the event.

After reading the account for the second time, the therapist sought to flush out details of the event that Tom had "glossed" over and to focus on what appeared to be the most difficult aspects of the situation.

THERAPIST: What part of what you just read to me is the most difficult?

TOM: It is all difficult. The whole thing is horrible.

THERAPIST: What is the worst of it, though?

TOM: I guess the worst of it is seeing that small girl in the backseat of the car.

THERAPIST: What did she look like when you saw her?

(*Tom describes his memory of the girl when he arrived at the car.*)

THERAPIST: Therapist: What are you feeling right now?

TOM: I feel sick to my stomach. I feel like I did at the time—that I want to throw up. I am also disgusted and sad. I killed an innocent child. There are so many things I could have done differently not to have taken her life.

(*The therapist is aware of the assimilation process in Tom's use of hindsight bias. She stores that information away for future reference, because she wants to make sure that Tom is feel-*

ing strongly as many of his natural emotions as possible about the traumatic event.)

THERAPIST: Continue to feel those feelings. Don't run away from them. Anything else that you're feeling?

TOM: I feel mad at myself and guilty.

THERAPIST: Were you feeling mad at yourself and guilty at the time?

TOM: No. I was horrified.

THERAPIST: OK, let's stay with that feeling.

TOM: (*Pauses.*) I don't want to feel this anymore.

THERAPIST: I know you don't want to feel this anymore. You're doing a great job of not avoiding your feelings here. In order to not feel like this for a long time, you need to feel these absolutely natural feelings. Let them run their course. They'll decrease if you stay with them.

After a period in which Tom experienced his feelings related to the situation and allowed them to dissipate, a discussion ensued regarding how hurtful it was to Tom to hear other people's reaction to the war. He expressed specific frustration with the presidential administration and its policy on the war. The therapist gently redirected Tom's more philosophical discussion of international policy to the effects of the trauma on him. He then told a story of how he had shared his traumatic experience with a high school friend. Tom felt that this person had a negative reaction to him as a result of sharing the story. Tom felt judged and unsupported by this friend. Since this experience with his friend, Tom had refrained from telling others about his combat experience. Using Socratic questioning, the therapist asked Tom if there might be any reason, outside of him, that someone might have a negative reaction to hearing about the shooting. Through this exchange, Tom was able to recognize that when others hear about traumatic events, they also are trying to make sense of these experiences in light of their existing belief systems. In other words, others around him might fall prey to the "just world" belief that bad things only happen to bad people. They also might not take into account the entire context in which Tom shot the passengers in the car. This recognition resulted in Tom feeling less angry at his friend for this perceived judgment. He was also somewhat willing to admit that his interpretation of his friend's reaction might have been skewed by his own judgment of himself. In fact, later in the therapy, when Tom was able to ask his friend directly about his reaction, the friend indicated that it had been hard for him to hear, but that he had not been judging Tom at all. In actuality, he was thinking about the terrible predicament Tom had endured at the time.

The therapist asked Tom what stuck points he had identified in writing and reading his account. The following dialogue then occurred:

TOM: I'm not sure what the stuck points are, but from what you've been asking me, I guess you question whether or not I murdered this family.

THERAPIST: That's true. I think it is worthwhile for us to discuss the differences between blame and responsibility. Let's start with responsibility. From your account, it sounds like you were *responsible* for shooting the family. It sounds like other people may have been responsible, too, given that you were not the only person who shot at them.

(*The therapist stores this fact in her mind to challenge Tom later about the appropriateness of his actions. This also provides a good opportunity to reinforce Tom for performing well in a stressful situation.*)

The bottom line is that responsibility is about your behavior causing a certain outcome. *Blame* has to do with your intentionality. It has to do with your motivations at the time. In this case, did you go into the situation with the motivation and intention to kill a family?

TOM: No, but the outcome was that they were murdered.

THERAPIST: Some *died*. From what you've shared, if we put ourselves back into the situation at the time, it was not at all your intention for them to die. They were barreling down the road, not responding to the very clear efforts to warn them to stop. Your own and others' intentions were to get them to stop at the checkpoint. Your intention at the time did not seem to be to kill them. In fact, wasn't your intention quite the opposite?

TOM: Yes (*begins to cry*).

THERAPIST: (*Pauses until Tom's crying subsides somewhat.*) Your intention was not to *kill* them at all. Thus, the word "blame" is not

appropriate. Murder or considering yourself a murderer is not appropriate in this situation. The reason I've questioned the term "murder" or "murderer" all along was because it doesn't seem like your intention at all was to have to shoot at them.

TOM: But why do I feel like I am to blame?

THERAPIST: That's a good question. What's your best guess about why that is?

TOM: (*Still crying*) If someone dies, someone should take responsibility.

THERAPIST: Do you think it is possible to take responsibility without being to blame? What would be a better word for a situation that is your responsibility, but that you didn't intend to happen? If a person shot someone but didn't intend to do that, what would we call that?

TOM: An accident, I guess.

THERAPIST: That's right. In fact, what would you call shooting a person when you are trying to protect something or someone?

TOM: Self-defense.

THERAPIST: Yes, very good. Weren't you responsible for guarding the checkpoint?

TOM: Yeah.

THERAPIST: So, if you were responsible for guarding that checkpoint, and they continued through, wouldn't that have put the area at risk?

TOM: Yes, but it was a family—not insurgents.

THERAPIST: How do you know that?

TOM: There was woman and child in the car.

THERAPIST: Did you know that at the time?

TOM: No.

THERAPIST: So only in hindsight do you know that it was a family that *might* have had no bad intention. We actually don't know the family's intention, do we? They didn't heed the several warnings, right?

TOM: Yes. (*pauses*) I hadn't thought that they would be looking to do something bad with a woman and child in the car.

THERAPIST: We don't know, and won't know, bottom line. However, what we do know is what *you* knew at the time. What you knew at the time is that they did not heed the warnings, that you were responsible for securing the checkpoint, and that you took action when you needed to take action to protect the post. Thinking about those facts of what happened and what you knew at the time, how do you feel?

TOM: Hmm . . . I guess I'd feel less guilty.

THERAPIST: Therapist: You'd feel less guilty, or you feel less guilty?

TOM: When I think through it, I do feel less guilty.

THERAPIST: There may be points when you start feeling guiltier again. It will be important for you to hold onto the facts of what happened versus going to your automatic interpretation that you've had for awhile now. Is there any part of it that makes you proud?

TOM: Proud?

THERAPIST: Yes. It seems like you did exactly what you were supposed to do in a stressful situation. Didn't you show courage under fire?

TOM: It's hard for me to consider my killing them as courageous.

THERAPIST: Sure. You haven't been thinking about it in this way before, but it is something to consider.

The therapist's Socratic questioning was designed to help Tom consider the entire context in which he was operating. She also began to plant seeds that Tom not only did nothing wrong but he also did what he was supposed to do to protect the checkpoint. Whenever possible, pointing out acts of heroism or courage can be powerful interventions with trauma survivors.

Prior to ending the session, the therapist checked Tom's emotional state to make sure he was calmer than he had been during the session. She also inquired about his reaction to the therapy session. He commented that it had been very difficult, but that he felt better than he expected in going into the "nitty-gritty" of what happened. He also noted that there were things that he had not considered about the event that were "food for thought." The therapist praised Tom for doing a great job on the writing assignment and reinforced the importance of not quitting now. She commented that he had completed one of the hardest steps of the therapy, which would help him recover.

The therapist took the first account of the trauma and gave Tom his next homework assignment: to write the entire account again.

The therapist asked Tom to add any details he might have left out of the first account and to provide even more sensory details. She also asked him to record any thoughts and feelings that he was having in the here and now in parentheses, along with his thoughts and feelings at the time of the event.

Session 5

Tom arrived at Session 5 looking brighter and making more eye contact with the therapist. He indicated that he had written the account again, right after the previous session. He commented that the writing was hard, but not as hard as the first time. The therapist used this as an opportunity to reinforce how natural emotions resolve *naturally* as they are allowed expression. Tom noted that he had talked with his wife more this week, avoiding her less. Their increased communication allowed Tom's wife to express her concerns about Tom's well-being. She shared that he seemed disinterested in her and in their unborn child. Tom had previously told his wife about the incident, but he had not shared the specific detail that the woman in the vehicle appeared to be pregnant. Tom perceived his wife as having a very good reaction to his disclosure about the pregnant woman. He noted that she asked him questions, and that her comments indicated that she did not blame him for his actions. For example, she asked, "How could you have known at the time that it was a family?" She also reportedly said, "It's hard to know with terrorism if they were actually just a family traveling." Tom laughed when he reported that their conversation sounded like his last psychotherapy session.

The therapist asked Tom to read his second account out loud, with as many emotions as possible. Tom had written more about the event, and the therapist noted that he had included more information about what he and the other guards had done to warn the passengers in the car to slow down for the checkpoint. Tom read the second account more slowly and was not as tense as he had been the first time he read aloud. Tom's second essay included much more detail and focused more on the vehicle and its occupants after he had fired upon them.

THERAPIST: I notice that you wrote more about the car and the family. What are you feeling about that right now?

TOM: I feel sad.

THERAPIST: Do you feel as sad as you felt the first time you wrote about it?

TOM: I think I may feel sadder about it now.

THERAPIST: Hmm . . . Why do you think that is?

TOM: I think it's like what I wrote in the parenthesis about what I'm thinking now. Now, instead of feeling so much guilt that I shot them, I think it's sad that they didn't heed the warnings.

THERAPIST: You mentioned that you're feeling less guilt now. Why is that?

TOM: I'm beginning to realize that I was not the only one there that was trying to stop them. Several of us were trying to get them to stop. There is still some guilt that *I* was the one who shot them.

THERAPIST: If one of the other guards had shot them, would you blame him or her for the shooting? Would you expect him or her to feel guilty for their behavior?

TOM: (*Laughs.*) I started thinking about that this week. It made me wonder if it was really me who shot them. As I was writing and thinking about it more, I realized that there is a possibility that another of the guards may have been shooting at the same time.

THERAPIST: What would it mean if he or she was shooting at the same time?

TOM: If he was shooting at the same time, it means that he thought that shooting at them might be the right thing to do in that situation.

THERAPIST: *Might* have been the right thing to do?

TOM: (*Smiling*) Yeah, I still have questions that we might have been able to do something else.

THERAPIST: It seems like you're still trying to "undo" what happened. I'm curious, what else could you have done?

TOM: Not have shot at them.

THERAPIST: Then what would have happened?

TOM: They might have stopped. *(pauses)* Or I guess they could have gone through the checkpoint and hurt other people past the checkpoint. I guess they could have also been equipped with a car bomb that could have hurt many other people. That seems hard to believe, though, because of the woman and child in the car.

THERAPIST: It is impossible for us to know their intentions, as we discussed before. The bottom line is that you've tended to assume that doing something different, or doing nothing, would have led to a better outcome.

TOM: That is true. I still feel sad.

THERAPIST: Sure you do—that's natural. I take it as a good sign that you feel sad. Sadness seems like a very natural and appropriate reaction to what happened—much more consistent with what happened than the guilt and self-blame that you've been manufacturing.

Tom and the therapist discussed how the goal of the therapy was not to forget what had happened, but to have the memory without all of the anxiety, guilt, and other negative emotions attached to it. Tom indicated that he was becoming less afraid and more able to tolerate his feelings, even when they were intense. Tom acknowledged that reading his account, talking about his trauma, and coming to psychotherapy sessions were becoming easier and that his negative feelings were beginning to diminish.

After discussing Tom's reactions to his memories, with a focus on how he had attempted to assimilate the memory into his existing beliefs, the therapist began to discuss areas of overaccommodation. One area of overaccommodation was Tom's beliefs about the U.S. military. He had entered the service with a very positive view of the military. Tom had a family history of military service and believed in service to the country and the "rightfulness" of the military. Subsequent to his traumatic event and military service in Iraq, he developed a negative view of the military that had extended to the Federal government in general. The therapist used this content to introduce the first series of tools to help challenge Tom's stuck points. She also emphasized how he would gradually be taking over as his own therapist, capable of challenging his own dysfunctional patterns of thinking that kept him "stuck."

THERAPIST: It seems that you have some very strong beliefs about the military and the U.S. government since your service. I'd like to use those beliefs to introduce some new material that will be helpful to you in starting to challenge stuck points on your own. You've done an outstanding job of considering the way that you think and feel about things. You've been very open to considering alternative interpretations of things. Starting in this session, I'm going to help you to become your own therapist and to attack your own stuck points directly.

TOM: OK.

THERAPIST: Today we will cover the first set of skills. We're going to be building your skills over the next few sessions. The first tool is a sheet called the Challenging Questions Sheet. Our first step is to identify a single belief that you have that may be a stuck point. As I mentioned before, I'd like us to use your beliefs about the Federal government now. So, if you were to boil down what you believe about the Federal government or the military, what is it?

TOM: I don't know. I'm not sure. I guess I'd say that the U.S. military is extremely corrupt.

THERAPIST: Good. That is very clear and to the point. So let's go over these questions and answer them as they relate to this belief. The first question you ask yourself is, "What's the evidence for and against this idea?"

TOM: The evidence for this is Abu Ghraib. Can you believe that they would do that? I would have also put my own shooting under the "for" list, but I'm beginning to question that.

THERAPIST: What other evidence is there of corruption?

TOM: Oh, and these defense contractors . . . what a scam! That leads me to the current administration and its vested interests in going to war to make money on defense contracting. And, oh, of course, to make money on the oil coming out of these countries!

THERAPIST: OK. Sounds like you have some "for" evidence. What about the "against" evidence?

TOM: Well, some of my fellow soldiers were very good. They were very committed in their service and to the mission. I also had mostly good leaders, although some of them were real pigs. Some were really power-hungry a- -holes, frankly.

THERAPIST: So, it sounds like you have some pros and cons that support your belief that the U.S. military is completely corrupt. In the process of changing, it is not uncommon to

have thoughts on both sides. That is great news! It means that you are considering different alternatives, and are not "stuck" on one way of seeing things. Let's take the next one. . . .

The therapist spent the balance of the session going over the list of questions to make sure that Tom understood them. Although most of the questions focused on the issue of corruption in the military, other issues were also brought in to illustrate the meaning of the questions. For example, the therapist introduced the probability questions with the example from Tom's life, in which he was shot by a sniper. These questions are best illustrated with regard to issues of safety. The therapist pointed out that perhaps not all of the questions applied to the belief on which Tom was working. The question "Are you thinking in all-or-none terms?" seemed to resonate with Tom the most, because it applied to his belief about the military. He commented that he was applying a few examples of what seemed to be corruption to the entire military. Tom also indicated that his description of the military as "extremely" corrupt was consistent with the question "Are you using words or phrases that are extreme or exaggerated?" Indicative of his grasp of the worksheet, Tom also noticed that the question "Are you taking selected examples out of context?" applied to his prior view of his behavior as a murder in the traumatic event.

For homework prior to Session 6, Tom agreed to complete one Challenging Questions Sheet each day. He and the therapist brainstormed about potential stuck points prior to the end of the session to facilitate homework compliance. These stuck points included "I don't deserve to have a family," "I murdered an innocent family," and "I am weak because I have PTSD."

Session 6

Tom completed Challenging Questions Sheets about all of the stuck points he and the therapist had discussed. The therapist reviewed these worksheets to determine whether Tom had used the questions as designed. She asked Tom which of the worksheets he had found *least* helpful. He responded that he had had the most difficulty completing the sheet about deserving to have a family. The therapist then reviewed this sheet in detail with Tom (see Figure 2.2).

Challenging Questions Sheet

Below is a list of questions to be used in helping you challenge your maladaptive or problematic beliefs. Not all questions will be appropriate for the belief you choose to challenge. Answer as many questions as you can for the belief you have chosen to challenge below.

Belief: _I don't deserve to have a family._

1. What is the evidence for and against this idea?
   FOR: _I took some other man's family._

   AGAINST: _I didn't want to have to shoot anyone. An "eye for an eye" does not apply here._

2. Is your belief a habit or based on facts?
   It is a habit for me to think this way. The facts are that I didn't do something wrong to deserve to be punished in this way.

3. Are your interpretations of the situation too far removed from reality to be accurate?
   My interpretation of the original situation has been fairly unrealistic, which is where I get this belief.

4. Are you thinking in all-or-none terms?
   _N/A_

5. Are you using words or phrases that are extreme or exaggerated? (i.e., always, forever, never, need, should, must, can't, and every time)
   I guess maybe "deserve" could be an extreme word.

6. Are you taking the situation out of context and only focusing on one aspect of the event?
   Yes, like #3, I tend to forget what all was going on at the time of my shooting.

7. Is the source of information reliable?
   No, I'm not very reliable these days.

8. Are you confusing a low probability with a high probability?
   _N/A_

9. Are your judgments based on feelings rather than facts?
   I'm feeling guilty like I did something wrong when the truth is that I did what I was supposed to do.

10. Are you focused on irrelevant factors?
    Maybe my deserving a family has nothing to do with someone else losing theirs?

FIGURE 2.2. Challenging Questions Sheet.

THERAPIST: So, I notice that in your answer about the evidence for and against this idea about deserving a family, you included as evidence that you took some other man's family. I'm glad to see that you didn't include the word "murder"—that's progress. But, how is that evidence for _you_ not deserving a family?

TOM: It is evidence, because I feel like I took someone else's; therefore, I don't deserve one for myself. It seems fair.

THERAPIST: Remind me to make sure and look what you put for item 9 about confusing feelings and facts. For now, though, help me understand the math of why you don't deserve your family, and your happiness about your family, because of what happened?

TOM: I don't know—it just seems fair.

THERAPIST: Fair? That implies that you did something bad that requires you to be punished.

TOM: As I've been thinking about it more, I don't think I did something wrong when I really look at it, but it still _feels_ like I did something wrong and that I shouldn't have something good like a wife and child in my life.

THERAPIST: Maybe we should look at your response to item 9 now. What did you put in response to the question "Are your judgments based on feelings rather than facts?"

TOM: I said that they were. I wrote, "I'm feeling guilty like I did something wrong when the truth is that I did what I was supposed to do." I try to remember what we talked about, and what my wife also has said to me about them not responding to the warnings and my shooting them, which may have prevented something else that was bad. I still feel bad—not as bad as I did—but I still feel like I did something wrong.

(*The therapist uses this as an opportunity to talk about the need for practicing new alternative thoughts in order to elicit emotional change.*)

THERAPIST: You are well on your way, Tom, to getting unstuck and recovering. Your head is starting to get it, and your feelings need to catch up. You've been thinking about what happened and what you did in a certain way for awhile now. You blamed yourself over and over and over again, telling yourself that you did something wrong. You gave yourself a steady diet of that type of thinking, which resulted in you feeling guilty about what happened. It is like a well-worn rut of thinking in your brain that automatically leads you down the path of feeling guilty. What you need to do now is start a new road of more realistic and truthful thinking about the situation that will eventually be a well-worn path. What is the more realistic view of your role in this event?

TOM: (*Tearfully*) I had to shoot at the car, and people died.

THERAPIST: That's right. And, let's pretend that you really do believe that thought. If so, what would you feel?

TOM: I'd feel so much lighter. I wouldn't feel guilty. I'd continue to feel sad about this horrible situation, but I wouldn't blame myself.

THERAPIST: Let's take it the next step. If you didn't blame yourself and feel guilty, then would you believe that you deserve to be happy with your wife and the baby that will soon be here?

TOM: Sure.

THERAPIST: So, Tom, your work is to practice, practice, practice this new and more accurate way of looking at what happened and your role in it. With practice, your feelings will start matching the truth about what happened and the fact that you are not to blame.

TOM: It is kind of like training to use a weapon. They made us do certain things with our guns over and over and over again, until it was automatic. It was very automatic after awhile.

THERAPIST: That's right. There are other questions on this sheet that might be helpful in convincing you of the truth about this in your practice. What did you put for the question "Is your belief a habit or based on a fact?"

This dialogue illustrates a common occurrence at this stage in the therapy. Tom was starting to experience cognitive change but his emotional change was lagging. The therapist reinforced the need to practice the new ways of thinking to feel different. It is also important to highlight clients' gains in changing their thinking, even if their feelings have not changed or are ambivalent. A change in thinking is framed as more than halfway to a change in feeling. In effect, changed thinking involves competing thoughts or learning, and with more repetitions of the new thought, the associated feeling follow and eventually win out.

In the latter portion of this session the therapist introduced the Patterns of Problematic Thinking Sheet and provided an explanation of how this list was different from the Challenging Questions Sheet (see Figure 2.3). More specifically, she indicated that the Patterns of Problematic Thinking Sheet pertains to more general patterns of thinking versus challenging individual thoughts that Tom might have. The Patterns of Problematic Thinking Sheet lists seven types of faulty thinking patterns (e.g., oversimplifying, overgeneralizing, and emotional reasoning). Tom and therapist went through the list and generated examples for each of the patterns. For example, for "Disregarding important aspects of a situation," the therapist pointed out something that Tom had brought up several times during therapy. Initially Tom had not included the important information that he and the other guards had attempted to stop the car before shooting at it.

Patterns of Problematic Thinking

Listed below are several types of patterns of problematic thinking that people use in different life situations. These patterns often become automatic, habitual thoughts that cause us to engage in self-defeating behavior. Considering your own stuck points, find examples for each of these patterns. Write in the stuck point under the appropriate pattern and describe how it fits that pattern. Think about how that pattern affects you.

1. **Jumping to conclusions** when the evidence is lacking or even contradictory.
   I tend to jump to the conclusion that I have done something wrong when bad things happen. I assume things are my fault.

2. **Exaggeratlng or minimizing** a situation (blowing things way out of proportion or shrinking their importance inappropriately).
   I minimize the things that I have done well in the military.

3. **Disregarding important aspects** of a situation.
   In the past I have tended to neglect the important aspect that several of us tried to stop the car from going through the checkpoint.

4. **Oversimplifying** things as good–bad or right–wrong.
   I can sometimes think of all Iraqis as all bad.

5. **Overgeneralizing** from a single incident (a negative event is seen as a never-ending pattern).
   I have assumed that because of my traumatic event, I could not be safe with my baby to be born.

6. **Mind reading** (you assume people are thinking negatively of you when there is no definite evidence for this).
   I assume that everyone thinks I am a terrible person, a murderer, because of what I did.

7. **Emotional reasoning** (you have a feeling and assume there must be a reason).
   This one is easy—I feel guilty, and therefore I must be.

FIGURE 2.3. Patterns of Problematic Thinking Sheet.

She also pointed out that emotional reasoning was similar to confusing a feeling with a fact, which had been a primary focus of the session.

When they got to the item "Overgeneralizing from a single incident," Tom said that he had noticed he was beginning to change his thoughts about the government and its leaders. He commented that it had been very powerful for him to consider that in a number of instances his fellow soldiers had operated with integrity and were committed to the mission, and to the safety and protection of others. Tom said spontaneously, "I guess that is also kind of like drawing conclusions when evidence is lacking or even contradictory." He said that he had started stereotyping after the traumatic event—applying negative attributes and opinions to everyone in the military and the government too broadly. Tom and the therapist discussed how the goal of the therapy was to have

a balanced and realistic view of things versus an overly ideal version he had pretrauma or the overly pessimistic version he had posttrauma. In other words, the goal was to find shades of gray and balance in his thinking about the government, the military, and their leadership. Tom added an example of this thinking: "There are at least some people in government who want to do good for others."

Tom was given the homework assignment to read over the list in the Patterns of Problematic Thinking Sheet and to note examples of times he used each of the problematic thinking patterns.

Session 7

Tom began the session stating that he was feeling better, and that his wife had also noted a difference in him and was feeling less concerned about the therapy making him worse rather than better. The therapist had given Tom a PCL and BDI to complete while he was waiting for his appointment. She quickly scored these assessment measures and gave Tom feedback about his scores at the beginning of this session. His PCL score had decreased from 68 to 39, which was a clear and clinically meaningful change in his PTSD symptomatology. She noticed that his avoidance and reexperiencing symptoms had decreased the most; his hyperarousal symptoms had also decreased, but less so. His score on the BDI had decreased from 28 to 14, clearly indicating a reduction in his depressive symptoms.

The therapist asked whether Tom had completed his practice assignment, the Patterns of Problematic Thinking Sheet. He indicated that he had not, but that he had thought about it over the week. He also laughed, and said that he had noticed the thinking patterns in his wife and others. The therapist asked Tom to complete some of the sheet in session. At this point in therapy, the therapist was sitting back more as Tom took on the role of challenging his own cognitions. The therapist provided both minimal clarification and also additional examples that she had noticed in working with Tom.

In this session, the therapist introduced the Challenging Beliefs Worksheet. She was careful to point out that the worksheet integrated all of the previous work that Tom had done and added a few new elements. The following dialogue illustrates the introduction of this sheet (see Figure 2.4).

THERAPIST: I want to show you the final worksheet that we're going to be using.

TOM: OK. Wow—that looks complicated!

THERAPIST: Actually, you've done pretty much everything on this worksheet already. This worksheet brings together into one place everything that we've been working on.

TOM: I'll take your word for it, Doc.

THERAPIST: Remember the A-B-C Sheets from way back when?

TOM: Yes.

THERAPIST: (*pointing to first three columns on the Challenging Beliefs Worksheet*) This is A, B, and C. You have in column A the situation, or "Activating Event" that you had on the A-B-C Sheet. In column B you have "Automatic Thoughts," which is the "Belief"

portion of the A-B-C Sheet. Last, column C, "Emotions," the "Consequence" portion of A-B-C Sheet.

TOM: OK. So far, so good.

THERAPIST: Column D is where you identify the "Challenging Questions" from that sheet that apply to the thought or stuck point that you're working on. In column E, you identify the type of "Patterns of Problematic Thinking" that apply to the thought or stuck point that you're working on. Make sense?

TOM: Yes.

THERAPIST: So, only column F, "Alternative Thought," is new. Here you identify alternative thoughts that you could have about the situation. In other words, we're looking for alternative statements that you tell yourself or different interpretations of the event. In columns G and H, you get to see how your belief in your original thoughts may change and how the new thoughts affect your feelings.

TOM: OK.

THERAPIST: So, let's pick a stuck point and start using this Challenging Beliefs Worksheet. We're going to be talking about safety as one of the first topics of the next few sessions. Can you think of a stuck point that relates to your ability to keep yourself safe or to how safe others are around you?

TOM: Well, I still wonder if there are people out in the world who want to hurt me, even if I now realize that no sniper is going to take me out.

THERAPIST: So, let's pick a specific event—the more specific, the better.

TOM: I was in the grocery store, and I had my uniform on. There was this guy who seemed to have a chip on his shoulder about it—like he hated me or something.

THERAPIST: So, write down the event in Column A. (*pauses*) What was your thought? You've already mentioned one of them.

TOM: This guy has a chip on his shoulder about me, because I'm in the military.

THERAPIST: Good. How strongly do you believe that thought?

TOM: 100%

THERAPIST: OK, let's write that next to the thought. We are now rating how much you believe in your thoughts, because you're go-

A. Situation	B. Thoughts	C. Emotion(s)	D. Challenging Thoughts	E. Problematic Patterns	F. Alternative Thought
Describe the event, thought, or belief leading to the unpleasant emotion(s).	Write thought(s) related to Column A. Rate belief in each thought below from 0–100%. (How much do you believe this thought?)		Use **Challenging Questions** to examine your automatic thoughts from Column B. Is the thought balanced and factual or extreme?	Use the **Problematic Thinking Patterns** sheet to decide if this is one of your problematic patterns of thinking.	What else can I say instead of Column B? How else can I interpret the event instead of Column B? Rate belief in alternative thought(s) from 0–100%.
At store in uniform	*"This guy has a chip on his shoulder because I am in the military."* (100%)		Evidence? **Habit or Fact?** *Habit to think everyone dislikes me because I was in Iraq.*	Jumping to conclusions	*"I don't know if he has chip on his shoulder."* (60%)
				Exaggerating or minimizing	
			Interpretations not accurate?	Disregarding important aspects	*"If he does have a chip on his shoulder, I don't know what it is about – maybe it isn't even about me, let alone having served in Iraq."* (80%)
			All or none?	Oversimplifying	
			Extreme or exaggerated?		
			Out of context?	Overgeneralizing	
		C. Emotion(s)	**Source unreliable?** *Me*	**Mind reading** *I am assuming that he is thinking the worst of me.*	**G. Rerate Old Thoughts**
		Specify sad, angry, etc., and rate how strongly you feel each emotion from 0–100%.	Low versus high probability?		Rerate how much you now believe the thought in Column B from 0–100%.
			Based on feelings or facts?	Emotional reasoning	35%
			Irrelevant factors?		**H. Emotion(s)**
		Anger (80%) ***Fear (30%)***			Now what do you feel? 0–100% ***Anger (20%)*** ***Fear (15%)***

FIGURE 2.4. Challenging Beliefs Worksheet completed in session.

ing to see at the end how much your thought has changed. What feeling or feelings are associated with that thought?

TOM: Definitely anger.

THERAPIST: Makes sense given your thought. How much anger from 0 to 100%, with 100% being as much anger as you could possibly imagine having?

TOM: Hmm . . . I'd say 80%.

THERAPIST: Any other feelings? You can have more than one.

TOM: I guess when I stop and think about it, there is some fear there, too.

THERAPIST: That makes sense, too. How much fear from 0 to 100%?

TOM: Oh, maybe 30%. It's not the strongest feeling, but it's there, because I'm wondering if he is going to say something or do something.

THERAPIST: Nice job. Let's move onto the next column that relates to the Challenging Questions Sheet you've already done. Take a look at this list. What questions might apply here?

TOM: I guess I might be confusing a habit with a fact. It seems like it is a habit for me to assume that everyone dislikes me because I was in Iraq. I really don't know if that is why he seemed to have a chip on his shoulder. I guess I also don't know for sure if he had a chip on his shoulder. He didn't say anything to me. (pauses) I guess that is also an example of the source of information being unreliable and that source is me! (Laughs.)

THERAPIST: While you were talking, I was thinking that the same things applied. So you'd write those in this column. You can also pick out other challenging questions that might apply, but usually two or three will do the trick. In the next column, we're going to refer to the Patterns of Problematic Thinking Sheet. What might fit here?

TOM: I guess one jumps out—mind reading.

THERAPIST: How so?

TOM: I'm assuming that he is thinking the worst about me and about my having served my country in this war. I'm good at that.

THERAPIST: Write that down. You can add others later if something seems to apply. The next column is very important. This is where you start coaching yourself to come up with alternative thoughts or perceptions about the situation. Based on having asked yourself these questions and noticing the problematic thinking patterns, what other ways might you think about this situation?

TOM: I guess one thing I could say to myself is, "I don't know if he has chip on his shoulder." I could also say, "If he does have a chip on his shoulder, I don't know what it is about—maybe it isn't even about me, let alone having served in Iraq."

THERAPIST: Wow! You're doing great at this. Let's get those written down. Let's also add how much you believe those two new thoughts. Below those alternative thoughts is the column that asks you to reconsider how much you believe your original thoughts over here in column B. How much do you believe them after walking through this process? Before you said 100%.

TOM: Oh, I'd say now it is only about 35%.

THERAPIST: That is a big change. You went from 100% certainty to 35% certainty that he had a chip on his shoulder, because you fought in the war.

TOM: I'm a little surprised by that myself.

THERAPIST: Let's take it the final step. How about your feelings now? Let's rerate those here.

TOM: My anger is way down—I'd say only about 20%. The anxiety is still there, because I really wouldn't want to have to protect myself, and he might have had a chip on his shoulder at me. It is down a little, though, because I realize I'm not 100% certain he was out to get me. I'd say maybe 15% on fear.

THERAPIST: Do you have questions about what we just did here?

TOM: Not at the moment. I'll get back to you.

THERAPIST: I'm going to ask that you do one of these sheets about stuck points per day, until I see you again. I'm also going to give you some example sheets other patients have done that might be helpful to you.

TOM: OK. Should be interesting. . . .

The therapist reminded Tom that he might find that he is not using problematic thinking, and in that case, no change in feelings would be expected. She also cautioned Tom that he should not expect his beliefs and feelings to change completely in the process of doing the sheet. The old thought would need to be completely dismantled and the new thought would need to become more habitual for him to see a more permanent change. The therapist suggested that Tom read the sheets he completed over to himself a number of times to facilitate the process.

The *Safety* module was then introduced. Safety is the first of five modules (two- to three-page handouts) that also include trust, power, esteem, and intimacy. The therapist oriented Tom to the format of the module, which included discussion about how beliefs about the self and others in this area can be "shattered" or seemingly confirmed after a traumatic event depending on one's history prior to the traumatic event. The modules describe how these problematic beliefs are manifested emotionally and behaviorally (e.g., not leaving one's home because of the belief that the world is unsafe). It also provides alternative self-statements that are more balanced and realistic in each area.

Tom had felt safe with others before the traumatic event occurred, and this sense of safety about others had been disrupted, as evidenced by his sense that others around him were out to get him. Pretrauma, Tom had also felt as though he was not a danger to others. Posttrauma, he believed that he could not be safe with others, which specifically manifested in his concerns about being around his pregnant wife. The therapist suggested that Tom complete at least one worksheet on his stuck points about others being safe, as well as his being a possible danger to others. The therapist also reminded Tom that he needed to finish the Patterns of Problematic Thinking Sheet homework from last session.

Session 8

Tom arrived at the session having completed the Patterns of Problematic Thinking Sheet, as well as two Challenging Beliefs Worksheets. The therapist spent a little time looking at his answers to the Patterns of Problematic Thinking Sheet, because she did not want to send the message inadvertently that completing homework was unimportant. She asked Tom to read the patterns that he had completed at home, as opposed to those in their previous session.

Tom completed two Challenging Beliefs Worksheets related to the topic of safety, as the therapist had instructed. He did one each on

self and other safety beliefs. He did not seem to understand that he could use the Challenging Beliefs Worksheets on everyday events that were distressing or even positive for him. Thus, the therapist emphasized how Tom might use this process more generally in his day-to-day life, and highlighted how more practice would lead to more results. She noted that using the process on less emotionally distressing topics could actually be very helpful in getting the process down. It is always easier to learn something when one is not dealing with the most challenging circumstances. She used a military analogy with Tom, about learning to load and shoot a gun—best learned in a nonconflict situation, so that it is a more rote behavior when under fire.

The therapist skimmed the two sheets Tom had completed and noticed that he had struggled most coming up with alternative statements related to his own sense of dangerousness related to his wife's impending delivery of their child. The following dialogue ensued (see Figure 2.5):

THERAPIST: I notice that you might have had the most trouble coming up with alternative thoughts about how safe you can be with your wife and your child that is about to be born.

TOM: Yeah, I don't really like to talk about it. It freaks my wife out. I'm uncomfortable being around my wife, which makes her feel bad, but I'm just afraid I'm going to hurt her or the child.

THERAPIST: Let's take your first thought, because it is kind of general. How is it that you think you're going to hurt them? Are we talking physically or mentally?

TOM: Oh, physically is what I mean. I don't know how exactly, but somehow, someway, I guess.

THERAPIST: That makes it a bit more concrete. How do you physically think you're going to hurt them? Do you think you'll shoot them, given your trauma history?

TOM: No. Absolutely not. There are no firearms in my house, and I don't go hunting or have friends or family that hunt—nothing that would make guns a part of our life.

THERAPIST: So, what have you considered in your mind?

A. Situation	B. Thoughts	D. Challenging Thoughts	E. Problematic Patterns	F. Alternative Thought
Describe the event, thought, or belief leading to the unpleasant emotion(s).	Write thought(s) related to Column A. Rate belief in each thought below from 0–100%. (How much do you believe this thought?)	Use **Challenging Questions** to examine your automatic thoughts from Column B. Is the thought balanced and factual or extreme?	Use the **Problematic Thinking Patterns** sheet to decide if this is one of your problematic patterns of thinking.	What else can I say instead of Column B? How else can I interpret the event instead of Column B? Rate belief in alternative thought(s) from 0–100%.
	"Out of nowhere, I'll get physically violent." (80%)	Evidence? Habit or fact? Interpretations not accurate? All or none?	Jumping to conclusions **Exaggerating or minimizing** *I'm exaggerating the likelihood that I'd be violent.* Disregarding important aspects	*"It is unlikely that I'll hurt my family, and even more unlikely that it will be sudden and unexpected."* (95%)
	C. Emotion(s)		Oversimplifying	**G. Rerate Old Thoughts**
Being around my wife and child	Specify sad, angry, etc., and rate how strongly you feel each emotion from 0–100%.	Extreme or exaggerated? Out of context? Source unreliable? **Low versus high probability?** *Given my history, it is actually a low probability not high.*	**Overgeneralizing** *I'm assuming because I shot once in a certain situation, I'll be violent in general.*	Rerate how much you now believe the thought in Column B from 0–100%. *10%*
	Fear (85%)	Based on feelings or facts? Irrelevant factors?	Mind reading Emotional reasoning	**H. Emotion(s)** Now what do you feel? 0–100% *Fear (< 10%)*

FIGURE 2.5. Challenging Beliefs Worksheet regarding safety.

TOM: I guess I'm worried that, out of nowhere, I'll get physically violent.

THERAPIST: OK, now we're cooking. Let's write that down. "Out of nowhere I'll get violent." I noticed that in column C you didn't mention anything about probabilities. Safety issues are almost always about gauging probabilities. The world is not a completely safe place, and every day we all make calculated risks about our safety based on the probability of bad things happening to us or to someone else. How do you think the probability questions might apply?

TOM: Are you getting at the idea that I'm confusing a low probability with a high probability?

THERAPIST: Precisely. How do you think that applies here?

TOM: I'm convinced that "somehow, someway" I'm going to hurt my family, so I believe that it is a high probability that it will happen and not a low probability. I think you think that the probability I will do that is low. But, I'm still concerned about it.

THERAPIST: Let's talk about the actual probability. How often have you hurt your family physically?

TOM: Never. Are you kidding?

THERAPIST: I thought as much, but you made it sound like it was very likely to happen. I guess that's part of the problem, right?

TOM: You're right.

THERAPIST: How often have you been physically violent against anyone?

TOM: I haven't. And it surely hasn't been unexpected. Now that we're talking through it, it feels a little silly.

THERAPIST: So, it sounds like figuring out the actual probability of this is right where we needed to go. Given what we've talked about, what is an alternative statement that you can tell yourself and how much do you believe it?

TOM: It is unlikely that I'll hurt my family, and even more unlikely that it will be sudden and unexpected given that it has never happened.

THERAPIST: Let's keep going to see how that might change how you feel. You wrote that you had 85% fear. What is that rating now?

TOM: Less than 10%. There is some fear now that I know that I am capable of hurting a family, but like we've talked about before—and what I have to remember—is that it occurred in a certain situation and not in my everyday life now as a civilian in my family.

This exchange between Tom and the therapist illustrates the hallmark role of probability in assessments and beliefs about safety. It is important to realize that there are some objectively unsafe situations or behaviors, and those should not be minimized or restructured. If there are unreasonable safety precautions or beliefs, the actual probability of harm should be carefully evaluated, keeping in mind that 100% safety is rarely, if ever, guaranteed.

The therapist transitioned the session to introduce the Trust module. Tom noted that he had pretty good trust of himself and others prior to his best friend committing suicide when they were in high school. Tom said that after that experience, he sometimes did not trust his judgments about other people and that he felt responsible for not anticipating his friend's suicide. The military traumatic event served to confirm his belief that he could not trust his judgments about others' intentions. Tom's concerns about his ability to be safe with his wife and unborn child also dovetailed with the issue of trust. The therapist and Tom went over the information in the Trust module handout, and Tom seemed to resonate with all of the potential effects. He reported that he had really been trying to open up with his wife and not avoid her. He noted that they were communicating more, and that made both of them more relaxed and comfortable in the final days of her pregnancy.

The therapist closed the session by assigning daily Challenging Beliefs Worksheets, asking Tom to do at least one on the topic of trust. She reminded him that, like other areas, the goal is to develop balanced alternative thoughts. In the case of trust, she noted that stuck points about trust often revolve around making all-or-none judgments, either trusting or not. The goal is to consider trust as multidimensional, with different types of issues resulting in different levels of trust in different situations.

Session 9

Tom arrived at this session having completed a number of Challenging Beliefs Worksheets. Several of them were about trust, including his level of trust of his government and trust of himself in being a father. He had also used the worksheets on non-trust-related topics relative to his daily life. He commented that the worksheets had been helpful in working out his thinking before he behaved impulsively or felt miserable.

The therapist praised Tom for completing the worksheets so well, and asked Tom whether he needed assistance on any of the worksheets he felt he could use some assistance on. Tom quickly responded that he wanted to focus on the sheet about fatherhood, because he was experiencing so much anxiety about his child's impending birth. In turning their attention to this worksheet, the therapist immediately noticed that Tom had probably struggled with this worksheet, because he had listed so many different types of thoughts that were fueling his anxiety about becoming a father. She used this as an opportunity to fine-tune Tom's use of the worksheets. The therapist's choice in thoughts to challenge first also illustrates the prioritization of treatment targets in the therapy. She chose to go after the more directly trauma-related thoughts that contained remnants of assimilation. Tom's thoughts about deserving to be happy about starting a family, given the death of the woman, fetus, and child, suggested that he had not fully accepted the traumatic event and the circumstances surrounding it. Thus, she addressed this first thought (see Figure 2.6).

THERAPIST: Wow, you've got lots of thoughts going on in your head about becoming a father, don't you? I'm going to suggest that we use different worksheets for each of the clusters of thoughts you're having on this topic. I think that will make your use of the Challenging Beliefs Worksheet better. It seems that some thoughts are directly related to your traumatic experience, others are specifically related to your wife's labor and delivery, and still others are related more generally to being a parent. Let's focus on those that are directly related to your trauma. You wrote that one of your feelings was guilt (85%), and I'm assuming that it is related to your thought that it isn't right that you're happy with a soon-to-be-born baby given what happened.

TOM: That's right. If I'm really honest, I still feel guilty that the Iraqi woman was pregnant and getting ready to have a child, and

the shooting deprived her of the ability to have that child and be happy, and I'm getting ready to have that happiness.

THERAPIST: We've talked about this before, but we've been more focused on the man involved in the situation.

TOM: Yeah, I think the closer my wife gets to delivery, the more I think about the Iraqi woman. I've been imagining that she wasn't part of a potential plot for terrorist activity and was more an innocent participant. Then, I go back and forth, thinking that she might have actually been involved and didn't care that she was pregnant. Or maybe it was just an accident, and they truly didn't understand that they needed to stop. Uggghhhh, it is exhausting.

THERAPIST: And you'll never know. If your friend were saying all of this to you, what would be your response to him?

TOM: I'd be telling him to quit beating himself up and feeling guilty.

THERAPIST: Easier said than done. Anything else? Maybe it would help to look at the Challenging Questions and Patterns of Problematic Thinking Sheets. I'm wondering if you are focusing on irrelevant factors—item 10 on the Challenging Questions Sheet.

TOM: Hmm . . . what is irrelevant in this case?

THERAPIST: How relevant are *her* intentions to deserving to be happy yourself about having a child?

TOM: (*Pauses*) I'm going to have to think about that for a second.

THERAPIST: Aren't *your* intentions in that situation what is relevant? Were your intentions at that time to deprive her of the right to bear her child and live happily ever after?

TOM: No, not at all.

THERAPIST: So, why the guilt? What did you do wrong that you should be punished about?

TOM: Oh, wow. I hadn't thought of that. Her intentions are irrelevant. It only makes me crazy to try to get in her head. I guess that would be mind reading, now wouldn't it?

THERAPIST: Very good—a different spin on mind reading. So what is the alternative, more balanced and realistic thought?

TOM: My intentions are what matter. I didn't intend for her to lose her own or her baby's life.

A. Situation	B. Thoughts	C. Emotion(s)	D. Challenging Thoughts	E. Problematic Patterns	F. Alternative Thought	G. Rerate Old Thoughts	H. Emotion(s)
Describe the event, thought, or belief leading to the unpleasant emotion(s).	Write thought(s) related to Column A. Rate belief in each thought below from 0–100%. (How much do you believe this thought?)		Use **Challenging Questions** to examine your automatic thoughts from Column B. Is the thought balanced and factual or extreme?	Use the **Problematic Thinking Patterns** sheet to decide if this is one of your problematic patterns of thinking.	What else can I say instead of Column B? How else can I interpret the event instead of Column B? Rate belief in alternative thought(s) from 0–100%.		
Killing a pregnant Iraqi woman and her son.	*"It isn't right that I'm happy with a baby on the way, given what happened."* (80%)		Evidence?	Jumping to conclusions	*"My intentions are what matter. I didn't intend to do anything to deprive someone else of family happiness."* (85%)		
			Habit or fact?	Exaggerating or minimizing			
			Interpretations not accurate?	Disregarding important aspects			
			All or none?	Oversimplifying			
	"She might not have been part of a terrorist plot, but just a passenger." (50%)		Extreme or exaggerated?	Overgeneralizing			
			Out of context?				
			Source unreliable?	**Mind reading** *I'm trying to figure out what was in her head.*			
		Specify sad, angry, etc., and rate how strongly you feel each emotion from 0–100%.	Low versus high probability?	Emotional reasoning	Rerate how much you now believe the thought in Column B from 0–100%.		
			Based on feelings or facts?			15% *(2nd doesn't matter)*	
		Guilt (85%)	**Irrelevant factors?** *Her intentions are not relevant. Mine are.*				Now what do you feel? 0–100% *Guilt (5%) Happy (10%)*

FIGURE 2.6. Challenging Beliefs Worksheet regarding trauma.

THERAPIST: Go on . . . don't you have every right in the world to experience happiness?

TOM: I guess so. It just feels weird.

THERAPIST: Sure it does. It is different than what you've been thinking about it for awhile. I'm curious—what would you feel if you said to yourself, "I did not intentionally do anything to deprive someone else of family happiness. I deserve to be happy in becoming a father."

TOM: I'd feel less guilty for sure, and even happy.

THERAPIST: Let's get this all written down. Now you have the job of holding on to these new insights and practicing them. Read over this worksheet every day until you see me again. I'd also like you to take these other thoughts on your original Challenging Beliefs Worksheet about this topic and put them on separate worksheets and work through them. Can you commit to doing that?

TOM: Yes, I already feel lighter.

THERAPIST: This is an exciting time—you've got to continue to work on this, so that you can have the enjoyment you deserve!

At this point, the therapist introduced the Power/Control module. Tom admitted that prior to the traumatic event, he was someone who liked to be in control. He did not like unpredictability, and he noticed that this tendency had gotten especially bad after his friend's suicide. The military lifestyle seemed to be congruent with this tendency. Tom indicated that he had not had authority issues prior to the traumatic event, but he had noticed himself questioning authority much more since his military trauma. As with previous sessions, Tom was given as homework to complete Challenging Beliefs Worksheets every day prior to the next session, and at least one was assigned on power/control.

Session 10

Tom began the session saying that his wife had gone to her obstetrician on the previous day, and that her labor would be induced in 1 week if she did not go into natural labor before then. Tom indicated that the last session had been very good in helping him to become happier about his child's impending birth, and that he had read the Challenging Questions Worksheet about deserving to be happy several times since the last session, and he believed it more and more. He stated that he was still having some anxiety about becoming a father, and about everything going OK with his wife's labor and delivery. The therapist normalized some of Tom's anxiety, stressing how it was very natural for a first-time father, and Tom was able to recognize the typicality of this anxiety in others he had witnessed becoming parents.

Tom stated that since reading the Power/Control module after the last session, he had started to realize that not everyone in authority over him had wielded his or her authority malevolently. This was very important in light of Tom's preexisting history of desiring to exert control; he had directly confronted his illusion of control. The therapist and Tom went over this worksheet.

Tom went on to describe how his belief that he could and *should* have control over everything had resulted in low self-esteem. In general, when things did not go as he desired, Tom felt as though he was a failure for not controlling the outcome. This belief structure led him to think that he should have been able to control his friend and stop him from committing suicide. It also led him to believe that he should have been able to create a positive outcome in the military traumatic event. This discussion served as a natural segue to the next topic— esteem. Tom admitted that he had become someone who thrived too much on accomplishment. This had affected his self-esteem and was especially relevant to his belief that he had not accomplished his goal in the military, because he had to be airlifted out of country after the traumatic event at the checkpoint.

After reviewing the Esteem module, the therapist asked Tom to complete Challenging Beliefs Worksheets on his remaining stuck points, as well as any stuck points relating to esteem. He was also given two other assignments: to practice giving and receiving compliments every day, and to do one nice thing for himself every day that was not contingent on "achieving" something. These assignments were to help him with his self- and other-esteem.

Session 11

Tom completed a worksheet on his self-esteem, related to his belief that he had not achieved his goal within the military. The therapist and Tom went over this worksheet, and both noted that he had made significant progress by using the worksheet to change the way that he thought and felt about himself. He asserted that he was beginning to see that people are much more than their professional accomplishments. They also have other activities and relationships with their families, friends, and themselves.

The therapist inquired about the homework of giving and receiving compliments. Tom replied that it had gone well, even though it felt a bit awkward and forced. He was even able to notice that when he gave compliments and was more positive toward other people, he seemed to get more positive responses back from them. The therapist noticed that several of the compliments were to his wife, and she pointed out that Tom seemed more connected to his wife. He said that he was actually beginning to feel glimmers of excitement about the birth of their child. He reported that he was still feeling some anxiety about becoming a father, and about how the labor and delivery would go, but that the anxiety was less and more manageable. When the therapist asked about Tom *receiving* compliments, he reported more difficulties. She asked what Tom typically did when he received compliments, and it became clear that he often deflected or minimized them. Correspondingly, Tom also said that he had only done one nice thing for himself since the last session, and that it had felt uncomfortable. This pattern seemed to fit with Tom's overall schema of being unworthy and undeserving. The following dialogue related to this:

THERAPIST: It seems like you have a hard time letting someone be nice to you and being nice to yourself.

TOM: Yes.

THERAPIST: Why do you think that is?

TOM: I don't know. *(pauses)* I don't like it. It feels like *they* shouldn't be nice to me, and *I* shouldn't be nice to me.

THERAPIST: Hmm . . . I wonder if there is anything "off" about that thinking? What do you think?

TOM: As I hear myself say it, it sounds a little weird. It sounds like I don't deserve to have nice things for me. Kind of like not deserving to have a family . . .

THERAPIST: This seems like a larger tendency in your life—one of those problematic thinking patterns. What pattern do you hear in your

thinking? Look at the worksheet if you want to.

TOM: Maybe emotional reasoning. I feel like I don't deserve it; therefore, I must not deserve it. That seems like the best one. Maybe I'm also drawing a conclusion when the evidence is lacking.

THERAPIST: I agree. Given how much you seem to follow this pattern of thinking, I'm betting it has been around for awhile—maybe even before the shooting occurred in Iraq.

TOM: It has. I think it had to do with my dad, his alcoholism, and not being close to me. As a kid, I always thought I had done something wrong, or that I was so bad that he didn't want to be around me.

THERAPIST: Now, with adult eyes, what do you think about your dad not being close to you?

TOM: I figure that he drank for a reason, and that it might have been me and my other brothers and sisters.

THERAPIST: Why do you assume that he drank because of you kids?

TOM: I don't know. I figure it was stressful having four kids.

THERAPIST: It probably was at times, but as you hear yourself talk about this, what is amiss in how you've made sense of his drinking and being close to you?

TOM: I know other people who have had four kids and didn't have drinking problems. There were a lot of big families where I grew up. Plus, I know that he and my mom had money problems when we were young, and that they fought a lot.

THERAPIST: So, again, why do you assume it was *you* then that caused his drinking and alienation?

TOM: When we talk about it, I guess I see that it might not have been me alone.

THERAPIST: Or not even you *at all*. Everybody has a choice about how they handle their stress, and it seems that he is distant from everyone, not just you.

TOM: True. It still *feels* that way.

THERAPIST: There seems to be a well-worn path in your brain to assume that when something goes wrong, you blame yourself. The next step is that you deserve to be punished, or at least you don't deserve anything good. I don't think this tendency is going to change overnight. You're going to need to work hard at talking to yourself more rationally to change how you feel. For that new path to get worn, you're going to have to walk down it a number of times. Pretty soon, the path will be more worn and automatic. It will take some effort, but you can change the way you automatically feel. I'd like you to do a Challenging Beliefs Worksheet about what we've just talked about. Once we get a good one about it, you can read and refer to it as part of forging that new path. Can you do that?

TOM: Yes. I think it would be good.

This exchange regarding Tom's dad dovetailed nicely with the final module, Intimacy. The therapist noted that people tend to think of intimacy as it relates to romantic relationships, and especially in terms of sexual intimacy. She stressed that there are all kinds of intimacy with different people. In essence, intimacy relates to how close and open we feel with other people. She went on to discuss the notion of self-intimacy, or how well we take care of, support, and soothe ourselves. In other words, it reflects how good a relationship we have with ourselves. Tom admitted that he struggled with being close to other people, which had most obviously manifested in the work he had done about his wife and child, who was to be born at any moment. As noted earlier, Tom also struggled with doing nice things and taking good care of himself. Both of these areas seemed to be affected by Tom's underlying schema that he was undeserving and unworthy. The therapist assigned daily Challenging Beliefs Worksheets and requested that he do worksheets on being nice to himself and being close to his wife. In addition, she asked Tom to write a final Impact Statement, specifically about his understanding of the trauma now, after all the work he had done. The therapist asked him to write about his current thoughts/beliefs in the areas of safety, trust, power/control, esteem, and intimacy.

Session 12

The day after Session 11, Tom left a message indicating that his wife had delivered a healthy baby girl. He indicated in his voice mail message that he felt happy and relieved. He went on about how beautiful the baby was, how well his wife had done in labor and delivery, and how he had enjoyed holding his daughter in his arms the first time. The 12th session was delayed an extra week because of the baby's arrival.

Tom's wife and new daughter accompanied him to the final session. The therapist spent some time admiring Tom's new baby and congratulating his wife before the final session started. Tom seemed genuinely proud and happy about his daughter, and noted that becoming a father had been more natural than he had anticipated. He commented that he had been worried that he would not want to hold the infant for fear of hurting her or because he would do something wrong. Instead, he found it almost "instinctual" to hold her, and that soothing her had come more naturally than he expected. Tom seemed surprised about how natural his role as a father had become.

The therapist inquired about how the homework had gone. Tom said that he had not done as much as he had hoped given the baby's arrival, but that he had done worksheets about his father and about being close to his wife. The therapist looked over these worksheets, which Tom had done very well. She asked Tom about how helpful they had been, and he reported that they had been very helpful. He added that he was still struggling about his father, but that he was beginning to think that it was not all about him, which had made him feel better about himself and less guilty in general. He mentioned that he was considering writing a letter to his father about his daughter's arrival, and that he was thinking about asking his father about why he drank and distanced himself from his family. The therapist reinforced Tom for considering this and for not blindly making assumptions about his role in his father's drinking. However, she also attempted to inoculate Tom to the possibility that his father could blame him or his siblings for his alcoholism (given that she did not know his father or his history), and that this did not necessarily mean that it was true. She reminded him that he needed to consider the source of information, and that any good detective would get multiple reporters. Tom seemed to like the idea of getting more information from others, mentioning that he and his siblings had never really talked about his belief that they were to blame for their father's alcoholism.

Tom also shared that he better understood the idea of having intimacy, without sex, in his relationship with his wife. He said that since the birth of their child, he felt closer to his wife and had generally been more open and present to her. The therapist asked him about doing nice things for himself, and Tom laughed and said that he was more open to that but was finding less time to do it with a new baby.

The therapist then asked Tom to read what he had written about the meaning of the event for him after the work that he had done. He wrote:

There is no doubt that this traumatic event has deeply impacted me. My thoughts about myself, others, and the world were changed. When I started therapy, I believed that I was a murderer. I blamed myself completely. Now, I believe that I shot a family, but I did not murder them. I realize that I and others around me had to do what we did at the time, and that we chose to shoot because we had to. I will never know what that man, or maybe even the family, was trying to do by going through that checkpoint, but I know now that I had no choice but to shoot to stop them. Regarding safety, I used to think that there were people out to get me, but now I realize that the probability of that is slim. I still feel a little anxious about myself, my wife, and now my daughter, getting hurt, but not by a sniper. That seems unlikely. Now I worry about the stuff that everyone worries about—like crazy drivers, illness, or some accident. About safety, I used to worry that I was going to go "off" and hurt my family. I don't believe that I will do that, because I've never done that before and basically this trauma messed with my head about how likely I would be to hurt someone unless I had to. I'm trusting myself more in terms of the decisions I make, and I have some more faith and trust in my government now that I realize I really needed to shoot in that situation. I think I may always struggle with wanting to have power and control over things, but I'm working on not having control over everything. The fact is, I don't have control, even though I like to think that I do. My self-esteem is improving. I have to remember that not every bad thing that happens is my fault, and that I deserve to be happy even if I don't fully believe it yet. One of the biggest things that seems to be chang-ing is that I'm enjoying being close to my wife and my new daughter. I used to avoid my wife, because I thought I didn't deserve to be happy and that I might hurt her. Slowly I'm realizing that it is not very likely that I'll hurt my wife or my new daughter, or at least hurt them intentionally. My wife seems much happier now. I want to hold on to this time in my life and provide a good life for my daughter and wife. I'm happy to know that my daughter is not going to know someone who thought that snipers were out to get him, and who was anxious, avoiding everything and everyone. It sounds silly, but I'm kind of glad that I went through this, because I think I'm going to be better because of it.

Tom was a bit teary as he finished reading. The therapist asked Tom whether he remembered what he wrote the first time. Tom said no, so the therapist read to him his first Impact Statement. She pointed out that Tom had come a long way, and he agreed. The therapist and Tom reviewed the whole therapy process, what they had covered, and the "stuck points" that Tom had challenged. Tom said that he was going to continue using the worksheets, because they had been so helpful in making him slow down to think about things instead of just reacting. They did some lapse planning, and the therapist asked Tom what he could do if he sensed that he was struggling with PTSD or depressive symptoms, or second-guessing his new ways of thinking. He mentioned that he was going to share the materials with his wife, because she was very good at helping him to "get his head on straight." He also included on his list a review of the materials he had completed during the course of therapy. The therapy session ended with a discussion of Tom's goal to write his father a letter and to increase his contact with his siblings. He was planning to use these contacts to discover more about the reasons his father was alcoholic and had seemed to abandon the family. Tom also shared his goals about the type of father and husband he hoped to be, and what his professional future held as he left the military. The therapist congratulated Tom on his willingness to do the hard work to recover from what happened to him and wished him the best with his family and future. Tom expressed his appreciation for the therapy.

REFERENCES

Amdur, R. L., & Liberzon, I. (2001). The structure of posttraumatic stress disorder symptoms in combat veterans: A confirmatory factor analysis of the Impact of Event Scale. *Journal of Anxiety Disorders, 15,* 345–357.

American Psychiatric Association. (1994). *Diagnostic and statistical manual of mental disorders* (4th ed.). Washington, DC: Author.

Andrews, B., Brewin, C. R., Rose, S., & Kirk, M. (2000). Predicting PTSD symptoms in victims of violent crime: The role of shame, anger, and childhood abuse. *Journal of Abnormal Psychology, 109,* 69–73.

Asmundson, G. J. G., Frombach, I., McQuaid, J., Pedrelli, P., Lenox, R., & Stein, M. B. (2000). Dimensionality of posttraumatic stress symptoms: A confirmatory factor analysis of DSM-IV symptom clusters and other symptom models. *Behaviour Research and Therapy, 38,* 203–214.

Astin, M. C., Layne, C. M., Camilleri, A. J., & Foy, D. W. (1994). Posttraumatic stress disorder in victimization-related traumata. In I. J. Briere (Ed.), *Assessing and treating victims of violence: New directions for mental health services* (pp. 39–51). San Francisco: Jossey-Bass.

Becker, J. V., Skinner, L. J., Abel, G. G., Axelrod, R., & Cichon, J. (1984). Sexual problems of sexual assault survivors. *Women Health, 9,* 5–20.

Beckham, J. C., Feldman, M. E., & Kirby, A. C. (1998). Atrocities exposure in Vietnam combat veterans with chronic posttraumatic stress disorder: Relationship to combat exposure, symptom severity, guilt, and interpersonal violence. *Journal of Traumatic Stress, 11,* 777–785.

Blake, D. D., Weathers, F. W., Nagy, L. M., Kaloupek, D. G., Gusman, F. D., Charney, D. S., et al. (1995). The development of a Clinician-Administered PTSD Scale. *Journal of Traumatic Stress, 8,* 75–90.

Blanchard, E. B., Hickling, E. J., Buckley, T. C., & Taylor, A. E. (1996). Psychophysiology of posttraumatic stress disorder related to motor vehicle accidents: Replication and extension. *Journal of Consulting and Clinical Psychology, 64,* 742–751.

Blanchard, E. B., Hickling, E. J., Devinei, T., Veazey, C. H., Galovski, T. E., & Mundy, E. (2003). A controlled evaluation of cognitive behavioral therapy for posttraumatic stress in motor vehicle accident survivors. *Behaviour Research and Therapy, 41,* 79–96.

Boudewyns, P. A., Hyer, L. A., Peralme, L., Touze, J., & Kiel, A. (1995, August). *Eye movement desensitization and reprocessing (EMDR) and exposure therapy in the treatment of combat-related PTSD: An early look.* Paper presented at the annual meeting of the American Psychological Association, New York.

Bowen, G. R., & Lambert, J. A. (1986). Systematic desensitization therapy with post-traumatic stress disorder cases. In C. R Figley (Ed.), *Trauma and its wake: Vol. II. Traumatic stress theory, research, and intervention* (pp. 280–291). New York: Brunner/Mazel.

Breslau, N., Davis, G. C., & Andreski, P. (1995). Risk factors for PTSD-related traumatic events: A prospective analysis. *American Journal of Psychiatry, 152,* 529–535.

Brewin, C. R., Dalgleish, T., & Joseph, S. (1996). A dual representation theory of posttraumatic stress disorder. *Psychological Review, 103,* 670–686.

Briere, J. (1995). *The Trauma Symptom Inventory (TSI): Professional manual.* Odessa, FL: Psychological Assessment Resources.

Brom, D., Kleber, R. J., & Defares, P. B. (1989). Brief psychotherapy for PTSD. *Journal of Consulting and Clinical Psychology, 57,* 607–612.

Bryant, R. A., Harvey, A. G., Dang, S. T., Sackville, T., & Basten, C. (1998). Treatment of acute stress disorder: A comparison of cognitive-behavioral therapy and supportive counseling. *Journal of Consulting and Clinical Psychology, 66,* 862–866.

Bryant, R. A., Moulds, M. L., Guthrie, R. M., Dang, S. T., & Nixon, R. D. V. (2003). Imaginal exposure alone and imaginal exposure with cognitive restructuring in treatment of posttraumatic stress disorder. *Journal of Consulting and Clinical Psychology, 71,* 706–712.

Buckley, T. C., Blanchard, E. B., & Hickling, E. J. (1998). A confirmatory factor analysis of posttraumatic stress symptoms. *Behaviour Research and Therapy, 36,* 1091–1099.

Burt, M. R. (1980). Cultural myths and supports for rape. *Journal of Personality and Social Psychology, 38,* 217–230.

Chard, K. M. (2005). An evaluation of cognitive processing therapy for the treatment of posttraumatic stress disorder related to childhood sexual abuse. *Journal of Consulting and Clinical Psychology, 73,* 965–971.

Chemtob, C., Roitblat, H. L., Hamada, R. S., Carlson, J. G., & Twentyman, C. T. (1988). A cognitive action theory of post-traumatic stress disorder. *Journal of Anxiety Disorders, 2,* 253–275.

Cloitre, M. (1998). Sexual revictimization: Risk factors and prevention. In V. M. Follette, J. I. Ruzek, & F. R. Abueg (Eds.), *Cognitive-behavioral therapies for trauma* (pp. 278–304). New York: Guilford Press.

Cloitre, M., Koenen, K. C., Cohen, L. R., & Han, H. (2002). Skills training in affective and interpersonal regulation followed by exposure: A phase-based treatment for PTSD related to childhood abuse. *Journal of Consulting and Clinical Psychology, 70,* 1067–1074.

Cloitre, M., Stovall-McClough, K. C., Miranda, R., & Chemtob, C. M. (2004). Therapeutic alliance, negative mood regulation, and treatment outcome in child abuse-related posttraumatic stress disorder. *Journal of Consulting and Clinical Psychology, 72,* 411–416.

Creamer, M., Burgess, P., & Pattison, P. (1992). Reactions to trauma: A cognitive processing model. *Journal of Abnormal Psychology, 101,* 452–459.

Creamer, M., Morris, P., Biddle, D., & Elliott, P. (1999). Treatment outcome in Australian veterans with combat-related posttraumatic stress disorder: A cause for cautious optimism? *Journal of Traumatic Stress, 12,* 545–558.

Dalgleish, T. (2004). Cognitive approaches to posttraumatic stress disorder: The evolution of multirepresentational theorizing. *Psychological Bulletin, 130,* 228–260.

Denny, N., Robinowitz, R., & Penk, W. (1987). Conducting applied research on Vietnam combat-related post-traumatic stress disorder. *Journal of Clinical Psychology, 43,* 56–66.

Derogatis, L. R. (1983). *SCL-90-R: Administration, scoring and procedures manual-II.* Towson, MD: Clinical Psychometric Research.

Devilly, G. J., & Spence, S. H. (1999). The relative efficacy and treatment distress of EMDR and a cognitive-behavior trauma treatment protocol in the amelioration of posttraumatic stress disorder. *Journal of Anxiety Disorders, 13,* 131–157.

Dohrenwend, B. P., Turner, J. B., Turse, N. A., Adams, B. G., Koenen, K. C., & Marshall, R. (2006). The psychological risks of Vietnam for U.S. veterans: A revisit with new data and methods. *Science, 313,* 979–982.

Ehlers, A., & Clark, D. M. (2000). A cognitive model of posttraumatic stress disorder. *Behaviour Research and Therapy, 38,* 319–345.

Ehlers, A., Clark, D. M., Hackmann, A., McManus, F., Fennell, M., Herbert, C., et al. (2003). A randomized controlled trial of cognitive therapy, a self-help booklet, and repeated assessments as early interventions for posttraumatic stress disorder. *Archives of General Psychiatry, 60,* 1024–1032.

Ehlers, A., Hackmann, A., Steil, R., Clohessy, S., Wenninger, K., & Winter, H. (2002). The nature of intrusive memories after trauma: The warning signal hypothesis. *Behaviour Research and Therapy, 40,* 995–1002.

Falsetti, S. A., Resnick, H. S., Resick, P. A., & Kilpatrick, D. G. (1993). The Modified PTSD Symptom Scale: A brief self-report measure of posttraumatic stress disorder. *Behavior Therapist, 16,* 161–162.

First, M. B., Spitzer, R. L., Williams, J. B. W., & Gibbon, M. (1995). *Structured Clinical Interview for DSM-IV—Patient Edition (SCID-P).* Washington, DC: American Psychiatric Press.

Foa, E. B. (1995). *Posttraumatic Stress Diagnostic Scale (manual).* Minneapolis, MN: National Computer Systems.

Foa, E. B. (1996, November). *Conceptualization of post-trauma psychopathology as failure in emotional processing.* Information Processing Theories: Variations on a Theme symposium conducted at the meeting of the International Society for Traumatic Stress Studies, San Francisco.

Foa, E. B., Dancu, C. V., Hembree, E. A., Jaycox, L. H., Meadows, E. A., & Street, G. P. (1999). A comparison of exposure therapy, stress inoculation training, and their combination for reducing posttraumatic stress disorder in female assault victims. *Journal of Consulting and Clinical Psychology, 67,* 194–200.

Foa, E. B., Hembree, E. A., Cahill, S. E., Rauch, S. A. M., Riggs, D. S., Feeny, N. C., et al. (2005). Randomized trial of prolonged exposure for posttraumatic stress disorder with and without cognitive restructuring: Outcome at academic and community clinics. *Journal of Consulting and Clinical Psychology, 73,* 953–964.

Foa, E. B., Riggs, D. S., Dancu, C. V., & Rothbaum, B. O. (1993). Reliability and validity of a brief instrument for assessing post-traumatic stress disorder. *Journal of Traumatic Stress, 6,* 459–473.

Foa, E. B., Rothbaum, B., Riggs, D., & Murdock, T. (1991). Treatment of posttraumatic stress disorder in rape victims: A comparison between cognitive-behavioral procedures and counseling. *Journal of Consulting and Clinical Psychology, 59,* 715–723.

Foa, E. B., & Rothbaum, B. O. (1998). *Treating the trauma of rape: Cognitive-behavioral therapy for PTSD.* New York: Guilford Press.

Foa, E. B., Steketee, G., & Rothbaum, B. O. (1989). Behavioral/cognitive conceptualizations of post-traumatic stress disorder. *Behavior Therapy, 20,* 155–176.

Frank, E., Anderson, B., Stewart, B. D., Dancu, C., Hughes, C., & West, D. (1988). Efficacy of cognitive behavior therapy and systematic desensitization in the treatment of rape trauma. *Behavior Therapy, 19,* 403–420.

Frank, E., & Stewart, B. D. (1983). Treating depression in victims of rape. *Clinical Psychologist, 36,* 95–98.

Frank, E., & Stewart, B. D. (1984). Depressive symptoms in rape victims: A revisit. *Journal of Affective Disorders, 1,* 269–277.

Glover, H., Pelesky, C. A., Bruno, R., & Sette, R. (1990). Post-traumatic stress disorder conflicts in Vietnam combat veterans: A confirmatory factor analytic study. *Journal of Traumatic Stress, 3,* 573–591.

Green, B. L. (1996). Trauma History Questionnaire. In B. H. Stamm (Ed.), *Measurement of stress, trauma, and adaptation* (pp. 366–369). Lutherville, MD: Sidran Press.

Griffin, M. G., Resick, P. A., & Mechanic, M. B. (1997). Objective assessment of peritraumatic dissociation: Psychophysiological indicators. *American Journal of Psychiatry, 154,* 1081–1088.

Griffin, M. G., Uhlmansiek, M. H., Resick, P. A., & Mechanic, M. B. (2004). Comparison of the Posttraumatic Stress Disorder Scale versus the Clinician-Administered Posttraumatic Stress Disorder Scale in domestic violence survivors. *Journal of Traumatic Stress, 17,* 497–504.

Gutner, C., Rizvi, S. L., Monson, C. M., & Resick, P. A. (2006). Changes in coping strategies, relationship to the perpetrator, and posttraumatic stress disorder in female crime victims. *Journal of Traumatic Stress, 19,* 813–823.

Hembree, E. A., Cahill, S. E., & Foa, E. B. (2004). Impact of personality disorders on treatment outcome for female assault survivors with chronic posttraumatic stress disorder. *Journal of Personality Disorders, 18,* 117–127.

Henning, K. R., & Frueh, B. C. (1997). Combat guilt and its relationship to PTSD symptoms. *Journal of Clinical Psychology, 53,* 801–808.

Hoge, C. W., Auchterlonie, J. L., & Milliken, C. S. (2006). Mental health problems, use of mental health services, and attrition from military service after returning from deployment to Iraq or Afghanistan. *Journal of the American Medical Association, 295,* 1023–1032.

Hoge, C. W., Castro, C. A., Messer, S. C., McGurk, D., Cotting, D. I., & Koffman, R. L. (2004). Combat duty in Iraq and Afghanistan, mental health problems, and barriers to care. *New England Journal of Medicine, 351,* 13–22.

Holmes, M. R., & St. Lawrence, J. S. (1983). Treatment of rape-induced trauma: Proposed behavioral conceptualization and review of the literature. *Clinical Psychology Review, 3,* 417–433.

Horowitz, M. J. (1986). *Stress response syndromes* (2nd ed.). New York: Aronson.

Horowitz, M. J., Wilner, N., & Alvarez, W. (1979). Impact of Event Scale: A measure of subjective stress. *Psychosomatic Medicine, 41,* 209–218.

Ironson, G., Freund, B., Strauss, J. L., & Williams, J. (2002). Comparison of two treatments for traumatic stress: A community-based study of EMDR and Prolonged Exposure. *Journal of Clinical Psychology, 58,* 113–128.

Janoff-Bulman, R. (1985). The aftermath of victimization: Rebuilding shattered assumptions. In C. R. Figley (Ed.), *Trauma and its wake: Vol. I. The study and treatment of posttraumatic stress disorder* (pp. 15–35). New York: Brunner/Mazel.

Janoff-Bulman, R. (1992). *Shattered assumptions: Towards a new psychology of trauma.* New York: Free Press.

Jensen, J. A. (1994). An investigation of eye movement desensitization and reprocessing (EMD/R) as a treatment for posttraumatic stress disorder (PTSD) symptoms of Vietnam combat veterans. *Behavior Therapy, 25,* 311–325.

Jordan, B. K., Marmar, C. R., Fairbank, J. A., Schlenger, W. E., Kulka, R. A., Hough, R. L., et al. (1992). Problems in families of male Vietnam veterans with posttraumatic stress disorder. *Journal of Consulting and Clinical Psychology, 60,* 916–926.

Keane, T. M., Brief, D. J., Pratt, E. M., & Miller, M. W. (2007). Assessment and its comorbidities in adults. In M. J. Friedman, T. M. Keane, & P. A. Resick (Eds.), *Handbook of PTSD: Science and practice* (pp. 279–305). New York: Guilford Press.

Keane, T. M., Caddell, J. M., & Taylor, K. L. (1988).

Mississippi Scale for Combat-Related Posttraumatic Stress Disorder: Three studies in reliability and validity. *Journal of Consulting and Clinical Psychology, 56,* 85–90.

Keane, T. M., Fairbank, J. A., Caddell, J. M., & Zimering, R. T. (1989). Implosive (flooding) therapy reduces symptoms of PTSD in Vietnam combat veterans. *Behavior Therapy, 20,* 245–260.

Keane, T. M., Kaloupek, D. G., & Kolb, L. C. (1998). VA Cooperative Study #334: I. Summary of findings on the psychological assessment of PTSD. *PTSD Research Quarterly, 9,* 1–4.

Keane, T. M., Kolb, L. C., Kaloupek, D. G., Orr, S. P., Blanchard, E. B., Thomas, R. G., et al. (1998). Utility of psychophysiology measurement in the diagnosis of posttraumatic stress disorder: Results from a Department of Veteran's Affairs cooperative study. *Journal of Consulting and Clinical Psychology, 66,* 914–923.

Keane, T. M., Malloy, P. F., & Fairbank, J. A. (1984). Empirical development of an MMPI subscale for the assessment of combat-related posttraumatic stress disorder. *Journal of Consulting and Clinical Psychology, 52,* 888–891.

Keane, T. M., Zimering, R. T., & Caddell, J. M. (1985). A behavioral formulation of posttraumatic stress disorder. *Behavior Therapist, 8,* 9–12.

Kessler, R. C., Berglund, P., Demler, O., Jin, R., Merikangas, K. R., & Walters, E. E. (2005). Lifetime prevalence and age-of-onset distributions of DSM-IV disorders in the National Comorbidity Survey Replication. *Archives of General Psychiatry, 62,* 593–602.

Kessler, R. C., Chiu, W. T., Demler, O., Merikangas, K. R., & Walters, E. E. (2005). Prevalence, severity, and comorbidity of 12-month DSM-IV disorders in the National Comorbidity Survey Replication. *Archives of General Psychiatry, 62,* 617–627.

Kessler, R. C., Sonnega, A., Bromet, E., Hughes, M., & Nelson, C. B. (1995). Posttraumatic stress disorder in the National Comorbidity Survey. *Archives of General Psychiatry, 52,* 1048–1060.

Kilpatrick, D. G. (1983). Rape victims: Detection, assessment and treatment. *Clinical Psychologist, 36,* 92–95.

Kilpatrick, D. G., & Amick, A. E. (1985). Rape trauma. In M. Hersen & C. Last (Eds.), *Behavior therapy casebook* (pp. 86–103). New York: Springer.

Kilpatrick, D. G., Edmunds, C. N., & Seymour, A. K. (1992). *Rape in America: A report to the nation.* Arlington, VA: National Victim Center.

Kilpatrick, D. G., Resnick, H. S., & Freedy, J. R. (1991). *The Potential Stressful Events Interview.* Unpublished instrument, National Crime Victims Research and Treatment Center, Medical University of South Carolina, Charleston.

Kilpatrick, D. G., Saunders, B. E., Veronen, L. J., Best, C. L., & Von, J. M. (1987). Criminal victimization: Lifetime prevalence, reporting to police, and psychological impact. *Crime and Delinquency, 33,* 479–489.

Kilpatrick, D. G., & Veronen, L. J. (1983). Treatment

for rape-related problems: Crisis intervention is not enough. In L. H. Cohen, W. L. Claiborn, & G. A. Specter (Eds.), *Crisis intervention* (pp. 165–185). New York: Human Sciences Press.

Kilpatrick, D. G., Veronen, L. J., & Best, C. L. (1985). Factors predicting psychological distress among rape victims. In C. R. Figley (Ed.), *Trauma and its wake: Vol. I. The study and treatment of posttraumatic stress disorder* (pp. 114–141). New York: Brunner/Mazel.

Kilpatrick, D. G., Veronen, L. J., & Resick, P. A. (1982). Psychological sequelae to rape: Assessment and treatment strategies. In D. M. Doleys, R. L. Meredith, & A. R. Ciminero (Eds.), *Behavioral medicine: Assessment and treatment strategies* (pp. 473–497). New York: Plenum Press.

King, D. W., Leskin, G. A., King, L. A., & Weathers, F. W. (1998). Confirmatory factor analysis of the Clinician-Administered PTSD Scale: Evidence for the dimensionality of posttraumatic stress disorder. *Psychological Assessment, 10*, 90–96.

Koss, M. P., & Harvey, M. R. (1991). *The rape victim: Clinical and community interventions* (2nd ed.). Thousand Oaks, CA: Sage.

Kubany, E. S., Abueg, F. R., Owens, J. A., Brennan, J. M., Kaplan, A. S., & Watson, S. B. (1995). Initial examination of a multidimensional model of trauma-related guilt: Applications to combat veterans and battered women. *Journal of Psychopathology and Behavioral Assessment, 17*, 353–376.

Kubany, E. S., Haynes, S. N., Abueg, F. R., & Manke, F. P. (1996). Development and validation of the Trauma-Related Guilt Inventory (TRGI). *Psychological Assessment, 8*, 428–444.

Kubany, E. S., Haynes, S. N., Leisen, M. B., Owens, J. A., Kaplan, A. S., Watson, S. B., et al. (2000). Development and preliminary validation of a brief broadspectrum measure of trauma exposure: The Traumatic Life Events Questionnaire. *Psychological Assessment, 12*, 210–224.

Kubany, E. S., Hill, E. E., Owens, J. A., Iannce-Spencer, C., McCaig, M. A., & Tremayne, K. J. (2004). Cognitive trauma therapy for battered women with PTSD (CTT-BW). *Journal of Consulting and Clinical Psychology, 72*, 3–18.

Kubany, E. S., Leisen, M. B., Kaplan, A. S., & Kelly, M. P. (2000). Validation of a brief measure of posttraumatic stress disorder: The Distressing Event Questionnaire (DEQ). *Psychological Assessment, 12*, 197–209.

Kulka, R. A., Schlenger, W. E., Fairbank, J. A., Hough, R. L., Jordan, B. K., Marmar, C. R., et al. (1990). *Trauma and the Vietnam war generation: Report of findings from the National Vietnam Veterans Readjustment Study.* New York: Brunner/Mazel.

Lang, P. J. (1968). Fear reduction and fear behavior: Problems in treating a construct. In J. M. Schlien (Ed.), *Research in psychotherapy* (pp. 90–102). Washington, DC: American Psychological Association.

Lang, P. J. (1977). Imagery in therapy: An information processing analysis of fear. *Behavior Therapy, 8*, 862–886.

Lauterbach, D., & Vrana, S. R. (1996). Three studies on the reliability and validity of a self-report measure of posttraumatic stress disorder. *Assessment, 3*, 17–25.

Lee, C., Gavriel, H., Drummond, P., Richards, J., & Greenwald, R. (2002). Treatment of PTSD: Stress inoculation training with prolonged exposure compared to EMDR. *Journal of Clinical Psychology, 58*, 1071–1089.

Leskela, J., Dieperink, M., & Thuras, P. (2002). Shame and posttraumatic stress disorder. *Journal of Traumatic Stress, 15*, 223–226.

Mahoney, M. J., & Lyddon, W. J. (1988). Recent developments in cognitive approaches to counseling and psychotherapy. *Counseling Psychologist, 16*, 190–234.

Marks, I., Lovell, K., Noshirvani, H., Livanou, M., & Thrasher, S. (1998). Treatment of posttraumatic stress disorder by exposure and/or cognitive restructuring: A controlled study. *Archives of General Psychiatry, 55*, 317–325.

McCann, I. L., & Pearlman, L. A. (1990). Vicarious traumatization: A framework for understanding the psychological effects of working with victims. *Journal of Traumatic Stress, 3*, 131–149.

McFall, M., Fontana, A., Raskind, M., & Rosenheck, R. (1999). Analysis of violent behavior in Vietnam combat veteran psychiatric inpatients with posttraumatic stress disorder. *Journal of Traumatic Stress, 12*, 501–517.

McNair, L. D., & Neville, H. A. (1996). African American women survivors of sexual assault: The intersection of race and class. In M. Hill & E. D. Rothblum (Eds.), *Classism and feminist therapy: Counting costs* (pp. 107–118). New York: Haworth Press.

Meichenbaum, D. H. (1985). *Stress inoculation training.* Elmsford, NY: Pergamon Press.

Miller, M. W., Kaloupek, D. G., Dillon, A. L., & Keane, T. M. (2004). Externalizing and internalizing subtypes of combat-related PTSD: A replication and extension using the PSY-5 scales. *Journal of Abnormal Psychology, 113*, 636–645.

Miller, M. W., Kaloupek, D. G., & Keane, T. M. (1999, October). *Antisociality and physiological hyporesponsivity during exposure to trauma-related stimuli in patients with PTSD.* Poster presented at the 39th Annual Meeting of the Society for Psychophysiological Research, Granada, Spain.

Monson, C. M., Price, J. L., & Ranslow, E. (2005, October). Treating combat PTSD through cognitive processing therapy. *Federal Practitioner, 75–83.*

Monson, C. M., Schnurr, P. P., Resick, P. A., Friedman, M. J., Young-Xu, Y., & Stevens, S. P. (2006). Cognitive processing therapy for veterans with military-related posttraumatic stress disorder. *Journal of Consulting and Clinical Psychology, 74*, 898–907.

Mowrer, O. H. (1947). On the dual nature of learning—a re-interpretation of "conditioning" and "problem-solving." *Harvard Educational Review, 14,* 102–148.

Neuner, F., Schauer, M., Klaschik, C., Karunakara, U., & Elbert, T. (2004). A comparison of narrative exposure therapy, supportive counseling, and psychoeducation for treating posttraumatic stress disorder in an African refugee settlement. *Journal of Consulting and Clinical Psychology, 72,* 579–587.

Norris, F. (1990). Screening for traumatic stress: A scale for use in the general population. *Journal of Applied Social Psychology, 20,* 1704–1718.

Norris, F. H. (1992). Epidemiology of trauma: Frequency and impact of different potentially traumatic events on different demographic groups. *Journal of Consulting and Clinical Psychology, 60,* 409–418.

Oquendo, M. A., Friend, J. M., Halberstam, B., Brodsky, B. S., Burke, A. K., Grunebaum, M. F., et al. (2003). Association of comorbid posttraumatic stress disorder and major depression with greater risk for suicidal behavior. *American Journal of Psychiatry, 160,* 580–582.

Orr, S. P., Lasko, N. B., Metzger, L. J., Berry, N. J., Ahern, C. E., & Pitman, R. K. (1998). Psychophysiologic assessment of women with posttraumatic stress disorder resulting from childhood sexual abuse. *Journal of Consulting and Clinical Psychology, 66,* 906–913.

Orr, S. P., Metzger, L. J., Miller, M. W., & Kaloupek, D. G. (2004). Psychophysiological assessment of PTSD. In J. P. Wilson & T. M. Keane (Eds.), *Assessing psychological trauma and PTSD* (2nd ed., pp. 289–343). New York: Guilford Press.

Paunovic, N., & Öst, L. G. (2001). Cognitive-behavior therapy versus exposure therapy in the treatment of PTSD in refugees. *Behaviour Research and Therapy, 39,* 1183–1197.

Pitman, R. K., Orr, S. P., Altman, B., Longpre, R. E., Poire, R. E., & Lasko, N. B. (1993, October). *A controlled study of eye movement desensitization/reprocessing (EMDR) treatment of post-traumatic stress disorder.* Presentation at International Society for Traumatic Stress Studies, San Antonio, TX.

Pitman, R. K., Orr, S. P., Forgue, D. F., & Altman, B. (1990). Psychophysiologic responses to combat imagery of Vietnam veterans with posttraumatic stress disorder versus other anxiety disorders. *Journal of Abnormal Psychology, 99,* 49–54.

Pitman, R. K., Orr, S. P., Forgue, D. F., de Jong, J., & Claiborn, J. M. (1987). Psychophysiologic assessment of posttraumatic stress disorder imagery in Vietnam combat veterans. *Archives of General Psychiatry, 44,* 970–975.

Power, K., McGoldrick, T., Brown, K., Buchanan, R., Sharp, D., & Swanson, V. (2002). A controlled comparison of eye movement desensitization and reprocessing versus exposure plus cognitive restructuring versus wait list in the treatment of posttraumatic stress disorder. *Clinical Psychology and Psychotherapy, 9,* 299–318.

Prins, A., Ouimette, P., Kimerling, R., Camerond, R. P.,

Hugelshofer, D. S., Shaw-Hegwer, J., et al. (2004). The Primary Care PTSD Screen (PC-PTSD): Development and operating characteristics. *Primary Care Psychiatry, 9,* 9–14.

Renfrey, G., & Spates, C. R. (1994). Eye movement desensitization: A partial dismantling study. *Journal of Behavior Therapy and Experimental Psychiatry, 25,* 231–239.

Resick, P. A., Jordan, C. G., Girelli, S. A., Hutter, C. K., & Marhoeder-Dvorak, S. (1988). A comparative outcome study of behavioral group therapy for sexual assault victims. *Behavior Therapy, 19,* 385–401.

Resick, P. A., & Markaway, B. E. (1991). Clinical treatment of adult female victims of sexual assault. In C. R. Hollin & K. Howells (Eds.), *Clinical approaches to sex offenders and their victims* (pp. 261–284). London: Wiley.

Resick, P. A., Nishith, P., & Griffin, M. G. (2003). How well does cognitive-behavioral therapy treat symptoms of complex PTSD?: An examination of child sexual abuse survivors within a clinical trial. *CNS Spectrums, 8,* 340–355.

Resick, P. A., Nishith, P., Weaver, T. L., Astin, M. C., & Feuer, C. A. (2002). A comparison of cognitive processing therapy, prolonged exposure and a waiting condition for the treatment of posttraumatic stress disorder in female rape victims. *Journal of Consulting and Clinical Psychology, 70,* 867–879.

Resick, P. A., & Schnicke, M. K. (1992). Cognitive processing therapy for sexual assault victims. *Journal of Consulting and Clinical Psychology, 60,* 748–756.

Resick, P. A., & Schnicke, M. K. (1993). *Cognitive processing therapy for rape victims: A treatment manual.* Newbury Park, CA: Sage.

Resnick, H. S., Kilpatrick, D. G., Dansky, B. S., Saunders, B. E., & Best, C. L. (1993). Prevalence of civilian trauma and posttraumatic stress disorder in a representative national sample of women. *Journal of Consulting and Clinical Psychology, 61,* 984–991.

Resnick, H. S., Kilpatrick, D. G., & Lipovsky, J. A. (1991). Assessment of rape-related posttraumatic stress disorder: Stressor and symptom dimensions [Special section: Issues and methods in assessment of posttraumatic stress disorder]. *Psychological Assessment, 3,* 561–572.

Robins, L. N., Helzer, J. E., Croughan, J., & Ratcliff, K. S. (1981). National Institute of Mental Health Diagnostic Interview Schedule: Its history, characteristics, and validity. *Archives of General Psychiatry, 38,* 381–389.

Rosenheck, R., & Fontana, A. (1996). PTSD and community-based treatment: A commentary on "PTSD diagnosis and treatment for mental health clinicians." *Community Mental Health Journal, 32,* 191–193.

Rosenheck, R., Fontana, A., & Cottrol, C. (1995). Effect of clinician–veteran racial pairing in the treatment of posttraumatic stress disorder. *American Journal of Psychiatry, 152,* 555–563.

Rothbaum, B. O. (1998, March). *Virtual reality expo-*

sure therapy for Vietnam veterans with PTSD: Pre-liminary results. Paper presented at the Lake George Conference on Posttraumatic Stress Disorder, Bolton Landing, NY.

Rothbaum, B. O., Astin, M. C., & Marsteller, F. (2005). Prolonged exposure versus eye movement desensitization and reprocessing (EMDR) for PTSD rape victims. *Journal of Traumatic Stress, 18,* 607–616.

Rothbaum, B. O., & Foa, E. B. (1992). Exposure therapy for rape victims with post-traumatic stress disorder. *Behavior Therapist, 15,* 219–222.

Rothbaum, B. O., & Foa, E. B. (1993). Subtypes of posttraumatic stress disorder and duration of symptoms. In J. R. T. Davidson & E. B. Foa (Eds.), *Posttraumatic stress disorder: DSM-IV and beyond* (pp. 23–35). Washington, DC: American Psychiatric Press.

Saunders, B. E., Arata, C. M., & Kilpatrick, D. G. (1990). Development of a crime-related posttraumatic stress disorder scale for women within the Symptom Checklist–90—Revised. *Journal of Traumatic Stress, 3,* 439–448.

Schindler, F. E. (1980). Treatment by systematic desensitization of a recurring nightmare of a real life trauma. *Journal of Behavior Therapy and Experimental Psychiatry, 11,* 53–54.

Schnurr, P. P., Friedman, M. J., Engel, C. C., Foa, E. B., Shea, T., Chow, B. K., et al. (2007). Cognitive-behavioral therapy for posttraumatic stress disorder in women: A randomized controlled trial. *Journal of the American Medical Association, 297*(8), 820–830.

Schnurr, P. P., Friedman, M. J., Foy, D. W., Shea, M. T., Hsieh, F. Y., Lavori, P. W., et al. (2003). Randomized trial of trauma-focused group therapy for posttraumatic stress disorder: Results from a Department of Veterans Affairs cooperative study. *Archives of General Psychiatry, 60,* 481–489.

Shalev, A. Y., Orr, S. P., & Pitman, R. K. (1992). Psychophysiologic response during script-driven imagery as an outcome measure in posttraumatic stress disorder. *Journal of Clinical Psychiatry, 53,* 324–326.

Shapiro, F. (1989). Eye movement desensitization: A new treatment for post-traumatic stress disorder. *Journal of Behavior Therapy and Experimental Psychiatry, 20,* 211–217.

Shapiro, F. (1995). *Eye movement desensitization and reprocessing: Basic principles, protocols, and procedures.* New York: Guilford Press.

Shay, J., & Munroe, J. (1999). Group and milieu therapy for veterans with complex posttraumatic stress disorder. In P. A. Saigh & J. D. Bremner (Eds.), *Posttraumatic stress disorder: A comprehensive text* (pp. 391–413). Needham Heights, MA: Allyn & Bacon.

Shin, L. M., Rauch, S. L., & Pitman, R. K. (2005). Structural and functional anatomy of PTSD: Findings from neuroimaging research. In J. J. Vasterling & C. R. Brewin (Eds.), *Neuropsychology of PTSD: Biological, cognitive, and clinical perspectives* (pp. 59–82). New York: Guilford Press.

Silverman, D. (1977). First do no more harm: Female rape victims and the male counselor. *American Journal of Orthopsychiatry, 47*(1), 91–96.

Simms, L. J., Watson, D., & Doebbeling, B. N. (2002). Confirmatory factor analyses of posttraumatic stress symptoms in deployed and nondeployed veterans of the Gulf War. *Journal of Abnormal Psychology, 111,* 637–647.

Smith, M. Y., Redd, W., DuHamel, K., Vicksberg, S. J., & Ricketts, P. (1999). Validation of the PTSD Checklist—Civilian version in survivors of bone marrow transplantation. *Journal of Traumatic Stress, 12,* 485–499.

Sutker, P. B., Uddo-Crane, M., & Allain, A. N. (1991). Clinical and research assessment of posttraumatic stress disorder: A conceptual overview [Special section: Issues and methods in assessment of posttraumatic stress disorder]. *Psychological Assessment, 3,* 520–530.

Tarrier, N., Pilgrim, H., Sommerfield, C., Faragher, B., Reynolds, M., Graham, E., et al. (1999). A randomized trial of cognitive therapy and imaginal exposure in the treatment of chronic posttraumatic stress disorder. *Journal of Consulting and Clinical Psychology, 67,* 13–18.

Tarrier, N., & Sommerfield, C. (2004). Treatment of chronic PTSD by cognitive therapy and exposure: 5 year follow-up. *Behavior Therapy, 35,* 231–246.

Taylor, S., Kuch, K., Koch, W. J., Crockett, D. J., & Passey, G. (1998). The structure of posttraumatic stress symptoms. *Journal of Abnormal Psychology, 107,* 154–160.

Taylor, S., Thordarson, D. S., Maxfield, L., Fedoroff, I. C., Lovell, K., & Orgodniczuk, J. (2003). Comparative efficacy, speed, and adverse effects of three PTSD treatments: Exposure therapy, EMDR, and relaxation training. *Journal of Consulting and Clinical Psychology, 71,* 330–338.

Tolin, D. F., & Foa, E. B. (2006). Sex differences in trauma and posttraumatic stress disorder: A quantitative review of 25 years of research. *Psychological Bulletin, 132,* 959–992.

Turner, S. M. (1979, December). *Systematic desensitization of fears and anxiety in rape victims.* Paper presented at the Association of Advancement of Behavior Therapy, San Francisco.

U.S. Department of Health and Human Services. (2001). *Mental health: A report of the Surgeon General.* Washington, DC: Author.

Vrana, S., & Lauterbach, D. (1994). Prevalence of traumatic events and post-traumatic psychological symptoms in a nonclinical sample of college students. *Journal of Traumatic Stress, 7,* 289–302.

Weathers, F., Litz, B. T., Herman, D. S., Huska, J. A., & Keane, T. M. (1993, October). *The PTSD Checklist (PCL): Reliability, validity, and diagnostic utility.* Presentation at the International Society for Traumatic Stress Studies, San Antonio, TX.

Weathers, F. W., & Keane, T. M. (1999). Psychological assessment of traumatized adults. In P. A. Saigh & J.

D. Bremner (Eds.), *Posttraumatic stress disorder: A comprehensive text* (pp. 219–247). Boston: Allyn & Bacon.

Weathers, F. W., Keane, T. M., & Davidson, J. R. (2001). Clinician-Administered PTSD Scale: A review of the first ten years of research. *Depression and Anxiety, 13*, 132–156.

Weathers, F. W., Ruscio, A. M., & Keane, T. M. (1999). Psychometric properties of nine scoring rules for the Clinician-Administered Posttraumatic Stress Disorder Scale. *Psychological Assessment, 11*, 124–133.

Weiss, D. S., & Marmar, C. R. (1997). The Impact of Event Scale—Revised. In J. P. Wilson & T. M. Keane (Eds.), *Assessing psychological trauma and PTSD* (pp. 399–411). New York: Guilford Press.

Wilson, A. E., Calhoun, K. S., & Bernat, J. A. (1999). Risk recognition and trauma-related symptoms among sexually revictimized women. *Journal of Consulting and Clinical Psychology, 67*, 705–710.

Wilson, D., Silver, S. M., Covi, W., & Foster, S. (1996). Eye movement desensitization and reprocessing: Effectiveness and automatic correlates. *Journal of Behavior Therapy and Experimental Psychiatry, 27*, 219–229.

Wong, M. R., & Cook, D. (1992). Shame and its contribution to PTSD. *Journal of Traumatic Stress, 5*, 557–562.

Zoellner, L. A., Feeny, N. C., Fitzgibbons, L. A., & Foa, E. B. (1999). Response of African American and Caucasian women to cognitive behavioral therapy for PTSD. *Behavior Therapy, 30*, 581–595.

CHAPTER 3

Social Anxiety Disorder

CYNTHIA L. TURK
RICHARD G. HEIMBERG
LEANNE MAGEE

Many people are very shy and somewhat inhibited. For this reason, the suffering associated with social anxiety disorder is often minimized as a common trait in the population that does not require a heavy artillery of formalized treatment interventions (either drugs or psychological treatments). Nothing could be further from the truth. For members of a very large segment of the population with debilitating social anxiety (over 12% and increasing), at some point in their lives the seemingly simple process of interacting with people or forming relationships provokes overwhelming terror and is often avoided. The effects on career and quality of life can be devastating. This chapter examines the latest iteration of an established psychological treatment for social anxiety disorder. As is increasingly true of our new generation of psychological interventions, cognitive-behavioral group therapy has proven to be significantly better than equally credible but less focused psychological interventions, and its effect is increasingly powerful over time. As such, this treatment is among the best of the new generation of psychological treatments characterized by power and specificity. The case of Josie, new to this edition, also illustrates the maturity and clinical sophistication of this remarkable approach to social anxiety.—D. H. B.

The National Comorbidity Survey Replication Study (NCS-R), which assessed over 9,000 noninstitutionalized individuals throughout the United States, found that 12.1% of people have social anxiety disorder at some point during their lives (Kessler et al., 2005). In this survey, social anxiety disorder (also known as social phobia; Liebowitz, Heimberg, Fresco, Travers, & Stein, 2000) was the fourth most common psychiatric disorder, with only major depressive disorder, alcohol abuse, and specific phobia being more prevalent. More conservative lifetime prevalence estimates suggest that clinically significant social anxiety affects a compelling but more modest 4% of the population (Narrow, Rae, Robins, & Regier, 2002).

When social anxiety disorder was first included as a diagnostic category in the third edition of the *Diagnostic and Statistical Manual of Mental Disorders* (DSM-III; American Psychiatric Association, 1980), it was thought to result in only minimal disruption in role functioning. Research has since revealed that social anxiety disorder can be quite incapacitating. The vast majority of individuals with social anxiety disorder report that their career, academic, and general social functioning have been seriously impaired by their fears

(Katzelnick et al., 2001; Schneier et al., 1994; Turner, Beidel, Dancu, & Keys, 1986). In one study, despite a mean age in the early 30s, 50% of the individuals with social anxiety disorder had never married, compared to 36% of individuals with panic disorder and agoraphobia, and 18% of those with generalized anxiety disorder (Sanderson, Di Nardo, Rapee, & Barlow, 1990). In another study, individuals with social anxiety disorder were more likely than their nonanxious counterparts to work at a job below their level of educational attainment and to believe that their supervisors did not think that they fit into the work environment (Bruch, Fallon, & Heimberg, 2003). Symptoms of social anxiety are also associated with low life satisfaction, even after taking into account the level of disability engendered by these symptoms (Hambrick, Turk, Heimberg, Schneier, & Liebowitz, 2003).

Social anxiety disorder most commonly begins during early childhood or adolescence (Schneier, Johnson, Hornig, Liebowitz, & Weissman, 1992) and typically follows an unremitting course (Chartier, Hazen, & Stein, 1998; Reich, Goldenberg, Vasile, Goisman, & Keller, 1994). Nevertheless, most individuals with social anxiety disorder do not seek treatment unless they develop an additional disorder (Schneier et al., 1992). Unfortunately, recognition of social anxiety disorder appears to be poor among health care professionals (Bisserbe, Weiller, Boyer, Lepine, & Lecrubier, 1996; Katzelnick et al., 2001; Weiller, Bisserbe, Boyer, Lepine, & Lecrubier, 1996).

Approximately 70–80% of individuals with social anxiety disorder meet criteria for additional diagnoses, and, in most cases, social anxiety disorder predates the onset of the comorbid condition (W. Magee, Eaton, Wittchen, McGonagle, & Kessler, 1996; Schneier et al., 1992). In community samples, the most common additional diagnoses include specific phobia, agoraphobia, major depression, and alcohol abuse and dependence (W. Magee et al., 1996; Schneier et al., 1992). Compared to individuals with uncomplicated social anxiety disorder, persons with social anxiety disorder and comorbid disorders have higher rates of suicide attempts, are more likely to report significant role impairment, and more often use medication to control their symptoms (W. Magee et al., 1996; Schneier et al., 1992). Comorbidity is also associated with more severe impairment before and after cognitive-behavioral therapy

(CBT), although individuals with and without comorbid conditions make similar gains (Erwin, Heimberg, Juster, & Mindlin, 2002). Comorbid mood disorders appear to be more strongly associated with impairment than do comorbid anxiety disorders (Erwin et al., 2002).

SUBTYPES OF SOCIAL ANXIETY DISORDER AND AVOIDANT PERSONALITY DISORDER

Socially anxious individuals are a heterogeneous group in terms of the pervasiveness and severity of their fears. In the current diagnostic system, the *generalized* subtype is specified for individuals who fear most social situations. These individuals often simultaneously have a variety of social interaction fears (e.g., dating, joining an ongoing conversation, being assertive), performance fears (e.g., public speaking, playing a musical instrument in front of others), and observation fears (e.g., working in front of others, walking down the street). The *nongeneralized* subtype is "a heterogeneous group that includes persons who fear a single performance situation as well as those who fear several, but not most, social situations" (American Psychiatric Association, 1994, p. 413). For example, individuals who fear public speaking or eating in front of others but otherwise feel comfortable interacting with and being observed by others would be assigned to the nongeneralized subtype.

Relative to the nongeneralized subtype, the generalized subtype has been associated with earlier age of onset, decreased educational attainment, higher rates of unemployment, and a greater likelihood of being unmarried (Heimberg, Hope, Dodge, & Becker, 1990b; Mannuzza et al., 1995). This group also experiences more depression, social anxiety, avoidance, fear of negative evaluation, and functional impairment (e.g., Brown, Heimberg, & Juster, 1995; Herbert, Hope, & Bellack, 1992; Turner, Beidel, & Townsley, 1992). Nevertheless, clients with generalized social anxiety disorder improve as much as clients with the nongeneralized subtype after CBT (Brown et al., 1995; Hope, Herbert, & White, 1995; Turner, Beidel, Wolff, Spaulding, & Jacob, 1996). However, because clients with generalized social anxiety disorder begin treatment with greater impairment, they remain more impaired after receiving the same number of treatment sessions. Therefore, clients with generalized social anxiety disorder may require a longer course of treatment to achieve outcomes similar to those of clients with nongeneralized social anxiety.

The generalized subtype of social anxiety disorder has many features in common with avoidant personality disorder (APD). In the current diagnostic system, APD is characterized by a long-standing pattern "of social inhibition, feelings of inadequacy, and hypersensitivity to negative evaluation" (American Psychiatric Association, 1994, p. 664). Given the similarity between the descriptions of the two disorders, it is not surprising that many individuals who meet criteria for generalized social anxiety disorder also meet criteria for APD. However, there is little scientific evidence to suggest that individuals meet criteria for APD without also meeting criteria for social anxiety disorder (Widiger, 1992). The most parsimonious description of the relationship between social anxiety disorder and APD is that they are not different disorders and that individuals meeting criteria for both disorders are simply the most severely impaired persons with social anxiety disorder (Heimberg, Holt, Schneier, Spitzer, & Liebowitz, 1993). With regard to treatment outcome, some studies have found that clients with and without comorbid APD make similar gains (Brown et al., 1995; Hofmann, Newman, Becker, Taylor, & Roth, 1995; Hope, Herbert, & White, 1995), although others have found that comorbid APD is associated with a poorer treatment response (Chambless, Tran, & Glass, 1997; Feske, Perry, Chambless, Renneberg, & Goldstein, 1996). As with individuals meeting criteria for generalized social anxiety disorder, clients with APD may require a longer course of treatment to achieve an optimal outcome.

OVERVIEW OF THE TREATMENT OUTCOME LITERATURE

Researchers have investigated the efficacy of a broad range of treatments for social anxiety disorder, including social skills training, cognitive therapy, relaxation training, exposure, interpersonal psychotherapy, dynamically oriented supportive psychotherapy, and various pharmacotherapies. This review examines only studies that have tested the efficacy of combined exposure and cognitive treatment. The combination of exposure and cognitive restructuring has been the most frequently studied form of psychosocial intervention for social anxiety disorder and represents the focus of the intervention described in this chapter (a broader review of the treatment outcome literature is provided by Rodebaugh, Holaway, & Heimberg, 2004).

Researchers have often sought to demonstrate that the efficacy of exposure is improved by the addition of cognitive restructuring. The data from such efforts are mixed. For example, in an early study, Butler, Cullington, Munby, Amies, and Gelder (1984) compared *in vivo* exposure to *in vivo* exposure plus an anxiety management program that comprised distraction, relaxation, and rational self-talk, and a waiting-list control. At posttest, both exposure treatments were more effective than the waiting-list control across a variety of measures, with few differences between the active treatments. However, at follow-up, participants who received exposure plus anxiety management training (which included a cognitive component) fared better than participants who received exposure alone. Similarly, Mattick and colleagues (Mattick & Peters, 1988; Mattick, Peters, & Clarke, 1989), in two studies examining the efficacy of a combined package of exposure and cognitive restructuring, provided evidence for a somewhat greater advantage for combined exposure and cognitive restructuring relative to exposure alone. However, Taylor et al. (1997a) found no differences between participants randomized initially to receive cognitive restructuring or a control therapy prior to both groups receiving exposure treatment; that is, exposure with and without prior cognitive restructuring produced similar improvement in outcomes for the socially anxious participants in this study.

Heimberg, Dodge, and colleagues (1990) conducted the first controlled trial of his group treatment for social anxiety disorder, which comprised integrated exposure, cognitive restructuring, and homework assignments (i.e., cognitive-behavioral group therapy [CBGT]). This treatment was compared to an attention control treatment that comprised education about social anxiety disorder and nondirective supportive group therapy. CBGT participants reported less anxiety during an individualized behavioral test and were more likely than control participants to be rated as improved by a clinical assessor. At 6-month follow-up, the internal dialogue of CBGT participants was characterized by a "positive dialogue," a state associated with good mental health according to Schwartz and Garamoni's (1989) states of mind (SOM) model. The internal dialogue of attention control participants, in contrast, represented a "negative monologue," the most pathological state of mind described in the SOM model (Bruch, Heimberg, & Hope, 1991). A 5-year follow-up of a subset of participants from the original sample indicated that individuals who had received CBGT were more likely than comparable attention control participants to maintain their gains (Heimberg, Salzman, Holt, & Blendell, 1993).

In a component analysis of CBGT, Hope, Heimberg, and Bruch (1995) reported that CBGT and exposure alone were both more effective than a waiting-list control. At posttest, there was evidence that the exposure-alone condition was more effective than CBGT, but these differences disappeared at 6-month follow-up.

In a two-site study, 133 clients were randomly assigned to receive CBGT, the monoamine oxidase inhibitor phenelzine, pill placebo, or the attention control psychotherapy developed by Heimberg, Dodge, and colleagues (1990, 1998). At posttest, independent assessors classified 21 of 28 CBGT completers (75%) and 20 of 26 phenelzine completers (77%) as treatment responders. The response rates for phenelzine and CBGT clients were significantly better than those for clients receiving pill placebo or the attention control psychotherapy. In the second phase of this study, clients who responded to CBGT or phenelzine were continued through 6 additional months of maintenance treatment and a 6-month follow-up period (Liebowitz et al., 1999). At study's end, 50% of previously responding clients who received phenelzine relapsed, compared to only 17% of clients who received CBGT.

A waiting-list controlled study of an individually administered version of this treatment was recently completed (Zaider, Heimberg, Roth, Hope, & Turk, 2003). The individual cognitive-behavioral treatment consistently outperformed the waiting list on both self-report and clinician-administered measures of social anxiety. Effect sizes were large, and little dropout occurred.

Controlled trials of Clark's (1997) version of cognitive-behavioral treatment for social anxi-

ety disorder have also yielded large effect sizes and appear promising (Clark et al., 2003, 2006; Stangier, Heidenreich, Peitz, Lauterbach, & Clark, 2003). Clark's protocol includes both cognitive restructuring and exposure elements. However, his treatment also emphasizes procedures derived from his theoretical work and basic research, such as identification of safety behaviors, shifting focus of attention away from the self (to the social situation), behavioral experiments in which safety behaviors are dropped, and video feedback on social performance.

In summary, it appears that a combined package of exposure and cognitive restructuring is an effective intervention for social anxiety disorder. Whether it is the most effective treatment, or more effective than exposure alone, is more difficult to determine given the limited number of studies and mixed results. However, more important to practitioners is the mounting evidence that three of four clients with social anxiety disorder are likely to realize clinically significant change after a reasonably intensive trial of combined exposure and cognitive restructuring.

AN INTEGRATED COGNITIVE-BEHAVIORAL MODEL OF SOCIAL ANXIETY DISORDER

Rapee and Heimberg (1997; see also Heimberg & Becker, 2002; Roth & Heimberg, 2001; Turk, Lerner, Heimberg, & Rapee, 2001) developed an integrated cognitive-behavioral model that describes how individuals with social anxiety disorder process information when confronted with a situation that holds the potential for negative evaluation (see Figure 3.1). The process begins when the socially anxious individual is in the presence of an audience. The term "audience" captures the sense that socially anxious individuals have of being "on stage" in the presence of others, whether the situation is a speech, social interaction, or another situation in which the person may be observed by others. Socially anxious persons perceive this audience as inherently critical (e.g., Leary, Kowalski, & Campbell, 1988) and as having standards that they are unlikely to meet (e.g., Wallace & Alden, 1991). Trower and Gilbert (1989; Gilbert, 2001) also suggest that socially anxious individuals view their audience as competitors. According to their

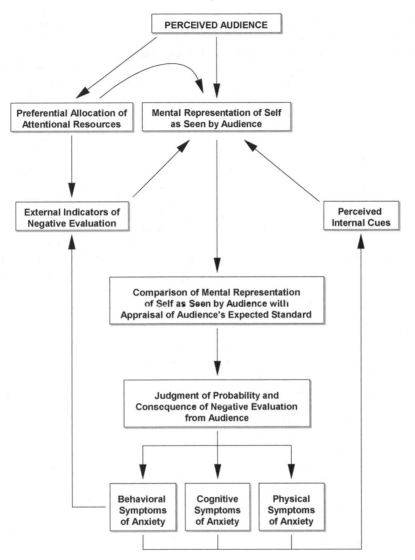

FIGURE 3.1. A model of the generation and maintenance of anxiety in social-evaluative situations. From Rapee and Heimberg (1997). Copyright 1997 by Elsevier Science Ltd. Reprinted by permission.

psychobiological/ethological theory, two systems have evolved that allow social groups to develop and maintain order. The defense system involves the establishment of dominant and subordinate roles within social groups. Individuals are ranked within hierarchies, and the ultimate goal is to have dominant status, because higher levels in the hierarchy are associated with greater access to resources (e.g., mates, food). In contrast, in the safety system, a more recent and highly evolved system of social interaction, group members offer signals of re-

assurance and positive reinforcement instead of threats to maintain structure. Inevitably, this creates less social anxiety between members, decreases the need to maintain a constant state of social comparison, and encourages a less threatening and more cooperative environment. Trower and Gilbert suggest that everyone has access to both of these systems, but socially anxious individuals are more prone to utilize the defense system, even when the social environment is nonthreatening. Thus, socially anxious individuals view others as threatening competitors who have the goal of dominating them. In fact, socially anxious individuals have been shown to perceive social interactions as more competitive than do their nonanxious counterparts and to view themselves as coming across to others as submissive (Hope, Sigler, Penn, & Meier, 1998). To illustrate, one client who avoided dancing in public made progress on this issue when he reconceptualized dancing as an opportunity for people to have fun together rather than a competition in which everyone judges and criticizes the skills of everyone else.

In the presence of an audience, socially anxious individuals construct a mental representation of how they appear to these other people. This mental representation of the self comprises negative and distorted images in which the self is viewed from an observer perspective (Hackmann, Surawy, & Clark, 1998). These images have been found to be related to memories of early adverse social events such as being bullied (Hackmann, Clark, & McManus, 2000). For example, one client described being mercilessly teased by her peers as a young adolescent for being tall and skinny. Although at the time of treatment she was an attractive adult, she still described her appearance as "gangly," "awkward," and "ugly." Research has also shown that socially anxious individuals rate their own social behavior more harshly than do objective observers (Rapee & Lim, 1992; Stopa & Clark, 1993) and overestimate the visibility of their anxiety relative to ratings by objective observers (Bruch, Gorsky, Collins, & Berger, 1989; Norton & Hope, 2001). Undoubtedly, these beliefs negatively impact their image of how they are coming across to others. The image of the self is further influenced by internal cues (e.g., somatic sensations of perspiration may produce images of sweat dripping down one's face) and external cues such as others' reactions (e.g., someone glancing at one's clothing and frowning might lead to images of appearing disheveled).

Beliefs that they are unacceptable to other people, that other people are inherently critical, and that the evaluation of others is extremely important motivate individuals with social anxiety disorder to be hypervigilant for early indications of disapproval from others (e.g., frowns, yawns) and aspects of their own behavior or appearance that might elicit negative evaluation from others (e.g., making an in-

ane comment, not being dressed appropriately, visibly shaking). The division of attentional resources among external social threats, the (distorted) mental representation of the self as seen by others, and the demands of the current social task *may* result in actual performance deficits (which may then elicit actual negative social feedback). In effect, socially anxious persons operate within the equivalent of a multiple-task paradigm, which increases the probability of disrupted social performance (MacLeod & Mathews, 1991). Therefore, complex social tasks are more likely than less complex tasks to result in poorer performance, due to limited processing resources.

Persons with social anxiety disorder also attempt to predict the standards that the audience holds for them in the situation. Characteristics of the audience (e.g., importance, attractiveness) and features of the situation (e.g., whether it is formal or informal) influence the projected standards of the audience. Individuals with social anxiety disorder then attempt to judge the extent to which their current mental representation of their appearance and behavior matches the predicted standards of the audience. Of course, given the negative bias present in their mental self-representation, they are likely to conclude that they are falling short of the audience's expectations, and painful outcomes such as loss of social status and rejection are likely follow. Negative predictions result in cognitive, behavioral, and physiological symptoms of anxiety that eventually feed back into the negatively biased mental representation of the self as seen by others and perpetuate the cycle of anxiety.

Clark and Wells (1995) emphasize that when in social situations, socially anxious individuals may engage in safety behaviors. Safety behaviors are essentially behaviors that the person performs in an attempt to avoid the negative outcomes that he or she fears. For example, a man who is afraid of his hand shaking while drinking coffee may grip the cup tightly, hoping to prevent any observable trembling. Such compensatory acts are viewed as helpful by the individual with social anxiety disorder, but these behaviors often make the feared outcome—in this case, shaking—more likely. Furthermore, they increase the likelihood that individuals with social anxiety disorder will conclude that they cannot make it through the social situation successfully in the absence of safety behaviors (Clark & Wells, 1995).

TREATMENT RATIONALE FROM A COGNITIVE-BEHAVIORAL PERSPECTIVE

The heart of our approach to treatment involves the integration of exposure and cognitive restructuring (Heimberg & Becker, 2002; Hope, Heimberg, Juster, & Turk, 2000). Exposure is beneficial for several reasons that are communicated to the client. From the perspective of the model, one of the most important aspects of exposure is the opportunity to test dysfunctional beliefs (e.g., "I will get too anxious to finish the speech") and to generate more realistic ways of understanding the self and others (e.g., "I can continue the speech even if I am anxious"). Exposure also allows clients to experience the natural reduction in anxiety that comes with staying in a feared situation for a prolonged period of time on several occasions (i.e., habituation). Last, exposure allows clients to practice perhaps long-avoided behavioral skills (e.g., asking someone for a date, being assertive) and to engage in behaviors consistent with their long-term, valued goals (e.g., engaging in small talk with new people today may lead to friendships in the future).

From the perspective of the model, cognitive restructuring is also important for several reasons communicated to the client. Clients learn to treat their anxiety-provoking thoughts and beliefs as hypotheses and to explore whether there are more helpful or realistic ways of viewing the situation, the self, and others. As clients come to view social situations as less threatening, they are often more willing to confront those situations in exposures. Furthermore, addressing dysfunctional cognitions often frees up attentional resources that can be used to increase focus on the social task at hand and potentially improve performance. Additionally, cognitive restructuring may help clients to take credit for successes and cope with disappointments after exposures. The use of cognitive skills to diffuse postevent rumination may be especially important given that more rumination following one anxiety-provoking event has been shown to be associated with greater initial anxiety prior to confronting another anxiety provoking event (Kocovski, Rector, & Denisoff, 2004). Last, as clients' cognitive assessments of the danger inherent in social situations become more realistic, their physiological symptoms of anxiety often diminish as well.

In-session exposures, with cognitive restructuring occurring before, during, and after each exposure, are viewed as particularly crucial. With the gentle encouragement and emotional support of the therapist, clients are often willing to engage in behaviors in session that they have avoided outside of session for many years. Successful in-session exposures can provide clients with the confidence and motivation to try out these behaviors in the real world. In-session exposures may also be more easily graduated than *in vivo* exposures. For example, a client who is terrified of formal public speaking might do an initial in-session exposure that comprises reading an article aloud from a magazine while sitting down. The next exposure might involve standing up while reading the article aloud, then taking questions from a small audience. In-session exposures also provide the therapist with the opportunity to teach clients about the principles of effective exposure, such as staying in a feared social situation for a prolonged period of time without avoiding, even if anxiety escalates. In-session exposures also allow the therapist to see firsthand any subtle avoidance behaviors (i.e., safety behaviors) that the client may be employing to manage anxiety. For example, a client who fears that other people might reject him if they got to know him personally may assail a conversation partner with questions and not reveal any personal information. A client who is afraid of the reaction of others to her speech might never look up from her notes, so that she never has to see any bored or critical faces (and, of course, also never has a chance to see any interested or approving faces). As noted by Clark and Wells (1995), such safety behaviors may have the unintended effect of making individuals appear socially awkward and increase the likelihood of negative reactions from others. Furthermore, clients do not learn that they might have managed the social situation as well, if not better, without engaging in the safety behaviors. In-session exposures provide the therapist with the opportunity to point out these behaviors and to set goals for the next exposure that involve fully confronting the feared situation (e.g., looking at the audience during the speech, revealing personal information during a conversation). In-session exposures also provide the opportunity for clients to receive direct feedback on their social performance in a way that is often not possible in real life. For example, a client who believes that she trembles so much during public speaking that others pity her can ask her exposure audience how noticeable the trembling was and what they thought of her (rarely will an audience reply that an anxious person was pitied). Last, in-session exposures provide the opportunity for the therapist to assist clients in applying cognitive restructuring skills to an actual anxiety-provoking situation. Once in-session exposures begin, homework involves confronting similar situations outside of session. As with in-session exposures, clients are asked to engage in cognitive restructuring activities before, during, and after each *in vivo* exposure.

TREATMENT-RELATED VARIABLES

Group versus Individual Treatment

Treatment of social anxiety disorder has most commonly been conducted in a group format (e.g., Heimberg, Dodge, et al., 1990; Heimberg et al., 1998), which has been conceptualized as having a number of advantages over the individual format. It provides opportunities for vicarious learning, support from others with similar problems, the availability of multiple role-play partners, informal exposure stemming from group participation, and a range of people to provide evidence to counter distorted thinking (Heimberg & Becker, 2002; Sank & Shaffer, 1984). Nevertheless, the group format has a number of potential disadvantages as well. Treatment cannot begin until a group of approximately six clients has been assembled, which means that the first few individuals joining the group may have to wait for an extended period before starting treatment. Some of these individuals lose motivation and drop out before the group begins. Group treatment also provides less flexibility in making up missed sessions. Although group treatment provides opportunities for vicarious learning, this benefit may be offset by the reduced time available for the idiosyncratic needs of each client. Clinically, some clients appear to get discouraged and lose motivation when they see other group members progressing at a more rapid pace than themselves. Additionally, even when efforts are made to screen potential group members, a group may include a client who is domineering, aggressive, or otherwise difficult to manage, and may have a negative impact on the group. Last, some individuals never fully habituate to the group setting, and their anxiety may interfere with their ability to process information during sessions.

Little available data speak to the issue of whether individual or group therapy provides better outcomes. In their meta-analysis, Gould, Buckminster, Pollack, Otto, and Yap (1997) reported that group and individual cognitive behavioral interventions for social anxiety disorder produced similar effect sizes. Group and individual formats have rarely been compared within the same study. Lucas and Telch (1993) found that group and individual versions of Heimberg's treatment resulted in similar gains, both superior to an educational-supportive control group. Scholing and Emmelkamp (1993) examined various combinations of exposure and cognitive restructuring delivered in group or individual formats and found no clear advantage for either treatment modality. Similarly, Wlazlo, Schroeder-Hartwig, Hand, Kaiser, and Münchau (1990) found no differences in outcome between group and individual exposure treatment. One study did find that an individual version of CBT for social anxiety disorder was superior to the group version, and that both formats were superior to a waiting list (Stangier et al., 2003). However, the data do not clearly suggest an advantage for either modality in the treatment for social anxiety disorder.

Heimberg and Becker (2002) provide a description of CBGT for social anxiety disorder. This chapter provides a description of the individual version of this treatment, which has been the focus of our research in recent years (see also Hope et al., 2000; Hope, Heimberg, & Turk, 2006).

Appropriate Clients

In anxiety studies to date, social anxiety disorder has been the primary diagnosis of the participants. As previously discussed, social anxiety disorder is often comorbid with other disorders (W. Magee et al., 1996; Schneier et al., 1992). In such cases, the clinician and client need to reach a joint decision that social anxiety will be the focus of treatment for a specified period of time (e.g., 16 weeks). Clinically, it is important to clarify this issue prior to beginning treatment, because some clients may express a desire to switch the focus of treatment to another problem area when it is time to begin exposures. In general, our policy is to remind the client of the original treatment contract and goals, and to encourage him or her to "avoid avoidance." In some cases, the best clinical decision is to change the focus of treatment due to changes in the client's life circumstances or symptoms. Nevertheless, we are especially wary of altering the treatment plan when the client's desire to change the focus of treatment coincides with the initiation of exposures. Therapists without a strong background in CBT or exposure therapy may be at risk for changing the focus of treatment too readily, partially due to their own discomfort with conducting in-session exposures. Sometimes a compromise can be reached in which exposures remain in the treatment plan but some session time is set aside to deal with other issues.

Appropriate Therapists

The ideal therapist has a strong background in the theoretical underpinnings of CBT for anxiety disorders, experience conducting exposures, good basic therapy skills, and experience with social anxiety in particular. Little is known about the effectiveness of manualized treatments when implemented by clinicians without extensive training in the manual's theoretical underpinnings and procedures (Chambless & Ollendick, 2001). Clearly, more research is needed on this issue. That said, our clinical experience suggests that with good supervision, this treatment can be successfully implemented by novice therapists seeing their very first clients (in fact, the case study presented later was treated by L. Magee, who at the time was a novice therapist) and experienced therapists with a theoretical orientation other than a cognitive-behavioral one. Experienced clinicians with a good cognitive-behavioral background are likely to do quite well working independently with this manualized treatment. Moreover, our client workbook (Hope et al., 2000) and therapist guide (Hope et al., 2006) were designed with the intention of being sufficiently detailed to allow therapists with a wide variety of backgrounds to provide this treatment, although supervision and/or consultation with an experienced cognitive-behavioral therapist on the first few cases and the more complex cases would be beneficial.

Medication and CBT for Social Anxiety Disorder

Many clients are already taking psychotropic medications when they present for therapy. Some take medication to control their social anxiety, whereas others take medications for comorbid conditions. We do not require clients to discontinue medications prior to starting CBT (unless dictated by a specific research protocol). However, we do ask clients to stabilize their dosage before starting treatment and to refrain from changing their dosage or trying any new medications during treatment. Clinically, we want clients to attribute positive changes in their symptoms to the work they are doing in therapy rather than to changes in their medication regimen. Individuals who take medication on an as-needed basis are asked to refrain from doing so before sessions or exposure homework assignments. The same request is made of individuals who use nonprescription drugs or alcohol to control their anxiety.

PRETREATMENT ASSESSMENT AND PREPARATION FOR TREATMENT

Assessment should play an integral part in diagnosis, case conceptualization, treatment planning, and termination decisions. Although administering all of the measures presented here is not practical in most clinical settings, we highly recommend administering a subset of the self-report and clinician-rated instruments described below, and a behavioral assessment, if at all possible (for a more thorough review of assessment of social anxiety disorder, see Heimberg & Turk, 2002).

Clinical Interview

The Anxiety Disorders Interview Schedule for DSM-IV (ADIS-IV; Brown, Di Nardo, & Barlow, 1994) and the ADIS-IV Lifetime Version (ADIS-IV-L; Di Nardo, Brown, & Barlow, 1994) provide a thorough diagnostic assessment of the anxiety disorders and include modules for mood disorders, substance use disorders, and disorders that overlap with anxiety disorders in terms of presenting symptoms (e.g., hypochondriasis, somatization disorder). There are screening questions for other major disorders (e.g., psychosis). A 0–8 clinician's severity rating (CSR) designates the degree of distress and interference associated with each diagnosis. A CSR of 4 or higher suggests that the client meets criteria for the specific DSM-IV diagnosis. When multiple disorders receive a CSR of 4 or higher, the disorder receiving the highest CSR is designated as the principal diagnosis and the other disorders are designated as additional. In a major reliability study of the ADIS-IV-L, 362 individuals seeking treatment at an anxiety specialty clinic received two independent administrations of the ADIS-IV (Brown, Di Nardo, Lehman, & Campbell, 2001). Social anxiety disorder evidenced good reliability when examined as a principal diagnosis (kappa = .77), as a clinical (principal or additional) diagnosis (kappa = .77), and as a past (lifetime) diagnosis (kappa = .72). The CSR for social anxiety disorder (r = .80) also evidenced good interrater reliability.

Our clinics routinely employ the ADIS-IV during the first client visit. Semistructured interviews such as the ADIS-IV assist with differential diagnosis and in providing systematic assessment for a broad range of comorbid conditions that may affect the course of treatment. Nevertheless, diagnostic interviews may be costly and time-consuming. Regardless of whether a semistructured or unstructured clinical interview is conducted, devoting time to a thorough and accurate diagnostic evaluation is crucial to appropriate treatment planning. Clients whose symptoms are better accounted for by another diagnosis may experience, among other things, little improvement with treatment targeting social anxiety, unnecessarily prolonged suffering as they go without the appropriate treatment, and increased hopelessness and financial hardship.

Self-Report Instruments

At the Adult Anxiety Clinic of Temple University and the Anxiety Clinic at Washburn University, clients complete a packet of questionnaires prior to treatment. Self-report instruments are an important complement to the diagnostic interview. In an interview, at a time when they may experience feelings of shame and embarrassment, clients may give descriptions of their problems that do not fully reflect the severity or pervasiveness of their social fear and avoidance. Furthermore, normative data on questionnaires allow the clinician to evaluate the severity of a client's symptoms relative to meaningful reference points. Importantly, pretreatment scores provide a baseline against which treatment progress can be assessed.

Measures of Social Anxiety

A number of questionnaires are available to assess social anxiety and avoidance. The Social Interaction Anxiety Scale (SIAS) and Social Phobia Scale (SPS) are commonly used companion measures designed specifically for the assessment of social anxiety disorder (Mattick & Clarke, 1998). The SIAS assesses fear of interacting in dyads and groups, and the SPS assesses fear of being observed by others (e.g., eating in front of others). In most published studies, the SIAS and SPS contain 20 items each. For each instrument, respondents rate how characteristic each statement is of them on a 5-point Likert-type scale (0, Not at all; 4, Extremely). Multiple studies suggest that the SIAS and SPS are reliable and valid measures, and sensitive to the effects of CBT (e.g., Brown et al., 1997; Cox, Ross, Swinson, & Direnfeld, 1998; Heimberg, Mueller, Holt, Hope, & Liebowitz, 1992; Ries et al., 1998).

Another commonly used instrument developed to assess social anxiety disorder, the Social Phobia and Anxiety Inventory (SPAI; Turner, Beidel, Dancu, & Stanley, 1989), comprises a Social Phobia subscale, an Agoraphobia subscale, and a derived Difference (or Total) score (i.e., Social Phobia–Agoraphobia subscales). The SPAI contains 45 items, 21 of which require multiple responses. For example, for the item that begins "I attempt to avoid social situations where there are . . . ," the client separately rates how frequently he or she avoids situations involving strangers, authority figures, the opposite sex, and people in general. The client makes a total of 109 responses, making the administration and scoring of the SPAI relatively time-consuming. Despite the disadvantages imposed by the length of the scale, the quantity and specificity of information that it elicits can be quite helpful in case formulation and treatment planning. The Social Phobia subscale assesses somatic, cognitive, and behavioral responses to a variety of interaction, performance, and observation situations. The Agoraphobia subscale assesses anxiety in situations commonly feared by individuals with panic disorder with agoraphobia (e.g., waiting in line). Respondents rate how frequently they feel anxious in each situation using a 7-point Likert-type scale (1, *Never*; 7, *Always*). The Difference score is intended to provide an index of social anxiety and avoidance distinct from the sometimes similar concerns of clients with agoraphobia. However, the very high correlation between the Difference score and the score of the Social Phobia subscale ($r = .91$) (Ries et al., 1998) suggests that there may be little benefit to this strategy. Multiple studies suggest that the SPAI is a reliable and valid instrument (e.g., Beidel, Turner, Stanley, & Dancu, 1989; Herbert, Bellack, & Hope, 1991; Turner et al., 1989), and sensitive to treatment-related change (e.g., Cox et al., 1998; Ries et al., 1998; Taylor, Woody, McLean, & Koch, 1997b).

Another scale that may prove to be quite useful is the 17-item Social Phobia Inventory, also known as the SPIN (Antony, Coons, McCabe, Ashbaugh, & Swinson, 2006; Connor et al., 2000), which has demonstrated good reliability, significant correlations with related measures, and the ability to discriminate between clients with social anxiety disorder and those with other anxiety disorders. A 3-item version of the SPIN, the Mini-SPIN, has also shown substantial utility as a screening device for social anxiety disorder in both general health care (Connor, Kobak, Churchill, Katzelnick, & Davidson, 2001) and anxiety specialty clinic (Weeks, Spokas, & Heimberg, in press) settings.

Although developed and validated with college students prior to the inclusion of social anxiety disorder in the DSM, the original Fear of Negative Evaluation scale (FNE; Watson & Friend, 1969) and the brief version of the scale (BFNE; Leary, 1983) continue to be widely used, because they target the core construct of the disorder. The FNE comprises 30 items and employs a true–false format. In treatment studies, changes on the FNE have been found to predict end-state functioning (Mattick & Peters, 1988; Mattick et al., 1989). The FNE appears to be sensitive to the effects of treatment, although changes are typically small in magnitude (Heimberg, 1994). The BFNE contains 12 items, uses a 5-point Likert-type format (1, *Not at all characteristic of me*; 5, *Extremely characteristic of me*), and correlates highly with the original scale ($r = .96$) (Leary, 1983). A recent study by Rodebaugh, Woods, and colleagues (2004) that utilized a large sample of undergraduates found that the BFNE was more sensitive than the FNE to differing degrees of fear of negative evaluation. A study by Weeks and colleagues (2005) that utilized a large sample of clients with social anxiety disorder found that the BFNE had high internal consistency, correlated with measures of social anxiety, showed good discriminant validity, and was sensitive to the effects of CBT. Both of these studies suggest quite compellingly that the reverse-scored items of the BFNE may detract from its validity, and we now score only the straightforwardly worded items. Others have taken a similar approach by rewording the reverse-scored items to be consistent with the straightforwardly worded items (e.g., Collins, Westra, Dozois, & Stewart, 2005).

In a recently developed measure for the assessment of session-by-session change in the treatment of social anxiety disorder, the Social Anxiety Session Change Index (SASCI; Hayes, Miller, Hope, Heimberg, & Juster, in press), clients use a 7-point Likert-type scale to indicate how much they feel that they have changed since the beginning of therapy on four dimensions: anxiety, avoidance, concern about humiliation and embarrassment, and interference. More specifically, the SASCI measures how *anxious* the respondent becomes in anticipation of or when he or she is in social or performance situations; how much the respondent *avoids* social or performance situations; how *concerned* the respondent is about embarrassing or humiliating him- or herself in front of others; and how much the respondent's anxiety *interferes* with work or social activities. A total score of 16 indicates no change since the beginning of treatment. Scores of 4–15 indicate improvement, whereas scores of 17–28 indicate deterioration. The internal consistency of the SASCI across sessions ranged from .84 to .94 across sessions ($M = .89$) in the study by Hayes, Miller, and colleagues (in press). Change on the SASCI was related to change in fear of negative evaluation and to clinician-rated improvement, but not to ratings of anxiety sensitivity or depression. The use of the SASCI and the BFNE as session-by-session measures is demonstrated in the case study reported later in this chapter.

Other Self-Report Measures

In addition to measures targeting social anxiety, we administer questionnaires assessing other constructs relevant to case conceptualization and treatment outcome. We routinely administer the Beck Depression Inventory–II

(BDI-II; Beck, Steer, & Brown, 1996), which assesses symptoms of depression, including the affective, cognitive, behavioral, somatic, and motivational components, as well as suicidal wishes. We also use the Liebowitz Self-Rated Disability Scale (Schneier et al., 1994), which assesses impairment across 11 domains (e.g., school, work, alcohol abuse), and the Quality of Life Inventory (Frisch, 1994), which assesses the client's overall sense of well-being and satisfaction with life.

Feedback and Treatment Contract Interview

At the session following the intake session, the interviewer reviews the assessment data with the client, explains diagnoses, answers questions, and offers treatment recommendations. For clients with comorbid diagnoses, the benefits of initially making social anxiety the primary focus of treatment for 12–16 weekly sessions is discussed, as noted earlier. Last, clients are assured that the severity of their social anxiety symptoms and any comorbid conditions will be reassessed following this initial course of treatment and, if necessary, additional treatment recommendations will be made at that time. Additional assessments may be conducted at this visit, or clients may be scheduled for one additional session to conduct further assessments before treatment formally begins. The additional assessments may include clinician-administered measures of social anxiety and behavior tests.

Clinician-Administered Measures of Social Anxiety

The two most commonly used clinician-administered measures of social anxiety are the Liebowitz Social Anxiety Scale (LSAS; Liebowitz, 1987) and the Brief Social Phobia Scale (BSPS; Davidson et al., 1991, 1997). Both measures have been shown to have good psychometric properties (Heimberg & Turk, 2002). Our clinics routinely utilize the LSAS, so we describe it here. This measure is completed at the second clinic visit largely to avoid making the initial intake session unduly lengthy. The LSAS separately evaluates Fear and Avoidance of 11 interaction (e.g., talking to people in authority) and 13 performance (e.g., working while being observed) situations using 4-point Likert-type scales. Summing the Fear and Avoidance ratings for all 24 items

yields an index of overall severity. The LSAS has been shown to have good reliability and convergent/discriminant validity (e.g., Cox et al., 1998; Heimberg et al., 1999). It discriminates well between clients with social anxiety disorder and generalized anxiety disorder (Heimberg & Holaway, in press). It has also demonstrated sensitivity to cognitive-behavioral and pharmacological treatment of social anxiety disorder (e.g., Heimberg et al., 1998). When the LSAS is accompanied by detailed instructions, it appears that it also has good reliability and validity as a self-report instrument (Fresco et al., 2001).

Behavioral Assessment

Behavior tests, or role-played re-creations of social situations relevant to the client, can be a very useful addition to the self-report and clinician-administered measures described here. Although these tests may be quite anxiety provoking for the client, the information obtained during a behavior test is unique and important in several ways. Individuals with social anxiety disorder are likely to describe their social behavior as inadequate (e.g., Rapee & Lim, 1992; Stopa & Clark, 1993) and their anxiety as highly visible to others (e.g., Norton & Hope, 2001). However, behavior tests often demonstrate that these reports are largely inaccurate and are essentially examples of distorted beliefs. Furthermore, level of anxiety and quality of performance exhibited by a client during behavior tests may be used to calibrate the difficulty of exposures and increase the likelihood that the therapist creates a first exposure that provides both a challenge and a successful experience for the client.

During behavior tests, the clinician may ask for anxiety ratings before, at several points during, and after the role play. Other assessments, such as asking clients to rate the quality of their performance or list the thoughts they had during the role play, are easily incorporated. Affordable ambulatory physiological equipment, particularly pulse monitors, is increasingly available and adds a useful dimension. The clinician can choose to test the limits of a client's ability to perform when anxious by asking him or her to remain in the situation for a certain period of time (typically 4–5 minutes). On the other hand, the clinician may give the client explicit permission to stop (e.g., Ries et al., 1998) when the anxiety is excessive, and latency to escape the situation becomes a measure of avoidance.

Behavior tests may either be standardized or individualized. Standardized role plays allow for the observation of differences across patients for a particular task. Commonly used tasks include a conversation with a same-sex stranger, a conversation with an opposite-sex stranger, a conversation with two or more people, and a speech to a small audience. In contrast, the advantage of individualized behavior tests is that they may be designed more precisely to target idiosyncratic fears. For example, a client with a fear of displaying a hand tremor when eating in front of others may experience little anxiety during a one-on-one conversation. However, if that client is asked to engage in a one-on-one conversation while eating a bowl of soup, his or her anxiety is more likely to be activated.

INDIVIDUAL CBT FOR SOCIAL ANXIETY DISORDER

Principles and Logistics

For our studies on individual treatment of social anxiety disorder, we have established guidelines to which our therapists must adhere (Hope et al., 2006). One issue facing manualized treatments is that it is unclear to what extent one may take liberties with how the treatment is carried out and still expect outcomes similar to those obtained during efficacy studies. Therefore, although we recognize that this treatment may be applied more flexibly in clinical settings, we present these guidelines to help therapists understand the treatment as it has been most thoroughly studied.

The treatment comprises 16 weekly 1-hour sessions within a period of 16–20 weeks. Although completing 16 sessions within 16 weeks might be ideal, up to 20 weeks are allowed to take into consideration sessions missed due to illness, vacations, holidays, and so forth. Taking longer than 20 weeks to complete 16 sessions may compromise the momentum of therapy. The two to three pretreatment sessions described earlier, as well as posttreatment assessment and feedback sessions, are not counted as part of the 16-session treatment phase.

Our individual treatment requires that the client use a workbook (Hope et al., 2000) as he or she works with the therapist during each

session and for homework assignments. This workbook comprises 14 chapters, but the treatment program does not follow a one-chapter-per-session format. Rather, treatment is divided into five segments, and the therapist has flexibility in terms of the pace and, to some extent, the content of these segments. The description of the treatment that follows is organized around these segments. We ask clients to read assigned chapters before coming to the session.

Clients are asked to bring their workbook to every session. Therapists typically bring their own copy of the workbook and/or a copy of the therapist guide to session as well. The therapist also makes sure that there is something to write on that the therapist and client can look at together during the session. In our clinics, a newsprint easel or a dry-erase board mounted to the wall is typically used (for ease, we refer to the use of an easel hereafter). However, at times, we have also just pulled two chairs side by side, so that both the therapist and client can write on and view the same piece of paper on a clipboard. Importantly, every session introduces key concepts that are written down (e.g., a therapist may draw a continuum of anxiety in Session 1; client automatic thoughts and rational responses are always recorded). Writing things down during session helps clients better to track and process the information being covered and is a required component of the treatment.

The therapeutic relationship is actively fostered throughout treatment. As Kendall, Chu, Gifford, Hayes, and Nauta (1998) have pointed out, some critics assume that the therapeutic relationship is not considered relevant when a manual is utilized. In fact, in our research studies, our therapist adherence manual (Hope, Van Dyke, Heimberg, Turk, & Fresco, 2002) includes explicit ratings of the therapeutic relationship within each segment of treatment. Therapists are rated on how well they engage in active listening, respond to verbal and nonverbal cues, facilitate the client's investment in treatment, and communicate support of and investment in the client. Additionally, contrary to the criticism that CBTs encourage blanket suppression of affect, therapists are expected to help clients to experience and deepen affect as appropriate to the situation at hand. For example, a therapist would be expected to help a client to be open to the experience of anxiety during exposures and to help the client process and grieve losses that are a consequence of many years of social avoidance. In other situations, the therapist would be expected to help the client use uncomfortable feelings as cues for additional cognitive coping practice. For example, the therapist would help a client who experiences a deep sense of shame or guilt after making a small social mistake (e.g., spilling a drink, calling someone by the wrong name) to engage in cognitive restructuring to change the meaning of the event eliciting such emotions. Therapists are actively supervised on these aspects of treatment and not attending to the therapeutic relationship or appropriately responding to what is going on in session is considered a serious failure to follow protocol.

Recent data suggest that the therapeutic relationship is indeed related to successful outcomes in our protocol (Hayes, Hope, Van Dyke, & Heimberg, 2007). Clients' ratings of the therapeutic alliance were positively related to their perceptions of session helpfulness. Interestingly, however, the relationship between the therapeutic alliance and anxiety reduction during in-session exposures was curvilinear; that is, when ratings of the alliance were higher or lower, clients showed less anxiety reduction than when the ratings of the alliance were moderate. The effect for low ratings of the alliance may not require explanation, but we have conjectured that if the client feels too comfortable with the therapist, then this may possibly interfere with anxiety evocation during exposures and thereby interfere with emotional processing. Maintaining the "right" therapeutic alliance is important in the CBT for social anxiety disorder (Hayes et al., 2007).

Therapists are also expected to engage in efficient time management. Our therapist adherence manual rates therapists' ability to cover required topics flexibly, without rushing or boring the client by belaboring various points (Hope et al., 2002). Two types of problems tend to crop up with regard to time management (and may negatively impact the therapeutic relationship as well). Some therapists fall into the trap of turning each session into a psychoeducational lecture, and this tendency may be aggravated if the therapist is working with a client who is very quiet in the early sessions. The primary recommendation in this situation is to ask open-ended questions that prompt the client to relate his or her personal experiences to the material. The client's verbalizations in response to these questions are then reinforced

through active listening skills, which elicit more client verbalizations. The other trap into which some therapists fall is allowing the client to dominate the session with long, detailed stories about experiences with social anxiety. In some cases, the therapist may have inadvertently taught the client to lead the session in this way, by indiscriminately using active listening skills and nonverbal cues, even when the client is discussing tangential or repetitive material. In other cases, clients may be accustomed to dominating sessions through prior experiences with traditional talk therapy, or they may even intentionally attempt to dominate the session to avoid threatening material, particularly in-session exposures. In this situation, gentle verbal redirection is required. In some cases, a straightforward discussion of time management issues and negotiation of session time may be beneficial.

Last, we want to emphasize our belief that manualized treatments such as this one do not represent an inflexible set of procedures applied in an indiscriminant fashion to all clients. Rather, we expect therapists to develop an individualized conceptualization of each client's particular presenting problem. This conceptualization is continually refined over the course of treatment and incorporates the unique characteristics of the client (e.g., cultural group, sex, educational background). Treatment procedures are then tailored to address the unique aspects of each case.

Segment 1: Psychoeducation

Segment 1 covers the material in Chapters 1–4 of the client workbook (Hope et al., 2000). Establishing a good working relationship is a critical goal for this segment of therapy. Therefore, if the therapist was not also the initial interviewer, three to four sessions are typically needed for the psychoeducation segment to allow adequate attention to building rapport. If a good working alliance has been established during the course of the initial assessment and if the client is especially bright and motivated, then it may be possible to cover two chapters per session, finishing this portion of treatment in as little as 2 weeks. Therapists should not assign more than two chapters per week at any point in therapy, because clients are unlikely to process the material fully and make the most of the associated exercises and self-monitoring homework.

With regard to homework during this segment, one or two chapters are assigned at the end of each session. Each chapter includes a variety of forms that the client attempts to complete as well. At the beginning of the next session, the therapist asks the client for reactions to and questions about the readings, and therapist and client review corresponding forms completed by the client. If the client has not made an attempt to complete a form, it is completed at the beginning of the session during homework review.

Therapists are required to review certain topics from each chapter in the client workbook in session; other topics are optional depending on the needs of the individual client. For Chapter 1, the therapist must review two topics: (1) normal versus problematic social anxiety, and (2) the investment that treatment will require. The discussion of normal and problematic social anxiety conveys to the client that social anxiety exists along a continuum, with some people rarely experiencing any social anxiety, other people frequently experiencing intense social anxiety, and most people falling somewhere between these extremes. People who fall in the middle of the continuum experience social anxiety in some situations, such as a first date or a job interview, but the anxiety is typically manageable and decreases as the person remains in the situation. Factors such as intensity and duration of anxiety before and during social situations, the number of situations eliciting anxiety, and the degree of life impairment differentiate between normal social anxiety and problematic social anxiety for which a diagnosis may be assigned. Therapists often engage clients in this material by asking what types of situations elicit social anxiety for many people and what purpose social anxiety might serve—to illustrate the notion that social anxiety has an adaptive value (e.g., caring about what other people think might cause anxiety, but it also helps people to treat each other more kindly). A therapist typically uses this opportunity to launch a discussion about what the client should expect in terms of treatment outcome. First, the therapist points out that social anxiety is part of the human condition; thus, it is impossible to remove it completely, even if this were a desirable goal. Therefore, total freedom from social anxiety is not a reasonable expectation for treatment. However, it is reasonable to expect to move down the continuum from problematic levels of social anxiety to a level of social anxiety that is more typical of most people. Not all clients are willing to accept that social anxiety exists on a continuum, or that it can have an adaptive value this early in treatment. This first session is merely an introduction to these concepts, and arguing with a client about these issues is likely to be unproductive. Rather, the therapist empathizes with the client's current worldview (e.g., "You feel you are either calm or extremely anxious, and that no middle ground is possible for you") but does not agree with it.

The discussion of the required investment in treatment involves instilling hope in the client that he or she will be able to make significant changes and conveying the time, effort, and emotional energy that treatment activities require. Research has shown that positive expectancies are associated with more favorable outcomes for CBT for social anxiety (Chambless et al., 1997; Safren, Heimberg, & Juster, 1997b). The therapist shares with the client that in studies of individuals who completed CBT, approximately 75–80% were rated by independent clinical interviewers as having experienced meaningful reductions in their social anxiety (e.g., Heimberg et al., 1998). The therapist also emphasizes that attending sessions regularly, doing homework, being willing to experience anxiety during exposures, and being open to new ways of looking at the world, other people, and oneself are factors that substantially influence whether someone becomes a treatment responder, and that these factors are largely under the client's control. During this time, clients are encouraged to speak about their fears regarding treatment and their goals for a better life after treatment.

Next, the therapist reviews with the client the three components of anxiety, which are presented in Chapter 2 of the client workbook (Hope et al., 2000). Each of the three components of anxiety is described: (1) the physiological component comprises bodily reactions, such as a pounding heart; (2) the cognitive component comprises what a person says to him- or herself, such as "I look foolish"; and (3) the behavioral component comprises what a person does when he or she is anxious, such as avoiding eye contact. When presenting the behavioral component, the therapist emphasizes how escape and avoidance behaviors may reduce anxiety in the short term but lead to a less satisfying life and to other negative feelings, such as guilt and shame, in the long term.

The therapist then helps the client to practice identifying each of these components with a hypothetical example. Over the years, we have found that using a hypothetical example initially is much more conducive to learning than starting with an example from the client's own experience. Issues such as fear of negative evaluation, defensiveness, anxiety, and lack of objectivity can result in a client having difficulty identifying the three components from a personal experience this early in treatment (e.g., "I wasn't thinking anything"). One option is for the therapist simply to review the hypothetical examples from the workbook that illustrate the three components, but we generally recommend using a different hypothetical example in session to give the client more practice. Often we use the example from the group treatment version (Heimberg & Becker, 2002), in which the client is asked to imagine a person waiting in the lobby for a job interview that is extremely attractive in terms of responsibilities, pay, and hours. The client is told that the person is feeling anxious about the interview, then is asked what that person might be experiencing as he or she anxiously waits to be called in to the office. Using the easel, the therapist writes the client's responses under the appropriate heading (e.g., "feeling nauseous" is written under "Physiological Component"). After classifying the client's spontaneous responses, the therapist then asks questions to elicit several examples of each of the three components (e.g., "Might the person have any thoughts relating to her sweaty palms? What might she say to herself about that?"). The therapist makes an effort to draw out how each of the three components interacts with the others, resulting in an escalating spiral of anxiety (e.g., sweaty palms might lead to the thought "The interviewer will think I am anxious," which might lead to a behavior of wiping sweaty hands on one's suit). The therapist concludes that treatment involves learning ways to disrupt this spiral of anxiety. Assuming that the client does reasonably well with this exercise, the therapist then helps the client to repeat the exercise with a recent, personal experience of social anxiety. At this point in therapy, the therapist makes no effort to help the client to challenge anxiety-provoking cognitions, only to identify the three components of anxiety and to understand how they interact with each other. In addition to readings from the workbook, the client is given the homework assignment of identifying all

three components of anxiety experienced during a social situation during the week.

Next, the therapist describes for the client factors that are thought to be related to the development of problematic social anxiety, which are also presented in Chapter 3 of the workbook. The therapist tells the client that research suggests that genetics play a role in the etiology of social anxiety disorder. The therapist emphasizes that what is inherited is probably a tendency to be a sensitive and emotionally reactive individual rather than a gene that inevitably results in social anxiety (Barlow, 2002). This inherited sensitivity might not be at all problematic, and it may even be a good thing. For example, the person might be especially empathic toward others and have a greater capacity to experience joy, as well as anxiety. However, if a biologically sensitive individual is exposed to important social experiences during development and learns that others are threatening and hurtful, then the biological vulnerability may contribute to the development of problematic social anxiety. The therapist might inquire whether other family members seem to have problems with social anxiety or other types of anxiety, suggesting a genetic predisposition. The therapist then presents experiences within the family as another potential factor contributing to social anxiety. For example, a socially anxious mother might teach a child that the opinions of others are extremely important, and that negative evaluation is to be avoided at all cost. Alternatively, a verbally abusive father might provide experiences that teach the child that other people are dangerous, and that avoidance is a good strategy for self-protection. Again, the therapist asks the client whether this information fits with his or her personal experiences. Last, the therapist describes how experiences outside of the family can similarly teach a person that others are a source of threat. For example, teasing by peers seems to be related to later social anxiety (Roth, Coles, & Heimberg, 2002). Moreover, throughout the discussion, the therapist emphasizes the idea that because social anxiety is largely learned through experience, it can be changed through experience.

This discussion of the etiology of social anxiety leads into a discussion of dysfunctional thoughts; that is, therapists might ask clients what lessons they learned about themselves and other people through a negative early-life social experience, such as being teased (e.g., "I learned that I don't fit in"). In this way, therapists educate clients about the origins of many of their automatic thoughts, which is important given that many clients view their tendency to have negative cognitions as a sign of inherent personal flaws rather than a logical consequence of their experiences. They then ask clients to think about how these dysfunctional ways of thinking color the kinds of thoughts and reactions they now have when confronting social situations (e.g., thoughts of not fitting in at parties, expecting to be made fun of by coworkers). At this point in therapy, clients are asked simply to consider the possibility that changing some of these automatic thinking biases might change the experience of anxiety. Therapists then set forth the rationale for primary interventions of cognitive restructuring, exposures, and homework.

Referring to the material covered in Chapter 4 of the client workbook, the therapist teaches the client how to use the Subjective Units of Discomfort Scale (SUDS; Wolpe & Lazarus, 1966) and to construct a fear and avoidance hierarchy. Self-monitoring of daily overall anxiety, overall depression, and social anxiety is also introduced and continued throughout treatment.

Segment 2:
Training in Cognitive Restructuring

Training in cognitive restructuring typically requires two to three sessions. The material is presented in Chapters 5 and 6 of the client workbook (Hope et al., 2000). After three sessions, a small minority of clients may still be struggling to master the cognitive concepts due to factors such as low educational attainment and/or poor abstract thinking skills. Our experience suggests that rather than forcing the issue with such clients, it is better simply to move on to the next segment of treatment after three sessions. In this circumstance, Heimberg and Becker (2002) recommend that, for the remainder of therapy, the cognitive portion of treatment be deemphasized in favor of relying more heavily on repeated exposure. Additionally, such clients may be able to generate realistic self-statements (e.g., "I have done this before") or self-instructions (e.g., "Start by introducing myself") informally, with help from the therapist, for use in anxiety-provoking situations rather than relying on more formal cognitive restructuring.

As in the previous segment, each session begins with a homework review and ends with homework assignment. Homework assignments include of readings from the client workbook, associated forms, and self-monitoring. Some clients begin to attempt *in vivo* exposures spontaneously at this point in treatment, without being specifically assigned to do so. If these exposures go well, then they may be beneficial to the client. However, therapists should not actively encourage exposures as homework until completion of training in cognitive restructuring and one in-session exposure. At this point in treatment, clients still have few adaptive strategies for managing anxiety or coping with social situations that have disappointing outcomes. They are also likely to escape a situation at the first sign of trouble. Therefore, the possibility of a less than positive exposure experience at this phase of treatment could lead to resistance to attempting future exposures.

In this segment of treatment, clients are explicitly introduced to the basic tenet of the cognitive-behavioral model, which proposes that emotional reactions occur as a result of *interpretations* of situations, not situations themselves. "Automatic thoughts" are defined as negative, distorted, or irrational thoughts about oneself, the world, or the future that lead to or increase the experience of problematic anxiety. These concepts are first demonstrated with a hypothetical example rather than an emotionally-charged example from the client's own life. The client workbook describes the very different thoughts of two young men after meeting a woman. Negative thoughts lead one man to give up any attempts to get to know the woman better and to experience several more unpleasant thoughts and emotions. The more neutral and realistic thoughts of the other man facilitate his continued efforts at making conversation. Additional examples are provided for the therapist and client to examine if the client appears to need further instruction on the concept of automatic thoughts. The client then completes an exercise, listing any automatic thoughts he or she may have about starting CBT for social anxiety. For homework, the client monitors his or her automatic thoughts and the emotions they cause in one or two naturally occurring situations during the week.

At the next session, "thinking errors" are defined as common categories into which automatic thoughts may fall. In other words, people often find that they are particularly prone to engage in certain types of distorted thinking (e.g., mind reading, fortune-telling, disqualifying the positive), and identifying these habitual thinking errors can assist in challenging automatic thoughts (e.g., "There I go, mind reading again. I have no reason to assume that they are thinking the worst"). Clients are introduced to an adaptation of the list of thinking errors outlined by Judith Beck (1995) in her book *Cognitive Therapy: Basics and Beyond*. Ideally, the client has reviewed this list in the course of doing the readings for homework, and the therapist and client can briefly discuss which thinking errors the client personally found most relevant. If the client has not done the homework, each thinking error is briefly reviewed by the therapist and client in session. The therapist and client can practice identifying both the thinking errors in workbook examples and the client's automatic thoughts recorded as part of self-monitoring homework, and further examine automatic thoughts the client might have about upcoming situations.

The next step in cognitive restructuring is to challenge the automatic thoughts and develop rational responses to them. The process of challenging automatic thoughts is begun with the assistance of disputing questions, originally adapted from the work of Sank and Shaffer (1984). These generic questions can be brought to bear on automatic thoughts (e.g., "Do I know for certain that _____?"; "What evidence do I have that _____?; What evidence do I have that the opposite is true?"; "What is the worst that could happen? How bad is that? How can I cope with that?"; "What does _____ mean? Does _____ really mean that I am a(n) _____?"). Before having the client attempt to apply these questions to his or her own thoughts, however, the therapist and client review two hypothetical examples from the client workbook. Thereafter, the client's automatic thoughts examined in the earlier discussion of thinking errors are addressed. Together the client and therapist question the automatic thoughts using the disputing questions and answer the disputing questions to arrive at alternative, more realistic ways of viewing the situation. The answers to the disputing questions are then summarized into one or two statements that serve as rational responses. Alternatively, the most compelling answer to one of the disputing questions may be adopted as a rational response. The

therapist explains that a rational response provides a realistic view of the situation that is more positive than that provided by the automatic thoughts. Rational responses are also relatively short and concise. For the next homework assignment, the client is now ready to record his or her automatic thoughts from an anxiety-provoking situation during the week, to identify the thinking errors, to dispute the automatic thoughts, and to develop a rational response.

Toward the end of the final session in this segment, the therapist informs the client that exposures will begin the following week. To the extent that beginning exposures causes the client to feel anxious, the client is encouraged to "avoid avoidance" by coming to the next session and to identify automatic thoughts related to the exposure, challenge them, and arrive at a rational response. The therapist reassures the client that a challenging, but not overwhelming, situation will be used for the first exposure. More experienced therapists often discuss a few possibilities for the first exposure during this session. Therapists new to this treatment approach often discuss details of the exposure with the client the following week, after the therapist has had supervision.

Segment 3: Exposures

Exposures should begin no later than Session 8 and may begin as early as Session 5, depending on the rate at which the earlier material was covered. Chapter 7 from the client workbook reviews the rationale for exposures and introduces the concept of setting achievable behavioral goals. The content of Chapter 7 is only briefly touched upon; many of these concepts have been covered earlier (e.g., why exposures are important), and the new material is demonstrated during the exposure itself. Similarly, when Chapter 8 (Ongoing Exposures) and one or more of the specific topic chapters (Chapter 9, Observational Fears; Chapter 10, Interaction Fears; Chapter 11, Public Speaking Fears) are assigned during this segment, therapists rarely devote an entire session to discussing each chapter. Rather, the content is only briefly addressed during the homework review and an in-session exposure is conducted; that is, during this phase of treatment, therapists strive for the goal of completing an exposure almost every session. To follow protocol in our research studies, a minimum of 4 in-session exposures must be completed. More commonly, at least six in-session exposures are completed, and the more the better. Therefore, although the protocol does allow the therapist the freedom to a use a couple of sessions during this segment to do cognitive restructuring alone or to review a topic chapter in detail, our belief is that the time is best devoted to repeated in-session exposures integrating cognitive restructuring.

All exposure sessions follow the same basic format (see Table 3.1). The session begins with a homework review and ends with a homework assignment. The homework assignment typically comprises self-monitoring and *in vivo* exposure tasks, and associated cognitive restructuring that logically build upon the in-session exposure. The first in-session exposure typically includes a role play with the therapist of a situation that the client assigned a SUDS

TABLE 3.1. Outline of Exposure Sessions

1. Review homework from previous week.

2. Complete in-session exposure.

   a. Exposure preprocessing
     • Briefly negotiate details of exposure
     • Elicit automatic thoughts
     • Client labels thinking errors in automatic thoughts
     • Client disputes one or two automatic thoughts
     • Client develops a rational response
     • Client sets nonperfectionistic, behavioral goals

   b. Conduct role play for approximately 10 minutes
     • Request SUDS and the rational response every minute
     • Track client's progress on behavioral goals

   c. Exposure postprocessing
     • Review whether goals were attained
     • Discuss how well the rational response worked
     • Discuss any unexpected or new automatic thoughts
     • Client, therapist, and role players react to client's performance
     • Graph and interpret SUDS ratings pattern
     • Client states what was learned from the exposure

3. Assignment of homework

   a. Related *in vivo* exposures with associated cognitive restructuring
   b. Continued self-monitoring of depression, general anxiety, and social anxiety
   c. Other assignments as appropriate

rating of at least 50. The rule of thumb is that clients should perceive exposures as challenging but not overwhelming or beyond their ability to use cognitive coping skills. Therapists make exposures as realistic as possible by rearranging furniture, using props, and instructing role-play partners (i.e., therapist assistants brought into session to assist with exposures) to behave in particular ways. A bit of effort in making the situation more realistic may mean the difference between an exposure that elicits significant anxiety and one that is too artificial to be relevant. Commonly used props include food or drink for individuals with fears of eating, drinking, or serving food in front of others, and client-prepared notes for presentations. Careful attention should be paid to aspects that make the situation more or less anxiety-provoking. For example, a client who fears eating in front of others may be more anxious when eating something that is easy to spill (e.g., soup) than when eating finger foods.

The essence of the treatment is the coordination between the cognitive restructuring work and the exposure (see Table 3.1). The therapist begins the exposure preprocessing by briefly describing an exposure situation. The client may suggest modifications or alternatives. However, the therapist needs to balance approaching the exposure task collaboratively with being highly vigilant for overly detailed discussions that largely serve to avoid getting started with the exposure. The therapist then elicits the client's automatic thoughts regarding the chosen situation and records the thoughts on the easel. The therapist picks one or two automatic thoughts to dispute rather than attempting to help the client to dispute all automatic thoughts. The client takes the lead in identifying thinking errors, challenging the thoughts with disputing questions, and developing a rational response. The therapist only assists as needed. The rational response is written on a fresh sheet of paper, so that the client may refer to it during the exposure, without being distracted by automatic thoughts listed on the same page.

Next, behavioral goals for the exposure are set. Without guidance, clients with social anxiety disorder tend to set unrealistic, perfectionistic goals (e.g., "I won't get anxious" or "I will never stumble over my words") or goals that are based on the reactions of other people and not under their control (e.g., to make a good impression). The therapist helps the client to develop two or three goals relating to what he or she wants to accomplish in the situation (e.g., asking at least three questions to get to know the person better, stating an opinion, talking about three different points during a speech). These goals are recorded below the rational response, so that the client can refer to them during the exposure.

During the exposure, the therapists requests SUDS ratings at 1-minute intervals and whenever anxiety appears to increase or decrease. At each SUDS prompt, the client also reads his or her rational response aloud. Clients quickly adjust to this disruption, particularly if the role player(s) help to reorient them with a verbal cue (e.g., "You were talking about . . . "). The exposure should continue until anxiety has begun to decrease or plateau and the goals have been met, typically at around 10 minutes. The therapist should be the one to end the exposure to help the client overcome any tendencies to escape the situation when it becomes difficult.

The postprocessing phase of the exposure includes a review of goal attainment, a discussion of the usefulness of the rational response, and identification of any unexpected automatic thoughts that should be addressed in the future. Rather than asking the client about how the role play went from his or her perspective, the therapist asks the whether the client's agreed-upon goals were accomplished, providing no opening for the client to revert to a discussion about failure to attain other goals, such as not becoming anxious. The therapist also shares his or her opinion on goal attainment and how well the exposure went, responding to concerns raised by the client and not allowing the client to disqualify the positive. In later exposures, outside role players may also be asked to share their reactions and answer any questions the client has about how the exposure went. Feedback from the therapist and any role players should emphasize information that counters the client's negative beliefs. For example, the client might believe that he blushes bright red, is boring, appears inadequate to others, and cannot carry on a 10-minute conversation. Perhaps, objectively, the client did blush at the beginning of the exposure, only responded to questions from the role player, and reported very high SUDS for the whole 10 minutes (90 or higher). However, the client met his goals of sharing something about himself and staying in the exposure until the therapist said to stop. In this situation, the therapist would point out how the client met his goals and how many of the client's feared consequences (e.g., being too anxious to carry on a conversation) did not occur. Additionally, only in rare cases do clients look as anxious as they think they do, so it is often quite appropriate to acknowledge that the client showed some symptoms of anxiety, but that the anxiety was not as noticeable as the client's SUDS ratings might suggest, the anxiety did not detract from enjoyment of the conversation, and so forth. Therapists who deny seeing any anxiety in a client who was obviously anxious risk damaging their credibility. Especially early in treatment, therapists should think seriously before providing a laundry list of client behaviors that detracted from the quality of the conversation (e.g., the client only responded to questions and did not ask any, the client could have engaged in more eye contact). Many clients discount the positive aspects of the exposure and focus only on the negative feedback. Therefore, it is better to set this information aside temporarily and to make sure that these behaviors are included as goals for the next role play—if the client does not spontaneously suggest one of these problematic behaviors as a goal. For clients who are self-critical during the postprocessing for an objectively poor behavior such as never asking any questions, the most common strategy is to share with the client the conceptualization of the problematic behavior as an avoidance response to significant anxiety (rather than as evidence of poor social skills or some other inadequacy within the client). Working from this conceptualization, the therapist may then inquire about automatic thoughts leading to the problematic behavior. The client's responses are often quite illuminating (e.g., "I might inadvertently ask a question about a sensitive subject that will offend the other person"). The therapist would then plan with the client to work on these automatic thoughts and approach the feared social behavior by including it as a goal in a future exposure.

Next, the pattern of SUDS ratings is quickly graphed for the client. Different SUDS patterns may be used to make different points. The most common pattern is for the initial SUDS ratings to be rather high, then to decline over time. In these cases, the therapist can point out that it seems like getting started is the hardest part, and that if the client hangs in there, things seem to get easier. If this pattern holds across future exposures, it can lead to a new rational response (e.g., "It gets easier"; "The hardest part is getting started"). For clients with high SUDS ratings throughout the entire exposure who still meet their goals, the therapist can point out that a person may simultaneously be quite anxious and still do what he or she needs to do in a given social situation (e.g., "I can be anxious and still share my opinion" might be a future rational response). The therapist also inquires about any automatic thoughts that may have interfered with habituation, so that these might be addressed prior to the next exposure. Another common pattern is decreasing or steady SUDS ratings that spike to a high level when the client perceives a difficulty arising during the exposure. Sometimes the therapist is able to observe what led to the spike in anxiety (e.g., a pause in the conversation). At other times, it may not be as obvious, and the client needs to explain what happened (e.g., there was no pause, but the client had an automatic thought that the discussion of the current topic had reached its limits, and feared that he or she would be unable to continue the conversation). Such discussions may lead to new goals (e.g., "Allow yourself to pause twice during the conversation, so that you can learn that you can recover from pauses and not to fear them") and targets for cognitive restructuring (i.e., the belief that pauses reflect social incompetence might be challenged and lead to a rational response, such as "Pauses are a normal part of conversations" or "I am only 50% responsible for ending a pause"). Finally, the client is asked what he or she has learned from the exposure that can be applied to life outside of the clinic.

Homework assignments are a very important part of treatment in this segment, because the client is asked to enter situations similar to those that have been targeted during in-session exposures. To assist them in engaging in cognitive restructuring prior to the actual conduct of the homework exposure, clients are provided copies of the Be Your Own Cognitive Coach worksheet (BYOCC), which is also discussed in session and exemplified in the client workbook. This form (or a slightly modified version of it from Heimberg & Becker, 2002) leads clients through each of the steps of cognitive restructuring described earlier and is often used for in-session exposures, as well as those assigned for homework. After the homework exposure is completed, the second portion of the BYOCC assists clients in completing a cognitive debriefing and consolidating the learning that has occurred during and after the homework experience.

Segment 4: Advanced Cognitive Restructuring

After three or four exposure sessions, the therapist and client should begin to notice common themes in the client's automatic thoughts. At this point, it is time to move on to advanced cognitive restructuring (Chapter 12 of the client workbook). This segment assists the client in moving beyond situation-specific automatic thoughts by applying the downward arrow technique (see J. S. Beck, 1995) to thoughts that have frequently recurred over the course of treatment. To accomplish this task efficiently, the client and therapist review all previous written homework assignments that involved the recording of automatic thoughts, as well as the thoughts recorded in advance of in-session exposures and work through the Peeling Your Onion worksheet from the client workbook. This worksheet provides a systematic approach to questioning automatic thoughts and further probing the responses to these questions, until the client's core belief(s) have been identified.

The beginning of advanced cognitive restructuring does not signal the end to exposures. Rather, the therapist and client create in-session and *in vivo* exposures to challenge core beliefs. For instance, if a client has a core belief along the lines of "I need to be perfect to be accepted by others," the client might be engaged in exposures that involve making mistakes or social missteps (e.g., spilling a drink, turning in a report with a typo) and noticing whether others continue to be accepting. Core beliefs may be challenged in other ways as well. For instance, in addition to exposures, the client may be asked to notice instances in which others' mistakes actually make them easy to identify with or more endearing. One session is typically devoted completely to helping the client utilize the downward arrow technique and challenge core beliefs. Additional sessions not only continue to explore core beliefs but also include an in-session exposure.

Segment 5: Termination

As treatment approaches Session 16, the issue of termination and/or reevaluation of the treatment contract will have been raised informally by the therapist several times. After Session 15,

Chapter 13 in the client workbook is assigned. Session 16 formally focuses on assessment of progress, relapse prevention, and the issue of termination. The therapist and client go over a worksheet in which the client reports things that he or she has learned during treatment (e.g., how to identify and challenge automatic thoughts, the importance of avoiding avoidance). The therapist asks the client to provide current ratings for all items from the fear and avoidance hierarchy developed earlier in treatment; a discussion follows regarding progress that has been made and where further work is needed. When the therapist and client mutually agree that termination is in order, risk factors for relapse are discussed (e.g., social pressure from others, new situations that arise as improvement continues). Plans to deal with signs of relapse are also made (e.g., the client can review chapters in the client workbook or call the therapist). Mixed emotions (e.g., pride, sadness over the termination of the therapeutic relationship) associated with termination are also processed.

In our clinics, the same self-report questionnaires, clinician-administered measures, and behavior tests that were administered at pretreatment are repeated after Session 16. The client is given feedback on these assessments, with data presented in the context of the initial pretreatment assessment results. At the end of 16 sessions, many clients still experience problematic social anxiety in a few domains. As we stated in the first session, elimination of social anxiety is not the criterion for termination. Instead, if the client has stopped avoiding key social situations, has experienced a meaningful reduction of anxiety in a few areas, and believes that he or she can use the skills gained in therapy to continue to work independently, then the client is ready to stop treatment. Most individuals who respond to treatment in this way are likely to continue to make progress after termination. Follow-up appointments are recommended to monitor the client's clinical status (e.g., 1- and 6-months posttreatment).

For some individuals, treatment gains will be evident, but the anxiety and avoidance continue to be too severe and pervasive for the client to continue on alone. This phenomenon is most common among clients with quite severe social anxiety at treatment onset, typically, clients with generalized social anxiety and/or APD. Clients with significant comorbidities may also take longer to make sufficient treatment gains. In such cases, continued treatment is recommended. The new treatment contract, as with the original one, should be for 16 sessions or less, at which point another assessment should occur. The treatment plan typically consists of more cognitive restructuring and exposures, although new domains are often introduced (e.g., moving from working on friendships to dating relationships).

CASE STUDY

To better illustrate how individual CBT for social anxiety disorder is implemented, a case example is presented. First, background and pretreatment assessment data are given, followed by a description of the client's progress through 16 weeks of treatment and her status 1-year posttreatment.

Josie, a 22-year-old woman, presented with significant anxiety concerning both social interaction and performance situations. She was studying music at a local college and living with a roommate. At the time she entered treatment, Josie was a full-time student. She was not employed despite significant financial need. Josie described herself as shy and having trouble connecting with others. Josie reported that she socialized with her roommate and her boyfriend, but she often turned down opportunities to socialize with their friends because of anxiety. Josie reported that she had no close friends of her own and that her anxiety kept her from forming close friendships, especially with women her age. Josie's social anxiety had also resulted in occupational and academic impairment. For example, although Josie had gone on numerous job interviews and had even been offered positions, she was currently unemployed because she had difficulty accepting job offers because of fears that she would get fired. She reported great anxiety in her classes and did not participate unless directly asked a question, even if participation was a significant part of her grade. She often declined to enroll in classes that interested her because of participation requirements. In addition, Josie was required to do recitals and in-class critiques of her music compositions several times a semester. Although she never avoided any of these recitals, she worried about them for weeks in advance and suffered through them with great anxiety. Josie feared that her social anxiety would cause her even greater difficulty after graduation, when she would need to go on job interviews and auditions.

Pretreatment Assessment

Josie came to the clinic seeking help for social anxiety, but she also had difficulties with general worry and tension, depression, and panic attacks. She was administered the ADIS-IV-L and a series of self-report measures. Based on this information, Josie was assigned a diagnosis of generalized social anxiety disorder, with an ADIS-IV-L clinician severity rating of 5, which indicates moderate to severe symptoms. She received additional diagnoses of generalized anxiety disorder, recurrent major depressive disorder of moderate severity, posttraumatic stress disorder related to a recent automobile accident, and panic disorder with agoraphobia.

With regard to measures of social anxiety, Josie's scores indicated significant fear in both social interaction and performance/observation situations (see Table 3.2). Heimberg and colleagues (1992) suggested cutoff scores of 34 for the SIAS (interaction fears) and 24 for the SPS (performance/observation fears) to differentiate between individuals with and without social anxiety disorder. Josie's scores on both measures exceeded these cutoffs. Similarly, on the LSAS, Josie reported fear and avoidance of both social interaction and performance situations, and her total score was well above the empirically derived cutoff score for the pres-

ence of social anxiety disorder (Mennin et al., 2002).

Ideally, treatment should result in symptom reduction and improved functionality, as well as promote the client's overall sense of well-being and life satisfaction. Safren, Heimberg, Brown, and Holle (1997) reported a mean score of 0.8 on the Quality of Life Inventory for clients with social anxiety disorder, which is significantly lower than the mean score of the nonclinical adult sample reported by Frisch (1994; $M = 2.6$, $SD = 1.3$). Josie's score indicated that her degree of life satisfaction was very low, but similar to that of others with social anxiety disorder.

The disruption in functioning caused by social anxiety and the associated poor quality of life frequently results in dysphoria. Josie's score on the BDI-II indicated a level of depression more severe than is typically seen among individuals in our treatment program (Elting, Hope, & Heimberg, 1997). Josie did not endorse having any thoughts of suicide. Based on clinical interview, we determined that Josie's current low mood was related to recurrent major depression. This most recent depressive episode had begun approximately 6 months prior to her assessment and was associated with negative social experiences while studying abroad. Josie reported that her depressed mood was slightly less distressing and impairing than her social anxiety. Thus, the depression was judged to be secondary to her social anxiety and unlikely to have an adverse impact on her treatment. Similarly, we determined that her other diagnoses, although clinically significant, did

TABLE 3.2. Self-Report and Clinician-Administered Assessments at Pretreatment and 1-Year Follow-Up

Measure	Pretreatment	1-year follow-up
Self-report		
Brief Fear of Negative Evaluation Scale	49	23
Social Interaction Anxiety Scale	48	22
Social Phobia Scale	38	12
Beck Depression Inventory–II	25	8
Quality of Life Inventory	–0.9	1.1
Clinician-rated		
ADIS-IV-L Clinician Severity Rating	5	3
Liebowitz Social Anxiety Scale—Total	48	37

Note. ADIS-IV-L, Anxiety Disorders Interview Schedule for DSM-IV—Lifetime Version.

not rise to a level of concern that might interfere with or derail the treatment of her social anxiety disorder.

Treatment

Psychoeducational Segment

SESSIONS 1–2

The first four sessions were devoted to laying the groundwork for treatment, establishing rapport, educating Josie about the cognitive-behavioral model of social anxiety disorder, and outlining her goals for treatment.

In the first two meetings, Josie was very soft-spoken and made little eye contact, and at times expressed feelings of hopelessness about her ability to get better. She asked many questions about how other clients had fared with the treatment program, and the therapist stressed that outcome is often dependent on the client's ability to put in consistent effort throughout treatment. The therapist used some of Josie's own experiences to parallel the challenges and rewards she might face in treatment. The therapist asked Josie how long she had been playing piano and whether she had noticed any changes over that time. Josie reported that when she started, the process was very effortful, challenging, and even disheartening, but that with ongoing practice and education, she had reached a point where it was enjoyable and easy for her. With this, Josie appeared to be very encouraged about her prognosis, reporting that she was eager to begin treatment and motivated to work very hard. The majority of the first session was spent establishing rapport and introducing psychoeducational material about social anxiety and the components of treatment. To encourage Josie to speak about her own experiences with social anxiety, the therapist employed open-ended questions, asked if the examples sounded familiar to Josie, and requested that she describe some situations in which her anxiety was better or worse than others. For example, although Josie felt she had a significant amount of anxiety when performing in front of an audience, she felt that this anxiety was typical for most people in that situation. However, her anxiety while interacting with others at receptions before and after performances was severe, and she often avoided these situations, arriving at recitals the last minute and leaving as soon as she finished. By

participating in this way, Josie demonstrated an understanding of the important concept that social anxiety exists on a continuum.

SESSION 3

In the third session, the development of Josie's social anxiety and how it was maintained over the years was explored. After asking her mother, Josie learned that she was very shy even as a young child, and that her mother often had to push her to participate in social activities with other children. Josie also reported that her mother always had a tendency to keep to herself and minimize interactions with others, which Josie may have modeled from a young age. In addition, Josie reported struggling with feelings of falling short from a young age. For example, she reported that she never qualified for elite youth soccer teams, although she was a skilled athlete and never received more than third place or honorable mention in recitals and competitions. The therapist discussed with Josie how such experiences may have shaped her beliefs that she is not good enough, and also highlighted how Josie's tendency to view the negative aspects of situations (e.g., not getting first place) often led her to disqualify other successes (e.g., being among the top five performers in a large competition).

SESSIONS 4–5

In the early part of the fourth session, the therapist and Josie completed a discussion from Session 3 on the role that perfectionistic standards and low self-efficacy played in Josie's experience of social anxiety. The remainder of this session and the next were spent developing and refining Josie's fear and avoidance hierarchy (see Table 3.3). Josie reported that interacting with people in person was easier than talking over the phone, because face-to-face contact allowed her to interpret body language and facial expressions to determine how the interaction was going for the other person. In addition, Josie felt that it was easier to interact with males than with females, who she believed were more critical. Josie was also more anxious around individuals she respected and admired than she was with strangers. She responded well to the rationale regarding the importance of self-monitoring her symptoms of anxiety, de-

TABLE 3.3. Fear and Avoidance Hierarchy with Pretreatment, Posttreatment, and 1-Year Follow-Up Ratings

	Situation	Pretreatment	Posttreatment	1-year follow-up
1	Riding public transportation alone			
	Fear	100	20	9
	Avoidance	100	20	6
2	Staying after recitals to socialize			
	Fear	95	7	3
	Avoidance	95	8	0
3	Going to recitals			
	Fear	90	7	3
	Avoidance	70	8	0
4	Making phone calls to people I used to be close with			
	Fear	75	5	3
	Avoidance	60	5	1
5	Class critiques and talking about my compositions in class			
	Fear	65	6	1
	Avoidance	50	1	0
6	Talking with professors and authority figures I respect			
	Fear	65	4	5
	Avoidance	50	2	5
7	Making/maintaining conversations with friends and people I respect			
	Fear	60	3	4
	Avoidance	60	1	2
8	Making the first phone call			
	Fear	55	2	4
	Avoidance	5	0	1
9	Hanging out with boyfriend's friends' girlfriends			
	Fear	50	6	3
	Avoidance	85	2	0
10	Talking with old friends I've lost touch with			
	Fear	40	7	4
	Avoidance	70	4	2

pression, and social anxiety in two situations. Josie decided to monitor her peak anxiety during class critiques of her music composition and casual conversations with friends.

Cognitive Restructuring Training Segment

SESSION 6

In this session, Josie was introduced to cognitive restructuring. Though she demonstrated an understanding of the importance of thoughts in producing feelings of anxiety, Josie reported having continued difficulty identifying her own automatic thoughts. Specifically, she tended to identify questions that passed through her mind in anticipation of or during

anxiety-provoking situations. For example, when recalling a recent anxiety-provoking situation in which she had to present her work to a class, Josie identified the thought, "What will other people think of me?" The therapist helped Josie to restate this question as a statement of what she feared, asking Josie to let her "anxious self" answer the question. She was able to come up with automatic thoughts, such as "Other people will think I'm a moron" and "Other people will think I am unprepared for this presentation." She identified other thoughts, such as "I am wasting their time," "They will get bored with me," and "My professor will be disappointed that I didn't do a better job." Many of the automatic thoughts appeared to be related to a general sense of letting others down. Regarding self-monitoring of anxiety, depression, and peak anxiety in two situations, Josie had only practiced self-monitoring for 1 day over the past week, reporting that she was overwhelmed with the amount of homework and struggling to "correctly" identify her automatic thoughts. Time was spent discussing the importance of regularly monitoring her anxiety and depression, along with her automatic thoughts, so that the therapist would be able to assess her anxiety and progress throughout treatment more accurately. The therapist encouraged Josie that, with continued practice, she would get better at recognizing automatic thoughts.

SESSION 7

In this session, Josie again struggled to identify automatic thoughts, but with prompting, was increasingly able to do so. She also had some difficulty identifying the thinking errors contained in her automatic thoughts, often insisting that all the thoughts qualified as maladaptive thoughts—that is, true but unhelpful. The therapist asked Josie some disputing questions to illustrate that the thoughts were not true or totally accurate, and that other thinking errors could apply. By the end of session, Josie had a better handle on thinking errors and was able to start using some disputing questions successfully. Josie reported that the cognitive restructuring work was much more challenging than she expected, but that she was eager to put the work into action during exposures.

SESSION 8

The therapist decided to take an additional session to continue work on cognitive restructuring before moving onto exposures, so that Josie was maximally prepared. Cognitive restructuring practice was focused on a recent situation in which Josie turned down tickets, offered by a professor at school, to a show by her favorite artist. Josie was much better able to identify her automatic thoughts related to this situation, which included the following:

1. "Other students will be mad at me if I take the tickets."
2. "I will be too scared to go and would waste the tickets."
3. "I will not be able to take public transportation to get there."

4. "If I do take public transportation, I will get lost and miss the show."
5. "Other students want the tickets more than I do."

Josie was able to identify thinking errors such as fortune-telling, mind reading, and catastrophizing, among others. However, there was evidence that Josie was critical of herself and her occasional difficulty grasping the concepts of cognitive restructuring. At first, Josie struggled with labeling her automatic thoughts as wrong, and trying to search for the right rational response. The therapist encouraged Josie that there was no right or wrong way to challenge automatic thoughts or to develop a rational response, but Josie continued to evaluate her suggestions as not good enough. Furthermore, Josie grew extremely frustrated and pessimistic when she used disputing questions to challenge her automatic thoughts. Specifically, she had trouble challenging the thought that getting lost on the subway would have to lead to missing the show entirely. She reported that she doubted her own ability to read the subway map or ask for help, and predicted that she would get so lost that she would either turn around and go home or arrive at the show after it had already started. Josie's anxiety about entering the performance late would then, she predicted, lead her to go home anyway. Josie reported that she would feel disappointed, embarrassed, and ashamed if she lost her way on public transportation, because it would mean she had failed to attend the performance and in doing so would anger her classmates, who she predicted would feel as though she wasted the opportunity. Josie grew increasingly frustrated with the strength of her anxious thoughts and reported that she felt "stupid" for not being able to challenge them successfully. This highlighted some patterns noted throughout treatment, including Josie's tendency to rely on perfectionist standards and all-or-nothing thinking (e.g., evaluating her thoughts and behavioral responses as all right or all wrong), and impatience with her own progress in treatment. Despite this, she reported being willing to keep practicing and move on to in-session exposures. The therapist worked with Josie for the remainder of session to challenge her automatic thoughts. It was particularly helpful for Josie to identify that she had no evidence that she would get lost and to recognize that even if she did get lost, it would be important enough for her to attend the performance that she would ask for additional help or directions.

Exposure Segment

SESSION 9

During homework review, Josie reported that she was able to use her cognitive restructuring skills when she ran into an old roommate at a coffee shop. Josie reported that the exchange had gone much more smoothly than she anticipated and had encouraged her to feel more confident in her understanding of and abilities to use cognitive restructuring skills actively in social situations. With regard to the in-session exposure, the therapist wanted to choose a situation that would seem relevant to her treatment goals, elicit a moderate amount of anxiety, and be one in which Josie was likely to perform reasonably well. The in-session exposure was a follow-up to Josie's recent interaction with her classmate Anne, who mentioned to Josie that some people from class would be getting together one weekend to hang out. However, Anne did not call Josie to make specific plans; neither did Josie follow through with making plans to attend the event, and she ended up missing it. Josie thought that Anne did not call because she might have interpreted Josie's anxiety symptoms (e.g., shyness, quietness, lack of eye contact) as disinterest in socializing. Josie's exposure involved her talking with Anne, whose role was played by the therapist, about this misunderstanding. The following excerpts are from the cognitive restructuring prior to the exposure.

THERAPIST: First, let's go to the BYOCC worksheet and work through the situation before the exposure happens. When you think about this situation happening now, what kind of automatic thoughts come up for you?

JOSIE: I'm not going to talk to her, because I won't know what to say. Also, I shouldn't say anything about her not calling me, because it would make everything awkward. I should be really friendly and smile the whole time.

THERAPIST: Are you making any predictions about how this interaction will go?

JOSIE: Oh, yeah. I'm going to choke up, and she is going to judge me. I think that's it.

THERAPIST: OK, good job identifying those automatic thoughts. Now what kinds of emotions come up when you think those thoughts?

JOSIE: I feel sad. The anxiousness almost goes away, and I just don't feel like talking to her. I also feel a little bit of anger and frustration at myself, because I can't confront her about this and I don't want to make her feel uncomfortable.

THERAPIST: So it sounds like that kind of thinking might lead to you not saying anything at all then, avoiding the interaction?

JOSIE: Yeah, I'd definitely avoid it.

THERAPIST: Well this exposure will allow us to practice confronting those automatic thoughts, but first we need to do some cognitive restructuring practice. Why don't we start by identifying some thinking errors?

JOSIE: Right away I see should statements and fortune-telling. And to think that she's judging me, that's mind reading.

THERAPIST: Good job. Now let's try to dispute some of these thoughts. Let's start with the automatic thought: "I'm not going to talk to her, because I won't have anything to say." Do you know this for certain?

JOSIE: (Smiling) No, actually I do want to talk with her, and I could always ask her little things. I have no evidence that I'll have nothing to say.

THERAPIST: So you could come up with something to say?

JOSIE: Yeah, even if it's just small talk, I could come up with something. I do want to ask her about what happened, but I don't want to come across as too aggressive or confrontational. I feel bad when I confront people.

THERAPIST: So let's figure out some ways you'd feel comfortable asking her to hang out, ways that allow you to get your message across without feeling aggressive or blunt. This can help us start to identify some behavioral goals for the exposure. Let's take a look at what it is you want to ask her or tell her.

JOSIE: Well, I want to ask her if we can hang out some other time, since she didn't call me last time. But I have the automatic thought that I shouldn't say anything, because it will make things awkward. I guess if I challenge that, I don't really know that I will make things awkward.

THERAPIST: What might be another outcome if you say something?

JOSIE: She might apologize and ask me if I want to come, and I can tell her that I'd love to come the next time she invites me. She did invite me in the first place. She just never called, because she thought I didn't want to go.

THERAPIST: Good. So we identified some automatic thoughts, and you said they made you feel sad and frustrated. Then we challenged them and came up with some coping thoughts. How do those thoughts make you feel?

JOSIE: That's better. I feel a lot better.

THERAPIST: How could we sum these up into a rational response? Does anything stand out to you?

JOSIE: "Saying something might have a positive outcome" really stands out to me. I'd feel better and things might turn out better if I remind myself of that. It will help me to challenge the thought that I'll choke up or run out of things to say.

The therapist selected that automatic thought for cognitive restructuring, because it had been a recurrent one for Josie in homework and seemed relevant to the upcoming exposure. Also, the therapist made an effort to take Josie through the cognitive restructuring relatively quickly, because the longer the exposure was delayed, the more anxious she would get and the more difficult it would be for her to focus on the cognitive restructuring because of her anxiety. The next step was to set goals for the exposure. Josie decided that her achievable behavioral goals for this exposure would include telling Anne that she was interested in the last social event, letting Anne know that she would be interested in hanging out some time soon, and giving Anne her phone number.

The exposure began with both Josie and the therapist standing up to simulate more closely the interaction that might occur as they passed each other in the hallway at school. Josie stood where she would be able to see her rational response and behavioral goals written on the easel.

THERAPIST: Josie, what is your initial SUDS rating?

JOSIE: About a 45.

THERAPIST: OK, and what is your rational response?

JOSIE: Saying something might have a positive outcome.

Josie and the therapist began to chat about class, and Josie soon brought up the recently past social event. The therapist let the exposure go on for approximately 5 minutes. Upon being prompted by the therapist, Josie gave SUDS ratings at 1-minute intervals throughout the interaction and read her rational response aloud. After the exposure had ended, postprocessing began.

THERAPIST: Did you reach your behavioral goals?

JOSIE: I told her I wanted to hang out and asked her to call me again.

THERAPIST: So you met your goals. Great job. Did any new automatic thoughts come up?

JOSIE: I noticed that I fidgeted a lot. I had the thought "This is scary," but also that she seemed pretty cool about the interaction. I thought I really shouldn't be nervous.

THERAPIST: Did the thoughts we identified earlier come up?

JOSIE: Yeah. I thought I wouldn't know what to say, and there was a pause in the conversation but it was fine when I said something. I worried that I'd make this awkward for her, but I think it was more awkward for me, because I was so nervous.

THERAPIST: How did your rational response work?

JOSIE: It worked pretty well; it got easier to remember and I believed it was true when I said it. It really seemed to help me think more about rational thoughts instead of anxious ones.

THERAPIST: Let's take a look at your SUDS. You started at a 45 and went up to 55 when conversation started. When you said something to her about wishing she'd call you, SUDS went up to a 60. By the time she told you what happened, the SUDS dropped to 40. After some small talk, it went down to a 20. That's a pretty significant drop.

JOSIE: It was a lot better after I got over that bump, when I told her I wanted to hang out.

THERAPIST: What thoughts do you remember having then?

JOSIE: I shouldn't say anything. I should walk away. I have to say something.

THERAPIST: So what happened then?

JOSIE: I said my rational response when you asked, right after I asked her about what happened, and I felt a lot better. It felt like things were going to be OK. I feel really good about how it went.

After processing the exposure, the therapist helped Josie to plan an *in vivo* exposure to do on her own that week. She planned to meet her old roommate for coffee, using the BYOCC forms to guide her cognitive restructuring, the exposure, and her own postprocessing of the experience.

SESSION 10

In the 10th session, Josie reported that she had a very challenging but rewarding week. She recalled an in-class critique of her work, and, though her anxiety was intense, she was able to manage it and remain in class by reminding herself of her rational response: "I can learn something from their feedback." Josie also noted that she had completed two *in vivo* exposures, including having coffee with her old roommate and a conversation with her classmate Anne, just as she practiced in last week's session. Josie seemed very encouraged by the outcomes of these situations and her ability to use cognitive restructuring techniques before and during anxiety-provoking events.

For exposure this session, Josie planned to interact with two women playing the roles of her boyfriend's friends' fiancées, to whom Josie felt she could not relate. The therapist anticipated that this exposure would be more difficult for Josie, because it involved a fairly unstructured interaction and likely a conversation about topics with which Josie was relatively unfamiliar, such as wedding planning. Josie reported the following automatic thoughts in anticipation of the exposure:

1. "I'm not married yet, so what do I know about relationships and weddings?"
2. "I will offend them with my views."

3. "They are going to think I am weird."
4. "They are going to think I act too young."
5. "I'm not going to give the right answers to their questions."

As with automatic thoughts in her first exposure, Josie was able to identify thinking errors, including fortune-telling, mind reading, labeling, and all-or-nothing thinking. By using the disputing questions, Josie was able to challenge the automatic thoughts she identified. In response to the first thought, Josie determined that although she was not married, she had been in a relationship for a number of years, so she would be able to relate to the other women on that level. In addition, she had helped her sister plan a wedding, so she was familiar with some aspects of wedding planning. Regarding her fear of being offensive, Josie noted that she was not sure she would offend them with her views, and that her different perspective might lead to an interesting conversation. The automatic thought, that the other women would think she was weird, was more difficult for Josie to challenge, but she was satisfied when she determined that she would be able to live with herself if they thought she was a little unusual, and that it was unlikely to affect her relationships with them. In reference to her fears that she would act too young, Josie used the challenge that she was only 2 years younger than these women, but she had chosen a different path for herself that involved continued education and saving marriage until she felt more settled in life, a decision she felt was very mature. In response to the automatic thought that she would not give the right answer to their questions, Josie argued that perhaps there was no right or wrong answer, and that even if she gave an answer that was inconsistent with the other women's views, she could recover from those mistakes, and differences of opinion could lead to interesting conversation.

Josie decided that an appropriate rational response would be one that helped her feel that she could relate to these two women despite their different circumstances. Her rational response for this exposure was "I'm not so different." Josie's goals were to talk about her own interests (e.g., music), ask a question, offer an opinion, and stay in the conversation until the exposure was over. Josie's SUDS ratings started out at 45, decreased to about 20 by the fourth minute of the exposure, and went as low as 15 by the final minute of the 8-minute exposure. Josie met all of her behavioral goals, and though she was quiet compared to the role players early in the conversation, she appeared to grow more at ease as time passed. Josie reported that the exposure went fairly well and was pleased that her sharing a story during the conversation led to a change of subject and additional conversation among the three women. Although Josie did not share their experiences and opinions, she was able to find a way to relate to them and to participate in the conversation. She reported having thoughts of leaving, but she convinced herself to stay by reminding herself that she would benefit from staying in the situation. Josie's homework was to call an old music composition classmate, have a conversation over the phone with him, and ask him to listen to her practice a piece she was working on for an upcoming show.

SESSION 11

Prior to this session, Josie had gotten very busy with class work and preparation for an upcoming recital of her compositions as part of a final exam. Consequently, she had missed several sessions. Josie reported that over the course of the past month, she had interviewed for a job at a local bookstore, was offered the position, and accepted it. She said she experienced a significant amount of anxiety on the interview and in the first few days of work, but that she was feeling much more confident about things now. Although she had made dramatic improvements in her self-reported anxiety and continued to improve during the 1-month hiatus from regular treatment, the therapist discussed the importance of completing the remaining 5–6 weeks of the treatment program. Josie committed to following through with treatment and doing her homework more consistently. Though Josie had not formally been doing her homework and an in-session exposure was not conducted, the therapist reviewed her progress so far in relation to her fear and avoidance hierarchy. Socializing with a group of friends and riding public transportation alone were identified as areas for continued work. For homework, Josie was assigned the task of handing out fliers to friends and family for the upcoming recital, which was to involve repeated social interactions and a discussion of her work. She was also given the assignment of reading the chapter in the client workbook re-

lated to social interactions and making small talk.

SESSION 12

In the Session 12 homework review, Josie said she interacted with many people on campus and around town, and that the conversations had gone much more smoothly than anticipated. She said it was helpful to remind herself that she was an expert on her own compositions, so she could talk at least some about the performance she was advertising. The third in-session exposure, completed in this session, was designed to help Josie work on some of her automatic thoughts related to her upcoming recital that weekend. The therapist had planned an exposure during which Josie was to interact with audience members at a reception following her recital, and staff members from the clinic volunteered to play these roles. Josie agreed that this exposure was very relevant to her current concerns and would make her very anxious. Josie reported the following automatic thoughts in anticipation of the exposure:

1. "I'm going to sound pretentious if I talk confidently about my performance."
2. "They are only talking to me because they feel bad for me."
3. "I have to impress them."
4. "They will think this is boring."
5. "I won't know what to say."

Josie was able to identify thinking errors, including all-or-nothing thinking, labeling, fortune-telling, and mind reading. During the cognitive restructuring, Josie was encouraged to look at her successful experiences in the two previous exposures as evidence that she had things to say that were of interest to others. With the help of the therapist, Josie arrived at this rational response: "I can talk about my performance, because I created it."

Josie's goals were to talk slowly, to provide information about herself, to answer questions posed to her, and to stay in a given interaction until the other person ended it. Josie's initial SUDS rating started out at 80, but it had decreased to 30 within 3 minutes. At the end of the 10-minute exposure, Josie's SUDS rating was below 20. Once again, Josie met her behavioral goals, and her performance was objectively skilled. Josie said that in addition to her rational response, it was helpful to tell herself that she did not have to take everything others said to heart. Josie thought the exposure went very well and even reported having fun interacting with the audience members and being the center of attention. She felt that this practice was going to be very helpful when she encountered the real situation at that weekend's recital. Josie's homework was to use the BYOCC forms before and after her actual recital to prepare herself to cope with anxious thoughts that might arise before, during, and after the performance.

SESSION 13

Josie came to the session, reporting that her anxiety at the reception following last week's recital was much more manageable than it had been in the past, and that she was actually able to enjoy conversations she had with family, music instructors, and fellow students. She reported feeling confident about her performance, which helped her to feel confident and comfortable while interacting with others at the reception. Though Josie did report experiencing significant anxiety as she began to socialize with family and friends after the recital, she said that her anxiety dropped substantially as she continued to interact with others about her performance, and at no point did she have thoughts of leaving the reception. Josie felt that the recital and reception were a success, and that her anxiety did not prevent her from enjoying these situations as it had in the past.

For an in-session exposure, Josie said it would be helpful to practice receiving feedback, both positive and negative, about her musical and academic performances. This situation was relevant because, as part of a final exam in Josie's music composition course, she was to perform an original composition in front of students and her instructor, then receive their feedback. Though her ability to do this had improved on a smaller scale during her coursework, this particular class critique elicited a considerable amount of anxiety for Josie, and she wanted some direct help with the cognitive restructuring and behavioral practice. The therapist decided to conduct two smaller exposures—one in which Josie received neutral or positive feedback from class members and her instructor, and another in which she received negative feedback. Each exposure was designed to go on for approximately 5–10 minutes to allow Josie to discuss her composition

and performance adequately and to receive and respond to feedback. A number of clinic staff members volunteered to assist with this exposure.

Prior to the exposure, Josie identified the following automatic thoughts for both exposures:

1. "I am going to mess this up."
2. "I must appear professional."
3. "I have to perform perfectly to impress them."
4. "I won't know what to say."
5. "I won't understand their questions."

Josie was able to identify thinking errors such as fortune-telling, all-or-nothing thinking, catastrophizing, and "should" statements. She also noted how her perfectionistic standards and feelings of low self-efficacy were quickly elicited by this situation involving overt evaluation of her performance and interaction skills. After challenging her automatic thoughts, Josie decided that a helpful rational response in each of the exposures would be "I know my work, because I did it," which she felt would encourage her to continue talking confidently about her own composition and performance, regardless of the feedback she received. Josie's behavioral goals were to answer questions posed to her and to ask follow-up questions, if she needed clarification.

The exposures were set up to take place immediately after a performance and began with Josie saying, "Thank you, I'd like to hear your thoughts about the piece." In the first exposure, she received a mix of neutral and positive feedback about her composition, her performance, and her ability to conduct herself during the critique. Josie's SUDS score started at 45 and dropped down to 15 within 3 minutes. She met all of her behavioral goals. The second exposure began the same way, but this time she received a mix of neutral and negative feedback; listeners pointed out mistakes she made in her performance, told her that she looked nervous, and indicated that they did not like the music she wrote. Josie's SUDS score again started at a 45 and went up as high as 60 when she received her first negative comment. By the fifth minute of the exposure, her SUDS score was 30, and by the end of the exposure, 20. Josie again met her behavioral goals and reported that she handled both situations very well. Josie noted that although her anxiety peaked when she received negative feedback, she felt she responded to the comments politely and was even able to learn from them. She felt the exposure was very helpful in preparing for her upcoming feedback sessions in class. For homework, Josie was asked to read the client workbook chapter on core beliefs and to do an *in vivo* exposure that would involve her taking public transportation to and from school with a friend. She was also asked to complete a BYOCC form before and after her in-class performance and evaluation.

Advanced Cognitive Restructuring Segment

SESSION 14

Josie completed her homework exposure of riding the bus to and from school with a friend and reported that she was not very anxious. She said that next time she would take the bus on her own and work toward going to places farther away and less familiar. Josie also reported that things went well with her in-class evaluation, that her performance of the music she composed went well, but that she thought she messed up once or twice. However, she noted that no students gave her feedback indicating that they noticed the mistake. Josie reported feeling incredibly anxious after she finished playing, and that right before the feedback session she even had thoughts of excusing herself for a few minutes. Reminding herself of her rational response, "I can learn something from their feedback," encouraged Josie to stay in class and complete the evaluation. Though she received some challenging questions about how she composed the music and who had influenced her, Josie thought she had done a decent job, although she had stumbled over her words a few times. She noted that a few students commented about not particularly liking the style of music she chose, but Josie said she was able not to take such comments personally. Overall Josie felt that she had learned a lot from the students' and instructor's feedback and that, although anxious, felt it was an acceptable level of anxiety given the performance and evaluation aspects of the situation.

Josie did not read the chapter on core beliefs, so the therapist spent time in session introducing this concept. Josie worked hard in this session to identify her core beliefs, using the Peeling Your Onion worksheet. She realized that her most common automatic thoughts across situations were related to labeling herself, feeling as though she would not live up to others' expectations, and fears that others would judge her negatively because of her social or performance skills. Josie felt that the theme of "not measuring up" was familiar and related potentially to her beliefs about never measuring up to her parents' standards and not doing anything right, which led to more generalized perfectionism. Josie identified the thought, "I'm not measuring up," as related to a fear that she would not be successful in life, and that to be successful, she felt she must be perfect. Identifying this chain of thinking left her feeling sad, frustrated, and disappointed. From here, Josie worked through the worksheet and identified the core belief, "If I'm not perfect, I'm worthless." Time was spent brainstorming exposures Josie could do on her own to test and challenge this core belief. For homework, the therapist asked Josie to mess up intentionally while playing the piano for some family members, so as to challenge her core belief that anything short of perfectionism represents a failure. Josie also identified another situation in which she could intentionally mess up, while using the intercom system at her job. The therapist also challenged Josie to identify ways that her imperfections might actually contribute to her value as a person. Josie was hesitant to do this but agreed when she reminded herself of the importance of facing feared situations.

SESSION 15

Josie arrived at the 15th session and reported that she had been unable to make a mistake intentionally in her musical performance in front of family members, but she was able to make a mistake while using the intercom system at work. The therapist continued to use cognitive restructuring to explore Josie's core belief, "If I'm not perfect, I'm worthless."

THERAPIST: So, last week we started to talk about some core issues, and I felt like you left here feeling a little overwhelmed. How are you feeling about things now?

JOSIE: It was a difficult session, because I was feeling really good about overcoming hard stuff in the beginning, like learning how to pick out automatic thoughts, see how they were wrong, then finding a really good, challenging response to them and actually believing it. I felt good because I can do that now, almost automatically, or at least without too much effort. I felt like I was done, and then we ended up having to face some really scary stuff again. I feel like I took a giant step up, to a harder level of work.

THERAPIST: The things we talked about last week were harder. That's a good sign that we've really worked our way to your core beliefs, because it feels so different. But remember all the work and practice that you put into identifying and challenging every other automatic thought or situation that we've worked on. It didn't all happen right away. In terms of core beliefs, we're going to do the same thing. All we've done is identify it. Now we will spend time challenging it and testing out the thought, "If I'm not perfect, I'm worthless." We'll start here in session today, but this is work you'll continue on your own. What might be some thinking errors? What's limiting in thinking that anything less than 100% is a failure?

JOSIE: That's catastrophizing. Probably also a "should" statement, because I feel like I must be perfect. And also maybe fortunetelling, because I feel like I'm assuming things will go wrong eventually. That's it.

THERAPIST: What about all-or-nothing thinking?

JOSIE: Oh yeah, definitely. In my mind, it's like there's 0% success or 100% success.

THERAPIST: So what are some ways we can challenge this? It won't be easy, but let's try.

JOSIE: Umm, I guess simple challenges, like "How do I know I'm going to be worthless if I'm not perfect?" I don't know. I guess not being perfect doesn't have to equal being worthless.

THERAPIST: Tell me more about that.

JOSIE: Some things are maybe valuable even when they're not perfect. Like people. Or art.

THERAPIST: So sometimes people's flaws, or quirks, make them more interesting?

JOSIE: Yeah, that's what I like best about my boyfriend. Those things other people are bothered by I find endearing. I like things that are imperfect, that have their own per-

sonality to them that's not quite right. I don't really have a problem when the imperfection is with someone else. But with me, it's different.

THERAPIST: Are you a harsher critic of yourself than others?

JOSIE: Definitely. Too bad I can't see myself the way I see others.

THERAPIST: Maybe you can, maybe we can try that. It's hard, because you've been looking at yourself critically for a long time. It's going to be a change, and it will take testing and practice. But what might be the reward for trying something besides being a harsher judge of yourself than others?

JOSIE: I guess the work will pay off, like it did with everything else. With practice, I even had fun at my show. I didn't believe that I was going to be a failure. I believed I could do it. It was a huge success.

THERAPIST: Were there any minor flaws with the evening? Things that went wrong, but that you coped with?

JOSIE: Oh, yeah, tons. Like I forgot my friend's name when I was introducing her to my parents. But it didn't ruin the evening. Overall things were good, and I felt good about it. I could skip over those flaws and just enjoy it.

THERAPIST: So when thinking about that situation, how true does it feel that if you are not perfect, you are worthless?

JOSIE: When I came in, I felt overwhelmed by everything; now that we can see all the work I've done, I feel better. I think I can challenge this. I don't think it feels totally true anymore.

THERAPIST: OK, so what's some evidence that this core belief may not be true?

JOSIE: Well, it's OK for everyone else to not be perfect. Maybe a little less OK for me, but I guess it's still somewhat OK. And some people are more valuable to me because of their imperfections. I guess being perfect is boring. Being perfect is impossible.

THERAPIST: So that seems like a high standard to hold yourself to.

JOSIE: (*Laughs.*) Yeah. I don't know anyone who's perfect. Everyone makes mistakes. Even me. Especially me. Everyone in the history of the world has been imperfect.

THERAPIST: Right. Now let's get back to you, not just others. Do we have evidence that you may be valuable even if you're imperfect? Are there upsides of imperfection?

JOSIE: I'll be more unique, more of an individual. It makes for interesting challenges; it could make for a really interesting life. I could learn a lot about different ways to do things, try out all kinds of new things. Make lots of mistakes, and just learn to do things better the next time. Not perfect, but just better. And make room for failure.

THERAPIST: So how much do you believe that if you're not perfect, you're worthless?

JOSIE: Maybe like 20%. Right now, at least, only 20%.

THERAPIST: So how can we sum up some of these challenges that have gotten you to believing this only about 20%? What might be a rational response to this core belief, "If I'm not perfect, I'm worthless."

JOSIE: I don't know; this is hard. If I'm not perfect, I'm worthy? I don't believe it, but it makes me laugh. I guess maybe it's OK if I'm not perfect.

THERAPIST: Does that feel convincing?

JOSIE: Not really. I'm drawing a blank with coming up with the right rational response.

THERAPIST: What if we recognized that this rational response won't be perfect? Maybe we need to find one that's good enough for now. So let's keep at this.

JOSIE: Oh I see, there's the perfectionistic thinking again. I guess really, it is not humanly possible to be perfect. And I don't think I would even want to be that person who finally was perfect.

THERAPIST: So it seems like a lot of work to be chasing perfection when it kind of doesn't exist. It sounds like no matter how hard you try, there would always be the attempt to do better than perfect.

JOSIE: Yeah, like no matter what, I'd never be able to be perfect. It's not humanly possible. I guess if I had to make this a rational response, I'd tell myself something like "There is no such thing as perfect." I like that. I think that will work for now. I'm going to think about this more. This is a challenge, but I want to spend time on this.

THERAPIST: Ok, so maybe we can try out this rational response this week by having you do some exposures that will allow you to challenge the core belief, "If I'm not perfect, I'm worthless."

JOSIE: Yeah. I need to do that every day, challenge this, become more accepting of my imperfections. It might be fun to mess up on purpose. But a lot of the time I mess up just naturally, but I guess even then I'm not worthless. Mistakes are going to happen, because there is no such thing as perfect.

For homework this session, Josie was assigned the task of intentionally making mistakes in conversation (e.g., forgetting people's names, asking them to repeat something they have said), at work (e.g., pressing the wrong button when using the intercom, asking for help with a task), and in performances (e.g., playing the wrong notes while playing the piano for her family and friends).

Termination Segment

SESSION 16

In the final session, Josie and the therapist discussed her progress and the challenges that lay ahead. Josie rerated her fear and avoidance hierarchy, and the decrease in her ratings was considered significant and meaningful (see Table 3.3). She reported that, over the course of treatment, she learned new skills such as recognizing and challenging automatic thoughts and seeing all aspects of herself—including imperfection—as acceptable. The most important change she noted was being able to get and to keep a job at a bookstore, where she must interact with customers and coworkers all day. Josie reported that as a result of her treatment, for the first time she was able to see herself as equal rather than inferior to others, and she was optimistic about her future goals, both personal and professional.

Session-by-Session Assessment

Figure 3.2 displays Josie's session-by-session scores on the SASCI and the BFNES. Recall that a score of 16 on the SASCI corresponds to no change, with lower scores indicative of increasingly greater improvement relative to baseline levels. Josie started to show modest improvement after Session 3. Her score spiked

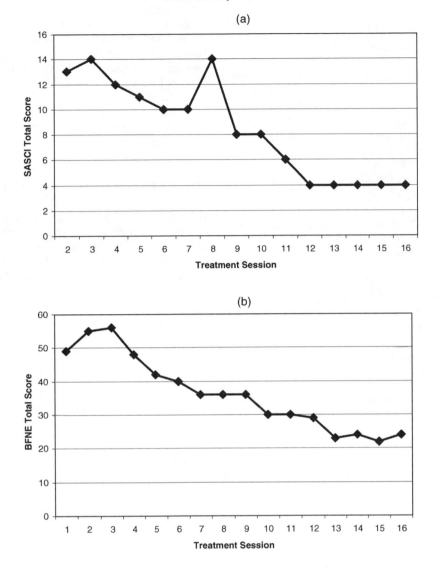

FIGURE 3.2. Weekly scores on the (a) Social Anxiety Session Change Index (SASCI) and (b) Brief Fear of Negative Evaluation Scale (BFNE).

at Session 8, then began a steady decline, reaching the minimum score of 4 by Session 12 and remaining there until the end of treatment. For the BFNE, Weeks and colleagues. (2005) reported a mean score of 46.91 (SD = 9.27) in a large sample with social anxiety disorder and a mean of 26.81 (SD = 4.78) among normal controls. Early in treatment, Josie's session scores exceeded the mean of the clinical sample by as much as 10 points. However, her scores declined consistently thereafter, and by the end of treatment were just below the mean of the control sample.

One-Year Follow-Up Assessment

After 1 year with no treatment, Josie showed considerable improvement on all self-report and clinician-administered measures compared to her pretreatment assessment (see Table 3.2). In fact, she no longer met diagnostic criteria for social anxiety disorder. She was considering applications to graduate programs to continue her study of music and had plans to audition for the local orchestra. Josie reported that she had been making friends at her job and felt that she now had a core of social supports on whom she could rely.

CLINICAL PREDICTORS OF SUCCESS AND FAILURE

Josie's treatment turned out well, as it does for many clients. However, treatment response is a variable phenomenon, and researchers have investigated a number of predictors of CBT outcome (see a more thorough review of this topic by L. Magee, Erwin, & Heimberg, in press).

Expectancy for improvement, subtype of social anxiety disorder, and comorbidity with other anxiety or mood disorders, as well as APD, have been discussed in other sections of this chapter. Here we briefly review three other variables—adherence to assigned CBT homework, anger, and cognitive change.

Adherence to prescribed homework assignments has been associated with positive treatment outcome, and evidence suggests that adherence to particular components of CBT homework assignments may be differentially predictive of outcome. For instance, adherence to between-session cognitive restructuring and exposure assignments predicts posttreatment outcome better than adherence to assignments related more to psychoeducation early in treatment (Leung & Heimberg, 1996). Other studies have not replicated these effects immediately after treatment (Edelmann & Chambless, 1995; Woody & Adessky, 2002). However, 6-month follow-up assessments revealed that homework-compliant individuals reported fewer avoidant behaviors, less fear of negative evaluation, and less anxiety when giving a speech compared to less compliant clients (Edelman & Chambless, 1995).

Anger is a significant predictor of CBT outcome as well. In a study by Erwin, Heimberg, Schneier, and Liebowitz (2003), individuals with high levels of trait anger were more likely to terminate treatment prematurely. Also, levels of state and trait anger and anger suppression before treatment were significantly correlated with posttreatment severity of social anxiety.

Finally, in a study comparing group CBT, exposure group therapy, and waiting-list control conditions, changes in estimated social cost, or negative cognitive appraisal, mediated pretreatment to posttreatment changes in both active treatment groups (Hofmann, 2004). Furthermore, only the group receiving cognitive techniques, in addition to exposure, continued to show improvement from posttreatment to the 6-month follow-up assessment. Continued benefit was associated with an overall reduction in estimated social cost from pre- to posttreatment assessments, suggesting that the cognitive-behavioral intervention is associated with greater treatment gains that are mediated through changes in estimated social cost (Hofmann, 2004).

SUMMARY AND CONCLUSIONS

Our primary purpose in this chapter was to provide a step-by-step analysis of the conduct of individual CBT for social anxiety disorder from initial assessment to long-term follow-up. Discussion of procedural difficulties that may arise in the conduct of CBT for social anxiety disorder were not be discussed in detail here because of space limitations but are discussed thoroughly by Heimberg and Becker (2002). Individuals like Josie, who make dramatic improvements in their lives, provide the impetus for continued research on the treatment of social anxiety disorder—a potentially debilitating disorder with an increasingly encouraging prognosis.

REFERENCES

American Psychiatric Association. (1980). *Diagnostic and statistical manual of mental disorders* (3rd ed.). Washington, DC: Author.

American Psychiatric Association. (1994). *Diagnostic and statistical manual of mental disorders* (4th ed.). Washington, DC: Author.

Antony, M. M., Coons, M. J., McCabe, R. E., Ashbaugh, A., & Swinson, R. P. (2006). Psychometric properties of the Social Phobia Inventory: Further evaluation. *Behaviour Research and Therapy, 44,* 1177–1185.

Barlow, D. H. (2002). *Anxiety and its disorders: The nature and treatment of anxiety and panic* (2nd ed.). New York: Guilford Press.

Beck, A. T., Steer, R. A., & Brown, G. K. (1996). *Beck Depression Inventory manual* (2nd ed.). San Antonio, TX: Psychological Corporation.

Beck, J. S. (1995). *Cognitive therapy: Basics and beyond.* New York: Guilford Press.

Beidel, D. C., Turner, S. M., Stanley, M. A., & Dancu, C. V. (1989). The Social Phobia and Anxiety Inventory: Concurrent and external validity. *Behavior Therapy, 20,* 417–427.

Bisserbe, J. C., Weiller, E., Boyer, P., Lepine, J.-P., &

Lecrubier, Y. (1996): Social phobia in primary care: Level of recognition and drug use. *International Clinical Psychopharmacology, 11,* 25–28.

Brown, E. J., Heimberg, R. G., & Juster, H. R. (1995). Social phobia subtype and avoidant personality disorder: Effect on severity of social phobia, impairment, and outcome of cognitive-behavioral treatment. *Behavior Therapy, 26,* 467–486.

Brown, E. J., Turovsky, J., Heimberg, R. G., Juster, H. R., Brown, T. A., & Barlow, D. H. (1997). Validation of the Social Interaction Anxiety Scale and the Social Phobia Scale across the anxiety disorders. *Psychological Assessment, 9,* 21–27.

Brown, T. A., Di Nardo, P. A., & Barlow, D. H. (1994). *Anxiety Disorders Interview Schedule for DSM-IV.* Albany, NY: Graywind.

Brown, T. A., Di Nardo, P. A., Lehman, S. L., & Cambell, L. A. (2001). Reliability of DSM-IV anxiety and mood disorders: Implications for the classification of emotional disorders. *Journal of Abnormal Psychology, 110,* 49–58.

Bruch, M. A., Fallon, M., & Heimberg, R. G. (2003). Social phobia and difficulties in occupational adjustment. *Journal of Counseling Psychology, 50,* 109–117.

Bruch, M. A., Gorsky, J. M., Collins, T. M., & Berger, P. (1989). Shyness and sociability reexamined: A multicomponent analysis. *Journal of Personality and Social Psychology, 57,* 904–915.

Bruch, M. A, Heimberg, R. G., & Hope, D. A. (1991). States of mind model and cognitive change in treated social phobics. *Cognitive Therapy and Research, 15,* 429–441.

Butler, G., Cullington, A., Munby, M., Amies, P., & Gelder, M. (1984). Exposure and anxiety management in the treatment of social phobia. *Journal of Consulting and Clinical Psychology, 52,* 642–650.

Chambless, D. L., & Ollendick, T. H. (2001). Empirically supported psychological interventions: Controversies and evidence. *Annual Review of Psychology, 52,* 685–716.

Chambless, D. L., Tran, G. Q., & Glass, C. R. (1997). Predictors of response to cognitive-behavioral group therapy for social phobia. *Journal of Anxiety Disorders, 11,* 221–240.

Chartier, M. J., Hazen, A. L., & Stein, M. B. (1998). Lifetime patterns of social phobia: A retrospective study of the course of social phobia in a nonclinical population. *Depression and Anxiety, 7,* 113–121.

Clark, D. M. (1997). *Cognitive therapy for social phobia: Some notes for therapists.* Unpublished manuscript, University of Oxford, Department of Psychiatry.

Clark, D. M., Ehlers, A., Hackmann, A., McManus, F., Fennell, M., Grey, N., et al. (2006). Cognitive therapy versus exposure and applied relaxation in social phobia: A randomized controlled trial. *Journal of Consulting and Clinical Psychology, 74,* 568–578.

Clark, D. M., Ehlers, A., McManus, F., Hackmann, A.,

Fennell, M., Campbell, H., et al. (2003). Cognitive therapy versus fluoxetine in generalized social phobia: A randomized placebo-controlled trial. *Journal of Consulting and Clinical Psychology, 71,* 1058–1067.

Clark, D. M., & Wells, A. (1995). The cognitive model of social phobia. In R. G. Heimberg, M. R. Leibowitz, D. A. Hope, & F. R. Schneier (Eds.), *Social phobia: Diagnosis, assessment, and treatment* (pp. 69–93). New York: Guilford Press.

Collins, K. A., Westra, H. A., Dozois, D. J. A., & Stewart, S. H. (2005). The validity of the brief version of the Fear of Negative Evaluation Scale. *Journal of Anxiety Disorders, 19,* 345–359.

Connor, K. M., Davidson, J. R. T., Churchill, E., Sherwood, A., Foa, E. B., & Weisler, R. H. (2000). Psychometric properties of the Social Phobia Inventory (SPIN): A new self-rating scale. *British Journal of Psychiatry, 176,* 379–386.

Connor, K. M., Kobak, K. A., Churchill, E., Katzelnick, D., & Davidson, J. R. T. (2001). Mini-SPIN: A brief screening assessment for generalized social anxiety disorder. *Depression and Anxiety, 14,* 137–140.

Cox, B. J., Ross, L., Swinson, R. P., & Direnfeld, D. M. (1998). A comparison of social phobia outcome measures in cognitive-behavioral group therapy. *Behavior Modification, 22,* 285–297.

Davidson, J. R. T., Miner, C. M., De Veaugh-Geiss, J., Tupler, L. A., Colket, J. T., & Potts, N. L. (1997). The Brief Social Phobia Scale: A psychometric evaluation. *Psychological Medicine, 27,* 161–166.

Davidson, J. R. T., Potts, N. L., Richichi, E. A., Krishnan, R. R., Ford, S. M., Smith, R. D., et al. (1991). The Brief Social Phobia Scale. *Journal of Clinical Psychiatry, 52,* 48–51.

Di Nardo, P. A., Brown, T. A., & Barlow, D. H. (1994). *Anxiety Disorders Interview Schedule for DSM-IV: Lifetime version (ADIS-IV-L).* Albany, NY: Graywind.

Edelmann, R. E., & Chambless, D. L. (1995). Adherence during session and homework in cognitive-behavioral group treatment of social phobia. *Behaviour Research and Therapy, 33,* 537–577.

Elting, D. T., Hope, D. A., & Heimberg, R. G. (1997). Inter-relationships among measures commonly used in research on social phobia. *Depression and Anxiety, 4,* 246–248.

Erwin, B. A., Heimberg, R. G., Juster, H. R., & Mindlin, M. (2002). Comorbid anxiety and mood disorders among persons with social phobia. *Behaviour Research and Therapy, 40,* 19–35.

Erwin, B. A., Heimberg, R. G., Schneier, F. R., & Liebowitz, M. R. (2003). Anger experience and expression in social anxiety disorder: Pretreatment profile and predictors of attrition and response to cognitive-behavioral treatment. *Behavior Therapy, 34,* 331–350.

Feske, U., Perry, K. J., Chambless, D. L., Renneberg, B., & Goldstein, A. J. (1996). Avoidant personality disorder as a predictor for severity and treatment out-come among generalized social phobics. *Journal of Personality Disorders, 10,* 174–184.

Fresco, D. M., Coles, M. E., Heimberg, R. G., Liebowitz, M. R., Hami, S., Stein, M. B., et al. (2001). The Liebowitz Social Anxiety Scale: A com-parison of the psychometric properties of self-report and clinician-administered formats. *Psychological Medicine, 31,* 1025–1035.

Frisch, M. B. (1994). *Manual and treatment guide for the Quality of Life Inventory.* Minneapolis, MN: Na-tional Computer Systems.

Gilbert, P. (2001). Evolution and social anxiety: The role of attraction, social competition, and social hier-archies. *Psychiatric Clinics of North America, 24,* 723–751.

Gould, R. A., Buckminster, S., Pollack, M. H., Otto, M. W., & Yap, L. (1997). Cognitive-behavioral and pharmacological treatment for social phobia: A meta-analysis. *Clinical Psychology: Science and Prac-tice, 4,* 291–306.

Hackmann, A., Clark, D. M., & McManus, F. (2000). Recurrent images and early memories in social pho-bia. *Behaviour Research and Therapy, 38,* 601–610.

Hackmann, A., Surawy, C., & Clark, D. M. (1998). Seeing yourself through others' eyes: A study of spon-taneously occurring images in social phobia. *Behav-ioural and Cognitive Psychotherapy, 26,* 3–12.

Hambrick, J. P., Turk, C. L., Heimberg, R. G., Schneier, F. R., & Liebowitz, M. R. (2003). The experience of disability and quality of life in social anxiety disorder. *Depression and Anxiety, 18,* 46–50.

Hayes, S. A., Hope, D. A., Van Dyke, M., & Heimberg, R. G. (2007). Working alliance for clients with social anxiety disorder: Relationship with session helpful-ness and within-session habituation. *Cognitive Be-haviour Therapy, 36,* 34–42.

Hayes, S. A., Miller, N. A., Hope, D. A., Heimberg, R. G., & Juster, H. R. (in press). Assessing client prog-ress session-by-session: The Social Anxiety Session Change Index. *Cognitive and Behavioral Practice.*

Heimberg, R. G. (1994). Cognitive assessment strategies and the measurement of outcome of treatment for so-cial phobia. *Behaviour Research and Therapy, 32,* 269–280.

Heimberg, R. G., & Becker, R. E. (2002). *Cognitive-behavioral group therapy for social phobia: Basic mechanisms and clinical strategies.* New York: Guilford Press.

Heimberg, R. G., Dodge, C. S., Hope, D. A., Kennedy, C. R., Zollo, L. J. & Becker, R. E. (1990). Cognitive-behavioral group treatment for social phobia: Com-parison with a credible placebo control. *Cognitive Therapy and Research, 14,* 1–23.

Heimberg, R. G., & Holaway, R. M. (in press). Exami-nation of the known-groups validity of the Liebowitz Social Anxiety Scale. *Depression and Anxiety.*

Heimberg, R. G., Holt, C. S., Schneier, F. R., Spitzer, R. L., & Liebowitz, M. R. (1993). The issues of sub-types in the diagnosis of social phobia. *Journal of Anxiety Disorders, 7,* 249–269.

Heimberg, R. G., Hope, D. A., Dodge, C. S., & Becker, R. E. (1990). DSM-III-R subtypes of social phobia: Comparison of generalized social phobics and public speaking phobics. *Journal of Nervous and Mental Disease, 178,* 172–179.

Heimberg, R. G., Horner, K. J., Juster, H. R., Safren, S. A., Brown, E. J., Schneier, F. R., et al. (1999). Psycho-metric properties of the Liebowitz Social Anxiety Scale. *Psychological Medicine, 29,* 199–212.

Heimberg, R. G., Liebowitz, M. R., Hope, D. A., Schneier, F. R., Holt, C. S., Welkowitz, L. A., et al. (1998). Cognitive behavioral group therapy vs. phenelzine therapy for social phobia: 12-week out-come. *Archives of General Psychiatry, 55,* 1133–1141.

Heimberg, R. G., Mueller, G. P., Holt, C. S., Hope, D. A., & Liebowitz, M. R. (1992). Assessment of anx-iety in social interaction and being observed by others: The Social Interaction Anxiety Scale and the Social Phobia Scale. *Behavior Therapy, 23,* 53–73.

Heimberg, R. G., Salzman, D. G., Holt, C. S., & Blendell, K. A. (1993). Cognitive-behavioral group treatment for social phobia: Effectiveness at five-year followup. *Cognitive Therapy and Research, 17,* 325–339.

Heimberg, R. G., with Turk, C. L. (2002). Assessment of social phobia. In R. G. Heimberg & R. E. Becker (Eds.), *Cognitive-behavioral group therapy for social phobia: Basic mechanisms and clinical strategies* (pp. 107–126). New York: Guilford Press.

Herbert, J. D., Bellack, A. S., & Hope, D. A. (1991). Concurrent validity of the Social Phobia and Anxiety Inventory. *Journal of Psychopathology and Behav-ioral Assessment, 13,* 357–368.

Herbert, J. D., Hope, D. A., & Bellack, A. S. (1992). Va-lidity of the distinction between generalized social phobia and avoidant personality disorder. *Journal of Abnormal Psychology, 101,* 332–339.

Hofmann, S. G. (2004). Cognitive mediation of treat-ment change in social phobia. *Journal of Consulting and Clinical Psychology, 72,* 392–399.

Hofmann, S. G., Newman, M. G., Becker, E., Taylor, C. B., & Roth, W. T. (1995). Social phobia with and without avoidant personality disorder: Preliminary behavior therapy outcome findings. *Journal of Anxi-ety Disorders, 9,* 427–438.

Hope, D. A., Heimberg, R. G., & Bruch, M. A. (1995). Dismantling cognitive-behavioral group therapy for social phobia. *Behaviour Research and Therapy, 33,* 637–650.

Hope, D. A., Heimberg, R. G., Juster, H., & Turk, C. L. (2000). *Managing social anxiety: A cognitive-behavioral therapy approach* (client workbook). New York: Oxford University Press.

Hope, D. A., Heimberg, R. G., & Turk, C. L. (2006). *Managing social anxiety: A cognitive-behavioral therapy approach* (therapist guide). New York: Oxford University Press.

Hope, D. A., Herbert, J. D., & White, C. (1995). Diagnostic subtype, avoidant personality disorder, and efficacy of cognitive behavioral group therapy for social phobia. *Cognitive Therapy and Research, 19,* 399–417.

Hope, D. A., Sigler, K. D., Penn, D. L., & Meier, V. (1998). Social anxiety, recall of interpersonal information, and social impact on others. *Journal of Cognitive Psychotherapy: An International Quarterly, 12,* 303–322.

Hope, D. A., Van Dyke, M., Heimberg, R. G., Turk, C. L., & Fresco, D. M. (2002). *Cognitive-behavioral therapy for social anxiety disorder: Therapist adherence scale.* Unpublished manuscript, available from Richard G. Heimberg, Adult Anxiety Clinic, Department of Psychology, Temple University, Philadelphia, PA 19122-6085.

Katzelnick, D. J., Kobak, K. A., DeLeire, T., Henk, H. J., Greist, J. H., Davidson, J. R. T., et al. (2001). Impact of generalized social anxiety disorder in managed care. *American Journal of Psychiatry, 158,* 1999–2007.

Kendall, P. C., Chu, B., Gifford, A., Hayes, C., & Nauta, M. (1998). Breathing life into a manual: Flexibility and creativity with manual-based treatments. *Cognitive and Behavioral Practice, 5,* 177–198.

Kessler, R. C., Berglund, P. D., Demler, O., Olga, J. R., Merikangas, K. R., & Walters, E. E. (2005). Lifetime prevalence and age-of-onset distributions of DSM-IV disorders in the National Comorbidity Survey Replication. *Archives of General Psychiatry, 62,* 593–602.

Kocvoski, N. L., Rector, N. A., & Denisoff, E. (2004, November). *Post-event processing during CBGT for social anxiety disorder.* Poster presented at the meeting of the Association for the Advancement of Behavioral Therapy, New Orleans, LA.

Leary, M. R. (1983). A brief version of the Fear of Negative Evaluation Scale. *Personality and Social Psychology Bulletin, 9,* 371–375.

Leary, M. R., Kowalski, R. M., & Campbell, C. D. (1988). Self-presentational concerns and social anxiety: The role of generalized impression expectancies. *Journal of Research in Personality, 22,* 308–321.

Leung, A. W., & Heimberg, R. G. (1996). Homework compliance, perceptions of control, and outcome of cognitive-behavioral treatment for social phobia. *Behaviour Research and Therapy, 34,* 423–432.

Liebowitz, M. R. (1987). Social phobia. *Modern Problems in Pharmacopsychiatry, 22,* 141–173.

Liebowitz, M. R., Heimberg, R. G., Fresco, D. M., Travers, J., & Stein, M. B. (2000). Social phobia or social anxiety disorder: What's in a name? *Archives of General Psychiatry, 57,* 191–192.

Liebowitz, M. R., Heimberg, R. G., Schneier, F. R., Hope, D. A., Davies, S., Holt, C. S., et al. (1999). Cognitive-behavioral group therapy versus

phenelzine in social phobia: Long-term outcome. *Depression and Anxiety, 10,* 89–98.

Lucas, R. A., & Telch, M. J. (1993, November). *Group versus individual treatment of social phobia.* Paper presented at the annual meeting of the Association for Advancement of Behavior Therapy, Atlanta, GA.

MacLeod, C., & Mathews, A. (1991). Biased cognitive operations in anxiety: Accessibility of information or assignment of processing priorities? *Behaviour Research and Therapy, 29,* 599–610.

Magee, L., Erwin, B. A., & Heimberg, R. G. (in press). Psychological treatment of social anxiety disorder and specific phobia. In M. M. Antony & M. B. Stein (Eds.), *Handbook of anxiety and the anxiety disorders.* New York: Oxford University Press.

Magee, W. J., Eaton, W. W., Wittchen, H.-U., McGonagle, K. A., & Kessler, R. C. (1996). Agoraphobia, simple phobia, and social phobia in the National Comorbidity Survey. *Archives of General Psychiatry, 53,* 159–168.

Mannuzza, S., Schneier, F. R., Chapman, T. F., Liebowitz, M. R., Klein, D. F., & Fyer, A. J. (1995). Generalized social phobia: Reliability and validity. *Archives of General Psychiatry, 52,* 230–237.

Mattick, R. P., & Clarke, J. C. (1998). Development and validation of measures of social phobia scrutiny fear and social interaction anxiety. *Behaviour Research and Therapy, 36,* 455–470.

Mattick, R. P., & Peters, L. (1988). Treatment of severe social phobia: Effects of guided exposure with and without cognitive restructuring. *Journal of Consulting and Clinical Psychology, 56,* 251–260.

Mattick, R. P., Peters, L., & Clarke, J. C. (1989). Exposure and cognitive restructuring for social phobia: A controlled study. *Behavior Therapy, 20,* 3–23.

Mennin, D. S., Fresco, D. M., Heimberg, R. G., Schneier, F. R., Davies, S. O., & Liebowitz, M. R. (2002). Screening for social anxiety disorder in the clinical setting: Using the Liebowitz Social Anxiety Scale. *Journal of Anxiety Disorders, 16,* 661–673.

Narrow, W. E., Rae, D. S., Robins, L. N., & Regier, D. A. (2002). Revised prevalence estimates of mental disorders in the United States: Using a clinical significance criterion to reconcile two surveys' estimates. *Archives of General Psychiatry, 59,* 115–123.

Norton, P. J., & Hope, D. A. (2001). Kernels of truth or distorted perceptions: Self and observer ratings of social anxiety and performance. *Behavior Therapy, 32,* 765–786.

Rapee, R. M., & Heimberg, R. G. (1997). A cognitive-behavioral model of anxiety in social phobia. *Behaviour Research and Therapy, 35,* 741–756.

Rapee, R. M., & Lim, L. (1992). Discrepancy between self- and observer ratings of performance in social phobics. *Journal of Abnormal Psychology, 101,* 728–731.

Reich, J., Goldenberg, I., Vasile, R., Goisman, R., & Keller, M. (1994). A prospective follow-along study of the course of social phobia. *Psychiatry Research*, 54, 249–258.

Ries, B. J., McNeil, D. W., Boone, M. L., Turk, C. L., Carter, L. E., & Heimberg, R. G. (1998). Assessment of contemporary social phobia verbal report instruments. *Behaviour Research and Therapy*, 36, 983–994.

Rodebaugh, T. L., Holaway, R. M., & Heimberg, R. G. (2004). The treatment of social anxiety disorder. *Clinical Psychology Review*, 24, 883–908.

Rodebaugh, T. L., Woods, C. M., Thissen, D. M., Heimberg, R. G., Chambless, D. L., & Rapee, R. M. (2004). More information from fewer questions: The factor structure and item properties of the original and Brief Fear of Negative Evaluation Scale. *Psychological Assessment*, 16, 169–181.

Roth, D. A., Coles, M. E., & Heimberg, R. G. (2002). The relationship between memories for childhood teasing and anxiety and depression in adulthood. *Journal of Anxiety Disorders*, 16, 149–164.

Roth, D. A., & Heimberg, R. G. (2001). Cognitive-behavioral models of social anxiety disorder. *Psychiatric Clinics of North America*, 24, 753–771.

Safren, S. A., Heimberg, R. G., Brown, E. J., & Holle, C. (1997). Quality of life in social phobia. *Depression and Anxiety*, 4, 126–133.

Safren, S. A., Heimberg, R. G., & Juster, H. R. (1997). Client expectancies and their relationship to pretreatment symptomatology and outcome of cognitive-behavioral group treatment for social phobia. *Journal of Consulting and Clinical Psychology*, 65, 694–698.

Sanderson, W. C., Di Nardo, P. A., Rapee, R. M., & Barlow, D. H. (1990). Syndrome comorbidity in patients diagnosed with a DSM-III-R anxiety disorder. *Journal of Abnormal Psychology*, 99, 308–312.

Sank, L. I., & Shaffer, C. S. (1984). *A therapist's manual for cognitive behavior therapy in groups*. New York: Plenum Press.

Schneier, F. R., Heckelman, L. R., Garfinkel, R., Campeas, R., Fallon, B. A., Gitow, A., et al. (1994). Functional impairment in social phobia. *Journal of Clinical Psychiatry*, 55, 322–331.

Schneier, F. R., Johnson, J., Hornig, C. D., Liebowitz, M. R., & Weissman, M. M. (1992). Social phobia: Comorbidity and morbidity in an epidemiologic sample. *Archives of General Psychiatry*, 49, 282–288.

Scholing, A., & Emmelkamp, P. M. G. (1993). Exposure with and without cognitive therapy for generalized social phobia: Effects of individual and group treatment. *Behaviour Research and Therapy*, 31, 667–681.

Schwartz, R. M., & Garamoni, G. L. (1989). Cognitive balance and psychopathology: Evaluation of an information processing model of positive and negative states of mind. *Clinical Psychology Review*, 9, 271–294.

Stangier, U., Heidenreich, T., Peitz, M., Lauterbach, W.,

& Clark, D. M. (2003). Cognitive therapy for social phobia: Individual versus group treatment. *Behaviour Research and Therapy*, 41, 991–1007.

Stopa, L., & Clark, D. M. (1993). Cognitive processes in social phobia. *Behaviour Research and Therapy*, 31, 255–267.

Taylor, S., Woody, S., Koch, W., McLean, P., Paterson, R., & Anderson, K. W. (1997a). Cognitive restructuring in the treatment of social phobia: Efficacy and mode of action. *Behavior Modification*, 21, 487–511.

Taylor, S., Woody, S., McLean, P. D., & Koch, W. J. (1997b). Sensitivity of outcome measures for treatments of generalized social phobia. *Assessment*, 4, 181–191.

Trower, P., & Gilbert, P. (1989). New theoretical conceptions of social anxiety and social phobia. *Clinical Psychology Review*, 9, 19–35.

Turk, C. L., Lerner, J., Heimberg, R. G., & Rapee, R. M. (2001). An integrated cognitive-behavioral model of social anxiety. In S. G. Hofmann & P. M. DiBartolo (Eds.), *From social anxiety to social phobia: Multiple perspectives* (pp. 281–303). Needham Heights, MA: Allyn & Bacon.

Turner, S. M., Beidel, D. C., Dancu, C. V., & Keys, D. J. (1986). Psychopathology of social phobia and comparison to avoidant personality disorder. *Journal of Abnormal Psychology*, 95, 389–394.

Turner, S. M., Beidel, D. C., Dancu, C. V., & Stanley, M. A. (1989). An empirically derived inventory to measure social fears and anxiety: The Social Phobia and Anxiety Inventory. *Psychological Assessment*, 1, 35–40.

Turner, S. M., Beidel, D. C., & Townsley, R. M. (1992). Social phobia: A comparison of specific and generalized subtype and avoidant personality disorder. *Journal of Abnormal Psychology*, 101, 326–331.

Turner, S. M., Beidel, D. C., Wolff, P. L., Spaulding, S., & Jacob, R. G. (1996). Clinical features affecting treatment outcome in social phobia. *Behaviour Research and Therapy*, 34, 795–804.

Wallace, S. T., & Alden, L. E. (1991). A comparison of social standards and perceived ability in anxious and nonanxious men. *Cognitive Therapy and Research*, 15, 237–254.

Watson, D., & Friend, R. (1969). Measurement of social-evaluative anxiety. *Journal of Consulting and Clinical Psychology*, 33, 448–457.

Weeks, J. W., Heimberg, R. G., Fresco, D. M., Hart, T. A., Turk, C. L., Schneier, F. R., et al. (2005). Empirical validation and psychometric evaluation of the Brief Fear of Negative Evaluation Scale in patients with social anxiety disorder. *Psychological Assessment*, 17, 179–190.

Weeks, J. W., Spokas, M. E., & Heimberg, R. G. (in press). Psychometric evaluation of the Mini–Social Phobia Inventory (Mini-SPIN) in a treatment-seeking sample. *Depression and Anxiety*.

Weiller, E., Bisserbe, J. C., Boyer, P., Lepine, J.-P., &

Lecrubier, Y. (1996). Social phobia in general health care: An unrecognised undertreated disabling disorder. *British Journal of Psychiatry, 168*, 169–174.

Widiger, T. A. (1992). Generalized social phobia versus avoidant personality disorder: A commentary on three studies. *Journal of Abnormal Psychology, 101*, 340–343.

Wlazlo, Z., Schroeder-Hartwig, K., Hand, I., Kaiser, G., & Münchau, N. (1990). Exposure *in vivo* vs. social skills training for social phobia: Long-term outcome and differential effects. *Behaviour Research and Therapy, 28*, 181–193.

Wolpe, J., & Lazarus, A. A. (1966). *Behavior therapy techniques*. New York: Pergamon.

Woody, S. R., & Adessky, R. S. (2002). Therapeutic alliance, group cohesion, and homework compliance during cognitive-behavioral group treatment of social phobia. *Behavior Therapy, 35*, 5–27.

Zaider, T. I., Heimberg, R. G., Roth, D. A., Hope, D., & Turk, C. L. (2003, November). *Individual cognitive-behavioral therapy for social anxiety disorder: Preliminary findings*. Paper presented at the Annual Meeting of the Association for Advancement of Behavior Therapy, Boston.

CHAPTER 4

Obsessive–Compulsive Disorder

MARTIN E. FRANKLIN
EDNA B. FOA

It will not take the reader long to see that successful therapy for obsessive–compulsive disorder (OCD) is markedly different in both structure and content from the usual therapeutic approaches. For this reason, regrettably, few therapists feel self-efficacious enough to undertake this therapy, yet this approach is clearly the treatment of choice for the most beneficial short- and long-term effects in OCD according to recent clinical trials. The information provided in this detailed chapter should be sufficient for any reasonably well-trained mental health professional to undertake this treatment, particularly if few other options are available. The suffering involved with OCD can be extraordinary, and even imperfect attempts at therapy can relieve much of this suffering. This chapter describes the detailed conduct of intensive daily sessions involving both imaginal and direct *in vivo* practice. Also noticeable is the ingenuity required of therapists (e.g., Where do you find dead animals?). The importance of involving significant others continues a theme first described by Craske and Barlow in Chapter 1 of this volume, where spouses/partners or other people close to the individual with the problem become an important and integral part of treatment. Finally, this chapter contains an up-to-date review of the current status of psychological and pharmacological approaches to OCD.—D. H. B.

Advances in cognitive-behavioral and pharmacological treatments in the last three decades have greatly improved the prognosis for patients with obsessive–compulsive disorder (OCD). In this chapter we first discuss diagnostic and theoretical issues of OCD and review the available treatments, then describe assessment procedures and illustrate in detail how to implement intensive cognitive-behavioral treatment (CBT) involving exposure and ritual prevention (EX/RP) for OCD. Throughout the chapter, we use case material to illustrate interactions that occur between therapist and patient to demonstrate the process that occurs during treatment.

DEFINITION

According to the text revision of the fourth edition of the *Diagnostic and Statistical Manual of Mental Disorders* (DSM-IV-TR; American Psychiatric Association, 2000), OCD is characterized by recurrent obsessions and/or compulsions that interfere substantially with daily functioning. Obsessions are "persistent ideas, thoughts, impulses, or images that are experienced as intrusive and inappropriate and cause marked anxiety or distress" (p. 457). Common obsessions are repeated thoughts about causing harm to others, contamination, and doubting whether one locked the front door. Compulsions are "repetitive behaviors or mental acts of which the goal is to prevent or reduce anxiety or distress" (p. 457). Common compulsions include handwashing, checking, and counting.

In DSM-IV-TR, the functional link between obsessions and compulsions is emphasized: "Obsessions" are defined as thoughts, images, or impulses that *cause* marked anxiety or distress, and "compulsions" are defined as overt (behavioral) or covert (mental) actions that are performed in an attempt to *reduce* the distress brought on by obsessions or according to rigid rules. This modification is supported by findings from the DSM-IV field trial on OCD, in which over 90% of participants reported that the aim of their compulsions was either to prevent harm associated with their obsessions or to reduce obsessional distress (Foa et al., 1995).

Data from the DSM-IV field study also indicated that the vast majority (over 90%) of individuals with OCD manifest both obsessions and behavioral rituals. When mental rituals are included, only 2% of the sample reported "pure" obsessions (Foa et al., 1995). Behavioral rituals (e.g., handwashing) are equivalent to mental rituals (e.g., silently repeating special prayers) in their functional relationship to obsessions: Both serve to reduce obsessional distress, to prevent feared harm, or to restore safety. Thus, whereas all obsessions are indeed mental events, compulsions can be either mental or behavioral. Identification of mental rituals is an especially important aspect of treatment planning, because obsessions and compulsions are addressed via different techniques. For example, we once treated a patient who described himself as a "pure obsessional," who would experience intrusive and unwanted images of harm coming to his girlfriend by an animal attack. The patient would quickly and intentionally insert his own image into the scene to become the victim of the animal mauling, thereby reducing his distress and, in his estimation, reducing the likelihood that some future harm would come to his girlfriend. The substitution of his own image into the scene constituted a mental ritual, and the success of imaginal exposure exercises required that the patient refrain from this form of compulsion.

A growing consensus about a continuum of insight in individuals with OCD (e.g., Foa et al., 1995; Insel & Akiskal, 1986) led to the inclusion in DSM-IV (American Psychiatric Association, 1994) of a subtype of OCD "with poor insight" to include individuals who indeed have obsessions and compulsions but fail to recognize their senselessness; this change was retained in DSM-IV-TR. Clinically it is important to evaluate the degree of insight prior to initiating CBT, because fixed belief about the consequences of refraining from compulsions and avoidance behaviors has been found to be associated with attentuated treatment outcome (e.g., Foa, Abramowitz, Franklin, & Kozak, 1999; Neziroglu, Stevens, Yaryura-Tobias, & McKay, 2000).

To be diagnosed with OCD, obsessions and/or compulsions must be found to be of sufficient severity to cause marked distress, be time-consuming, and interfere with daily functioning. If another Axis I disorder is present, the obsessions and compulsions cannot be restricted to the content of that disorder (e.g., preoccupation with food in the presence of eating disorders). There continues to be much discussion about the presence of an obsessive–compulsive spectrum that includes a wide variety of compulsive and impulsive disorders (e.g., pathological gambling, trichotillomania; see Hollander & Stein, 2006), but current DSM-IV-TR nosology still specifies that such disorders should not be diagnosed as OCD.

PREVALENCE AND COURSE OF OCD

Once thought to be an extremely rare disorder, the 12-month prevalence of OCD was estimated at 1.0% in the recent National Comorbidity Survey Replication involving over 9,000 adult participants in the United States (Kessler et al., 2005). Epidemiological studies with children and adolescents suggest similar lifetime prevalence rates in these samples (e.g., Flament et al., 1988; Valleni-Basille et al., 1994). Slightly more than half of adults suffering from OCD are female (Rasmussen & Tsuang, 1986), whereas a 2:1 male to female ratio has been observed in several pediatric clinical samples (e.g., Hanna, 1995; Swedo, Rapoport, Leonard, Lenane, & Cheslow, 1989). Age of onset of the disorder typically ranges from early adolescence to young adulthood, with earlier onset in males; modal onset is ages 13–15 in males, and ages 20–24 in females (Rasmussen & Eisen, 1990). However, cases of OCD have been documented in children as young as age 2 (Rapoport, Swedo, & Leonard, 1992).

Development of the disorder is usually gradual, but acute onset has been reported in some cases. Although chronic waxing and waning of symptoms are typical, episodic and deteriorating courses have been observed in about 10% of patients (Rasmussen & Eisen, 1989). In some cases of pediatric OCD and tic disorders, onset is very sudden and associated with strep infection; treatment of the infection is associated with substantial reduction of symptoms, but recurrence of infection is again associated with symptom exacerbation (Swedo et al., 1998). Presentation of OCD in these cases is much more typical in males than in females and has come to be known as pediatric autoimmune neuropsychiatric disorders (PANDAS); the prevalence of PANDAS has yet to be determined. OCD is frequently associated with impairments in general functioning, such as disruption of gainful employment (Koran, 2000; Leon, Portera, & Weissman, 1995), and interpersonal relationship difficulties (Emmelkamp, de Haan, & Hoogduin, 1990; Riggs, Hiss, & Foa, 1992). Adolescents identified as having OCD (Flament et al., 1988) reported in a subsequent follow-up study that they had withdrawn socially to prevent contamination and to conserve energy for obsessive–compulsive behaviors (Flament et al., 1990).

Many individuals with OCD suffer for years before seeking treatment. In one study, individuals first presented for psychiatric treatment over 7 years after the onset of significant symptoms (Rasmussen & Tsuang, 1986). The disorder may cause severe impairment in functioning, resulting in job loss and disruption of marital and other interpersonal relationships. Marital distress is reported by approximately 50% of married individuals seeking treatment for OCD (Emmelkamp et al., 1990; Riggs et al., 1992).

COMORBIDITY

Convergent epidemiological and clinical data indicate that OCD rarely occurs in isolation: Although the rates of comorbidity differ across studies due to selection of population and methodology, comorbidity is generally high. For example, Weissman and colleagues (1994) found that 49% of individuals diagnosed with OCD suffered from a comorbid anxiety disorder and 27% from comorbid major depressive disorder (MDD). Among studies conducted

specifically within anxiety clinics, there is great variability, but comorbid conditions are generally common (for a review, see Ledley, Pai, & Franklin 2007). In the largest of the studies conducted in the context of an anxiety clinic, Brown, Campbell, Lehman, Grisham, and Mancill (2001) found that 57% of 77 adults with a principal diagnosis of OCD had a current comorbid Axis I condition; the rate rose to 86% for lifetime comorbid Axis I conditions. Notably, when OCD co-occurs with other anxiety disorders, it is typically the principal diagnosis (e.g., the diagnosis of greatest severity; see Antony, Downie, & Swinson, 1998). It also appears to be the case that MDD onset tends to follow that of OCD, suggesting that depression might be a response to OCD symptoms (Bellodi, Sciuto, Diaferia, Ronchi, & Smeraldi, 1992; Diniz et al., 2004).

The data are equivocal with respect to the influence of comorbidity on OCD presentation. In one study, Denys, Tenney, van Megen, de Geus, and Westenberg (2004) found that comorbidity did not influence OCD symptom severity, whereas others (Angst, 1993; Tukel, Polat, Ozdemir, Aksut, & Turksov, 2002) found a relationship between comorbidity and OCD symptom severity. A more consistent finding is that comorbidity is associated with poorer quality of life, particularly in the case of comorbid depression (Lochner & Stein, 2003; Masellis, Rector, & Richter, 2003).

With respect to the effect of comorbid anxiety and depression on treatment outcome, the influence of depression has received more empirical attention to date. Some studies have found that higher levels of depression at pretreatment are related to poorer outcome (e.g., Keijsers, Hoogduin, & Schaap, 1994; Steketee, Chambless, & Tran, 2001), whereas others have found little or no effect (Mataix-Cols, Marks, Greist, Kobak, & Baer, 2002; O'Sullivan, Noshirvani, Marks, Monteiro, & Lelliot, 1991; Steketee, Eisen, Dyck, Warshaw, & Rasmussen, 1999). Some have suggested that, more specifically, the *severity* of the comorbid depression might influence its effects on OCD treatment outcome: Abramowitz, Franklin, Street, Kozak, and Foa (2000) found that only severely depressed patients were less likely to respond to EX/RP therapy for OCD. Similarly, highly depressed OCD patients seem to be at greater risk for relapse following treatment discontinuation (Abramowitz & Foa, 2000; Basoglu, Lax, Kasvikis, & Marks,

1998). The influence of comorbid anxiety disorders on outcome has received less attention thus far: One study reported that patients with OCD and comorbid generalized anxiety disorder (GAD) terminate OCD treatment at higher rates than other patients (Steketee et al., 2001), and another found that the presence of posttraumatic stress disorder (PTSD) in patients with OCD attenuated response to EX/RP (Gershuny, Baer, Jenike, Minichiello, & Wilhelm, 2002). The mechanisms by which these comorbid conditions influence outcome have yet to be explored.

Tourette syndrome and other tic disorders also appear to be related to OCD. Estimates of the comorbidity of Tourette syndrome and OCD range from 28 to 63% (Comings, 1990; Kurlan et al., 2002; Leckman & Chittenden, 1990; Pauls, Towbin, Leckman, Zahner, & Cohen, 1986). Conversely, up to 17% of patients with OCD are thought to have Tourette syndrome (Comings, 1990; Kurlan et al., 2002; Rasmussen & Eisen, 1989). In a recent report, tic comorbidity was associated with poorer treatment outcome in general (Matsunaga et al., 2005), yet in a recent pediatric study was found to influence pharmacotherapy treatment outcome but not CBT response (March et al., 2007).

DIFFERENTIAL DIAGNOSIS

The high comorbidity of OCD with other disorders noted earlier, as well as the similarity between the criteria for OCD and other DSM-IV disorders, can pose diagnostic quandaries. Below we review some of the more common diagnostic difficulties likely to confront clinicians, and provide recommendations for making these difficult diagnostic judgments.

Obsessions versus Depressive Rumination

It is sometimes difficult to differentiate between depressive ruminations and obsessions. The distinction rests primarily on thought content and the patient's reported resistance to such thoughts. Unlike obsessions, ruminations are typically pessimistic ideas about the self or the world, and ruminative content frequently shifts. Additionally, depressive ruminators tend to not make repeated attempts to suppress their ruminations the way individuals with OCD try to suppress obsessions. When depression and

OCD co-occur, both phenomena may be present, but only obsessions should be targeted with exposure exercises. We have also found clinically that the generally pessimistic presentation of depressed patients can undermine hopefulness about improvement during EX/RP; thus, these beliefs may require therapeutic intervention even though they are not obsessional.

Other Anxiety Disorders

OCD often co-occurs with other anxiety disorders, and diagnostic criteria are sometimes similar among anxiety disorders, but the symptoms associated with each diagnosis can usually be distinguished. For example, the excessive worries characteristic of GAD may appear similar to those in OCD but, unlike obsessions, worries are excessive concerns about real-life circumstances and are experienced by the individual as appropriate (ego-syntonic). In contrast, obsessive thinking is more likely to be unrealistic or magical, and obsessions are usually experienced by the individual as inappropriate (ego-dystonic). There are, however, exceptions to this general rule: Individuals with either GAD or OCD may worry about everyday matters, such as their children getting sick. However, when worried about their children catching cold, parents with GAD might focus their concern on the long-term consequences (e.g., falling behind in school, development of a lifelong pattern of debilitation), whereas parents with OCD might focus more on the contamination aspect of illness (e.g., their child being infested with "cold germs"). The problem of distinguishing between obsessions and worries in a particular patient is most relevant when the patient exhibits no compulsions, but, as we mentioned earlier, pure obsessionals comprise only about 2% of individuals with OCD (Foa et al., 1995).

In the absence of rituals, the avoidance associated with specific phobias may also appear similar to OCD. For example, excessive fear of germs and specific phobia both may result in persistent fear of dogs. However, unlike an individual with OCD, a person with a specific phobia can successfully avoid dogs for the most part, or reduce distress quickly by escaping dogs when avoidance is impractical. In contrast, the individual with OCD who is obsessed with "dog germs" continues to feel contaminated even after the dog is gone, and sometimes knowing that a dog was in the vicinity several hours earlier can also produce obsessional distress even if there is no possibility that the dog will return. This distress often prompts subsequent avoidance behaviors (e.g., taking off clothing that might have been near the contaminating dog) not typically observed in specific phobias.

Hypochondriasis and Body Dysmorphic Disorder

The health concerns that characterize hypochondriasis and the preoccupation with imagined physical defects of body dysmorphic disorder (BDD) are both formally similar to the obsessions of OCD. The best way to differentiate between these disorders and OCD is to examine for content specificity of the fear-provoking thoughts. Most individuals with hypochondriasis or BDD are singly obsessed, whereas most individuals with OCD have multiple obsessions. Moreover, patients with OCD typically obsess about contracting diseases or becoming ill in the future, whereas patients with hypochondriasis focus on physical and psychological symptoms that lead them to fear they have already contracted diseases or illnesses.

Tourette Syndrome and Tic Disorders

To differentiate the stereotyped motor behaviors that characterize Tourette syndrome and tic disorders from compulsions, the functional relationship between these behaviors and any obsessive thoughts must be examined. Motor tics are generally experienced as involuntary and are not aimed at neutralizing distress brought about by obsessions. There is no conventional way to differentiate them from "pure" compulsions, but OCD with "pure" compulsions is extremely rare (Foa et al., 1995). As noted earlier, there appears to be a high rate of comorbidity between OCD and tic disorders (e.g., Pauls et al., 1986); thus, both disorders may be present simultaneously in a given patient. Interestingly, recent research indicated that tics were similarly responsive to an exposure plus response prevention protocol when compared in a randomized study to habit-reversal training in which a competing response is substituted for the tic; this finding suggests that the conceptual model underlying the treatment of tics might require modifica-

tion (Verdellen, Keijsers, Cath, & Hoogduin, 2004).

Delusional Disorder and Schizophrenia

Individuals with OCD may present with obsessions of delusional intensity (for a review, see Kozak & Foa, 1994). Approximately 5% of patients with OCD report complete conviction that their obsessions and compulsions are realistic, with an additional 20% reporting strong but not fixed conviction. Therefore, it is important to consider the diagnosis of OCD "with poor insight" even if these beliefs are very strongly held. The differentiation between delusional disorder and OCD can depend on the presence of compulsions in OCD (Eisen et al., 1998). In OCD, obsessions of delusional intensity are usually accompanied by compulsions.

It is also important to recognize that the content of obsessions in OCD may be quite bizarre, as in the delusions of schizophrenia, but bizarreness in and of itself does not preclude a diagnosis of OCD. For example, one patient seen at our center was fearful that small bits of her "essence" would be forever lost if she passed too close to public trash cans. This patient did not report any other symptoms of formal thought disorder, such as loose associations, hallucinations, flat or grossly inappropriate affect, and thought insertion or projection. Following a course of EX/RP that focused on exercises designed to expose the patient to the loss of her "essence" (e.g., driving by the city dump), her OCD symptoms were substantially reduced. On occasion patients do meet diagnostic criteria for both OCD and schizophrenia, and a dual diagnosis is appropriate under these circumstances. Importantly, EX/RP with such patients should proceed only if the associated treatment exercises do not exacerbate the comorbid thought disorder symptoms.

COGNITIVE AND BEHAVIORAL MODELS

Mowrer's (1939) two-stage theory for the acquisition and maintenance of fear and avoidance behavior has been commonly adopted to explain phobias and OCD. As elaborated by Mowrer (1960), this theory proposes that in the first stage, a neutral event becomes associated with fear by being paired with a stimulus that by its nature provokes discomfort or anxiety. Through conditioning processes, objects, as well as thoughts and images, acquire the ability to produce discomfort. In the second stage of this process, escape or avoidance responses are developed to reduce the anxiety or discomfort evoked by the various conditioned stimuli and are maintained by their success in doing so. Dollard and Miller (1950) adopted Mowrer's two-stage theory to explain the development of phobias and obsessive–compulsive neurosis. As noted earlier, because of the intrusive nature of obsessions, many situations that provoke obsessions cannot readily be avoided. Passive avoidance behaviors, such as those utilized by phobics, are also less effective in controlling obsessional distress. Active avoidance patterns in the form of ritualistic behaviors are then developed and maintained by their success in alleviating this distress.

In light of equivocal empirical support for the two-stage theory and its limitations in explaining the etiology of obsessions, several cognitive explanations have been offered to account for the development and maintenance of OCD symptoms. Carr (1974) proposed that individuals with OCD have unusually high expectations of negative outcome; they overevaluate the negative consequences for a variety of actions. He noted that obsessional content typically includes exaggerations of the concerns of normal individuals: health, death, welfare of others, sex, religion, and the like. According to this theory, the sources of obsessive–compulsive concerns are identical to those found in GAD, agoraphobia, and social phobia. In this way, Carr's explanation of OCD is similar to that offered by Beck (1976), who suggested that the content of obsessions is related to danger in the form of doubt or warning. However, neither account distinguishes between threat-related obsessions and threat-related thoughts in phobics.

Salkovskis (1985) offered a more comprehensive cognitive analysis of OCD. He posited that intrusive obsessional thoughts are stimuli that may provoke certain types of negative automatic thoughts. Accordingly, an intrusive thought leads to mood disturbances only if it triggers negative automatic thoughts through interaction between the unacceptable intrusion and the individual's belief system (e.g., only bad people have sexual thoughts). According to Salkovskis, exaggerated senses of responsibility and self-blame are the central themes in the belief system of a person with OCD.

Neutralization, in the form of behavioral or cognitive compulsions, may be understood as an attempt to reduce this sense of responsibility and to prevent blame. In addition, frequently occurring thoughts regarding unacceptable actions may be perceived by the individual with OCD as equivalent to the actions themselves, so, for example, even if the person has not sinned, the thought of sinning is as bad as sinning itself.

Salkovskis (1985) further proposed that five dysfunctional assumptions characterize individuals with OCD and differentiate them from persons without OCD:

> (1) Having a thought about an action is like performing the action; (2) failing to prevent (or failing to try to prevent) harm to self or others is the same as having caused the harm in the first place; (3) responsibility is not attenuated by other factors (e.g., low probability of occurrence); (4) not neutralizing when an intrusion has occurred is similar or equivalent to seeking or wanting the harm involved in that intrusion to actually happen; (5) one should (and can) exercise control over one's thoughts. (p. 579)

Thus, while the obsession may be ego-dystonic, the automatic thought it elicits will be ego-syntonic. By extension, this model suggests that treatment of OCD should largely focus on identifying the erroneous assumptions and modifying the automatic thoughts. This theory paved the way for various elaborations on the cognitive models, experimental studies of the model, and the development of cognitive therapies that derive from the central role of these key cognitive factors.

Salkovskis's (1985) theory sparked examination of the role of responsibility in the psychopathology of OCD (Ladoucer et al., 1995; Rachman, Thordarson, Shafran, & Woody, 1995; Rhéame, Freeston, Dugas, Letarte, & Ladoucer, 1995). Further attention has been paid to what Rachman (1998) referred to as thought–action fusion (TAF), wherein individuals believe that simply having an unacceptable thought increases the likelihood of the occurrence of a feared outcome, and that thoughts of engaging in repugnant activities are equivalent to actually having done so. Contemporary cognitive theorists would then suggest that obsessive–compulsive beliefs such as TAF, exaggerated responsibility, and intolerance of uncertainty likely result in increased and ultimately futile efforts at thought suppression and other ill-advised mental control strategies, which would then yield increased frequency of such thoughts and associated distress (Purdon & Clark, 2002). Hence a vicious cycle of avoidance maintains and strengthens the OCD, and the cognitive therapies that derive from these contemporary models would directly target these obsessive–compulsive beliefs in an effort to break the cycle.

In an integrated cognitive-behavioral account, Foa and Kozak (1985) conceptualized anxiety disorders in general as specific impairments in emotional memory networks. Following Lang (1979), they view fear as an information network existing in memory that includes representation about fear stimuli, fear responses, and their meaning. With regard to the fear content, Foa and Kozak suggested that fear networks of individuals with anxiety disorders are characterized by the presence of erroneous estimates of threat, unusually high negative valence for the feared event, and excessive response elements (e.g., physiological reactivity), and are resistant to modification. This persistence may reflect failure to access the fear network, because of either active avoidance or because the content of the fear network precludes spontaneous encounters with situations that evoke anxiety in everyday life. Additionally, anxiety may persist because of some impairment in the mechanism of extinction. Cognitive defenses, excessive arousal with failure to habituate, faulty premises, and erroneous rules of inference are all impairments that would hinder the processing of information necessary for modifying the fear structure to reduce fear behavior.

Foa and Kozak (1985) suggested several forms of fear occur in individuals with OCD. The patient who fears contracting venereal disease from public bathrooms and washes to prevent such harm has a fear structure that includes excessive associations between the stimuli (e.g., bathroom) and the anxiety/distress responses, as well as mistaken beliefs about the harm related to the stimulus. For other individuals with OCD, fear responses are associated with mistaken meaning rather than with a particular stimulus. For example, some patients who are disturbed by perceived asymmetry, and who reduce their distress by rearranging objects, do not fear the objects themselves, nor do they anticipate disaster from the asymmetry. Rather, they are upset by their view that certain arrangements of stimuli are "improper."

Like Reed (1985), Foa and Kozak (1985) proposed that in addition to the pathological content of the obsessions, OCD is distinguished from other disorders by pathology in the mechanisms underlying information processing. Specifically, they suggested that patients with OCD experience impairments in considering the rules for making inferences about harm, often concluding that a situation is dangerous based on the absence of evidence for safety, and that they often fail to make inductive leaps about safety from information about the absence of danger. Consequently, rituals performed to reduce the likelihood of harm can never provide safety and must be repeated. In an elaboration on emotional processing theory and the mechanism by which exposure works, Foa, Huppert, and Cahill (2006) suggested that in vivo exposure to the feared stimulus in the absence of the anticipated harm corrects the exaggerated probability estimates; imaginal exposure not only corrects the exaggerated cost but also strengthens the discrimination between "thoughts about harm" and "real harm," thus altering the associations between threat meaning of stimulus and/or response elements in the fear structure.

In contrast to the more general theories of OCD described earlier, some theorists have posed more specific hypotheses to account for the pathology observed in certain OCD subtypes. For example, clinical observations led some investigators to hypothesize that memory deficits for actions underlie compulsive checking (e.g., Sher, Frost, & Otto, 1983). However, the results of experimental investigations of this hypothesis are equivocal. Some support for an action–memory deficit was found in nonclinical individuals with checking rituals (e.g., Rubenstein, Peynircioglu, Chambless, & Pigott, 1993; Sher et al., 1983). In contrast, a study using a clinical sample found that compared to nonpatients, OCD patients with checking rituals *better* recalled their fear-relevant actions (e.g., plugging in an iron, unsheathing a knife), but not fear-irrelevant actions (e.g., putting paper clips in a box; Constans, Foa, Franklin, & Mathews, 1995). From these data, it appears that checking is not motivated primarily by memory problems; hence, teaching mnemonic strategies to OCD patients with checking rituals is probably not the optimal clinical strategy; rather, having patients repeatedly confront the low-risk situations that provoke obsessional distress, while simultaneously refraining from checking behavior or mental reviewing of actions, is preferred.

TREATMENTS

Exposure and Ritual Prevention

The prognostic picture for OCD has improved dramatically since Victor Meyer (1966) first reported on two patients who responded well to a treatment that included prolonged exposure to obsessional cues and strict prevention of rituals. This procedure, known at the time as exposure and ritual prevention (EX/RP), was later found to be extremely successful in 10 of 15 cases and partly effective in the remainder. Patients treated with this regimen also appeared to maintain their treatment gains: At a 5-year follow-up only two of these patients had relapsed (Meyer & Levy, 1973; Meyer, Levy, & Schnurer, 1974).

As was the case with Meyer's program, current EX/RP treatments typically include both prolonged exposure to obsessional cues and procedures aimed at blocking rituals. Exposure exercises are often done in real-life settings (*in vivo*), for example, by asking the patient who fears accidentally causing a house fire by leaving the stove on, to leave the house without checking the burners. When patients report specific feared consequences of refraining from rituals, these fears may also be addressed via imaginal exposure. In fact, *in vivo* and imaginal exposure exercises are designed specifically to prompt obsessional distress. It is believed that repeated, prolonged exposure to feared thoughts and situations provides information that disconfirms mistaken associations and evaluations held by the patients and thereby promotes habituation (Foa & Kozak, 1986). Exposure is usually done gradually by confronting situations that provoke moderate distress before confronting more upsetting ones. Exposure homework is routinely assigned between sessions, and patients are also asked to refrain from rituals.

Since Meyer's (1966) initial positive report of the efficacy of EX/RP, many subsequent studies of EX/RP have indicated that most EX/RP treatment completers make and maintain clinically significant gains. Randomized controlled trials (RCTs) have indicated that EX/RP is superior to a variety of control treatments, including placebo medication (Marks, Stern, Mawson, Cobb, & McDonald, 1980), relaxation (Fals-Stewart, Marks, & Schafer, 1993), and anxiety management training (Lindsay, Crino, & Andrews, 1997). Foa and Kozak's (1996) review of 12 outcome studies (*N* = 330) that reported treatment responder rates indicated that 83% of EX/RP treatment completers were classified as responders at posttreatment. In 16 studies reporting long-term outcome (*N* = 376; mean follow-up interval of 29 months), 76% were responders. Moreover, several studies have now indicated that these encouraging findings for EX/RP are not limited to highly selected RCT samples (Franklin, Abramowitz, Kozak, Levitt, & Foa, 2000; Rothbaum & Shahar, 2000; Valderhaug, Larsson, Gotestam, & Piacentini, 2006; Warren & Thomas, 2001).

In general, EX/RP has been found quite effective in ameliorating OCD symptoms and has produced great durability of gains following treatment discontinuation. In our review of the literature, it also was apparent that among the many variants of EX/RP treatment, some are relevant for outcome and others are not. We review the literature on the relative efficacy of the ingredients that comprise EX/RP to help clinicians decide which EX/RP components are most essential.

EX/RP Treatment Variables

EXPOSURE VERSUS RITUAL PREVENTION VERSUS EX/RP

To separate the effects of exposure and ritual prevention on OCD symptoms, Foa, Steketee, Grayson, Turner, and Latimer (1984) randomly assigned patients with washing rituals to treatment by exposure only (EX), ritual prevention only (RP), or their combination (EX/RP). Each treatment was conducted intensively (15 daily 2-hour sessions conducted over 3 weeks) and followed by a home visit. Patients in each condition were found to be improved at both posttreatment and follow-up, but EX/RP was superior to the single-component treatments on almost every symptom measure at both assessment points. In comparing EX and RP, patients who received EX reported lower anxiety when confronting feared contaminants than patients who had received RP, whereas the RP group reported greater decreases in urge to ritualize than did the EX patients. Thus, it appears that EX and RP affected different OCD symptoms. The findings from this study clearly suggest that EX and RP should be implemented concurrently; treatments that do not include both components yield inferior outcome. It is important to convey this information to patients, especially when they are experiencing difficulty either refraining from rituals or engaging effectively in exposure exercises during and between sessions.

IMPLEMENTATION OF RITUAL PREVENTION

Promoting abstinence from rituals during treatment is thought to be essential for successful treatment outcome, but the preferred method of RP has changed over the years. In Meyer's (1966) EX/RP treatment program, hospital staff physically prevented patients from performing rituals (e.g., turning off the water supply in a patient's room). However, physical intervention by staff or family members to prevent patients from ritualizing is no longer typical nor recommended. It is believed that such prevention techniques are too coercive to be an accepted practice today. Moreover, physical prevention by others may actually limit generalizability to nontherapy situations in which others are not present to intercede. Instead, instructions and encouragement to refrain from ritualizing and avoidance are now recommended. As noted earlier, although exposure in itself can reduce obsessional distress, it is not so effective in reducing compulsions. To maximize treatment effects, the patient needs to voluntarily refrain from ritualizing while engaging in systematic exposure exercises. The therapist should strongly emphasize the importance of refraining from rituals and help the patient with this difficult task by providing support, encouragement, and suggestions about alternatives to ritualizing.

USE OF IMAGINAL EXPOSURE

Treatment involving imaginal plus *in vivo* EX/RP was superior at follow-up to an *in vivo* EX/RP program that did not include imaginal exposure (Foa, Steketee, Turner, & Fischer, 1980; Steketee, Foa, & Grayson, 1982). However, a second study did not find that the addition of

imaginal exposure enhanced long-term efficacy compared to *in vivo* exposure only (De Araujo, Ito, Marks, & Deale, 1995). The treatment program in the former study differed from that of De Araujo and colleagues (1995) on several parameters (e.g., 90-minute vs. 30-minute imaginal exposures, respectively); thus, the source of these studies' inconsistencies cannot be identified.

In our clinical work, we have found imaginal exposure to be helpful for patients who report that disastrous consequences will result if they refrain from rituals. Because many of these consequences cannot be readily translated into *in vivo* exposure exercises (e.g., burning in hell), imaginal exposure allows the patient an opportunity to confront these feared thoughts. Also, the addition of imagery to *in vivo* exposure may circumvent the cognitive avoidance strategies used by patients who intentionally try not to consider the consequences of exposure while confronting feared situations *in vivo*. In summary, although imaginal exposure does not appear essential for immediate outcome, it may enhance long-term maintenance and be used as an adjunct to *in vivo* exercises for patients who fear disastrous consequences. For patients who only report extreme distress as a consequence of refraining from rituals and avoidance behaviors, imaginal exposure may not be needed.

GRADUAL VERSUS ABRUPT EXPOSURES

No differences in OCD symptom reduction were detected in a study comparing patients who confronted the most distressing situations from the start of therapy to those who confronted less distressing situations first, yet patients preferred the more gradual approach (Hodgson, Rachman, & Marks, 1972). Because patient motivation and agreement with treatment goals are core elements of successful EX/RP, situations of moderate difficulty are usually confronted first, followed by several intermediate steps, before the most distressing exposures are attempted. Thus, we emphasize that exposure will proceed at a pace that is acceptable to the patient, and that no exposure will ever be attempted without the patient's approval. At the same time, it is preferable to confront the highest item on the treatment hierarchy relatively early in treatment (e.g., within the first week of intensive treatment) to allow sufficient time to repeat these difficult exposures over the later sessions.

DURATION OF EXPOSURE

Duration of exposure was once believed to be important for outcome in that prolonged, continuous exposure was found more effective than short, interrupted exposure (Rabavilas, Boulougouris, & Perissaki, 1976). Indeed, reduction in anxiety (habituation) across sessions has been associated with improvement following exposure-based treatments for OCD and for PTSD (e.g., Jaycox, Foa, & Morral, 1998; Kozak, Foa, & Steketee, 1988; van Minnen & Hagenaars, 2002). However, several studies have not found a strong relationship between within-session habituation and fear and symptom reduction (Jaycox et al., 1998; Kozak et al., 1988; Mathews, Johnston, Shaw, & Gelder, 1974; Rowe & Craske, 1998). In an elaboration on emotional processing theory, Foa and colleagues (2006) found that the recent deemphasis on the relationship between within-session habituation and outcome is not critical to emotional processing theory, because the proposed mechanism underlying symptom reduction is the modification of the relevant erroneous associations through disconfirming information, not through habituation per se. In practical terms, this means patients should be instructed that although, optimally, they should persist with exposure until the anxiety is substantially reduced, the more important factor is repeating the same exposures, to promote reduction of associated anxiety over time. Patients with OCD might be particularly vulnerable to fears of ending exposures "too soon," hence, doing the treatment incorrectly, so this new instruction might help encourage patients to go about their business without ritualizing or avoiding, regardless of whether anxiety still lingers on from an exposure task.

FREQUENCY OF EXPOSURE SESSIONS

Optimal frequency of exposure sessions has yet to be established. Intensive exposure therapy programs that have achieved excellent results (e.g., Foa, Kozak, Steketee, & McCarthy, 1992) typically involve daily sessions over the course of approximately 1 month, but quite favorable outcomes have also been achieved with more widely spaced sessions (e.g., Abram-owitz, Foa, & Franklin, 2003; De Araujo et al., 1995; Franklin et al., 1998). A recent RCT in pediatric OCD found no difference between intensive and weekly treatment (Storch, Geffken, et al., in press). Clinically, we have found that less frequent sessions may be sufficient for highly motivated patients with mild to moderate OCD symptoms, who readily understand the importance of daily exposure homework. Patients with very severe symptoms or those who for various reasons cannot readily comply with EX/RP tasks between sessions, are typically offered intensive treatment.

THERAPIST-ASSISTED VERSUS SELF-EXPOSURE

Evaluations of the presence of a therapist during exposure have yielded inconsistent results. In one study, patients with OCD receiving therapist-assisted exposure were more improved immediately posttreatment than those receiving clomipramine and self-exposure, but this difference was not evident at follow-up (Marks et al., 1988). However, these results are difficult to interpret in light of the study's complex design. A second study using patients with OCD also indicated that therapist-assisted treatment was not superior to self-exposure at posttreatment or at follow-up (Emmelkamp & van Kraanen, 1977), but the number of patients in each condition was too small to render these findings conclusive. In contrast to the negative findings of Marks and colleagues (1988) and Emmelkamp and van Kraanen (1977), therapist presence yielded superior outcome of a single, 3-hour exposure session compared to self-exposure for persons with specific phobia (Ost, 1989). Because specific phobias are, on the whole, less disabling and easier to treat than OCD, one may surmise that therapist presence should also influence treatment outcome with OCD. Moreover, using meta-analytic procedures, Abramowitz (1996) found that therapist-controlled exposure was associated with greater improvement in OCD and GAD symptoms compared to self-controlled procedures. A recent study found comparable outcome for patients receiving EX/RP with therapist assistance and those who received teletherapy (Lovell et al., 2006), which further raises the question of whether therapist assistance is required for good outcome. In light of these inconsistent findings, no clear answer is available on the role of therapist assistance with exposure tasks in OCD treatment. However, we have found clinically that the presence of a therapist can be useful in helping patients remain engaged in exposures while anxiety is high, to avoid subtle rituals or avoidance behaviors during exposure (e.g., distraction, mental rituals), and to remain sufficiently motivated despite distress.

EX/RP versus Other Treatment Approaches

In this section we review the literature on the efficacy of standard individual EX/RP treatment versus other therapeutic approaches, including group treatment, family-based EX/RP treatment, cognitive therapy, and pharmacotherapy.

INDIVIDUAL VERSUS GROUP EX/RP

Intensive individual EX/RP, although effective, can pose practical obstacles such as high cost for treatment, and scheduling problems for patient and therapist alike. Additionally, because experts in EX/RP treatment are few and far between, patients may need to wait for long periods of time or travel substantial distances to be treated. Thus, some researchers have begun to examine the efficacy of more affordable and efficient treatment modalities. One such alternative is group treatment. Fals-Stewart and colleagues (1993) conducted a controlled study in which patients with OCD were randomly assigned to individual EX/RP, group EX/RP, or a psychosocial control condition (relaxation). Each of the active treatments was 12 weeks long, with sessions held twice weekly, and included daily exposure homework. Significant improvement in OCD symptoms was evident in both active treatments, with no differences detected between individual and group EX/RP immediately posttreatment or at 6-month follow-up. Profile analysis of OCD symptom ratings collected throughout treatment did indicate a faster reduction in symptoms for patients receiving individual treatment. These results offer evidence for the efficacy of group treatment. However, because patients were excluded from this study if they were diagnosed with *any* personality disorder or with comorbid depression, it may be that the sample was somewhat atypical. In addition, none of the participants had received previous OCD treatment, which is also unusual for this population and suggestive of a less symptomatic sample.

Thus, inferences about the broader OCD population merit caution until these results are replicated.

More recently, Barrett, Healy-Farrell, and March (2004) found that individual and group CBT were highly and similarly efficacious for children and adolescents with OCD relative to a wait-list control; this raises the possibility that group interventions might hold particular promise in the treatment of youth with OCD. Also in youth, Asbahr and colleagues (2005) found group CBT and sertraline comparable at posttreatment but less relapse in the former condition. More recently, another Australian research group found comparable outcomes for group treatment compared to individual treatment, both of which were superior to a waiting-list control (Anderson & Rees, 2007); not surprisingly, though, individual treatment was associated with more rapid response.

FAMILY INVOLVEMENT VERSUS STANDARD EX/RP TREATMENT

Emmelkamp, de Haan, and Hoogduin (1990) examined whether family involvement in treatment would enhance the efficacy of EX/RP for OCD. Patients who were married or living with a romantic partner were randomly assigned to receive EX/RP either with or without partner involvement in treatment. Results indicated that OCD symptoms were significantly lowered following treatment for both groups. No differences between the treatments emerged, and initial marital distress did not predict outcome. However, the reduction in anxiety/distress reported for the sample as a whole was modest (33%), which may have resulted from the relatively short treatment sessions and absence of *in vivo* exposure exercises in treatment sessions.

Mehta (1990) also examined the effect of family involvement on EX/RP treatment outcome. To adapt the treatment to serve the large numbers of young unmarried people seeking OCD treatment and the "joint family system" prevalent in India, Mehta used a family-based rather than spouse-based treatment approach. Patients who did not respond to previous pharmacotherapy were randomly assigned to receive treatment by systematic desensitization and EX/RP, either with or without family assistance. Sessions in both conditions were held twice per week for 12 weeks; response prevention was described as "gradual." In the family condition, a designated family member (parent, spouse, or adult child) assisted with homework assignments, supervised relaxation therapy, participated in response prevention, and was instructed to be supportive. On self-reported OCD symptoms, a greater improvement was found for the family-based intervention at posttreatment and 6-month follow-up. Although this study had methodological problems that complicate interpretation of findings (e.g., use of self-report OCD measures only, unclear description of treatment procedures), it offers some preliminary evidence that family involvement may be helpful in OCD treatment. Clinically, we routinely enlist the support of family members in EX/RP, providing psychoeducation about the illness and its consequences during the early stages of treatment planning, and advice and encouragement in managing the patient's request for assurances, avoidant behaviors, and violation of EX/RP rules between sessions. We also try to reduce family members' criticism of the patient and unconstructive arguing about OCD and related matters when these issues arise in the therapy.

Published randomized studies of CBT for OCD with youth have each included parents at least to some extent in treatment (Barrett et al., 2004; de Haan, Hoogduin, Buitelaar, & Keijsers, 1998; Pediatric OCD Treatment Study Team, 2004), and a direct comparison of CBT, with and without a family component, using an otherwise identical protocol has yet to be conducted in pediatric OCD. Research on whether family involvement enhances individual CBT outcomes in other anxiety disorders has generally yielded mixed findings, however, and a large, recently completed RCT indicated that both forms of treatment are both efficacious and essentially equivalent to one another (Bogels & Bodden, 2005). Higher family dysfunction was associated with poorer long-term outcome in a recent study (Barrett, Farrell, Dadds, & Boulter, 2005), and at this point it might be clinically prudent to include a more comprehensive family component when the family is very directly involved in the patient's rituals (e.g., reassurance seeking) or when family psychopathology threatens generalizability of treatment gains to a chaotic home environment. It also may be that greater family involvement in treatment is needed when the patient is very young (Freeman et al., 2003, 2007).

EX/RP VERSUS COGNITIVE THERAPIES

Increased interest in cognitive therapy (e.g., Beck, 1976; Ellis, 1962), coupled with dissatisfaction with formulations of treatment mediated by processes such as extinction (Stampfl & Levis, 1967) or habituation (Watts, 1973), prompted examination of the efficacy of cognitive procedures for anxiety disorders in general and for OCD in particular. A number of early studies found few differences between standard behavioral treatments and behavioral treatments enhanced with various cognitive approaches (e.g., Emmelkamp & Beens, 1991; Emmelkamp, Visser, & Hoekstra, 1988). Recent advances in cognitive conceptualizations of OCD have apparently yielded more efficacious and durable cognitive treatments. Freeston and colleagues (1997) found a cognitive-behavioral intervention efficacious compared to a wait-list control group for patients with "pure" obsessions. Several other recent studies (Cottraux et al., 2001; McLean et al., 2001; Vogel, Stiles, & Götestam, 2004; Whittal, Thordarson, & McLean, 2005) have suggested equivalent results for CBT and EX/RP, respectively, although some procedural overlap between the two conditions in these studies makes their findings difficult to interpret. In concert with studies attesting to the utility of cognitively oriented approaches for conditions that are quite similar to OCD, such as hypochondriasis (Barsky & Ahern, 2004; Warwick, Clark, Cobb, & Salkovskis, 1996), it does appear that cognitive therapies hold promise for the treatment of OCD and might be an efficacious potential alternative to EX/RP.

The question of whether cognitive therapy improves the efficacy of EX/RP is generally difficult to discern, because both exposure therapy and cognitive therapy are intended to modify mistaken cognitions. A randomized controlled study that compared "pure" forms of CT or EX/RP, with or without medication, found similar, yet somewhat attenuated outcomes relative to what might typically be expected from either treatment (van Balkom et al., 1998). Foa and Kozak (1986) argued that the disconfirmation of erroneous associations and beliefs is a crucial mechanism underlying the efficacy of exposure treatments, hence disputing discussions that mistaken cognitions from EX/RP might be expected to hamper outcome. For example, a patient and therapist sitting on the bathroom floor in a public restroom conducting an exposure to contaminated surfaces routinely discuss risk assessment, probability overestimation, and so forth, as the therapist helps the patient achieve the cognitive modification necessary for improvement. The practical issue of interest is how to maximize efficacy: Is informal discussion of cognitive distortions during the exposure exercises sufficient, or should the therapist engage in formal Socratic questioning of hypothesized distortions, such as inflated responsibility? Notably, in a meta-analytic review, cognitive therapies for OCD that included some form of exposure to feared stimuli were superior to those that did not, suggesting that exposure may be necessary to maximize outcomes (Abramowitz, Franklin, & Foa, 2002).

To further expand upon this point, Hiss, Foa, and Kozak (1994) investigated whether formal relapse prevention techniques following intensive EX/RP enhanced maintenance of gains. Notably, all discussions about cognitive factors typically included during the core treatment (e.g., discussion of lapse vs. relapse, posttreatment exposure instructions, themes of guilt and personal responsibility, and feared consequences) were removed. Patients received this modified EX/RP, followed by either a relapse prevention treatment or a psychosocial control treatment (associative therapy). All patients in both conditions were classified as responders at posttreatment (defined as 50% or greater reduction in OCD symptoms), with treatment gains better maintained in the relapse prevention group than in the associative therapy condition at 6-month follow-up. The percentages of responders at follow-up were 75% in the relapse prevention condition and 33% in associative therapy. The higher than usual observed relapse rate in the associative therapy may have resulted from the removal of cognitive techniques typically utilized during the core treatment, such as discussion of feared consequences. These findings, and those discussed earlier, further underscore our belief that blended treatment designed to provide patients the opportunity to disconfirm their erroneous cognitions makes the most sense clinically. Accordingly, our approach clearly incorporates informal cognitive procedures, and discussions of the outcome of exposures are geared toward challenging mistaken beliefs; this is accomplished in the context of a treatment approach that still emphasizes the importance of EX/RP in bringing about such changes.

Serotonergic Medications

Effectiveness of Medications

The use of serotonergic medications in the treatment of OCD has received a great deal of attention in the past 25 years. Of the tricyclic antidepressants, clomipramine (CMI) has been studied most extensively. In controlled trials, CMI has consistently been found to be superior to placebo (e.g., DeVeaugh-Geiss, Landau, & Katz, 1989). Similar results have been obtained with the selective serotonin reuptake inhibitors (SSRIs) fluoxetine, fluvoxamine, and sertraline (see Greist, Jefferson, Kobak, Katzelnick, & Serlin, 1995). Accordingly, each of these medications has been approved by the U.S. Food and Drug Administration (FDA) as treatments for adult OCD. On the whole, these studies suggest that up to 60% of patients show some response to treatment with SSRIs. However, even the average treatment gain achieved by treatment responders is moderate at best (Greist, 1990). In addition, amelioration of obsessive–compulsive symptoms is maintained only as long as the drug is continued: For example, in an early controlled, double-blind discontinuation study, 90% of patients relapsed within a few weeks after being withdrawn from CMI (Pato, Zohar-Kadouch, Zohar, & Murphy, 1988). More recent discontinuation studies with slower taper periods have not yielded such dramatic results, but they nevertheless converge to suggest that maintenance treatment is necessary to sustain achievements attained with pharmacotherapy alone for OCD (Dougherty, Rauch, & Jenike, 2002).

EX/RP versus Pharmacotherapy

Many controlled studies have indicated that serotonergic antidepressants are superior to placebo in ameliorating OCD symptoms (for a review, see Greist et al., 1995). However, only a few controlled studies have directly compared the relative or combined efficacy of antidepressant medications and EX/RP, and several studies that have made such a comparison included complex designs that make it difficult to draw confident conclusions about relative and combined efficacy (e.g., Marks et al., 1980, 1988).

Cottraux and colleagues (1990) compared fluvoxamine (FLV) with antiexposure instructions, FLV plus weekly EX/RP, and pill placebo (PBO) plus EX/RP, and found FLV + EX/RP and FLV + antiexposure instructions superior to PBO + EX/RP; there was a trend toward an advantage for combined treatment, but it failed to reach significance. Hohagen and colleagues (1998) compared EX/RP + FLV to EX/RP + PBO and found that both groups improved significantly and comparably on compulsions, but the patients who received EX/RP + FLV were significantly better at posttreatment on obsessions than those who received EX/RP + PBO. Subanalyses indicated that patients with secondary depression also fared better if they were receiving EX/RP + FLV.

The relative and combined efficacy of CMI and intensive EX/RP was examined in a multicenter, RCT conducted at our center (Penn) and at Columbia University. Findings with both treatment completer and intention-to-treat (ITT) data indicated at posttreatment that the active treatments were superior to placebo, EX/RP was superior to CMI, and the combination of the two treatments was not superior to EX/RP alone (Foa et al., 2005); relapse was more evident following treatment discontinuation in the CMI group than in either treatment that included intensive EX/RP (EX/RP, EX/RP + CMI; Simpson et al., 2004). However, the design used in the Penn–Columbia study may not have optimally promoted an additive effect for CMI, because the intensive portion of the EX/RP program was largely completed before patients reached their maximum dose of CMI. In addition, combined treatment effects may be more evident when intensive EX/RP is not used (Foa, Franklin, & Moser, 2002). Notably, an additive effect for combined treatment was found in a recent study in pediatric OCD at Penn, Duke, and Brown (Pediatric OCD Treatment Study Team, 2004), although examination of effect sizes by site indicated that the CBT monotherapy effect at Penn was very large, and no additive effect for combined treatment was found at this site.

In summary, although there is clear evidence that both pharmaceutical treatment with serotonergic medications and EX/RP treatments are effective for OCD, information about their relative and combined efficacy remains scarce, because most of the studies that examined these issues have been methodologically limited. Nevertheless, no study has found clear,

long-term superiority for combined pharmacotherapy plus EX/RP over EX/RP alone. The absence of conclusive findings notwithstanding, many experts continue to advocate combined procedures as the treatment of choice for OCD (e.g., Greist, 1992). In clinical practice, it is common to see patients in EX/RP treatment who are taking SSRIs concurrently. In uncontrolled examinations of EX/RP treatment outcome for adults (Franklin, Abramowitz, Bux, Zoellner, & Feeny, 2002) and youth (Franklin et al., 1998; Piacentini, Bergman, Jacobs, McCracken, & Kretchman, 2002) treated in OCD outpatient clinics, no posttreatment differences in OCD symptom severity were detected between patients who received EX/RP alone and those who received SSRI medication when receiving EX/RP. From these data we can surmise that concomitant pharmacotherapy is not required for every patient to benefit substantially from EX/RP, and that concomitant pharmacotherapy does not appear to inhibit EX/RP treatment response. More definitive conclusions about the effects of augmenting pharmacotherapy with EX/RP await a more carefully controlled examination, however.

ASSESSMENT

Following a diagnostic interview to ascertain the presence of OCD, it is advisable to quantify the severity of the OCD symptoms with one or more of the instruments described below. Quantification of symptom severity assists the therapist in evaluating how successful treatment was for a given patient. In our clinic, we use several assessment instruments. As in most OCD clinical research studies, however, the primary measure of OCD symptom severity used in our center is the Yale–Brown Obsessive–Compulsive Scale (Goodman et al., 1989a, 1989b).

Yale–Brown Obsessive–Compulsive Scale

The Yale–Brown Obsessive–Compulsive Scale (Y-BOCS; Goodman et al., 1989a, 1989b), a standardized, semistructured interview, takes approximately 30 minutes to complete. The Y-BOCS severity scale includes 10 items (five assess obsessions and five compulsions), each of which is rated on a 5-point scale ranging from 0 (*No symptoms*) to 4 (*Severe symptoms*). Assessors rate the time occupied by the obsessions and compulsions, the degree of interference with functioning, the level of distress, attempts to resist the symptoms, and level of control over the symptoms. The Y-BOCS has shown adequate interrater agreement, internal consistency, and validity (Goodman et al., 1989a, 1989b). The Y-BOCS served as the primary measure of outcome in most of the published OCD pharmacotherapy and CBT treatment studies conducted during the 1990s.

Self-Report Measures

Obsessive–Compulsive Inventory—Revised

The Obsessive–Compulsive Inventory—Revised (OCI-R; Foa, Huppert, et al., 2002) is an 18-item, self-report measure that assesses the distress associated with obsessions and compulsions. In addition to the total score, six separate subscale scores are calculated by adding the three items that comprise each subscale: Washing, Checking, Ordering, Obsessing, Hoarding, and Neutralizing. Foa, Huppert, and colleagues (2002) reported good internal consistency, test–retest reliability, and discriminant validity in clinical patients with OCD, PTSD, generalized social phobia, and non-anxious controls. The total score ranges from 0 to 72, and each subscale ranges from 0 to 12.

Other Self-Report Measures

A few self-report instruments for assessing OCD symptoms, such as the Leyton Obsessional Inventory (Kazarian, Evans, & LeFave, 1977) and the Lynfield Obsessional/Compulsive Questionnaire (Allen & Tune, 1975), are also available. These instruments are limited in that they assess only certain forms of obsessive–compulsive behavior and/or they include items that are unrelated to OCD symptoms. More recently, Storch, Murphy, and colleagues (in press) have developed the Children's Florida Obsessive–Compulsive Inventory, which is intended primarily for screening purposes.

INITIAL INTERVIEW

After a diagnosis of OCD has been established, and before actually beginning treatment, the therapist should schedule 4–6 hours of ap-

pointments with the patient. In these sessions, the therapist needs to accomplish three important tasks. First, the sessions are used to collect the information necessary to develop a treatment plan. Specifically, the therapist must first identify specific cues that cause the patient distress (threat cues), avoidance, rituals, and feared consequences. Second, the therapist should develop a good rapport with the patient, because the patient will engage in exposure exercises designed to elicit anxiety and distress during intensive EX/RP, and the lack of a good relationship between the therapist and the patient may compromise outcome. Third, the therapist needs to explore the patient's beliefs about OCD and the perceived consequences of refraining from rituals and avoidance, because this information guides the informal discussions of cognitive processes that take place throughout EX/RP.

Threat cues may be either (1) tangible objects in the environment or (2) thoughts, images, or impulses that the person experiences (for lack of better terms, we have labeled them "external cues" and "internal cues," respectively). Passive avoidance and ritualistic behavior (sometimes called "active avoidance") both serve to reduce the distress associated with the threat cues. Rituals may be further divided into overt or covert (mental) forms. It is essential that patients understand the difference between obsessions and mental compulsions, because obsessions are treated with systematic exposure and mental compulsions, with ritual preventions. During treatment, patients should be instructed to report any mental compulsions to the therapist, because performing such compulsions during exposure exercises attenuates the effects of these exercises in the same way that behavioral compulsions do.

External Fear Cues

Most individuals with OCD experience fear in reaction to specific environmental cues (objects, persons, or situations), but each patient will have his or her own idiosyncratic threat cues. For example, individuals who fear contamination from toilets may differ as to whether all toilets are feared or only those open to the public. One patient may fear only the toilet itself, whereas another patient also fears bathroom floors, doorknobs, and faucets. Similarly, two individuals may experience distress at the prospect of a fire burning down their home, but whereas one experiences the distress only when she is the last person to leave the house, the other experiences distress before going to bed at night when his children are present.

The therapist needs to gather specific information about cues that elicit the patient's distress to identify the basic sources of the fear. Identification of the basic source is important for planning the treatment program. Confronting the source of the fear is essential for successful behavioral treatment of OCD. Often, when such exposure does not take place during treatment, relapse will occur. For example, a patient who feared contamination by her hometown was treated with EX/RP 3,000 miles away from the town. Because of the distances involved, direct exposure to the town was impossible, so treatment comprised exposure to objects contaminated directly or indirectly by contact with the town. Although the patient habituated to the objects used in the exposure sessions, she continued to fear her hometown. Within 1 year after treatment, she had developed fears to new objects related to her hometown. Not until she engaged in repeated exposures to the town itself did she experience lasting improvement.

It is important that the therapist conduct a thorough investigation of objects, situations, and places that evoke obsessional distress for the patient at the time of presentation and at onset. Such information helps to identify the source of the distress. To facilitate communication with the patient about situations that evoke distress, a Subjective Units of Discomfort Scale (SUDS) ranging from 0 to 100 is introduced. Patients are asked to rate each situation with respect to the level of distress that they expect to experience upon exposure. The source of the distress is expected to be 100. The following dialogue between therapist and patient illustrates the process of gathering information about distressing situations.

THERAPIST: When do you get the urge to wash your hands?

PATIENT: In a lot of places. There are so many places.

THERAPIST: Are there any places where the urges are particularly strong?

PATIENT: Well when I am sitting in my living room, particularly near the fireplace. Also in the laundry room, which I never go to. Also, when I walk in the park.

THERAPIST: Let's talk about your living room. How upset are you when you are sitting next to your fireplace?

PATIENT: That's bad. I guess about a 90.

THERAPIST: Can you tell me what makes you so upset in your living room?

PATIENT: Well that is a long story . . . and I know it doesn't make sense.

THERAPIST: Go on. It's important that we understand what makes you uncomfortable and fearful in your living room.

PATIENT: About 2 years ago, I got up in the morning and went into the living room, and I saw a dead squirrel in the fireplace. I guess he got in through the chimney. So, I figured that if the squirrel was dead, he must have been sick. I know that a lot of squirrels have rabies, so I thought that if the squirrel died of rabies, then there are germs all over the chimney.

THERAPIST: Have you tried to have the chimney and the fireplace cleaned?

PATIENT: Yes, we did have a company come in and clean the whole area, but I'm not sure that they can clean away the germs.

THERAPIST: I understand. How about the laundry room, how upsetting is it to be in the laundry room?

PATIENT: That would be a 100; that's why I don't go in there.

THERAPIST: How did the laundry room become dangerous?

PATIENT: Oh, that's another story. Until a year ago, my children used to keep their guinea pigs in the laundry room. One day we found the female guinea pig dead. So I thought that it probably died of rabies too.

THERAPIST: Oh, I understand. So you are generally afraid that you will contract rabies if you come in contact with things that you think are contaminated with rabies germs. Is this true?

PATIENT: Exactly. That's why I don't like to walk in the woods or the park. You know those places have all kind of animals, and you can never tell where the germs might be.

It is clear from this conversation that it was not living rooms, laundry rooms, or parks per se that the patient feared. Rather, any situation or object that, in her mind, had some probability of being infested with rabies germs became a source of contamination. Some contamination-fearful patients, however, cannot specify feared consequences of coming into contact with stimuli they perceive to be contaminated. For these patients, the primary fear is that they will not be able to tolerate the extreme emotional distress generated by being contaminated. With such patients, it is also important to probe further to discern whether the patient has fears about the long-term health consequences of experiencing high and unremitting anxiety in response to stimuli that prompt obsessions.

Internal Fear Cues

Anxiety and distress may also be generated by images, impulses, or abstract thoughts that the individual finds disturbing, shameful, or disgusting. Examples of such cues include impulses to stab one's child, thoughts of one's spouse injured in an accident, or images of religious figures engaged in sexual activity. Clearly, internal threat cues may be produced by external situations, such as the sight of a knife triggering the impulse to stab one's child. Some patients may become distressed when they experience certain bodily sensations, such as minor pains triggering the fear of having cancer.

In many cases, patients may be reluctant to express their obsessive thoughts, because they are either ashamed of them or fear that expressing them will make the consequence more likely to occur. In these cases, the therapist needs to encourage the expression of these thoughts through direct questioning and a matter-of-fact attitude. Sometimes it helps to tell the patient that many people with and without OCD have unwanted thoughts (as many as 85% of normal individuals) (Rachman & DeSilva, 1978). It may also be helpful to remind the patient that talking about the obsessions will be a part of therapy; the evaluation session provides an opportunity to begin this process.

THERAPIST: So tell me, when is it that you feel the urge to count?

PATIENT: It seems like I'm always counting something, but it's mostly when I think about certain things.

THERAPIST: What kind of things?

PATIENT: I don't know. Bad things.

THERAPIST: Can you give me some examples of bad thoughts that will make you want to count?

PATIENT: (*brief silence*) I really prefer not to talk about them. It makes things worse.

THERAPIST: You mean it makes the counting worse?

PATIENT: Yes.

THERAPIST: All right, I know now that when you think or talk about certain bad things, you have an urge to count, but I still don't know what those bad things are. How about you tell me so that I can help you with them?

PATIENT: I'd really rather not. Can't we talk about something else?

THERAPIST: It is important that I know what the thoughts are to plan your treatment. I'll try to help you. Do the thoughts involve someone being hurt?

PATIENT: Yes.

THERAPIST: Do the thoughts involve only certain people getting hurt or could it be anyone?

PATIENT: Mostly my family.

THERAPIST: OK, what else can you tell me about the thoughts?

PATIENT: I really don't want to say any more.

THERAPIST: I know this is scary, but remember that facing your fears is what this treatment is all about.

PATIENT: OK. It's not always thoughts. Sometimes I see pictures in my mind, where my brother or my mom and dad are killed. I'm afraid when I talk about these thoughts and pictures that they really will die.

THERAPIST: A lot of people have thoughts that they don't like to have. Even people without OCD. Just because you have these thoughts, or talk about them, doesn't mean that bad things will actually happen or that you want them to come true.

It is important to reassure the patient that unpleasant thoughts occur often and to emphasize the distinction between thoughts and reality. Many patients with OCD have magical ideas in which the distinction between "thinking about" and "making things happen" is blurred, a process labeled by Salkovskis (1985) as "thought–action fusion" (TAF). It is important to point out to the patient that thoughts are different from actions. Also, many patients think that if negative thoughts enter their mind, then it means they wish the bad thing will happen. The therapist should assure the patient that thinking about bad things does not mean that one wants them to happen. These sorts of informal discussions of mistaken beliefs are an integral part of correct implementation of EX/RP. Such discussions should accompany the treatment planning process, and should be reiterated as needed during exposure exercises. It is, however, important that such discussions accompany EX/RP exercises rather than replace them.

Feared Consequences

Many individuals with OCD are afraid that something terrible will happen if they fail to perform their rituals. Such patients with washing rituals, for example, typically fear that they and/or someone else will become ill or disabled, or die as a result of being contaminated. Many patients with checking rituals fear that, because of their negligence, certain catastrophes will occur, such as their homes burning down or that they might kill someone while driving. Some patients have only a vague notion of what these negative consequence might be (e.g., "I don't know exactly what will happen, but I feel that if I don't count to seven, something bad will happen to my family"). Others do not fear catastrophes at all, but they cannot tolerate the emotional distress they experience if they do not perform rituals. Some fear that unless they ritualize, anxiety will increase continually, until they have a nervous breakdown. Data from the DSM-IV field trial indicated that approximately two-thirds of patients with OCD could clearly identify consequences other than emotional distress that would follow from refraining from rituals, whereas the remainder could report no such consequences (Foa et al., 1995).

It is important to identify the specific details of the patient's feared consequences to plan an effective exposure program. For example, the content of the imaginal exposure of a patient who checks while driving for fear of having hit a pedestrian and being sent to jail differs from that of a patient who fears that hitting a pedestrian will result in punishment by God. Similarly, patients who ritualistically place objects in a specific order may differ with respect to

their feared catastrophes. Some perform the ritual to prevent catastrophic consequences (e.g., death of parents), whereas others do so only to reduce distress elicited by disordered objects. The former would benefit from treatment that includes both imaginal and *in vivo* exposure, whereas the latter is likely to profit from *in vivo* exposure alone.

Strength of Belief

Clinical observations have led to suggestions that individuals with OCD who have poor insight do not respond well to exposure and response prevention, although two later studies failed to find a linear relationship between strength of belief in feared catastrophes and improvement following exposure and response prevention (Foa et al., 1999; Lelliott, Noshirvani, Basoglu, Marks, & Monteiro, 1988). Two issues need to be considered in evaluating these collective findings. First, the reliability and validity of the strength of belief measures used in previous studies are unknown. Second, the relationship between overvalued ideation and treatment outcome may not be linear. Clinical observation suggests that only patients who express extreme belief in their obsessional ideation show poor outcome. Indeed, Foa and colleagues (1999) found that only extremely strong belief (fixed belief) was associated with attenuated outcome. Such patients may appear delusional when discussing their feared catastrophes. We hypothesize that the effect of fixed belief on outcome may be mediated by treatment compliance: Patients who are convinced that feared disasters will ensue if they engaged in prescribed exercises probably will not complete the tasks as assigned.

When assessing the strength of belief, it is important to remember that a patient's insight into the senselessness of his or her belief often fluctuates. Some patients readily acknowledge that their obsessional beliefs are irrational, but they still cause marked distress. A few individuals firmly believe that their obsessions and compulsions are rational. In most patients, though, the strength of belief fluctuates across situations, making it difficult to ascertain the degree to which they believe the obsessions are irrational. The following example is an inquiry into the strength of a patient's belief in her obsessional fear of contracting acquired immune deficiency syndrome (AIDS).

THERAPIST: How likely is it that you will contract AIDS from using a public restroom?

PATIENT: I'm really terrified that I will get AIDS if I use a bathroom in a restaurant.

THERAPIST: I know that you are afraid of getting AIDS, but if you think logically, how likely do you think you are to get AIDS by sitting on a public toilet?

PATIENT: I think I will get AIDS if I use a public toilet.

THERAPIST: So do you mean to say that there is a 100% chance of you getting AIDS if you sit on a public toilet once?

PATIENT: Well, I don't know about once, but if I did it again and again I would.

THERAPIST: What about other people? Will they get AIDS if they use a public toilet?

PATIENT: I guess so. I'm not sure.

THERAPIST: Since most people use public bathrooms, almost everyone should have AIDS by now. How do you explain the fact that a relatively small number of people have AIDS?

PATIENT: Maybe not everybody is as susceptible to AIDS as I am.

THERAPIST: Do you think that you are more susceptible than other people?

PATIENT: I don't know for sure. Maybe the likelihood of my getting AIDS is only 50%.

Based on the interaction just described, the therapist concluded that the patient was not an "overvalued ideator"; thus, the prognosis for this patient is brighter than it would be if she continued strongly to hold her original belief. Accordingly, the implementation of EX/RP for this patient would follow the standard guidelines.

Avoidance and Rituals

To maximize treatment efficacy, all avoidance and ritualistic behaviors, even seemingly minor ones, should be prevented. Therefore, the therapist should gather complete information about all passive avoidance and rituals. When the therapist is in doubt as to whether a particular avoidance behavior is related to OCD, he or she might suggest an "experiment" in which the patient is exposed to the avoided situation. If the patient experiences anxiety or distress, the avoidance behavior should be prevented as part of treatment. Similarly, if it is unclear whether a given action constitutes a ritual, a response prevention "experiment" may be implemented. If refraining from performing the action evokes distress, the action is identified as a ritual and should be addressed in therapy.

Individuals with OCD, like those with specific phobias, often attempt to avoid anxiety-evoking situations. Most passive avoidance strategies are fairly obvious (e.g., not entering public rest rooms, not preparing meals, and not taking out the trash). However, the therapist also needs to be attentive to subtle forms of avoidance, such as carrying money in one's pockets to avoid opening a wallet, wearing slip-on shoes to avoid touching laces, and using drinking straws to avoid contact with a glass or a can. Patients with obsessive–compulsive checking rituals also engage in subtle avoidance behaviors that are important to explore, such as arranging their work schedules to ensure that they are rarely, if ever, the last person to leave the business, thus ensuring that the responsibility for checking the safe falls on a coworker.

Active rituals, such as passive avoidance, may be explicit (e.g., prolonged washing, repeated checks of the door, and ordering of objects) and/or subtle (e.g., wiping hands on pant legs, blinking, and thinking "good" thoughts). It is important that the therapist identify both explicit and subtle rituals, so they both may be addressed during treatment.

Although compulsive rituals are intended to reduce the distress associated with obsessions, patients sometimes report that the performance of these rituals is aversive in itself. For example, Ms. S, who was obsessed with the orderliness of objects on her shelves, found reordering the shelves aversive, because she was unable to find the "perfect" place for everything. Similarly, Mr. J, who felt contaminated by chemicals, found the act of decontaminating himself by repeated handwashing aversive, because he was unable to decide when his hands were sufficiently clean; therefore, he washed until his hands became raw. Rituals may also become aversive because of their intrusion into other aspects of the person's life. For example, Mr. J, who would take 2-hour-long showers to feel adequately clean, was reprimanded repeatedly by his supervisor for arriving late to work.

When certain compulsions become aversive, some patients decrease the time they spend performing the ritual by increasing avoidance behaviors, or by substituting other, less time-consuming rituals. For example, Ms. E, who was obsessed with fears of contamination by funeral-related objects (e.g., cemeteries and people returning from a funeral), responded with hours of showering and handwashing. She eventually retreated into her bedroom and avoided all contact with the outside world. Mr. J, described earlier, avoided taking a shower for days at a time, but between showers he wiped his hands compulsively and avoided touching his wife. In some cases, seemingly "new" rituals may develop during the course of treatment to function in the place of those previously identified and eliminated. For example, Mr. F, who was concerned about his hands becoming contaminated, successfully resisted the urge to wash his hands, but soon after response prevention was implemented, he started to rub his hands together vigorously to "decontaminate" them. When such a substitute ritual is identified, it also needs to be addressed in treatment with ritual prevention. Therapists must not only remain alert to such shifts in ritualistic behaviors but also alert patients to the possibility of such shifts.

History of Main Complaint and Treatment History

Many individuals with OCD are unable to give a detailed account of the onset of their symptoms, because the symptoms began subtly, many years ago. Nevertheless, therapists should attempt to collect as much information as possible about the onset and course of the disorder. Such information may provide clues about aspects of the fear network and variables associated with the maintenance of symptoms, and may help to anticipate difficulties that may arise during treatment (e.g., old obsessions or rituals that may resurface as more prominent ones diminish).

Many such individuals also have an extensive history of psychological and pharmacological treatments, and it is important to make a detailed inquiry about the outcome of previous treatments. If the patient has been treated with EX/RP, the therapist should assess whether the treatment was implemented appropriately and the patient was compliant with treatment demands. Knowledge that a patient experienced difficulty complying with response prevention instructions, or that previous therapy failed to provide adequate exposure experiences or re-

sponse prevention instructions, is important for designing the behavioral program. Other factors that may have prevented successful outcome or caused relapse, such as job stress, death in the family, or pregnancy, should be discussed. At the same time, a prior failed course of EX/RP should not necessarily be viewed as prognostic, especially if the patient recognizes why the therapy was less successful in the past. One of our patients, who had failed multiple trials of less intensive EX/RP, came to our center with the knowledge that his noncompliance with exposure exercises between weekly sessions greatly reduced the effects of treatment. He also noted that the slow progress he observed in these previous therapies demoralized him and caused further disengagement from the treatment. When offered a choice of daily versus twice-weekly sessions, he opted for the daily treatment, noting that the more intensive approach might decrease the chance of similar lapses. He has now successfully completed the intensive regimen.

In our clinic we have observed that a substantial majority of our outpatients have been treated, or are currently being treated, with serotonergic medications. Some seek EX/RP to augment the partial gains they have achieved with the medication. Others wish to discontinue the medication because it was ineffective, because of side effects, or because they do not want to continue taking medicine indefinitely. Assessment of the patient's treatment goals is necessary for planning his or her treatment program.

Social Functioning

Obsessive–compulsive symptoms may severely disrupt the daily functioning of patients. Therapists should assess the impact of OCD symptoms on the various areas of functioning. Where appropriate, this information should be used to design suitable exposure exercises. For example, Ms. D experienced difficulties completing assignments at work because she repeatedly checked each task. Treatment included exposures to performing tasks at work without checking. Even if the client is not currently working, exposures simulating work situations may be necessary if symptoms created difficulties in previous jobs.

OCD clearly has a deleterious effect on the intimate relationships of many patients. About half of married individuals seeking treatment for OCD experience marital distress (Emmelkamp et al., 1990; Riggs et al., 1992). Other family and social relationships may also suffer as a result of OCD symptoms. The impairment in social functioning may arise either because social contact is perceived as threatening (e.g., "I may spread germs to other people") or because so much of the patient's time and energy is invested in performing rituals and planning ways to avoid distressing situations. Again, information about the relation of social dysfunction to OCD symptoms may lead the therapist to include specific exposures aimed at ameliorating these social difficulties.

The assessment of social functioning should also include an evaluation of what role, if any, other people play in the patient's compulsive rituals. If the patient relies on others for reassurance or compliance with rituals (e.g., family members must remove their shoes before entering the house), the therapist should instruct family members how to respond appropriately when asked to participate in the patient's rituals. A careful analysis of the relationship is called for before specific instructions are given to significant others. Moreover, if family members tend to criticize the patient when obsessional distress arises, it is important to address these negative exchanges in treatment. We have often addressed this issue with a combination of empathic discussion of the frustration experienced by the family member and role playing of more effective responses.

Mood State

Although some patients with serious depression and OCD may benefit from behavioral therapy for OCD (Foa et al., 1992), research suggests that severe depression may limit the extent to which the OCD symptoms are reduced and the maintenance of those gains (e.g., Abramowitz et al., 2000). Therefore, it is important to assess the mood state of the patient prior to beginning behavioral therapy. Patients with severe depression should be treated with antidepressant medication or cognitive therapy to reduce the depressive symptoms prior to implementing behavioral therapy for the OCD. Treatment with serotonergic antidepressants may reduce OCD symptoms, as well as depression. Because the effects of such medication on OCD symptoms may not be evident until 3 months after treatment begins, the therapist needs to use his or her clinical judgment to decide whether to begin EX/RP when the depression decreases or to wait until the effects of the medication on OCD symptoms can be assessed.

Choice of Treatment

How should a therapist determine the most suitable treatment for a given patient? As discussed earlier, exposure and response prevention, as well as serotonergic medications, have demonstrated efficacy for OCD. The therapist and patient are faced with the choice of EX/RP, pharmacotherapy, or a combination of the two. Neither treatment is effective with all patients, and no consistent predictors of who will benefit most from which treatment modality have been identified. Therefore, unless the patient has been particularly successful or unsuccessful with some previous course of treatment, the decision should be based on factors such as availability of treatment, amount of time the patient is able or willing to invest in treatment, and his or her motivation and willingness to tolerate side effects.

The intensive treatment requires a considerable investment of time over a period of several weeks. Many patients are unable, or unwilling, to devote 4 to 5 hours a day to treatment. These patients should be advised to try pharmacological treatment, which does not require the same extensive time commitment. Recent investigations of the effects of a twice-weekly EX/RP regimen compared to intensive treatment suggested comparable outcomes at follow-up (Abramowitz et al., 2003; Storch, Geffken, et al., 2007); thus, in our center, we routinely offer either program to patients considering EX/RP. Some patients may be unwilling (sometimes expressed as "I can't do that") to experience the temporary discomfort caused by EX/RP. These patients, too, may be advised to try medications. The need to develop "readiness programs" designed to prepare such patients to accept EX/RP treatment is often cited in light of the relatively high refusal rate among patients offered EX/RP. Such programs may include testimonials from previously treated patients, cognitive strategies designed to help the patient calculate objective risks more accurately, psychoeducation about OCD and EX/RP, and a review of the outcome literature for various treatments (Tolin, Maltby, Diefenbach, Hannan, & Worhunsky, 2004). Manualizing such programs and investigating their effectiveness in increasing the acceptance rate and the efficacy of EX/RP for patients who enter such programs await controlled studies.

Patients who are concerned about the potential (or have already experienced) side effects of medications or their unknown long-term effects often prefer EX/RP. Other patients are concerned with the prospect of entering an "endless" treatment because, according to present knowledge, relapse occurs when medication is withdrawn (Pato et al., 1988; Thoren, Asberg, Chronholm, Journestedt, & Traskman, 1980). This concern is particularly relevant for women who plan to bear children and would need to withdraw from the medication during pregnancy. EX/RP should be recommended to these patients because its effects are more enduring.

As discussed earlier, the long-term effects of combining EX/RP and medication are unclear; therefore, it is premature to recommend treatment programs that combine the two therapies. However, some patients who present for treatment are already on antidepressant medication. Because these medications were found not to interfere with the effectiveness of EX/RP (Franklin et al., 2000), it is recommended that patients continue to take the medication if they have experienced some improvement in either obsessive–compulsive symptoms or depression. However, if the patient has not experienced improvement with medication, withdrawal of the medication before or during EX/RP should be considered. Special consideration should be given to patients with severe depression concurrent with their OCD. It is recommended that these patients be treated with antidepressants or with cognitive therapy for the depression prior to entering intensive EX/RP for the OCD, given recent findings of somewhat attenuated outcome for severely depressed patients (Abramowitz et al., 2000).

INTENSIVE EX/RP

The intensive treatment program comprises four phases: (1) information gathering, (2) intensive EX/RP, (3) a home visit, and (4) a maintenance and relapse prevention phase.

Information Gathering and Treatment Planning

The first stage of information gathering consists of a thorough diagnostic evaluation to determine that the patient's main psychopathology is OCD. The second step is to assess whether the patient is appropriate for EX/RP. We recommend that individuals who are abusing drugs or alcohol should be treated for the substance abuse prior to intensive treatment for OCD. Patients who have clear delusions and hallucinations are also poor candidates for intensive treatment. Individuals with severe MDD should be treated for depression before beginning treatment for OCD. The patient's motivation to comply with the demands of intensive treatment should be carefully evaluated. It is important to describe the treatment program in enough detail that the patient is not surprised when treatment begins. If the patient does not express strong motivation and commitment to treatment, it might be preferable to delay implementation of intensive treatment or to offer alternative treatments, such as medication. As noted earlier, a study of less intensive EX/RP for patients who appear otherwise motivated, yet cannot accommodate the daily regimen into their schedules, suggested comparable outcome compared to intensive treatment; future research with much larger samples is needed to determine whether patient factors predict differential outcome to either treatment schedule.

Once a patient is judged to be appropriate for intensive treatment, information gathering for treatment planning begins. This phase typically comprises 4–6 hours of contact with the patient over a period of 2–3 days. During this phase, the therapist collects information about the patient's obsessive–compulsive symptoms, general history, and the history of treatment for OCD, as described earlier. During these sessions, the therapist discusses the rationale for treatment, describes the program in detail, teaches patients to monitor their rituals, and develops a treatment plan.

First Information-Gathering Session

It is very important to discuss the rationale for treatment and to describe the treatment program in detail. The program requires that the patient abandon his or her obsessive–compulsive habits, therefore temporarily experiencing substantial discomfort. If patients do not understand why they are asked to suffer this short-term distress or are not convinced that treatment will work, they are unlikely to comply with treatment instructions. The treatment rationale is explained as follows:

"You have a set of habits that, as you know, are called obsessive–compulsive symptoms. These are habits of thinking, feeling, and acting that are extremely unpleasant, wasteful, and difficult to get rid of on your own. Usually, these habits involve thoughts, images, or impulses that habitually come to your mind, even though you don't want them. Along with these thoughts you have unwanted feelings of extreme distress or anxiety and strong urges to do something to reduce the distress. To try to get rid of the anxiety, people get into the habit of engaging in various special thoughts or actions, which we call 'rituals.'

"Unfortunately, as you know, the rituals do not work all that well, and the distress decreases for a short time only, then comes back again. Eventually, you may find yourself doing more and more ritualizing to try to reduce anxiety, but even then the relief is temporary and you have to do the ritual all over again. Gradually, you find yourself spending so much time and energy ritualizing—which does not work that well anyway—that other areas of your life are seriously disrupted.

"The treatment we are about to begin is called exposure and response prevention. It is designed to break two types of associations. The first association is between sensations of anxiety and the objects, situations, or thoughts that produce this distress. [The therapist uses information collected as examples, e.g., 'Every time you touch anything associated with urine you feel anxious, distressed, or contaminated.'] The second association we want to break is that between carrying out ritualistic behavior and the feeling of less anxiety or less distress. In other words, after you carry out [specifies the identified rituals], you temporarily feel less distress. Therefore, you continue to engage in this behavior frequently. The treatment we offer breaks the automatic bond between the feelings of discomfort/anxiety/contamination of [specifies the obsession] and your rituals. It will also train you not to ritualize when you are anxious."

After presenting the treatment rationale, the therapist should begin to collect information about the patient's OCD symptoms. The rationale for information gathering and a description of the treatment is presented as follows:

"In the next two sessions, I will ask you specific questions about the various situations and thoughts that generate discomfort or anxiety in you. We will order them according to the degree of distress they generate in you on a scale from 0 to 100, where 0 means *No anxiety* and 100 means *Maximum anxiety or panic*. The exposure treatment program involves confronting you with situations and thoughts that you avoid because they generate anxiety and urges to carry out ritualistic behavior. Why do we want to expose you to places and objects that will make you uncomfortable, situations that you have attempted to avoid even at much cost? We know that when people are exposed to situations that they fear, anxiety gradually declines. Through exposure, then, the association between anxiety and [specifies the obsession] weaken, because you are repeatedly exposed to these situations, so that the previously evoked anxiety decreases with time.

"For many people with OCD the obsessions occur within their imagination and rarely take place in reality. This makes it impossible to practice exposure by actually confronting those situations for prolonged periods. For example, if a person fears that her home will burn down, we certainly do not wish to have her house catch on fire in order to practice exposure. Similarly, someone who fears that he has run over a person who is now lying in the road cannot in reality be exposed to such a situation.

"If confrontation with the feared situation is necessary to reduce obsessions, how can you improve without directly confronting the situation? You can confront these fears through imagery, in which you visualize the circumstances that you fear will happen. In imagery practice, you create in your mind detailed pictures of the terrible consequences that you are afraid will occur if you do not engage in the ritualistic behavior. During prolonged exposure to these images, the distress level associated with them gradually decreases.

"When people with OCD encounter their feared situations or their obsessional thoughts, they become anxious or distressed and feel compelled to perform the ritualistic behavior as a way to reduce their distress. Exposure practices can cause this same distress and urge to ritualize. Usually, performing rituals strengthens the pattern of distress and rituals. Therefore in treatment, ritual prevention is practiced to break the habit of ritualizing. This requires that you stop ritualizing, even though you are still having urges to do so. By facing your fears without resorting to compulsions, you gradually become less anxious. Behavior therapists call this process 'habituation.' Therefore, during the 3 weeks of intensive exposure, the association between relief from anxiety and carrying out [specifies the patient's rituals] will become weaker, because you will not be allowed to engage in such behaviors; therefore, you will find out that your anxiety decreases even if you do not resort to these activities."

The initial information-gathering session is also used to begin training the patient to monitor his or her rituals accurately. Accurate reports of the frequency and duration of ritualistic behavior are important to evaluate the progress of treatment and to demonstrate the reality of changes to the patient. In some cases, the monitoring also serves an active role in treatment. Patients begin to recognize that rituals do not truly occur "all day long" and the act of monitoring the rituals may decrease their frequency and duration.

"It is very important for the treatment program that we have an accurate picture of the extent to which you engage in obsessive thinking and compulsive behavior. Having a clear picture of how much of your time is taken up by your problem will help us to monitor your progress and adjust the treatment program accordingly. Therefore, during this week while I am still collecting information to form a treatment program, I would like you to record your symptoms every day. It is not easy to report accurately on how much you engage in your obsessive–compulsive behavior; therefore, we will spend some time now and in the next session going over some rules for how to record your symptoms. Here are some monitoring forms on which you will record your thoughts and rituals."

The therapist should specify which ritual(s) the patient is to record, go over the instructions carefully with the patient, and practice filling out the form with the patient using an "imaginary day" of his or her life. The following rules are helpful in monitoring rituals:

1. Use your watch to monitor the time you spend on your rituals.
2. Do not guess the time of ritualizing; be exact.
3. Write the time immediately on your monitoring form.
4. Do not save the recording to the end of the day or the beginning of the next day.
5. Write a short sentence to describe the trigger for ritualizing.

Prior to beginning treatment, the patient identifies an individual (e.g., parent, spouse, or close friend) who can serve as a support person during the intensive treatment program. The patient is instructed to rely on this person for support during exposures, and the support person is asked to help monitor compliance with response prevention instructions. If the patient experiences difficulty resisting the urge to ritualize, then the support person is contacted for support. Because the support person is involved in the therapy, the therapist allocates time during the information-gathering phase to describe the treatment and discuss its rationale with him or her.

The therapist makes an effort to ensure that the support person and the patient mutually agree that the support person will offer constructive criticism and observations. In making these suggestions, the support person should be sensitive to any difficulties that have arisen in the past. For example, Mr. B, who served as his wife's primary source of reassurance, also criticized her severely when he "caught" her performing her handwashing ritual. To prevent these responses from hampering treatment, to help the husband supervise his wife's response prevention, the therapist spent time with the couple negotiating appropriate, uncritical responses to the wife's requests for reassurance.

The support person is in regular (at least twice weekly) contact with the therapist and is not only informed about the specific homework exposures that the patient has to accomplish but also relays his or her observations about the patient's behavior outside the therapy session. In addition, with the consent of the patient, the support person should contact the therapist if major treatment violations occur (e.g., refusing to do homework or engaging in ritualistic behavior).

Second Information-Gathering Session

At the beginning of the second information-gathering session, the therapist devotes time to the patient's self-monitoring form, which includes examining the descriptions of situations that trigger ritualistic behavior and offering constructive comments when necessary. The therapist reminds the patient to use short phrases or sentences to describe the trigger situations, assesses the accuracy of the patient's time estimates, and emphasizes the need for accurate measurements.

Generating a Treatment Plan

The bulk of the second information-gathering session is allotted to gathering detailed information about the patient's symptoms and, based on what is learned about the symptoms, developing a treatment with the patient. It is important to explain to the patient how the exposure exercises that comprise his or her treatment will reduce the OCD symptoms. For, example, the patient with religious obsessions is told that the imaginal exposure to burning in hell in excruciating detail is designed to reduce his obsessional distress when a less elaborate image of burning in hell comes into his mind. It is important that patients understand the rationale underlying the central concept in EX/RP, that confronting obsession-evoking stimuli during treatment increases their suffering in the short run but will reduce it in the long run. We often tell patients that the difficulties they experience during the first week of exposure sessions are likely to diminish with proper implementation of EX/RP.

Describing Homework

At the end of the second information-gathering session, the therapist describes the homework assignments included in the treatment program. The homework, which usually requires 2–3 hours, in addition to the 2-hour treatment session, consists of additional exposure exercises to be done between treatment sessions at the patient's home or elsewhere (e.g., a shopping mall or a relative's home). We suggest that the patient monitor his or her SUDS level every 10 minutes during the homework exposures. In some cases, when it is impossible for the patient to maintain an exposure for 45–60 minutes, the therapist works with the patient to develop a plan that allows the exposure to be prolonged. For example, instead of asking the patient to spend 45 minutes sitting in the restroom of a local restaurant, the therapist might suggest that he or she contaminate a handkerchief on the toilet seat and carry this "contamination rag" in a pocket.

Treatment Period

The treatment program at our center typically comprises fifteen 2-hour treatment sessions conducted daily for 3 weeks. Clinical observation suggests that massed sessions produce better results than do sessions spread out over time; therefore, we recommend a minimum of three sessions per week. Each session begins with a 10- to 15-minute discussion of homework assignments and the previous day's ritual monitoring. The next 90 minutes are divided into 45 minutes each of imaginal and *in vivo* exposure. The final 15 minutes are spent discussing the homework assignment for the following day. This format may be adjusted when necessary. For example, if an *in vivo* exposure requires that the therapist and patient travel to a local shopping mall to contaminate children's clothing, the entire session is devoted to this activity. Some patients have difficulty engaging emotionally in imaginal exposures (i.e., the images fail to elicit distress). In these cases, treatment should focus exclusively on *in vivo* exercises.

We recommend that the therapist discuss the plan for that session with the patient in the beginning of the session. Barring any unusual circumstances (e.g., patient's stated objection to proceeding with the planned exposure), it is important to limit these discussions to no more than 15 minutes. Patients with OCD are usually very fearful of engaging in exposure tasks, and elaborate discussion of the task at hand may serve as a form of avoidance of going ahead with the exposure. These preexposure discussions are also fertile ground for assurance seeking (i.e., the patient asking the therapist if he or she is certain that the proposed exercise is safe). The therapist should answer such questions carefully, avoiding either extreme (i.e., neither providing compulsive reassurance nor of conveying to the patient that the proposed exposure is objectively dangerous).

Imaginal exposure exercises are typically conducted prior to *in vivo* exercises in each session, often as a prelude to the scheduled *in vivo* exercise. During imaginal exposure the patient is seated in a comfortable chair and is given the following instructions:

"Today you will be imagining [describes scene]. I'll ask you to close your eyes so that you won't be distracted. Please try to picture this scene as fully and vividly as possible, not like your being told a story, but as if you were experiencing it now, right here. Every few minutes I will ask you to rate your anxiety level on a scale from 0 to 100. Please answer quickly and try not to leave the image."

The imaginal exposure sessions are audiotaped, and the patient is asked to repeat the exposure by listening to the tape as part of that day's homework.

The situations included in *in vivo* exposure vary greatly from patient to patient (particularly with patients with prominent checking rituals). Below are some examples of instructions that might be offered to patients during *in vivo* exposure exercises.

For patients with prominent washing rituals:

"Today, you will be touching [specifies item(s)]. This means that I will ask you to touch it with your whole hand, not just the fingers, and then to touch it to your face, hair, and clothing, all over yourself, so you feel that no part of you has avoided contamination. Then I'll ask you to sit and hold it and repeatedly touch it to your face, hair, and clothes during the rest of the session. I know that this is likely to make you upset, but remember the anxiety will eventually decrease. I also want you to go ahead and let yourself worry about the harm you are afraid will occur—for example, disease—since you won't he washing or cleaning after this exposure. I am sorry that this treatment has to be difficult and cause so much discomfort, but I'm sure you can do it. You'll find it gets easier as time goes on. OK, here it is, go ahead and touch it."

The therapist should give the patient the object to hold, ask him or her to touch it, and then ask the patient to touch the object or the "contaminated" hands directly to his or her face, hair, and clothing. Every 10 minutes the patient should be asked, "What is your level of anxiety or discomfort from 0 to 100 right now as you focus on what you're touching?" This can be shortened to "What is your SUDS?" once the patient understands the question.

For patients with prominent checking rituals:

"Now, I'd like you to [e.g., write out your checks to pay your monthly bills without looking at them after you've finished; just put them in the envelope and then we will mail them right away without checking even once after you've done it]. Then we will go on and do [e.g., drive on a bumpy road without looking in the rearview mirror] in the same way. While doing this, I would like you to worry about what harm might occur because you aren't checking your actions, but don't let the thoughts interfere with actually doing those activities."

Patients should be reminded of the specific instructions for response prevention on the first day of treatment and periodically during treatment. We have found that giving patients a printed copy of the rules for response prevention can help them to understand and remember the rules. If the rules as outlined for the patient do not adequately cover the type of ritual(s) the patient exhibits, the therapist should provide a written set of instructions modeled after these forms.

During the last few sessions of treatment, the patient should be introduced to rules of "normal" washing, cleaning, or checking. Response prevention requirements should be relaxed to enable the patient to return to what is considered a normal routine.

Home Visit

It is important to ensure that the patient's gains from the treatment program generalize to the home environment. Usually homework assignments function to produce this generalization, but we have found that visits by the therapist to the patient's home can be quite helpful, especially in cases where the patient is not able to return home daily during the intensive treatment phase (e.g., patients who are from out of town or are hospitalized). The home visit also offers the therapist and patient an opportunity to discuss guidelines for "normal" behavior. The therapist should discuss the plans for these visits with the patient and his or her family before the treatment ends. It is also important to note that, in some cases, the majority of the treatment sessions need to be conducted at the patients home, such as when treating a hoarder. The frequency of home visiting during the core treatment should be determined based on whether the patient's OCD symptoms are readily "transportable" to situations outside the home, or whether they are specific to the home. For patients with prominent washing rituals, with "safe" rooms and areas in their houses, contamination of these areas is imperative and also quite difficult; it is often advisable that the therapist assist directly with these home-based exposures when it is questionable whether the patient can contaminate these "sanctuaries" successfully on his or her own.

Typically, the home visit comprises 4-hour sessions held on each of 2 days at the end of the treatment program. The bulk of the time in these sessions is used to conduct additional exposures to obsessive stimuli in and around the patient's home or workplace. For example, the therapist might accompany the patient as he/ she contaminates objects around the house or at the local grocery store. Similarly, the patient might be asked to turn the stove on and off without checking and leave the house with the therapist. Most patients, particularly those who were able to return home during treatment, will report little or no discomfort when doing these exposures, because they represent repetition of homework assignments. In some cases, though, the therapist will discover areas that the patient has not contaminated, or some areas at home that continue to generate distress despite previous exposures. The home visit should focus on exposure to situations or objects that remain problematic.

Maintenance Period

In addition to prescribing continued self-exposure tasks to help the patient maintain therapy gains, the therapist may wish to schedule regular maintenance sessions. These sessions may be used to plan additional exposures, to refine guidelines for normal behavior, and to address issues that arise as the patient adjusts to life without OCD.

There is some evidence that patients benefit from continued contact with the therapist following the intensive therapy sessions. In one study, 12 weekly supportive therapy sessions (no exposure exercises) appeared to reduce the number of relapses in a sample of individuals with OCD treated with 3 weeks of intensive EX/RP (Foa et al., 1992). In another study, following the intensive treatment with 1 week of daily cognitive-behavioral sessions followed by eight brief (10-minute) weekly telephone contacts resulted in better long-term outcome than following intensive treatment with 1 week of treatment with free association (Hiss et al., 1994).

Therapeutic Setting

It is advisable for patients to remain in their normal environments during intensive treatment. This is particularly important for patients whose fears are cued mainly by stimuli in their home environment. The hospital may be an artificially protected setting, particularly for patients with prominent checking rituals, who may not feel responsible for their surroundings and as a result do not experience their usual urges to check. If patients live too far away to commute for daily sessions, we recommend that they rent an apartment or hotel room near the clinic. When this is not possible, hospitalization should be considered. Hospitalization is recommended for patients deemed to be at risk for suicide or psychotic breakdown, and for those who need close supervision but lack a support system sufficient to aid them during treatment.

If a patient is employed and his or her OCD symptoms are work related, he or she should be encouraged to continue working, so that relevant exposures can he included in treatment. However, since treatment requires 5 to 6 hours per day, the patient may opt to work half-days during the intensive treatment.

When the patient's symptoms are unrelated to work, he or she may decide not to continue working during intensive treatment. Because of the time-consuming nature of the treatment, we often suggest that patients take some time off from work. If it is not possible for the patient to take 3 full weeks off from work, the therapist might suggest that the patient work half-days or take time off from work during the first and second weeks of the treatment program.

Therapist Variables

Intensive treatment with exposure to feared situations and response prevention of ritualistic behavior provoke considerable stress for patients. Their willingness to undergo such "torture" attests to their strong motivation to rid themselves of the OCD symptoms. The intensive treatment regimen requires that the therapist maintain a delicate balance between pressuring the patient to engage in the treatment and empathizing with his or her distress. Clinical observations and findings from a study by Rabavilas and colleagues (1979) suggest that a respectful, understanding, encouraging, explicit, and challenging therapist is more likely to achieve a successful outcome than a permissive, tolerant therapist. Notably, patients of well-supervised, nonexpert EX/RP therapists appear to fare well with EX/RP (Franklin, Abramowitz, Furr, Kalsy, & Riggs, 2003; Valderhaug et al., 2007).

During treatment, patients' behavior may range from extreme cooperation and willingness to participate in exposures to blatant manipulation and refusal to follow the therapist's instructions. An individual patient may fluctuate depending on what exposure is conducted during a particular session. To a great extent, the "art" of conducting behavioral therapy for OCD involves knowing when to push, when to confront, and when to be more flexible. Such decisions require that the therapist carefully observe the patient's reactions and make a judgment based on his or her experience. As much as possible, the therapist should display an attitude that counteracts the harshness of the treatment program, while maintaining the rules for therapy established at the beginning of the program. The therapist should assure the patient that he or she would not use force to implement exposure and that no exposure will be planned without the patient's consent. If the patient cannot trust that the therapist will adhere to these essential guidelines, the treatment is likely to be compromised. We also assure the patients that family members will be asked not to present unplanned exposures to the patient (e.g., taking out the garbage) without discussing it.

Patient Variables

A primary factor that influences a patient's potential for benefiting from intensive behavioral treatment is the level of his or her motivation.

Because EX/RP causes high distress, patients need to be highly motivated to undertake the treatment. Often the level of motivation is related to the severity of the patient's symptoms. When symptoms are sufficiently intolerable, patients are more likely to tolerate considerable discomfort for a short period to gain relief from their symptoms in the long run. Tolin and colleagues (2004) have also discussed the importance of motivational readiness in EX/RP (Tolin et al., 2004), and have suggested specifically how best to prepare patients for the often grueling treatment regimen.

Sometimes individuals are pressured into entering therapy by their families, and they agree to participate in treatment only to appease a spouse or a parent. These patients are unlikely to follow the therapist's instructions strictly; therefore, they are less likely to make lasting gains in therapy. In light of these observations, we do not recommend that patients enter into EX/RP if they are not committed to follow such instructions; alternative treatment strategies are typically recommended in such circumstances.

It is important that the therapist clearly explain to the patient that 1 month of therapy, albeit intensive, is unlikely to eliminate all OCD symptoms. Rather, patients should expect that their anxiety and the urges to ritualize will diminish and become more manageable. An expectation of becoming symptom free at the end of treatment may lead to disappointment and can potentiate relapse, because maintenance of treatment gains usually requires continued effort over time following the intensive treatment. Thus, in the initial interview we tell patients that we do not have a "cure" for OCD; rather, we have a treatment that is likely to help them substantially reduce their symptoms in both the short and the long run.

It is also important to explain to patients that EX/RP treatment is not a panacea for all of their psychological and interpersonal problems. This treatment is aimed specifically at reducing the patient's obsessions and urges to ritualize. Problems that existed prior to treatment (e.g., marital discord or depression) are likely to remain, although they may be somewhat alleviated after treatment.

As mentioned earlier, patients with severe depression and/or an extremely strong belief in the reality of the obsessive fear may not benefit from EX/RP. An additional factor that has been identified as a potential hindrance to the cognitive-behavioral and pharmacological treatment of OCD is concurrent schizotypal personality disorder (Jenike, Baer, Minichiello, Schwartz, & Carey, 1986). Although some questions have been raised about the method used to diagnose schizotypy (see Stanley, Turner, & Borden, 1990), therapists should be alerted to the probability that schizotypal patients may respond poorly to treatment for OCD.

CASE STUDY

In this section we demonstrate through verbatim material the process of gathering information relevant to treatment, planning the treatment program, and conducting exposure sessions.

Case Description

"June," a 26-year-old married woman who had just completed her bachelor's degree in nursing, sought treatment for a severe washing and cleaning problem. She was extremely agitated in the first interview and described herself as "crying a whole lot" during the previous 6 weeks. She arrived in the company of her husband of 6 months and her sister-in-law, whom she considered a good friend. Previous treatment by systematic desensitization, antidepressants, tranquilizers, and cognitive restructuring had proven ineffective. June had been unable to seek employment as a nurse due to her symptoms.

This information was collected at June's initial evaluation for participation in EX/RP treatment. After ascertaining the absence of psychosis, drug and alcohol abuse, and organic disorders, June was assigned a therapist.

Information Gathering

Current Symptoms

First, the therapist sought information from June about the obsessional content, including external and internal fear cues, and beliefs about consequences, and information about passive avoidance patterns and types of rituals. Because rituals are the most concrete symptom, it is often convenient to begin the inquiry by asking for a description of this behavior.

THERAPIST: I understand from Dr. F that you are having a lot of difficulty with washing and cleaning. Can you tell me more about the problem?

JUNE: I can't seem to control it at all recently. I wash too much. My showers are taking a long time, and my husband is very upset with me. He and my sister-in-law are trying to help, but I can't stop it. I'm upset all the time and I've been crying a whole lot lately (*on the verge of tears*). Nothing seems to help.

THERAPIST: I see. You look upset right now. Please try to explain what your washing has been like in the past few days, so I can understand. How much washing have you been doing?

JUNE: Much too much. My showers use up all the hot water. And I have to wash my hands, it seems like, all the time. I never feel clean enough.

THERAPIST: About how long does a shower take? How many minutes or hours would you say?

JUNE: About 45 minutes, I guess. I try to get out sooner. Sometimes I ask Kenny to make me stop.

THERAPIST: And how often do you take one?

JUNE: Usually only twice, once in the morning and once at night before bed, but sometimes, if I'm really upset about something, I could take an extra one.

THERAPIST: And what about washing your hands? How much time does that take?

JUNE: You mean how many times do I wash?

THERAPIST: How long does it take each time you wash your hands, and how often do you wash your hands in a day?

JUNE: Umm, maybe 20 times a day. It probably takes me five minutes each time, maybe more sometimes. I always have the feeling they're not really clean, like maybe I touched them to the side of the sink after I rinsed and then I think they're dirty again.

The therapist now had some basic information about the most prominent rituals. Some further questioning clarified whether other compulsions were also in evidence.

THERAPIST: Do you do anything else to make your self feel clean?

JUNE: Yes, I alcohol things. I wipe with alcohol, like the car seat before I sit down.

THERAPIST: Do you wipe yourself with alcohol?

JUNE: No, only things that I think are dirty.

THERAPIST: Can you tell me how much you do that?

JUNE: I use about a bottle of alcohol a week.

Here the therapist had to choose whether to inquire about what objects June cleans or to ask about possible additional rituals. The therapist chose to continue the inquiry about ritualistic actions, and to turn to the subject of "contaminants" as soon as the inquiry was completed.

THERAPIST: OK, can you think of any other things that you do to clean yourself, or other things around you that you feel are dirty?

JUNE: That's all I can think of right now.

THERAPIST: What about other kinds of what we call "compulsive" type of activities? Do you have to check or repeat things over and over?

JUNE: No, except when I wash, if I don't feel it's enough. Then I wash again.

THERAPIST: No other repetitive actions besides washing?

Since this patient did not appear to have multiple types of ritualistic behaviors, the therapist turned to the obsessional content. External cues are usually solicited first.

THERAPIST: What are the things that make you feel you want to wash? For instance, why do you wipe the car seat with alcohol?

JUNE: I think that maybe I got dog dirt on it when I got in from before, or Kenny might have.

THERAPIST: From your shoes?

JUNE: Yes, I also worry about the hem of my dress touching the seat. I've been worrying that my shoe could kick my skirt hem or when I step up a step, like to go in a building, the dress could touch the step.

THERAPIST: A dress like this? June was wearing a dress that came to just below her knee. [The likelihood that it could have touched a curb or sole of her shoe was very slim.]

JUNE: Yes.

THERAPIST: Has your skirt ever had dog dirt on it?

JUNE: I don't think so, but in my mind I think that maybe it could have gotten some on it. I suppose it would be hard for that to happen, wouldn't it?

Thoughts that highly improbable events might have occurred are common in OCD. Such distortions may be the result of intense anxiety. Doubts about "safety" often lead to requests for reassurance or to rituals. Reassuring June that her dress is unlikely to be soiled would have been countertherapeutic, because it perpetuates the neurotic fears. Rather, the therapist inquired further about the obsessional content.

THERAPIST: Is dog "dirt" the most upsetting thing that you worry about?

JUNE: Probably. Yes, I think so, but bathroom germs are pretty bad too.

THERAPIST: What sort of germs?

JUNE: From toilets. You know, when you go to the bathroom.

THERAPIST: Urine and feces?

JUNE: Yes, urine doesn't bother me as much as the other.

THERAPIST: Why?

JUNE: Because I learned in nursing school that it's almost sterile. I had a hard time in the course about microbiology, because it upset me to try to learn about bacteria and microorganisms. They make it sound like there are all kinds of germs everywhere that are real dangerous. I didn't learn it very well; I tried to avoid thinking about it.

June's concerns with both dog dirt and bathroom germs suggested that her fear structure includes apprehension about potential illness. The therapist questioned her to better understand the nature of the feared consequences of contamination.

THERAPIST: Are you afraid of diseases that could come from feces?

JUNE: Yes, I guess so. The thing of it is, though, I know other people don't worry about it like I do. To them, you know, they just go to the bathroom and wash their hands and don't even think about it. But I can't get it out of my head that maybe I didn't get clean enough.

THERAPIST: If you didn't wash enough, would you get sick or would you cause someone else to get sick?

JUNE: Mostly I worry that I'll get sick, but sometimes I worry about Kenny too.

THERAPIST: Do you worry about a particular kind of disease?

JUNE: I'm not sure. Some kind of illness.

It is not uncommon for patients who fear harm that may ensue from not ritualizing to be unable to identify a specific feared consequence. Patients with prominent checking rituals often fear they will forget or throw out something important, but they do not always know exactly what this will be. Repeaters may fear that something bad will happen to a loved one but often cannot specify what particular disaster will befall them. However, many individuals with OCD do fear specific consequences (e.g., blindness or leukemia). At this point, the therapist may either choose to complete the inquiry about external threat cues or pursue the investigation about the feared consequences and the belief that such harm is indeed likely to occur. The latter course was selected here.

THERAPIST: Let's say that you did actually touch dog feces or human feces, and you weren't aware of it, so you didn't wash to remove it. What is the likelihood that you or Kenny would really get seriously ill?

JUNE: Well, I feel like it really could happen.

THERAPIST: I understand that when it happens and you become very distressed, it feels like you will actually become sick, but if I ask you to judge objectively, right now, how likely is it that you will get sick from touching feces and not washing? For example, if you were to touch feces 10 times, how many times would you get sick?

JUNE: Oh, I know it's pretty unlikely, but sometimes it seems so real.

THERAPIST: Can you put a number on it? What's the percent chance that if you touched a small amount of feces and didn't wash that you'd get sick?

JUNE: I'd say low, less than 25%.

THERAPIST: That means that one time in every four, you'd get sick.

JUNE: No, that's not right. I guess it's really less than 1%.

From this dialogue it is clear that June did not strongly believe that her feared disasters would actually occur, although her initial estimate of the likelihood was high. A person with poor insight regarding the senselessness of his or her OCD symptoms would have assigned higher probabilities (usually over 80%) and would insist on the accuracy of his or her estimate even in the face of persistent questioning. Note also that this exchange is an example of the informal cognitive restructuring accompanying EX/RP that we discussed earlier. The therapist may need to repeat this discussion during subsequent exposure sessions when June, highly anxious about confronting contaminants, readjusts her likelihood estimates when anxious. Strength of belief can change in a given patient but is stronger when the patient perceives threat.

THERAPIST: OK. Now, besides disease, what else could happen if you got feces on you?

JUNE: I suppose I'm also afraid of what other people might think if I got dog feces on my shoe or on my dress. Somebody would see it or smell it and think it was really disgusting, and I was a dirty person. I think I'm afraid they would think I'm not a good person.

The therapist then questioned June further about this feared consequence, inquiring about the possibility of others evaluating her character negatively because she had feces on her dress. The material regarding feared consequences was collected for later inclusion in the imaginal exposure scenes. To conclude the inquiry about the nature of the obsessions, the therapist further elucidated the external feared stimuli.

THERAPIST: Besides dog and human feces and toilets, what else can "contaminate" you? Is it OK if I use the word "contaminated" to describe how you feel if you handle these things?

JUNE: Yes, it's like I can feel it on my skin, even if I can't see it. Umm, I also get upset if I see "bird doo" on my car.

THERAPIST: Bird droppings? The whitish spots?

JUNE: Yeah, I have to hold my skirt close to me so that I don't touch any of these spots with my clothes.

THERAPIST: OK, bird doo, what else?

JUNE: Dead animals, like on the roadside. I feel like the germs, or whatever it is, get on the tires from the pavement and get on the car. Even if I don't run over it. Like it's spread around the street near it.

THERAPIST: What do you do if you see a dead animal?

JUNE: I swerve wide around it. Once I parked the car and as I got out, I saw this dead cat right behind the car. I had to wash all my clothes and take a shower right away. It was really a mess that day.

THERAPIST: It sounds like that was very difficult for you. Is there anything else besides dead animals that contaminates you?

JUNE: I can't think of any. There are lots of places I avoid now, but that's because of what we just talked about.

The therapist questions June further about other items that are likely to be contaminated, because of their potential relationship to the ones she has already noted.

THERAPIST: What about trash or garbage?

JUNE: Yeah, that bothers me. And I also avoid gutters on the street.

THERAPIST: What's in the gutter that upsets you?

JUNE: Dead animals, I guess. And then the rain spreads the germs down the street. Also rotten garbage. It's really dirty. Sometimes the gutters are really disgusting.

THERAPIST: Um hmm. Are you afraid you could get sick from dead animals and garbage?

JUNE: Yes, it's like the toilets or dog dirt.

To prepare for an exposure program in which objects are presented hierarchically with respect to their ability to provoke discomfort, June was asked to rank her major contaminants. Here she also provided information about avoidance behaviors associated with her contaminants.

THERAPIST: Now, let's make a list of the main things that upset you. I'm going to ask you how distressed you would be on a 0- to 100-point scale if you touched the thing I'll name. Zero indicates no distress at all and 100 means you'd be extremely upset, the most you've ever felt.

JUNE: OK.

THERAPIST: What if you touched dog dirt?

JUNE: And I could wash as much as I wanted?

THERAPIST: No, let's say you couldn't wash for a while.

JUNE: 100.

THERAPIST: A dead animal.

JUNE: Also 100.

THERAPIST: Bird doo on your car.

JUNE: That depends on whether it is wet or dry.

THERAPIST: Tell me for both.

JUNE: 100 wet and 95 dry.

THERAPIST: Street gutter.

JUNE: 95.

THERAPIST: Garbage in your sink at home.

JUNE: Not too bad. Only 50. But, the trash can outdoors would be 90.

THERAPIST: Why the difference?

JUNE: Because the inside of the trash can is dirty from lots of old garbage.

THERAPIST: I see. What about a public toilet seat?

JUNE: That's bad. 95.

THERAPIST: Car tires?

JUNE: Usually 90. But if I just passed a dead animal, they'd be 99.

THERAPIST: What about a doorknob to a public bath room?

JUNE: The outside knob is low, like 40. But the inside knob is 80, because people touch it right after they've used the bathroom, and I've seen that some don't wash their hands.

THERAPIST: I understand. How about grass in a park where dogs are around?

JUNE: If I did walk in the grass, it would be about 80 or 85, but I don't usually do it. I also have a lot of trouble on sidewalks. You know, the brown spots on the concrete. I guess most of it is just rust or other dirt, but I think maybe it could be dog dirt.

THERAPIST: How much does that bother you?

JUNE: To step on a brown spot? About 90. I always walk around them.

The therapist should continue in this manner until a list of 10–20 items is formed. More items may be necessary for patients with multiple obsessional fears or rituals. The items are ordered from low- to high-level fear in preparation for treatment by exposure. Items equivalent with regard to their level of disturbance are grouped together. Moreover, it is important to probe the rationale for one stimulus differing from another, because it provides further information about the patient's particular "OCD logic." This information is highly relevant for the construction of the exposure hierarchy and for the informal cognitive discussions about risk assessment, responsibility, and so forth.

Considerable information about avoidance patterns and rituals emerged from the previous interview about external threat cues. More details may be obtained by asking the patient to provide a step-by-step description of a typical day's activities from the time he/she awakens until he/she goes to sleep. Usually, patients are not entirely accurate when describing their compulsive behaviors during the interview, because, as one patient told us, they have not "thought of their OCD in that way before." Thus, the self-monitoring tasks assist patients in raising their awareness about the OCD patterns and provide the therapist with more accurate data about rituals and avoidant behaviors.

We were particularly concerned by June's bathroom routines, her shower, use of the toilet, handling of towels and dirty clothes, and dressing and putting on shoes. Additional information about avoidance patterns may be ascertained by inquiring about other routine activities, such as shopping, eating out, housecleaning, preparing meals, working, and so on. The following dialogue exemplifies the degree of detail desired.

THERAPIST: June, for us to plan your treatment carefully, I need to know what you avoid in your daily routine. Why don't you start by describing what you do first when you wake up.

JUNE: I go to use the bathroom first.

THERAPIST: Nightgown on or off?

JUNE: I take off my nightgown because I don't want it to touch the toilet. That way it's clean at night after I shower.

THERAPIST: Go on.

JUNE: I go to the toilet. I suppose I use a lot of toilet paper because I don't want to get anything on my hand. Then I have to shower after a bowel movement.

THERAPIST: How do you get ready to shower?

JUNE: I have to put a new towel on the rod near the shower. I don't like it to touch anything before I use it. Oh, and I put my slippers facing the door, near the shower, so I can put them on without stepping on the bathroom floor when I get out of the shower. Then I get into the shower.

THERAPIST: You said you shower for 45 minutes. Why does it take so long?

JUNE: I have to wash myself in a special order and I count how many times I wash each part. Like I wash my arm four times. That's why it takes so long.

THERAPIST: What is the order you use?

JUNE: First I wash my hands, then my face and hair and then I go from the top down.

THERAPIST: What about the genital and anal area? [This area should disturb this patient most, because she fears contamination from fecal "germs."]

JUNE: Oh yes, those are last, after my feet.

Such a detailed description helps the therapist to anticipate possible avoidance by the patient during treatment and to plan specific exposure instructions. Supervision of normal washing behavior at the end of treatment will address June's tendency to count and to order her washing. During the initial session of information gathering, June was instructed to self-monitor the frequency and duration of her compulsions.

THERAPIST: Between now and our next session, I'd like you to record all the washing and cleaning that you do, including wiping things with alcohol. You can use this form (*hands her a self-monitoring of rituals form*). Please write down every time you wash, how long you washed, what made you wash, and how anxious you were before you washed. This kind of record will help us identify any sources of contamination you've forgotten to mention, and we can also use it to measure your progress during treatment.

JUNE: Do you want me to write in each space for each half hour?

THERAPIST: No, only when you wash or use alcohol.

JUNE: OK.

History of Symptoms and Treatment History

After assessing the patient's current symptoms, the therapist sought information about the onset of the problem, with particular reference to the presence of specific stressors at the time and whether these stressors are still present.

THERAPIST: How long have you been washing like this?

JUNE: It started about 2 years ago in my first year of nursing school. It wasn't real bad right away. It started with the city. I had to go into the city to classes, and the city seemed real dirty.

THERAPIST: Did nursing have something to do with it?

JUNE: Maybe. I was under a lot of tension. I had to quit working as a secretary and it was pretty hard without an income and a lot of school bills. My mother and dad weren't much help. And then we started to learn all the sterilizing techniques, and I already told you about the course in microbiology.

THERAPIST: Did it gradually get worse?

JUNE: Mostly, but I did notice that it was a lot worse after a rotation on surgery, where I was really worried about germs contaminating the instruments. That's when I started to wash more than usual.

THERAPIST: Did you seek help at that time?

JUNE: I was already seeing Dr. W at the university, and he tried to help.

THERAPIST: You were already in treatment with him? For what reason?

JUNE: He was helping me with an eating problem. I had anorexia. I'd been seeing him for about a year when the washing started.

THERAPIST: Anorexia? Did treatment help?

JUNE: Yes. I was down to 85 pounds and I'm up around 105 now. He mostly asked me to increase my weight every week and he did "cognitive therapy," I think its called.

THERAPIST: I see. What about the washing problem?

JUNE: He tried the same type of therapy, but it didn't work for that. That's why I'm here. My sister-in-law heard about it, and Dr. W said I should come.

THERAPIST: What about drugs? Were you ever given medication for this problem?

JUNE: Yes, I tried Anafranil [clomipramine] for a while and it helped a little, but it made me dizzy and sleepy, so I decided to stop taking it. Also, I heard that you can't take the medication when you are pregnant, and Kenny and I want to have a baby soon. Before that, I took Xanax [alprazolam]; it calmed me down but didn't stop the washing.

THERAPIST: Have you tried any other treatments?

JUNE: Only for the anorexia. I went to another counseling center at the university for about a year, but that didn't really help at all.

June's history was unusual only in the relatively recent onset of her symptoms. Typically, patients in our clinic present a much longer duration of symptoms, with the mean around 8 years. Other centers in England and Holland report similar figures. June's treatment history of trying various psychotherapeutic and pharmacological treatments prior to seeking EX/RP was quite typical. Since previous failure with nonbehavioral treatments has not been found to influence outcome with exposure and response prevention, the clinician should not be discouraged by such a history. However, because of a possible skeptical attitude about the value of treatment, the therapist should provide the patient with a clear rationale for EX/RP treatment along the lines discussed earlier and demonstrated below.

THERAPIST: Before I continue to collect more information about your problem, let me tell you about our treatment.

JUNE: Well, Dr. F told me something about it, but I'm still not sure what this treatment is going to be like.

THERAPIST: The treatment is called exposure and ritual prevention. I'll be asking you to confront situations and things that frighten you or make you feel contaminated. We will do this gradually, working up to the hardest things. For example, we may begin with the outside door handles of bathrooms and work our way up to toilet seats and bird doo. We'll do this together, and I'll be there to help you. The sessions will last 1½ or 2 hours, and we'll meet every weekday. In addition, I'll assign you homework to do similar things between the therapy sessions.

JUNE: You mean I have to touch them, even dog dirt?

THERAPIST: Yes, to get over these kind of fears, people must learn to confront what they're afraid of and stay with it until the discomfort decreases.

JUNE: Even if I did, it would probably take me a year to get used to it.

THERAPIST: Remember, you didn't always feel like this about dog dirt. When you were younger, did you ever step in dog dirt and just wipe it off on the grass and go on playing?

JUNE: Yeah, I forget that. It seems such a long time ago. I used to not think twice about this stuff.

THERAPIST: To get you back to how you used to feel, we need to expose you directly to what you're afraid of. Now, there's a second part to treatment. I'm also going to ask you not to wash for 3 days at a stretch. No hand-washing or showering for 3 days. Then you can take a shower, but you will have to limit it to 10 minutes. After the shower, you will have to contaminate yourself again, then wait another 3 days for your next shower.

JUNE: I can't believe it! I'll never be able to do that. If I could, I wouldn't be here. How can I not wash? Every day I resolve to stop, but I always give in. You mean I wouldn't be able to wash after I use the bathroom or before I eat? Other people wash after they use the toilet. Why can't I just wash less, like normal people do?

THERAPIST: Other people don't have OCD. Remember for you, washing makes you feel less "contaminated" and less anxious. Right?

JUNE: Yes.

THERAPIST: If you wash, even briefly, whenever you feel "contaminated," you never get a chance to learn that the feeling of contamination would go away by itself without washing. If you are really very anxious, it might take a while, even several hours, be-

fore you feel better, but it will eventually happen. On the other hand, if you wash, even briefly, every few hours, it will reinforce your idea that you have to wash to feel better.

JUNE: But why 3 days? Couldn't I shower once a day like other people?

THERAPIST: For the same reason. You'd still feel relief, even if you waited 24 hours between washings. And that would strengthen your belief that you need to "decontaminate" by washing yourself. You must learn to use soap and water to feel clean and fresh but not to "decontaminate" yourself.

JUNE: I think I understand. I know I shower now to get the things I'm afraid of off my body. I used to shower just to get sweat and dirt off, and feel nice. I'm still not sure I could stand it though, not washing for that long.

THERAPIST: The treatment is very demanding. Before we start the treatment program you will need to make a commitment to yourself that even though you will feel very uncomfortable and even quite upset at times, you won't wash. I'll try to help you as much as I can by planning the treatment so you know what to expect each day and by supporting you whenever you need it. Someone will have to be available to help supervise and support you any time you need it. Between sessions you can always call me here or at home if a problem comes up. I know the treatment won't be easy for you, but I'm sure you can do it if you make up your mind.

At this point, a firm commitment should not be requested. Rather, the patient should be made aware of what will be required of him or her so that he or she can adjust to these expectations and plan activities during the treatment period accordingly. The patient should make the arrangements necessary to attend daily treatment sessions for 3 to 4 weeks. As we discussed earlier, two to three sessions per week may be sufficient for patients with less severe symptoms. It is important that the therapist not minimize the difficulty of the treatment regimen, so that the patient is prepared to struggle and enters treatment with a readiness to mobilize inner resources and emotional support from family and friends.

The history of the patient is usually taken in the first session. Because collecting histories of individuals with OCD does not differ from collecting histories of other psychiatric patients, details are not provided here.

Treatment Planning

The therapist began the second session by briefly reviewing the patient's self-monitoring of rituals form. The remainder of the session was devoted to developing a treatment plan.

THERAPIST: OK, now I want to discuss our plan for each day during the first week of therapy. We need to expose you both in imagination and in reality to the things that bother you, which we talked about in our first sessions. As I said already we'll also limit your washing. The scenes you imagine will focus on the harm that you fear will occur if you do not wash. The actual exposures will focus on confronting the things that contaminate you. Restricting your washing will teach you how to live without rituals. In imaginal exposure, you will picture yourself touching something you're afraid of, like toilet seats, and not washing and then becoming ill. We can have you imagine going to a doctor who can't figure out what's wrong and can't fix it. That's the sort of fear you have, right?

JUNE: Yes, that and Kenny getting sick, and it being my fault.

THERAPIST: OK, so in some scenes you'll be sick, and in others Kenny will get sick. Should I add that other people blame you for not being careful? Is this what you're afraid of?

JUNE: Yes, especially my mother.

THERAPIST: OK. We'll have her criticize you for not being careful enough. Can you think of anything else we should add to the image?

JUNE: No, that's about it.

THERAPIST: We can compose the scenes in detail after we plan the actual exposures. Let's review the list of things you avoid or are afraid to touch and make sure that we have listed them in the right order. Then we'll decide what to work on each day. OK?

JUNE: OK.

June reviewed the list, which included items such as trash cans, kitchen floor, bathroom floor, public hallway carpet, plant dirt, puddles, car tires, dried dog "dirt," and bird "doo." Changes were made as needed.

THERAPIST: Good. Now let's plan the treatment. On the first day we should start with things that you rated below a 60. That would include touching this carpet, doorknobs that are not inside bathrooms, books on my shelves, light switches, and stair railings. On the second day, we'll do the 60- to 70-level items, like faucets, bare floors, dirty laundry, and the things on Kenny's desk. [The therapist continued to detail Sessions 3 to 5, increasing the level of difficulty each day.] In the second week, we will repeat the worse situations like gutters, tires, public toilets, bird doo, and dog dirt, and we'll also find a dead animal to walk near and touch the street next to it.

On rare occasions, direct confrontation with a feared object (e.g., pesticides or other chemicals) may have some likelihood of producing actual harm. In such cases, the therapist's judgment should be exercised to find a middle ground between total avoidance and endangerment. With chemicals, for example, patients are exposed to small quantities that are objectively nonharmful. In June's case the therapist decided that direct contact with a dead animal was not called for, and that stepping on the animal's fur with her shoe and then touching the shoe sole constituted sufficient exposure. In general, the therapist must weigh the level of obsessional distress that will be evoked by a given exposure with the objective risks entailed in completing that exposure. Patients with OCD have difficulty assessing such risks realistically; thus, it is the responsibility of the therapist to evaluate whether exposure is warranted. For example, patients with fears of contracting HIV would certainly be highly distressed if asked to handle a dirty hypodermic needle found in a city gutter, but because exposure to such stimuli is objectively risky, they should not be included on the treatment hierarchy.

THERAPIST: How does this plan sound?

JUNE: The first week is OK, but I'm really scared about the second week. I'm not sure I'll be ready to do the bathrooms and dog dirt by then.

THERAPIST: Many people feel this way at the beginning, but by the end of the first week, you won't be as frightened as you are now about touching tires or public toilets. Remember, I will be here to help you, because it will probably be difficult in the beginning.

JUNE: Yes, I know it. I feel like I don't really have a choice anyhow. This washing is crazy and I'm disgusted with myself. I suppose I'm as ready as I'll ever be.

THERAPIST: Good. Now remember, I'll ask you to keep working on these things for 2 to 3 hours at home after each session, but you will already have done them with me, so I don't think it will be too hard. I take it that you talked to Kenny about assisting us with supervising, since I saw him out in the waiting room.

JUNE: Yes, he said that's fine. He wanted to know what he should do.

THERAPIST: Let's call him in. Did you talk to your sister-in-law about being available when Kenny is at work during the day?

JUNE: Yes, she was really good about it, but she couldn't come today because of the kids.

THERAPIST: If it's difficult for her to come, I could talk to her on the phone. Why don't you go get Kenny now?

Treatment

June was seen for 15 treatment sessions, held every weekday for 3 weeks. During the fourth week the therapist visited her twice at her home for 4 hours each time. During these visits, under the therapist's supervision, June contaminated her entire house and exposed herself to objects at home and in her neighborhood that provoked distress. Thereafter, once-weekly follow-up sessions were instituted to ensure maintenance of gains and to address any other issues of concern to her.

As discussed earlier, treatment begins with exposure to moderately difficult items on the hierarchy and progresses to the most disturbing ones by the beginning of the second week. The most distressing items are repeated during the remainder of the second and third weeks. The following sequence, which occurred on the sixth day of treatment, exemplifies this process.

THERAPIST: How was your weekend?

JUNE: Not that great. I suppose it was as good as I could expect. I took my shower Sunday

night and I was so nervous about finishing in time I don't even know if I washed right.

THERAPIST: Most people feel the same way. Remember though, you aren't supposed to wash "right," just to wash. Did Kenny time it?

JUNE: Yes, he called out the minutes like you said, "5, 7, 9," and then "stop."

THERAPIST: You stopped when he said to?

JUNE: Yes, but it still wasn't easy.

THERAPIST: I know. I'm really pleased that you were careful to follow the rules.

JUNE: I have pretty much decided that this is my chance to get better, so I'm trying my best.

THERAPIST: Good. I am glad you feel so positive. How was the homework?

JUNE: I touched the floor and the soles of my shoes and the cement. It is all written on the daily sheet there. On Saturday, I went to my sister's, so I could play with the kids like we said. They stepped on me when I lay on the floor and I tried to touch their bottoms when I held them. On Sunday, Kenny and I went to the park. I didn't sit in the grass but I did walk around and touched my shoes afterward.

THERAPIST: The soles?

JUNE: Yeah. We also went downtown and I threw some things in the trash cans and pushed them down, and tried to touch the sides. It's sort of hard because I felt conspicuous, but I did it anyway.

THERAPIST: That sounds really good. I'm glad to hear it. How about your doormat and going into the garden?

JUNE: I did the doormat and I stood in the garden, but I couldn't touch the dirt. The neighbor's dog always runs all over. I know I should have touched it, but I just couldn't get up the courage.

THERAPIST: Well, you did do many other things. Let's plan to go outside today and do it together, so it will be easier for you to walk in the garden when you go home.

JUNE: OK.

June was very compliant with the treatment regimen. Some patients occasionally lapse on response prevention, particularly during the first week of the treatment program. The therapist should reinforce the patient for partial compliance but emphasize the need to comply fully with treatment instructions. With regard to exposure homework, it is not uncommon for patients to neglect completing some assignments. Again, they should be reinforced for what they have achieved and encouraged to complete all of the assignments.

THERAPIST: How are you and Kenny doing?

JUNE: He got mad on Sunday night after the shower because I started to ask him how he showered and if I was clean enough. I think I nagged him too much, so he lost his temper. We just watched TV, and after a while we talked a bit and he sort of apologized for getting mad. But I understand; I ask too many questions. Otherwise, the rest of the weekend was OK.

THERAPIST: Well, it's unfortunate that Kenny got mad, but it's good that he didn't answer your questions. He's not supposed to reassure you about cleanliness.

JUNE: I think he has a hard time knowing when to answer me and when not to. I am not real sure either. Could you talk to him before Wednesday when I shower again?

THERAPIST: That's a good idea. I'll call him after we're done with today's session. Now, today we'll start with the scene about you driving your car to an appointment with me, and you get a flat tire and have to change it. The cars splash water in the puddle near you, and it lands on the car and on you. Then you notice a dead animal when you walk behind the car, and it's right behind you. You really feel contaminated. You walk to the gas station nearby to see if they can fix the tire and you have to urinate so badly that you have to use their rest room. They agree to fix the tire if you remove it and bring it to them, because otherwise they are too busy. Of course, that means you will have to handle the tire that is contaminated by the dead animal. We'll add some bird doo on the street and on the sidewalk too. Then, later you start to feel sick, and you feel like it's from the dead animal. Sound awful enough?

JUNE: Yeah. Ugh. That one is really bad. Do I have to? Never mind, I know the answer.

THERAPIST: OK. I want you to close your eyes now and imagine that you are driving your car on West Avenue.

Note that the therapist checked the patient's assignment from the previous day to verify that she completed it and did not engage in avoidance and rituals. This provided an opportunity to reinforce efforts at self-exposure. It is important to keep track of completion of homework, because patients do not always volunteer information about omissions. They will, however, admit failure to comply if directly asked and are likely to carry out the next assignment if reinforced adequately.

With regard to the conflict between June and Kenny, it is our experience that, like Kenny, most family members are quite willing to help. Difficulty may, however, arise when they are unable to help without becoming upset, thereby increasing the patient's tension. Providing them with an opportunity to ventilate their frustration by contacting the therapist, who also may coach them in alternative reactions, may reduce familial tension.

That same sessions also included imaginal exposure to do a scenario planned in advance. Since that scenario had already been discussed in detail with the patient, it posed no surprises for her. It is presented for up to 1 hour, or until a substantial decrease in anxiety is evident. Next, the patient is confronted *in vivo* with situations like those included in the fantasized scene.

THERAPIST: It's time to do the real thing now. I looked for a dead animal by the side of the road yesterday and I found one about a mile away. I think we should go there.

JUNE: Yuck, that's terrific. Just for me you had to find it.

THERAPIST: Today's our lucky day. You knew we were going to have to find one today anyhow. At least it's close.

JUNE: Great.

Humor is encouraged and can be quite helpful if the patient is capable of responding to it. At the same time, it is important that the therapist laugh *with* rather than *at* the patient. Patients and therapists often develop a shorthand lexicon for discussing OCD and its treatment that is specific to them and aimed at promoting compliance with treatment. For example, one patient–therapist pair began to discuss exposure homework as "swallowing the frog," based on a proverb that the patient introduced.

When the therapist asked the patient if she had, "swallowed the frog" that morning, it conveyed the difficulty of the exposure tasks she needed to do between sessions. It is important for the therapist to observe the patient's interpersonal style to determine whether such banter is likely to promote the therapeutic goals.

THERAPIST: (*outside the office*) There it is, behind the car. Let's go and touch the curb and street next to it. I don't think that you need to touch it directly, because it's a bit smelly, but I want you to step next to it, then touch the sole of your shoe.

JUNE: Yuck! It's really dead. It's gross!

THERAPIST: Yeah, it is a bit gross, but it's also just a dead cat if you think about it plainly. What harm can it cause?

JUNE: I don't know. Suppose I get germs on my hand?

THERAPIST: What sort of germs?

JUNE: Dead cat germs.

THERAPIST: What kind are they?

JUNE: I don't know. Just germs.

THERAPIST: Like the bathroom germs that we've already handled?

JUNE: Sort of. People don't go around touching dead cats.

THERAPIST: They also don't go running home to shower or alcohol the inside of their car. It's time to get over this. Now, come on over and I'll do it first. (*June follows.*) OK. Touch the curb and the street. Here's a stone you can carry with you and a piece of paper from under its tail. Go ahead, take it.

JUNE: (*looking quite uncomfortable*) Ugh!

THERAPIST: We'll both hold them. Now, touch it to your front and your skirt, and your face and hair. Like this. That's good. What's your anxiety level?

JUNE: Ugh! 99. I'd say 100, but it's just short of panic. If you weren't here, it'd be 100.

THERAPIST: You know from past experience that this will be much easier in a while. Just stay with it and we'll wait here. You're doing fine.

JUNE: (*A few minutes pass in which she looks very upset.*) Would you do this if it weren't for me?

THERAPIST: Yes, if this were my car and I

dropped my keys here, I'd just pick them up and go on.

JUNE: You wouldn't have to wash them?

THERAPIST: No. Dead animals aren't delightful, but they're part of the world we live in. What are the odds that we'll get ill from this?

JUNE: Very small, I guess. I feel a little bit better than at first. It's about 90 now.

THERAPIST: Good! Just stay with it now.

The session continued for another 45 minutes or until anxiety decreased substantially. During this period conversation focused generally on the feared situations and the patient's reaction to them. The therapist inquired about June's anxiety level approximately every 10 minutes. It is important to note that June and the therapist have engaged in conversation throughout the exposure task, discussing issues such as habituation, risk, responsibility, and long-term outcomes. At the same time it is imperative to refocus the patient on the exposure task at hand to ensure that he or she remains engaged with it. Thus, asking for SUDS ratings serves two purposes: It provides data about fear reduction, and it refocuses the patient on the exposure. However, if the informal discussion serves as a distractor, helping the patient "not think about" what he or she is doing, the therapist should limit such conversations.

THERAPIST: How do you feel now?

JUNE: Well, it is easier, but I sure don't feel great.

THERAPIST: Can you put a number on it?

JUNE: About 55 or 60, I'd say.

THERAPIST: You worked hard today. You must be tired. Let's stop now. I want you to take this stick and pebble with you so that you continue to be contaminated. You can keep them in your pocket and touch them frequently during the day. I want you to contaminate your office at work and your apartment with them. Touch them to everything around, including everything in the kitchen, chairs, your bed, and the clothes in your dresser. Oh, also, I'd like you to drive your car past this spot on your way to and from work. Can you do that?

JUNE: I suppose so. The trouble is going home with all of this dirt.

THERAPIST: Why don't you call Kenny and plan to get home after he does, so he can be around to help you. Remember, you can always call me if you have trouble.

JUNE: Yeah. That's a good idea. I'll just leave work after he does. See you tomorrow.

This scenario illustrates the process of *in vivo* exposure. The therapist answered clearly the questions raised without detouring from the essential purpose of the session, exposure to the feared contaminant. After the initial increase, for some patients the anxiety may begin to drop relatively quickly and may require longer for others. As noted previously, it is advisable to continue the exposure until the patient appears visibly more at ease and reports a substantial decrease in anxiety (40 or 50%).

After 10–15 sessions, the patient's reported anxiety level is expected to decrease considerably. At the 15th session, June reported a maximum discomfort of 70 SUDs (still somewhat high, although reduced from 99 SUDs), that lasted for a few minutes. Her minimal anxiety was 35 SUDs. Her average anxiety level during this session was 45 SUDs. Ideally, by the end of treatment the highest level should not exceed 50 SUDs and should drop below 20 SUDs at the end of the session. In June's case, more follow-up sessions were required because her anxiety was still quite high.

To facilitate a transition to normal washing and cleaning behavior, the therapist instituted a normal washing regimen during the third week of treatment. The patient was allowed one 10-minute shower daily and no more than five 30-second handwashes when there was visible dirt on her hands or when they were sticky.

When the therapist arrived for a home treatment session the next week, the following conversation ensued:

THERAPIST: How did it go over the weekend?

JUNE: Not too bad. But I got sort of upset Saturday. We went to a picnic and there were several piles of dog dirt around. I had on my flip-flops and I wanted to play volleyball. You can't in flip-flops, so I went barefoot.

THERAPIST: That's great! I'm glad to hear it.

JUNE: Yeah, but then I got really upset about going home and carrying it into the apartment. I did it. I walked all over barefoot and

with the flip-flops, but I worried about it for another whole day, till I talked to Kenny about my thoughts on Sunday around noon. I felt better when he said he wouldn't worry about it. It seems like I feel guilty or something, like the house isn't clean enough. But lately if he says it is clean, I've been able to take his word for it.

THERAPIST: Well, in time you'll be able to make this kind of judgment yourself. How about your washing and cleaning?

JUNE: It was all right. I washed for half a minute before I ate, because I was dusty from playing volleyball. I deliberately didn't wash when I got home, because I felt bad and I knew that if I did, it would be to "decontaminate" myself. I showered Saturday night and I did feel relieved, but I knew I should go and walk around barefoot and touch the floors I'd walked on. So I did that.

THERAPIST: That's great! It sounds like you handled it fine. I'm really pleased. You avoided washing when it would mean reducing feelings of contamination, and you exposed yourself when you felt concerned about germs. That's excellent. Now, let's go over the problem situations that still need work here at home. What things still disturb you?

JUNE: The basement. I haven't done much with the kitty litter box and old shoes that I threw down there a year ago because they got contaminated. The closet still has some contaminated clothes. And I still worry about the backyard some. Also the porch. Pigeons have been perching on the roof and there are droppings on the railing now, so I thought I'd wait until you came to do that.

THERAPIST: OK. Let's start low and work up. Which is easiest?

JUNE: The basement and closets.

THERAPIST: Fine, down we go.

Exposure to contaminants during the home visit is conducted in the same manner as that during treatment sessions. Typically, home sessions last longer, from 2 to 4 hours, until all "dirty" items are touched and "clean" places are contaminated. These visits should be repeated if the patient expresses considerable concern about his or her ability to adopt a permanent regimen of nonavoidance.

Follow-Up Sessions

June was seen weekly for 3 months, until she experienced a setback following the development of a new obsession. She became concerned about hitting a pedestrian while driving. Thoughts that she "might have hit someone" intruded, particularly after turning a corner or glancing in the mirror to change lanes. Once evoked, they persisted for several hours. To overcome this new problem, the therapist directed her to increase her driving and refrain from retracing her path or looking in the mirror to check for casualties. June was told that she could stop her car only if she knew for certain that she hit someone. Thoughts that it "might" have occurred were to be ignored. To reduce June's anxiety about having obsessions (e.g., "Oh, my God, here it is again. This is terrible"), she was advised to expect occasional recurrences of obsessive thoughts. The frequency of obsessions about hitting someone decreased from several each day to once weekly after 3 weeks of self-exposure; the associated anxiety diminished from 95 to 50 SUDs or less.

Of June's germ-related obsessions, only that of dog feces partially recurred. Fears of public bathrooms and dead animals remained low. The therapist felt that June's fear of dog feces had received insufficient attention during treatment. To address this return of fear, June was seen three times a week for 1-hour exposure sessions, in which she touched brown spots on the sidewalk and walked near, and eventually stepped on, dog feces. Homework included going to parks, walking on sidewalks without looking, stepping on dog feces, and stepping on the grass where she thought dogs had been. This treatment continued for 4 weeks and was reduced to twice a week for an additional 3 weeks. Thereafter, June came once weekly for another 6 weeks, during which the therapist assigned self-exposure and dealt with June's everyday concerns. News media coverage of herpes led to a brief concern about public toilets, but this dissipated within a few days.

In the dialogue below, the therapist reviewed with June her progress at a 9-month follow-up.

THERAPIST: I'd like to know how you feel compared to when you first came here 9 months ago.

JUNE: I'm definitely a lot better. But, I still have some bad days when I worry a lot about something, and I get down on myself. But when I remember how upset I was last summer and all that washing I did, it's really a whole lot better. Maybe about 80% better. I'm not ready to be a floor nurse yet, but the job I got after treatment is pretty good for now. Kenny and I are doing fine, except he's real sensitive if I bring up one of my fears. I wish he'd just listen and say "OK" or something instead of looking worried about me. It's like he's afraid I'm going to get upset again. It makes it hard for me to talk freely, but sometimes he does handle it fine. I really can't complain. He's been through a lot too, when I was really a mess last year and before that.

THERAPIST: I'm glad to hear you feel so much better. You look a lot more at ease. You laugh more now. I don't know if you recall, but you never did in the beginning.

JUNE: I remember.

THERAPIST: What's left now, the other 20%?

JUNE: Obsessions, I guess. I can still work on my fear of driving over someone. Mostly it lasts less than 15 minutes, but now and then it hangs on through an evening.

THERAPIST: How often?

JUNE: Once every week or two, I think. And I still have an urge to avoid walking on the grass in parks. Like I'm hyperalert. I do it pretty often, but I'm self-conscious.

THERAPIST: You mean you have to remind yourself not to avoid dog feces?

JUNE: Yeah. And I tend to see things in black and white, all good or all bad. I catch myself feeling guilty for dumb things like eating dessert after a full meal. I can stop, but it's like I'm out to punish myself or think badly about what I did. I have to watch out for it. Still, the thoughts are nothing like they used to be. I can have fun now. And work is pretty absorbing, so I can go whole days without getting down on myself for something. Will I always do that?

THERAPIST: Maybe to some extent. We know that you have a tendency to obsess. Most people who have had an obsessive–compulsive problem say that the rituals and urges to do them decrease more quickly than the obsessive ideas. You might have disturbing thoughts for a while, but you can expect them to become less frequent if you're careful not to attempt to control them through rituals or by avoiding things. Can you handle that?

JUNE: I suppose so. They're not a lot of fun, but I feel like I'm living a normal life again. I suppose everyone has some problems to deal with.

Rarely do patients report complete remission of all obsessions. It is unrealistic to lead a patient to expect that 4 weeks of treatment will result in a total absence of obsessions and rituals. Patients should expect some continued struggle with obsessions and urges to ritualize. Strategies for coping with such occasional difficulties should be rehearsed.

COMPLICATIONS DURING BEHAVIORAL TREATMENT

Obviously, difficulties may arise during implementation of EX/RP treatment for OCD. Several of these are described below and possible solutions are discussed.

Noncompliance with Response Prevention

Individuals with OCD often report engaging in rituals despite the response prevention instructions. In most cases these represent brief "slips" that the therapist addresses by reiterating the rationale for the treatment regimen and the need to follow the response prevention instructions strictly. The therapist also may offer ways the ritual might be "undone" (e.g., recontaminating or turning the stove on and off again).

Sometimes the patient's support person reports violations of response prevention to the therapist. The therapist should discuss the violations with the patient, emphasizing the fact that continued failure to comply with the response prevention instructions may result in treatment failure. The following is an example of how violations of response prevention may be presented to the patient.

"I understand from your father that on three occasions this weekend he saw you checking the front door lock five or six times before you left the house. As we agreed in the first session, he called to inform me about your checking. I am sure you remember that we agreed that you would check the doors only once, and that if you had a problem, you would discuss it with your father or me right away, so we could help you overcome your urge to ritualize. Will you explain to me what happened?"

If the patient acknowledges the slip and responds with a renewed agreement to follow instructions, the therapist need not pursue the issue further. However, if a second significant infraction of the response prevention instructions occurs, the therapist should again remind the patient of the therapy rules and the rationale for these rules, and "troubleshoot" with the patient how to successfully implement ritual prevention. During the course of this discussion, if it becomes evident that the patient is unwilling to consider these recommendations and remains committed to rituals and avoidance as a means to reduce obsessional distress, then the therapist may broach the subject of discontinuing treatment unless the patient is ready to comply.

"It seems that right now you aren't able to stop ritualizing. For treatment to be successful, it is essential that you *completely* stop your rituals. Every time that you relieve your discomfort by ritualizing, you prevent yourself from learning that anxiety would have declined eventually without rituals, and you don't permit your obsessional fears to be disconnected from distress and anxiety. Exposing you to feared situations without stopping your rituals won't be helpful. If you cannot follow the no-rituals rule quite strictly, then we ought to stop treatment now and wait until you are really prepared to follow through with all the requirements. It is very hard for people to resist the urge to ritualize, and it may be that you are just not ready yet and will feel more able to do so in the future. It is much better for us to stop treatment now than to continue under conditions where you are unlikely to benefit from treatment. That would only leave you feeling more hopeless about future prospects for improvement."

As discussed earlier, patients sometimes replace identified rituals with less obvious avoidance patterns. For example, a patient may use hand lotion to "decontaminate" the hands instead of the excessive washing that was done originally. If this occurs, the therapist should immediately instruct the patient to stop the new ritual. Other examples of replacement washing rituals include brushing off one's hands or blowing off "germs"; extensive checks are often replaced with quick glances. Direct questioning of the patient to solicit such information should proceed as follows:

"Now that you've stopped your washing rituals, do you find yourself doing other things to relieve your anxiety? For example, some people start to wipe their hands with paper towels or tissues as a substitute for washing with soap and water. Are you doing anything like this?"

If the answer is "yes," the therapist should identify these new behaviors as rituals and instruct the patient to resist engaging in them in the same manner as he or she resists other compulsions.

Continued Passive Avoidance

Patients who continue to avoid situations likely to evoke obsessional distress are also likely to experience attentuated outcome in EX/RP. For example, a patient may put "contaminated" clothing back in the closet as instructed, but in doing so he/she may ensure that the contaminated clothes do not touch clean garments. Such avoidance reflects an ambivalent attitude toward treatment and hinders habituation of anxiety to feared situations. Because such processes may hinder outcome, the presence of continued and frequent avoidance behavior calls for the therapist and patient to reevaluate whether the patient should continue treatment.

THERAPIST: Jim, let's make sure that you are doing your homework the right way. I know that you had a problem putting your dirty underwear in with your other dirty clothes. How are you doing with it now?

PATIENT: Well, I was afraid you might ask that. I still haven't mixed them up. I was too scared to do it.

THERAPIST: We discussed this several days ago and you were instructed to do it that night. It would have been better had you told me the next day that you weren't able to. What I'd like you to do for tomorrow is to bring in some dirty clothes. Bring in the underwear and the other clothes in separate bags, and

we will mix them here in the office. Are there any other things you have been avoiding that you haven't told me about?

PATIENT: I don't think so.

THERAPIST: I want you to pay careful attention to things you are doing, or not doing, and make a list of anything you are avoiding, particularly things that you are supposed to do for therapy. It is very important that you don't protect yourself by avoiding distressing situations, since if you don't face these situations, your obsessive–compulsive symptoms won't get better. Let's give it another try, but if you can't bring yourself to confront these problematic situations without these little avoidances, perhaps you would be better off delaying your treatment to a later time when you will be more ready to comply with the treatment program.

Arguments

Some individuals who carry out the required exposure without ritualizing may attempt to engage the therapist in arguments about the assignments. It is quite tempting to get involved in arguments with patients over what they will or will not do during treatment. To avoid this, it is important for the therapist and the patient to agree on some ground rules before the intensive program begins. Patients must agree to follow the treatment plan that they developed in conjunction with the therapist, and to expose themselves to the distressing situations without argument. New, feared situations that are discovered should be discussed, and a new exposure program should be developed and agreed to, before exposures to the new situations are carried out. If a patient balks at or attempts to alter a planned exposure, the therapist should acknowledge and empathize with the patient's the discomfort, inquire about the reasons for the hesitation, and encourage the patient to proceed in the following manner:

"I'm sorry to see that you are having so much trouble sitting on the floor. I know it's difficult and that you're frightened, but it won't do you any good if we delay the exposure for another day or let you skip it all together. You really need to touch the floor, so let's go ahead and do it now. We have agreed that today is the 'floor' day, and I wouldn't be doing you a favor if I allowed you to avoid it.

Remember, though, I am here to support you as much as I can when you become upset."

In some instances, difficulties may be overcome by first exposing the patient to similar items that generate a lower level of distress. For example, if a patient refuses to touch a toilet seat, then the therapist may ask him or her to first touch the bathroom floor or the door to the bathroom stall. Thereafter, the patient might touch the walls of the stall and the toilet handle before proceeding to the toilet seat itself.

Emotional Overload

Occasionally during treatment a patient will become overwhelmed by fear or another emotion that is not directly related to his or her OCD symptoms. For example, a patient may be upset by a recent event (e.g., the death of a relative) or by fears of facing future plans (e.g., living on one's own or getting a job). Implementing exposure exercises is inadvisable when the patient is extremely upset, because it is unlikely that the patient will adequately attend to the exposure stimulus; therefore, anxiety is unlikely to habituate. Instead, the therapist should discuss the distressing situation with the patient and proceed with exposure only when the patient is calmer. On rare occasions, exposure may be postponed altogether until the next day's session. If this becomes a repetitive pattern, it may be advisable to interrupt treatment until the crisis is over.

Nonanxious Reactions to Exposures

Occasionally patients respond to exposures with emotions other than anxiety or distress, such as anger or depression. Clinical observations suggest that anger often serves as a means for the patient to avoid the distress or anxiety that is the target of exposure. If this happens, the anger should be viewed as an avoidance. The therapist should refocus the patient on the anxiety-evoking aspects of the situation and point out to the patient that the anger only stands in the way of progress.

Sometimes during imaginal exposure, when patients are exposed to the feared consequences of their behaviors, they become depressed. Such depression and other emotional reactions may reduce the efficacy of treatment, and the therapist needs to help the patient to focus on the anxiety-evoking cues. This may be done by directing the content of the imaginal exposure away from the feared consequences and toward the external threat cues. In some cases, such redirection does not resolve the problem, and the patient continues to display a depressive reaction to the exposure. When this happens, alternative scenarios that do not elicit depression should be developed.

Emergent Fears and Rituals

As mentioned earlier, sometimes patients develop "new" fears or rituals during treatment. Often, the content of these new symptoms is closely related to the original fears and may be treated by extending to these fears the EX/RP instructions given earlier in treatment. For example, following the successful implementation of response prevention for his compulsive handwashing, Mr. F began to rub his hands together to decontaminate them. The therapist identified this as another ritual and instructed Mr. F to resist the urge to rub his hands together. Next, Mr. F began subtly to rub his fingers against the palms of his hands to cleanse his hands and to reduce anxiety. The therapist asked Mr. F to stop this ritual as he had the others and was again successful.

Some emergent fears may not be as clearly connected to the patient's original fears. For example, the fear that June developed of hitting someone while driving was not obviously related to her fears of contamination. Further assessment often results in the discovery of a conceptual link between the two reported fears. In June's case, her fear of being blamed for causing someone to become ill or die, and her concern about being thought of as a "bad person" because she killed someone, or because she smelled of dog feces, may have been the connection between her two identified fears. In such cases, it is important for the therapist to develop exposures that include cues for this more general fear. June's therapist might conduct imaginal exposures that include images of people criticizing June or blaming her for causing someone to die.

Negative Family Reactions

Because family members have typically experienced years of frustration with the patient's symptoms, it is not surprising that some are impatient, expecting treatment to progress smoothly and to result in total symptom remission. It is not uncommon for family members to become disappointed or angry when they perceive that the symptoms are not subsiding quickly enough. In such cases, the therapist should assure family members that occasional strong anxiety reactions are to be expected and do not reflect failure. The family should be encouraged to respond calmly and be supportive should the patient experience a burst of anxiety.

Often, families have developed patterns of behavior designed to reduce the patient's distress. Some family members may continue these patterns either in an attempt to protect the patient from upsetting situations or because it is difficult to break habits established over years of accommodating the patient's requests. For example, Mr. P, who was accustomed to entering his home through the basement, immediately removing his clothes, and showering for his wife's sake, was instructed to enter through the front door and toss his overcoat on the couch. Similarly, family members may find themselves continuing to perform a variety of household activities that they have come to regard as their responsibility because of the patient's wishes to avoid the distress that the activity caused. For instance, Mr. P was responsible for preparing all the family meals, because his wife was distressed by the possibility that she might inadvertently contaminate the food. Because such familiar patterns may hinder progress in treatment, the therapist should ask both the patient and family members about such habits and prescribe appropriate alternative behaviors that maximize the patient's exposure and minimize avoidance.

Functioning without Symptoms

At the end of treatment, many individuals with OCD find themselves left with a considerable void in their daily routines. The fact that they no longer need to allocate a large portion of their day to performing rituals leaves them wondering what to do. The therapist should be sensitive to these issues and aid in planning new social or occupational goals to be achieved following therapy. If needed, the therapist should conduct additional sessions or refer the patient to another therapist who will focus on adjustment-related issues. It may also be the case that behavioral treatments such as acceptance and commitment therapy (ACT) are directly applicable to this problem given the ex-

plicit focus on functioning; patients with OCD might be especially vulnerable to the belief that they cannot move forward successfully in their lives unless their obsessions are gone, and ACT is particularly well suited to address these kinds of problems. Preliminary evidence from a case series suggests the applicability of ACT to OCD (Twohig, Hayes, & Masuda, 2006); RCTs, direct comparisons to other established treatments, and further examination of the putative mechanisms that underlie symptom reduction are now needed.

Because they have spent years performing their rituals, patients may be unsure about what constitutes normal behavior. The therapist should offer guidelines for appropriate washing, checking, repeating, or ordering. If rituals are still present, the therapist needs to give instructions to continue the response prevention of some behaviors to ensure maintenance of treatment gains. A patient may also develop a fear that the OCD symptoms will return. The therapist should reassure the patient that a single washing of his or her hands does not signal the beginning of a relapse.

CONCLUSION

In this chapter we have reviewed the literature on OCD and its treatment, and provided verbatim dialogue from patient–therapist interactions to demonstrate how EX/RP is implemented. Our review illustrates clearly that much is already known about CBT and pharmacotherapy for OCD. In our clinical practice with adults, we are guided by the empirical research summarized in this chapter, although not all of our clinical decisions are unequivocally supported by empirical studies. For example, no controlled, direct comparison study has indicated that intensive EX/RP yields superior outcome to less intensive treatment, yet we typically provide intensive treatment to our adult patients with at least moderately severe OCD. Although our clinical experience suggests that weekly sessions are probably insufficient to produce meaningful gains in most adult patients with OCD, it has yet to be established whether two or three weekly sessions would yield results comparable to daily sessions both immediately after treatment and at follow-up. Future research should examine this important issue to establish a "dose–response" curve for EX/RP. Another important issue is how to best combine EX/RP with medication. Future research will allow us to identify the optimal treatment course for a particular patient.

Empirical results and clinical observations converge to indicate that psychosocial treatment for OCD must involve both exposure and ritual prevention instructions, and that failure to conduct exposures to the most anxiety-evoking situations is likely to compromise outcome. With respect to the therapist-assisted versus self-exposure issue, we routinely choose therapist-assisted exposure in our clinical practice. At present, eliminating therapist assistance with exposure exercises seems premature, because existing studies have methodological problems such as insufficient sample sizes. With respect to the role of cognitive interventions in the treatment of OCD, the EX/RP program described in this chapter is a "cognitive-behavioral" treatment in that it targets both cognitions and behaviors; however, we do not typically include formal cognitive restructuring. Future research needs to delineate which cognitive and behavioral procedures are most effective for correcting particular pathological emotions. Cognitive procedures may also be utilized in "readiness programs" designed to help patients who are highly ambivalent about EX/RP realize that the treatment is both tolerable and effective. Empirical research to date suggest that although antidepressant medications for OCD do not interfere with the efficacy of CBT, combination treatment is not necessarily more effective than EX/RP alone. However, the partial symptom reduction typically found in pharmacotherapy studies for OCD may render some patients more willing to tolerate the distress associated with EX/RP; thus, premedication may be helpful in promoting readiness in such cases.

What factors seem to enhance long-term efficacy of EX/RP for OCD? Studies suggest that patients with OCD who show great improvement immediately after CBT are more likely to retain their gains at follow-up than those who make only moderate posttreatment gains (e.g., Simpson et al., 2004). Thus, emphasis on procedures that are likely to lead to maximal short-term efficacy also serves to yield superior maintenance of gains. In our clinical experience, understanding of the treatment rationale, active engagement in exposure exercises, strict adherence to ritual prevention instructions, willingness to design and implement exposure exercises between sessions, and willingness to confront even the most difficult tasks on the fear hierarchy are all factors associated with positive treatment outcome. Thus, verbal reinforcement of patients when they accomplish these goals, and reinstruction when they do not, are important in promoting lasting improvement. In addition, relapse prevention techniques designed specifically for OCD have been found effective in promoting maintenance of gains at follow-up (Hiss et al., 1994). In clinical practice we begin discussing relapse prevention procedures long before treatment is completed, and focus on maintaining gains in the last few active treatment sessions. Some continuing contact with the treating clinician is also thought to be of benefit; thus, brief follow-up sessions are held in the first few months after the active treatment is completed, with contact as needed following the formal follow-up phase. As part of relapse prevention, we often ask our patients to plan EX/RP exercises for hypothetical obsessions they might encounter in the future (e.g., "If you became obsessed in 6 months that touching tree bark would result in your contracting a terrible illness, what exercises should you do?") to encourage them to problem-solve around OCD issues for themselves rather than relying on the therapist's instruction. We also emphasize that the occasional occurrence of obsessions should not be a cause of great alarm, provided that patients implement exposure and ritual prevention to combat these recurring obsessions and urges to ritualize. The patients who are accepting of this reality are often the ones most able to apply what they have learned in treatment, and this process enables them to keep their OCD symptoms under control long after treatment has terminated.

REFERENCES

Abramowitz, J. S., (1996). Variants of exposure and response prevention in the treatment of obsessive compulsive disorder: A meta-analysis. *Behavior Therapy*, 27, 583–600.

Abramowitz, J. S., & Foa, E. B. (2000). Does major depressive disorder influence outcome of exposure and response prevention for OCD? *Behavior Therapy*, 31, 795–800.

Abramowitz, J. S., Foa, E. B., & Franklin, M. E. (2003). Exposure and ritual prevention for obsessive–compulsive disorder: Effects of intensive versus twice-weekly sessions. *Journal of Consulting and Clinical Psychology*, 71, 394–398.

Abramowitz, J. S., Franklin, M. E., & Foa, E. B. (2002). Empirical status of cognitive-behavioral therapy for obsessive compulsive disorder: A meta-analytic review. *Romanian Journal of Cognitive and Behavior Psychotherapies, 2,* 89–104.

Abramowitz, J. S., Franklin, M. E., Street, G. P., Kozak, M. J., & Foa, E. B. (2000). Effects of comorbid depression on response to treatment for obsessive-compulsive disorder. *Behavior Therapy, 31,* 517–528.

Allen, J. J., & Tune, G. S. (1975). The Lynfield Obsessional/Compulsive Questionnaire. *Scottish Medical Journal, 20,* 21–24.

American Psychiatric Association. (1994). *Diagnostic and statistical manual of mental disorders* (4th ed.). Washington, DC: Author.

American Psychiatric Association. (2000). *Diagnostic and statistical manual of mental disorders* (4th ed., text rev.). Washington, DC: Author.

Angst, J. (1993). Comorbidity of anxiety, phobia, compulsion and depression. *International Clinical Psychopharmacology, 8*(Suppl. 1), 21–25.

Anderson, R. A., & Rees, C. S. (2007). Group versus individual cognitive-behavioural treatment for obsessive–compulsive disorder: A controlled trial. *Behaviour Research and Therapy, 45*(1), 123–137.

Antony, M. M., Downie, F., & Swinson, R. P. (1998). Diagnostic issues and epidemiology in obsessive–compulsive disorders. In R. P. Swinson, M. M. Antony, S. Rachman, & M. A. Richter (Eds.), *Obsessive–compulsive disorder: Theory, research and treatment* (pp. 3–32). New York: Guilford Press.

Asbahr, F. R., Castillo, A. R., Ito, L. M., Latorre, R. D., Moreira, M. N., & Lotufo-Neto, F. (2005). Group cognitive-behavioral therapy versus sertraline for the treatment of children and adolescents with obsessive–compulsive disorder. *Journal of the American Academy of Child and Adolescent Psychiatry, 44*(11), 1128–1136.

Barrett, P., Farrell, L., Dadds, M., & Boulter, N. (20050. Cognitive-behavioral family treatment of childhood obsessive–compulsive disorder: Long-term follow-up and predictors of outcome. *Journal of the American Academy of Child and Adolescent Psychiatry, 44,* 1005–1014.

Barrett, P., Healy-Farrell, L., & March, J. S. (2004). Cognitive-behavioral family treatment of childhood obsessive–compulsive disorder: A controlled trial. *Journal of the American Academy of Child and Adolescent Psychiatry, 43,* 46–62.

Barsky, A. J., & Ahern, D. (2004). Interventions for hypochondriasis in primary care: In reply. *Journal of the American Medical Association, 292*(1), 42–43.

Basoglu, M., Lax, T., Kasvikis, Y., & Marks, I. M. (1988). Predictors of improvement in obsessive–compulsive disorder. *Journal of Anxiety Disorders, 2,* 299–317.

Beck, A. T. (1976). *Cognitive therapy and the emotional disorders.* New York: International Universities Press.

Bellodi, L., Scuito, G., Diaferia, G., Ronchi, P., & Smeraldi, E. (1992). Psychiatric disorders in the families of patients with obsessive–compulsive disorder. *Psychiatry Research, 42*(2), 111–120.

Bogels, S. M., & Bodden, D. (2005, November). *Family versus child CBT for childhood anxiety disorders: Short and long-term results of a multicenter study.* In S. M. Bogels (Chair), Family-based prevention and treatment of childhood anxiety disorders. Symposium presented at the annual meeting of the Association for Behavioral and Cognitive Therapies, Washington, DC.

Brown, T., Campbell, L., Lehman, C., Grisham, J., & Mancill, R. (2001). Current and lifetime comorbidity of the DSM-IV anxiety and mood disorders in a large clinical sample. *Journal of Abnormal Psychology, 110*(4), 585–599.

Carr, A. T. (1974). Compulsive neurosis: A review of the literature. *Psychological Bulletin, 81,* 311–318.

Comings, D. E. (1990). *Tourette syndrome and human behavior.* Duarte, CA: Hope Press.

Constans, J. I., Foa, E. B., Franklin, M. E., & Mathews, A. (1995). Memory for actions in obsessive compulsives with checking rituals. *Behaviour Research and Therapy, 33,* 665–671.

Cottraux, J., Mollard, L., Bouvard, M., Marks, L., Sluys, M., Nury, A. M., et al. (1990). A controlled study of fluvoxamine and exposure in obsessive–compulsive disorder. *International Clinical Psychopharmacology, 5,* 17–30.

Cottraux, J., Note, I., Yao, S. N., Lafont, S., Note, B., Mollard, E., et al. (2001). A randomized controlled trial of cognitive therapy versus intensive behavior therapy in obsessive compulsive disorder. *Psychotherapy and Psychosomatics, 70*(6), 288–297.

De Araujo, L. A., Ito, L. M., Marks, I. M., & Deale, A. (1995). Does imaginal exposure to the consequences of not ritualising enhance live exposure for OCD?: A controlled study: I. Main outcome. *British Journal of Psychiatry, 167,* 65–70.

de Haan, E., Hoogduin, K. A., Buitelaar, J. K., & Keijsers, G. P. (1998). Behavior thearpy versus clomipramine for the treatment of obsessive–compulsive disorder. *Journal of the American Academy of Child and Adolescent Psychiatry, 37,* 1022–1029.

Denys, D., Tenney, N., van Megen, J. G., de Geus, F., & Westernberg, H. G. (20040. Axis I and II comorbidity in a large sample of patients with obsessive–compulsive disorder. *Journal of Affective Disorders, 80,* 155–162.

DeVeaugh-Geiss, J., Landau, P., & Katz, R. (1989). Treatment of OCD with clomipramine. *Psychiatric Annals, 19,* 97–101.

Diniz, J. B., Rosario-Campos, M. C., Shavitt, R. G., Curi, M., Hounie, A. G., Brotto, S. A., et al. (2004). Impact of age at onset and duration of illness on the expression of comorbidities in obsessive–compulsive disorder. *Journal of Clinical Psychiatry, 65,* 22–27.

Dollard, J., & Miller, N. L. (1950). *Personality and psychotherapy: An analysis in terms of learning, thinking and culture.* New York: McGraw-Hill.

Dougherty, D. D., Rauch, S. L., & Jenike, M. A. (2002). Pharmacological treatments for obsessive compulsive disorder. In P. E. Nathan & J. M. Gordon (Eds.), *A guide to treatments that work* (2nd ed., pp. 387–410). New York: Oxford University Press.

Eisen, J. L., Phillips, K. A., Baer, L., Beer, D. A., Atala, K. D., & Rasmussen, S. A. (1998). The Brown Assessment of Beliefs Scale: Reliability and validity. *American Journal of Psychiatry, 155,* 102–108.

Ellis, A. (1962). *Reason and emotion in psychotherapy.* New York: Lyle Stuart.

Emmelkamp, P. M. G., & Beens, H. (1991). Cognitive therapy with obsessive–compulsive disorder: A comparative evaluation. *Behaviour Research and Therapy, 29,* 293–300.

Emmelkamp, P. M. G., de Haan, E., & Hoogduin, C. A. L. (1990). Marital adjustment and obsessive–compulsive disorder. *British Journal of Psychiatry, 156,* 55–60.

Emmelkamp, P. M. G., & van Kraanen, J. (1977). Therapist-controlled exposure *in vivo:* A comparison with obsessive–compulsive patients. *Behaviour Research and Therapy, 15,* 491–495.

Emmelkamp, P. M. G., Visser, S., & Hoekstra, R. J. (1988). Cognitive therapy vs. exposure *in vivo* in the treatment of obsessive–compulsives. *Cognitive Therapy and Research, 12,* 103–114.

Fals-Stewart, W., Marks, A. P., & Schafer, J. (1993). A comparison of behavioral group therapy and individual behavior therapy in treating obsessive compulsive disorder. *Journal of Nervous and Mental Disease, 181,* 189–193.

Flament, M., Koby, E., Rapoport, J. L., Berg, C., Zahn, T., Cox, C., et al. (1990). Childhood obsessive compulsive disorder: A prospective follow-up study. *Journal of Child Psychology and Psychiatry, and Allied Disciplines, 31,* 363–380.

Flament, M., Whitaker, A., Rapoport, J. L., Davies, M., Berg, C., Kalikow, K., et al. (1988). Obsessive compulsive disorder in adolescence: An epidemiological study. *Journal of the American Academy of Child and Adolescent Psychiatry, 27,* 764–771.

Foa, E. B., Abramowitz, J. S., Franklin, M. E., & Kozak, M. J. (1999). Feared consequences, fixity of belief, and treatment outcome in patients with obsessive compulsive disorder. *Behavior Therapy, 30,* 717–724.

Foa, E. B., Franklin, M. E., & Moser, J. (2002). Context in the clinic: How well do CBT and medications work in combination? *Biological Psychiatry, 51,* 989–997.

Foa, E. B., Huppert, J. D., & Cahill, S. P. (2006). Emotional processing theory: An update. In B. O. Rothbaum (Ed.), *Pathological anxiety: Emotional processing in etiology and treatment* (pp. 3–24). New York: Guilford Press.

Foa, E. B., Huppert, J. D., Leiberg, S., Langner, R.,

Kichic, R., & Hajcak, G., et al. (2002). The Obsessive–Compulsive Inventory: Development and validation of a short version. *Psychological Assessment, 14*(4), 485–495.

Foa, E. B., & Kozak, M. J. (1985). Treatment of anxiety disorders: Implications for psychopathology. In A. H. Tuma & J. D. Maser (Eds.), *Anxiety and the anxiety disorders* (pp. 421–452). Hillsdale, NJ: Erlbaum.

Foa, E. B., & Kozak, M. J. (1986). Emotional processing of fear: Exposure to corrective information. *Psychological Bulletin, 99,* 20–35.

Foa, E. B., & Kozak, M. J. (1996). Psychological treatments for obsessive compulsive disorder. In M. R. Mavissakalian & R. P. Prien (Eds.), *Long-term treatments of anxiety disorders* (pp. 285–309). Washington, DC: American Psychiatric Press.

Foa, E. B., Kozak, M. J., Goodman, W. K., Hollander, E., Jenike, M. A., & Rasmussen, S. (1995). DSM-IV filed trial: Obsessive compulsive disorder. *American Journal of Psychiatry, 152,* 90–96.

Foa, E. B., Kozak, M. J., Steketee, G., & McCarthy, P. R. (1992). Treatment of depressive and obsessive–compulsive symptoms in OCD by imipramine and behavior therapy. *British Journal of Clinical Psychology, 31,* 279–292.

Foa, E. B., Liebowitz, M. R., Kozak, M. J., Davies, S. O., Campeas, R., Franklin, M. E., et al. (2005). Treatment of obsessive compulsive disorder by exposure and ritual prevention, clomipramine, and their combination: A randomized, placebo-controlled trial. *American Journal of Psychiatry, 162,* 151–161.

Foa, E. B., Steketee, G., Grayson, J. B., Turner, R. M., & Latimer, P. (1984). Deliberate exposure and blocking of obsessive–compulsive rituals: Immediate and long-term effects. *Behavior Therapy, 15,* 450–472.

Foa, E. B., Steketee, G., Turner, R. M., & Fischer, S. C. (1980). Effects of imaginal exposure to feared disasters in obsessive–compulsive checkers. *Behaviour Research and Therapy, 18,* 449–455.

Franklin, M. E., Abramowitz, J. S., Bux, D. A., Zoellner, L. A., & Feeny, N. C. (2002). Cognitive-behavioral therapy with and without medication in the treatment of obsessive compulsive disorder. *Professional Psychology: Research and Practice, 33,* 162–168.

Franklin, M. E., Abramowitz, J. S., Furr, J., Kalsy, S., & Riggs, D. S. (2003). A naturalistic examination of therapist experience and outcome of exposure and ritual prevention for OCD. *Psychotherapy Research, 13,* 153–167.

Franklin, M. E., Abramowitz, J. S., Kozak, M. J., Levitt, J., & Foa, E. B. (2000). Effectiveness of exposure and ritual prevention for obsessive compulsive disorder: Randomized compared with non-randomized samples. *Journal of Consulting and Clinical Psychology, 68,* 594–602.

Franklin, M. E., Kozak, M. J., Cashman, L., Coles, M., Rheingold, A., & Foa, E. B. (1998). Cognitive behavioral treatment of pediatric obsessive compulsive disorder: An open clinical trial. *Journal of the American*

Academy of Child and Adolescent Psychiatry, 37, 412–419.

Freeman, J. B., Choate-Summers, M. L., Moore, P. S. Garcia, A. M., Sapyta, J. J., Leonard, H. L., et al. (2007). Cognitive behavioral treatment of young children with obsessive compulsive disorder. Biological Psychiatry, 61, 337–343.

Freeman, J. B., Garcia, A. M., Fucci, C., Karitani, M., Miller, L., & Leonard, H. L. (2003). Family-based treatment of early-onset obsessive–compulsive disorder [Special issue: Obsessive–compulsive disorder]. Journal of Child and Adolescent Psychopharmacology, 13(2), 71–80.

Freeston, M. H., Ladouceur, R., Gagnon, F., Thibodeau, N., Rhéaume, J., Letarte, H., et al. (1997). Cognitive-behavioral treatment of obsessive thoughts: A controlled study. Journal of Consulting and Clinical Psychology, 65, 405–413.

Gershuny, B. S., Baer, L., Jenike, M. A., Minichiello, W. E., & Wilhelm, S. (2002). Comorbid posttraumatic stress disorder: Impact on treatment outcome for obsessive–compulsive disorder. American Journal of Psychiatry, 159, 852–854.

Goodman, W. K., Price, L. H., Rasmussen, S. A., Mazure, C., Delgado, P., Heninger, G. R., et al. (1989b). The Yale–Brown Obsessive–Compulsive Scale: II. Validity. Archives of General Psychiatry, 46, 1012–1016.

Goodman, W. K., Price, L. H., Rasmussen, S. A., Mazure, C., Fleischmann, R. L., Hill, C. L., et al. (1989a). The Yale–Brown Obsessive–Compulsive Scale: I. Development, use, and reliability. Archives of General Psychiatry, 46, 1006–1011.

Greist, J. H. (1990). Treatment of obsessive–compulsive disorder: Psychotherapies, drugs, and other somatic treatments. Journal of Clinical Psychiatry, 51, 44–50.

Greist, J. H. (1992). An integrated approach to treatment of obsessive compulsive disorder. Journal of Clinical Psychiatry, 53(Suppl.), 38–41.

Greist, J. H., Jefferson, J. W., Kobak, K. A., Katzelnick, D. J., & Serlin, R. C. (1995). Efficacy and tolerability of serotonin reuptake inhibitors in obsessive compulsive disorder: A meta-analysis. Archives of General Psychiatry, 46, 53–60.

Hanna, G. L. (1995). Demographic and clinical features of obsessive compulsive disorder in children and adolescents. Journal of the American Academy of Child and Adolescent Psychiatry, 34, 19–27.

Hiss, H., Foa, F. B., & Kozak, M. J. (1994). A relapse prevention program for treatment of obsessive compulsive disorder. Journal of Consulting and Clinical Psychology, 62, 801–808.

Hodgson, R. J., Rachman, S., & Marks, L. M. (1972). The treatment of chronic obsessive–compulsive neurosis: Follow-up and further findings. Behaviour Research and Therapy, 10, 181–189.

Hohagen, F., Winkelmann, G., Rasche-Raeuchle, H., Hand, I., Konig, A., Munchau, N., et al. (1998). Combination of behaviour therapy with fluvoxamine

in comparison with behaviour therapy and placebo: Results of a multicentre study. British Journal of Psychiatry, 173, 71–78.

Hollander, E., & Stein, D. J. (2006). Clinical manual of impulse-control disorders. Arlington, VA: American Psychiatric Publishing.

Insel, T. R., & Akiskal, H. (1986). Obsessive–compulsive disorder with psychotic features: A phenomenologic analysis. American Journal of Psychiatry, 12, 1527–1533.

Jaycox, L. H., Foa, E. B., & Morral, A. R. (1998). Influence of emotional engagement and habituation on exposure therapy for PTSD. Journal of Consulting and Clinical Psychology, 66, 185–192.

Jenike, M., Baer, L., Minichiello, W., Schwartz, C., & Carey, R. (1986). Concomitant obsessive–compulsive disorder and schizotypal personality disorder. American Journal of Psychiatry, 143, 530–532.

Kazarian, S. S., Evans, D. L., & Lefave, K. (1977). Modification and factorial analysis of the Leyton Obsessional Inventory. Journal of Clinical Psychology, 33, 422–425.

Keijsers, G. P., Hoogduin, C. A., & Schaap, C. P. (1994). Predictors of treatment outcome in the behavioural treatment of obsessive–compulsive disorder. British Journal of Psychiatry, 165, 781–786.

Kessler, R. C., Demier, O., Frank, R. G., Olfson, M., Pincus, H. A., Walters, E. E., et al. (2005). Prevalence and treatment of mental disorders, 1990 to 2003. New England Journal of Medicine, 352(24), 2515–2523.

Koran, L. M. (2000). Quality of life in obsessive–compulsive disorder. Psychiatric Clinics of North America, 23, 509–517.

Kozak, M. J., & Foa, E. B. (1994). Obsessions, overvalued ideas, and delusions in obsessive compulsive disorder. Behaviour Research and Therapy, 32, 343–353.

Kozak, M. J., Foa, E. B., & Steketee, G. (1988). Process and outcome of exposure treatment with obsessive-compulsives: Psychophysiological indicators of emotional processing. Behavior Therapy, 19, 157–169.

Kurlan, R., Como, P. G., Miller, B., Palumbo, D., Deeley, C., Andersen, E. M., et al. (2002). The behavioral spectrum of tic disorders: A community-based study. Neurology, 59, 414–420.

Ladoucer, R., Rhéame, J., Freeston, M. H., Aublet, F., Jean, K., Lachance, S., et al. (1995). Experimental manipulations of responsibility: An analogue test for models of obsessive–compulsive disorder. Behaviour Research and Therapy, 33, 937–946.

Lang, P. J. (1979). A bio-informational theory of emotional imagery. Psychophysiology, 6, 495–511.

Leckman, J. F., & Chittenden, E. H. (1990). Gilles de la Tourette syndrome and some forms of obsessive-compulsive disorder may share a common genetic diathesis. L'Encephale, 16, 321–323.

Ledley, D. R., Pai, A., & Franklin, M. E. (2007). Treating comorbid presentations: Obsessive compulsive disorder, anxiety, and depression. In M. M. Antony, C. Purdon, & L. Summerfeldt (Eds.), *Psychological treatment of OCD: Fundamentals and beyond* (pp. 281–293). Washington, DC: American Psychological Association Press.

Lelliott, P. T., Noshirvani, H. F., Basoglu, M., Marks, I. M., & Monteiro, W. O. (1988). Obsessive–compulsive beliefs and treatment outcome. *Psychological Bulletin, 18,* 697–702.

Leon, A. C., Portera, L., & Weissman, M. M. (1995). The social costs of anxiety disorders. *British Journal of Psychiatry, 166*(Suppl.), 19–22.

Lindsay, M., Crino, R., & Andrews, G. (1997). Controlled trial of exposure and response prevention in obsessive compulsive disorder. *British Journal of Psychiatry, 171,* 135–139.

Lochner, C., & Stein, D. J. (2003). Heterogeneity of obsessive–compulsive disorder: A literature review. *Harvard Review of Psychiatry, 11*(3), 113–132.

Lovell, K., Cox, D., Haddock, G., Jones, C., Raines, D., Garvey, R., et al. (2006). Telephone administered cognitive behaviour therapy for treatment of obsessive compulsive disorder: Randomised controlled non-inferiority trial. *British Medical Journal.com, 333,* 883.

March, J. S., Franklin, M. E., Leonard, H., Garcia, A., Moore, P., Freeman, J., et al. (2007). Tics moderate the outcome of treatment with medication but not CBT in pediatric OCD. *Biological Psychiatry, 61,* 344–347.

Marks, I. M., Lelliott, P., Basoglu, M., Noshirvani, H., Monteiro, W., Cohen, D., et al. (1988). Clomipramine self-exposure, and therapist-aided exposure for obsessive–compulsive rituals. *British Journal of Psychiatry, 152,* 522–534.

Marks, I. M., Stern, R. S., Mawson, D., Cobb, J., & McDonald, R. (1980). Clomipramine and exposure for obsessive–compulsive rituals—I. *British Journal of Psychiatry, 136,* 1–25.

Masellis, M., Rector, N. A., & Richter, M. A. (2003). Quality of life in OCD: Differential impact of obsessions, compulsions, and depression comorbidity. *Canadian Journal of Psychiatry, 48*(2), 72–77.

Mataix-Cols, D., Marks, I. M., Greist, J. H., Kobak, K. A., & Baer, L. (20020. Obsessive–compulsive symptoms dimensions as predictors of compliance with and response to behaviour therapy: Results from a controlled trial. *Psychotherapy and Psychosomatics, 71,* 255–262.

Mathews, A. M., Johnston, D. W., Shaw, P. M., & Gelder, M. G. (1974). Process variables and the prediction of outcome in behavior therapy. *British Journal of Psychiatry, 125,* 256–264.

Matsunaga, H., Kiriike, N., Matsui, T., Oya, K., Okino, K., & Stein, D. (2005). Impulsive disorders in Japanese adult patients with obsessive–compulsive disorder. *Comprehensive Psychiatry, 46,* 43–49.

McLean, P. L., Whittal, M. L., Thordarson, D. S., Taylor, S., Sochting, I., Koch, W. J., et al. (2001).

Cognitive versus behavior therapy in the group treatment of obsessive–compulsive disorder. *Journal of Consulting and Clinical Psychology, 69,* 205–214.

Mehta, M. (1990). A comparative study of family-based and patients-based behavioural management in obsessive–compulsive disorder. *British Journal of Psychiatry, 157,* 133–135.

Meyer, V. (1966). Modification of expectations in cases with obsessional rituals. *Behaviour Research and Therapy, 4,* 273–280.

Meyer, V., & Levy, R. (1973). Modification of behavior in obsessive–compulsive disorders. In H. E. Adams & P. Unikel (Eds.), *Issues and trends in behavior therapy* (pp. 77–136). Springfield, IL: Charles C. Thomas.

Meyer, V., Levy, R., & Schnurer, A. (1974). A behavioral treatment of obsessive-compulsive disorders. In H. R. Beech (Ed.), *Obsessional states.* London: Methuen.

Mowrer, O. H. (1939). A stimulus–response analysis of anxiety and its role as a reinforcing agent. *Psychological Review, 46,* 553–565.

Mowrer, O. H. (1960). *Learning theory and behavior.* New York: Wiley.

Neziroglu, F., Stevens, K. P., Yaryura-Tobias, J. A., & McKay, D. (2000). Predictive validity of the Overvalued Ideas Scale: Outcome in obsessive–compulsive and body dysmorphic disorder. *Behaviour Research and Therapy, 39,* 745–756.

Ost, L. G. (1989). One-session treatment for specific phobias. *Behaviour Research and Therapy, 27,* 1–7.

O'Sullivan, G., Noshirvani, H., Marks, I., Monteiro, W., & Lelliott, P. (1991). Six-year follow-up after exposure and clomipramine therapy for obsessive–compulsive disorder. *Journal of Clinical Archives, 52,* 150–155.

Pato, M. T., Zohar-Kadouch, R., Zohar, J., & Murphy, D. L. (1988). Return of symptoms after discontinuation of clomipramine in patients with obsessive–compulsive disorder. *American Journal of Psychiatry, 145,* 1521–1525.

Pauls, D. L., Towbin, K. E., Leckman, J. F., Zahner, G. E., & Cohen, D. J. (1986). Gilles de la Tourette syndrome and obsessive–compulsive disorder. *Archives of General Psychiatry, 43,* 1180–1182.

Pediatric OCD Treatment Study Team. (2004). Cognitive-behavioral therapy, sertraline, and their combination for children and adolescents with obsessive–compulsive disorder: The Pediatric OCD Treatment Study (POTS) randomized controlled trial. *Journal of the American Medical Association, 292,* 1969–1976.

Piacentini, J., Bergman, R. L., Jacobs, C., McCracken, J. T., & Kretchman, J. (2002). Open trial of cognitive behavior therapy for childhood obsessive–compulsive disorder. *Journal of Anxiety Disorders, 16,* 207–219.

Purdon, C., & Clark, D. A. (2002). The need to control thoughts. In R. Frost & G. Steketee (Eds.), *Cognitive approaches to obsessions and compulsions: Theory, research, and treatment* (pp. 29–43). Oakland, CA: New Harbinger.

Rabavilas, A. D., Boulougouris, J. C., & Perissaki, C. (1979). Therapist qualities related to outcome with exposure *in vivo* in neurotic patients. *Journal of Behavior Therapy and Experimental Psychiatry, 10,* 293–299.

Rachman, S. (1998). A cognitive theory of obsessions: Elaborations. *Behaviour Research and Therapy, 36,* 385–401.

Rachman, S., & DeSilva, P. (1978). Abnormal and normal obsessions. *Behaviour Research and Therapy, 16,* 233–248.

Rachman, S., Thordarson, D. S., Shafran, R., & Woody, S. R. (1995). Perceived responsibility: Structure and significance. *Behaviour Research and Therapy, 33*(7), 779–784.

Rapoport, J. L., Swedo, S. E., & Leonard, H. L. (1992). Childhood obsessive compulsive disorder (144th Annual Meeting of the American Psychiatric Association: Obsessive compulsive disorder: Integrating theory and practice [1991, New Orleans, LA]). *Journal of Clinical Psychiatry, 53*(Suppl. 4), 11–16.

Rasmussen, S. A., & Eisen, J. L. (1989). Clinical features and phenomenology of obsessive–compulsive disorder. *Psychiatric Annals, 19,* 67–73.

Rasmussen, S. A., & Eisen, J. L. (1990). Epidemiology of obsessive–compulsive disorder. *Journal of Clinical Psychiatry, 51,* 10–14.

Rasmussen, S. A., & Tsuang, M. T. (1986). Clinical characteristics and family history in DSM III obsessive–compulsive disorder. *American Journal of Psychiatry, 1943,* 317–382.

Reed, G. E. (1985). *Obsessional experience and compulsive behavior: A cognitive structural approach.* Orlando, FL: Academic Press.

Rhéaume, J., Freeston, M. H., Dugas, M. J., Letarte, H., & Ladouceur, R. (1995). Perfectionism, responsibility, and obsessive compulsive symptoms. *Behaviour Research and Therapy, 36,* 385–402.

Riggs, D. S., Hiss, H., & Foa, E. B. (1992). Marital distress and the treatment of obsessive–compulsive disorder. *Behavior Therapy, 23,* 585–597.

Rothbaum, B. O., & Shahar, F. (2000). Behavioral treatment of obsessive–compulsive disorder in a naturalistic setting. *Cognitive and Behavioral Practice, 7,* 262–270.

Rowe, M. K., & Craske, M. G. (1998). Effects of an expanding-space vs. massed exposure schedule on fear reduction and return of fear. *Beahviour Research on Therapy, 36,* 701–717.

Rubenstein, C. S., Peynircioglu, Z. F., Chambless, D. L., & Pigott, T. A. (1993). Memory in sub-clinical obsessive–compulsive checkers. *Behaviour Research and Therapy, 31*(8), 759–765.

Salkovskis, P. M. (1985). Obsessional compulsive problems: A cognitive-behavioral analysis. *Behaviour Research and Therapy, 23,* 571–583.

Sher, K. J., Frost, R. O., & Otto, R. (1983). Cognitive deficits in compulsive checkers: An exploratory study. *Behaviour Research and Therapy, 21,* 357–364.

Simpson, H. B., Liebowitz, M. R., Foa, E. B., Kozak, M. J., Schmidt, A. B., Rowan, V., et al. (2004). Post-treatment effects of exposure therapy and clomipramine in obsessive–compulsive disorder. *Depression and Anxiety, 19,* 225–233.

Stampfl, T. G., & Levis, D. J. (1967). Essentials of implosive therapy: A learning-based psychodynamic behavioral therapy. *Journal of Abnormal Psychology, 72,* 496–503.

Stanley, M. A., Turner, S. M., & Borden, J. W. (1990). Schizotypal features in obsessive–compulsive disorder. *Comprehensive Psychiatry, 31,* 511–518.

Steketee, G., Chambless, D. L., & Tran, G. Q. (2001). Effects of Axis I and II comorbidity on behavior therapy outcome for obsessive–compulsive disorder and agoraphobia. *Comprehensive Psychiatry, 42,* 76–86.

Steketee, G., Eisen, J., Dyck, I., Warshaw, M., & Rasmussen, S. (1999). Predictors of course in obsessive-compulsive disorder. *Psychiatry Research, 89,* 229–238.

Steketee, G. S., Foa, E. B., & Grayson, J. B. (1982). Recent advances in the treatment of obsessive-compulsives. *Archives of General Psychiatry, 39,* 1365–1371.

Storch, E., Geffken, G., Merlo, L., Mann, G., Duke, D., Munson, M., et al. (2007). Family-based cognitive-behavioral therapy for pediatric obsessive–compulsive disorder: Comparison of intensive and weekly approaches. *Journal of American Academy of Child and Adolescent Psychiatry, 46,* 469–478.

Storch, E. A., Murphy, T. K., Geffken, G. R., Soto, O., Sajid, M., Allen, P., et al. (in press). Development of the Children's Florida Obsessive–Compulsive Inventory (C-FOCI). *Journal of Behavior Therapy and Experimental Psychiatry.*

Swedo, S. E., Leonard, H. L., Garvey, M., Mittleman, B., Allen, A. J., Perlmutter, S., et al. (1998). Pediatric autoimmune neuropsychiatric disorders associated with streptococcal infections: Clinical description of the first 50 cases. *American Journal of Psychiatry, 155,* 264–271.

Swedo, S. E., Rapoport, J. L., Leonard, H. L., Lenane, M., & Cheslow, D. (1989). Obsessive compulsive disorder in children and adolescents: Clinical phenomenology of 70 consecutive cases. *Archives of General Psychiatry, 46,* 335–341.

Thoren, P., Asberg, M., Chronholm, B., Jornestedt, L., & Traskman, L. (1980). Clomipramine treatment of obsessive–compulsive disorder: I. A controlled clinical trial. *Archives of General Psychiatry, 37,* 1281–1285.

Tolin, D. F., Maltby, N., Diefenbach, G. J., Hannan, S. E., & Worhunsky, P. (2004). Cognitive-behavioral therapy for medication nonresponders with obsessive–compulsive disorder: A wait-list-controlled open trial. *Journal of Clinical Psychiatry, 65,* 922–931.

Tukel, R., Polat, A., Ozdemir, O., Aksut, D., & Turksov, N. (2002). Comorbid conditions in obsessive–compulsive disorder. *Comprehensive Psychiatry, 43,* 204–209.

Twohig, M. P., Hayes, S. C., & Masuda, A. (2006). Increasing willingness to experience obsessions: Acceptance and commitment therapy as a treatment for obsessive compulsive disorder. *Behavior Therapy, 37,* 3–13.

Valderhaug, R., Larsson, B., Gotestam, K. G., & Piacentini, J. (2007). An open clinical trial of cognitive-behaviour therapy in children and adolescents with obsessive–compulsive disorder administered in regular outpatient clinics. *Behaviour Research and Therapy, 45,* 577–589.

Valleni-Basille, L. A., Garrison, C. Z., Jackson, K. L., Waller, J. L., McKeown, R. E., Addy, C. L., et al. (1994). Frequency of obsessive–compulsive disorder in a community sample of young adolescents. *Journal of the American Academy of Child and Adolescent Psychiatry, 33,* 782–791.

van Balkom, A. J., de Haan, E., van Oppen, P., Spinhoven, P., Hoogduin, K. A., Vermeulen, A. W. A., et al. (1998). Cognitive and behavioral therapies alone and in combination with fluvoxamine in the treatment of obsessive compulsive disorder. *Journal of Nervous and Mental Disease, 186,* 492–499.

van Minnen, A., & Hagenaars, M. (2002). Fear activation and habituation patterns as early process predictors of response to prolonged exposure treatment in PTSD. *Journal of Traumatic Stress, 15,* 359–367.

Verdellen, C. W., Keijsers, G. P., Cath, D. C., & Hoogduin, C. A. (2004). Exposure with response prevention versus habit reversal in Tourette syndrome: A controlled study. *Behaviour Research and Therapy, 42,* 501–511.

Vogel, P. A., Stiles, T. C., & Götestam, K. G. (20040. Adding cognitive therapy elements to exposure therapy for obsessive–compulsive disorder: A controlled study. *Behavioural and Cognitive Psychotherapy, 32,* 275–290.

Warren, R., & Thomas, J. C. (2001). Cognitive-behavior therapy of obsessive–compulsive disorder in private practice: An effectiveness study. *Journal of Anxiety Disorders, 15,* 277–285.

Warwick, H. M., Clark, D. M., Cobb, A. M., & Salkovskis, P. M. (1996). A controlled trial of cognitive-behavioural treatment of hypochondriasis. *British Journal of Psychiatry, 169*(2), 189–195.

Watts, F. N. (1973). Desensitization as an habituation phenomenon: II. Studies of interstimulus interval length. *Psychological Reports, 33,* 715–718.

Weissman, M. M., Bland, R. C., Canino, G. J., Greenwald, S., Hwu, H. G., Lee, C. K., et al. (1994). The cross national epidemiology of obsessive compulsive disorder: The Cross National Collaborative Group. *Journal of Clinical Psychiatry, 55*(Suppl.), 5–10.

Whittal, M. L., Thordarson, D. S., & McLean, P. D. (2005). Treatment of obsessive–compulsive disorder: Cognitive behavior therapy vs. exposure and response prevention. *Behaviour Research and Therapy, 43,* 1559–1576.

CHAPTER 5

Emotional Disorders

A UNIFIED PROTOCOL

LAURA B. ALLEN
R. KATHRYN McHUGH
DAVID H. BARLOW

In this chapter we describe the most recently developed treatment protocol from the Center for Anxiety and Related Disorders at Boston University. In this "unified" protocol, therapeutic principles common to psychological treatment of the various emotional disorders have been distilled and integrated into a single protocol that is, in theory, applicable to the full range of emotional disorders. Unlike protocols for specific problems or disorders described in other chapters, this new approach has not yet benefited from efforts to establish extensive empirical validation. But the components that make up this treatment have achieved wide and deep empirical support, and what is new about this approach is the interaction of these components and the systematic manner in which they are applied across disorders. The major advantage, of course, in addition to greatly simplifying dissemination by eliminating numerous overlapping single-disorder protocols, is that this approach also takes into consideration the extensive comorbidity often found among emotional disorders. This approach is illustrated in the treatment of "Oscar."—D. H. B.

When the first edition of this book was published in 1985 it was the dawn of evidence-based psychological treatments. Descriptions of only those treatments with sufficient empirical support that were broadly applicable to large numbers of individuals with various forms of psychopathology at that time were included. Over succeeding editions of this book new treatment approaches with wide appeal and strong empirical support have been added, whereas others have been deleted. In addition, the field has matured to the point where public health services around the world have directed that evidence-based psychological treatments

become an integral part of health care delivery systems due to their effectiveness, efficiency, and durability (British Psychological Society, 2004; Nathan & Gorman, 2002). It is also a sign of the maturity of a field to examine closely the limitations of existing evidence. Obviously, a considerable number of patients still do not respond as well as would be desirable to our current arsenal of psychological (or drug) treatments, and there is plenty of room for improvement. Another problem that has become apparent, particularly in the context of emotional disorders, is that there now exists a plethora of treatment protocols for each of the discrete anxiety and mood disorders. Although these protocols, by and large, have proven useful and been well received, it takes a significant amount of training to become sufficiently familiar with the distinct protocols to integrate them into clinical practice. For example, in the area of depression, a recent National Institute of Mental Health (NIMH) Task Force specified three priorities for treatment development, including more efficacious psychological treatments and more "user-friendly" protocols (Hollon et al., 2002). Unless these treatments become more "user-friendly" as recommended, clinicians are less likely to have a sufficient understanding of, or access to, these evidence-based treatments for the emotional disorders. In this chapter, we present, for the first time (the fourth edition) in this book, a unified treatment protocol for the emotional disorders. "Emotional disorders" in our conception include not only the anxiety and mood disorders but also other classes of disorders in which emotional dysregulation plays a prominent role, such as the somatoform disorders, dissociative disorders, and, to some extent, the eating disorders. Borderline personality disorder also may be conceptualized as a disorder of extreme emotional dysregulation (Linehan & Dexter-Mazza, Chapter 9, this volume). Although readers should be forewarned that this protocol is still a "work in progress," our science and practice have advanced sufficiently that there are now several strong arguments for developing such an approach, in addition to the very practical advantage of substantially reducing the number of existing protocols. We touch on these arguments here before describing the latest iteration of this protocol in some detail, in keeping with the long-standing format of this book.

RATIONALE FOR A UNIFIED APPROACH

Perhaps the strongest argument for a unified treatment approach to emotional disorders is an emerging body of evidence supporting commonalities in the etiology of these disorders that we have summarized recently in the form of a new etiological model referred to as "triple vulnerability" (Barlow, 1991, 2000, 2002; Suárez, Bennett, Goldstein, & Barlow, in press). Nevertheless, it is important to note that shared etiological pathways or pathophysio-

logical processes are not yet firmly established, and that emotional disorders and their subtypes may each turn out to be associated with unique underlying pathology (reflecting a true categorical organization) with identifiable *taxa*. Yet we believe that the evidence on shared pathological processes is sufficiently strong at present to provide further justification for developing and testing a unified treatment approach, even if its mechanisms of action, provided they are proven efficacious, do not turn out to be associated with fundamental changes in hypothetical specific pathophysiology.

A second argument focuses on conceptions of the major emotional disorders that emphasize their commonalities rather than their differences. The "spectrum" approach is one manifestation of this conception. For example, high rates of comorbidity suggest considerable overlap among disorders. The observed effects of current psychological treatments on comorbid conditions also point to at least a partial nonspecificity of treatment response. From a phenomenological perspective, emerging research on the latent structure of dimensional features of emotional disorders is revealing a hierarchical structure that can accommodate these disorders. The sections to follow briefly review evidence relevant to these arguments.

Etiology

We have described in some detail an interacting set of vulnerabilities or diatheses relevant to the development of anxiety, anxiety disorders, and related emotional disorders. This "triple vulnerability" theory encompasses a generalized biological vulnerability, a generalized psychological vulnerability, and a specific psychological vulnerability emerging from early learning (Barlow, 2000, 2002; Suárez et al., in press). A generalized biological vulnerability involves nonspecific genetic contributions to the development of anxiety and negative affect. Much of the research on this generalized biological vulnerability has focused on temperaments labeled "neuroticism," "negative affect," or "behavioral inhibition." Although the relationships among these closely related traits and temperaments have yet to be worked out fully, it seems that they substantially overlap, and that each (partially) represents a common theme associated with a biological vulnerability to develop emotional disorders generally (Barlow, 2000, 2002; Campbell-Sills, Liverant, & Brown,

2004; Suárez et al., in press). Additionally, early life experiences fostering a sense that events, particularly negative events, are unpredictable or uncontrollable and are accompanied by weak or nonexistent coping mechanisms, contribute to a generalized psychological vulnerability, or diathesis, to experience anxiety and related negative affective states later on. This sense of uncontrollability seems to be at the core of negative affect and derivative states of anxiety (and depression). If a generalized biological and a generalized psychological vulnerability happen to line up, and are potentiated by the influence of life stress, the likely result is the clinical syndromes of generalized anxiety disorder and/or depressive disorders. Notice that false alarms (panic attacks) may also occur as a function of stressful life events, facilitated by high levels of baseline anxiety. But these false alarms seem to have a different heritability than anxiety/negative affect and are not necessarily implicated in a clinical disorder. For that to occur, an additional layer of a more specific psychological vulnerability must be considered. In particular, certain learning experiences seem to focus anxiety on specific life circumstances, and these circumstances or events are associated with a heightened sense of threat or danger. For example, specific early learning experiences seem to determine whether individuals may view somatic sensations, intrusive thoughts, or social evaluation as specifically dangerous (Barlow, 2002; Bouton, Mineka, & Barlow, 2001); that is, to take one example, individuals with social anxiety often have in their background admonitions from parents or family always to be on their best behavior and to look their best to avoid the dreaded consequence of being "disapproved" by others. It is this specific psychological vulnerability that, when coordinated with the generalized biological and psychological vulnerabilities mentioned earlier, seems to contribute to the development of discrete anxiety disorders such as social phobia, obsessive–compulsive disorder, panic disorder, and specific phobias. Existing evidence for this "triple vulnerability" model has been reviewed in detail elsewhere (Barlow, 2000, 2002; Bouton et al., 2001; Chorpita & Barlow, 1998; Suárez et al., in press). Whereas confirmation of this model awaits further research, it is consistent with the overriding importance of common factors in the genesis and presentation of emotional disorders.

Latent Structure of the Emotional Disorders

Whereas the *Diagnostic and Statistical Manual of Mental Disorders*, fourth edition (DSM-IV; American Psychiatric Association, 1994), represents the zenith of a "splitting approach" to nosology in an attempt to achieve high rates of diagnostic reliability, this achievement may have come at the expense of diagnostic validity; that is, the current system may be highlighting categories that are minor variations of more fundamental, underlying syndromes. New quantitative approaches using structural equation modeling are capable of examining the full range of anxiety and mood disorders without the constraints of existing (possibly) artificial categories (Brown, Chorpita, & Barlow, 1998; Chorpita, Albano, & Barlow, 1998; Clark, 2005; Clark & Watson, 1991; Watson, 2005; Watson, Clark, & Harkness, 1994) as recently articulated in DSM-V research planning committees (Kupfer, First, & Regier, 2002). Indeed, a recent special issue of the Journal of Abnormal Psychology is devoted to this topic (Krueger, Watson, & Barlow, 2005). We have been studying this question for over a decade. For example, Brown and colleagues (1998), using a sample of 350 patients with DSM-IV anxiety and mood disorders, confirmed a hierarchical structure to the emotional disorders. In this structure, negative affect and positive affect were identified as crucial, higher-order factors to the DSM-IV disorder factors, with significant paths from negative affect to each of the five DSM-IV factors. Interestingly, low positive affect emerged with significant paths to the mood disorders and social phobia only. In this model, autonomic arousal represents the phenomenon of panic, and this arousal emerges as a lower-order factor with significant paths to panic disorder and generalized anxiety disorder (where the relationship was negative). From these findings it seems safe to conclude that what is common to emotional disorders outweighs what is not (DSM-IV factors). We have concluded from this research that DSM-IV emotional disorder categories are best considered as useful concepts or constructs that emerge as "blips" on a general background of neuroticism/behavioral inhibition, but may not be the best way to organize nosology. It is likely that DSM-V will turn to a more dimensional description of these phenomena that would reinforce conceptions of common underlying components (Krueger et al., 2002, 2005).

Overlap among Disorders

Anxiety and mood disorders are overlapping and strongly related. We have reviewed the genetic and neurobiological evidence on the commonalities among anxiety and depressive states in some detail (Barlow, 2002, Chapters 3, 6, 7, and 8; Bouton, 2005; Brown, 2007; Suárez et al., in press). For example, most work on genetic contributions to anxiety and depression supports the early dictum of Ken Kendler (1996; Kendler et al., 1995) "same genes, different environment" (e.g., Eley & Brown, 2007; Hettema, Neale, & Kendler, 2001; Rutter, Moffit, & Caspi, 2006; Smoller & Tsuang, 1998). Davidson and colleagues have reported robust findings supporting increased relative right-hemisphere interior electroencephalographic (EEG) activation linked to heightened negative affect and decreased positive affect in individuals who are either depressed or anxious (Davidson, 2000; Wiedemann, Pauli, & Dengler, 1999). Nemeroff and his colleagues (Cameron, Champagne, & Parent, 2005; Heim & Nemeroff, 1999; Sullivan, Kent, & Coplan, 2000) are focusing on whole-brain systems associated with stress, anxiety, and depression, in which corticotropin-releasing factor (CRF) plays an essential role, with implications for common neurobiological underpinnings. Of course, this is work in progress, and many of its nuances and qualifications are beyond the scope of these few brief summary sentences.

At the diagnostic level, this is most evident in the high rates of current and lifetime comorbidity (e.g., Brown, Campbell, Lehman, Grisham, & Mancill, 2001; Kessler et al., 1996, 1998; Roy-Byrne, Craske, & Stein, 2006; Tsao, Mystowski, Zucker, & Craske, 2002, 2005). Results from Brown, Campbell, and colleagues (2001) indicate that 55% of patients with a principal anxiety disorder had at least one additional anxiety or depressive disorder at the time of assessment. But if one examines for the presence of a disorder over the lifetime of the patient, whether it is present or not at the time of interview, this rate increases to 76%. To take one example, 60% of 324 patients diagnosed with panic disorder with or without agoraphobia (PDA/PD) were determined to meet criteria for either an additional anxiety or mood disor-

der, or both. Specifically 47% presented with an additional anxiety disorder and 33% with an additional mood disorder. When lifetime diagnoses are considered, the percentages rise to 77% experiencing any anxiety or mood disorder, breaking down to 56% for any anxiety disorder and 60% for any mood disorder. If posttraumatic stress disorder (PTSD) or generalized anxiety disorder (GAD) were the principal (most severe) diagnoses, comorbidity rates were highest. Merikangas, Zhang, and Aveneoli (2003) followed almost 500 individuals for 15 years and found that relatively few people suffer from anxiety or depression alone. When a single disorder did occur at one point in time, the additional mood state would almost certainly emerge later.

Several possible explanations for these high rates of comorbidity have been reviewed extensively elsewhere (Brown & Barlow, 2002). Among these are relatively trivial issues with overlapping definitional criteria; artifactual reasons, such as differential base rates of occurrence in our setting; and the possibility that disorders are sequentially related, and that the features of one disorder act as risk factors for another disorder. For example, depression seems to follow PDA, and PDA seems to follow PTSD. But the more intriguing explanation, for our purposes, offered by individuals such as Gavin Andrews or Peter Tyrer (Andrews, 1990, 1996; Tyrer, 1989; Tyrer et al., 1998) is that this pattern of comorbidity argues for the existence of what has been called a "general neurotic syndrome." Andrews and Tyrer have suggested that differences in the expression of emotional disorder symptoms (individual variation in the prominence of social anxiety, panic attacks, anhedonia, etc.) is simply a trivial variation in the manifestation of a broader syndrome. This, in turn, is consistent with "triple vulnerability" models mentioned earlier, that anxiety (and mood) disorders emerge from shared psychosocial and biological/genetic diatheses. If this is the case, then a unified treatment protocol cutting across current diagnostic categories to address core features of the anxiety and mood disorders could be a more parsimonious, and, perhaps, powerful option.

The Broad Effects of Psychological Treatments for Emotional Disorders

Other findings that may support our contention of an emerging "general neurotic syndrome" or "negative affect syndrome" include the observation that specific psychological treatments for a given anxiety disorder produce significant improvement in additional comorbid anxiety or mood disorders that are not specifically addressed in treatment (Borkovec, Abel, & Newman, 1995; Brown, Antony, & Barlow, 1995; Tsao, Lewin, & Craske, 1998; Tsao et al., 2002, 2005). In our own center, we examined the course of additional diagnoses in a sample of 126 patients being treated for PDA. At pretreatment, 26% had an additional diagnosis of GAD, but the rate of comorbid GAD declined significantly to 9% after treatment for PDA and remained at this level at a 2-year follow-up (Brown et al., 1995). More recently, a multisite study examining second-stage treatments for PDA found that patients who were considered treatment responders after receiving 11 sessions of cognitive-behavioral therapy (CBT) for PDA showed significant reductions in both number and frequency of comorbid diagnoses, whereas those who were considered "nonresponders" showed no reductions in comorbidity (Allen et al., 2007). This could represent either the generalization of elements of treatment to independent facets of both disorders or a way of effectively addressing "core" features of emotional disorders. In both cases, the efficiency of a unified treatment protocol is suggested.

In summary, the existing literature supports several arguments for stepping back from individual DSM-IV diagnostic categories and associated specific psychological protocols, and considering a more unified approach based on new findings on the nature of emotion regulation and dysregulation. In addition, current CBT protocols for emotional disorders have much in common and reduce to three broad principles of change: altering emotion-based misappraisals of salient events; preventing avoidance of negative, emotionally charged internal or external triggers; and modifying emotion-driven behaviors. A full explanation of this protocol and a description of the application of the protocol with a patient follows.

TREATMENT VARIABLES

Setting

All assessments and treatments of patients are conducted in the Center for Anxiety and Related Disorders at Boston University. Our clinic receives over 500 new admissions per year, with many patients being offered treatment after their initial intake assessments. The Center for Anxiety and Related Disorders, in addition to housing staff psychologists and a psychiatrist, is also a training center for doctoral students and psychiatric residents. At any given time, numerous NIMH-funded treatment and research studies are ongoing at the Center. Regarding diagnostic breakdown of treatment-seeking patients, the most common diagnosis assigned is GAD, followed by social phobia, PDA, specific phobia, obsessive–compulsive disorder (OCD), and PTSD. A small percentage of patients are assigned "coprincipal diagnoses," referring to cases where two separate diagnoses are judged to be of equal severity.

Individuals seeking assessments and/or treatment at the Center are typically given a brief screening over the telephone or in person to determine eligibility for services. Individuals who appear to be eligible due to reports of emotional dysfunction of some type are then scheduled for an intake assessment. The assessment is conducted as soon as possible, although it is required that patients currently taking psychoactive medications or in therapy be medication and/or psychotherapy stable for 3 months prior to the date of the assessment (1 month stabilization is required for use of benzodiazepines); that is, they cannot have recently begun a treatment that could make their assessment unreliable due to a rapid change in their condition. For individuals tapering off a medication or psychotherapy, the "wash out" period is 1 month.

Prior to the intake evaluation, each patient is mailed a packet of questionnaires to bring to the assessment, which are scored and interpreted subsequent to the interview. The questionnaires provide additional self-report data in examining hypothesized underlying symptoms and factors associated with diagnostic categories. The intake evaluation includes the administration of two semistructured interviews, typically conducted during a single 4-hour appointment. The UCLA Life Stress Interview (Hammen, 1991) is a short interview designed to assess for chronic and episodic stressors occurring over the past 6 months. The majority of the intake appointment comprises administration of the Anxiety Disorders Interview Schedule for DSM-IV—Lifetime Version (ADIS-IV-L; Di Nardo, Brown, & Barlow, 1994). Following completion of the entire assessment process, consensus diagnoses are determined during a weekly staff meeting, after which the patient is provided with diagnostic feedback and treatment recommendations. Based on the information from the interview, the patient may be offered one of several treatment options at the Center, or a referral in the community.

Format

Treatment with the unified protocol (UP) is typically conducted in an individual format, although it has been successfully conducted in a group format with patients with mixed principal diagnoses (anxiety and mood disorders). The treatment described in this chapter reflects the individual treatment protocol, which allows for greater attention to the description and application of treatment components during each session. However, when administered in a group setting, patients were easily able to see the commonalities among their diverse presenting complaints, and this understanding often created a strong bond among group members. Therefore, it may be useful to consider adapting the protocol for group treatment in the future.

Therapist Variables

Thus far, the UP has been administered by therapists of varying degrees of clinical experience and expertise with the protocol. To our knowledge, both junior therapists (even therapists who have never had experience with cognitive-behavioral treatments) and senior therapists (i.e., therapists with at least 4 or more years of treatment experience) have been able to adapt to the UP without significant difficulty. Certainly, a background in cognitive-behavioral techniques may be helpful when utilizing the protocol (e.g., facilitating cognitive reappraisal, and designing and conducting exposures). Recent evidence suggests some benefit to therapist experience, at least when treating PDA with a highly structured CBT protocol (Huppert et al., 2001).

The UP is an emotion-focused treatment approach; that is, the focus of every exercise is on eliciting and changing behavioral responses to a variety of emotions and emotional cues. Perhaps one of the most challenging aspects for the therapist is to be able to create and utilize emotion-provoking exposures effectively, which often begin at the first treatment session. Most importantly, the therapist must have a sense of when a patient is avoiding the process of experiencing, expressing, or accepting emotions, and this is often signaled by very subtle behavioral cues, such as avoiding eye contact, changing the topic of discussion, arriving late for session, and not completing (or "overdoing") homework assignments. Each of these behaviors represents attempts to control uncomfortable emotions either through direct avoidance or overcontrol. It is essential that the therapist be able to recognize and address such behaviors when they occur, thereby allowing the opportunity for an effective emotion exposure and discussion of avoidance to facilitate emotional processing.

A second challenge for the therapist is to be able to tolerate and experience the expression of emotion by the patient. It is common for less experienced therapists to quickly "rationalize away" the patient's emotional reactions; however, this only feeds into the cycle of emotions and avoidance. At every step, the therapist should encourage the expression and acceptance of emotion, while guiding the patient in how to "examine" it, without letting the emotion "take over." In such cases, modeling from a senior therapist and/or extensive supervision may be helpful instruction for less experienced therapists in how to allow their patients to be "emotional."

Client Variables

As previously mentioned, the rate of comorbidity among patients with a principal anxiety or mood disorder is approximately 55% (Brown, Campbell, et al., 2001), depending on the principal diagnosis. In most CBT protocols, comorbid diagnoses are never a focus of treatment, although successful treatment of a principal anxiety disorder often results in decreases in comorbidity (e.g., Allen et al., 2007; Brown et al., 1995). One advantage of a unified treatment approach is that symptoms related to comorbid diagnoses can be discussed in treatment sessions, and may even be the focus of an emotion exposure. For example, a patient with GAD who experiences chronic worry about daily matters may also feel anxious in social situations. Therefore, that patient's in-session emotion exposure might consist of a conversation with a stranger or giving a speech to a small group of people. Contrary to traditional protocols, it is the experience of any emotion that is the target of treatment, which may be particularly beneficial for patients with significant comorbidity or for those who would like to address multiple concerns during the course of treatment.

Concurrent Drug Treatment

Many patients who present for treatment are also taking some form of psychoactive medication. As described earlier, patients are required to have stabilized on the dosage of medication prior to the intake interview, so that the therapist has a clear picture of actual symptoms (as opposed to symptoms that may be caused by the initial addition or removal of a medication). Whereas concurrent use of medications such as tricyclic antidepressants and selective serotonin reuptake inhibitors (SSRIs) does not appear to have a negative impact on treatment outcome initially, once the medications are removed, evidence suggests that patients who received medication alone or CBT in addition to medication are more likely to relapse (e.g., Barlow, Gorman, Shear, & Woods, 2000; Heimberg et al., 1998; Liebowitz et al., 1999). The exact mechanisms underlying the return of symptoms are unclear, although some authors have suggested that patients may attribute the success of the treatment to the use of medication and, once it is withdrawn, no longer believe they have the ability to manage their symptoms. However, in a recent investigation using the data from a multisite comparative study for the treatment of panic disorder, results indicated that patients who received CBT plus pill placebo were equally likely to believe they had received medication as patients who had actually received the medication (Raffa et al., in press). Yet those in the CBT plus placebo condition were less likely to relapse compared to those who had received either CBT plus medication or medication alone. Therefore, it appears unlikely that the higher relapse rates in the medication conditions were due solely to this "attribution hypothesis." One other hypothesis to explain greater relapse in patients receiving psychopharmacological treatment is that the medication provides an unintended "protective" effect against increased physiological arousal and anxiety. However, eliciting anxiety and panic is a core component of CBT protocols, so patients taking medication (1) may have experienced greater physical sensa-

tions when the medication was removed and/or (2) were never able fully to confront the physiological arousal and panic during the course of treatment. However, these hypotheses have yet to be fully investigated.

One additional consideration is the use of benzodiazepines on a prn, or "as needed," basis during the course of treatment. Following conceptions outlined in the UP, any strategy used to reduce the intensity of emotions in the moment is considered an avoidance strategy, and ultimately contributes to increasing levels of anxiety and emotional reactivity. Therefore, the use of benzodiazepines (or other fast-acting medications) is discouraged, particularly if the medications are carried with the person as a "safety signal."

ASSESSMENT

Case Study

Oscar is a 28-year-old graduate student in the sciences, studying at a university in the United States. He is engaged to be married and living with his fiancée. Several months prior to referral to the Clinic, he encountered a difficult situation while working under a vent in a chemistry laboratory when a distinct odor of a toxic gas produced noticeable tingling in his nose. Knowing this chemical well, he was aware that the physical consequences of contact with the gas would be delayed for up to 48 hours but could then result in potentially serious cardiovascular and pulmonary complications. Oscar immediately visited the health clinic, where he was cleared of any obvious toxic reactions, and returned again 5 days later and, once again, was given a clean bill of health.

Despite these reassurances, Oscar continued to experience recollections of the event, particularly upon the occurrence of any physical sensations resembling those that occurred during the event, such as tingling in his nose, slight headache, or dizziness. As a result, he had largely stopped the laboratory work that was important to his progress toward his doctoral degree and spent a great deal of time monitoring his body for physical symptoms and worrying about his health. If certain physical sensations occurred, particularly nasal obstruction or tingling, combined with slight headache, he would call his mother, who was a physician in South America and, if these symptoms persisted, possibly visit the university health clinic.

Oscar had been prescribed 0.5 mg of clonaze-pam, which he took upon experiencing anxiety due to physical symptoms that lasted more than several hours. At the time of referral, he was taking 1 to 2 pills approximately once a week.

Contact with any substances that might be toxic was also sufficient to trigger Oscar's health concerns. For example, while shopping in a department store he picked up a plate and, after putting it down, noticed a bit of residue on his fingers. Hypothesizing the source of this substance as something utilized in the manu-facture and/or shipping of this plate, he experi-enced a surge of anxiety, left the store, and pro-ceeded to the nearest public men's room in a nearby restaurant to wash his hands thor-oughly. This was followed by additional anxi-ety as he continued to notice mild somatic sen-sations in various systems in his body over the next several days.

In fact, Oscar reported that although the in-cident several months earlier was perhaps the most "traumatic," he had experienced health-related worries for approximately 5 years, dur-ing which he would focus on various somatic sensations and report them to his mother or take other steps to ensure that these sensations did not represent an incipient illness. Typically, these episodes would occur every 2–3 months and were not connected with any specific trig-gering event that Oscar could remember. Con-cern and worry about his health had occupied a significant portion of most of Oscar's days for the past 5 years.

In addition, he reported intrusive thoughts of varying content, including crashing his car into an abutment or driving onto the sidewalk; stabbing himself or his fiancée, if he was hold-ing a knife; drinking acid that he might be holding in the laboratory; as well as jumping off high places. Objective assessment of his emotional state via questionnaires resulted in score of 9 on the Beck Depressive Inventory–II (BDI-II; Beck, Steer, & Brown, 1996); a score of 51 on the Penn State Worry Questionnaire (PSWQ; Meyer, Miller, Metzger, & Borkovec, 1990), reflecting mild to moderate worry; and a score of 20 on the Anxiety Sensitivity Index (ASI; Peterson & Reiss, 1992), reflecting mild concern over somatic symptoms. Diagnoses re-vealed a principal diagnosis of hypochondriasis with a comorbid diagnosis of OCD at a lower level of clinical severity (less than necessary for a DSM-IV diagnosis).

Interviews

A number of structured and semistructured clinical interviews may be appropriate for diag-nosing Axis I disorders. The Structured Clinical Interview for DSM-IV (SCID; First, Spitzer, Gibbon, & Williams, 1996) is widely used and assesses for Axis I disorders. Because this inter-view is highly structured and focuses only on current symptom count, it achieves a high de-gree of interrater reliability for many diagno-ses. However, this interview does not include dimensional ratings of frequency and severity of symptoms, so it may be less useful for re-search projects examining treatment outcome.

The Anxiety Disorders Interview Schedule for DSM-IV—Lifetime Version (ADIS-IV-L; Di Nardo et al., 1994), a semistructured, diagnos-tic clinical interview, focuses on DSM-IV diag-noses of anxiety disorders and their accompa-nying mood states, somatoform disorders, and substance and alcohol use. The information de-rived from the interview using the ADIS-IV-L allows clinicians to determine differential diag-noses and gain a clear understanding of the level and severity of each diagnosis. Principal and additional diagnoses are assigned a clini-cian severity rating (CSR) on a scale from 0 (*No symptoms*) to 8 (*Extremely severe symp-toms*), with a rating of 4 or above (*Definitely disturbing/disabling*) passing the clinical threshold for DSM-IV diagnostic criteria. In-quiries about suicidal ideation are part of this interview. This measure has demonstrated ex-cellent to acceptable interrater reliability for the anxiety and mood disorders (Brown, Di Nardo, Lehman, & Campbell, 2001). The full ADIS-IV-L (focusing on current and lifetime di-agnoses) is typically administered at the initial intake. An abbreviated version of the ADIS that focuses only on current symptomatology (Mini-ADIS-IV; Brown, Di Nardo, & Barlow, 1994) is used for posttreatment and follow-up assessments. Because the CSR assigned for each diagnosis does not follow a normal curve (due to a "cutoff" score of 4 to indicate diagnoses of clinical severity), it is typically not used for sta-tistical analyses. However, the CSR is a dimen-sional measure, so it can assess improvement in symptoms over treatment, even if a patient is still given the diagnosis at posttreatment.

Two additional clinician-rated measures that provide a wider range of scores are the (1) Structured Interview Guide for the Hamilton Anxiety Rating Scale (SIGH-A; Shear, Vander

Bilt, & Rucci, 2001) and (2) Structured Interview Guide for the Hamilton Depression Rating Scale (SIGH-D; Williams, 1988). The SIGH-A was developed to create a structured format for administering the Hamilton Anxiety Rating Scale (HARS; Hamilton, 1959). Respondents are asked to indicate the presence and severity of a number of symptoms that may have been present over the past week, including anxious mood, tension, sleep problems, irritability, and so forth. The rater is also asked to rate the interview behavior of the patient. The SIGH-A includes specific instructions on administration and anchor points for assigning severity ratings. This measure demonstrated good interrater and test–retest reliability. In addition, scores are similar to (although consistently higher than) the HARS.

Similar to the SIGH-A, the SIGH-D was developed to provide more specific instructions for administration and scoring of the Hamilton Depression Rating Scale (HDRS; Hamilton, 1960). Again, patients are questioned about the presence and severity of a range of depressive symptoms over the past week, including depressed mood, suicidal ideation, fatigue, feelings of hopelessness, weight loss, and so forth. The SIGH-D also demonstrated good interrater and test–retest reliability and produces scores similar to the HDRS.

Medical Evaluations

Medical evaluations are generally recommended prior to assignment of diagnoses and initiation of treatment to rule out organic causes for symptoms of emotional disorders. Some conditions such as hypothyroidism, hyperthyroidism, hypoglycemia, mitral valve prolapse, or alcohol or substance withdrawal may elicit symptoms similar to those associated with GAD or PDA. Although the diagnosis of such medical conditions does not preclude the need for a psychological treatment, it is generally recommended that such conditions be examined by a medical doctor, because an alternative treatment may be clinically indicated.

Self-Monitoring

Self-monitoring forms are an important part of the treatment protocol for several reasons. First, the therapist is able to discuss specific situations or events that occurred over the past week and may have contributed to emotional reactions. Such records can facilitate discussions of concepts presented during the treatment sessions and help the therapist integrate the general treatment components into the patient's specific symptoms. Second, some evidence suggests that patients' retrospective recall of past episodes of anxiety may be inflated, particularly when recalling panic attacks (Margraf, Taylor, Ehlers, Roth, & Agras, 1987; Rapee, Craske, & Barlow, 1990). Self-monitoring forms allow for a prospective, and possibly more accurate, account of anxiety episodes, and may therefore be more useful therapeutically. In addition, consistent with the themes outlined in the UP, practicing awareness of emotions in the present moment is believed to be an important component of changing the cycle of emotions. The very nature of self-monitoring requires the patient to disengage, even briefly, from the habitual anxious process to write down concrete thoughts, feelings, behaviors, and reactions. Developing this habit ultimately aids the patient in beginning to change emotional reactions and resulting behaviors.

Self-monitoring forms used in the UP include standardized forms for automatic thoughts, avoidance, interoceptive and situational exposure, and emotion (e.g., Weekly Record of Anxiety and Depression [WRAD]; see Barlow & Craske, 2000; Barlow, Rapee, & Reisner, 2001; Craske, Barlow, & O'Leary, 1992). Figure 5.1 illustrates the WRAD used in the UP. This form is given for several weeks at the beginning of treatment, in the middle of treatment, and in the final weeks of treatment to allow for comparison of rates of anxiety and depression of the course of the therapy. Once the concept of emotion-driven behaviors (EDBs) is introduced, patients are asked to monitor situations and change EDBs on the Changing EDBs form (see Figure 5.2).

Several problems may arise with the introduction and completion of self-monitoring forms. First, some patients may not be compliant with completion of monitoring forms and homework assignments, which is an important issue to be addressed in the therapy session. The therapist must identify cognitive misappraisals and emotional reasons contributing to the lack of completion of monitoring forms, and help the patient understand that the avoidance is part of the cycle of emotions he or she is trying to break. Therapeutic strategies such as cognitive reappraisal may be used to increase

WEEKLY RECORD OF ANXIETY AND DEPRESSION

Each evening, please make the following ratings, using the scale below:

1. Your AVERAGE level of anxiety (taking all things into consideration).
2. Your MAXIMUM level of anxiety, experienced at any one point in the day.
3. Your AVERAGE level of depression (taking all things into consideration).
4. Your AVERAGE level of pleasantness (taking all things into consideration).

Level of Anxiety/Depression/Pleasantness

0————1————2————3————4————5————6————7————8
None   Slight   Moderate   A lot   As much
                                                                 as I can imagine

Date	Average anxiety	Maximum anxiety	Average depression	Average pleasantness

FIGURE 5.1. Weekly Record of Anxiety and Depression (WRAD) monitoring form.

patients' willingness to complete homework forms. In addition, successful completion of homework forms may become an emotion exposure in and of itself.

One other common problem with the completion of self-monitoring may be the tendency for some patients (particularly those with more obsessive or "perfectionistic" features, such as in GAD and OCD) to "overdo" the homework forms; that is, the patient may write an extremely long and involved description of a situation and his or her reactions to it. This is common with patients who feel a need to "unload" every piece of information about the event. Although the patient is doing the homework, his or her overengagement may also be facilitating the anxious/worry process. If this becomes evident, the therapist may want to discuss the tendency to overengage in the homework as an emotional avoidance strategy and encourage the patient to monitor situations and events using one- or two-word descriptions.

Questionnaires

A number of self-report questionnaires are used over the course of treatment. General questionnaires (measures designed to assess a range of symptoms associated with anxiety and mood disorders, as well as symptoms associated with emotion regulation difficulties) are administered at pretreatment, midtreatment, posttreatment, and follow-up, and are designed to provide a broad picture of a patient's overall functioning and life satisfaction, in addition to interference from anxiety and depression. Symptom-specific measures are designed to track symptoms associated with each patient's

CHANGING EDBs

Situation/trigger	Emotion	EDB	New (incompatible) response	Consequence

FIGURE 5.2. Changing EDBs monitoring form.

particular principal diagnosis and are administered at each of these assessment points, as well as on a weekly basis, prior to each session.

General Measures

The Positive and Negative Affect Scale (PANAS; Watson, Clark, & Tellegen, 1988), a brief, reliable, and valid measure of positive and negative affect, comprises 20 feeling or emotion words. The PANAS assesses core negative affect and deficits in positive affect in those disorders (e.g., social phobia) with this characteristic, and is useful in determining changes in positive and negative affect over the course of treatment. The BDI-II (Beck et al., 1996) and the Beck Anxiety Inventory (BAI; Beck & Steer, 1990; Steer, Ranieri, Beck, & Clark, 1993) are widely used measures assessing current depressive and anxious symptomatology, respectively. Both measures contains 21 items, each focusing on severity of particular symptoms occurring over the past week. In an effort to establish degree of interference from symptoms in various domains of living, the Work and Social Adjustment Scale (WSAS; modification of a scale introduced by Hafner & Marks, 1976) includes five items that ask participants to rate the degree of interference caused by their symptoms in work, home management, private leisure, social leisure, and family relationships. The WSAS, a descriptive measure of subjective interference in various domains of living, has been successfully used in previous studies (e.g., Brown & Barlow, 1995). In addition, the RAND-modified Medical Outcomes Study 36-Item Short Form Health Survey (RAND MOS-SF-36; Hays, Sherbourne, & Mazel, 1993; Ware & Sherbourne, 1992) is a well-validated, comprehensive, self-administered instrument that is widely used in medical and psychiatric settings to provide a multidimensional assessment of mental and physical health-related status. The SF-36 measures several health-related dimensions, including physical functioning, bodily pain, role limitations due to physical health problems, general mental health, social functioning, energy/fatigue, and general health perceptions. This measure allows for a detailed analysis of psychiatric and medical health changes over treatment. Finally, the Quality of Life Inventory (QOLI; Frisch, Cornell, & Villaneuva, 1992) consists of 32 items relevant to overall life satisfaction, including items related to work, love relationships, friendships, self-regard, standard of living, recreation, community, home, and so forth.

Emotion Regulation Measures

Measures designed to assess general concepts related to emotion regulation, emotion dysregulation, and related variables may also be useful tools to assess treatment outcome. Although a number of instruments exist, the following are examples that are commonly used in psychological research. The abbreviated version of the Trait Meta-Mood Scale (TMMS; Salovey, Mayer, Goldman, Turvey, & Palfai, 1995) is a 30-item questionnaire that measures attention to moods, clarity of emotions, and ability to repair emotional experiences. The subscales of the TMMS demonstrate good reliability and validity (Salovey et al., 1995), and have been shown to be consistent with physiological indicators of stress (Salovey, Stroud, Woolery, & Epel, 2002). The Anxiety Control Questionnaire—Revised (ACQ-R; Brown, White, Forsyth, & Barlow, 2004) is a measure of perceived control over emotional reactions and stressful events. Participants rate how much each statement is typical of their experience on a 0 (*Strongly disagree*) to 5 (*Strongly agree*) scale. Also, the Affective Control Scale (ACS; Williams, Chambless, & Ahrens, 1997), a 42-item scale, examines fear of losing control while experiencing strong emotional reactions such as anxiety, depression, anger, and positive affective states. These measures may be helpful in assessing the degree to which patients are better able to manage a variety of emotional experiences, in addition to the emotions that are a target of treatment.

Symptom-Specific Measures

Given the variability in treatment strategies addressed at each session, in addition to life stressors that occur during treatment, it is important to have repeated measures for each patient at every treatment session. These repeated measures typically focus on the patient's principal diagnosis and related symptoms, although the therapist may want to select specific measures to address additional concerns (e.g., if a patient's principal diagnosis is an anxiety disorder but he or she is also experiencing a significant depressive episode, the therapist may also want to administer a measure of depression at each session).

The Obsessive–Compulsive Inventory—Revised version (OCI-R; Foa et al., 2002), an 18-item self-report instrument that measures the frequency of and distress caused by a variety of obsessions and compulsions, is used in patients with a principal diagnosis of OCD. The Panic Disorder Severity Scale—Self-Report Version (PDSS-SR; adapted from Shear et al., 1997) is a 7-item measure adapted from the original, clinician-administered version (PDSS; Shear et al., 1997). This questionnaire for use with individuals already diagnosed with PDA measures the frequency, interference of, and distressed caused by panic attacks. Scores range from 0 to 21, with higher scores reflecting more severe panic symptomatology. This measure has been used successfully in treatment outcome research for patients with PDA/PD (Shear et al., 1997). For patients with a principal diagnosis of GAD, the PSWQ (Meyer et al., 1990) is a 16-item measure to assess general anxiety and worry; scores on the PSWQ are significantly higher for those diagnosed with GAD compared to other anxiety disorders or depression (Brown, Antony, & Barlow, 1992; Molina & Borkovec, 1994). The Social Interaction Anxiety Scale (SIAS; Mattick & Clarke, 1998) measures the extent of an individual's anxiety in a variety of social settings and is primarily used for patients who are being treated for social phobia. The SIAS has shown good convergent and divergent validity (Heimberg, Mueller, Holt, Hope, & Liebowitz, 1992; Mattick & Clarke, 1998) and adequately discriminates between individuals diagnosed with social phobia and other anxiety disorders (Brown et al., 1997). Finally, the Health Anxiety Inventory, short version (HAI; Salkovskis, Rimes, & Warwick, 2002), a measure designed to assess anxiety about one's health, is typically used for individuals with a principal diagnosis of hypochondriasis. For individuals with a principal diagnosis of a mood disorder such as major depressive disorder (MDD) or dysthymia, the BDI-II (described earlier) may be used as a weekly measure. The Brief Posttraumatic Diagnostic Scale (BPDS), designed to measure PTSD symptoms, can also be administered on a weekly basis (Foa, Cashman, Jaycox, & Perry, 1997).

Functional Analysis

Regardless of the diagnosis, a clear functional analysis of the patient's behavior is essential prior to beginning treatment. Several components are important to consider when diagnosing a patient based on a functional analysis. These include a close examination of symptom topography (including duration of illness, physical sensations, level of distress and interference from symptoms), triggers (situations, physical symptoms, places, thoughts, etc.), cognitions (beliefs about symptoms and misappraisals), behavioral responses to emotions (including avoidance of situations, places, people, or triggers, as well as escape behaviors), and the consequences of behavioral reactions (limiting quality of life, reduced "comfort zone," etc.).

In this case, Oscar presented with anxiety and avoidance of cues that were reminders of the lab accident. Many of his symptoms mimicked those associated with a PTSD reaction, and because Oscar believed his life was in danger at the time of the accident (the gas to which he was exposed was potentially life-threatening), the therapist considered assigning a diagnosis of PTSD (although Oscar did not meet full symptom criteria for the diagnosis). Oscar also presented with significant worry and anxiety about his work and several other topics, which may have been consistent with a diagnosis of GAD. However, after further investigation, it appeared that all the topics of worry were in some way related to the lab accident, which therefore precluded a diagnosis of GAD. After exploring Oscar's lifelong history of health-related anxiety, as well as his strong belief that he had been physically hurt by the exposure to the toxic gas (despite reassurance from medical personnel that he was physically fine) and his engagement in excessive reassurance-seeking from family members, the therapist assigned a diagnosis of hypochondriasis.

For Oscar, this functional analysis was particularly important in guiding treatment planning and application of the UP. Beyond diagnostic considerations, functional analyses are an essential aspect of determining which procedures may be most helpful for patients. Oscar's extensive avoidance of both the laboratory, where he was originally exposed to toxic gas, and somatic sensations associated with what he believed would indicate toxic poisoning provided several important contexts for developing and creating emotion exposures. As we have mentioned, one noteworthy difference when comparing the UP and traditional CBT protocols is that the focus of treatment techniques in the UP is on an individual's particular emotional symptoms, whereas CBT protocols apply the same strategies to all individuals in a specific diagnostic category. This difference allows the UP techniques to be tailored individually to each patient and further highlights the necessity of a clear functional analysis rather than reliance on diagnostic categories for treatment planning.

COMPONENTS OF TREATMENT

The structure of the UP outlines fifteen 45- to 50-minute individual treatment sessions, held on a weekly basis. However the final three sessions (Sessions 13, 14, and 15) may be held every other week to allow patients to consolidate gains and to provide somewhat of a "taper" off the intensive weekly therapy. However, this format for the final sessions is not a requirement, and it may be more beneficial for the patient to continue to have weekly sessions if he or she might potentially have trouble using the treatment concepts consistently without the weekly reinforcement of sessions. Therefore, spacing of the final sessions is determined by the therapist, who takes into consideration the patient's progress and any anticipated difficulties after treatment.

Currently, the UP comprises four basic components: (1) psychoeducation about emotions, including a review of the functional nature of emotions and how emotions become disordered; (2) alteration of antecedent cognitive misappraisals, an intensive antecedent-based emotional regulation procedure that directly facilitates the next two steps in treatment; (3) prevention of emotional avoidance; a broad-based effort that goes well beyond traditional attempts to prevent behavioral avoidance in phobic disorders by targeting cognitive, behavioral, and somatic experiential avoidance; and (4) modification of EDBs, which implements specific behaviors not associated with the emotion that is disordered. This treatment takes place in the context of provoking emotional expression (emotion exposure) through situational, internal, and somatic (interoceptive) cues, as well as through standard mood induction exercises, and differs from patient to patient only in the situational cues and exercises utilized. In addition, "exposure" is not concep-

tualized as a mechanism of action. Rather, successfully provoking emotions creates a setting condition to implement the essential treatment components. Emotion exposures begin with general stimuli (e.g., mood induction and interoceptive provocation) and are later tailored to address each patient's particular concerns and symptoms. Although each session addresses a specific component of the protocol, the expectation is that patients then "carry through" to future sessions the strategies they learn (e.g., patients learn cognitive reappraisal strategies in Session 3 but are expected to continue to use cognitive reappraisal for emotion exposures conducted throughout the remainder of the treatment).

Psychoeducation

Psychoeducation about the nature and function of emotions is directly addressed in the first session. This component is common to most CBT protocols, although the focus is expanded to include the function of many different emotions (anger, sadness, etc.), in addition to the function of anxiety. Patients are provided with information about the cognitive, physiological, and behavioral sequelae of emotional reactions and how these three components interact. It is important that the patient begin to consider that his or her reactions are functional and serve the purpose of providing information about the environment, in addition to protection from harm. This three-component model is then applied to a recent situation or event that the patient experienced, so that he or she may better understand the aspects of each component and how they interact.

Another important aspect of psychoeducation is a discussion of negative reinforcement. Specifically, this is a detailed discussion of how the patient's behavioral response to an emotional episode (usually escape or some form of emotional avoidance) is problematic, because it reduces the emotion in the short term (i.e., by removing the person from the emotional stimulus) but reinforces the cycle of emotions in the long term (i.e., by teaching the person that escape/avoidance is the only way to manage these feelings in the future). It is extremely important that the patient understand the connection between behavioral responses and reinforcement of emotion, so that he or she is better able to appreciate the purpose and function of emotion exposures introduced in future sessions.

Antecedent Cognitive Reappraisal

Cognitive therapy, initially developed by Aaron T. Beck to treat depression (Beck, 1967/1972; Beck, Rush, Shaw, & Emery, 1979), has become a fundamental part of psychological treatments. Particularly common in individuals with emotional disorders are tendencies toward appraisals and interpretations of external events that are characterized by cognitive biases, such as the tendency to overestimate the likelihood of the occurrence of negative events and to underestimate the ability to cope with these events. Thus, the aim of cognitive therapy is to evaluate objectively the likelihood of these negative appraisals and to incorporate more realistic, evidence-based appraisals of the outcome of a situation. On the surface, this technique may appear to be a way to suppress or control negative thoughts by "rationalizing" them, and occasionally, this is how cognitive therapy is incorrectly used, as noted by Hayes, Strosahl, and Wilson (1999). However, this strategy can also be conceptualized from an emotion regulation perspective, if reappraisals of threat and negativity are made *prior to* the emotionally arousing situation. Data from the emotion regulation literature have demonstrated that use of antecedent cognitive reappraisals prior to experiencing heightened levels of emotional arousal can have a salutary effect on the later expression of negative emotions (Gross, 1998; Richards & Gross, 2000; Thayer, 2000). Antecedent cognitive reappraisal has also been shown to reduce the subjective experience of negative emotion (Gross, 1998).

The UP has identified two fundamental antecedent misappraisals: the probability of a negative event happening (probability overestimation) and the consequences if the negative event did happen (catastrophizing) (Barlow & Craske, 2000; Craske et al., 1992). Although a number of other misappraisals are noted in other, traditional CBT protocols, most misappraisals can be condensed into one of the two appraisals listed here. The patient must first begin to identify misappraisals that occur in anxiety- or emotion-provoking situations. He/she may be able to list a variety of misappraisals occurring in a situation, although initially the therapist may choose to focus on just one appraisal. Generally, the therapist can elicit appraisals by discussing a situation from either the self-monitoring forms from the previous week or a hypothetical situation. If the patient has trouble identifying misappraisals (or any appraisals at all), the therapist uses standard cognitive therapy techniques, such as questioning what the patient feared would happen in the situation and identifying *any* thoughts or reaction he or she might have had at the time. The goal of this process is to help the patient recognize that his or her emotional reactions are due, at least in part, to the appraisals or interpretations made about the situation. It is also important to note that interpretations of situations are based on past experience (e.g., it is very likely that a person who was teased by another person for giving an incorrect answer in class will appraise similar situations as negative and anxiety-provoking).

One other strategy used in the UP to identify and illustrate misappraisals is to present an ambiguous picture and ask the patient to interpret what is happening. Typically, the interpretation will in some way be related to the patient's primary symptoms, and it is useful for the patient to know that he or she is likely to appraise even neutral situations in a biased way, because his or her attention is focused on specific cues and/or threats.

The next step is to assist the patient in reappraising interpretations of situations by examining the evidence for and against each interpretation and generating an alternative appraisal. Again, standard cognitive restructuring strategies may be used, although the focus of cognitive reappraisal is slightly different. First, the patient is not encouraged to "change" his or her thoughts to "more realistic" ones; rather, he or she is asked to allow for other possible interpretations that may be more likely based on the evidence, while allowing all possible appraisals to exist in his or her mind, without attaching too much significance to any particular one. The goal of antecedent cognitive reappraisal is flexibility in thinking and acknowledging that many possible outcomes may exist.

In addition, it is important that the therapist utilize cognitive strategies to help the patient identify his or her "core" cognitive misappraisal. This misappraisal, usually a statement about the patient's self or self-worth (i.e., "I am worthless" or "I am incompetent"), may underlie many of his or her surface appraisals in various situations. Once the core misappraisal has been identified, the therapist illustrates how this misappraisal triggers emotional reactions in various situations and helps the patient examine whether the misappraisal is actually accurate.

As mentioned earlier, the emotion-regulating properties of cognitive reappraisal are present only when reappraisal strategies are used *prior* to engagement in an emotionally salient task. Patients have a strong tendency to use the reappraisal techniques at the height of emotional experiences, in an attempt to minimize uncomfortable emotions. However, this is incorrect, and the therapist must be aware when a patient attempts to use reappraisal strategies in this way. Using reappraisal techniques prior to a task may help the patient be more willing to engage in the task and allow for greater emotion provocation during the task, as opposed to using the techniques at the height of emotion, which is best conceptualized as a form of emotional avoidance.

Prevention of Emotional Avoidance

Evidence now points to a key concept in understanding emotional disorders, attempts to down-regulate or avoid unexpected, excessive emotions leading to the development of increasingly intense emotional experiences—a process that is central to depression, anger, and excitement (mania), in addition to fear (Barlow, 1988; Gross, 2002; Gross & Levenson, 1997). For example, Roemer, Litz, Orsillo, and Wagner (2001) found that veterans with PTSD were more likely to withhold negative *and* positive emotions compared to veterans without PTSD. Evidence on the deleterious consequences of avoidance strategies also extends to the calming and relaxation techniques that were a significant part of earlier treatment protocols (Barlow & Cerny, 1988). When relaxation strategies are used specifically for the purpose of reducing uncomfortable emotions in the moment, these techniques can actually become counterproductive. Similar results have been obtained in examinations of the impact of distraction techniques (Craske, Street, & Barlow, 1989; Craske, Street, Jayaraman, & Barlow, 1991; Kamphuis & Telch, 2000) and safety signals (Salkovskis, Clark, Hackmann, Wells, & Gelder, 1999; Sloan & Telch, 2002; Wells et al., 1995).

The concept of emotional avoidance is likely to be particularly important for patients who do not physically avoid or escape situations but still experience high levels of anxiety without much relief. The therapist should convey that even if the person stays physically in the situation, he or she is likely to engage in a number of other subtle behaviors to prevent full emotional arousal. In the UP, emotional avoidance strategies are behaviors that prevent the full experience of emotion in a situation, as opposed to EDBs, which are behavioral consequences of the experience of emotion (described later in the chapter). *Any* technique or strategy the patient uses to reduce or to down-regulate emotions may be conceptualized as an emotional avoidance strategy, and it is essential that emotional avoidance be eliminated prior to engagement in emotion exposures, to allow for full emotional processing. Therefore, a very detailed description of individual emotional avoidance strategies must be obtained for each patient.

We have identified three general categories of emotional avoidance strategies: (1) subtle behavioral avoidance, (2) cognitive avoidance, and (3) safety signals (see Table 5.1 for examples). Subtle behavioral avoidance strategies may consist of a number of different behaviors, with certain behaviors occurring more frequently with particular disorders. For example, the avoidance of caffeine in panic disorder or social phobia (prior to a social engagement) is an attempt to keep physiological symptoms from becoming strong in anxiety-provoking situations. Patients with social phobia may also avoid eye contact or wear sunglasses when interacting in social settings. Individuals with GAD may excessively plan, prepare, or write "to do" lists in an attempt to control potentially negative outcomes. At the same time, procrastination is also a form of subtle behavioral avoidance, if a particular task or project seems too emotionally arousing for the patient. It is very important to conduct a functional analysis of the subtle behaviors to determine which ones are avoidance strategies, that is, behaviors that serve to reduce or avoid emotional experience and are functional responses to situations. And, notably, what may be an avoidance strategy for one person may be a functional response for another.

Cognitive avoidance strategies are typically more difficult to identify, because they tend to occur outside of the patient's awareness. Some of these strategies include distraction, "tuning out," and mentally checking lists or reviewing past conversations. However, data also suggest that worry and rumination actually function as a way to down-regulate and avoid emotions (e.g.,

TABLE 5.1. Examples of Emotional Avoidance Strategies

Emotional Avoidance Strategy	Disorder most usually associated
1. Subtle behavioral avoidance	
• Avoid eye contact	Social phobia
• Avoid drinking caffeine	PDA
• Attempt to control breathing	PDA
• Avoid exercise/physiological arousal (interoceptive avoidance)	PDA/depression
• Avoid touching sink/toilet	OCD
• Procrastination (avoiding emotionally salient tasks)	GAD
2. Cognitive avoidance	
• Distraction (reading a book, watching television)	Depression/PDA
• "Tune out" during a conversation	Social phobia
• Reassure self that everything is OK	GAD
• Try to prevent thoughts from coming into mind	OCD
• Distraction from reminders of trauma	PTSD
• Force self to "think positive"	Depression
• Worry	GAD
• Rumination	Depression
• Thought suppression	All disorders
3. Safety signals	
• Carry cell phone	PDA/GAD
• Carry empty medication bottles	PDA
• Hold onto "good luck" charms	OCD
• Carry items that are associated with positive experiences (e.g., teddy bears, pictures)	GAD/depression
• Have mace at all times	PTSD
• Carry water bottle	PDA
• Have reading material/prayer books on hand	GAD
• Carry sunglasses or item to hide face/eyes	Social phobia

Borkovec, 1994). The function of worry is to enable the person to prepare for a possible threat. However, when someone experiences chronic worry and associated anxiety, his or her attention is focused on the future as opposed to the present moment. Research has shown that when confronted with an emotionally arousing event, chronic worriers do not experience the full emotional impact of that event, because (1) they have been "bracing" themselves for something bad to happen, and (2) their focus has already shifted to other, future negative outcomes (Borkovec, Hazlett-Stevens, & Diaz, 1999). Therefore, the worry functions as a cognitive avoidance strategy and only serves as a maladaptive attempt to gain control over seemingly uncontrollable future events. Obsessions, common to individuals with OCD, may also function in a similar manner.

Safety signals are most common to patients with PDA, although may also be present in individuals with GAD, OCD, or other emotional disorders. Safety signals include any object that

the patient carries to feel more safe or "comfortable," particularly if he or she is entering an emotionally arousing situation. Safety signals can range from actual medication (such as benzodiazepines for reducing physiological arousal or medications for gastrointestinal distress) to empty medication bottles, to "lucky" objects (e.g., a talisman, teddy bear, "lucky" pen, etc.). Regardless of the object itself, if its function is to help the patient reduce emotional arousal in the moment, then it also is problematic, because it feeds into the cycle of negative reinforcement.

To combat the problems associated with emotional avoidance, the therapist introduces the concept of "emotional awareness training" to assist the patient in preventing the emotional avoidance strategies he/she uses regularly. Emotional awareness training comprises several components, which include staying in the present moment, relinquishing behavioral avoidance strategies and safety signals, and fully engaging with emotions as they come and go. This requires some practice for the patient, and an in-session emotion provocation and practice of emotional awareness is often helpful. After identifying the range of strategies, the therapist asks the patient to begin to monitor (and attempt to prevent) the use of the strategies for the remainder of the treatment sessions.

Modifying EDBs

As noted by Izard (1971), data and hypotheses from emotion theory suggest that the most efficient and effective way to change emotions is by changing responses to them; thus, it is conceivable that the mechanism of change during an exposure is to prevent the action tendency associated with a particular emotional experience. Over the past several decades, research has focused on these action tendencies, and changing action tendencies has become an important treatment component for anxiety, as well as for other emotional disorders (Barlow, 1988). For example, Beck and colleagues (1979) based a large part of their treatment for depression on changing the action tendencies of their patients to behave in a "passive, retarded, and apathetic manner" (p. 312). More recently, behavioral activation strategies have become a central feature of newer treatments for depression (Dimidjian, Martell, Addis, & Herman-Dunn, Chapter 8, this volume; Dimidjian et al., 2006; Jacobson, Martell, & Dimidjian, 2001).

In fact, these strategies go well beyond simply preventing escape from fearful situations. Laughter, humor, and related facial expressions have been induced during successful paradoxical intention strategies (Frankl, 1960). These strategies have also effectively counteracted fear (Ascher, 1980). Originally, the proposed mechanism of action was thought to be the induction of cognitive changes, although it seems plausible that these strategies may have worked through the prevention of behavioral responses and modification of action tendencies (facial expressions) previously associated with the emotion. Linehan (1993) adapted the strategy of modifying action tendencies with much success in her treatment for individuals with borderline personality disorder. Hayes's acceptance and commitment therapy (ACT; Hayes et al., 1999) emphasizes the importance of behaviorally active responses to emotions, with the purpose of implementing a sense of control over one's responses to emotions, as opposed to decreasing the occurrence of unwanted internal events.

To distinguish action tendencies from avoidance strategies (described earlier), the UP has termed these behavioral responses to emotions as "emotion-driven behaviors" (EDBs). Whereas the function of emotional avoidance strategies is to down-regulate or suppress emotions, EDBs include a specific set of "reactive" behaviors associated with each emotion. For example, the EDB for a panic attack is escape (fight or flight), whereas that for anxiety is hypervigilance. Similarly, the emotion of anger elicits an EDB of attacking/defending, and the EDB for sadness is cognitive, emotional, and physical slowing and withdrawal (see Table 5.2 for examples of EDBs associated with different emotional disorders). It is important to note, however, that the therapist must focus on changing EDBs, in addition to preventing emotional avoidance. For example, a patient with social phobia may be able to maintain eye contact and fully engage in social situations, but he may escape the situation when his anxiety rises to the level of panic. On the contrary, this same patient may be able to stay in the situation as long as needed, but he may be distracting himself the whole time or avoiding conversations with people. Clearly, both scenarios are problematic, because the patient is preventing himself from learning that he can experience emotions at their fullest without leaving the situation. It should also be noted that, in practice, avoidance and EDBs may be difficult to distinguish, and this distinction can be downplayed with a given patient, if necessary or clinically relevant.

After the concept of EDBs is introduced, patients begin to track EDBs on the self-monitoring forms and eventually focus on changing EDBs. This can be a very concrete exercise for the patient, because he or she is instructed to "do something different than he or she would typically do." The Changing EDBs monitoring form is illustrated in Figure 5.2.

These concepts are extended during the in-session emotion exposures created by the therapist and individually tailored to the patient's presenting symptoms. In-session exposures can range from an imaginal exposure to a past emotional event (for PTSD or GAD), a conversation with a stranger (for social phobia), going into a dirty bathroom (for OCD), or watching a sad movie or movie clip (for MDD or

TABLE 5.2. Examples of Emotion-Driven Behaviors and Incompatible Behaviors

EDBs	Disorder most usually associated	Incompatible behaviors
Calling relatives to check on safety	GAD	Restricting contact/calling relatives
Perfectionistic behavior at work or home	GAD	Leaving things untidy or unfinished
Checking locks, stove, or other appliances	OCD	Repeatedly locking–unlocking and turning on–off until memory is unclear
Leaving (escaping from) a theater, religious service, or other crowded area	PDA	Move to the center of the crowd. Smile or produce nonfearful facial expressions
Social withdrawal	Depression	Behavioral activation
Leaving (escaping) a social situation	Social phobia	Staying in situation and approaching people
Verbally/physically attacking someone when in an argument	PTSD	Remove self from situation and/or practice relaxation techniques
Hypervigilance	All disorders	Focus attention on specific task at hand; meditation; relaxation

dysthymia). The goal of the emotion exposure is to elicit any emotion, so that the patient has the opportunity to practice the techniques taught in treatment (antecedent cognitive reappraisal, modifying EDBs, and prevention of emotional avoidance). With this new conceptualization, the exposure to the emotion is the necessary mechanism of action for emotional change. Thus, the actual situational context of the exposure becomes less important. Therapists must be creative in the design of the exposure to maximize the emotion provocation for the patient.

DETAILED DESCRIPTION OF PROTOCOL

The following session descriptions and accompanying transcripts are from the case of "Oscar," described earlier, treated by one of the authors (D. H. B).

Session 1

In the first session, the therapist reviews treatment logistics, including session length and structure, the therapist's role, and the importance of prioritizing treatment. Sessions are approximately 45–50 minutes in duration and occur weekly for the first 12 weeks and 2 weeks apart for Sessions 13–15. The collaborative na-

ture of treatment is emphasized, including the importance of feedback from the patient. Following this introduction is a detailed review of the presenting complaint. In this review, the therapist focuses on emotions experienced and any strategies the patient uses to manage these emotions. Below, Oscar describes situational avoidance resulting from the lab accident.

THERAPIST: Let's review a couple of these things. When exactly was it that the incident occurred?

OSCAR: It was at the very end of May.

THERAPIST: Of course, it was an extraordinarily distressing incident. Would you say that over the last 6 months you've noticed any change in the level of distress?

OSCAR: For a few different reasons the incident does not come up in my mind as often as it did in the beginning. It could be because it happened a while ago, or it could be that I currently do no acid work in these labs. In fact, somebody else does it for me.

THERAPIST: So that's something that was arranged then?

OSCAR: Yes, my advisors arranged it, by my request. It wasn't a big deal. There is another person in my group that was happy to do it. I help her with something else. I know that given your recommendations it is probably not the way to proceed, but at the time it seemed like a good idea.

THERAPIST: Oh sure. It may be, and of course everything we do will be fully collaborative, no surprises, but it may be that we talk about the possibility of getting you back into some of these situations.

OSCAR: I do encounter situations in the lab that I work in now where I get anxious. It could be a small thing like walking past someone working with acids, and wondering "Did some liquid get on me?" You get little itches here and there, and then you attribute them to something instead of just dismissing it.

After reviewing the presenting problem, the therapist discusses the treatment model, with a focus on normative emotional experience and how emotions can become disordered. Emotions are presented as natural reactions to the environment that motivate adaptive behavior. The therapist describes that the goal of treatment is to help the patient increase awareness and control of emotions that are excessive. Negative reinforcement is introduced as a way that cognitions and behaviors can serve to maintain emotional disorders. The therapist describes this as an effective strategy that decreases emotion in the short term but contributes further to the disorder in the long run. For Oscar, health-related anxiety had become so pervasive that even minor physical sensations led to fear of serious illness or death. In this discussion, the therapist emphasized the concept that emotions themselves do not present a threat or danger, and that any emotion passes with time.

The three-component model is described as a framework for examining emotions by dividing them into components (cognitions, behaviors, and physiological sensations), thereby making them more manageable. The therapist uses an example relevant to the patient's experience to demonstrate the contribution of each component to his or her emotional experience. The therapist guides the patient in identifying each component in this example and presents the model as the structural basis for treatment. Each component is addressed separately over the course of treatment as contributing to the overall emotion and interacting with the other components. A brief introduction to the necessity of provoking emotions as part of treatment is also presented.

THERAPIST: You may know that emotion is a good thing. It helps us to function, and it is very adaptive evolutionarily. It motivates us to engage in a behavior that would protect us or sustain the species. And it is absolutely fine as long as it occurs at the right time, but sometimes it occurs at the wrong time, such as when the danger is not present or should be tolerable. And in that case emotions can keep you, to some extent, from doing what you want to do, such as, in your case, getting into the lab.

OSCAR: Right, among other things.

THERAPIST: We deal with these emotions by trying to break them down into different components. Emotions, as you have pointed out, can be very overwhelming. They grab you and can feel like a big blob. You can be overwhelmed by these feelings and the necessity to do what the emotion is telling you to do. And to get away from this big blob, it will be much easier to deal with it one piece at a time. Now in order to do that, we are going to have you monitor your emotions, and we want you to actually elicit some of these emotions. We want to train you to be an expert observer of your emotions.

In this session, the therapist provides a rationale for homework assignments, including prospective emotion monitoring, which provides a means of recording ongoing experiences throughout treatment and increasing awareness of emotions, as well as exercises designed to elicit emotion outside of the treatment session. General emotion monitoring with the WRAD is employed beginning in Session 1. This session's exercise includes assigning a mood induction CD we put together that includes selections such as the theme from the movie *Schindler's List* and the *Forrest Gump* soundtrack to listen to before Session 2. The patient is asked to listen to one or two songs at a time and to record emotional reactions to the music. This exercise introduces the concepts of provoking emotion and developing emotional awareness. Additionally, the patient is provided with a worksheet on which he or she is asked to break down an emotion from the week into the three-component model presented in session, by recording the thoughts, behaviors, and feelings specific to that example. The therapist should spend sufficient time in the first session to ensure that the patient understands the rationale for and importance of homework, and how to complete each of the forms.

Session 2

The therapist begins Session 2 with a review of the treatment model presented in Session 1. Any reservations or concerns about the treatment should be validated, and the rationale is reinforced in the context of the lack of success the patient has had with current emotion regulation strategies. Homework forms are then discussed in detail, and any difficulties in completion (e.g., procrastination) are addressed as needed. After reviewing the WRAD, the therapist reviews the three-component model worksheet and addresses any questions that arise. Particular attention is paid to the patient's understanding of the model and ability to identify the distinct components. The therapist then reviews the mood induction exercise in detail with the patient, focusing on identifying emotions experienced, and determining the patients level of awareness and ability to induce emotion.

THERAPIST: What were your reactions to the mood induction CD? Let's start with the first song.

OSCAR: For this one, I remember feeling anger.

THERAPIST: Are you aware of any thoughts you were having at the time? How did you know you were angry?

OSCAR: I'm not sure. It is kind of a feeling of relief in a way. It's kind of like when you're angry and you scream. It's as if I'm letting out some anger through the music, like the music is doing it for me.

THERAPIST: Any thoughts?

OSCAR: Not that I'm aware of.

THERAPIST: A lot of people have difficulty identifying these kinds of things. But the point of this and future exercises is to get you to be more introspective and aware of your emotions.

The therapist then introduces cognitive reappraisal. "Appraisals" are described as important aspects of the experience of emotion, which often occur automatically. "Cognitive errors," or "thinking traps," are defined as appraisals that are repeatedly and automatically

assigned to situations at the expense of other possible interpretations. When these appraisals limit the flexibility of interpretation, they can contribute to the cycle of negative emotion. With this background, the therapist guides the patient in generating examples from his or her experience. For Oscar, physical sensations were frequently interpreted as signs of serious medical problems that might lead to death.

An in-session exercise is used to demonstrate the concept of cognitive flexibility. The therapist shows the patient an "ambiguous" picture (we use a card from the Thematic Apperception Test [TAT]; Morgan & Murray, 1935) to which many cognitive appraisals can be assigned. The therapist instructs the patient to look at the picture for approximately 30 seconds, then elicits both the patient's primary interpretation and at least two or three alternative interpretations. Additionally, the patient is asked what specifically may have contributed to the automatic appraisal (e.g., memories of similar situations, specific details in the picture). This exercise is used to demonstrate the way that situations can be interpreted in many ways, if all available information is considered. Probability overestimation, or the tendency to assume a high likelihood of the occurrence of a negative event, and catastrophizing, or assuming that the consequences of an event will be beyond the individual's ability to cope, are presented as two cognitive errors common to all emotional disorders. The therapist guides the patient in beginning to identify these errors in the context of his or her experience. Below, the therapist discusses both of these cognitive errors based on the example described earlier in which Oscar touched a residue on a plate at a department store.

THERAPIST: Sitting here now, what is the probability that the residue was the acid?

OSCAR: Maybe, one in a million—very, very small.

THERAPIST: One in a million?

OSCAR: No, there are millions of plates. Probably zero. Vanishingly small.

THERAPIST: When you are right in front of it, feeling emotional, what do you think the probability is?

OSCAR: That's not something that came into my mind. Like a number or something?

THERAPIST: Well, that's typically not the way we would think about it. But thinking back on it in your emotional mind, what do you think you may have estimated as the probability at that moment?

OSCAR: Maybe 25%.

THERAPIST: So you can see the interplay of the two: "This residue is the acid, then I'm going to die." Both thinking the worst—"I'm going to die," and overestimating the probability—"this is an acid." What we want to do is to make it crystal clear what your automatic thoughts are, and second, what the alternatives are, just as you know there are many truths to a situation, including the rational one in the front of your head and the emotional one in the back of your head. One of the ways we approach this is to try to weaken the irrational, strengthen the rational, and give you multiple perspectives.

General strategies to address cognitive errors are presented, including identification of thinking traps and generation of alternative appraisals, with more specific reappraisal techniques introduced in the next session. Over the next week, the patient is asked to begin monitoring automatic appraisals by identifying the emotional trigger, the subsequent appraisal, and whether the appraisal represents probability overestimation or catastrophizing, in addition to monitoring daily emotions with the WRAD.

Session 3

This session begins with a review of reactions to the previous session and addresses lingering questions about automatic appraisals. The WRAD is reviewed for the remainder of the treatment as needed, with more focus on the more specific monitoring forms. In reviewing the cognitive appraisals monitoring form, the therapist provides guidance on identifying thinking traps and tries to focus the patient's attention on the "core" appraisal through the use of Socratic questioning. The excerpt below is from a discussion of an example in which Oscar suspected he had been exposed to a chemical in the lab.

THERAPIST: So you were worried about being exposed to this chemical, but what specifically were you thinking about the chemical?

OSCAR: It's toxic.

THERAPIST: And what does that mean?

OSCAR: It's dangerous to me.

THERAPIST: And what?

OSCAR: And, I might die.

THERAPIST: Now that is what we want, the real core of it, what is driving this interpretation. A lot of these anxious thoughts often do come down to dying. So you think, "I'm going to die and I need to start looking for the signs of impending death"—the scratchy throat and such. Of course, anyone would be scared or anxious with that type of appraisal.

The therapist then engages the patient in a more detailed discussion of cognitive reappraisal, focusing on flexible thinking. The importance of identifying core appraisals is emphasized as the level at which reappraisal will be focused. Countering probability overestimation and decatastrophizing strategies are presented as a way to generate alternative appraisals and to place less focus on the automatic appraisal. Countering probability estimation involves drawing on past evidence to examine how realistic the patient's estimation is when experiencing an emotion. The therapist guides the patient in making concrete estimations and comparing the original estimation to a more realistic one. Decatastrophizing involves helping the patient to identify his or her ability to cope with the feared situation using past evidence and specific examples (e.g., similar experiences in the past). It is important to communicate that these strategies do not eliminate negative appraisals, but they provide greater flexibility and allow the patient to gain perspective on the feared situations.

Over the next three sessions, the patient is asked to continue to monitor automatic appraisals and to note the strategies used to improve interpretive flexibility. The patient is asked to generate at least one additional interpretation for each automatic appraisal identified. The therapist again emphasizes that there is no "correct" interpretation; rather, the range of possibilities should be considered.

Session 4

In Session 4, the therapist reviews the cognitive reappraisal monitoring form in detail and clarifies any residual questions or problems. At this time, the therapist ensures the patient's ability to identify automatic appraisals and to generate alternatives before moving on to the next topic of treatment, which focuses on the behavioral component of emotion. First, EDBs are described. A description of the adaptive nature of emotion as a strong motivator for behavior is provided, followed by how EDBs can become maladaptive and serve to maintain disordered emotional experiences. The therapist also distinguishes between EDBs and emotional avoidance in this session. The patient is asked to generate examples of EDBs from his or her experience. In the transcript below, Oscar describes personal examples of EDBs, including seeking reassurance regarding physical symptoms from his mother, a physician.

THERAPIST: Given the past examples we've talked about, what would you say are some of the behaviors these emotions cause you to do?

OSCAR: One would be to leave where I am, so that's different than not going in the first place.

THERAPIST: And how do you feel when you get out?

OSCAR: Well, a little better, but then I start worrying again.

THERAPIST: But for the moment you feel a little better, and certainly better than you would imagine feeling if you had stayed in the situation. What are some others?

OSCAR: Calling my mother?

THERAPIST: Right. Particularly when you call to check in about physical symptoms. What effect do you think this has on your emotions?

OSCAR: Well, I've been trying to think about that and I'm not sure. Sometimes when I call my mother, for example, while I'm speaking to her, it certainly makes me a little calmer. Other times it does not. But has it ever made the problem completely go away? Probably not.

THERAPIST: So it does make you feel better in the short term? You feel reassured, you escape. Do you do other checks?

OSCAR: Yeah, like scanning my body internally. Or if there are other people around, I'll ask them if they smell anything.

THERAPIST: What happens is when you call your mother or engage in these other behaviors and feel better temporarily, that strengthens that relationship. It's a very powerful concept. So what will you do next time? Something that you know will make you feel better. But the problem is, that increases the probability that the next time a little trigger occurs, the whole sequence will follow.

OSCAR: So you're saying that after a while, the behavior will be connected with even smaller triggers, which will seem bigger?

The therapist also guides the patient in understanding that EDBs may decrease the emotional experience in the short term but maintain or heighten the emotion in the long term. Though EDBs have helped the patient to attenuate the emotional experience to some degree, they have not been working as a long-term strategy to control emotions. Following this discussion, Oscar was able to identify an example of this concept.

OSCAR: I'm not sure if this is related, but at the beginning of the semester I was forced to be in the lab 2 days straight and I was really anxious, but I forced myself to stay. Now, being in that lab is not as big a deal.

THERAPIST: There, you broke the cycle. Because the fact is, those things you've been doing haven't been working and in fact make it worse. And you yourself found that if you don't do those things and stay in the situation, it works.

OSCAR: It feels a lot worse for a while.

THERAPIST: But in the long run it feels better.

OSCAR: Right.

THERAPIST: So things you do in the short run—wrestling with the emotion, trying to get rid of it—haven't worked.

OSCAR: Does it mean that I should try not to do these things?

THERAPIST: We want to get to a point that it is OK to have these emotions. Your emotions are going to happen. With you, they're not always happening at the right time, so what are we going to do? We need to pay a little less attention to them. And we also want to stop these behaviors that haven't been working.

Session 4 concludes with a brief introduction to emotion exposure. The therapist describes the rationale for emotion exposures and introduces an in-session exercise. Four slides designed to elicit emotion, selected from the International Affective Picture System (IAPS) slides (Center for the Study of Emotion and Attention, 2001), are presented sequentially to the patient on a computer screen. The slides we use are: a young child crying, a woman being held at knifepoint, a mutilated body, and a ski-jumper about to descend a ramp. The patient is instructed to attend to each slide for approximately 30 seconds and to notice any emotions that he or she experiences. After the presentation of each slide, the therapist asks the patient what emotions he or she is experiencing and for any reactions to the slide. During this exercise, the therapist emphasizes awareness of the emotion and minimization of any avoidance strategies. Additionally, the therapist demonstrates that many situations can trigger an emotion, including the slides from the exercise. It is important for the patient to be able to identify these reactions and their triggers. In the following sequence, the slide used was the photo of the mutilated body.

THERAPIST: (*following the presentation of the slide*) What is your reaction to this image?

OSCAR: Kind of disturbing.

THERAPIST: OK, let the emotion wash over you, just take it in.

OSCAR: I guess some anxiety, also not wanting to look at it.

THERAPIST: That's important, you wanted to turn away to . . . ?

OSCAR: To not see it anymore.

THERAPIST: To decrease the emotion?

OSCAR: Yeah.

THERAPIST: Any physical sensations?

OSCAR: I guess the anxiety comes along with maybe with a feeling of adrenaline rush. And the kind of feeling of tension. Like something I want to get out. I feel like there's something building up.

THERAPIST: OK. We can take the picture away now.

OSCAR: I feel like I'm almost going to cry at this point. (*Begins to cry.*)

THERAPIST: That's OK. And, now the emotion probably feels a little more intense.

OSCAR: Yeah, but the tension loosens up a bit.

THERAPIST: Thoughts going through your head?

OSCAR: It's interesting, I was really more aware of myself than actually thinking about the picture.

THERAPIST: What about yourself?

OSCAR: It's almost like my muscles are hurting, from being tense.

THERAPIST: You see, all of these feelings, some of which might even seem a bit strange, are part of your emotion.

For homework, in addition to continuing with cognitive reappraisal, the patient is asked to begin designing emotion exposures for the coming week. At this stage in treatment, general instructions are given, but the therapist is not yet helping the patient to design exposures. The patient is encouraged to enter situations that may elicit unwanted emotions. The patient is asked to monitor progress and obstacles that arise. Additionally, the patient is given a form to monitor EDBs over the next week.

Session 5

This session begins with a review of the homework, with a particular focus on the EDBs monitoring form. The therapist then reviews emotion exposures completed in the past week. It is important to validate any concerns about the exposures and to encourage the patient to seek out opportunities to experience emotion. In the excerpt below, Oscar experienced a high level of anxiety following identification of a strange smell in a chemistry lab. The day after this incident, he entered the same lab and did not experience the expected anxiety.

THERAPIST: What are some other possibilities as to why you didn't have a spike of anxiety this morning?

OSCAR: I had already taken the clonazepam.

THERAPIST: Anything else?

OSCAR: I didn't smell anything. I went through a different door.

THERAPIST: Did you expect to have a difficult time going back into the lab today?

OSCAR: Yes.

THERAPIST: But you didn't?

OSCAR: Right. Or was the anxiety from that not sufficient to make a noticeable difference from the already high anxiety? So throughout the day, I wonder every time I cough a little bit.

THERAPIST: Is there the possibility also that having survived yesterday with nothing more than a suspicious scratchy throat, your thoughts about the danger lessened a bit?

OSCAR: Yeah, maybe a little bit. But I'm still waiting for the delayed reaction. But there is the constant internal discussion.

THERAPIST: Tell me about that.

OSCAR: First, there is no reason for it to smell in that part of the room. That's one thing. The other thing is, if it were actually this chemical and it were enough to be dangerous, I should have had a more immediate reaction in terms of much more coughing and wheezing, that type of thing. Then I come back saying, "But I'm feeling this or that, and what if it's some other type of chemical?"

THERAPIST: OK, the one good thing about this incident, although clearly distressing to you, is that it really gives us something to work with. These thoughts and behaviors that have been maintaining these emotions have become so automatic that in order to change them, we need you to fully experience these emotions.

Following the homework review, the therapist introduces the concept of emotional avoidance, describing how avoidance is harmful in both maintaining negative emotion and preventing the patient from engaging in certain situations. Types of avoidance, including subtle behavioral (e.g., procrastination), cognitive (e.g., distraction) and safety signals (e.g., carrying a medication bottle), are introduced. The patient is asked to generate personally relevant examples of avoidance. As with the description of EDBs, the therapist emphasizes that avoidance can work in the short term but is not a long-term solution.

THERAPIST: There are also a number of things you do to avoid even getting these emotional reactions. For example, you didn't go to the lab on Friday.

OSCAR: A better example is the lab where the incident happened. Even on a day that I'm feeling good, I avoid it.

THERAPIST: Those are the easy ones to see,

when you flat out don't go there. There are some other things that are often so subtle that we're not even aware of them. For example, some people will give up caffeine.

OSCAR: Yeah, I found myself doing that. In the past few months I have stopped drinking coffee. And I try to avoid things that will make me uncomfortable, like taking the stairs.

THERAPIST: Your tendency right now is to seek to avoid and to try to suppress or make emotions less intense. Attempts to control, diminish, or decrease them have the paradoxical effect of increasing them in the long run. There are a variety of these subtle and less subtle ways to avoid and try to get rid of emotions.

An in-session exercise to demonstrate emotional avoidance is then completed. An image intended to evoke emotion is chosen by the therapist from the IAPS slides and presented on a computer screen. The patient is instructed to look at the image for approximately 30 seconds and to attempt to not think about the image during that time. The patient can use any avoidance strategy he or she chooses but must continue looking at the image. The therapist then takes the image away and asks what strategies the patient used and how successful they were. This exercise demonstrates that avoiding a situation or trigger entails thinking about it in some respect, which prevents avoidance from being successful.

At the end of the session, a brief "emotional awareness training" is provided. Awareness is framed as "not avoiding" or as allowing emotions to occur without attempts to suppress or control them. An Awareness of Emotions handout (see Figure 5.3) is provided and reviewed. The handout includes specific instructions to guide the patient in accepting and understanding emotions to interrupt the cycle of negative emotion. The therapist emphasizes that rather than eliminating emotion, awareness and acceptance of emotion will the patient help to gain greater control over disordered emotions.

Homework includes monitoring any emotional avoidance strategies that the patient engages in over the week, continuing to monitor EDBs, and engaging in general emotion exposures. The patient is asked this week also to note the degree of emotional awareness during each exposure by rating awareness on a scale

Components of "Emotional Awareness"

1. Allowing oneself to *fully experience* emotions as they happen.

2. Focusing on being in the *present moment*, not "living" in the future or in the past.

3. *Allowing emotions to come and go*, without trying to push away feelings or trying to hold on to certain feelings. When you allow yourself to experience a negative emotion, then you are able to process it and move forward. If you don't give yourself permission to experience the emotion but push it away, then it becomes a "tidal wave" of emotion that feels very out of control.

4. *Being aware of your emotions does not always "feel good."* However, if will allow you to move past the experience, instead of getting stuck trying to push it away, which only reinfoces its power.

5. Awareness does *not necessarily mean acceptance of the situation or environment. Instead, we are focusing on acceptance of one's emotional reaction to it, before possibly acting in a different way.*

6. Having some *understanding* for one's own emotional experience. Getting "mad" or "frustrated" with yourself or saying "I'm so stupid for feeling this way" will only make you want to control and resist emotional experiences even more. This treatment focuses on increasing the range of emotional experience, instead of keeping it restricted. This includes allowing oneself to be sad, frustrated, and anxious, as well as *letting it pass* when emotions have changed. Occasionally, it may also mean substituting a different behavior, such as smiling or laughing when afraid— or getting up and doing something when all you feel like doing is going to your room and going to sleep. But, again, these new actions must be coming from a place of really trying to change what you are doing, instead of "forcing" or "punishing" yourself into a new way of behaving.

FIGURE 5.3. Awareness of emotions.

from 0 (*No awareness*) to 100 (*Complete awareness*).

Session 6

Following a detailed homework review, Session 6 introduces the third component of emotion by focusing on physical sensations. Following an introduction to the rationale for interoceptive exposure, the therapist and patient work through a list of exercises designed to elicit emotion through physical activation. Some examples include hyperventilating, spinning, and running in place. In addition, any exercises that are particularly relevant to the patient may be added. Prior to each exercise, the therapist demonstrates the exercise, and following the patient's completion of the exercise asks the patient to rate the intensity, distress, and similarity to physical sensations typically experiences during an emotion, each on a scale of 0 (*Not at all*) to 8 (*Very much*).

THERAPIST: So today we'll do a number of exer-cises to induce some of these physical sensations that are often the trigger for your anxiety and look at the intensity, distress, and whether it's similar to your experience. So the first one I'm going to ask you to do is the hyperventilation exercise. (*following the exercise*) What sensations are you feeling?

OSCAR: My legs are tingling, and I'm feeling a little dizzy. My throat is dry, for obvious reasons.

THERAPIST: Scan your body and notice any sensations.

OSCAR: A little tingling in the fingers and in the head. I feel like my eyes are kind of . . . not just dizziness, but a little unsteady, almost like they're vibrating.

THERAPIST: How intense were these sensations in totality from 0 to 8, with 8 being the most intense?

OSCAR: Maybe a 6?

THERAPIST: How distressing?

OSCAR: Maybe a 4, because I knew I was doing it myself?

THERAPIST: What about similarity? Any similarity to what you experience in the lab or other situations?

OSCAR: I wasn't able to describe it well, but definitely the eye thing.

THERAPIST: How similar would that be to your naturally occurring symptoms?

OSCAR: Well, I would give it a 4 just because the fingers and the legs tingling are not typically things that I experience, but the dizziness and the eye vibration are.

Following this exercise, the therapist and patient choose the most relevant exercises to engage in regularly over the next week. The patient is asked to complete the exercise several times a day, until the associated distress decreases. Additionally, for homework, the patient is asked to complete an Avoidance Hierarchy (see Figure 5.4) in which situations that the patient fears and avoids are listed. The therapist provides instructions on how to complete the form, which will be used to guide future emotion exposures. The patient is asked to continue with the general emotion exposures and to monitor EDBs.

AVOIDANCE HIERARCHY

Rate the degree to which you avoid each of the following situations due to the unpleasant feelings associated with them. For each, write the applicable number in the space provided.

Do not avoid		Hesitate to enter but rarely avoid		Sometimes avoid		Usually avoid		Always avoid
0	1	2	3	4	5	6	7	8
No distress		Slight distress		Definite distress		Strong distress		Extreme distress

	Description	Avoid	Distress
1 WORST			
2			
3			
4			
5			
6			
7			
8			
9			
10			

FIGURE 5.4. Example of an Avoidance Hierarchy.

Session 7

Session 7 serves as a review of the concepts presented in the first six sessions and a transition to the second half of treatment, which focuses on emotion exposures. The therapist reviews any interoceptive exercises done in the past week and encourages the patient to continue these exercises, if they were helpful. Because many of Oscar's symptoms involve physical sensations these exercises are continued outside of session. In particular, exercises that induced respiratory symptoms (e.g., hyperventilation) were encouraged because of his sensitivity to these symptoms. The Avoidance Hierarchy is also reviewed in detail to ensure that it can be used to guide treatment. It is important to have an appropriate range of avoidant situations to structure exposures, such that a graded exposure framework can be utilized. After discussing the homework, the therapist reviews treatment concepts in the context of the three-component model, and how cognition, behavior (including avoidance and EDBs), and physical sensations all contribute to the experience of emotion. At this stage in treatment, the review of concepts should be more idiographic, reflecting back on the patient's experience, and cover the concepts most relevant to the individual. After addressing any lingering questions, the therapist provides a rationale for situational emotion exposures.

THERAPIST: You want to get to a point where you can invite these emotions to come on and almost stand aside and watch them. The only way to do this is to experience the emotion, even at extreme levels. So now we're going to start purposefully engaging in exercises to provoke these emotions, with the goal of your being able to let an emotion wash over you, stand beside it, and cut out these emotion-driven behaviors, stripping away these procedures that prevent you from experiencing emotions.

OSCAR: In terms of distress, every time I go into one of the labs I get some anxiety, but I don't worry so much about it, because I feel now that I'm able to make it go away. Sometimes I feel that if I just went into the lab where the incident happened, I could handle it.

THERAPIST: We want to turn this around now. We want you to invite the emotion, not

thinking about whether you can handle it. And we also don't want you to talk yourself out of it. The process of experiencing emotion is harmless.

The therapist also describes the process of designing emotional exposures by using the Avoidance Hierarchy. Beginning with this session through the end of treatment, the patient is asked to monitor emotion exposures prospectively, including the situation, intensity of emotion prior to, during, and following the exposure, and any automatic appraisals and reappraisals identified. Three exposures are assigned by the therapist for homework, beginning at the bottom of the patient's hierarchy. The therapist and patient work together to design emotion exposures that are more challenging than the general exposures done thus far. Oscar's three chosen situations were entering a lab that contained hazardous chemicals, going to a challenging class at a gym (which he anticipated would lead to strong cardiovascular activation), and performing his lab work without the "extra" precautions he had utilized since the lab accident.

Sessions 8–12

Sessions 8–12 focus on both processing the emotion exposures completed outside of session and completing in-session exposures. The therapist begins by reviewing assigned exposures in detail, paying close attention to any obstacles or avoidance behaviors that may have prevented the patient from completing assigned exposures. An exposure near the top of Oscar's hierarchy was to use a public drinking fountain in the lab. Since the lab incident, he had been unable to use the fountain for fear that a dangerous substance might have contaminated the water. As is evident below, this proved very difficult for Oscar at first.

OSCAR: So the first one was the drinking fountain, which ended up pretty intense. I was really anticipating that it was going to be bad. I drank. In fact, I drank twice and felt fine, and a few hours later the anxiety started coming and lasted for about 3 days. It was pretty bad. And I really felt like calling my mother. Sometimes instead of worrying, I would try to really focus on the physical sensation and it helped, but it wouldn't go 100% away.

THERAPIST: Remember the goal is not to make it go 100% away. We are working toward not trying to make it go away. In *not* looking to make it go away, that is where the change can be made.

Oscar was encouraged to continue this exposure outside of session. Below is an excerpt from the following session.

THERAPIST: How was drinking from the water fountain?

OSCAR: The anxiety kind of came and went, and it really felt like this time around I was able to be really aware and pay attention to the feelings. And then it went away, and by the time I went to sleep, it had dissipated a lot, and it didn't come back the next day. And since then I've been drinking there every day, and it hasn't been a problem except maybe for some anticipatory anxiety. But, of course, going from there back to working with acids, you know, it feels like a slightly different beast.

THERAPIST: In what way does it feel different?

OSCAR: Because it feels like a real danger. With the water fountain there is no danger, but with the acid if I made a mistake, there is a real danger.

THERAPIST: What is the probability of a mistake?

OSCAR: One serious enough to be dangerous? Low, well, very low. They are very uncommon.

THERAPIST: And in the event of such a mistake, what safety procedures are available?

OSCAR: We have excellent safety precautions in place for just that reason. So if a mistake like that is made, there are built in safeties. Unless I really purposefully did something stupid, it couldn't produce any real danger.

In-session exposures are also employed in these sessions, which can be either situational or imaginal. Situational exposures relevant to the patient are chosen by the therapist and/or designed collaboratively with the patient. Imaginal exposures can be utilized when situational exposures are not appropriate for the patient or are prevented by logistics. Because Os-

car's feared situations were difficult to recreate in session, imaginal exposures were helpful. In these types of exposures, the patient describes an emotion exposure in a very detailed manner, trying to recreate the situation in as much detail as possible and to experience the emotion as fully as possible. The therapist leaves at least 15 minutes after the exposure to process the emotions experienced. Prior to attempting the exposure at the top of his hierarchy (entering the lab where the incident took place), the therapist guided Oscar through an imaginal exposure, allowing him to visualize this situation and to imagine any physical sensations that he might experience. Throughout these sessions, additional exposures assigned for homework should be based on both the Avoidance Hierarchy and other potential situations discussed in session. The exposures increase in difficulty over time, and as the sessions progress, the patient begins to take more responsibility for designing the exposures and the therapist provides less guidance. Exposures done outside of the session are monitored so that they may be discussed and processed in session.

Sessions 13–14

In Sessions 13 and 14 the therapist revisits the patient's continuing need for emotional exposures. If he or she determines that the patient would benefit from additional emotion exposures, they can be continued both in session and for homework at this time. Additionally, the therapist can focus on any events or emotional reactions over the past week that can be processed in session. In these sessions, Oscar continues to enter difficult situations, proceeding to his most feared situations following Session 13. Obstacles to exposure completion and reactions to exposures are discussed in session. The patient continues prospectively to monitor emotions, emotional exposures, and EDBs throughout Session 14.

Session 15

In this session the therapist reviews both the major concepts presented in treatment and the patient's progress. The therapist reviews the three-component model, focusing on cognitive reappraisals, modifying EDBs, and preventing emotional avoidance strategies. The therapist then discusses the inevitability of future stressors and potential reoccurrence of symptoms.

The continuation of informal emotion exposures and use of techniques to think more flexibly and to modify EDBs are encouraged. At this time the therapist provides to the patient handouts reviewing the treatment concepts and may at his or her discretion show the patient the results of process or outcome measures collected over the course of treatment.

OUTCOME AND CONCLUSION

Oscar received follow-up assessments at the termination of treatment and at 3-months posttreatment. These included the Mini-ADIS-IV (Brown et al., 1994), the SIGH-A (Shear et al., 2001) and SIGH-D (Williams, 1998), and a battery of self-report questionnaires. Additionally, the HAI (Salkovskis et al., 2002) was administered prior to each session to measure progress. During treatment, Oscar's HAI score decreased from 24 at Session 2 to 17 at Session 12. At the 3-month follow-up assessment, Oscar was assigned a diagnosis of anxiety disorder not otherwise specified at a CSR of 4, just meeting the DSM-IV diagnostic threshold. His symptoms of hypochondriasis and OCD were both noted to be at subclinical levels (CSR = 3 and 2, respectively). By 3 months posttreatment, Oscar was back in the laboratory full-time and was on track to complete his graduate degree as scheduled. At the next follow-up, 6 months posttreatment, he was assigned no clinical diagnoses, with hypochondriasis and OCD noted to be in partial remission, both with a CSR of 2.

REFERENCES

Allen, L. B., White, K. S., Barlow, D. H., Gorman, J. M., Shear, M. K., & Woods, S. W. (2007). *Effects of cognitive-behavioral therapy (CBT) for panic disorder on comorbid depression and anxiety*. Manuscript submitted for publication.

American Psychiatric Association. (1994). *Diagnostic and statistical manual of mental disorders* (4th ed.). Washington, DC: Author.

Andrews, G. (1990). Classification of neurotic disorders. *Journal of the Royal Society of Medicine, 83*, 606–607.

Andrews, G. (1996). Comorbidity in neurotic disorders: The similarities are more important than the differences. In R. M. Rapee (Ed.), *Current controversies in the anxiety disorders* (pp. 3–20). New York: Guilford Press.

Ascher, L. M. (1980). Paradoxical intention. In A. Goldstein & E. B. Foa (Eds.), *Handbook of behavioral interventions: A clinical guide* (pp. 266–321). New York: Wiley.

Barlow, D. H. (1988). *Anxiety and its disorders: The nature and treatment of anxiety and panic*. New York: Guilford Press.

Barlow, D. H. (1991). Disorders of emotion. *Psychological Inquiry, 2*, 58–71.

Barlow, D. H. (2000). Unraveling the mysteries of anxiety and its disorders from the perspective of emotion theory. *American Psychologist, 55*, 1247–1263.

Barlow, D. H. (2002). *Anxiety and its disorders: The nature and treatment of anxiety and panic* (2nd ed.). New York: Guilford Press.

Barlow, D. H., & Cerny, J. A. (1988). *Psychological treatment of panic*. New York: Guilford Press.

Barlow, D. H., & Craske, M. G. (2000). *Mastery of your anxiety and panic: Client workbook for anxiety and panic* (3rd ed.). Boulder, CO: Graywind.

Barlow, D. H., Gorman, J. M., Shear, M. K., & Woods, S. W. (2000). Cognitive-behavioral therapy, imipramine, or their combination for panic disorder: A randomized controlled trial. *Journal of the American Medical Association, 283*, 2529–2536.

Barlow, D. H., Rapee, R. M., & Reisner, L. C. (2001). *Mastering stress 2001: A lifestyle approach*. Dallas, TX: American Health.

Beck, A. T. (1972). *Depression: Causes and treatment*. Philadelphia: University of Pennsylvania Press. (Original work published 1967)

Beck, A. T., Rush, A. J., Shaw, B. F., & Emery, G. (1979). *Cognitive therapy of depression*. New York: Guilford Press.

Beck, A. T., & Steer, R. A. (1990). Beck Self-Concept Test. *Psychological Assessment, 2*, 191–197.

Beck, A. T., Steer, R. A., & Brown, G. K. (1996). *Beck Depression Inventory manual* (2nd ed.). San Antonio, TX: Psychological Corporation.

Borkovec, T. D. (1994). The nature, functions, and origins of worry. In G. C. L. Davey & F. Tallis (Eds.), *Worrying: Perspectives on theory, assessment, and treatment* (pp. 5–34). New York: Wiley.

Borkovec, T. D., Abel, J. L., & Newman, H. (1995). Effects of psychotherapy on comorbid conditions in generalized anxiety disorder. *Journal of Consulting and Clinical Psychology, 63*, 479–483.

Borkovec, T. D., Hazlett-Stevens, H., & Diaz, M. L. (1999). The role of positive beliefs about worry in generalized anxiety disorder and its treatment. *Clinical Psychology and Psychotherapy, 6*, 126–138.

Bouton, M.E. (2005). Behavior systems and the contextual control of anxiety, fear, and panic. In L. Feldman Barrett, P. M. Niedenthal, & P. Winkielman (Eds.), *Emotion and consciousness* (pp. 205–227). New York: Guilford Press.

Bouton, M. E., Mineka, S., & Barlow, D. H. (2001). A modern learning-theory perspective on the etiology of panic disorder. *Psychological Review, 108*, 4–32.

British Psychological Society. (2004). *English survey of*

applied psychologists in health and social care and in the probation and prison service. Leicester, UK: Author.

Brown, E. J., Turovsky, J., Heimberg, R. G., Juster, H. R., Brown, T. A., & Barlow, D. H. (1997). Validation of the Social Interaction Anxiety Scale and the Social Phobia Scale across the anxiety disorders. *Psychological Assessment, 9,* 21–27.

Brown, T. A. (2007). Temporal course and structural relationships among dimensions of temperament and DSM-IV anxiety and mood disorders. *Journal of Abnormal Psychology, 116,* 313–328.

Brown, T. A., Antony, M. M., & Barlow, D. H. (1992). Psychometric properties of the Penn State Worry Questionnaire in a clinical anxiety disorders sample. *Behaviour Research and Therapy, 30,* 33–38.

Brown, T. A., Antony, M. M., & Barlow, D. H. (1995). Diagnostic comorbidity in panic disorder: Effect on treatment outcome and course of comorbid diagnoses following treatment. *Journal of Consulting and Clinical Psychology, 63,* 408–418.

Brown, T. A., & Barlow, D. H. (1995). Long-term outcome in cognitive-behavioral treatment of panic disorder: Clinical predictors and alternative strategies for assessment. *Journal of Consulting and Clinical Psychology, 63,* 754–765.

Brown, T. A., & Barlow, D. H. (2002). Classification of anxiety and mood disorders. In D. H. Barlow (Ed.), *Anxiety and its disorders: The nature and treatment of anxiety and panic* (2nd ed., pp. 292–327). New York: Guilford Press.

Brown, T. A., Campbell, L. A., Lehman, C. L., Grisham, J. R., & Mancill, R. B. (2001). Current and lifetime comorbidity of the DSM-IV anxiety and mood disorders in a large clinical sample. *Journal of Abnormal Psychology, 110,* 49–58.

Brown, T. A., Chorpita, B. F., & Barlow, D. H. (1998). Structural relationships among dimensions of the DSM-IV anxiety and mood disorders and dimensions of negative affect, positive affect, and autonomic arousal. *Journal of Abnormal Psychology, 107,* 179–192.

Brown, T. A., Di Nardo, P. A., & Barlow, D. H. (1994). *Anxiety Disorders Interview Schedule for DSM-IV: Treatment follow-up version (Mini-ADIS-IV).* San Antonio, TX: Psychological Corporation.

Brown, T. A., Di Nardo, P. A., Lehman, C. L., & Campbell, L. A. (2001). Reliability of DSM-IV anxiety and mood disorders: Implications for the classification of emotional disorders. *Journal of Abnormal Psychology, 110,* 49–58.

Brown, T. A., White, K. S., Forsyth, J. P., & Barlow, D. H. (2004). The structure of perceived emotional control: Psychometric properties of a revised Anxiety Control Questionnaire. *Behavior Therapy, 35,* 75–99.

Cameron, N. M., Champagne, F. A., & Parent, C. (2005). The programming of individual differences in defensive responses and reproductive stratifies in the rat through variations in maternal care. *Neuroscience and Biobehavioral Reviews, 29,* 843–865.

Campbell-Sills, L., Liverant, G. I., & Brown, T. A. (2004). Psychometric evaluation of the behavioral inhibition/behavioral activation scales in a large sample of outpatients with anxiety and mood disorders. *Psychological Assessment, 16,* 244–254.

Center for the Study of Emotion and Attention (CSEA-NIMH). (2001). *The International Affective Picture System: Digitized photographs.* Gainsville: Center for Research in Psychophysiology, University of Florida.

Chorpita, B. F., Albano, A. M., & Barlow, D. H. (1998). The structure of negative emotions in a clinical sample of children and adolescents. *Journal of Abnormal Child Psychology, 107,* 74–85.

Chorpita, B. F., & Barlow, D. H. (1998). The development of anxiety: The role of control in the early environment. *Psychological Bulletin, 124,* 3–21.

Clark, L. A. (2005). Temperament as a unifying basis for personality and psychopathology. *Journal of Abnormal Psychology, 114,* 505–521.

Clark, L. A., & Watson, D. (1991). Tripartite model of anxiety and depression: Psychometric evidence and taxonomic implications. *Journal of Abnormal Psychology, 103,* 103–116.

Craske, M. G., Barlow, D. H., & O'Leary, T. (1992). *Mastery of your anxiety and worry.* San Antonio, TX: Psychological Corporation/Graywind.

Craske, M. G., Street, L., & Barlow, D. H. (1989). Instructions to focus upon or distract from internal cues during exposure treatment for agoraphobic avoidance. *Behaviour Research and Therapy, 27,* 663–672.

Craske, M. G., Street, L. L., Jayaraman, J., & Barlow, D. H. (1991). Attention versus distraction during *in vivo* exposure: Snake and spider phobias. *Journal of Anxiety Disorders, 5,* 199–211.

Davidson, R. J. (2000). *Anxiety, depression, and emotion.* New York: Oxford University Press.

Di Nardo, P. A., Brown, T. A., & Barlow, D. H. (1994). *Anxiety Disorders Interview Schedule for DSM-IV.* Albany, NY: Graywind.

Dimidjian, S., Hollon, S. D., Dobson, K. S., Shmaling, K. B., Kohlenberg, R. J., Addis, M. E., et al. (2006). Randomized trial of behavioral activation, cognitive therapy, and antidepressant medication in the acute treatment of adults with major depression. *Journal of Consulting and Clinical Psychology, 74,* 658–670.

Eley, T. C., & Brown, T. A. (2007). *Phenotypic and genetic/environmental structure of anxiety and depressive disorder symptoms in adolescence.* Manuscript submitted for publication.

First, M. B., Spitzer, R. L., Gibbon, M., & Williams, J. B. W. (1996). *Structured Clinical Interview for DSM-IV Axis I Disorders—Patient Edition* (SCID-I/P, Version 2.0). New York: Biometrics Research Department, New York State Psychiatric Institute.

Foa, E., Cashman, L., Jaycox, L., & Perry, K. (1997). The validation of a self-report measure of posttraumatic stress disorder: The Posttraumatic Diagnostic Scale. *Psychological Assessment, 9,* 445–451.

Foa, E. B., Huppert, J. D., Leiberg, S., Langer, R., Kichic, R., Hajcak, G., et al. (2002). The Obsessive–Compulsive Inventory: Development and validation of a short version. *Psychological Assessment, 14,* 485–495.

Frankl, V. E. (1960). Paradoxical intention: A logo-therapeutic technique. *American Journal of Psychotherapy, 14,* 520–535.

Frisch, M. B., Cornell, J., & Villaneuva, M. (1992). Clinical validation of the Quality of Life Inventory: A measure of life satisfaction for use in treatment planning and outcome assessment. *Psychological Assessment, 4,* 92–101.

Gross, J. J. (1998). Antecedent- and response-focused emotion regulation: Divergent consequences for experience, expression, and physiology. *Journal of Personality and Social Psychology, 74,* 224–237.

Gross, J. J. (2002). Emotion regulation: Affective, cognitive, and social consequences. *Psychophysiology, 9,* 281–291.

Gross, J. J., & Levenson, R. W. (1997). The acute effects of inhibiting negative and positive emotion. *Journal of Abnormal Psychology, 106,* 95–103.

Hafner, J., & Marks, I. M. (1976). Exposure *in vivo* of agoraphobics: Contributions of diazepam, group exposure, and anxiety evocation. *Psychological Medicine, 6,* 71–88.

Hamilton, M. (1959). The assessment of anxiety states by rating. *British Journal of Medical Psychology, 32,* 50–55.

Hamilton, M. (1960). A rating scale for depression. *Journal of Neurology, Neurosurgery, and Psychiatry, 23,* 56–62.

Hammen, C. L. (1991). The generation of stress in the course of unipolar depression. *Journal of Abnormal Psychology, 100,* 555–561.

Hayes, S. C., Strosahl, K. D., & Wilson, K. G. (1999). *Acceptance and commitment therapy: An experiential approach to behavior change.* New York: Guilford Press.

Hays, R. D., Sherbourne, C. D., & Mazel, R. M. (1993). The RAND 36-Item Health Survey 1.0. *Health Economics, 2,* 217–227.

Heim, C., & Nemeroff, C. B. (1999). The impact of early adverse experiences on brain systems involved in the pathophysiology of anxiety and affective disorders. *Biological Psychiatry, 46,* 1509–1522.

Heimberg, R. G., Liebowitz, M. R., Hope, D. A., Schneier, F. R., Holt, C. S., Welkowitz, L. A., et al. (1998). Cognitive behavioral group therapy vs phenelzine therapy for social phobia: 12-week outcome. *Archives of General Psychiatry, 55,* 1133–1141.

Heimberg, R. G., Mueller, G. P., Holt, C. S., Hope, D. A., & Liebowitz, M. R. (1992). Assessment of anxiety in social interaction and being observed by others: The Social Interaction Anxiety Scale and the Social Phobia Scale. *Behavior Therapy, 23,* 53–73.

Hettema, J. M., Neale, M. C., & Kendler, K. S. (2001). A review and meta-analysis of the genetic epidemiol-ogy of anxiety disorders. *American Journal of Psychiatry, 158,* 1568–1578.

Hollon, S. D., Munoz, R. F., Barlow, D. H., Beardslee, W. R., Bell, C. C., Guillermo, B., et al. (2002). Psychosocial intervention development for the prevention and treatment of depression: Promoting innovation and increasing access. *Biological Psychiatry, 52,* 610–630.

Huppert, J. D., Bufka, L. F., Barlow, D. H., Gorman, J. M., Shear, M. K., & Woods, S. W. (2001). Therapists, therapist variables and cognitive-behavioral therapy outcome in a multicenter trial for panic disorder. *Journal of Consulting and Clinical Psychology, 69,* 747–755.

Izard, C. E. (1971). *The face of emotion.* New York: Appleton–Century–Crofts.

Jacobson, N. S., Martell, C. R., & Dimidjian, S. (2001). Behavioral activation treatment for depression: Returning to contextual roots. *Clinical Psychology: Science and Practice, 8,* 255–270.

Kamphuis, J. H., & Telch, M. J. (2000). Effects of distraction and guided threat reappraisal on fear reduction during exposure based treatments for specific fears. *Behaviour Research and Therapy, 38,* 1163–1181.

Kendler, K. S. (1996). Major depression and generalized anxiety disorder: Same genes, (partly) different environments—revisited. *British Journal of Psychiatry, 30*(Suppl.), 68–75.

Kendler, K. S., Walters, E. E., Neale, M. C., Kessler, R. C., Heath, A. C., & Eaves, L. J. (1995). The structure of genetic and environmental risk factors for six major psychiatric disorders in women: Phobia, generalized anxiety disorder, panic disorder, bulimia, major depression, and alcoholism. *Archives of General Psychiatry, 52,* 374–382.

Kessler, R. C., Nelson, C. B., McGonagle, K. A., Lui, J., Swartz, M., & Blazer, D. G. (1996). Comorbidity of DSM-III-R major depressive disorder in the general population: Results from the National Comorbidity Survey. *British Journal of Psychiatry, 168,* 17–30.

Kessler, R. C., Stang, P. E., Wittchen, H. U., Ustan, T. B., Roy-Byrne, P. P., & Walters, E. E. (1998). Lifetime panic–depression comorbidity in the National Comorbidity Survey. *Archives of General Psychiatry, 55,* 801–808.

Krueger, R. F., Watson, D., & Barlow, D. H. (Eds.). (2005). Introduction to the special section: Towards a dimensionally based taxonomy of psychopathology. *Journal of Abnormal Psychology, 114,* 491–493.

Kupfer, D. J., First, M. B., & Regier, D. A. (Eds.). (2002). *Research agenda for DSM-V.* Washington, DC: American Psychiatric Press.

Liebowitz, M. R., Heimberg, R. G., Schneier, F. R., Hope, D. A., Davies, S., Holt, C. S., et al. (1999). Cognitive-behavioral group therapy versus phenelzine in social phobia: Long term outcome. *Depression and Anxiety, 10,* 89–98.

Linehan, M. M. (1993). *Cognitive behavioral treatment*

of borderline personality disorder. New York: Guilford Press.

Margraf, J., Taylor, C. B., Ehlers, A., Roth, W. T., & Agras, W. S. (1987). Panic attacks in the natural environment. *Journal of Nervous and Mental Disease, 175*, 558–565.

Mattick, R. P., & Clarke, J. C. (1998). Development and validation of measures of social phobia scrutiny fear and social interaction anxiety. *Behaviour Research and Therapy, 36*, 455–470.

Merikangas, K. R., Zhang, H., & Aveneoli, S. (2003). Longitudinal trajectories of depression and anxiety in a prospective community study. *Archives of General Psychiatry, 60*, 993–1000.

Meyer, T. J., Miller, M. L., Metzger, R. L., & Borkovec, T. D. (1990). Development and validation of the Penn State Worry Questionnaire. *Behaviour Research and Therapy, 28*, 487–495.

Molina, S., & Borkovec, T. D. (1994). The Penn State Worry Questionnaire: Psychometric properties and associated characteristics. In G. C. L. Davey & F. Tallis (Eds.), *Worrying: Perspectives on theory, assessment and treatment* (pp. 265–284). New York: Wiley.

Morgan, C. D., & Murray, H. A. (1935). A method for investigating fantasies: The Thematic Apperception Test. *Archives of Neurology and Psychiatry, 34*, 289–306.

Nathan, P. E., & Gorman, J. M. (Eds.). (2002). *A guide to treatments that work.* London: Oxford University Press.

Peterson, R. A., & Reiss, S. (1987). *Anxiety Sensitivity Index manual.* Worthington, OH: IDS.

Raffa, S. D., Stoddard, J. A., White, K. S., Barlow, D. H., Gorman, J. M., Shear, M. K., et al. (in press). Relapse following combined-treatment discontinuation in a placebo-controlled trial for panic disorder. *Journal of Nervous and Mental Disease.*

Rapee, R. M., Craske, M. G., & Barlow, D. H. (1990). Subject described features of panic attacks using a new self-monitoring form. *Journal of Anxiety Disorders, 4*, 171–181.

Richards, J. M., & Gross, J. J. (2000). Emotion regulation and memory: The cognitive costs of keeping one's cool. *Journal of Personality and Social Psychology, 79*, 410–424.

Roemer, L., Litz, B. T., Orsillo, S. M., & Wagner, A. W. (2001). A preliminary investigation of the role of strategic withholding of emotions in PTSD. *Journal of Traumatic Stress, 14*, 143–150.

Roy-Byrne, P. P, Craske, M. G., & Stein, M. B. (2006). Panic disorder. *Lancet, 368*, 1023–1032.

Rutter, M., Moffit, T. E., & Caspi, A. (2006). Gene–environment interplay and psychopathology: Multiple varieties but real effects. *Journal of Child Psychology and Psychiatry, 47*, 226–261.

Salkovskis, P. M., Clark, D. M., Hackmann, A., Wells, A., & Gelder, M. G. (1999). An experimental investigation of the role of safety-seeking behaviors in the maintenance of panic disorder with agoraphobia. *Behaviour Research and Therapy, 37*, 559–574.

Salkovskis, P. M., Rimes, K. A., & Warwick, H. M. C. (2002). The Health Anxiety Inventory: Development and validation of scales for the measurement of health anxiety and hypochondriasis. *Psychological Medicine, 32*, 843–853.

Salovey, P., Mayer, J. D., Goldman, S., Turvey, C., & Palfai, T. P. (1995). Emotional attention, clarity, and repair: Exploring emotional intelligence using the Trait Meta-Mood Scale. In J. Pennebaker (Ed.), *Emotion, disclosure, and health* (pp. 125–153). Washington, DC: American Psychological Association.

Salovey, P., Stroud, L. R., Woolery, A., & Epel, E. S. (2002). Perceived emotional intelligence, stress reactivity, and symptom reports: Further explorations using the Trait Meta-Mood Scale. *Psychology and Health, 17*, 611–627.

Shear, M. K., Brown, T. A., Barlow, D. H., Money, R., Sholomskas, D. E., Woods, S. W., et al. (1997). Multicenter Collaborative Panic Disorder Severity Scale. *American Journal of Psychiatry, 154*, 1571–1575.

Shear, M. K., Vander Bilt, J., & Rucci, P. (2001). Reliability and validity of a structured interview guide for the Hamilton Anxiety Rating Scale (SIGH-A). *Depression and Anxiety, 13*, 166–178.

Sloan, T., & Telch, M. J. (2002). The effects of safety-seeking behavior and guided threat reappraisal on fear reduction during exposure: An experimental investigation. *Behaviour Research and Therapy, 40*, 235–251.

Smoller, J. W., & Tsuang, M. T. (1998). Panic and phobic anxiety: Defining phenotypes for genetic studies. *American Journal of Psychiatry, 155*, 1152–1162.

Steer, R. A., Ranieri, W. F., Beck, A. T., & Clark, D. A. (1993). Further evidence for the validity of the Beck Anxiety Inventory with psychiatric disorders. *Journal of Anxiety Disorders, 7*, 195–205.

Suárez, L., Bennett, S. M., Goldstein, C., & Barlow, D. H. (in press). Understanding anxiety disorders from a "triple vulnerability" framework. In M. M. Antony & M. B. Stein (Eds.), *Handbook of anxiety and the anxiety disorders.* New York: Oxford University Press.

Sullivan, G. M., Kent, J. M., & Coplan, J. D. (2000). The neurobiology of stress and anxiety. In D. I. Mostofsky & D. H. Barlow (Eds.), *The management of stress and anxiety in medical disorders* (pp. 15–35). Needham Heights, MA: Allyn & Bacon.

Thayer, R. E. (2000). Mood regulation and general arousal systems. *Psychological Inquiry, 11*, 202–204.

Tsao, J. C. I., Lewin, M. R., & Craske, M. G. (1998). The effects of cognitive-behavior therapy for panic disorders on comorbid conditions. *Journal of Anxiety Disorders, 12*, 357–371.

Tsao, J. C. I., Mystkowski, J. L., Zucker, B. G., & Craske, M. G. (2002). Effects of cognitive-behavior therapy for panic disorder on comorbid conditions:

Replication and extension. *Behavior Therapy, 33,* 493–509.

Tsao, J. C. I., Mystkowski, J. L., Zucker, B. G., & Craske, M. G. (2005). Impact of cognitive-behavioral therapy for panic disorder on comorbidity: A controlled investigation. *Behaviour Research and Therapy, 43,* 959–970.

Tyrer, P. J. (1989). *Classification of neurosis.* Chichester, UK: Wiley.

Tyrer, P. J., Seivewright, N., Murphys, S., Ferguson, B., Kingdon, D., Barczak, B., et al. (1998). The Nottingham study of neurotic disorder: Comparison of drug and psychological treatments. *Lancet, 2,* 235–240.

Ware, J. E., & Sherbourne, C. D. (1992). The MOS 36-Item Short-Form Health Survey (SF-36): I. Conceptual framework and item selection. *Quality of Life Research, 1,* 235–246.

Watson, D. (2005). Rethinking the mood and anxiety disorders: A quantitative hierarchical model for DSM-V. *Journal of Abnormal Psychology, 114,* 522–536.

Watson, D., Clark, L. A., & Harkness, A. R. (1994). Structures of personality and their relevance to psychopathology. *Journal of Abnormal Psychology, 103,* 18–31.

Watson, D., Clark, L. A., & Tellegen, A. (1988). Development and validation of brief measures of positive and negative affect: The PANAS scales. *Journal of Personality and Social Psychology, 54,* 1063–1070.

Wells, A., Clark, D. M., Salkovskis, P. M., Ludgate, J., Hackmann, A., & Gelder, M. (1995). Social phobia: The role of in-situation safety behaviors in maintaining anxiety and negative beliefs. *Behavior Therapy, 26,* 153–161.

Wiedemann, G., Pauli, P., & Dengler, W. (1999). Frontal brain asymmetry as a biological substrate of emotions in patients with panic disorders. *Archives of General Psychiatry, 56,* 78–84.

Williams, J. B. (1988). A structured interview guide for the Hamilton Depression Rating Scale. *Archives of General Psychiatry, 45,* 742–747.

Williams, K. E., Chambless, D. L., & Ahrens, A. (1997). Are emotions frightening?: An extension of the fear of fear construct. *Behaviour Research and Therapy, 35,* 239–248.

CHAPTER 6

Cognitive Therapy for Depression

JEFFREY E. YOUNG
JAYNE L. RYGH
ARTHUR D. WEINBERGER
AARON T. BECK

One of the most important developments in psychosocial approaches to emotional problems has been the success of cognitive therapy for depression. Evidence for the powerful efficacy of this approach has increased steadily over the years, particularly in regard to successful long-term outcome. Employing a variety of well-specified cognitive and behavioral techniques, cognitive therapy is also distinguished by the detailed structure of each session with its specific agendas, and by the very deliberate and obviously effective therapeutic style of interacting with the patient through a series of questions. Moreover, the authors underscore very clearly the importance of the collaborative relationship between therapist and patient and outline specific techniques to achieve this collaborative state so that patient and therapist become an investigative team. In this chapter, the authors present a second important phase of treatment that represents an interesting variation of cognitive therapy. This phase, called the "schema-focused" phase of treatment, concentrates on identifying and modifying early maladaptive or "core" schemas that developed during childhood in severely depressed and treatment-resistant patients. These schemas may make the patient vulnerable to relapse. Detailed explication of this second phase of treatment will be invaluable to experienced cognitive therapists, as well as to those becoming acquainted with cognitive therapy for depression for the first time. Two compelling cases, new to this edition, illustrate each approach.—D. H. B.

OVERVIEW AND RESEARCH

Depression and the Emergence of Cognitive Therapy

Depression is one of the most common disorders encountered by mental health professionals. Recent research from the U.S. National Comorbidity Survey Replication (NCS-R) studies and data provided by the National Institute of Mental Health (NIMH) indicate the following:

- The lifetime prevalence estimate for a DSM-IV mood disorder is 20.8% (Kessler, Beglund, et al., 2005).
- The 12-month prevalence estimate for a DSM-IV mood disorder is 9.5% (Kessler, Chiu, Demler, Merikangas, & Walters, 2005).
- Major depressive disorder is associated with 27.2 lost workdays and bipolar disorder (I or II) with 65.5 lost workdays for each ill worker per year (Kessler, Akiskal, et al. 2006).

- Depression increases the risk of heart attacks and is a frequent and serious complicating factor in stroke, diabetes, and cancer (NIMH, 1999).
- Major depressive disorder is the leading cause of disability in the United States for ages 15–44 (NIMH, 2006).
- The associated costs are more than $30 billion per year (NIMH, 1999).

The high risk of relapse (Scott, 2000), high resource utilization (Howland, 1993), and loss of human capital (Berndt et al., 2000) associated with depression reveal the seriousness of the problem. Current estimates suggest that by 2010, depression will be the second most costly of all illnesses worldwide; in 1990 it was ranked fourth (Keller & Boland, 1998). As these reports indicate, depression is widespread, debilitating, and costly.

No amount of data can adequately capture or convey the personal pain and suffering experienced in depression. Many depressed people do not get professional help (Frank & Thase, 1999; Jarrett, 1995) and although the number seeking help has increased over the last decade, undertreatment has remained a serious problem (Olfson et al., 2002). The social stigma still attached to people with depression is no doubt one factor, but the obstacles encountered while looking for appropriate care can be another stumbling block in getting help. Obtaining the right type of help can be at once inhibiting and overwhelming, especially to those already impaired:

> Americans who do seek treatment for depressive symptoms must decide where to seek which treatment and from what type of practitioner. . . . The clinician must select a somatic, psychological, or combination of treatment, at a given dose and/or schedule of appointments. . . . Throughout this procedure, the patient decides to what extent he/she will comply with the recommendations, for how long, against recognized and unrecognized economic, practical, physical, and emotional costs. . . . Sadly, the lack of information as well as the continued social stigma of psychiatric illness and treatment influence decision-making. Simultaneously, the decisions occur in an environment filled with social, political, and economic debate, and tension among policy makers, third-party payers, and clinicians, as well as among different types of practitioner guilds. (Jarrett, 1995, p. 435)

When care is provided, it is frequently inadequate, reflecting a public health crisis (Keller & Boland, 1998). The need for delivery of treatments with proven and rapid efficacy remains paramount.

One of the major developments in the treatment of depression has been the emergence of cognitive therapy, developed by Aaron T. Beck over the past 40-plus years. His work and that of his colleagues (Beck, 1967, 1976; Beck, Rush, Shaw, & Emery, 1979) has led to a paradigm shift within psychotherapy (Salkovskis, 1996). Due in part to Beck's development of testable hypotheses and clinical protocols, cognitive therapy has received an enormous amount of professional attention (Hollon, 1998; McGinn & Young, 1996; Rehm, 1990). Of all the cognitive-behavioral treatment approaches to depression, Beck's paradigm (Beck, 1967; Beck et al., 1979) has received the greatest amount of empirical study, validation, and clinical application (Barlow & Hofmann, 1997; de Oliveira, 1998; Dobson & Pusch, 1993; Hollon, 1998; Hollon, Thase, & Markowitz, 2002; Rehm, 1990; Roberts & Hartlage, 1996; Scott, 1996a). There are many excellent books for practitioners that teach cognitive therapy procedures (e.g., J. S. Beck, 1995).

Along with this attention, however, has come confusion about what is actually meant by the term "cognitive therapy." The actual cognitive therapeutic strategies employed in "cognitive" treatments may differ in many ways from one another and from those explicitly prescribed by Beck and colleagues (1979) in their manual for cognitive therapy of depression. Thus, the reader should be aware that common use of the term "cognitive therapy" does not necessarily imply uniformity in procedures. The therapy described by Beck and colleagues involves the use of both cognitive and behavioral techniques, and can therefore be accurately labeled "cognitive-behavioral"; however, in the literature, both terms have been applied in describing the Beck and colleagues procedures, with some articles utilizing the term "cognitive therapy" (Sacco & Beck, 1995, p. 345).

Research on Treatment of the Acute Phase

Outcome research has found cognitive therapy to be effective with clinical populations in a number of controlled trials (Hollon & Shelton, 2001). Although some early studies (Blackburn, Bishop, Glen, Whalley, & Christie,

1981; Rush, Beck, Kovacs, & Hollon, 1977) suggested that cognitive therapy may be superior to drug treatment for depression at termination, Meterissian and Bradwejn (1989) noted that psychopharmacological interventions often were not adequately implemented. In research where interventions have been adequate, cognitive therapy generally has been shown to be equivalent in efficacy to antidepressant medications, including tricyclic antidepressants (TCAs) and selective serotonin reuptake inhibitors (SSRIs) in the treatment of outpatients with nonbipolar depression (DeRubeis et al., 2005; Hollon et al., 1992; Murphy, Simmons, Wetzel, & Lustman, 1984) and a monoamine oxidase inhibitor (MAOI) in the treatment of outpatients with atypical depression (Jarrett et al., 1999). Although many studies have not included pill-placebo conditions, the studies by Jarrett and colleagues (1999) and DeRubeis and colleagues (2005) found the active treatments superior to pill-placebos. In a mega-analysis by DeRubeis, Gelfand, Tang, and Simons (1999) of treatment outcome in four studies with severely depressed outpatients, cognitive therapy was equivalent to antidepressant medication (imipramine or nortriptyline).

Only two studies that included a pill-placebo have found cognitive therapy to be less effective than psychopharmacological intervention. The first was the NIMH Treatment of Depression Collaborative Research Program (TDCRP) with moderate to severe depression in adults. The second was the multisite Treatment for Adolescents with Depression Study (TADS) for reduction of depressive symptoms in adolescents.

The NIMH TDCRP was the first major study to include a pill-placebo condition. The initial results (Elkin et al., 1989) suggested lower rates of improvement with cognitive-behavioral therapy (CBT) than did earlier studies. It also appeared that with more severely depressed patient groups, interpersonal psychotherapy and antidepressant drugs might be superior to CBT. The high visibility and prestige of the NIMH TDCRP study generated a great deal of debate (Hollon, DeRubeis, & Evans, 1996; Wolpe, 1993), because it appeared that the benefits of CBT in the acute treatment phase might have been overestimated in previous studies. However, on later examination of the data, Elkin, Gibbons, Shea, and Shaw (1996) acknowledged Jacobson and Hollon's

(1996) observation that the outcome results varied across sites, with cognitive therapy performing as well as medication at one of the three sites with severely depressed clients. Jacobson and Hollon noted that the best results were obtained at the site with the most experienced therapists. Hollon and colleagues (2002) "suspect that the explanation is not that cognitive therapy cannot be effective with such patients, but that the therapist's expertise makes a greater difference the more difficult the depression is to treat" (p. 62). Additionally, a study by Albon and Jones (2003) raises the question of the distinctness of the two types of psychotherapy treatments in the TDCRP. In this study, Albon and Jones, expert therapists in CBT and interpersonal psychotherapy, developed prototypes of ideal regimens of their own respective treatments. Then, actual transcripts of treatment sessions from the TDCRP were compared to these expert prototypes. Albon and Jones found that both CBT and interpersonal psychotherapy sessions conformed most closely to the cognitive-behavioral prototype, and that closer adherence to the cognitive-behavioral prototype produced more positive correlations with outcome measures across both types of treatment.

The multisite TADS study (2004) for reduction of depressive symptoms in adolescents found that the combination of medication (fluoxetine) and CBT produced the most positive outcome, medication alone was superior to pill-placebo but CBT alone did not significantly differ from pill-placebo. However, as noted by Weisz, McCarty, and Valeri (2006, p. 144) "the CBT ES (effect size) generated in TADS is not characteristic of most CBT," raising questions about the administration of CBT in this study.

Several studies have not found the combination of CBT and drugs to be superior to either treatment alone with depressed outpatients (Biggs & Rush, 1999; Evans et al., 1992; Hollon, Shelton, & Loosen, 1991; Scott, 1996a; Shaw & Segal, 1999). The increment in efficacy appears to be modest in the acute phase of treatment at best, with increases in efficacy from 10 to 20% (Conte, Plutchik, Wild, & Karasu, 1986). Studies regarding treatment with depressed inpatients suggest beneficial results when CBT is combined with medication (Bowers, 1990; Miller, Norman, Keitner, Bishop, & Dow, 1989; Stuart & Bowers, 1995; Wright, 1996). Although cognitive therapy appears to be a useful adjunct to standard care with inpatients, it remains unclear whether cognitive therapy alone is sufficient (Hollon et al., 2002).

Research on Relapse Prevention

Even though the vast majority of patients recover from an episode of depression, they nevertheless remain vulnerable to future depression.[1]

> Recurrence is a major problem for many individuals suffering from depression: at least 50% of individuals who suffer from one depressive episode will have another within 10 years. Those experiencing two episodes have a 90% chance of suffering a third, while individuals with three or more lifetime episodes have relapse rates of 40% within 15 weeks of recovery from an episode. (Kupfer, Frank, & Wamhoff, 1996, p. 293)

Other investigators have estimated that 85% of patients with unipolar depression are likely to experience recurrences (Keller & Boland, 1998, p. 350). As these numbers clearly show, there is an urgent need for treatments capable of minimizing and preventing relapse.

What we consider a very exciting finding in the treatment of depression with cognitive therapy is the consistent observation that patients treated with cognitive therapy alone or with a combination of cognitive therapy and medication fare far better in terms of relapse than do patients treated with medication alone (when both treatments are stopped at termination). Despite differences in sample characteristics and methodologies across studies, cognitive therapy appears to have important prophylactic properties. After a 1-year follow-up, numerous studies have reported lower relapse rates for patients treated with cognitive therapy than for patients treated with antidepressants. For examples, Simons, Murphy, Levine, and Wetzel (1986) found relapse rates of 12% with cognitive therapy versus 66% with antidepressants; Bowers (1990) found relapse rates of 20% with cognitive therapy versus 80% with antidepressants; Shea and colleagues (1992) reported 9% relapse with cognitive therapy versus 28% with antidepressants; Hollon and colleagues (2005) reported rates of 31% relapse with cognitive therapy versus 76% with antidepressants. Results from the most extensive meta-analysis to date revealed that "on average, only 29.5% of the patients treated with cognitive therapy

relapsed versus 60% of those treated with antidepressants" (Gloaguen, Cottraux, Cucherat, & Blackburn, 1998, p. 68). The prophylactic benefits of cognitive therapy are all the more significant because "there is no evidence that pharmacotherapy confers any protection against the return of symptoms after treatment has been terminated.[2] Since the majority of depressed individuals will experience multiple episodes, the capacity of an intervention to prevent the return of symptoms after treatment may be at least as important as its ability to treat the current episode" (Evans et al., 1992, p. 802).

A related concern—and one of the most salient with psychotropic agents—is the presence of residual symptoms after treatment: "Treatment of depression by pharmacological means is likely to leave a substantial amount of residual symptoms in most patients" (Fava, Rafanelli, Grandi, Conti, & Belluardo, 1998b, p. 820). Inevitably, patients who improve on antidepressants continue to manifest some of the symptoms of depression, and, as numerous investigators have concluded, unless patients achieve full recovery, residual symptoms increase the risk of relapse (Evans et al., 1992; Fava et al., 1998b; Keller & Boland, 1998).

A group of investigators concerned about the risk of relapse associated with residual symptoms looked at the lingering symptoms after treatment with fluoxetine (Prozac). They found that

> even among subjects who are considered full responders to fluoxetine 20 mg for 5 weeks, more than 80% had 1 or more residual DSM-III-R symptoms of major depressive disorder, more than 30% had 3 or more symptoms, and 10.2% met formal criteria for either minor or subsyndromal depression. . . . These findings imply that minimal depressive symptoms are prodromal and increase the risk of developing an initial full-blown episode of major depression. (Nierenberg et al., 1999, pp. 224–225)

Cognitive therapy has been found to be effective in reducing both residual symptoms and relapse after the termination of medication: "Short-term CBT after successful antidepressant drug therapy had a substantial effect on relapse rate after discontinuation of antidepressant drugs. Patients who received CBT reported a substantially lower relapse rate (25%) during the 2-year follow-up than those assigned to [clinical management] (80%)" (Fava et al., 1998b, p. 818). The protective benefits of cognitive therapy were still noticeable in a 4-year follow-up study, although the benefits faded after a 6-year period (Fava, Rafanelli, Grandi, Canestrari, & Morphy, 1998a). Another study found that only 5% of the "CBT treated and recovered" group sought additional treatment compared with 39% of the antidepressant group (see Williams, 1997). Paykel and colleagues (1999) found significantly lower cumulative relapse rates at 68 weeks in patients who received 16 sessions of CBT following a partial response to pharmacotherapy. Bockting and colleagues (2005) compared treatment as usual (TAU, which included continuation of medication) with TAU augmented with brief cognitive therapy and found relapse significantly reduced in patients with five or more previous episodes of depression. The relapse rates were 72% for TAU versus 46% for TAU augmented with brief cognitive therapy.

A preventive strategy used by psychiatrists to deal with high relapse rates associated with antidepressant medication is "continuation medication," which is long-term (and in many cases lifelong) maintenance treatment (Evans et al., 1992; Fava et al., 1998b; Thase, 1999)—usually at the same dosage provided during the acute phase of treatment. Some researchers have pointed out the tautological nature of this solution: "Drug treatment results in a higher relapse rate than cognitive-behavioral therapy; therefore patients should be maintained on drugs to prevent relapse" (Antonuccio, Danton, & DeNelsky, 1995, p. 578). In any case, research comparing relapse rates in patients continuing medication over the long term versus those treated and then withdrawn from cognitive therapy does not suggest a significant advantage to this practice. For example, DeRubeis and colleagues (2005) found that both groups had equivalent relapse rates (40%); Hollon and colleagues (2005) found that 31% relapsed when treated and then withdrawn from cognitive therapy compared to 47% who relapsed when treated with continuation medication.

What is the optimum frequency and duration of sessions for cognitive therapy to be effective, both at termination and at long-term follow-up? According to Sacco and Beck (1995),

General guidelines suggest 15 to 25 (50-minute) sessions at weekly intervals, with more seriously depressed clients usually requiring twice-weekly meetings for the initial 4–5 weeks. To avoid an abrupt termination, a "tapering off" process is recommended, with the last few sessions occurring once every 2 weeks. After termination, some clients may also need a few booster sessions (four or five are common). (p. 332)

Some writers have noted that longer treatment may be necessary for a full and more lasting recovery (Elkin et al., 1996; Thase, 1992). Research by Jarrett and colleagues (2001) suggests that relapse rates in high-risk patients with an early age of onset or unstable remission might possibly be reduced further with "continuation-phase cognitive therapy" (C-CT), which consists of 10 sessions (biweekly during the first 2 months and once a month for the following 6 months) following the acute phase of treatment. The focus in the continuation phase is on relapse prevention and the generalization of skills (across responses, settings, stimuli, and times).

Another alternative for relapse prevention is mindfulness-based cognitive therapy (MBCT), developed by Teasdale, Segal, and Williams (1995). MBCT draws from the acceptance and meditation strategies from dialectical behavior therapy for borderline personality (Linehan, 1993a, 1993b). "MBCT aims at developing participant's awareness of, and changing their relationship to, unwanted thoughts, feelings, and body sensations, so that participants no longer avoid them or react to them in an automatic way but rather respond to them in an intentional and skilful manner" (Ma & Teasdale, 2004, p. 32). Teasdale and colleagues (Ma & Teasdale, 2004; Teasdale, 1997a, 1997b; Teasdale et al., 1995, 2002) have argued that the primary mechanism of therapeutic change in cognitive therapy is in distancing or decentering from cognition rather than changing the content of thought. The two studies conducted on MBCT found that TAU in comparison with TAU followed by MBCT significantly reduced relapse in patients with three or more episodes of depression: 66% relapsed with TAU versus 37% with TAU followed by MBCT (Teasdale et al., 2000), 78% relapsed with TAU versus 36% with TAU followed by MBCT (Ma & Teasdale, 2004). The potential for lower costs associated with this treatment, in that it can be implemented in a group format, make it an attractive alternative.

Research Related to Chronic versus Nonchronic Depression

Although much progress has been made in the treatment of depression with cognitive therapy and/or psychopharmacological interventions, it is important to note that fully a third of patients in some studies do not respond to either treatment (Blackburn & More, 1997), and a much higher percentage do not achieve lasting improvements (Evans et al., 1992; Shaw & Segal, 1999). McCullough (2003) has proposed, on the basis of existing research, that there are qualitative differences between chronic and nonchronic forms of depression that require different treatment strategies. According to McCullough, research "shows that the chronic disorders, when compared with acute/episodic major depression (both single and recurrent episodes with interepisode full recovery), differ significantly in terms of age of onset, clinical course patterns, developmental history, modal Axis II comorbidity profiles, characteristic response-to-treatment rates, predictable relapse percentages, and need for long-term treatment" (p. 243). He notes that these differences largely have not been addressed in the treatment literature and, consequently, therapeutic work by psychologists, psychiatrists, and social workers has been conducted as if this is an undifferentiated population. Young, Klosko, and Weishaar (2003) also have noted that although traditional CBT is highly effective for many patients with Axis I disorders, those with Axis II disorders "either went largely unhelped or were helped with their Axis I disorders but still experienced significant emotional distress and impaired functioning— that is significant character psychopathology" (p. 271). Fortunately, two promising CBT-based treatments have been developed specifically to address chronic populations. These treatments are McCullough's (2000) cognitive-behavioral analysis system of psychotherapy (CBASP) and Young's (1990/1999; Young et al., 2003) schema therapy.

Before briefly introducing these newer treatments, we describe the general characteristics of this population. An early age of onset (usually in midadolescence, before age 20) in the form of dysthymia tends to differentiate between the chronic and nonchronic forms of depression in 70–75% of clinical populations (Keller & Boland, 1998; Keller & Hanks, 1995; McCullough, 2000). Early life trauma or adverse family relations (loss of parent in childhood; sexual, physical, and/or verbal abuse; neglect; and overprotection) is more evident in those with chronic depression (Chapman et al., 2004; Dube et al., 2001; Heim & Nemeroff, 2001; Kendler et al., 1995; Lizardi et al., 1995; Randolph & Dykman, 1998; Sachs-Ericsson, Verona, Joiner, & Preacher, 2006). In patients with early-onset dysthymia who experience chronic stress, those with the addition of an adverse family history evidence an increase in depression severity over time compared to those without such adverse family histories, but with familial loadings for dysthymic disorder (Dougherty, Klein, & Davila, 2004). Cluster C personality disorders are associated with chronic depression (Hayden & Klein, 2001). Maladaptive schemas (identified with the Schema Questionnaire (Young, 1990/1999) in the domains of Impaired Autonomy and Overvigilance significantly differentiate between chronic and nonchronic depression, although elevations across all schema domains are evident when comparing both types of depression and never-ill controls (Riso et al., 2003).

McCullough's (2000) CBASP is an integrative, time-limited treatment that contains elements of cognitive, behavioral, interpersonal, and psychodynamic psychotherapies. McCullough (2003) states:

> Treatment begins with a cognitive-emotionally retarded adult child who brings a negative "snapshot" view of the world to the session. The chronic patient functions, at least in the social–interpersonal arena, with the structural mindset of a 4–6 year old preoperational (Piaget) child. . . . The patient must be taught to function formally, to perceive that his or her behavior has consequences, be taught to generate authentic empathy, and to learn to assert himself or herself effectively. Psychotherapy begins with an "adult child" who must be assisted to mature developmentally in the cognitive–emotive sphere. (pp. 247, 248)

Change is brought about through a contingency program that relies on negative reinforcement. First, contingencies between behaviors and consequences are exposed. Then, as the result of positive changes in behavior, discomfort and distress are reduced or eliminated. Three techniques are used to bring about change: situational analysis, interpersonal discrimination exercise, and behavioral skill training/rehearsal. Two studies have used CBASP with chronically depressed outpatients. The first (Keller et al., 2000) compared the effects of CBSAP alone, Serzone (nefazodone) alone, and combined treatment after a 12-week acute phase of treatment. The overall response rate was 48% for both monotherapies and 73% for the combined treatment. Among the 76% (519 out of 681) completers of the study, 52% responded to CBSAP, 55% responded to Serzone, and 85% responded to combined treatments. The second (Klein et al., 2004), a 1-year follow-up to this initial study, examined relapse and depressive symptoms over time in the CBSAP responders by comparing the effects of continuation CBSAP therapy (16 sessions over 52 weeks) with assessment only. There were significantly fewer relapses and depressive symptoms for those in the continuation CBSAP therapy.

Schema therapy also is an integrative therapy (Young et al., 2003), with elements of cognitive, behavioral, and emotion-focused therapies. The focus of treatment is on the relationship with the therapist, daily life events, and early life trauma or adverse family relationships. The treatment incorporates the notion of "limited reparenting" for the purpose of bringing about corrective emotional experiences with respect to the patient's early unmet basic human needs for safety, nurturance, autonomy, self-expression, and/or limits. According to Young, when basic needs are not met, early maladaptive schemas (EMSs) within the individual (child or adolescent) are likely to develop. EMSs "refer to extremely stable and enduring themes that develop and are elaborated upon throughout the individual's lifetime and that are dysfunctional to a significant degree" (Young, 1990/1999, p. 9). Schemas are constructions of reality (which are deeply held emotion-based beliefs) that develop as the result of concrete experiences with the environment, particularly those early in life with significant others. Once developed, they are mostly outside of awareness and remain dormant until a life event stimulates one or more schemas. Once schema(s) are activated, the individual automatically processes information (cognitive, behavioral, affective, and interpersonal) in ways accordant with the schema(s). Young has identified 18 EMSs in five hypothesized domains (see Figure 6.1 on pages 261–263). Most of these schemas have been supported by subsequent research (Lee, Taylor, & Dunn, 1999; Schmidt, 1994; Schmidt, Joiner, Young, & Telch, 1995). Once the schema(s) have become

activated, Young has also observed specific characteristic modes of responding: child modes, maladaptive coping modes, and/or dysfunctional parent modes (see Figures 6.2a–c on pages 264–265). A mode is "the set of schemas or schema operations—adaptive or maladaptive—that are currently active for an individual" (Young et al., 2003, p. 271). The automatic processing and responses that occur when one is caught in a maladaptive mode preserve the underlying maladaptive schema(s). The focus of schema therapy is to increase the patient's awareness of the schemas and modes, understand the origin (and possible prior adaptive value) of the modes, link the modes to current experience, and to modify and/or incorporate new, more adaptive modes. This is accomplished by accessing the vulnerable child mode through imagery and helping the patient to reconstruct or alter the historical record of events by bringing in a newly developed or strengthened "healthy adult mode" to guide, support, set limits, and/or protect that vulnerable child. A recent study by Giesen-Bloo and colleagues (2006) found surprisingly strong and significant results in favor of schema-focused therapy over transference-focused therapy with the chronic disorder of borderline personality. After 3 years of treatment (sessions twice per week), 45% of the patients in schema-focused therapy (vs. 24% in transference-focused therapy) completely recovered. One year later, over half (52%) in schema-focused therapy fully recovered (vs. 29% in transference-focused therapy) and two-thirds (70%) in schema-focused therapy showed significant improvement. In addition, patients in schema-focused therapy were significantly less likely to drop out of therapy (27% dropped out of schema-focused therapy vs. 50% dropped out of transference-focused therapy). Given the high degree of similarities between patients with chronic disorders (adverse childhood histories, early-onset depression, and a multitude of schemas), we believe that schema-focused therapy is very likely to be an effective treatment for the chronically depressed population as well.

Research on Pharmacological Interventions and Cognitive Therapy

Despite the findings cited earlier, drugs are still the initial and most frequently prescribed form of treatment for unipolar depression in the

United Stares (Antonuccio et al., 1995) and the most commonly used method to maintain treatment gains (Geddes et al., 2003). Several factors likely have contributed to this treatment bias. The government's Depression Guideline Panel (1993) recommended that two trials of antidepressants, both unsuccessful, should be completed before recommending psychotherapy for depression. Although a later report from the Surgeon General (Mental Health: A report of the Surgeon General, 1997, Chapter 4) summarized research indicating the effectiveness of CBT for depression, specific treatment recommendations were not made. As such, the only recommendations made by the government have remained unrevised. Additionally, the most recent White House Conference on Mental Health continued to reveal a psychopharmacological treatment bias (Saeman, 1999). Treatment guidelines, such as the one issued by the American Psychiatric Association (2000), also continue to recommend that antidepressants be used to treat moderate to severe depression. Apart from the contribution of the political environment to this bias is that of the managed care environment. Managed care companies often use medical doctors as gatekeepers to the type of care a patient receives. Obvious professional allegiance is built into this system. Although psychotropic medications clearly provide enormous benefit and relief to a substantial portion of depressed patients, research does not support this bias toward medication. Three important points have not been adequately considered: premature termination and iatrogenic effects of pharmacotherapy, patient preference, and cost-effectiveness.

Research has shown that "a sizeable group of patients either chooses not to continue long-term pharmacotherapy in the absence of any depressive symptoms, cannot take medication due to a medical condition that precludes the use of antidepressants, or suffer from side effects that are intolerable to them" (Spanier, Frank, McEachran, Grochocinski, & Kupfer, 1999, p. 250). In fact, one group of researchers concluded that "there is much evidence that antidepressant medications are not benign treatments. . . . Many antidepressants are cardiotoxic, have dangerous side effects, and are often used in suicide attempts. . . . [They also] result in relatively poorer compliance than psychotherapy, have a higher dropout rate, and result in as much as a 60% non-

response rate with some patient populations" (Antonuccio et al., 1995, p. 581). (Of course, psychotherapy may also have unintended and undesirable side effects [Mohr, 1995], but very little is known about any negative effects associated with cognitive therapy.)

Another consideration is the preference of patients, the "consumers." Research suggests that consumers seem to have a preference for psychotherapy over medication for depression: "The results of treatment acceptability studies show that, as treatments for depression in adults, psychotherapies are perceived by potential consumers as more acceptable than pharmacotherapy alone as well as combinations of psychotherapy and pharmacotherapy" (Hall & Robertson, 1998, p. 271). This is not surprising given that most people attribute their depressions to negative life experiences, with stress and environmental factors playing major roles (Antonuccio et al., 1995; Brown, 1996; Eifert, Beach, & Wilson, 1998).

A final consideration is the cost-effectiveness of treatment. The research on this topic is surprisingly limited (Johnsson & Bebbington, 1994; Rosenbaum & Hylan, 1999; Scott & Freeman, 1992). Antonuccio, Thomas, and Danton (1997) conducted a cost-effectiveness analysis on several outcome studies on depression and found that over a 2-year period the cost of fluoxetine alone was 33% higher than individual CBT and that combined treatment of flouxetine and CBT was 23% higher than CBT alone. A recent Australian study (Vos, Corry, Haby, Carter, & Andrews, 2005) examined the cost and benefits of CBT and drugs in the episodic and maintenance treatment of depression. They found maintenance treatment with SSRIs to be the most expensive option, nearly double that of bibliotherapy, group CBT, individual CBT, and TCAs. Scott, Palmer, Paykel, Teasdale, and Hayhurst (2003) compared the cost-effectiveness of relapse prevention in depression by comparing CBT as an adjunctive treatment to antidepressants and clinical management, and with antidepressants and clinical management alone, over a 17-month period. They found the addition of CBT was not only more expensive but also more effective in reducing cumulative relapse rates (relapse rates were 29% with adjunctive CBT vs. 47% without adjunctive CBT). Importantly, they noted that the costs associated with adjunctive CBT in their study were a "worst-case" scenario, because the follow-up extended only 17 months; other research (as noted in the previous section) has demonstrated maintenance of gains and lowered relapse rates up to 6 years with CBT. Scott and colleagues argued that the incrementally adjusted costs over time to relapse should be considered in decision making on the value of various treatments. These initial findings suggest that CBT, either alone or in combination with drugs, can enhance cost-effectiveness, particularly when higher short-term costs of combined treatments are balanced by better outcomes and lower marginal costs in the long term.

Research Controversy and Criticism

Despite the fact that cognitive therapy is the most empirically tested psychotherapy for depression currently available, it has not been unequivocally embraced. Some have questioned the validity of the findings on the basis of methodological flaws or insufficient data (Gelder, 1994; Klein, 1996; Scott, 1996a), whereas others have attempted to temper the results by attributing them to "experimental allegiance"—the preference by the researcher for one therapy over others (Gaffan, Tsaousis, & Kemp-Wheeler, 1995; Luborsky et al., 1999). Some behaviorists have tried to dismiss cognitive therapy altogether by claiming that it is based on "cognitivist oversell" and "self-deception" (Wolpe, 1993, p. 143).

Parker, Roy, and Eyers (2003) conducted a review of meta-analyses and major studies, and concluded that CBT was less effective than suggested by adherents. However, Butler, Chapman, Forman, and Beck (2006, p. 20) noted that Parker and colleagues (2003)

> excluded . . . high quality clinical trials showing cognitive-behavioral therapy to be superior to alternative treatments at follow-up (see Shapiro et al., 1994, for a comparison with psychodynamic therapy; Blatt, Zuroff, Bondi, & Sanislow, 2000, for a comparison with antidepressant medication). Since Parker et al. did not report the criteria by which they selected research studies for their review, it is difficult to interpret their conclusions.

In the most extensive and methodologically rigorous meta-analysis to date, Gloaguen and colleagues (1998) found that CBT was superior to waiting-list or placebo controls, modestly superior (ES = 0.24) to a miscellaneous group of psychotherapies, and equivalent to behavior therapy. Wampold, Minami, Baskin, and

Tierney (2000) noted that some of the therapies included in the miscellaneous group were not comprehensive treatments for depression (e.g., progressive muscular relaxation). After categorizing these miscellaneous therapies into established and nonestablished treatments for depression, they found CBT only marginally superior (ES = 0.16) to other established treatments. As Butler and colleagues (2006) noted,

> a heterogeneous collection of miscellaneous therapies, as done by Gloaguen et al., can at best provide limited information. Future meta-analyses are needed that provide direct comparisons between CBT and specific alternative therapies. . . . There are relatively few direct comparisons and not enough to provide the basis for a meaningful meta-analysis. (pp. 22–23)

A recent meta-analysis of treatment outcome research on child and adolescent depression (Weisz et al., 2006) found that CBT performed no better than noncognitive psychotherapy treatments, all of which produced effects that were "significant but modest in their strength, breadth, and durability" (p. 132). The results of this meta-analysis stand in stark contrast to two prior meta-analyses published on CBT with depressed youth (Lewinsohn & Clarke, 1999; Reinecke et al., 1998), which indicated large treatment effects. The Weisz and colleagues (2006) meta-analysis included both peer-reviewed and non-peer-reviewed studies, and included results from the TADS (2004) study. Excluding the TADS results, the mean ES of the other 23 CBT studies (out of a total of 44 studies) was in the medium range (0.48). Weisz and colleagues noted a broad range of ESs across the studies (including the CBT studies) in their meta-analysis. They stated: "Indeed, five different treatment programs generated effects exceeding 1.0. Thus, some treatments in the current armamentarium may already have strong potential"; however, they also noted that "the strongest potential may not attach to the most popular treatments. In the current *zeitgeist*, treatments that focus on altering unrealistic, negative cognitions, have particularly prominent status" (p. 144).

There has been some debate as to whether the cognitive components of treatment are necessary for treating depression. Some researchers have argued that the behavioral aspects of cognitive therapy are primarily responsible for improvement. For example, the results from Gloaguen and colleagues' (1998) meta-analysis, based on clinical trials conducted between 1977 and 1996, indicated that cognitive therapy was equal to behavior therapy. In another study, a component analysis conducted by Jacobson and colleagues (1996), behavioral activation (BA) alone produced as much change as cognitive therapy. Additionally, Dimidjian and colleagues (2006) found a more comprehensive version of BA (Martell, Addis, & Jacobson, 2001) to be equivalent to medication, outperforming cognitive therapy for individuals with moderate to severe depression at both 8 weeks and 16 weeks of treatment. Dimidjian and colleagues noted:

> A. T. Beck and colleagues (1979) have long suggested that therapists focus on behavioral strategies early in treatment when patients are more depressed and return to that emphasis later if patients start to worsen. Although the current data do not specifically address whether change in cognition is a mediator of symptom change, they provide strong evidence that behavioral methods are sufficient to produce symptom change irrespective of whether improvement is mediated by cognitive change or not. (cf. Bandura, 1977) (p. 667)

It is important to note that length of treatment in the Dimidjian and colleagues study was on the short end (15–25 weeks) of the recommended length of CBT treatment and did not examine long-term efficacy. A study by Gortner, Gollan, Dobson, and Jacoboson (1998), which followed up the Jacobson and colleagues research, however, found that patients exposed to the behavioral components of treatment were no more likely to relapse following termination than those treated with both cognitive and behavioral components. These findings raise important questions for further research regarding parsimony of treatment.

Current Status and Future Research on Treating Depression

There is now a considerable body of research on antidepressant and cognitive treatments for depression. Certainly there are still enough inconsistencies in the literature to warrant continued debate and research regarding the relative merits of different treatments for depression (Agosti & Ocepek, 1997; Gortner et al., 1998; Oei & Free, 1995; Robinson, Berman, & Neimeyer, 1990; Stewart, Garfinkel, Nunes, Donovan, & Klein, 1998;

Thase et al., 1997). Nevertheless, the efficacy of cognitive therapy for depression is clearly a replicable and robust finding.

Our own hope, however, is that we will see a movement away from the current "horse race" approach so prevalent in the research literature (Williams, 1997). Many important, unanswered questions make it impossible, in our opinion, for proponents of any one treatment to make firm recommendations favoring one treatment for depression over another. In the spirit of Beck's testable hypotheses and clinical protocols, and through more sophisticated research studies, we hope that it will be possible to assess which types of depressed patients will benefit most from which type of treatment, or combination of treatments, and in what sequence.

The remainder of this chapter is devoted to detailing the basic characteristics of cognitive therapy and demonstrating applications of cognitive therapy to depression in clinical practice.

COGNITIVE MODEL OF DEPRESSION

The cognitive model assumes that cognition, behavior, and biochemistry are all important components of depressive disorders. We do not view them as competing theories of depression but as different levels of analysis. Each treatment approach has its own "focus of convenience." The pharmacotherapist intervenes at the biochemical level; the cognitive therapist intervenes at the cognitive, affective, and behavioral levels. Our experience suggests that when we change depressive cognitions, we simultaneously change the characteristic mood, the behavior, and, as some evidence suggests (Free, Oei, & Appleton, 1998; Joffe, Segal, & Singer, 1996), the biochemistry of depression. Although the exact mechanism of change remains a target of considerable investigation, speculation, and debate (Barber & DeRubeis, 1989; Castonguay, Goldfried, Wiser, Raue, & Hayes, 1996; Crews & Harrison, 1995; DeRubeis et al., 1990; DeRubeis & Feeley, 1990; Hayes & Strauss, 1998; Oei & Free, 1995; Oei & Shuttlewood, 1996; Shea & Elkin, 1996; Sullivan & Conway, 1991; Whisman, 1993), "there are indications that cognitive therapy works by virtue of changing beliefs and information-processing proclivities and that different aspects of cognition play different roles in the process of change" (Hollon et al., 1996, p. 314).

Our focus in this chapter is on the cognitive disturbances in depression. Cognitive science research emphasizes the importance of information processing in depressive symptomatology (Ingram & Holle, 1992). According to these theories, negatively biased cognition is a core process in depression. This process is reflected in the "cognitive triad of depression": Depressed patients typically have a negative view of themselves, of their environment, and of the future. They view themselves as worthless, inadequate, unlovable, and deficient. Depressed patients view the environment as overwhelming, as presenting insuperable obstacles that cannot be overcome, and that continually result in failure or loss. Moreover, they view the future as hopeless; they believe their own efforts will be insufficient to change the unsatisfying course of their lives. This negative view of the future often leads to suicidal ideation and actual suicide attempts.

Depressed patients consistently distort their interpretations of events, so that they maintain negative views of themselves, the environment, and the future. These distortions represent deviations from the logical processes of thinking typically used by people. For example, a depressed woman whose husband comes home late one night may conclude that he is having an affair with another woman, even though there is no other evidence supporting this conclusion. This example illustrates an "arbitrary inference," reaching a conclusion that is not justified by the available evidence. Other distortions include all-or-nothing thinking, overgeneralization, selective abstraction, and magnification (Beck et al., 1979).

According to subsequent developments within the cognitive model, an important predisposing factor for many patients with depression is the presence of early schemas (Stein & Young, 1992; Young, 1990/1999).[3] Beck (1976) emphasized the importance of schemas in depression and provided the following definition:

> A schema is a cognitive structure for screening, coding, and evaluating the stimuli that impinge on the organism. . . . On the basis of this matrix of schemas, the individual is able to orient himself in relation to time and space and to categorize and interpret experiences in a meaningful way. (p. 233)

Furthermore, Beck, Freeman, and Associates (1990) noted:

> In the field of psychopathology, the term "schema" has been applied to structures with a highly personalized idiosyncratic content that are activated during disorders such as depression, anxiety, panic attacks, and obsessions, and become prepotent. . . . Thus, in clinical depression, for example, the negative schemas are in ascendancy, resulting in a systematic negative bias in the interpretation and recall of experiences as well as in short-term and long-term predictions, whereas the positive schemas become less accessible. It is easy for depressed patients to see the negative aspects of an event, but difficult to see the positive. They can recall negative events much more readily than positive ones. They weigh the probabilities of undesirable outcomes more heavily than positive outcomes. (p. 32)

It is also becoming increasingly recognized that "focusing on core schemas is a key to effective short-term therapy" (Freeman & Davison, 1997, p. 8).

Through clinical observation, Young has identified a subset of schemas that he terms "early maladaptive schemas." The 18 EMSs in five hypothesized domains identified by Young can be seen in Figure 6.1. According to Young's (1990/1999) schema approach, children learn to construct reality through early experiences with the environment, especially with significant others. EMSs likely develop when the environment does not meet core needs for safety, stability or predictability, love, nurturance and attention, acceptance and praise, empathy, realistic limits, and validation of feelings and needs. Sometimes these early experiences lead children to accept attitudes and beliefs that later prove maladaptive. For example, a child may develop the schema that no matter what he or she does, his or her performance will never be good enough. These schemas usually occur outside of awareness and may remain dormant until a life event (e.g., being fired from a job) stimulates the schema. Once the schema is activated, the patient categorizes, selects, and encodes information in such a way that the failure schema is maintained. EMSs therefore predispose depressed patients to distort events in a characteristic fashion, leading to a negative view of themselves, the environment, and the future.

EMSs have several defining characteristics that are (1) a priori truths about oneself and/or

DISCONNECTION AND REJECTION
Expectation that one's needs for security safety, stability, nurturance, empathy, sharing of feelings, acceptance, and respect will not be met in a predictable manner. Typical family origin is detached, cold, rejecting, withholding, lonely, explosive, unpredictable, or abusive.

1. ABANDONMENT/INSTABILITY
   The perceived *instability* or *unreliability* of those available for support and connection. Involves the sense that significant others will not be able to continue providing emotional support, connection, strength, or practical protection because they are emotionally unstable and unpredictable (e.g., angry outbursts). unreliable or erratically present; because they will die imminently; or because they will abandon the patient in favor of someone better.

2. MISTRUST/ABUSE
   The expectation that others will hurt, abuse, humiliate, cheat, lie, manipulate, or take advantage. Usually involves the perception that the harm is intentional or the result of unjustified and extreme negligence. May include the sense that one always ends up being cheated relative to others or "getting the short end of the stick."

3. EMOTIONAL DEPRIVATION
   Expectation that one's desire for a normal degree of emotional support will not be adequately met by others. The three major forms of deprivation are:
   A. *Deprivation of nurturance:* Absence of attention, affection, warmth, or companionship.
   B. *Deprivation of empathy:* Absence of understanding, listening, self-disclosure, or mutual sharing of feelings from others.
   C. *Deprivation of protection:* Absence of strength, direction, or guidance from others.

4. DEFECTIVENESS/SHAME
   The feeling that one is defective, bad, unwanted, inferior, or invalid in important respects; or that one would be unlovable to significant others it exposed. May Involve hypersensitivity to criticism, rejection, and blame; self-consciousness, comparisons, and insecurity around others; or a sense of shame regarding one's perceived flaws. These flaws may be *private* (e.g., selfishness, angry impulses, unacceptable sexual desires) or *public* (e.g., undesirable physical appearance, social awkwardness).

5. SOCIAL ISOLATION/ALIENATION
   The feeling that one is isolated from the rest of the world, different from other people, and/or not part of any group or community.

IMPAIRED AUTONOMY AND PERFORMANCE
Expectations about oneself and the environment that interfere with one's perceived ability to separate, survive, function independently, or perform successfully. Typical family origin is enmeshed, undermining of child's confidence, overprotective, or failing to reinforce child for performing competently outside the family.

6. DEPENDENCE/INCOMPETENCE
   Belief that one is unable to handle one's *everyday responsibilities* in a competent manner, without considerable help from others (e.g., take care of oneself, solve daily problems, exercise good judgment, tackle new tasks, make good decisions). Often presents as helplessness.

7. VULNERABILITY TO HARM OR ILLNESS
   Exaggerated fear that *imminent* catastrophe will strike at any time and that one will be unable to prevent it. Fears focus on one or more of the following: (A) *medical catastrophes* (e.g., heart attacks, AIDS); (B) *emotional catastrophes* (e.g., going crazy); (C) *external catastrophes* (e.g., elevators collapsing, victimized by criminals, airplane crashes, earthquakes).

(continued)

FIGURE 6.1. Early maladaptive schemas with associated schema domains (revised November 1998). Copyright 1999 by Jeffrey E. Young, PhD. Reprinted with permission. Unauthorized reproduction without written consent of the author is prohibited. For more information, write Cognitive Therapy Center of New York, 36 West 44th Street, Suite 1007, New York, NY 10036.

8. ENMESHMENT/UNDEVOLOPED SELF

Excessive emotional involvement and closeness with one or more significant others (often parents), at the expense of full individuation or normal social development. Often involves the belief that at least one of the enmeshed individuals cannot survive or be happy without the constant support of the other. May also include feelings of being smothered by, or fused with, others OR insufficient individual identity. Often experienced as a feeling of emptiness and floundering, having no direction, or in extreme cases questioning one's existence.

9. FAILURE

The belief that one has failed, will inevitably fail, or is fundamentally inadequate relative to one's peers, in areas of *achievement* (school, career, sports, etc.) Often involves beliefs that one is stupid, inept, untalented. ignorant, lower in status, less successful than others, etc.

IMPAIRED LIMITS
Deficiency in internal limits, responsibility to others, or long-term goal orientation. Leads to difficulty respecting the rights of others, cooperating with others making commitments, or setting and meeting realistic personal goals. Typical family origin is characterized by permissiveness, overindulgence, lack of direction, or a sense of superiority—rather than appropriate confrontation discipline and limits in relation to taking responsibility, cooperating in a reciprocal manner and setting goals. In some cases, child may not have been pushed to tolerate normal levels of discomfort, or may not have been given adequate supervision, direction or guidance.

10. ENTITLEMENT/GRANDIOSITY

The belief that one is superior to other people; entitled to special rights and privileges; or not bound by the rules of reciprocity that guide normal social interaction. Often involves insistence that one should be able to do or have whatever one wants regardless of what is realistic, what others consider reasonable, or the cost to others; OR an exaggerated focus on superiority (e.g., being among the most successful, famous, and wealthy) in order to achieve *power or control* (not primarily for attention or approval). Sometimes includes excessive competitiveness toward, or domination of others: asserting ones power, forcing one's point of view, or controlling the behavior of others in line with one's own desires—without empathy or concern for others' needs or feelings.

11. INSUFFICIENT SELF-CONTROL/SELF-DISCIPLINE

Pervasive difficulty or refusal to exercise sufficient self-control and frustration tolerance to achieve one's personal goals, or to restrain the excessive expression of one's emotions and impulses. In its milder form, patient presents with an exaggerated emphasis on discomfort avoidance: avoiding pain, conflict, confrontation, responsibility, or overexertion—at the expense of personal fulfillment, commitment, or integrity.

OTHER-DIRECTEDNESS
An excessive focus on the desires, feelings and responses of others, at the expense of one's own needs—in order to gain love and approval, maintain one's sense of connection or avoid retaliation. Usually involves suppression and lack of awareness regarding one's own anger and natural inclinations. Typical family origin Is based on conditional acceptance: Children must suppress important aspects of themselves in order to gain love, attention, and approval. In many such families, the parents' emotional needs and desires—or social acceptance and status—are valued more than the unique needs and feelings of each child.

12. SUBJUGATION

Excessive surrendering of control to others because one feels coerced—usually to avoid anger, retaliation, or abandonment. The two major forms of subjugation are:
A. *Subjugation of needs*: Suppression of one's preferences, decisions, and desires.
B. *Subjugation of emotion:* Suppression of emotional expression, especially anger.
Usually involves the perception that one's own desires, opinions, and feelings are not valid or important to others. Frequently presents as excessive compliance, combined with hypersensitivity to feeling trapped. Generally leads to a buildup of anger, manifested in maladaptive symptoms (e.g., passive–aggressive behavior, uncontrolled outbursts of temper, psychosomatic symptoms, withdrawal of affection, "acting out," substance abuse).

(continued)

FIGURE 6.1. *(continued)*

13. SELF-SACRIFICE

Excessive focus on *voluntarily* meeting the needs of others in daily situations, at the expense of one's own gratification. The most common reasons are to prevent causing pain to others; to avoid guilt from feeling selfish; or to maintain the connection with others perceived as needy. Often results from an acute sensitivity to the pain of others. Sometimes leads to a sense that one's own needs are not being adequately met and to resentment of those who are taken care of. (Overlaps with concept of codependency.)

14. APPROVAL SEEKING/RECOGNITION SEEKING

Excessive emphasis on gaining approval, recognition or attention from other people or fitting in, at the expense of developing a secure and true sense of self. One's sense of esteem is dependent primarily on the reactions of others rather than on one's own natural inclinations. Sometimes includes an overemphasis on status, appearance, social acceptance, money, or achievements—as a means of gaining *approval, admiration,* or *attention* (not primarily for power or control). Frequently results in major life decisions that are inauthentic or unsatisfying, or in hypersensitivity to rejection.

OVERVIGILANCE AND INHIBITION

Excessive emphasis on suppressing one's spontaneous feelings, impulses, and choices OR on meeting rigid, internalized rules and expectations about performance and ethical behavior—often at the expense of happiness, self-expression, relaxation, close relationships, or health. Typical family origin is grim, demanding, and sometimes punitive: Performance, duty, perfectionism—following rules, hiding emotions, and avoiding mistakes predominate over pleasure, joy, and relaxation. There is usually an undercurrent of pessimism and worry that things could fall apart if one fails to be vigilant and careful at all times.

15. NEGATIVITY/PESSIMISM

A pervasive, lifelong focus on the negative aspects of life (pain, death, loss, disappointment, conflict, guilt, resentment, unsolved problems, potential mistakes, betrayal, things that could go wrong, etc.) while minimizing or neglecting the positive or optimistic aspects. Usually includes an exaggerated expectation—in a wide range of work, financial, or interpersonal situations—that things will eventually go seriously wrong, or that aspects of one's life that seem to be going well will ultimately fall apart. Usually involves an inordinate fear of making mistakes that might lead to financial collapse, loss, humiliation or being trapped in a bad situation. Because potential negative outcomes are exaggerated, these patients are frequently characterized by chronic worry, vigilance, complaining, or indecision.

16. EMOTIONAL INHIBITION

The excessive inhibition of spontaneous action, feeling, or communication—usually to avoid disapproval by others, feelings of shame, or losing control of one's impulses The most common areas of inhibition involve (A) inhibition of *anger* and aggression; (B) inhibition of *positive impulses* (e.g., joy, affection, sexual excitement, play); (C) difficulty expressing *vulnerability* or *communicating* freely about one's feelings, needs, etc.; or (D) excessive emphasis on *rationality* while disregarding emotions.

17. UNRELENTING STANDARDS/HYPERCRITICALNESS

The underlying belief that one must strive to meet very high *internalized standards* of behavior and performance usually to avoid criticism. Typically results in feelings of pressure or difficulty slowing down and in hypercriticalness toward oneself and others. Must involve significant impairment in pleasure, relaxation, health, self-esteem sense of accomplishment, or satisfying relationships. Unrelenting standards typically present as (A) *perfectionism*, inordinate attention to detail, or an underestimate of how good one's own performance is relative to the norm; (B) *rigid rules* and "shoulds" in many areas of life, including unrealistically high moral, ethical, cultural or religious precepts; or (C) preoccupation with *time and efficiency* so that more can be accomplished.

18. PUNITIVENESS

The belief that people should be harshly punished for making mistakes. Involves the tendency to be angry, intolerant, punitive, and impatient with those people (including oneself) who do not meet one's expectations or standards. Usually includes difficulty forgiving mistakes in oneself or others because of a reluctance to consider extenuating circumstances, allow for human imperfection, or empathize with feelings.

FIGURE 6.1. *(continued)*

the environment; (2) self-perpetuating and re-sistant to change; (3) dysfunctional; (4) often triggered by some environmental change (e.g., loss of a job or mate); (5) tied to high levels of affect when activated; and (6) usually result from an interaction of the child's innate tem-perament with dysfunctional developmental experiences with family members or caretakers (Young, 1990/1999).

When a multitude of EMSs develop, and are deeply entrenched, or the patient is highly avoidant or tends to be stuck in overcompen-sating for EMSs, as is likely in patients with chronic depression, the additional concept of "schema modes" or "modes" (Young et al., 2003) becomes therapeutically useful. Young's notion of a mode is similar to that of an ego state. A mode is defined as "those schemas or schema operations—adaptive or maladaptive—that are currently active for an individual" (p. 271). A dysfunctional mode is activated when specific maladaptive schemas or coping responses have erupted into distressing emo-tions, avoidance responses, or self-defeating behaviors that take over and control an indi-vidual's functioning at a given point in time. An individual also may shift from one dysfunction-al mode into another; as that shift occurs, dif-ferent schemas or coping responses, previously

dormant, become active (Young et al., 2003). Rapid shifts are referred to as "flipping" modes. Young and colleagues (2003) identified four main types of modes: Child modes (Figure 6.2a), Maladaptive Coping modes (Figure 6.2b), Dysfunctional Parent modes (Figure 6.2c), and Healthy Adult mode. The Healthy Adult mode is

> the healthy, adult part of the self that serves an "executive" function relative to the other modes. The Healthy Adult helps meet the child's basic emotional needs. Building and strengthening the patient's Healthy Adult to work with the other modes more effectively is the overarching goal of mode work in schema therapy. (p. 277)

In the following sections we present infor-mation about the general characteristics and nature of cognitive therapy, a discussion of the process of cognitive therapy, then two cases that illustrate cognitive therapy in action. The patient in the first case has a nonchronic form of depression and is treated with standard cog-nitive therapy. The focus of standard cognitive therapy is on changing depressive thinking. The patient in the second case has chronic de-pression and is treated with schema therapy. The focus of schema therapy, in this case, is on

Child Mode	Description	Common associated schemas
Vulnerable Child	Experiences dysphoric or anxious affect, especially fear, sadness, and helplessness, when "in touch" with associated schemas.	Abandonment, Mistrust/Abuse, Emotional Deprivation, Defectiveness, Social Isolation, Dependence/Incompetence, Vulnerability to Harm or Illness, Enmeshment/Undeveloped Self, Negativity/Pessimism.
Angry Child	Vents anger directly in response to perceived unmet core needs or unfair treatment related to core schemas.	Abandonment, Mistrust/Abuse, Emotional Deprivation, Subjugation (or, at times, any of the schemas associated with the Vulnerable Child).
Impulsive/Undisciplined Child	Impulsively acts according to immediate desires for pleasure without regard to limits or others' needs or feelings (not linked to core needs).	Entitlement, Insufficient Self-Control/Self-Discipline.
Happy Child	Feels loved, connected, content, satisfied.	None. Absence of activated schemas.

FIGURE 6.2a. Child modes. From Young, Klosko, and Weishaar (2003). Copyright 2003 by The Guilford Press. Reprinted by permission.

Maladaptive Coping Modes	Description
Compliant Surrenderer	Adopts a coping style of compliance and dependence.
Detached Protector	Adopts a coping style of emotional withdrawal, disconnection, isolation, and behavioral avoidance.
Overcompensator	Adopts a coping style of counterattack and control. May overcompensate through semiadaptive means, such as workaholism.

FIGURE 6.2b. Maladaptive Coping modes. From Young, Klosko, and Weishaar (2003). Copyright 2003 by The Guilford Press. Reprinted by permission.

identifying and modifying the patient's underlying schemas through mode work. Mode work strengthens and develops healthy modes and weakens dysfunctional modes, thereby increasing control over one's responding.

CHARACTERISTICS OF THERAPY

Cognitive therapy with adult depressed outpatients is usually undertaken in the therapist's office. It has most frequently been applied in a one-to-one setting. However, group cognitive therapy has also been shown to be successful with many depressed outpatients (Beutler et al., 1987; Jarrett & Nelson, 1987), although it may not be as effective as individual treatment (Wierzbicki & Bartlett, 1987). Additionally, computer-assisted cognitive therapy for depression (50-minute vs. 25-minute sessions with computer assistance) also has been found effective (Wright et al., 2005). It is not unusual to involve spouses, partners, parents, and other family members during treatment. They may be used, for example, to provide information

that helps patients test the validity of their thinking with respect to how other family members view them. Moreover, couple therapy based on the cognitive model is often very effective in relieving depression related to chronic interpersonal problems (Beck, 1988; O'Leary & Beach, 1990).

In our clinical experience, a number of therapist characteristics contribute to effective cognitive therapy. First, cognitive therapists ideally should demonstrate the "nonspecific" therapy skills identified by other writers (see, e.g., Truax & Mitchell, 1971): They should be able to communicate warmth, genuineness, sincerity, and openness. Second, the most effective cognitive therapists seem to be especially skilled at seeing events from their patients' perspective (accurate empathy). They are able to suspend their own personal assumptions and biases while listening to depressed patients describe their reactions and interpretations. Third, skilled cognitive therapists can reason logically and plan strategies; they are not "fuzzy" thinkers. In this respect they resemble good trial lawyers, who can spot the sometimes

Dysfunctional Parent Mode	Description	Common associated schemas
Punitive/Critical Parent	Restricts, criticizes, or punishes the self or others.	Subjugation, Punitiveness, Defectiveness, Mistrust/Abuse (as abuser).
Demanding Parent	Sets high expectations and high level of responsibility toward others; pressures the self or others to achieve them.	Unrelenting Standards, Self-Sacrifice.

FIGURE 6.2c. Dysfunctional Parent modes. From Young, Klosko, and Weishaar (2003). Copyright 2003 by The Guilford Press. Reprinted by permission.

subtle flaws in another individual's reasoning and skillfully elicit a more convincing interpretation of the same events. Skilled cognitive therapists plan strategies several steps ahead, anticipating the desired outcome. Fourth, the best practitioners of this approach are active. They have to be comfortable taking the lead, providing structure and direction to the therapy process.

Although patient characteristics have received some empirical attention (Eifert et al., 1998; Padesky & Greenberger, 1995; Persons, Burns, & Perloff, 1988; Shea et al., 1990), we do not yet have adequate knowledge of which patient characteristics are related to success in cognitive therapy. Our experience suggests that patients with major depressive disorder (single episode or recurrent)[4] and dysthymic disorder (with or without major depressive disorder) respond well to the cognitive therapy approach described in this chapter. To the extent that the patient is diagnosed with Axis II personality disorders and/or the patient's depression is chronic, schema therapy treatment may be significantly longer in duration and more crucial in obtaining a more complete and lasting positive response to treatment.

Cognitive therapy can serve an important adjunctive role to pharmacotherapy for bipolar disorders (Ball et al., 2006; Basco & Rush, 1996; Colom, Vieta, Martinez, Jorquera, & Gastó, 1998; Craighead, Miklowitz, Vajk, & Frank, 1998; Lam, Hayward, Watkins, Wright, & Sham, 2005; Scott, 1996b), and is effective in treating patients with severe endogenous depression (Thase, Bowler, & Harden, 1991; Whisman, 1993). Preliminary evidence also suggests that cognitive therapy is effective in the treatment of women with postpartum depression (Bledsoe & Grote, 2006).

It is advisable to assess patients' suitability for cognitive therapy (Padesky & Greenberger, 1995; Safran & Segal, 1990; Safran, Segal, Vallis, Shaw, & Samstag, 1993). In our experience, certain patient characteristics are predictive of a more rapid response: Patients who are appropriately introspective and can reason abstractly; who are well organized, good planners, and conscientious about carrying out responsibilities; who are employed; who are not excessively angry, either at themselves or at other people; who are less dogmatic and rigid in their thinking; who can identify a clear precipitating event for the depressive episode; and who have close relationships with others often show faster improvement in depressive symptoms through cognitive therapy. Age is not an obstacle, because both younger patients (Harrington, Wood, & Verduyn, 1998; Reinecke et al., 1998) and older adults (Beutler et al., 1987; Floyd, Scogin, McKendree-Smith, Floyd, & Rokke, 2004; Gallagher-Thompson, Hanley-Peterson, & Thompson, 1990; Koder, Brodaty, & Anstey, 1996; Levendusky & Hufford, 1997) seem to benefit from cognitive therapy. Many studies have indicated that children and adolescents show significant clinical improvement following CBT (Curry, 2001). Studies of older patients show that "various forms of cognitive and behavioral psychotherapy can be as effective in treating geriatric depression as depressions occurring earlier in life" (Futterman, Thompson, Gallagher-Thompson, & Ferris, 1995, p. 511).

COLLABORATION

Basic to cognitive therapy is a collaborative relationship between patient and therapist. When therapist and patient work together, the learning experience is enhanced for both, and the cooperative spirit that is developed contributes greatly to the therapeutic process. Equally important, the collaborative approach helps to ensure compatible goals for treatment, and to prevent misunderstandings and misinterpretations between patient and therapist. Because of the importance of the collaborative relationship, we place great emphasis on the interpersonal skills of the therapist, the process of joint selection of problems to be worked on, regular feedback, and the investigative process we call "collaborative empiricism."

Interpersonal Qualities

Because collaboration requires that the patient trust the therapist, we emphasize those interpersonal qualities that contribute to trust. As noted earlier, warmth, accurate empathy, and genuineness are desirable personal qualities for the cognitive therapist, as well as for all psychotherapists. It is important that the cognitive therapist not seem to be playing the *role* of therapist. The therapist should be able to communicate both verbally and nonverbally that he or she is sincere, open, concerned, and direct. It is also important that the therapist not seem to be withholding impressions or information, or evading questions. The therapist should be careful not to seem critical or disapproving of the patient's perspective.

Rapport between patient and therapist is crucial in the treatment of depressed patients. When rapport is optimal, patients perceive the therapist as someone who is tuned in to their feelings and attitudes, who is sympathetic and understanding, and with whom they can communicate without having to articulate feelings in detail or qualify statements. When the rapport is good, both patient and therapist feel comfortable and secure.

A confident, professional manner is also important in cognitive therapy. A therapist should convey relaxed confidence in his or her ability to help a depressed patient. Such confidence can help to counteract the patient's initial hopelessness about the future. Because the cognitive therapist must sometimes be directive and impose structure, especially in the early stages of treatment, it is helpful to maintain a clear sense of professionalism.

Joint Determination of Goals for Therapy

The patient and therapist collaboratively work together to set therapeutic goals, determine priorities among them, and create an agenda for each session. Problems to be addressed over the course of therapy include specific depressive symptoms (e.g., hopelessness, crying, and difficulty concentrating) and external problems (e.g., couple difficulties, career issues, child-rearing concerns). Priorities are then jointly determined in accordance with how much distress is generated by a particular problem and how amenable that particular problem is to change. During the agenda-setting portion of each therapy session (discussed in detail in the next section), therapist and patient together determine the items to be covered in that session. Through this collaborative process, target problems are selected on a weekly basis.

The process of problem selection often presents difficulties for the novice cognitive therapist, including failure to reach agreement on specific problems on which to focus, selection of peripheral concerns, and the tendency to move from problem to problem instead of persistently seeking a satisfactory solution to only one problem at a time. Because the problem selection process entails both structuring and collaboration on the part of the therapist, considerable skill is necessary.

Regular Feedback

Feedback is especially important in therapy with depressed patients; it is a crucial ingredient in developing and maintaining the collaborative therapeutic relationship. First, as part of the regular feedback process, it is important to share the rationale for each intervention mode. This serves to demystify the therapy process and facilitates the patient's questioning the validity of a particular approach. When the patient understands how a technique or assignment is related to the solution of a problem, he or she is more likely to participate conscientiously. The cognitive therapist initiates the feedback component early in therapy by eliciting the patient's thoughts and feelings about many aspects of the therapy, such as the handling of a particular problem, the therapist's manner, and homework assignments. Since many patients misconstrue therapists' statements and questions, only through regular feedback can the therapist ascertain whether he or she and the patient are on the same "wavelength." Second, the therapist must be alert for verbal and nonverbal clues to a patient's covert negative reactions, and address these reactions in an empathic manner. Sometimes these problems can be resolved through clarification of the rationale for a particular technique or assignment.

The third element of the feedback process is for the therapist to check regularly to determine whether the patient understands his or her formulations. Patients sometimes agree with a formulation simply out of compliance, and depressed patients frequently exhibit both compliance and reluctance to "talk straight" with their therapists for fear of being rejected or criticized, or of making a mistake. Therefore, the therapist must make an extra effort to elicit the patient's feelings or wishes relevant to compliance (e.g., anxiety about rejection, wish to please) and be alert for verbal and nonverbal clues that the patient may indeed not understand the explanations.

As a regular part of the feedback process, at the close of each session the cognitive therapist provides a concise summary of what has taken place, and asks the patient to abstract and write down the main points from the session. The patient keeps this summary for review during the week. In practice, the therapist uses capsule summaries at least three times during a standard therapeutic interview: in preparing the agenda, in a midpoint recapitulation of the material covered up to that point, and in the final summary of the main points of the interview. Patients generally respond favorably to the elicitation of feedback and presentation of capsule summaries. We have observed that the development of empathy and rapport is facilitated by these techniques.

Collaborative Empiricism

When the collaborative therapeutic relationship has been successfully formed, patient and therapist act as an investigative team. Though we elaborate on the investigative process later, it is appropriate to introduce it in the context of the collaborative relationship. As a team, patient and therapist approach the patient's automatic thoughts and schemas in the same manner that scientists approach questions: Each thought or schema becomes a hypothesis to be tested, and evidence is gathered that supports or refutes the hypothesis. Events in the past, circumstances in the present, and possibilities in the future are the data that constitute evidence, and the conclusion to accept or reject the hypothesis is jointly reached as patient and therapist subject the evidence to logical analysis. Experiments may also be devised to test the validity of particular cognitions. Cognitive therapists need not persuade patients of illogicality or inconsistency with reality, because patients "discover" their own inconsistencies. This guided discovery process, a widely accepted educational method, is one of the vital components of cognitive therapy.

THE PROCESS OF COGNITIVE THERAPY

Here we attempt to convey a sense of how cognitive therapy sessions are structured and a sense of the course of treatment. Detailed discussion of particular techniques follows this section.

The Initial Sessions

A main therapeutic goal of the first few sessions is to produce some symptom relief. Reducing the patient's suffering helps to increase rapport, collaboration, and confidence in the therapeutic process. Symptom relief, however, should be based on more than rapport, sympa-

thy, and implied promise of "cure." In the first few sessions, the cognitive therapist starts the process of defining the patient's problems and demonstrating some of the strategies that will be used in the therapy to deal with those problems.

Problem definition is a primary goal in the early stages of therapy. The therapist collaboratively works with the patient to define the specific problems on which they will focus during therapy sessions. The cognitive therapist does this by obtaining as complete a picture as possible of the patient's psychological and life situation difficulties. The therapist also seeks details concerning the depth of depression and particular symptomatology. Cognitive therapists are especially concerned with how patients see their problems.

Once the specific problems have been defined, patient and therapist establish priorities among them. Decisions are made on the basis of amenability to therapeutic change and centrality of the life problem or cognition to the patient's emotional distress. To help establish priorities effectively, the therapist must see the relationships among particular thoughts, particular life situations, and particular distressing emotions.

Another goal of the initial session is to illustrate the close relationship between cognition and emotion. When the therapist is able to observe the patient's mood change (e.g., crying), he or she points out the alteration in affect and asks for the patient's thoughts just before the mood shift. The therapist then labels the negative thought and points out its relationship to the change in mood. He or she initially gears homework assignments toward helping the patient see the close connection between cognition and emotion.

A frequent requirement in the early stage of therapy is to socialize the patient to cognitive therapy. A patient who has previously undertaken analytically oriented or Rogerian therapies may begin cognitive therapy expecting a more insight-oriented, nondirective therapeutic approach. The cognitive therapist can facilitate the transition to a more active and structured approach by maintaining a problem-oriented stance, which often entails gently interrupting a patient who tends to speculate about the sources of the problems and seeks interpretations from the therapist.

Finally, the therapist must communicate the importance of self-help homework assignments during the initial session by stressing that doing the homework is actually more important than the therapy session itself. The therapist also can enhance motivation by explaining that patients who complete assignments generally improve more quickly. The nature and implementation of self-help homework assignments are considered in further detail in a later section of this chapter.

The Progress of a Typical Therapy Session

Each session begins with the establishment of an agenda for that session. This ensures optimal use of time in a relatively short-term, problem-solving therapeutic approach. The agenda generally begins with a short synopsis of the patient's experiences since the last session, including discussion of the homework assignment. The therapist then asks the patient what he or she wants to work on during the session, and often offers topics to be included.

When a short list of problems and topics has been completed, the patient and therapist determine the order in which to cover them and, if necessary, the time to be allotted to each topic. There are several issues to consider in establishing priorities, including stage of therapy, severity of depression, likelihood of making progress in solving the problem, and potential pervasiveness of the effect of a particular theme or topic. The cognitive therapist is sensitive to a patient's occasional desire to talk about something that seems important to him or her at the moment, even if such discussion seems not to be productive in terms of other goals. This kind of flexibility characterizes the collaborative therapeutic relationship.

After these preliminary matters have been covered, patient and therapist move on to the one or two problems to be considered during the session. The therapist begins the discussion of a problem by asking the patient a series of questions designed to clarify the nature of the patient's difficulty. In doing so, the therapist seeks to determine whether early maladaptive schemas, misinterpretations of events, or unrealistic expectations are involved. The therapist also seeks to discover whether the patient had unrealistic expectations, whether the patient's behavior was appropriate, and whether all possible solutions to the problem were considered. The patient's responses suggest to the therapist a cognitive-behavioral conceptualization of why the patient is having difficulty in the area

of concern. The therapist by now has discerned the one or two significant thoughts, schemas, images, or behaviors to be worked on. When this target problem has been selected, the therapist chooses the cognitive or behavioral techniques to apply and shares their rationale with the patient. The specific techniques used in cognitive therapy are explained in the following sections of this chapter.

At the close of the session, the therapist asks the patient for a summary, often in writing, of the major conclusions drawn during the session. The therapist asks for the patient's reactions to the session to ascertain whether anything disturbing was said and to forestall any delayed negative reactions following the interview. Finally, the therapist gives a homework assignment designed to assist the patient in applying the particular skills and concepts from the session to the problem during the following week.

Progression of Session Content over Time

Although the structure of cognitive therapy sessions does not change during the course of treatment, the content often changes significantly. Treatment with both nonchronic and chronic patients begins with a focus on symptom reduction, behavioral activation, overcoming hopelessness, identifying problems, setting priorities, socializing the patient to cognitive therapy, establishing the collaborative relationship, demonstrating the relationship between cognition and emotion, and working toward progress on the targeted problems. Therapy is initially centered on the patient's symptoms, with attention given to behavioral and motivational difficulties. Once the patient shows some significant changes in these areas, the emphasis shifts to the content and pattern of the patient's thinking.

Once the patient is feeling less depressed, therapist and patient explore the patient's specific thoughts and assumptions about particular situations and/or problems, and underlying schemas that may be related. Schemas are deep-seated core beliefs about the self, relationships, and life. Schemas develop as the result of specific experiences within an individual's lifetime, mostly during childhood and/or adolescence. When schemas are identified, they reveal rules and formulas that the individual uses to "make sense" of the world. They are the overriding principles by which the individual organizes his or her perceptions and/or behavior. Maladaptive schemas often underlie many of the patient's problems. Cognitive therapy aims to counteract the effects of maladaptive schemas. If the schemas themselves can be changed, we believe that the patient will become less vulnerable to future depressions.

Over the course of therapy, the patient assumes increased responsibility for identifying problems, coming up with solutions, and implementing the solutions through homework assignments. The therapist increasingly assumes the role of advisor or consultant as the patient learns to implement therapeutic techniques without constant support. As the patient becomes a more effective problem solver, the frequency of sessions is reduced, and therapy is eventually discontinued.

The remainder of this chapter is devoted to a detailed description of traditional cognitive therapy and schema therapy strategies.

SYMPTOM REDUCTION

Behavioral Techniques

Behavioral techniques are used throughout the course of cognitive therapy, but they are generally concentrated in the earlier stages of treatment. Behavioral techniques are especially necessary for those more severely depressed patients who are passive, anhedonic, socially withdrawn, and unable to concentrate for extended periods of time. By engaging such a patient's attention and interest, the cognitive therapist tries to induce the patient to counteract withdrawal and become more involved in constructive activity. From a variety of behavioral techniques, the therapist selects those that will help the patient cope more effectively with situational and interpersonal problems. Through homework assignments, the patient implements specific procedures for dealing with concrete situations or for using time more adaptively.

The cognitive therapist uses behavioral techniques, with the goal of modifying automatic thoughts. For example, a patient who believes "I can't get anything done any more" can modify this thought after completing a series of graded tasks designed to increase mastery. The severely depressed patient is caught in a vicious cycle in which a reduced activity level leads to a negative self-label, which in turn results in even further discouragement and consequent inactivity. Interven-tion with behavioral techniques can change this self-destructive pattern.

The most commonly used behavioral techniques include scheduling activities that include both mastery and pleasure exercises, cognitive rehearsal, self-reliance training, role playing, and diversion techniques. The scheduling of activities is frequently used in the early stages of cognitive therapy to counteract loss of motivation, hopelessness, and excessive rumination. The therapist uses the Weekly Activity Schedule for planning activities hour by hour, day by day (see Figure 6.3). Patients maintain an hourly record of the activities in which they engaged. Activity scheduling also helps patients obtain more pleasure and a greater sense of accomplishment from activities on a daily basis. The patients rate each completed activity (using a 0- to 10-point scale) for both mastery and pleasure. The ratings usually contradict patients' beliefs that they cannot accomplish or enjoy anything any more. To assist some patients in initiating mastery and pleasure activities, the therapist may sometimes find it necessary to subdivide an activity into segments, ranging from the simplest to the most difficult and complex aspects of the activity. We call this the "graded task" approach. The subdivision enables depressed patients to undertake tasks that were initially impossible, thus providing proof of success.

Cognitive rehearsal entails asking a patient to picture or imagine each step involved in the accomplishment of a particular task. This technique can be especially helpful with those patients who have difficulty carrying out a task that requires successive steps for its completion. Sometimes impairment in the ability to concentrate creates difficulties for the patient in focusing attention on the specific task. The imagery evoked by the cognitive rehearsal technique helps the patient to focus and helps the therapist to identify obstacles that make the assignment difficult for the particular patient.

Some depressed patients rely on others to take care of most of their daily needs. With self-reliance training, patients learn to assume increased responsibility for routine activities such as showering, making their beds, cleaning the house, cooking their own meals, and shopping. Self-reliance involves gaining increased control over emotional reactions.

Role playing has many uses in cognitive therapy. First, it may be used to bring out automatic thoughts through the enactment of particular interpersonal situations, such as an

		Mon.	Tues.	Wed.	Thurs.	Fri.	Sat.	Sun.
Morning	6–7							
	7–8							
	8–9							
	9–10							
	10–11							
	11–12							
Afternoon	12–1							
	1–2							
	2–3							
	3–4							
	4–5							
	5–6							
Evening	6–7							
	7–8							
	8–9							
	9–10							
	10–11							
	11–12							
	12–6							

Note: Grade activities *M* for mastery and *P* for pleasure 0–10.

FIGURE 6.3. Weekly Activity Schedule.

encounter with a supervisor at work. Second, it may also be used, through homework assignments, to guide the patient in practicing and attending to new cognitive responses in problematic social encounters. A third use of role playing is to rehearse new behaviors. Thus, role playing may be used as part of assertiveness training and is often accompanied by modeling and coaching.

Role reversal, a variation of role playing, can be very effective in helping patients test how other people might view their behavior. This is well illustrated by a patient who had a "humiliating experience" while buying some clothes in a store. After playing the role of the clerk, the patient had to conclude that she had insufficient data for her previous conclusion that she appeared clumsy and inept. Through role reversal, patients begin to view themselves less harshly as "self-sympathy" responses are elicited.

Finally, the therapist may introduce various distraction techniques to assist the patient in learning to reduce the intensity of painful affects. The patient learns to divert negative thinking through physical activity, social contact, work, play, and visual imagery. Practice with diversion techniques also helps the patient gain further control over emotional reactivity.

Cognitive Techniques

The specific cognitive techniques provide points of entry into the patient's cognitive organization. The cognitive therapist uses techniques for eliciting and testing automatic thoughts, and identifying schemas to help both therapist and patient understand the patient's construction of reality. In applying specific cognitive techniques in therapy, it is important that the therapist work within the framework of the cognitive model of depression. Each set of techniques is discussed in turn.

Eliciting Automatic Thoughts

"Automatic thoughts" are those thoughts that intervene between outside events and the individual's emotional reactions to them. They often go unnoticed, because they are part of a repetitive pattern of thinking, and because they occur so often and so quickly. People rarely stop to assess their validity, because they are so believable, familiar, and habitual. The patient in cognitive therapy must learn to recognize these automatic thoughts for therapy to proceed effectively. The cognitive therapist and the patient make a joint effort to discover the particular thoughts that precede emotions such as anger, sadness, and anxiety. The therapist uses questioning, imagery, and role playing to elicit automatic thoughts.

The simplest method to uncover automatic thoughts is for therapists to ask patients what thoughts went through their minds in response to particular events. This questioning provides patients with a model for introspective exploration that they can use on their own, when the therapist is not present, and after the completion of treatment.

Alternatively, when a patient is able to identify those external events and situations that evoke a particular emotional response, the therapist may use imagery by asking the patient to picture the situation in detail. The patient is often able to identify the automatic thoughts connected with actual situations when the image evoked is clear. In this technique, therapists ask patients to relax, close their eyes, and imagine themselves in the distressing situation. Patients describe in detail what is happening as they relive the event.

If a distressing event is an interpersonal one, cognitive therapists also can utilize role playing. The therapist plays the role of the other person in the encounter, while the patient plays him- or herself. The automatic thoughts can usually be elicited when the patient becomes sufficiently engaged in the role play.

In attempting to elicit automatic thoughts, the therapist is careful to notice and point out any mood changes that occur during the session, and to ask the patient his or her thoughts just before the shift in mood. Mood changes include any emotional reaction, such as tears or anger. This technique can be especially useful when the patient is first learning to identify automatic thoughts.

Once patients become familiar with the techniques for identifying automatic thoughts, they are asked to keep a Daily Record of Dysfunctional Thoughts (Beck et al., 1979; see Figure 6.4), in which they record the emotions and automatic thoughts that occur in upsetting situations between therapy sessions. In later ses-

DATE	SITUATION Describe: 1. Actual even leading to unpleasant emotion, or 2. Stream of thoughts, daydream, or recollection, leading to unpleasant emotion.	EMOTION(S) 1. Specify sad/ anxious/ angry, etc. 2. Rate degree of emotion, 1–100.	AUTOMATIC THOUGHT(S) 1. Write automatic thought(s) that preceded emotion(s). 2. Rate belief in automatic thought(s), 0–100%.	RATIONAL RESPOSNE 1. Write rational response to automatic thought(s). 2. Rate belief in rational response, 0–100%	OUTCOME 1. Rerate belief in automatic thought(s), 0–100%. 2. Specify and rate subsequent emotions, 0–100.

Explanation: When you experience an unpleasant emotion, note the situation that seemed to stimulate the emotion. (If the emotion occurred while you were thinking, daydreaming, etc., please note this.) Then note the automatic thought associated with the emotion. Record the degree to which you believe this thought: 0% = not at all; 100% = completely. In rating degrees of emotion: 1 = a trace; 100 = the most intense possible.

FIGURE 6.4. Daily Record of Dysfunctional Thoughts.

sions, patients are taught to develop rational responses to their dysfunctional automatic thoughts and to record them in the appropriate column. Therapist and patient generally review the daily record from the preceding week, near the beginning of the next therapy session. In sessions with chronic patients, the therapist also teaches patients to recognize modes. Various affective exercises are then used to bring about change in the underlying schemas associated with those modes.

Eliciting automatic thoughts should be distinguished from the interpretation process of other psychotherapies. In general, cognitive therapists work only with those automatic thoughts mentioned by patients. Suggesting thoughts to patients may undermine collaboration and inhibit patients from learning to continue the process on their own. As a last resort, however, when nondirective strategies fail, a cognitive therapist may offer several possible automatic thoughts, then ask the patient whether any of these choices fit.

Even when many efforts to elicit automatic thoughts have been made by the therapist, sometimes the thought remains inaccessible. When this is the case, the cognitive therapist tries to ascertain the particular meaning of the event that evoked the emotional reaction. For example, one patient began to cry whenever she had an argument with her roommate, who was a good friend. Efforts to elicit automatic thoughts proved unsuccessful. Only after the therapist asked a series of questions to determine the meaning of the event did it become clear that the patient associated having an argument or fight with ending the relationship. Through this process, therapist and patient were able to see the meaning that triggered the crying.

Testing Automatic Thoughts with Nonchronic Patients

When therapist and patient have managed to isolate a key automatic thought, they approach the thought as a testable hypothesis. In this "scientific" approach, which is fundamental to cognitive therapy, the patient learns to think in a way that resembles the investigative process. Through the procedures of gathering data, evaluating evidence, and drawing conclusions, patients learn firsthand that their view of reality can be quite different from what actually takes place. By designing experiments that sub-

ject their automatic thoughts to objective analysis, patients learn how to modify their thinking, because they learn the *process* of empirical thinking. Patients who learn to think this way during treatment are better able to continue the empirical approach after the end of formal therapy.

The cognitive therapist approaches the testing of automatic thoughts by asking the patient to list evidence from his or her experience for and against the hypothesis. Sometimes, after considering the evidence, the patient immediately rejects the automatic thought, recognizing that it is either distorted or actually false.

When previous experience is not sufficient or appropriate to test a hypothesis, the therapist asks the patient to design an experiment for that purpose. The patient then makes a prediction and proceeds to gather data. If the data contradict the prediction, the patient can reject the automatic thought. The outcome of the experiment may, of course, confirm the patient's prediction. It is therefore very important for the therapist not to *assume* that the patient's automatic thought is distorted.

Some automatic thoughts do not lend themselves to hypothesis testing through the examination of evidence. In these cases, two options are available: The therapist may produce evidence from his or her own experience and offer it in the form of a question that reveals the contradiction; or the therapist can ask a question designed to uncover a logical error inherent in the patient's beliefs. The therapist might say, for example, to a male patient who is sure he cannot survive without a close personal relationship, "You were alone last year, and you got along fine; what makes you think you can't make it now?"

In testing automatic thoughts, it is sometimes necessary to refine the patient's use of a word. This is particularly true for global labels such as "bad," "stupid," or "selfish." What is needed in this case is an operational definition of the word. To illustrate, a patient at our clinic had the recurring automatic thought, "I'm a failure in math." Therapist and patient had to narrow down the meaning of the word before they could test the thought. They operationalized "failure" in math as "being unable to achieve a grade of C after investing as much time studying as the average class member." Now they could examine past evidence and test the validity of the hypothesis. This process can help patients to see the overinclusiveness of their negative self-assessments and the idiosyncratic nature of many automatic thoughts.

Reattribution is another useful technique for helping the patient to reject an inappropriate, self-blaming thought. It is a common cognitive pattern in depression to ascribe blame or responsibility for adverse events to oneself. Reattribution can be used when the patient unrealistically attributes adverse occurrences to a personal deficiency, such as lack of ability or effort. Therapist and patient review the relevant events and apply logic to the available information to make a more realistic assignment of responsibility. The aim of reattribution is not to absolve the patient of all responsibility, but to examine the many factors that contribute to adverse events. Through this process, patients gain objectivity, relieve themselves of the burden of self-reproach, and can then search for ways to solve realistic problems or prevent their recurrence.

Another strategy involving reattribution is for therapists to demonstrate to patients that they use stricter criteria for assigning responsibility to their own unsatisfactory behavior than they use in evaluating the behavior of others. Cognitive therapists also use reattribution to show patients that some of their thinking or behavior problems can be symptoms of depression (e.g., loss of concentration) and not signs of physical decay.

When a patient is accurate in identifying a realistic life problem or skills deficit, the cognitive therapist can use the technique of generating alternatives, in which therapist and patient actively search for alternative solutions. Because a depressed person's reasoning often becomes restricted, an effort to reconceptualize the problem can result in the patient's seeing a viable solution that he or she may previously have rejected.

It should be noted that the cognitive techniques outlined here all entail the use of questions by the therapist. A common error we observe in novice cognitive therapists is an exhortative style. We have found that therapists help patients to change their thinking more effectively by using carefully formed questions. If patients are prompted to work their own way through problems and reach their own conclusions, they learn an effective problem-solving process. We elaborate on the use of questioning in cognitive therapy later in the chapter.

Questioning

As we have stressed throughout this chapter, questioning is a major therapeutic device in cognitive therapy. A majority of the therapist's comments during the therapy session are questions. Single questions can serve several purposes at one time, whereas carefully designed series of questions can help patients consider a particular issue, decision, or opinion. The cognitive therapist seeks through questioning to elicit what patients are thinking, instead of telling patients what he or she believes they are thinking.

In the beginning of therapy, questions are employed to obtain a full and detailed picture of a patient's particular difficulties. They are used to obtain background and diagnostic data; to evaluate the patient's stress tolerance, capacity for introspection, coping methods, and so on; to obtain information about the patient's external situation and interpersonal context; and to modify vague complaints by working with the patient to arrive at specific target problems on which to work.

As therapy progresses, the therapist uses questioning to explore approaches to problems, to help the patient to weigh advantages and disadvantages of possible solutions, to examine the consequences of staying with particular maladaptive behaviors, to elicit automatic thoughts, and to demonstrate EMSs and their consequences. In short, the therapist uses questioning in most cognitive therapeutic techniques.

Although questioning is itself a powerful means of identifying and changing automatic thoughts and schemas, it is important that the questions be carefully and skillfully posed. If questions are used to "trap" patients into contradicting themselves, patients may come to feel that they are being attacked or manipulated by the therapist. Too many open-ended questions can leave patients wondering what the therapist expects of them. Therapists must carefully time and phrase questions to help patients recognize their thoughts and schemas, and to weigh issues objectively.

Self-Help Homework Assignments

Rationale

Regular homework assignments are very important in cognitive therapy. When patients systematically apply what they have learned during therapy sessions to their outside lives, they are more likely to make significant progress in therapy and to be able to maintain their gains after termination of treatment. Burns and Spangler (2000) found that patients who did the most homework showed large and significant decreases in depression in comparison with those who were less compliant. Homework assignments are often the means through which patients gather data, test hypotheses, and begin to modify their thoughts and schemas. In addition, the data provided through homework assignments help to shift the focus of therapy from the subjective and abstract to more concrete and objective concerns. When a patient and therapist review the previous week's activities during the agenda-setting portion of the interview, they may do so quickly, and the therapist can draw relationships between what takes place in the session and specific tasks, thereby avoiding tangents and side issues. Homework assignments further the patient's self-reliance and provide methods for the patient to continue working on problems after the end of treatment. Cognitive therapists emphasize the importance of homework by sharing with patients their rationale for assigning homework in therapy. They are also careful to explain the particular benefits to be derived from each individual assignment.

Assigning and Reviewing Homework

The cognitive therapist designs each assignment for the particular patient. The assignment should be directly related to the content of the therapy session, so that the patient understands its purpose and importance. Each task should be clearly articulated and very specific in nature. Near the end of each session, the assignment is written in duplicate, with one copy going to the therapist and one to the patient.

Some typical homework assignments include reading a book or article about a specific problem, practicing distraction or relaxation techniques, counting automatic thoughts on a wrist counter, rating activities for pleasure and mastery on the Weekly Activity Schedule, maintaining a Daily Record of Dysfunctional Thoughts, and listening to a tape of the therapy session.

During the therapy session, the therapists ask for the patient's reactions to homework assignments, for example, whether the assignment is clear and manageable. To determine potential impediments, the therapist may ask the patient to imagine taking the steps involved in the assignment. This technique can be especially helpful during the earlier stages of therapy. The patient assumes greater responsibility for developing homework assignments as therapy progresses through the middle and later stages.

It is essential that patient and therapist review the previous week's homework during the therapy session itself. If they do not, the patient may conclude that the homework assignments are not important. During the first part of the therapy sessions, therapist and patient discuss the previous week's assignment, and the therapist summarizes the results.

Difficulties in Completing Homework

When a patient does not complete homework assignments, or does them without conviction, the cognitive therapist elicits automatic thoughts, schemas, or behavioral problems that may help both therapist and patient understand where the difficulty resides. The therapist does not presuppose that the patient is being "resistant" or "passive–aggressive." When the difficulties have been successfully identified, therapist and patient work collaboratively to surmount them. It is, of course, common for patients to have difficulties in completing homework, and here we consider some of the typical problems and ways to counteract them.

When patients do not understand the assignment completely, the therapist should explain it more fully, specifying his or her expectations in detail. Sometimes using the behavioral technique of cognitive rehearsal (described earlier) can be helpful in such situations.

Some patients believe that they are naturally disorganized and cannot maintain records and follow through on detailed assignments. Therapists can usually help to invalidate such general beliefs by asking patients about other circumstances in which they make lists—for example, when planning a vacation or shopping trip. Therapists can also ask these patients whether they could complete the assignment if there were a substantial reward entailed. This kind of question helps such patients recognize that self-control is not the problem; rather, they do not believe that the reward is great enough. When patients realize that the problem is an attitudinal one, therapist and patient can proceed to enumerate the advantages of completing the assignment.

More severely depressed patients may need assistance to structure their time, so that homework becomes a regular activity. This can generally be accomplished by setting a specific time each day for the homework assignment. If necessary, patient and therapist can set up a reward or punishment system to make sure the homework gets done. For example, patients can reward themselves for doing the assignment with a special purchase, or punish themselves for failing to do it by not watching a favorite television program.

Some patients are afraid of failing the assignments or of doing them inadequately. In these cases, the therapist can explain that self-help assignments cannot be "failed": Doing an assignment partially is more helpful than not doing it at all, and mistakes provide valuable information about problems that still need work. In addition, because performance is not evaluated, patients cannot lose if they view the activity from a more adaptive perspective.

Sometimes patients believe their problems are too deeply embedded and complex to be resolved through homework assignments. The therapist can explain to these patients that even the most complex undertakings begin with and consist of small, concrete steps. A writer, for example, may resolve "writer's blocks" by taking the attitude, "If I can't write a book, I can at least write a paragraph." When enough paragraphs have been written, the result is a book. A therapist and patient can consider the advantages and disadvantages of the patient's believing that problems cannot be solved by doing homework. Or the therapist can ask the patient to experiment before reaching such a conclusion. In instances in which a patient believes that he or she has not made enough progress and, therefore, that the homework is not helpful, the therapist can detail the progress the patient has made or can help the patient see that it may take more time before substantial change can be perceived.

When patients seem to resent being given assignments, the therapist can encourage them to develop their own assignments. The therapist might also offer the patients alternative assignments from which to choose, making one of the alternatives noncompliance with homework assignments. If patients choose noncompliance,

the therapist can help to examine the consequences of that choice. Still another strategy is to present patients with a consumer model of therapy: Patients have a certain goal (overcoming depression), and the therapist offers a means to achieve that goal; patients are free to use or reject the tools, just as they are free to buy or not to buy in the marketplace.

Some patients believe that they can improve just as readily without homework. In this case, therapists have two options. First, they can offer their own clinical experience, which is supported by existing empirical evidence that most patients who do not actively engage with and complete therapeutic homework progress more slowly in therapy. The other option is to set up an experiment for a given period of time, during which patients do not have to complete assignments. At the end of the predetermined period, therapists and patients can evaluate the patients' progress during that time interval. Once again, it is important for cognitive therapists to keep an open mind: Some patients do indeed effect significant change without formally completing homework assignments.

Special Problems

The novice cognitive therapist often errs by staying with the standard method we have outlined here, even if it is not working very well. The cognitive therapist should be flexible enough to adapt to the needs of patients and to the several special problems that commonly arise in therapy. We have grouped these special problems into two categories: difficulties in the therapist–patient relationship and problems in which the therapy itself seems not to be working.

Therapist–Patient Relationship Difficulties

The first set of problems concerns the therapist–patient relationship itself. When the therapist first perceives a patient to be dissatisfied, oppositional, angry, or hostile, it is imperative that he or she present these observations to the patient in an empathic manner. It is important that the therapist refrain from responding to the patient simply with an increased and rigid adherence to prescribed techniques or the therapeutic rationale. It also is important that the therapist refrain from self-critical statements. Research indicates that such responses have detrimental effects on the therapeutic relationship (Castonguay et al., 1996; Henry, Strupp, Butler, Schact, & Binder, 1993; Piper et al., 1999). Instead, preliminary research (Castonguay et al., 2004; Safran, Muran, Samstag, & Stevens, 2002) indicates that the therapist's use of metacommunication skills (open discussion about the patient's negative reaction, exploration of the patient's experience, recognition and acknowledgement of any therapist contribution to those negative reactions) is significantly more likely to repair and restore—and even improve—the therapeutic bond.

It is essential for therapists to be aware that many interventions can be misinterpreted in a negative way by depressed patients. Therapists approach problems of misinterpretation in the same way that they approach other thoughts: They work with the patient to gather data and search for alternative accounts of the evidence. Difficulties in the therapist–patient relationship can generally be resolved through dialogue. There are times when a therapist may need to tailor behavior to the particular needs of an individual patient. For instance, a therapist may become freer with appropriate self-disclosure and personal reactions to meet the needs of a patient who persist in seeing the therapist as impersonal. Similarly, the therapist can make a point of checking formulations of the patient's thoughts more frequently to meet the needs of a patient who continues to believe that the therapist does not understand him or her.

It is imperative in situations like these for the therapist not to assume that the patient is being stubbornly resistant or irrational. In fact, therapeutic reactance ("a motivational state characterized by the tendency to restore or re-assert one's ability to engage in freedoms perceived as lost or threatened" [Arnow et al., 2003, p. 1026]) was found to be a positive predictor of treatment outcome in directive therapy with chronically depressed patients when therapists responded in a flexible manner to such patient behaviors. Cognitive therapists collaborate with patients to achieve a better understanding of patients' responses. The reactions themselves often provide data regarding the kinds of distortions patients make in their other social and personal relationships. Therefore, patients' responses give the therapists the opportunity to work with them on their maladaptive interpretations in relationships.

Unsatisfactory Progress

A second set of problems occurs when the therapy appears not to be working, even when the patient conscientiously completes homework assignments and the collaborative relationship seems successful. Sometimes problems stem from inappropriate expectations on the part of the patient—or unrealistic expectations on the part of the therapist—regarding the rapidity and consistency of change. When therapy seems not to be progressing as quickly as it "should," both patient and therapist must remember that ups and downs are to be anticipated in the course of treatment. It is important for therapists to keep in mind that some patients simply progress more slowly than others. The therapist or patient, or both, may be minimizing small changes that have indeed been taking place. In this case the therapist can emphasize the small gains that have been made and remind the patient that large goals are attained through small steps toward them.

At times, patients' hopelessness can lead them to invalidate their gains. Therapists should seek to uncover the thoughts and maladaptive assumptions that contribute to the pervasive hopelessness. In these cases, therapists must work to correct mistaken notions about the process of change and about the nature of depression before further progress in therapy can occur.

In some cases in which therapy seems not to be working successfully, it may be that some of the therapeutic techniques have not been correctly used. Problems often arise when patients do not really believe the rational responses or are not able to remember them in times of emotional distress. It is important for a therapist to determine the amount of a patient's belief in the rational responses and help him or her use the new responses as closely as possible to the moment when the automatic thoughts occur. To the patient who does not fully believe a rational response, the therapist can suggest an experimental stance—taking the new belief and "trying it on for size." The patient who cannot think of answers because of emotional upset should be told that states of emotional distress make reasoning more difficult, and that thoughts such as "If this doesn't work, nothing will" can only aggravate the problem. Patients should be assured that they will be able to think of rational responses more readily with practice.

Another problem deriving from the misapplication of cognitive therapy techniques occurs when the therapist uses a particular technique inflexibly. It is often necessary for the therapist to try out several behavioral or cognitive techniques before finding an approach to which a patient responds well. The cognitive therapist must stay with a particular technique for a while to see whether it works, but he or she must also be willing to try an alternative technique when it becomes apparent that the patient is not improving. To give a specific example, behavioral homework assignments are sometimes more helpful with particular patients, even though the therapist has every reason to predict in advance that cognitive assignments will be more effective.

In some instances in which it appears that little progress is being made in therapy, it turns out that the therapist has selected a tangential problem. The cognitive therapist should be alert to this possibility, especially during the early stages of therapy. When there appears to be little or no significant change in depression level, even when the patient seems to have made considerable progress in a problem area, the therapist should consider the possibility that the most distressing problem has not yet been uncovered. A typical example of this kind of difficulty is the patient who presents difficulty at work as the major problem, when it turns out that couple problems are contributing significantly to the work difficulties. The real issue may be withheld by the patient because it seems too threatening.

Finally, cognitive therapy is not for everyone. If the therapist has tried all available approaches to the problem and has consulted with other cognitive therapists, it may be best to refer the patient to another therapist with either the same or a different orientation.

Regardless of why therapy is not progressing satisfactorily, cognitive therapists should attend to their own affect and cognitions. They must maintain a disciplined, problem-solving stance. If the cognitive therapist finds him- or herself unduly influenced by a patient's despair or begins to notice that his or her own schemas are triggered by therapeutic interactions, he or she should seek supervision. Hopelessness in patients or therapists is an obstacle to problem solving. If therapists can effectively counteract their own negative self-assessments and other dysfunctional thoughts, they will be better able to concentrate on helping patients find solutions to their problems.

Case Study of Denise: Nonchronic Depression

In the case study that follows, we describe the course of treatment for a nonchronically depressed woman seen at our center. Through the case study, we illustrate many of the concepts described earlier in this chapter, including elicitation of automatic thoughts, the cognitive triad of depression, collaborative empiricism, structuring a session, and feedback.

Assessment and Presenting Problems

At the initial evaluation, Denise reported that she was a 59-year-old widow, who had been living alone for the last year. Denise's husband had been diagnosed with brain cancer three years prior and died approximately one year ago. She had two grown unmarried children (27 and 25 years old) who were pursuing careers in other parts of the country. Denise had an undergraduate degree and had worked until age 30 but stopped after marrying. Denise described her major problems as depression (over the last year and a half), difficulty coping with daily life, and loneliness. She reported one prior episode of major depression around age 25, following the death of her father.

Denise said she had become increasingly socially isolated with the onset of her husband's illness (brain cancer). She reported having had normal friendships as a child, teenager, and young adult. She and her husband had led a relatively quiet life together, mostly focused on raising their children and respective work. When they had free time, they had enjoyed intellectual and cultural activities together (museums, lectures, concerts, and fine restaurants). They had a few close friends with whom they socialized but those friends had retired in Florida and Arizona during the time of the husband's illness.

Denise was diagnosed with a major depressive disorder, recurrent, on Axis I. Her test scores verified the diagnosis of depression. Denise's Beck Depression Inventory (BDI) score was 28, placing her in the moderate to severe range of depression. Her most prominent depressive symptoms included loss of pleasure, irritability, social withdrawal, inability to make decisions, fatigue, guilt, difficulty motivating herself to perform daily functions, and loneliness.

Session I

The session began with Denise describing the "sad feelings" she was having. The therapist almost immediately started to elicit Denise's automatic thoughts during these periods.

THERAPIST: What kind of thoughts go through your mind when you've had these sad feelings this past week?

DENISE: Well, I guess I'm thinking what's the point of all this. My life is over. It's just not the same. I have thoughts like, "What am I going to do? Sometimes I feel mad at him, you know, my husband. How could he leave me? . . . Isn't that terrible of me? What's wrong with me? How can I be mad at him? He didn't want to die a horrible death. I should have done more. I should have made him go to the doctor when he first started getting headaches. . . . Oh, what's the use?

THERAPIST: It sounds like you are feeling quite bad right now. Is that right?

DENISE: Yes.

THERAPIST: Keep telling me what's going through your mind right now?

DENISE: I can't change anything. It's over. I don't know. . . . It all seems so bleak and hopeless. What do I have to look forward to . . . sickness and then death?

THERAPIST: So one of the thoughts is that you can't change things, and that it's not going to get any better?

DENISE: Yes.

THERAPIST: And sometimes you believe that completely?

DENISE: Yeah, I believe it, sometimes.

THERAPIST: Right now do you believe it?

DENISE: I believe it—yes.

THERAPIST: Right now you believe that you can't change things and it's not going to get better?

DENISE: Well, there is a glimmer of hope, but it's mostly . . .

THERAPIST: Is there anything that you kind of look forward to in terms of your own life from here on?

DENISE: Well, what I look forward to . . . I enjoy seeing my kids, but they are so busy right now. My son is a lawyer and my daughter is in medical school. So, they are very busy. They don't have time to spend with me.

By inquiring about Denise's automatic thoughts, the therapist began to understand her perspective—that she would go on forever, mostly alone. This illustrates the hopelessness about the future that is characteristic of most depressed patients. A second advantage to this line of inquiry is that the therapist introduced Denise to the idea of looking at her own thoughts, which is central to cognitive therapy.

As the session continued, the therapist probed Denise's perspective regarding her daily life. The therapist chose to focus on her inactivity and withdrawal. This is frequently the first therapeutic goal in working with a severely depressed patient.

In the sequence that follows, the therapist guided Denise to examine the advantages and disadvantages of staying in her house all day.

DENISE: Usually I don't want to leave my house. I want to stay there and just keep the shades closed; you know, I don't want to do anything. I just want to keep everything out, keep everything away from me.

THERAPIST: Now do you feel better when you stay in the house all day trying to shut everything out?

DENISE: Sort of . . .

THERAPIST: What do you mean?

DENISE: Well, I can watch TV all day and just lose myself in these silly shows. I feel better when I see other people and their problems on these shows. It makes me feel less lonely and like my problems aren't so bad.

THERAPIST: And so how much time do you spend doing that?

DENISE: Now, lately? . . . Most of the time. Staying inside and watching TV feels safe, sort of secure, everything . . . like my loneliness, feels more distant.

THERAPIST: Now after you have spent some time like this, how do you feel about yourself?

DENISE: Afterwards? I usually try not to pay much attention to how I'm feeling.

THERAPIST: But when you do, how do you feel?

DENISE: I feel bad. I feel bad for wasting the day. I don't get to things that I need to take care of . . . like my bills, like cleaning, like taking a shower. I usually end up feeling kind of pathetic . . . and guilty.

THERAPIST: On the one hand you seem to feel soothed and on the other hand, afterwards, you're a bit critical of yourself?

Note that the therapist did not try to debate or exhort Denise to get out of the house or become involved with necessary daily tasks. Rather, through questioning, the therapist encouraged her to examine more closely her assumption that she was really better off watching TV all day in her house. This is the process we call "collaborative empiricism." By the second session, Denise had reexamined her hypothesis about watching TV and remaining in the house all day.

DENISE: About watching TV in the house versus getting out, I thought about that the other day. I remember telling you that it made me feel better to stay there. When I paid attention to what I really felt, it didn't make me feel better. It just kind of blocked out feeling bad, but I didn't feel better.

THERAPIST: It is funny then that when you talked about it, your recollection of the experience was more positive than it actually was, but that sometimes happens with people. It happens to me too. I think that something is good that's not so hot when I actually check it out.

We now return to the first session. After some probing by the therapist, Denise mentioned that it sometimes feels like cognitive therapy "is my last hope." The therapist used this as an opportunity to explore her hopelessness and suicidal thinking.

THERAPIST: What was going through your mind when you said, "This is my last hope"? Did you have some kind of vision in your mind?

DENISE: Yeah, that if this doesn't work, I feel like I couldn't take living like this the rest of my life.

THERAPIST: If it doesn't work out, then what?

DENISE: Well, I don't really care what happens to me . . .

THERAPIST: Did you have something more concrete in mind?

DENISE: Well, right this minute I don't think I could commit suicide, but if I keep feeling this way for a long time, maybe I could. I don't know, though—I've thought about suicide before, but I have never really thought about how I would do it. I know certain things stop me, like my kids. I think it would really hurt them and some other people too, like my mother. My mom is in good health now, but she may need me some day. . . . Yeah, those are the two things that stop me, my children and my mother.

THERAPIST: Now those are the reasons for not committing suicide. Now what are some of the reasons why you might want to, do you think?

DENISE: Because sometimes it just feels so empty and hopeless. There's nothing to look forward to—every day is the same. My life is such a waste, so why not just end it?

The therapist wanted Denise to feel as free as possible to discuss suicidal thoughts; thus, he tried hard to understand both the reasons for her hopelessness and the deterrents to suicide. After determining that she had no imminent plans to make an attempt, the therapist said that he would work with her to make some changes. He then asked her to select a small problem that they could work on together.

THERAPIST: Now are there any small things that you could do that would affect your life right away?

DENISE: I don't know. Well, I guess just calling my friend Diane in Florida. She called about a month ago and then again last week. Both times I told her I was busy and would call her back, but I haven't. I've felt so down. I have nothing to say to her.

THERAPIST: Well, when she lived in the area, what kinds of things did you talk about?

DENISE: We have kids about the same age, so we would talk about our kids. We both like to read and we used to go to a book club together—so we would talk about the books we were reading. Both of us liked art. We used to attend lectures at the museum during the week, so we would talk about art and the lectures. We would spend time making plans to do things together in our free time. It always was very interesting when I spent time and with her. We had so much in common. I do miss her.

THERAPIST: It sounds like you used to be involved in a number of interesting activities. What about now?

DENISE: After my husband got sick and then my friends moved, I just stopped. I haven't done any of those things in quite a while.

THERAPIST: What do you think about attending a lecture series now?

DENISE: I don't know.

THERAPIST: Well, what do you think about that idea?

DENISE: It's an OK idea, but it just seems like too much. I don't think I'll enjoy it . . . the way I feel . . . I don't know.

THERAPIST: Would you be willing to test out that thought that you won't be able to enjoy it now?

DENISE: I don't know . . . I guess so.

THERAPIST: Is that a "yes"?

DENISE: Yes, but I don't see how I'm going to get myself to do it.

THERAPIST: Well, how would you go about finding out about a lecture series?

DENISE: You look online at the museum's website to see what's available.

THERAPIST: OK. Do you have a computer?

DENISE: Yes.

THERAPIST: Is it working?

DENISE: Yes.

THERAPIST: How do you feel about doing that?

DENISE: I guess I could do that. . . . I'm so pathetic, I know what to do. I don't need you to spell it out for me. Why didn't I just do this before?

THERAPIST: Well, you probably had good reasons for not doing it before. Probably you were just so caught up in the hopelessness.

DENISE: I guess so.

THERAPIST: When you are hopeless you tend to deny, as it were, or cut off possible options or solutions.

DENISE: Right.

THERAPIST: When you get caught up in hopelessness then, there is nothing you can do. Is that what you think?

DENISE: Yeah.

THERAPIST: So, then, rather than be down on yourself because you haven't looked this up online before, why don't we carry you right through?

This excerpt illustrates the process of graded tasks that is so important in the early stages of therapy with a depressed patient. The therapist asked the patient a series of questions to break down the process of attending a lecture series into smaller steps. Denise realized that she had known all along what to do, but, as the therapist pointed out, her hopelessness prevented her from seeing the options.

DENISE: Taking this step is going to be hard for me.

THERAPIST: First steps are harder for everybody, but that's why there is an old expression: "A journey of a thousand miles starts with the first step."

DENISE: That's very true.

THERAPIST: It's the first step that is so very important, and then you can ready yourself for the second step, and then the third step, and so on. Eventually, you build up some momentum, and each step begins to follow more naturally. But first, all you have to do is take one small step. You don't have to take giant steps.

DENISE: Well, yeah, I can see that. I guess I was thinking every step was just as hard as the first. Maybe it will get easier.

In the second session, Denise reported success.

DENISE: I checked online about the lecture series and I surprised myself. One actually sounded interesting, and I'm thinking that I might just register for it online. I really didn't think any of those feelings were still there. I'm kind of looking forward to that next step.

At the end of the first session, the therapist helped Denise fill out the Weekly Activity Schedule for the coming week. The activities were quite simple, such as getting up and taking a shower, fixing meals, going out shopping, and checking out the lecture series online. Finally, the therapist asked Denise for feedback about the session and about her hopelessness.

THERAPIST: Do you have any reactions?

DENISE: I'm still feeling down, but I'm also feeling a little better. It's interesting that just the idea of looking at what lecture's might be available is making me feel a little lighter. I even had the thought of calling Diane to talk over the options. . . . Is this a sign of better things to come?

THERAPIST: What do you think?

DENISE: Maybe.

Session 2

In the second session, the therapist began by collaborating with Denise to set an agenda. Denise wanted to discuss the fact that she had not been attending to her bills or to her housework and was still spending a good part of the day alone in front of the TV; the therapist utilized this as an opportunity to discuss the issue of activity versus inactivity on the agenda. They then reviewed the previous homework. Denise had carried out all the scheduled activities and had also listed some of her negative thoughts in between sessions. Her BDI score had dropped somewhat. (Patients routinely fill out the BDI before each session, so that both the patient and the therapist can monitor the progress of treatment.)

Denise then shared her list of negative thoughts with the therapist. One concern was that she had expressed angry feelings about her husband during the first session.

DENISE: I don't like revealing things about myself, but you told me to write down my thoughts. So here it is. When I went to bed the night after of our first session, I thought about what I said to you, you know, about being angry at my husband. I was thinking that you probably think I am this really harsh and cold person. I mean, here my husband died this horrible death and I have this hard, insensitive reaction. I started thinking that now you probably feel really negatively toward me because of that statement and that you don't want to work with me.

THERAPIST: I'm really glad you're telling me these thoughts. Let me start by asking you who is having these negative thoughts?

DENISE: You? Well, no. Actually, it's me.

THERAPIST: Right. Do you think that someone

like me might have another reaction to what you said?

DENISE: I don't know. I mean it is pretty harsh being angry at someone who had no control over what was happening.

The therapist then offered Denise an alternative perspective:

THERAPIST: Do you think that someone might react to your statements with empathy?

DENISE: How could they?

THERAPIST: I imagine it would be very upsetting and annoying to have lost both your husband and your friends—all around the same time. Even though you love and care about all of them, feeling angry is understandable. It sounds like a basic human reaction to some very difficult life events.

DENISE: Yeah, I guess that does make sense. Thanks.

This illustrates how a cognitive therapist can utilize events during the session to teach a patient to identify automatic thoughts and to consider alternative interpretations. In addition, the therapist provided a summary of a key theme he had identified from listening to Denise's automatic thoughts about her husband and about therapy. The theme was her fear of being harshly judged and potentially punished for her statement (punitiveness schema). Cognitive therapists often identify and begin to correct EMSs during the first phase of treatment. More intensive work on changing schemas in a later phase of treatment may be required to inoculate against relapse. We elaborate on this process in the next section of this chapter. In the segment that follows, the therapist explained how he arrived at the conclusion that punitiveness was an important schema for Denise.

THERAPIST: When you said that you thought I would have a negative opinion about you and not want to work with you because you said you felt angry at your husband, it sounded as though you were really concerned that you would be harshly judged and punished for your statements.

DENISE: Yes, that's right.

THERAPIST: I don't want to make too much out of this at the moment, but you also said that after your friends had moved, you felt angry at them and judgmental of their decision. Even though you knew that each set of friends had to move for specific financial or health reasons and they had been in the process of completing their moves over several years, part of you still felt very angry with them. You mentioned that you strongly believe that friends should be there for each other, especially in times of great need, and if a friend lets another friend down, that relationship should end. Is that right?

DENISE: Right.

THERAPIST: So here, you largely have withdrawn from these important relationships and now you're feeling quite lonely. The thought of talking to these friends again brings fears that they will now be angry and punitive with you for your reaction to them. You're caught in a no-win situation. Is that right?

DENISE: Yes, that sounds right.

THERAPIST: So one of the things that can really grab hold of you—and make you feel terrible—is this notion that people, including yourself, should behave in specific ways, and if they or you don't behave the "right" way, then harsh punishment should result. Is that correct?

DENISE: Yes, that sounds right. But hearing you say it makes me realize that it doesn't really sound right.

THERAPIST: What do you mean?

DENISE: It's too extreme. It's too harsh. People are human and they have limitations and they make mistakes sometimes.

THERAPIST: It's good that you are starting to notice and evaluate these thoughts rather than just responding to them automatically. What this tells us is that you have to be alert for whenever you have the sense that either you or others should be strongly punished for not behaving in a specified way. The idea that people should not be cut a break, even under very difficult circumstances, may not work very well in real life with real people. You mentioned that both friends told you they felt terrible about leaving you at this time, and both have called you regularly since leaving the area. Do you think that if you begin to respond to and return their calls, they might react differently—in the

same way that I reacted differently from what you expected?

DENISE: Yes, that is very likely.

About halfway through the session, the therapist asked the patient for feedback thus far:

THERAPIST: Now at this point, is there anything that we have discussed today that bothered you?

DENISE: That bothered me?

THERAPIST: Yeah.

DENISE: I feel like I'm a bit of a freak.

THERAPIST: That is important. Can you . . .

DENISE: Well, I'm trying not to feel that way, but I do.

THERAPIST: Well, if you are, you are. Why don't you just let yourself feel like a freak and tell me about it?

DENISE: Well, I'm feeling like I'm just so different from everyone else. Other people don't seem to have my problems. They're still happily married and carrying on with life. I just feel so different from everyone.

This comment led to identification of a third theme, the social isolation/alienation schema. Denise had been viewing herself as increasingly different for the past couple of years. By this point, however, she was beginning to catch on to the idea of answering her thoughts more rationally. After the therapist pointed out the negative thought in the preceding excerpt, the patient volunteered:

DENISE: I know what to do with the thought "I'm a freak."

THERAPIST: What are you going to do with it right this minute?

DENISE: I am going to say to myself, "I'm not so different from other people. Other people have lost their mates. I'm not the only one. I'm just the first one in my group of friends. Eventually, they will all have the same situation as me. It's just a part of life." Seeing you for help doesn't mean I'm a freak. You probably see lots of people and help them with problems like mine.

THERAPIST: Right.

The same automatic thoughts arose later in the session, when Denise noticed the therapist's wedding ring. In the extended excerpt below, the therapist helped her set up an experiment to test the thought "I'm so different from him."

THERAPIST: OK, now let's just do an experiment and see if you yourself can respond to the automatic thought, and let's see what happens to your feeling. See if responding rationally makes you feel worse or better.

DENISE: OK.

THERAPIST: OK. " 'I'm so different from him." What is the rational answer to that? A realistic answer?

DENISE: You are wearing a wedding ring and that is different from me, because I'm alone, without a mate.

THERAPIST: Yes. And?

DENISE: And? . . . I don't really know much about you, other than you're married. I guess from what I do know, that information could also be viewed as a similarity. We both have gotten married and know what it's like to be married. I assume that you've never lost a mate, but maybe that is not true. You may have lost a mate as well.

THERAPIST: So, is it that you're different or that I'm different? Or is it that we just have different situations with respect to our mates at this point in time?

DENISE: We just have different situations right now.

The preceding exchange demonstrates the use of reattribution. At first, Denise interpreted the therapist's ring as evidence that they were very different. As a result of the guided discovery approach, she reattributed the difference to one of two factors: Either she or the therapist was different or that the situation with respect to mates was different for each. At the end of the experiment, Denise expressed satisfaction that she was finally recognizing this tendency to distort her appraisals.

DENISE: Right now I feel glad. I'm feeling a little better that at least somebody is pointing these things out to me. I never realized I was so judgmental of myself and other people and that I'm assuming I'm so different from everyone.

THERAPIST: So you feel good that you have made this observation about yourself?

DENISE: Yes.

After summarizing the main points of the second session, the therapist assigned homework for the coming week: to fill out the Daily Record of Dysfunctional Thoughts (see Figure 6.4) and the Weekly Activity Schedule (with mastery and pleasure ratings; see Figure 6.3).

Session 3

By the beginning of the third session, Denise's mood had visibly improved. She had registered for a lecture series at the museum and was looking forward to attending the first lecture. She also had called her friend Diane with very positive results. She was catching negative and punitive thoughts toward others and herself and was challenging these thoughts. The primary agenda item Denise chose to work on was "how I back away from other people," an aspect of her unrelenting standards, punitiveness, and social isolation/alienation schemas.

DENISE: I want to stop withdrawing from people. I want to be more accepting and engaged with others.

THERAPIST: What holds you back?

DENISE: I guess I believe that I have to be a bit removed and strict in relation to others or they'll just behave in whatever way they want. People have to know my rules and abide by them if they want to have a relationship with me.

The therapist continued probing to understand why Denise believed she had to have others adhere to such a strict set of rules to have a relationship. As the discussion progressed, it became obvious that, in the abstract, she could see that such hard and fast rules were not necessarily conducive to having a good relationship—in fact, such rules sometimes put others off. But in real-life situations, Denise never felt she was wrong. The therapist's next task was to help Denise bring her rational thinking to bear on her distorted thinking *in the context of a concrete event*. At the therapist's request, Denise then described a conversation with her friend Diane, and how her intolerance for Diane's deviation from her rules created distance. Denise had wanted Diane and her husband to come for a visit the following summer. Diane, however, told her that their dog had been quite sick, and that if the dog was still alive she could not leave it. Denise thought this was ridiculous. She believed a relationship with a pet should never take precedence over a human relationship. This occurred when Denise actually had wanted and hoped to get closer to Diane again. The therapist helped her use logic to evaluate her maladaptive schema.

THERAPIST: You had the thought "I'm right to set the record straight with her. She can't put me in second place to her dog. She can't do that without consequence." It seems likely that you believed that thought, and that you believed the thought was right. And since you believed that thought was right, you then felt you had to withdraw your affection from her if she didn't abide by your wishes.

DENISE: Right.

THERAPIST: Now, let's look at it. Do you think that thought is correct?

DENISE: Well, yes, it's insulting.

THERAPIST: What's insulting?

DENISE: She's putting her dog in a higher priority position.

THERAPIST: Have you ever had a pet?

DENISE: No.

THERAPIST: Do you think that maybe Diane feels like her dog is a part of her family?

DENISE: I never thought of it that way.

THERAPIST: If you look at the situation from that perspective, how do you feel?

DENISE: I feel like I'm being a little insensitive. . . . That's not right. I'm not allowing for any other perspective. I've never had a pet, so I don't really know what it's like to have a pet. It's not right for me to be so judgmental of Diane. I need to be more understanding. I wasn't very caring. I am actually behaving in a way that goes directly against my deepest values.

THERAPIST: So, according to your own values, was this right?

DENISE: No, it's not right. I wasn't respecting her feelings. I was just demanding that she respect mine. That wasn't right.

THERAPIST: OK, now this is one of the problems. If you want to get over this sense that you should never give in or bend your rules for others, one of the things you can do is look for this thought, "I'm right and you

should have a negative consequence for your 'wrong' decision"—and refer back to this conversation we are having now and decide for yourself whether, indeed, you were right. Now, if every time you approach a conflict in a relationship and allow for the possibility that you might not fully understand, but really think underneath, "But I know I'm right," you are going to feel put out, and then you are not going to want to engage with that person. Is that right?

DENISE: Yeah, that sounds right.

THERAPIST: So we have to decide here and now. Do you indeed think that you are right to suspend your initial negative judgment to leave open the possibility of reevaluating your reaction to her behavior?

DENISE: Yes.

THERAPIST: Now, the next time you get the thought, "I'm right and I'm going to make sure this other person knows it," how are you going to answer that thought?

DENISE: If I'm right? But I'm not necessarily right. I need to consider the other person's perspective. I need to try to understand them and then see if what I'm thinking fits.

THERAPIST: Now are you saying that because that is the correct answer, or because you really believe it?

DENISE: No, I really believe it.

The therapist followed this discussion with a technique called "point–counterpoint" to help Denise practice rational responses to her automatic thoughts even more intensively. In this excerpt, the therapist expressed Denise's own negative thinking as Denise tried to defend herself more rationally.

THERAPIST: Now I am going to be like the prosecuting attorney, and I'll say, "Now I understand you let your friend violate one of your rules of friendship. Is that true?"

DENISE: Yes.

THERAPIST: "Now it seems to me that that was a very bad thing for you to do."

DENISE: No, it wasn't.

THERAPIST: "You don't think it was?"

DENISE: No, I should try to understand her perspective.

THERAPIST: "Well, you can sit there and say you

should be more understanding, but I thought you said before that you wanted people to respect you."

DENISE: I do, but I also need to respect others.

THERAPIST: "I know, but now you are saying that you are going to let her get away with this. What's next?"

DENISE: What's next can only be a better understanding of one another. We'll feel closer.

THERAPIST: "But how can you feel closer if she's not respecting your rules of friendship?"

DENISE: Maybe my rules are not appropriate in this situation. I need to learn to be more understanding, flexible, and tolerant of some deviations from my rules.

THERAPIST: "But then you'll lose control of the situation."

DENISE: No, that's an exaggeration. I don't need to control the whole situation. I can still decide what makes sense. I am still in control of what's important.

THERAPIST: "How can that be?"

DENISE: Because I can respect myself and respect my friend, as well. I don't have to turn everything into an either–or situation to try to make her see and do it my way. That just makes it difficult for her to get along with me, and I'll lose out on the relationship in the long run if I keep on insisting that she either do it my way or we do nothing.

Finally, the therapist returned to the schema and asked the patient how much she believed the new perspective.

THERAPIST: If you're flexible, you'll lose control. Now do you believe that?

DENISE: No.

THERAPIST: Do you believe it partially?

DENISE: No. In fact, I'm more likely to lose control of any possibility of getting what I want if I'm so inflexible. It's like I lose sight of the importance of the relationship when I get so stuck on thinking that I have to be in control and that the other person has to do it my way.

THERAPIST: OK, so right now, how much do you believe that?

DENISE: Completely.

THERAPIST: 100%?

DENISE: Yes.

THERAPIST: You are sure 100%, not 90 or 80%?

DENISE: No, 100%.

For the remainder of Session 3, Denise and the therapist reviewed other instances in which she noticed that her standards were not flexible and felt the urge to be punitive when her rules were not met. The session ended with a summary of the main issues raised in the first three sessions.

Summary of Initial Sessions

In the first three sessions, the therapist laid the groundwork for the remainder of treatment. He began immediately by teaching Denise to identify her negative automatic thoughts. By doing this, the therapist began to understand her feelings of hopelessness and to explore her isolation. By identifying her thoughts in a variety of specific situations, he was able to deduce several key schemas that later proved central to Denise's thinking: (1) unrelenting standards, (2) punitiveness, and (3) social isolation/alienation. All appeared to be contributing to Denise's social isolation and depression. The therapist made especially skillful use of Denise's thoughts during the second therapy session to help her see that she was distorting evidence about the therapeutic interaction and coming to the inaccurate conclusion that the therapist would be judgmental and punitive with her and withdraw positive feelings for her, in the same way that Denise tends to respond to others.

Beyond identifying thoughts and distortions, the therapist guided Denise to take concrete steps to overcome her inactivity and withdrawal. He asked her to weigh the advantages and disadvantages of staying in the house all day watching TV; he broke down the task of attending a lecture series at the museum into small, manageable steps; and he worked with her to develop an activity schedule to follow during the week.

Finally, the therapist employed a variety of strategies to demonstrate to Denise that she could test the validity of her thoughts, develop rational responses, and feel better. For example, during the course of the three sessions the therapist set up an experiment, used reattribution, offered alternative perspectives, and practiced the point–counterpoint technique.

One final point we want to emphasize is that the primary therapeutic mode was questioning. Most of the therapist's comments were in the form of questions. This helped Denise to evaluate her own thoughts outside of the session and prevented her from feeling attacked by the therapist.

By the end of these initial sessions, Denise reported being more optimistic that her life could change.

Later Sessions

Denise continued to fill out the Daily Record of Dysfunctional Thoughts and gathered evidence that she could relax her standards and be more tolerant of others' viewpoints and foibles. She discovered that she felt happier, both with herself and others, as a result.

The therapist set up several experiments with Denise to test a series of beliefs: that her friends would become punitive with her when she did not behave perfectly, and that her relationships would become unpleasant and undesirable if she relaxed any of her rigid standards regarding how others should behave in relationships. Through graded tasks, Denise counteracted her tendency to withdraw by gradually approaching new and sometimes unfamiliar situations. When she noticed herself imposing her standards of behavior on others, or noticed in herself the urge to become punitive, Denise practiced more open and accepting behaviors (by asking open-ended questions that reflected back her understanding of others' responses, and by inhibiting harsh and judgmental statements). She practiced tolerating the discomfort associated with these new behaviors until they began to feel more comfortable and natural.

When Denise terminated therapy, her BDI score was in the normal range. The symptom reduction phase of treatment was successfully completed in 20 sessions.

The next section describes and illustrates a case example of schema-focused therapy for chronic depression.

SCHEMA THERAPY FOR CHRONIC DEPRESSION

Schema therapy, developed by Young (1990/1999; Young et al., 2003), can be used with patients who present with recurrent depressive episodes, an early age of onset (before age 20)

of depression, early life trauma or adverse family relations (loss of parent in childhood, sexual, physical and/or verbal abuse, neglect, and overprotection), comorbid personality disorder(s), and a large number of EMSs (identified with the Young Schema Questionnaire; Young & Brown, 1990/1994), particularly in the domains of Impaired Autonomy and Overvigilance. Young (1990/1999; Young et al., 2003) has written extensively about the schema therapy approach. Young and Klosko (1994) have published a self-help book for patients to guide them.

Beck and colleagues (1990) have noted that

> schemas are difficult to alter. They are held firmly in place by behavioral, cognitive, and affective elements. The therapeutic approach must take a tripartite approach. To take a strictly cognitive approach and try to argue patients out of their distortions will not work. Having the patients abreact within the session to fantasies or recollections will not be successful by itself. A therapeutic program that addresses all three areas is essential. A patient's cognitive distortions serve as signposts that point to the schema. (p. 10)

As a result, schema therapy is significantly different from traditional CBT. It places more emphasis on early developmental patterns and origins, long-term interpersonal difficulties, the patient–therapist relationship, and emotive or experiential exercises.

Case Study of Barbara

The second case study demonstrates the use of schema therapy with a chronically depressed patient. We shifted to schema therapy because Barbara's depression was not lifting with standard cognitive therapy. Although Barbara had learned how to challenge automatic thoughts with rational responses and had followed through on graded behavioral assignments to test her thoughts, she never believed the rational responses. Barbara had remained convinced that she was worthless, useless, and hopeless. Additionally, many of the behavioral assignments presented "catch-22" scenarios within her current life situation. It was necessary to add various emotive and experiential techniques that are part of schema therapy to access Barbara's core beliefs. Core beliefs are the cognitive components of schemas. Schemas are deeply held emotionally based beliefs or EMSs that are unquestioningly experienced as true and impervious to rational challenges. The treatment was concentrated on schema mode work. Before presenting the specifics of the schema therapy treatment, we present Barbara.

History and Presenting Problems

The patient "Barbara" was a very physically attractive 46-year-old woman who had been married for the past 20 years to George, a functional alcoholic working on Wall Street in investment banking. It was the first marriage for both, but it had been extremely rocky throughout. Barbara had wanted children in the marriage but had been unable to conceive naturally. Although fertility treatments and adoption had been discussed, Barbara reported that George resisted following through on these options, because he questioned her ability to be an adequate parent. At the beginning of George and Barbara's relationship, Barbara reported extremely strong sexual chemistry. However, she stated that the chemistry had been erratic and often disappeared for long periods over the course of their relationship. She said that she had only felt real happiness with George in the first few months of the relationship, when he was extremely generous and attentive. Her decision to marry George was based on a feeling that they were meant for each other. They initially met at a high-end bar, where Barbara had worked as a cocktail waitress. Once their relationship was established, however, George continued to spend most of his free time in cocktail lounges without her, as she did not like to drink.

At the time she came in for her first interview, Barbara was spending most of her time in bed or watching TV. She rarely left the house except to go shopping. Outings with her mom or friends "to lift her spirits" often culminated in shopping sprees, followed by extended verbal berating by George, drunk upon his return home from the bar, because of what he perceived as her lack of taste, judgment, and intelligence regarding purchases. Barbara entered treatment because her husband told her that she "was driving him crazy with all her ridiculous behavior" and that she should "go get fixed." Barbara acknowledged feeling very depressed. She stated that this latest episode of depression started after a particularly upsetting fight with her husband over adopting a child.

Barbara reported having mild to moderate depression most of her life, interspersed with multiple episodes of major depression. She first became aware of feeling moderately depressed around age 11. An only child, she initially described her childhood family as "fine." Barbara described her mother as extremely attentive and devoted, a "very good mother who did everything for me." She stated that her mother lived for her, but also remembered her mother occasionally falling into depressions. She recalled that when her mother was depressed, she was emotionally unavailable. An imagery exercise brought up a memory of her mother during one of these periods, in which Barbara, at around the age of 6, felt very scared and lost. Barbara described her father as a workaholic who was almost never home. When he did come home, he was remote, preferring the solitude of his study over interacting with her and her mother. If Barbara tried to engage him as a child, he would upbraid her by calling her "an annoying simpleton" and demand that she leave him alone. An imagery exercise of her father revealed his intolerant, demeaning, and rejecting behavior toward Barbara as a young child. Barbara described her first major depressive episode, which occurred around age 16, after a breakup with her first serious boyfriend. Later episodes were triggered by other breakups and the fertility problems.

Barbara scored 29 on the BDl, placing her in the moderate to severe range of depression. She also completed the Young Schema Questionnaire (Young & Brown, 1990/1994), and received very high scores on Emotional Deprivation, Defectiveness, Abandonment, Dependence/Incompetence, Entitlement, Failure, Subjugation, Approval Seeking, and Negativity/Pessimism. Her Schema Mode Questionnaire (Young, Atkinson, Arntz, Weishaar, & Weishaar, 2004) indicated that she primarily functioned in the following modes: Detached Protector, Compliant Surrender, Punitive Parent, and Vulnerable Child. On the Multimodal Life History Inventory (Lazarus & Lazarus, 1991), a 15-page assessment tool covering a wide range of issues dealing with feelings, thoughts, behaviors, and a variety of other psychotherapeutic issues, Barbara reported her main problems as depression, being unhappy with herself, feeling empty and unloved, and feeling unappreciated. She also listed the following behaviors as applicable: procrastination, withdrawal, concentration difficulties, sleep disturbance, crying, and occasional outbursts of temper. She further indicated that she often felt sad, depressed, unhappy, hopeless, useless, and lonely. She endorsed the following statements: "I don't know what to do with my life," "Life is empty, a waste," and "There is nothing to look forward to."

Based on the initial interview, Barbara was diagnosed with major depressive disorder, recurrent episode on Axis I and dependent personality disorder on Axis II.

This section demonstrates schema therapy, or, more specifically, schema mode work with Barbara. The general overview is as follows. As noted earlier in this chapter, there are four main types of modes: child modes, maladaptive coping modes, dysfunctional parent modes, and the healthy adult modes (see Figures 6.2a–c, on pages 264–265). To understand the patient's current problems in terms of modes, first it is important to identify with the patient the primary modes in which he or she is functioning. Then, it is necessary to help the patient recognize and understand the origins of the maladaptive and dysfunctional modes (with their embedded EMSs), then heal and/or strengthen the healthy modes (child and adult). Once maladaptive modes are fully exposed and the healthy modes are sufficiently strengthened, the patient is assisted in seriously challenging the early maladaptive schemas with accompanying negative cognitions and the dysfunctional coping styles. Depression lifts as the patient more firmly establishes the healthy modes as his or her primary modes. To summarize, there are seven general steps in mode work: (1) increase awareness of modes by identifying and labeling modes with the patient; (2) explore origins of modes in childhood and/or adolescence and reveal their adaptive value when relevant; (3) link current problems and symptoms to maladaptive modes; (4) uncover the advantages and disadvantages of each mode; (5) use imagery to access the vulnerable child mode; (6) conduct dialogues between modes; and (7) generalize the results from mode work to real life. The following sections illustrate the therapeutic process with each step.

Step 1: Increase Awareness of Modes by Identifying and Labeling Modes with the Patient

This first step helps both the therapist and the patient conceptualize the problems in terms of different parts of the self or modes. From the Schema Mode Questionnaire, the therapist already was aware that Barbara primarily functioned in the Detached Protector, Compliant Surrenderer, Punitive/Critical Parent, and Vulnerable Child modes. The session reveals how the therapist queries the patient so that she can begin to recognize and differentiate these parts within herself. Throughout this section, the patient is encouraged to label modes with terms that feel right—rather than simply applying generic terms from the Schema Mode Questionnaire. Patients are encouraged to find terms that best capture the thoughts, emotions, and/or behaviors associated with each mode. A primary goal with this first step is to help the patient observe these parts, and decenter him- or herself from these parts. This step begins the process of interrupting the automaticity of the modes.

THERAPIST: I'm noticing in our sessions that sometimes you seem very sad and upset and critical of yourself, and other times you seem a bit distracted from what you're feeling, like when you were telling me about the great pair of shoes that you found on your shopping trip.

BARBARA: Yeah, I guess that's true. Talking about my purchases makes me feel better.

THERAPIST: When you say better, what do you mean?

BARBARA: I feel good.

THERAPIST: Like happy, peaceful, and content?

BARBARA: I feel pleasure.

THERAPIST: In what way is it pleasurable?

BARBARA: I feel pleasure when I look at pretty things with my mom or my friends, and I like buying those things. It takes my mind off of everything else.

THERAPIST: Like you're temporarily distracted from other feelings?

BARBARA: Yeah, that's right.

THERAPIST: What are those other feelings?

BARBARA: Just feeling real bad. I can't stand those feelings.

THERAPIST: So, sometimes there is this one part of you that just wants distance from this other part of you that feels bad?

BARBARA: Yes.

THERAPIST: Are there other things you do besides shopping that help you distance from bad feelings?

BARBARA: Well, yeah, I sleep a lot.

THERAPIST: Anything else?

BARBARA: I watch TV, but TV doesn't always work.

THERAPIST: This part of you that wants distance from feeling bad—what could we call that part of you?

BARBARA: That part of me? I don't know. I don't know what to call it.

THERAPIST: What does it feel like?

BARBARA: It feels like I'm escaping.

THERAPIST: OK. So should we call that part "the Escapist" [Detached Protector mode]?

BARBARA: I guess so. . . . That sounds right.

THERAPIST: And the part of you that you've escaped from—can you tell me more about that part of you?

BARBARA: That part feels bad . . . really bad and terrible.

THERAPIST: Let me hear that part speak about those feelings.

BARBARA: I'm just a bad person (*Starts to cry.*) . . . I'm a useless good for nothing. I feel so hopeless. I don't know what to do. I can't figure anything out. I'm such a zero, such a failure. . . . Do we really have to talk about this?

THERAPIST: Barbara, I know if feels bad to be in touch with this part of yourself, but if you can hang in there for just a bit, it will help me to understand why you're feeling so bad. Do you know what this part of you wants?

BARBARA: I want to feel good.

THERAPIST: What do you think would help you feel better?

BARBARA: I don't know. I really don't know. I just want you to fix me. My husband is right, I am a ridiculous person.

THERAPIST: It sounds like there is one part of you that feels really bad, like there is something really wrong with you, and then there is another part that agrees with what your husband says about you—that "you're ridiculous." I want you to hold back the part that is agreeing with your husband, and I want to hear more about the part of you that feels bad—the part of you who wants everything fixed. That part . . . do you feel it?

BARBARA: Yes, I feel it.

THERAPIST: Tell me more. What are the things you want to fix?

BARBARA: I don't know. I just want to feel good about myself, proud of myself, but I just don't. I want to have a child, but my husband doesn't think I can handle it. He's probably right. I need so much help with just everyday living. I don't know how to handle anything.

THERAPIST: So this part of you, this part that feels bad and helpless but also wants to feel better, what could we call this part?

BARBARA: I don't know. What do you think?

THERAPIST: Well, what does it feel like?

BARBARA: It feels helpless, bad and helpless.

THERAPIST: How old do you feel when you're in touch with this part of yourself?

BARBARA: I feel young, very young.

THERAPIST: Do you want to call that part "Bad Little Barbara" [Vulnerable Child mode with associated EMSs of defectiveness, dependence/incompetence, and enmeshment/undeveloped self]?

BARBARA: Sure.

THERAPIST: OK. And now this other part—the one that is agreeing with your husband and calling yourself ridiculous . . .

BARBARA: Well, I am ridiculous and silly. I can't cope with anything.

THERAPIST: Before you agree with that part, I want you to just notice how that part sounds. How does that part sound to you? Does it sound critical?

BARBARA: Yes, but I deserve it. I'm so useless.

THERAPIST: It sounds like you are having a hard time just listening to that part without automatically agreeing with it?

BARBARA: Yeah, I guess that's true.

THERAPIST: So, what do you want to call that part?

BARBARA: I don't know . . . But . . . you're not going to tell me what to call it, are you?

THERAPIST: Right.

BARBARA: OK. I guess "The Critic" [Punitive/Critical Parent mode with associated EMSs of defectiveness and subjugation].

In this part of the session, the therapist has helped Barbara begin to recognize and label the

Detached Protector, Punitive/Critical Parent, and Vulnerable Child modes. Although not fully illustrated here, the therapist also used a similar sequence of questions to help Barbara identify other modes. From this portion of the session, it is clear that "the Critic" (or Punitive/Critical Parent mode) is generating a tremendous amount of negative affect in Barbara. Barbara's only apparent way to cope with the onslaught of criticism from this mode is "the Escapist" (Detached Protector mode), in which she sleeps away much of her life. Otherwise, Barbara's primary experience of herself rests with the "Bad Little Barbara" (Vulnerable Child mode), where she feels defective, useless, hopeless, and helpless.

Step 2: Explore Origins of Modes in Childhood and/or Adolescence

This section illustrates how the therapist helps Barbara recognize the origins of these modes. In addition, the therapist assesses the strength of a Healthy Parent mode.

THERAPIST: Does "the Critic" sound like anyone else you know or have known in your life?

BARBARA: Yes, it sounds like George.

THERAPIST: Anyone else?

BARBARA: Yeah, it also sounds like my Dad . . . just like my Dad.

THERAPIST: In what way?

BARBARA: My Dad used to talk like that to me . . . whenever I tried to get his attention.

THERAPIST: How old were you?

BARBARA: Young, very young . . . 3 or 4 . . . as far back as I remember.

THERAPIST: Can you close your eyes and try to let yourself feel like that young child again with your dad?

BARBARA: (*Closes eyes.*)

THERAPIST: Tell me what's happening.

BARBARA: He's yelling at me because I pulled on his coat jacket.

THERAPIST: Let me hear what he's saying to you.

BARBARA: "Stop it, you little pest. You're such a simpleton. Can't you find anything better to do than pull on my coat? Get out of here!"

THERAPIST: And how are you feeling as he is yelling these things at you?

BARBARA: I feel stupid, like I'm a jerk. I'm nothing—a useless pest, an annoyance.

THERAPIST: Does it feel like he's right, or are you angry at him?

BARBARA: No. I don't feel angry. I just feel bad (*starts to cry*)—I'm just bad.

THERAPIST: So there is part of you agreeing with him, becoming critical of yourself—like your dad—thinking you're bad.

BARBARA: Yeah.

THERAPIST: And where is your mom?

BARBARA: She's telling me to shush and leave him alone. She says he's tired from working so hard all day.

THERAPIST: And what are you thinking and feeling when she says this?

BARBARA: I'm thinking that I'm a terrible person.

THERAPIST: So, you're getting the message that you are the problem from both of your parents. It feels like both parents are being critical of you, and there is a part of you that believes your parents' criticisms. Is that right?

BARBARA: Yes, that's right.

THERAPIST: So there is also this critical part of you, this part that has accepted your "Critical Parents" message, that you're bad and a problem—a pest.

BARBARA: Yes.

THERAPIST: What is your mom doing?

BARBARA: She whisks me away and tries to make me feel better by giving me something, like a toy or something to eat. A lot of times she takes me out shopping and buys me something special.

THERAPIST: And how do you feel when she does this?

BARBARA: I feel a little better, but deep down I know I'm bad and useless. I still have that bad and useless feeling inside.

THERAPIST: So there is still the "Bad Little Barbara" underneath?

BARBARA: Yes. That is it.

THERAPIST: If you could have rewritten the script for your family, a family with ideal parents, what would you have happen?

BARBARA: I have no idea. They weren't bad. They were doing their best.

THERAPIST: Yes, but what if you had had a daddy who was excited to see you at the end of his work day . . . a daddy who enjoyed coming home to his family . . . who found pleasure in talking with you and getting to know you, and played with you?

BARBARA: You mean . . . a daddy who loved me?

THERAPIST: Yes. I mean a daddy who was able to show you his love through all sorts of actions.

BARBARA: Wow . . . that would have been so different.

THERAPIST: Do you feel any angry feelings at him now as you think about how he spoke to you—this very young child simply trying to get his attention?

BARBARA: No, I was in his way. He worked hard. I had to leave him alone.

THERAPIST: What you just said—does that sound like anyone you know?

BARBARA: Yes. It sounds like my mother.

THERAPIST: And what do you think of that now?

BARBARA: Well. She was just trying to keep the peace and fill in for him.

THERAPIST: But what about you, Little Barbara?

BARBARA: It's sad. I feel sad for me.

THERAPIST: Right. It is sad for you. You are a child doing what children do—children try to get their parents' attention, children want to know they are loved, valued, appreciated. You were no different from any other child, but what is happening here?

BARBARA: (Cries.)

THERAPIST: No one's calling your dad on his poor behavior toward you. Everyone's accommodating *him* and speaking to you as if *you* are the problem, when all that you are doing is what every young child does. And yet your father and your mother are responding as if you are the problem.

BARBARA: Yeah. You're right. Why did they do that?

THERAPIST: Do you think there was something wrong with you, or do you think there was

something wrong with the way they were behaving with you?

BARBARA: The way they were behaving with me. . . . It's a problem with the way they treated me.

In the preceding section, the therapist helps Barbara to realize the origin of "the Critic," that part of her self that has accepted her "Critical Parent" message that she is bad and a useless pest. The therapist's questions and comments also help Barbara realize that the problem was actually a problem with her parents' behavior toward her rather than an inherent defect in herself.

The therapist now turns Barbara's attention to the origin of "the Escapist," that part that was seeking relief from these terrible feelings about herself as a child. The therapist also helps Barbara become more aware that "the Escapist" was only able to provide short-term relief.

THERAPIST: Now when you had this bad feeling about yourself as a child, the "Bad Barbara" feeling, how did you cope with that feeling? What did you do?

BARBARA: A lot of the time I did nothing. I just sat on my bed in my room daydreaming, wishing everything was different. I would fantasize being a star, a beautiful person that everyone adored. People would dote on me and give me expensive gifts and clothes that made me look even more beautiful. Sometimes when my mom would take me out and buy me things, it kind of felt like she was making this dream come true.

THERAPIST: Is that the "the Escapist" part of you trying to help you feel better?

BARBARA: Yes, it definitely is.

THERAPIST: And then what would happen?

BARBARA: I would feel better, especially as I got older and I got a lot of attention from the way I looked, but eventually my dad always would start yelling again. I remember him yelling at my mom for "spending too much money" simply to turn me into "a pretty Bimbo."

THERAPIST: So the efforts to feel better eventually backfired.

BARBARA: Right. I never felt very good for long. I never felt good inside.

Step 3: Link Current Problems and Symptoms to Maladaptive Modes

In this section, the therapist asks Barbara questions that help her to recognize how these modes that developed in childhood are still operating in the present. Barbara begins to connect these modes with why she is feeling so depressed, and she begins to see the repetitive patterns in her life.

THERAPIST: Let's look at what is happening now in your life. Do you recognize any relationship between what we have been talking about—these different parts of you—and how you are thinking and feeling about yourself and coping with your life now?

BARBARA: Yeah, I'm still trying to feel good—or just not feel—by being "the Escapist." When I go on these shopping sprees and let my mom and my friends dress me up, it still doesn't work any better than it ever did. And sleeping all the time doesn't work either.

THERAPIST: What do you mean?

BARBARA: Well, I only feel good for a short while. Then, instead of my dad coming home, now I'm coming home to George or he's coming home to me. George is just as critical of me and just as unavailable as my Dad.

THERAPIST: And then what happens?

BARBARA: I start to feel really bad again, really depressed. I feel like I'm not worth spending time with, like I'm boring and useless. I'm saying all sorts of bad things about myself and I agree with everything George says about me. I'm my worst "Critic." In the end, I still feel like the same old "Bad Little Barbara" inside who never ever really feels better. Then, I just want to go to sleep to get away from it all. I'm finally starting to see it more clearly, going around and around the same old circle—nothing has changed and nothing changes. I've been miserable my whole life.

THERAPIST: But there is one very important change.

BARBARA: What is that?

THERAPIST: You're starting to see and understand what's been happening for a long time instead of just being on the treadmill without any awareness.

Step 4: Uncover Advantages and Disadvantages of Each Mode

The therapist now begins to ask Barbara questions regarding the advantages and disadvantages of listening and acting on these different parts of her self. This helps Barbara to gain more distance from the modes and to reduce further automatically responding to them.

THERAPIST: When these different parts of yourself or modes developed, they served a purpose. Why don't we talk about each of them and explore their advantages and/or disadvantages both in the past and present? Let's start with "the Escapist."

BARBARA: Well, that part lets me feel good—or at least not feel bad.

THERAPIST: For how long?

BARBARA: For a while.

THERAPIST: And in the long run? Does that part help you feel better?

BARBARA: No, not really. I can't really escape feeling bad. I can't say I feel any better in the long run.

THERAPIST: So, is there any advantage to this part of you—"the Escapist"?

BARBARA: I'm mixed about it.

THERAPIST: Sure. I can understand that. If you don't know of any other way to feel better, any relief is better than no relief at all.

BARBARA: Yeah.

THERAPIST: But sometimes it is good to let yourself feel bad, because when you let yourself stay in touch with your feelings, you often can begin to recognize what feels better in the long run . . . like finding activities that are truly interesting to you or that give you a sense of accomplishment and purpose, or that bring out a feeling of deep enjoyment.

BARBARA: That makes sense, but I have no idea how to find those things.

THERAPIST: Well, that is something we can work on together.

BARBARA: That sounds good.

THERAPIST: And what about "the Critic"? Is there any advantage to listening to "the Critic"?

BARBARA: That part tells me what's wrong with me.

THERAPIST: And what does "the Critic" say is wrong with you?

BARBARA: That I'm stupid and silly, useless and annoying.

THERAPIST: Do you think "the Critic" is right?

BARBARA: Of course.

THERAPIST: But if you put the words of "the Critic" back in your dad's mouth and listen to him speak to little 3-year-old Barbara as she excitedly greets him coming home from work, what do you think?

BARBARA: When you put it that way, I think he's a jerk. I mean, what does he think he is doing to this poor little girl? What's wrong with him?

THERAPIST: Right. So is there any advantage to listening to these critical words?

BARBARA: No . . . no, definitely not.

THERAPIST: Are there any disadvantages of listening to "the Critic"?

BARBARA: Yes. It's getting clearer now why that part is making me feel so bad. I have to stop listening to that part. When I accept what my dad said as the truth, I feel bad, really bad, about myself.

THERAPIST: You mean it brings up that "Bad Little Barbara" feeling?

BARBARA: Yes.

THERAPIST: And what about her? Is there any advantage to listening to her?

BARBARA: I don't think anyone has ever really listened or paid attention to her, and what she needs to feel happy. There's a big advantage and no disadvantage to listening to that part of me.

THERAPIST: I agree.

Step 5: Use Imagery
to Access the Vulnerable Child Mode

The therapist now begins to engage Barbara in the Vulnerable Child mode. By accessing this mode, therapist and patient can begin to work on the core schemas that are part of Little Barbara: her feelings, needs, and beliefs.

THERAPIST: I know it's sometimes unpleasant to let yourself be in touch with "Bad Little Barbara," but would you be willing to go there, so that we can get to know that part of you to find out what you need to truly feel better and to find out what is getting in the way?

BARBARA: I guess . . . (*Closes eyes.*)

THERAPIST: Tell me what you are feeling and thinking right now.

BARBARA: It's the same old feelings—I feel bad . . . and useless. (*Visibly begins to look upset, then opens her eyes.*)

THERAPIST: Can you go back there to "Little Barbara," can you let yourself feel her?

BARBARA: OK (*Closes her eyes again.*)

THERAPIST: Where are you? What are you doing?

BARBARA: I'm sitting on my bed in my room. My daddy just told me to go away.

THERAPIST: And how are you feeling?

BARBARA: Awful.

THERAPIST: And what do you want?

BARBARA: I want my mommy to come in and make me feel better.

THERAPIST: Where is she?

BARBARA: She's in her room, lying on her bed. She doesn't feel good either.

THERAPIST: If you could bring in a healthy mommy to be with you right now, what would she say to you? Let me hear her speak to Little Barbara.

BARBARA: You know he's just tired from work. If you just leave him alone, everything will be all right.

THERAPIST: Let me hear what Little Barbara thinks of this?

BARBARA: That doesn't help much. I still feel upset and bad.

THERAPIST: How about if I come in to help?

BARBARA: OK.

THERAPIST: You are such a loving little girl. So many fathers would relish coming home to such a greeting from their little girl. Something is wrong with your Daddy. Why doesn't he recognize that you're offering him something that is precious—so special? . . . How does little Barbara feel as she hears this?

BARBARA: Better.

THERAPIST: Let me talk to your father now.

BARBARA: OK.

THERAPIST: How can you speak to your daughter that way? She's done nothing but welcome you home with joy and love. And look at how you are responding. Your response to her is completely inappropriate. You are so closed off and removed from everything. What is going on with you? Why can't you see that you have a beautiful, creative, and loving daughter? Barbara does not deserve this type of treatment. I'm not going to stand for this and let you hurt her anymore. . . . How does little Barbara feel as she hears this?

BARBARA: A lot better. I wish my mom would have spoken to my dad that way. But you know, if you really tried to say anything like that to him, he wouldn't listen. He never listened to my mom. He'd probably just say something mean to you and then shut the door.

THERAPIST: OK. Well if that happened, what would you want to happen next?

BARBARA: I don't know.

THERAPIST: Let me step in again and say this to him through the door. Whether or not you choose to listen, there is a limit, a limit as to how long we will stay here for you. If you choose not to be here for us, we will not stay here for you.

BARBARA: I don't think he'll change.

THERAPIST: Then you and I, together, will leave him and create a better life.

BARBARA: Is that really possible?

THERAPIST: Do you want to make it happen?

BARBARA: Yes, but what about him? He'll be so lonely.

THERAPIST: Who will be lonely?

BARBARA: He will, unless we stay.

THERAPIST: But if you stay, who will be lonely then?

BARBARA: Me.

THERAPIST: Do you want to continue to be there for someone who chooses not to be there for you?

BARBARA: Well, no—no, that isn't right.

THERAPIST: So what do you want to do?

BARBARA: I want to leave.

In this part of the session, the therapist has taken on the "Healthy Parent" mode for Barbara, because she does not have a strong template for this mode. This is one example of what is meant by "limited reparenting." In this role, the therapist temporarily steps in to support the client in relation to unmet basic needs for safety; stability or predictability; love, nurturance, and attention; acceptance and praise; empathy; realistic limits; and validation of feelings and needs. The therapist also counters and challenges any unreasonable messages or beliefs that such needs should remain unfulfilled.

Step 6: Conduct Dialogues between Modes

Once the patient clearly identifies and is able to evoke the Healthy Adult and the Vulnerable Child in imagery, the next step is to have the patient begin dialogues between the various modes. For example, the Healthy Adult can have a dialogue with the Vulnerable Child; the Critical Parent, with the Healthy Adult; and the Detached Protector, with the Vulnerable Child.

THERAPIST: How about having "Little Barbara" talk with "the Escapist" about things that she really enjoys?

BARBARA: OK . . . but how do we do that?

THERAPIST: First, I want you to sit on this side of the couch. When you're on this side of the couch, I want you to let yourself get in touch with and speak for "Little Barbara." Have "Little Barbara" talk about all those things that interest her—those things that help her feel alive. And then, I want you to get up and sit on the other side of the couch. When you're on this side of the couch, I want you to let yourself get in touch with and speak for "the Escapist." We'll go back and forth between those two parts of your self to see what comes out. I'll help out "Little Barbara" if she needs me.

BARBARA: [as "Little Barbara"] You know, I once made a dress at school, and I noticed that I really liked sewing. It was a really simple pattern, nothing special, but I had so much fun making it. I think I might want to take a class to try sewing again.

[as "the Escapist"] Why do you want to do that? If it doesn't turn out, you'll just feel bad about yourself. People might think you're ridiculous at this age, trying to learn to sew. Why take the chance that you'll feel bad or stupid? Why don't you just lie down and forget about it?

[as "Little Barbara"] But I might like it. If I don't start trying the things that I think I might enjoy, I'll never know what I like or what makes me happy . . . If I keep listening to you, I'll do nothing but sleep away the rest of my life. I want to have a life.

[as "the Escapist"] I don't know if it's worth the risk of feeling bad.

[as "Little Barbara"] Even if I feel bad at first, it will only be temporary. Either I'll get good at sewing or I can find something else that I'm good at. I'll eventually find something if I just keep at it.

[as "the Escapist"] Well OK, suit yourself.

[as "Little Barbara"] I will.

Part of the therapy at this point is focused on helping Barbara discover what gives her an inner sense of joy and accomplishment. This quest is complicated by the fact that Barbara spent so many of her early years dependent upon her mother, not developing any special skills or talents, and compliantly surrendering to what others wanted of her. At this point in her life, she is developmentally delayed in many areas. In the previous segment, however, Barbara has begun to acknowledge and is learning how to tolerate better the short-term discomfort of exposing these delays to herself and others to grow and feel more comfortable in the long term. The final step in therapy is to take these lessons into her everyday experiences.

Step 7: Generalize Results from Mode Work to Real Life

Barbara tried taking one sewing class and surprised herself by doing quite well. She then decided to take two more classes, a more advanced sewing class and another class in costume design. Following these classes, she started to volunteer for a local theater group, working on costumes. Barbara received much attention, praise, and appreciation from her teachers and theater friends. About 1½ years into treatment, Barbara commented to her therapist, "You know, I think this is the first time I have ever really felt good and proud of myself."

As Barbara's confidence and her network of friends grew, she became less accepting and less tolerant of George's neglectful and demeaning behaviors. She also became increasingly an-noyed with her mom's tendencies to excuse George's behavior for the sake of "being financially comfortable." This was in stark contrast to Barbara's unquestioning acceptance of her relationship with George at the beginning of treatment. As she began to see parallels between how she felt with George and how she felt as a child in her parents' home, Barbara began to question whether this was a good marriage for her. She recognized that many of George's behaviors were harmful in a similar way that her parent's behaviors had been harmful. Although Barbara continued to want to adopt a child, she began questioning George's ability to be a good parent. The following vignette is from a session 2 years into Barbara's treatment.

BARBARA: I'm noticing that when George speaks to me in such a condescending tone, I feel like a little girl with my father again. I don't want this. I want to be treated with love and respect, and as an equal. It isn't right for me to accept his behavior—being ignored and demeaned by someone who is supposed to love me.

THERAPIST: So what do you want to do?

BARBARA: I think I am ready to confront George about his drinking and abusive behavior. I can't even imagine adopting a child and bringing that child into our home if he continues to behave this way.

THERAPIST: What do you want to happen?

BARBARA: I want him to stop drinking and start treating me with love and respect.

THERAPIST: And if he doesn't? Then what?

BARBARA: I guess I will leave him and seek a divorce.

THERAPIST: And how will that be for you—in the worst case scenario?

BARBARA: In the worst case . . . you know, I think I will be OK. I mean, I have my own life now. I have my own friends. And I have you, if things really get rough.

THERAPIST: I'll be here for you whenever you need support. And financially?

BARBARA: Money is not everything. In any case, there will be a divorce settlement. Yeah, I think I will be OK.

At this point in treatment, Barbara has fully incorporated the Healthy Adult and has nurtured and is protecting the Vulnerable Child within. Along with these changes, Barbara's depression went into complete remission. Soon after this session, Barbara confronted her husband. Despite couple therapy, George refused to make any changes, and Barbara filed for divorce.

Barbara did experience one relapse of major depression as her divorce was finalized. "Bad Little Barbara" and "the Escapist" temporarily returned during this period. Barbara, however, was eventually able to empathize with and forgive herself, and to mourn the lost opportunity to have her own family. She also decided to go back to school to become a certified teacher at the high school level, teaching costume design and drama in the theater department. She eventually achieved this goal, and also met a single and emotionally available man who shared her passion for theater. Her chronic depression lifted, and Barbara has been relatively symptom free since.

CONCLUSION

Evidence demonstrating the efficacy of cognitive therapy in the treatment of unipolar and bipolar depression continues to mount. Adolescents, adults, and geriatric patients have all been shown to benefit from cognitive therapy.

Cognitive therapy helps patients understand the relationship among their thoughts, behaviors, and feelings. Cognitions are "put to the test" by examining evidence, setting up *in vivo* experiments, weighing advantages and disadvantages, trying graded tasks, and employing other intervention strategies. Through this process, patients begin to view themselves and their problems more realistically, to feel better, to change their maladaptive behavior patterns, and to take steps to solve real-life difficulties. These changes take place as a direct result of carefully planned, self-help homework assignments—one of the hallmarks of cognitive treatment. Cognitive therapy reduces symptoms by helping patients to identify and modify automatic thoughts, and the behaviors associated with them.

Another type of cognitive therapy—called schema therapy—has been developed to deal with the deeper psychological structures that predispose patients to chronic depression. After utilizing interventions aimed at initial symptom reduction, a great deal of subsequent at-

tention and effort are directed toward identifying and modifying the underlying schemas and schema modes that often predispose individuals to chronic depression. Following a thorough assessment, an extensive change component is developed and implemented. During this treatment, patients come to understand their own schemas and schema modes, their developmental origins, and the way they are triggered, reinforced, and maintained.

Throughout the treatment, cognitive therapists maintain a collaborative alliance with their patients. They are very active in structuring sessions, yet go to considerable lengths to help patients reach conclusions on their own. A therapist serves as a guide, helping a patient maneuver through a labyrinth of dysfunctional cognitions including EMSs and schema modes. As a result, patients attain the necessary psychological tools to become more proactive on their own behalf and are able to make the necessary cognitive, affective, interpersonal, and behavioral changes necessary to minimize further episodes of depression.

NOTES

1. Researchers have found it useful to differentiate between "relapse" (the return of symptoms within 6 months after termination of treatment) and "recurrence" (a whole new episode of depression, occurring at least 12 months after treatment has ended; Gelder, 1994; see also Overholser, 1998b). However because this distinction has not been uniformly incorporated into the literature (and for clarity of presentation), we have elected to use the term "relapse" to indicate the return of symptoms, regardless of the time frame.
2. Reported relapse rates for patients treated with medication have varied, depending on the definition of "relapse," the duration of the follow-up period, and the severity of depression within the patient population (Williams, 1997). Because of these differences, some of the estimates have ranged from 34 to 92% (Frank, 1996; Overholser, 1998b; Versiani, 1998; Williams, 1997), though lower rates have also been reported (Keller & Boland, 1998).
3. The book by Young (1990/1999) cited here and throughout the chapter, *Cognitive Therapy for Personality Disorders: A Schema-Focused Approach*, refers to the third edition. However, the ideas expressed were developed in 1990, for the original edition. Similarly, the Young Schema Questionnaire was developed in 1990, then reprinted in the third edition.
4. In this chapter, diagnoses are generally based on the *Diagnostic and Statistical Manual of Mental Disor-*

ders, fourth edition (DSM-IV; American Psychiatric Association, 1994). However, diagnoses for patients described in the case materials are based on DSM-III-R (American Psychiatric Association, 1987), the system in effect at the time of assessment.

REFERENCES

Agosti, V., & Ocepek, W. K. (1997). The efficacy of imipramine and psychotherapy in early-onset chronic depression: A reanalysis of the National Institute of Mental Health Treatment of Depression Collaborative Research Program. *Journal of Affective Disorders*, 43(3), 181–186.

Albon, J. S., & Jones, E. E. (2003). Validity of controlled clinical trials of psychotherapy: Findings from the NIMH Treatment of Depression Collaborative Research Program. *American Journal of Psychiatry*, 159(5), 775–783.

American Psychiatric Association. (1987). *Diagnostic and statistical manual of mental disorders* (3rd ed., rev.). Washington, DC: Author.

American Psychiatric Association. (1994). *Diagnostic and statistical manual of mental disorders* (4th ed.). Washington, DC: Author.

American Psychiatric Association. (2000). Practice guideline for the treatment of patients with major depressive disorder (revision). *American Journal of Psychiatry*, 157(Suppl. 4).

Antonuccio, D. O., Danton, W. G., & DeNelsky, G. Y. (1995). Psychotherapy versus medication for depression: Challenging the conventional wisdom with data. *Professional Psychology: Research and Practice*, 26(6), 574–585.

Antonuccio, D. O., Thomas, M., & Danton, W. G. (1997). A cost-effectiveness analysis of cognitive behavior therapy and fluoxetine (Prozac) in the treatment of depression. *Behavior Therapy*, 28, 187–210.

Arnow, B. A., Manber, R., Blasey, C., Klein, D. N., Blalock, J. A., Markowitz, J. C., et al. (2003). Therapeutic reactance as a predictor of outcome in the treatment of chronic depression. *Journal of Consulting and Clinical Psychology*, 71(6), 1025–1035.

Ball, J. R., Mitchell, P. B., Corry, J. C., Skillecorn, A., Smith, M., & Malhi, G. S. (2006). A randomized controlled trial of cognitive therapy for bipolar disorder: Focus on long-term change. *Journal of Clinical Psychiatry*, 67, 277–286.

Bandura, A. (1977). Self-efficacy: Toward a unifying theory of behavioral change. *Psychological Review*, 84, 181–215.

Barber, J. P., & DeRubeis, R. J. (1989). On second thought: Where the action is in cognitive therapy for depression. *Cognitive Therapy and Research*, 13(5), 441–457.

Barlow, D. H., & Hofmann, S. G. (1997). Efficacy and dissemination of psychological treatments. In D. M. Clark & C. G. Fairburn (Eds.), *Science and practice of cognitive behaviour therapy* (pp. 95–117). Oxford, UK: Oxford University Press.

Basco, M. R., & Rush, A. J. (1996). *Cognitive-behavioral therapy for bipolar disorder*. New York: Guilford Press.

Beck, A. T. (1967). *Depression: Causes and treatment*. Philadelphia: University of Pennsylvania Press.

Beck, A. T. (1976). *Cognitive therapy and the emotional disorders*. New York: International Universities Press.

Beck, A. T. (1988). *Love is never enough*. New York: Harper & Row.

Beck, A. T., Freeman, A., & Associates. (1990). *Cognitive therapy of personality disorders*. New York: Guilford Press.

Beck, A. T., Rush, A. J., Shaw, B. F., & Emery, G. (1979). *Cognitive therapy of depression*. New York: Guilford Press.

Beck, J. S. (1995). *Cognitive therapy: Basics and beyond*. New York: Guilford Press.

Berndt, E. R., Koran, L. M., Finkelstein, S. N., Gelenberg, A. J., Kornstein, S. G., Miller, I. M., et al. (2000). Lost human capital from early-onset chronic depression. *American Journal of Psychiatry*, 157, 940–947.

Beutler, L. E., Scogin, F., Kirkish, P., Schretlen, D., Corbishley, A., Hamblin, D., et al. (1987). Group cognitive therapy and alprazolam in the treatment of depression in older adults. *Journal of Consulting and Clinical Psychology*, 55(4), 550–556.

Biggs, M. M., & Rush, A. J. (1999). Cognitive and behavioral therapies alone or combined with antidepressant medication in the treatment of depression. In D. S. Janowsky (Ed.), *Psychotherapy indications and outcomes* (pp.121–172). Washington, DC: American Psychiatric Press.

Blackburn, I. M., Bishop, S., Glen, A. I. M., Whalley, L. J., & Christie, J. E. (1981). The efficacy of cognitive therapy in depression: A treatment trial using cognitive therapy and pharmacotherapy, each alone and in combination. *British Journal of Psychiatry*, 139, 181–189.

Blackburn, I. M., & Moore, R. G. (1997). Controlled acute and follow-up trial of cognitive therapy and pharmacotherapy in out-patients with recurrent depression. *British Journal of Psychiatry*, 171, 328–334.

Blatt, S. J., Zuroff, D. C., Bondi, C. M., & Sanislow, C. A. (2000). Short- and long-term effects of medication and psychotherapy in the brief treatment of depression: Further analysis of data from the NIMH TDCRP. *Psychotherapy Research*, 10(2), 215–234.

Bledsoe, S. E., & Grote, N. K. (2006). Treating depression during pregnancy and the postpartum: A preliminary meta-analysis. *Research on Social Work Practice*, 16(2), 109–120.

Bockting, C. L. H., Schene, A. H., Spinhoven, P., Koeter, M. W. J., Wouters, L. F., Huyser, J., et al. (2005). Preventing relapse/recurrence in recurrent depression with cognitive therapy: A randomized controlled trial. *Journal of Consulting and Clinical Psychology*, 73, 647–657.

Bowers, W. A. (1990). Treatment of depressed inpatients: Cognitive therapy plus medication, and medication alone. *British Journal of Psychiatry*, 156, 73–58.

Brown, G. W. (1996). Onset and course of depressive disorders: Summary of a research programme. In C. Mundt, M. J. Goldstein, K. Hahlweg, & P. Fiedler (Eds.), *Interpersonal factors in the origin and course of affective disorders.* (pp. 151–167). London: Gaskell/Royal College of Psychiatrists.

Burns, D. D., & Spangler, D. L. (2000). Does psychotherapy homework lead to improvements in depression in cognitive-behavioral therapy or does improvement lead to increased homework compliance? *Journal of Consulting and Clinical Psychology*, 68(1), 46–56.

Butler, A. C., Chapman, J. E., Forman, E. M., & Beck, A. T. (2006). The empirical status of cognitive-behavioral therapy: A review of meta-analyses. *Clinical Psychology Review*, 26, 17–31.

Castonguay, L. G., Goldfried, M. R., Wiser, S., Raue, P. J., & Hayes, A. M. (1996). Predicting the effect of cognitive therapy for depression: A study of unique and common factors. *Journal of Consulting and Clinical Psychology*, 64(3), 497–504.

Castonguay, L. G., Schut, A. J., Aikens, D., Constantino, M. J., Laurenceau, J. P., Bolough, L., et al. (2004). Integrative cognitive therapy: A preliminary investigation. *Journal of Psychotherapy Integration*, 14(1), 4–20.

Chapman, D. P., Whitfield, C. L., Felitti, V. J., Dube, S. R., Edwards, V. J., & Anda, R. F. (2004). Adverse childhood experiences and the risk of depressive disorders in adulthood. *Journal of Affective Disorders*, 82(2), 217–225.

Colom, F., Vieta, E., Martinez, A., Jorquera, A., & Gastó, C. (1998). What is the role of psychotherapy in the treatment of bipolar disorder? *Psychotherapy and Psychosomatics*, 67, 3–9.

Conte, H. R., Plutchik, R., Wild, K. V., & Karasu, T. B. (1986). Combined psychotherapy and pharmacotherapy for depression. *Archives of General Psychiatry*, 43, 471–479.

Craighead, W. E., Miklovitz, D. J., Vajk, F. C., & Frank, E. (1998). Psychological treatments for bipolar disorder. In P. E. Nathan & J. M. Gorman (Eds.), *A guide to treatments that work* (pp. 240–248). New York: Oxford University Press.

Crews, W. D., Jr., & Harrison, D. W. (1995). The neuropsychology of depression and its implications for cognitive therapy. *Neuropsychology Review*, 5(2), 81–123.

Curry, J. F. (2001). Specific psychotherapies for childhood and adolescent depression. *Biological Psychiatry*, 49, 1091–1100.

de Oliveira, I. R. (1998). The treatment of unipolar major depression: Pharmacotherapy, cognitive behaviour therapy or both? *Journal of Clinical Pharmacy and Therapeutics*, 23, 467–475.

Depression Guideline Panel. (1993). *Depression is a treatable illness: A patient's guide* (AHCPR Publication No. 93-0553). Rockville, MD: U.S. Department of Health and Human Services, Public Health Service, Agency for Health Care Policy and Research.

DeRubeis, R. J., & Feeley, M. (1990). Determinants of change in cognitive therapy for depression. *Cognitive Therapy and Research*, 14(5), 469–482.

DeRubeis, R. J., Gelfand, L. A., Tang, T. Z., & Simons, A. D. (1999). Medications versus cognitive behavior therapy for severely depressed outpatients: Mega-analysis of four randomized comparisons. *American Journal of Psychiatry*, 156(7), 1007–1013.

DeRubeis, R. J., Hollon, S. D., Amsterdam, J. D., Shelton, R. C., Young, P. R., Salomon, R. M., et al. (2005). Cognitive therapy vs. medications in the treatment of moderate to severe depression. *Archives of General Psychiatry*, 62, 409–416.

DeRubeis, R. J., Hollon, S. D., Grove, W. M., Evans, M. D., Garvey, M. J., & Tuason, V. B. (1990). How does cognitive therapy work?: Cognitive change and symptom change in cognitive therapy and pharmacotherapy for depression. *Journal of Consulting and Clinical Psychology*, 58(6), 862–869.

Dimidjian, S., Hollon, S. D., Dobson, K. S., Schmaling, K. B., Kohlenberg, R. J., Addis, M. E., et al. (2006). Randomized trial of behavioral activation, cognitive therapy, and antidepressant medication in the acute treatment of adults with major depression. *Journal of Consulting and Clinical Psychology*, 74(4), 658–670.

Dobson, K. S., & Pusch, D. (1993). Towards a definition of the conceptual and empirical boundaries of cognitive therapy. *Australian Psychologist*, 28(3), 137–144.

Dougherty, L. R., Klein, D. N., & Davila, J. (2004). A growth curve analysis of the course of dysthymic disorder: The effects of chronic stress and moderation by adverse parent-child relationships and family history. *Journal of Consulting and Clinical Psychology*, 72(6), 1012–1021.

Dube, S. R., Anda, R. F., Felitti, V. J., Chapman, D. P., Williamson, D. F., & Giles, W. H. (2001). Childhood abuse, household dysfunction, and the risk of attempted suicide throughout the life span: Findings from the adverse childhood experiences study. *Journal of the American Medical Association*, 286, 3089–3096.

Eifert, G. H., Beach, B. K., & Wilson, P. H. (1998). Depression: Behavioral principles and implications for treatment and relapse prevention. In J. J. Plaud & G. H. Eifert (Eds.), *From behavior theory to behavior therapy* (pp. 68–97). Boston: Allyn & Bacon.

Elkin, I., Gibbons, R. D., Shea, M. T., & Shaw, B. F. (1996). Science is not a trial (but it can sometimes be a tribulation). *Journal of Consulting and Clinical Psychology*, 64(1), 92–103.

Elkin, I., Shea, M. T., Watkins, J. T., Imber, S. D., Sotsky, S. M., Collins, J. F., et al. (1989). National Institute of Mental Health Treatment of Depression Collaborative Research Program: General effectiveness of treatments. *Archives of General Psychiatry, 46,* 971–982.

Evans, M. D., Hollon, S. D., DeRubeis, R. J., Piaseki, J. M., Grove, W. M., Garvey, M. J., et al. (1992). Differential relapse following cognitive therapy and pharmacotherapy for depression. In D. S. Janowsky (Ed.), *Psychotherapy indication and outcomes* (pp. 802–808). Washington, DC: American Psychiatric Press.

Fava, G. A., Rafanelli, C., Grandi, S., Canestrari, R., & Morphy, M. A. (1998a). Six-year outcome for cognitive behavioral treatment of residual symptoms in major depression. *American Journal of Psychiatry, 155*(10), 1443–1445.

Fava, G. A., Rafanelli, C., Grandi, S., Conti, S., & Belluardo, P. (1998b). Prevention of recurrent depression with cognitive behavioral therapy: Preliminary findings. *Archives of General Psychiatry, 55*(9), 816–820.

Floyd, M., Scogin, F., McKendree-Smith, N. L., Floyd, D. L., & Rokke, P. D. (2004). Cognitive therapy for depression: A comparison of individual psychotherapy and bibliotherapy for depressed older adults. *Behavior Modification, 28*(2), 297–318.

Frank, E. (1996). Long-term treatment of depression: interpersonal psychotherapy with and without medication. In C. Mundt & M. J. Goldstein (Eds.), *Interpersonal factors in the origin and course of affective disorders* (pp. 303–315). London: Gaskell/Royal College of Psychiatrists.

Frank E., & Thase, M. E. (1999). Natural history and preventative treatment of recurrent mood disorders. *Annual Review of Medicine, 50,* 453–468.

Free, M. L., Oei, T. P. S., & Appleton, C. (1998). Biological and psychological processes in recovery from depression during cognitive therapy. *Journal of Behavior Therapy and Experimental Psychiatry, 29,* 213–226.

Freeman, A., & Davison, M. R. (1997). Short-term therapy for the long-term patient. In L. Vandecreek, S. Knapp, & T. L. Jackson (Eds.), *Innovations in clinical practice: A source book* (pp. 5–24). Sarasota, FL: Professional Resource Press.

Futterman, A., Thompson, L., Gallagher-Thompson, D., & Ferris, R. (1995). Depression in later life: Epidemiology, assessment, etiology, and treatment. In E. E. Beckham & W. R. Leber (Eds.), *Handbook of depression* (2nd ed., pp. 494–525). New York: Guilford Press.

Gaffan, E. A., Tsaousis, J., & Kemp-Wheeler, S. M. (1995). Researcher allegiance and meta-analysis: The case of cognitive therapy for depression. *Journal of Consulting and Clinical Psychology, 63*(6), 966–980.

Gallagher-Thompson, D., Hanley-Peterson, P., & Thompson, L. W. (1990). Maintenance of gains versus relapse following brief psychotherapy for depression. *Journal of Consulting and Clinical Psychology, 58*(3), 371–374.

Geddes, J. R., Carney, S. M., Davies, C., Furukawa, T. A., Kupfer, D. J., Frank, E., et al. (2003). Relapse prevention with antidepressant drug treatment in depressive disorders: A systematic review. *Lancet, 361,* 653–661.

Gelder, M. G. (1994). Cognitive therapy for depression. In H. Hippius & C. N. Stefanis (Eds.), *Research in mood disorders: An update* (Vol. 1, pp. 115–124). Goettingen, Germany: Hogrefe & Huber.

Giesen-Bloo, J., van Dyck, R., Spinhoven, P., van Tilburg, W., Dirksen, C., van Asselt, T., et al. (2006). Outpatient psychotherapy for borderline personality disorder: A randomized trial of schema-focused therapy vs. transference-focused therapy. *Archives of General Psychiatry, 63,* 649–658.

Gloaguen, V., Cottraux, J., Cucherat, M., & Blackburn, I. M. (1998). A meta-analysis of the effects of cognitive therapy in depressed patients. *Journal of Affective Disorders, 49,* 59–72.

Gortner, E. T., Gollan, J. K., Dobson, K. S., & Jacobson, N. S. (1998). Cognitive-behavioral treatment for depression: Relapse prevention. *Journal of Consulting and Clinical Psychology, 2,* 377–384.

Hall, L. H., & Robertson, M. H. (1998). Undergraduate ratings of the acceptability of single and combined treatments for depression: A comparative analysis. *Professional Psychology: Research and Practice, 3,* 269–272.

Harrington, R., Wood, A., & Verduyn, C. (1998). Clinically depressed adolescents. In P. J. Graham (Ed.), *Cognitive-behaviour therapy for children and families* (pp. 156–193). New York: Cambridge University Press.

Hayden, E. P., & Klein, D. N. (2001). Predicting outcome of dysthymic disorder at a 5-year follow-up: The impact of familial psychopathology, early adversity, personality, comorbidity, and chronic stress. *American Journal of Psychiatry, 158,* 1864–1870.

Hayes, A. M., & Strauss, J. L. (1998). Dynamic systems theory as a paradigm for the study of change in psychotherapy: An application to cognitive therapy for depression. *Journal of Consulting and Clinical Psychology, 66*(6), 939–947.

Heim, C., & Nemeroff, C. B. (2001). The role of childhood trauma in the neurobiology of mood and anxiety disorders: Preclinical and clinical studies. *Biological Psychiatry, 49,* 1023–1039.

Henry, W. P., Strupp, H. H., Butler, S. F., Schacht, T. E., & Binder, J. L. (1993). The effects of training in time-limited dynamic psychotherapy: Changes in therapist behavior. *Journal of Consulting and Clinical Psychology, 61,* 434–440.

Hollon, S. D. (1998). What is cognitive behavioural therapy and does it work? *Current Opinion in Neurobiology, 8,* 289–292.

Hollon, S. D., DeRubeis, R. J., & Evans, M. D. (1996). Cognitive therapy in the treatment and prevention of depression. In P. M. Salkovskis (Ed.), *Frontiers of* cognitive therapy (pp. 293–317). New York: Guilford Press.

Hollon, S. D., DeRubeis, R. J., Evans, M. D., Weimer, M. J., Garvey, M. J., Grove, W. M., et al. (1992). Cognitive therapy and pharmacotherapy: Singly and in combination. Archives of General Psychiatry, 49, 774–781.

Hollon, S. D., DeRubeis, R. J., Shelton, R. C., Amsterdam, J. D., Salomon, R. M., O'Reardon, J. P., et al. (2005). Prevention of relapse following cognitive therapy vs. medications in moderate to severe depression. Archives of General Psychiatry, 62, 417–422.

Hollon, S. D., & Shelton, R. C. (2001). Treatment guidelines for major depressive disorder. Behavior Therapy, 32, 235–258.

Hollon, S. D., Shelton, R. C., & Loosen, P. T. (1991). Cognitive therapy and pharmacotherapy for depression. Journal of Consulting and Clinical Psychology, 59(1), 88–99.

Hollon, S. D., Thase, M. E., & Markowitz, J. C. (2002). Treatment and prevention of depression. Psychological Science in the Public Interest, 3, 39–77.

Howland, R. H. (1993). Chronic depression. Hospital and Community Psychiatry, 44, 633–639.

Ingram, R. E., & Holle, C. (1992). Cognitive science of depression. In D. J. Stein & J. E. Young (Eds.), Cognitive science and clinical disorders (pp. 187–209). San Diego, CA: Academic Press.

Jacobson, N. S., Dobson, K. S., Truax, P. A., Addis, M. E., Koerner, K., Gollan, J. K., et al. (1996). A component analysis of cognitive-behavioral treatment for depression. Journal of Consulting and Clinical Psychology, 64, 295–304.

Jacobson, N. S., & Hollon, S. D. (1996). Cognitive-behavior therapy versus pharmacotherapy: Now that the jury's returned its verdict, it's time to present the rest of the evidence. Journal of Consulting and Clinical Psychology, 64(1), 74–80.

Jarrett, R. B. (1995). Comparing and combining short-term psychotherapy and pharmacotherapy for depression. In E. E. Beckham & W. R. Leber (Eds.), Handbook of depression (2nd ed., pp. 435–464). New York: Guilford Press.

Jarrett, R. B., Basco, M. R., Risser, R., Ramanan, J., Marwill, M., Kraft, D., et al. (1998). Is there a role for continuation phase cognitive therapy for depressed outpatients? Journal of Consulting and Clinical Psychology, 66(6), 1036–1040.

Jarrett, R. B., Kraft, D., Doyle, J., Foster, B. M., Eaves, G. G., & Silver, P. C. (2001). Preventing recurrent depression using cognitive therapy with and without continuation phase. Archives of General Psychiatry, 58(4), 381–388.

Jarrett, R. B., & Nelson, R. O. (1987). Mechanisms of change in cognitive therapy of depression. Behavior Therapy, 18, 227–241.

Jarrett, R. B., Schaffer, M., McIntire, D., Witt-Browder, A., Kraft, D., & Risser, R. C. (1999). Treatment of atypical depression with cognitive therapy or phenelzine: A double-blind, placebo-controlled trial. Archives of General Psychiatry, 56, 431–437.

Joffe, R., Segal, Z., & Singer, W. (1996). Change in thyroid hormone levels following response to cognitive therapy for major depression. American Journal of Psychiatry, 153(3), 411–413.

Johnsson, B., & Bebbington, P. E. (1994). What price depression?: The cost of depression and the cost effectiveness of pharmacological treatment. British Journal of Psychiatry, 164, 665–673.

Keller, M. B., & Boland, R. J. (1998). Implications of failing to achieve successful long-term maintenance treatment of recurrent unipolar major depression. Biological Psychiatry, 44(5), 348–360.

Keller, M. B., & Hanks, D. L. (1995). Course and natural history of chronic depression. In J. H. Kocsis & D. N. Klein (Eds.), Diagnosis and treatment of chronic depression (pp. 58–72). New York: Guilford Press.

Keller, M. B., McCullough, J. P., Klein, D. F., Arnow, B., Dunner, D. L., Gelenberg, A. J., et al. (2000). A comparison of nefazodone, the cognitive behavioral-analysis system of psychotherapy, and their combination for the treatment of chronic depression. New England Journal of Medicine, 342, 1462–1470.

Kendler, K. S., Kessler, R. C., Walters, E. E., MacLean, C., Neale, M. C., Heath, A. C., et al. (1995). Stressful life events, genetic liability, and onset of an episode of major depression in women. American Journal of Psychiatry, 152, 833–842.

Kessler, R. C., Akiskal, H. S., Ames, M., Birnbaum, H., Greenberg, P. A., Jin, R., et al. (2006). Prevalence and effects of mood disorders on work performance in a nationally representative sample of U.S. workers. American Journal of Psychiatry, 163(9), 1561–1568.

Kessler, R. C., Berglund, P., Demler, O., Jin, R., Merikangas, K. R., & Walters, E. E. (2005). Lifetime prevalence and age-of-onset distributions of DSM-IV disorders in the National Comorbidity Survey Replication. Archives of General Psychiatry, 62(6), 593–602.

Kessler, R. C., Chui, W. T., Demler, O., Merikangas, K. R., & Walters, E. E. (2005). Prevalence, severity, and comorbidity of 12-month DSM-IV disorders in the National Comorbidity Survey Replication. Archives of General Psychiatry, 62(6), 617–627.

Klein, D. F. (1996). Preventing hung juries about therapy studies. Journal of Consulting and Clinical Psychology, 64, 81–87.

Klein, D. N., Santiago, N. J., Vivian, D., Blalock, J. A., Kocsis, J. H., Markowitz, J. C., et al. (2004). Cognitive-behavioral analysis system of psychotherapy as a maintenance treatment for chronic depression. Journal of Consulting and Clinical Psychology, 72, 681–688.

Koder, D. A., Brodaty, H., & Anstey, K. J. (1996). Cognitive therapy for depression in elderly. International Journal of Geriatric Psychiatry, 11(2), 97–107.

Kupfer, D. J., Frank, E., & Wamhoff, J. (1996). Mood disorders: Update on prevention of recurrence. In C.

Mundt, M. M. Goldstein, K. Hahlweg, & P. Fiedler (Eds.), *Interpersonal factors in the origin and course of affective disorders* (pp. 289–302). London: Gaskell.

Lam, D. H., Hayward, P., Watkins, E. R., Wright, K., & Sham, P. (2005). Relapse prevention in patients with bipolar disorder: Cognitive therapy outcome after 2 years. *American Journal of Psychiatry, 162*(2), 324–329.

Lazarus, A. A., & Lazarus, C. N. (1991). *Multimodal Life History Inventory* (2nd ed.). Champaign, IL: Research Press.

Lee, C. W., Taylor, G., & Dunn, J. (1999). Factor structure of the Schema Questionnaire in a large clinical sample. *Cognitive Therapy and Research, 23*(4), 441–451.

Levendusky, P. G., & Hufford, M. R. (1997). The application of cognitive-behavior therapy to the treatment of depression and related disorders in the elderly. *Journal of Geriatric Psychiatry, 30*(2), 227–238.

Lewinsohn, P. M., & Clarke, G. N. (1999). Psychosocial treatments for adolescent depression. *Clinical Psychology Review, 19*(3), 329–342.

Linehan, M. M. (1993a). *Cognitive-behavioral treatment of borderline personality disorder.* New York: Guilford Press.

Linehan, M. M. (1993b). *Skills training manual for treating borderline personality disorder.* New York: Guilford Press.

Lizardi, H., Klein, D. N., Ouimette, P. C., Riso, L. P., Anderson, R. L., & Donaldson, S. K. (1995). Reports of the childhood home environment in early onset dysthymia and episodic major depression. *Journal of Abnormal Psychology, 104*, 132–139.

Luborsky, L., Diguer, L., Seligman, D. A., Rosenthal, R., Krause, E. D., Johnson, S., et al. (1999). The researcher's own therapy allegiances: A "wild card" in comparisons to treatment efficacy. *Clinical Psychology: Science and Practice, 6*(1), 95–106.

Ma, S. H., & Teasdale, J. D. (2004). Mindfulness-based cognitive therapy for depression: Replication and exploration of differential relapse prevention effects. *Journal of Consulting and Clinical Psychology, 72*(1), 31–40.

Martell, C. R., Addis, M. E., & Jacobson, N. S. (2001). *Depression in context: Strategies for guided action.* New York: Norton.

McCullough, J. P., Jr. (2000). *Treatment for chronic depression: Cognitive behavioral analysis system of psychotherapy (CBASP).* New York: Guilford Press.

McCullough, J. P., Jr. (2003). Treatment for chronic depression: Cognitive behavioral-analysis system of psychotherapy. *Journal of Psychotherapy Integration, 13*(3/4), 241–263.

McGinn, L. K., & Young, J. E. (1996). Schema-focused therapy. In P. M. Salkovskis (Ed.), *Frontiers of cognitive therapy* (pp. 182–207). New York: Guilford Press.

Mental health: A report of the Surgeon General. (1997,

September 30). Available at *www.surgeongeneral.gov/library/mentalhealth.*

Meterissian, G. B., & Bradwejn, J. (1989). Comparative studies on the efficacy of psychotherapy, pharmacotherapy, and their combination in depression: Was adequate pharmacotherapy provided? *Journal of Clinical Psychopharmacology, 9*, 334–339.

Miller, I. W., Norman, W. H., Keitner, G. I., Bishop, S., & Dow, M. G. (1989). Cognitive-behavioral treatment of depressed inpatients. *Behavior Therapy, 20*, 25–47.

Mischoulon, D., Fava, M., & Rosenbaum, J.F. (1999). Strategies for augmentation of SSRI treatment: A survey of an academic psycopharmacology practice. *Harvard Review of Psychiatry, 6*(6), 322–326.

Mohr, D. C. (1995). Negative outcome in psychotherapy: A critical review. *Clinical Psychology: Science and Practice, 2*, 1–27.

Murphy, G. E., Simmons, A. D., Wetzel, R. D., & Lustman, P. J. (1984). Cognitive therapy and pharmacotherapy, singly and together, in the treatment of depression. *Archives of General Psychiatry, 41*, 33–41.

National Institute of Mental Health. (2006). *The numbers count: Mental disorders in America* (Publication No. 06-4584). Retrieved April 6, 2007, from *www.nimh.nih.gov/publicat/numbers*

Nierenberg, A. A., Keefe, B. R., Leslie, V. C., Alpert, J. E., Pava, J. A., Worthington, J. J., III, et al. (1999). Residual symptoms in depressed patients who respond acutely to fluoxetine. *Journal of Clinical Psychiatry, 60*(4), 221–225.

Oei, T. P. S., & Free, M. L. (1995). Do cognitive behaviour therapies validate cognitive models of mood disorders?: A review of the empirical evidence. *International Journal of Psychology, 30*(2), 145–180.

Oei, T. P. S., & Shuttlewood, G. J. (1996). Specific and nonspecific factors in psychotherapy: A case of cognitive therapy for depression. *Clinical Psychology Review, 16*(2), 83–103.

O'Leary, K. D., & Beach, S. R. H. (1990). Marital therapy: A viable treatment for depression and marital discord. *American Journal of Psychiatry, 147*(2), 183–186.

Olfson, M., Marcus, S. C., Druss, B., Elinson, L., Tanielian, T., & Pincus, H. A. (2002). National trends in the outpatient treatment of depression. *Journal of the American Medical Association, 287*, 203–209.

Overholser, J. C. (1998). Cognitive-behavioral treatment of depression, part X: Reducing the risk of relapse. *Journal of Contemporary Psychotherapy, 28*(4), 381–396.

Padesky, C. A., with Greenberger, D. (1995). *A clinician's guide to mind over mood.* New York: Guilford Press.

Parker, K., Roy, K., & Eyers, K. (2003). Cognitive behavior therapy for depression?: Choose horses for courses. *American Journal of Psychiatry, 160*, 825–834.

Paykel, E. S., Scott, J., Teasdale, J. D., Johnson, A. L., Garland, A., Moore, R., et al. (1999). Prevention of relapse in residual depression by cognitive therapy. *Archives of General Psychiatry, 56*, 829–835.

Persons, J. B., Burns, D. D., & Perloff, J. M. (1988). Predictors of dropout and outcome in cognitive therapy for depression in a private practice setting. *Cognitive Therapy and Research, 12*(6), 557–575.

Piper, W. E., Ogrodniczuk, J. S., Joyce, A. S., McCallum, M., Rosie, J. S., O'Kelly, J. G., et al. (1999). Prediction of dropping out in time-limited, interpretive psychotherapy. *Psychotherapy, 36*, 114–122.

Randolph, J. J., & Dykman, B. M. (1998). Perceptions of parenting and depression-proneness in the offspring: Dysfunctional attitudes as a mediating mechanism. *Cognitive Depressive Disorders, 21*, 401–449.

Rehm, L. P. (1990). Cognitive and behavioral theories. In B. B. Wolman & G. Stricker (Eds.), *Depressive disorders: Facts, theories, and treatment methods* (pp. 64–91). New York: Wiley.

Reinecke, M. A., Ryan, N. E., & DuBois, D. L. (1998). Cognitive-behavioral therapy of depression and depressive symptoms during adolescence: A review and meta-analysis. *Journal of the American Academy of Child and Adolescent Psychiatry, 37*(1), 26–34.

Riso, L. P., du Toit, P. L., Blandino, J. A., Penna, S., Dacey, S., Duin, J. S., et al. (2003). Cognitive aspects of chronic depression. *Journal of Abnormal Psychology, 112*(1), 72–80.

Roberts, J. E., & Hartlage, S. (1996). Cognitive rehabilitation interventions for depressed patients. In P. W. Corrigan & S. C. Yudofsky (Eds.), *Cognitive rehabilitation for neuropsychiatric disorders* (pp. 371–392). Washington, DC: American Psychiatric Press.

Robinson, L. A., Berman, J. S., & Neimeyer, R. A. (1990). Psychotherapy for the treatment of depression: A comprehensive review of controlled outcome research. *Psychological Bulletin, 108*, 30–49.

Rush, A. J., Beck, A. T., Kovacs, M., & Hollon, S. (1977). Comparative efficacy of cognitive therapy and imipramine in the treatment of depressed outpatients. *Cognitive Therapy and Research, 1*, 17–37.

Sacco, W. P., & Beck, A. T. (1995). Cognitive theory and therapy. In E. E. Beckham & W. R. Leber, *Handbook of depression* (2nd ed., pp. 329–351). New York: Guilford Press.

Sachs-Ericsson, N., Verona, E., Joiner, T., & Preacher, K. J. (2006). Parental abuse and mediating role of self-criticism in adult internalizing disorders. *Journal of Affective Disorders, 93*(1–3), 71–78.

Saeman, H. (1999). Psychotherapy gets short shrift at White House MH meeting. *National Psychologist, 8*(4), 21.

Safran, J. D., Muran, J. C., Samstag, L. W., & Stevens, C. (2002). Repairing alliance ruptures. In J. C. Norcross (Ed.), *Psychotherapy relationships that work: Therapists contributions and responsiveness to patients* (pp. 235–254). New York: Oxford University Press.

Safran, J. D., & Segal, Z. V. (1990). *Interpersonal processes in cognitive therapy.* New York: Basic Books.

Safran, J. D., Segal, Z. V., Vallis, T. M., Shaw, B. F., & Samstag, L. W. (1993). Assessing patient suitability for short-term cognitive therapy with an interpersonal focus. *Cognitive Therapy and Research, 17*(1), 23–38.

Salkovskis, P. M. (1996). *Frontiers of cognitive therapy: The state of the art and beyond.* New York: Guilford Press.

Schmidt, N. B. (1994). The schema questionnaire and the schema avoidance questionnaire. *Behavior Therapist, 17*(4), 90–92.

Schmidt, N. B., Joiner, T. E., Young, J. E., & Telch, M. J. (1995). The Schema Questionnaire: Investigation of psychometric properties and the hierarchical structure of a measure of maladaptive schemata. *Cognitive Therapy and Research, 19*(3), 295–321.

Scott, A. I., & Freeman, C. P. (1992). Edinburgh primary care depression study: Treatment outcome, patient satisfaction, and cost after 16 weeks. *British Medical Journal, 304*, 883–887.

Scott, J. (1996a). Cognitive therapy of affective disorders: A review. *Journal of Affective Disorders, 37*, 1–11.

Scott, J. (1996b). The role of cognitive behaviour therapy in bipolar disorders. *Behavioural and Cognitive Psychotherapy, 24*(3), 195–208.

Scott, J. (2000). New evidence in the treatment of chronic depression. *New England Journal of Medicine, 342*, 1518–1520.

Scott, J., Palmer, S., Paykel, E., Teasdale, J., & Hayhurst, H. (2003). Use of cognitive therapy for relapse prevention in chronic depression. *British Journal of Psychiatry, 182*, 221–227.

Shapiro, D. A., Barkman, M., Rees, A., Hardy, G. E., Reynolds, S., & Startup, M. (1994). Effects of treatment duration and severity of depression on the effectiveness of cognitive-behavioral and psychodynamic-interpersonal psychotherapy. *Journal of Consulting and Clinical Psychology, 62*, 522–534.

Shaw, B. F., & Segal, Z. V. (1999). Efficacy, indications, and mechanisms of action of cognitive therapy of depression. In D. S. Janowsky (Ed.), *Psychotherapy indications and outcomes* (pp. 173–196). Washington, DC: American Psychiatric Press.

Shea, M. T., & Elkin, I. (1996). The NIMH Treatment of Depression Collaborative Research Program. In C. Mundt, M. J. Goldstein, K. Hahlweg, & P. Fiedler (Eds.), *Interpersonal factors in the origin and course of affective disorders* (pp. 316–328). London: Gaskell/Royal College of Psychiatrists.

Shea, M. T., Elkin, I., Imber, S. D., Sotsky, S. M., Watkins, J. T., Collins, J. F., et al. (1992). Course of depressive symptoms over follow-up: Findings from the National Institute of Mental Health Treatment of

Depression Collaborative Research Program. *Archives of General Psychiatry, 49*(10), 782–787.

Shea, M. T., Pilkonis, P. A., Beckham, E., Collins, J. F., Elkin, I., Sotsky, S. M., et al. (1990). Personality disorders and treatment outcome in the NIMH Treatment of Depression Collaborative Research Program. *American Journal of Psychiatry, 147*(6), 711–718.

Simons, A. D., Murphy, G. D., Levine, J. L., & Wetzel, R. D. (1986). Cognitive therapy and pharmacotherapy for depression: Sustained improvement over 1 year. *Archives of General Psychiatry, 43*, 43–48.

Spanier, C. A., Frank, E., McEachran, A. B., Grochocinski, V. J., & Kupfer, D. J. (1999). Maintenance interpersonal psychotherapy for recurrent depression: Biological and clinical correlates and future directions. In D. S. Janowsky (Ed.), *Psychotherapy indications and outcomes* (pp. 249–273). Washington, DC: American Psychiatric Press.

Stein, D. J., & Young, J. E. (1992). Schema approach to personality disorders. In D. J. Stein & J. E. Young (Eds.), *Cognitive science and clinical disorders* (pp. 271–288). San Diego, CA: Academic Press.

Stewart, J. W., Garfinkel, R., Nunes, E. V., Donovan, S., & Klein, D. F. (1998). Atypical features and treatment response in the National Institute of Mental Health Treatment of Depression Collaborative Research Program. *Journal of Clinical Psychopharmacology, 18*(6), 429–434.

Stuart, S., & Bowers, W. A. (1995). Cognitive therapy with inpatients: Review and meta-analysis. *Journal of Cognitive Psychotherapy, 9*(2), 85–92.

Sullivan, M. J. L., & Conway, M. (1991). Dysphoria and valence of attributions for others' behavior. *Cognitive Therapy and Research, 15*(4), 273–282.

Teasdale, J. D. (1997a). Assessing cognitive mediation of relapse prevention in recurrent mood disorders. *Clinical Psychology and Psychotherapy, 4*, 145–156.

Teasdale, J. D. (1997b). The relationship between cognition and emotion: The mind-in-place in mood disorders. In D. M. Clark & C. G. Fairburn (Eds.), *Science and practice of cognitive behavior therapy* (pp. 67–93). Oxford, UK: Oxford University Press.

Teasdale, J. D., Moore, R. G., Hayhurst, H., Pope, M., Williams, S., & Segal, Z. V. (2002). Metacognitive awareness and prevention of relapse in depression: Empirical evidence. *Journal of Consulting and Clinical Psychology, 70*(2), 275–287.

Teasdale, J. D., Segal, Z. V., & Williams, J. M. G. (1995). How does cognitive therapy prevent depressive relapse and why should attentional control (mindfulness) training help? *Behaviour Research and Therapy, 33*, 25–39.

Teasdale, J. D., Segal, Z. V., Williams, J. M. G., Ridgeway, V. A., Soulsby, J. M., & Lau, M. A. (2000). Prevention of relapse/recurrence in major depression by mindfulness-based cognitive therapy. *Journal of Consulting and Clinical Psychology, 68*(4), 615–623.

Thase, M. E. (1992). Long-term treatments of recurrent depressive disorders. *Journal of Clinical Psychiatry, 53*(Suppl. 9), 32–44.

Thase, M. E. (1999). How should efficacy be evaluated in randomized clinical trials of treatments for depression? *Journal of Clinical Psychiatry, 60*(Suppl. 4), 23–32.

Thase, M. E., Bowler, K., & Harden, T. (1991). Cognitive behavior therapy of endogenous depression: Part 2. Preliminary findings in 16 unmedicated inpatients. *Behavior Therapy, 22*, 469–477.

Thase, M. E., Greenhouse, J. B., Frank, E., Reynolds, C.F., III, Pilkonis, P. A., Hurley, K., et al. (1997). Treatment of major depression with psychotherapy or psychotherapy–pharmacotherapy combinations. *Archives of General Psychiatry, 54*(11), 1009–1015.

Treatment for Adolescents with Depression Study (TADS) Team, U.S. (2004). Fluoxetine, cognitive-behavioral therapy, and their combination for adolescents with depression: Treatment for adolescents with depression study (TADS) randomized controlled trial. *Journal of the American Medical Association, 292*(7), 807–820.

Truax, C. B., & Mitchell, K. M. (1971). Research on certain therapist interpersonal skills in relation to process and outcome. In A. E. Bergin & S. L. Garfield (Eds.), *Handbook of psychotherapy and behavior change: An empirical analysis* (pp. 299–344). New York: Wiley.

Versiani, M. (1998). Pharmacotherapy of dysthymic and chronic depressive disorders: Overview with focus on moclobemide. *Journal of Affective Disorders, 51*(3), 323–332.

Vos, T., Corry, J., Haby, M. M., Carter, R., & Andrews, G. (2005). Cost-effectiveness of cognitive-behavioural therapy and drug interventions for major depression. *Australian and New Zealand Journal of Psychiatry, 39*(8), 683–692.

Vocisano, C., Klein, D., Arnow, B., Rivera, C., Blalock, J. A., Rothbaum, B., et al. (2004). Therapist variables that predict symptom change in psychotherapy with chronically depressed outpatients. *Psychotherapy: Theory, Research, Practice, Training, 41*(3), 255–265.

Wampold, B. E., Minami, T., Baskin, T. W., & Tierney, S. C. (2002). A meta-(re)analysis of the effects of cognitive therapy versus "other therapies" for depression. *Journal of Affective Disorders, 68*, 159–165.

Weisz, J. R., MacCarty, C. A., & Valeri, S. M. (2006). Effects of psychotherapy for depression in children and adolescents: A meta-analysis. *Psychological Bulletin, 132*, 132–149.

Whisman, M. A. (1993). Mediators and moderators of change in cognitive therapy of depression. *Psychological Bulletin, 114*, 248–265.

Wierzbicki, M., & Bartlett, T. S. (1987). The efficacy of group and individual cognitive therapy for mild depression. *Cognitive Therapy and Research, 11*(3), 337–342.

Williams, J. M. G. (1997). Depression. In D. M. Clark

& C. G. Fairburn (Eds.), *Science and practice of cognitive behaviour therapy* (pp. 259–283). Oxford, UK: Oxford University Press.

Wolpe, J. (1993). Commentary: The cognitivist oversell and comments on symposium contributions. *Journal of Behavior Therapy and Experimental Psychiatry, 24*(2), 141–147.

Wright, J. H. (1996). Inpatient cognitive therapy. In P. M. Salkovskis (Ed.), *Frontiers of cognitive therapy* (pp. 208–225). New York: Guilford Press.

Wright, J. H., Wright, A. S., Albano, A. M., Basco, M. R., Goldsmith, L. J., Raffield, T., et al. (2005). Computer-assisted cognitive therapy for depression: Maintaining efficacy while reducing therapist time. *American Journal of Psychiatry, 162*, 1158–1164.

Young, J. E. (1994). *Cognitive therapy for personality disorders: A schema-focused approach* (rev. ed.). Sarasota, FL: Professional Resource Press.

Young, J. E. (1999). *Cognitive therapy for personality disorders: A schema-focused approach* (3rd ed.). Sarasota, FL: Professional Resource Exchange. (Original work published 1990)

Young, J. E., Atkinson, T., Arntz, A., Weishaar, E., & Weishaar, M. (2004). *Schema Mode Questionnaire.* New York: Cognitive Therapy Center of New York.

Young, J. E., & Brown, G. (1994). Young Schema Questionnaire (2nd ed.). In J. E. Young (Ed.), *Cognitive therapy for personality disorders: A schema-focused approach* (pp. 63–76). Sarasota, FL: Professional Resource Press. (Original work published 1990)

Young, J. E., & Klosko, J. S. (1994). *Reinventing your life: How to break free of negative life patterns.* New York: Plume.

Young, J. E., Klosko, J. S., & Weishaar, M. E. (2003). *Schema therapy: A practitioner's guide.* New York: Guilford Press.

CHAPTER 7

Interpersonal Psychotherapy
for Depression

Kathryn L. Bleiberg
John C. Markowitz

Much evidence has emerged over the past decade supporting the clinical effectiveness of interpersonal psychotherapy (IPT) for a variety of problems, particularly depression. A substantial advantage of IPT is the relative ease with which clinicians can learn to administer this protocol with integrity. In this chapter, the process of IPT is illustrated in some detail in the context of the treatment of "Sara," who was suffering from a major depressive episode associated with grief following the death of her baby girl *in utero* at 27 weeks' gestation, some 2 months earlier. The lead author, Kathryn L. Bleiberg, an international authority on training in IPT, was the therapist. Although IPT is relatively easy to comprehend, the twists and turns encountered in the administration of IPT (or any therapeutic approach) are particularly evident in this chapter. Here the therapist skillfully focuses on resolving grief, as well as on the patient's social isolation and conflicts with her husband over emotional reactions to the loss. Also notable about IPT is the finding that the treatment is more successful when administered with fidelity to the goals of IPT and adherence to the protocol. The power of a therapist and patient working well together and staying on task provides some good evidence for the specific effects of an interpersonal focus to psychotherapy.—D. H. B.

Interpersonal psychotherapy (IPT) is a time-limited, diagnosis-targeted, pragmatic, empirically supported treatment that was originally developed to treat outpatients with major depression. IPT focuses on current or recent life events, interpersonal difficulties, and symptoms. Through the use of the medical model and by linking mood symptoms to recent life events, the IPT therapist helps the patient to feel understood. IPT aids recovery from depression by relieving depressive symptoms and by helping the patient to develop more effective strategies for dealing with current interpersonal problems related to the onset of symptoms (Bleiberg & Markowitz, 2007).

IPT's success as an individual treatment for major depression has led to its adaptation for subpopulations of patients with mood disorders including depressed older patients (Sholomskas, Chevron, Prusoff, & Berry, 1983), depressed adolescents (Mufson, Moreau, & Weissman, 1993; Mufson, Weissman, Moreau, & Garfinkel, 1999), depressed HIV-positive patients (Markowitz, Klerman, Perry,

Clougherty, & Mayers, 1992; Markowitz, Kocsis, et al., 1998), patients with antepartum (Spinelli & Endicott, 2003) and postpartum depression (O'Hara, Stuart, Gorman, & Wenzel, 2000), dysthymic disorder (Markowitz, 1998), and bipolar disorder (Frank, 2005). IPT has been adapted for anxiety disorders, including social phobia (Lipsitz, Fyer, Markowitz, & Cherry, 1999) and posttraumatic stress disorder (Bleiberg & Markowitz, 2005), bulimia nervosa (Fairburn, Jones, Peveler, Hope, & O'Connor, 1993; Fairburn et al., 1995), and, recently borderline personality disorder (Markowitz, Skodol, & Bleiberg, 2006). This chapter describes the principles, characteristics, and techniques of individual IPT for major depression and illustrates how a clinician implements IPT techniques with an actual patient.

MAJOR DEPRESSION

Major depressive disorder (MDD), the most common depressive illness, affects millions of Americans each year. The Global Burden of Disease Study, initiated by the World Health Organization (Murray & Lopez, 1996), estimated that depression is the fourth leading cause of disability and will become the second leading cause worldwide by the year 2020. Epidemiological studies of mood disorders have provided estimates of the prevalence and correlates of MDD. The National Comorbidity Survey Replication (NCS-R; Kessler et al., 2003) found a 16.2% lifetime and 6.6% annual prevalence of MDD in the United States, with the majority of cases of MDD associated with substantial symptom severity and impairment in functioning. National and international studies have consistently found a higher prevalence of MDD in women than in men; women are twice as likely as men to experience an episode of MDD. The average age of onset of MDD is between ages 20 and 40 years (Blazer, 2000).

The *Diagnostic and Statistical Manual of Mental Disorders*, fourth edition, text revised (DSM-IV-TR; American Psychiatric Association, 2000) defines MDD as a mood disorder characterized by one or more major depressive episodes. A major depressive episode entails a period of at least 2 weeks during which a person experiences depressed mood or loss of interest or pleasure in nearly all activities most of the day, nearly every day, accompanied by at least four additional symptoms of depression present nearly every day. Symptoms of depression include the following:

- Significant weight loss (not related to dieting), or weight gain or decrease or increase in appetite.
- Insomnia or hypersomnia.
- Psychomotor agitation or retardation severe enough to be observable by others.
- Fatigue or loss of energy.
- Feelings of worthlessness, or excessive or inappropriate or excessive guilt.
- Diminished ability to think or concentrate, or indecisiveness.
- Recurrent thoughts of death, recurrent suicidal ideation without a specific plan, or a suicide attempt or a specific plan to commit suicide.

To meet full criteria for a major depressive episode, the patient's symptoms must cause clinically significant distress or impairment in social, occupational, or other important areas of functioning. Depression is associated with social withdrawal and difficulty in social and occupational functioning. The diagnosis cannot be made if the symptoms meet criteria for a mixed episode, in which symptoms of both a manic episode and major depressive episode coexist. Nor may the symptoms be due to the direct physiological effects of a substance or a general medical condition. Finally, the symptoms may not be better accounted for by the death of a loved one, unless they persist 2 months beyond the loss or include marked functional impairment or include intense feelings of worthlessness, suicidal ideation, psychotic symptoms or psychomotor retardation.

THE DEVELOPMENT OF IPT

Klerman, Weissman, and colleagues developed IPT in the 1970s as a treatment arm for a pharmacotherapy study of depression. Being researchers, they developed a psychotherapy based on research data. Post–World War II research on psychosocial life events and the development of mental disorders had shown relationships between depression and complicated bereavement, role disputes (i.e., bad relationships), role transitions (e.g., a losing or getting a new job, or any meaningful life change), and interpersonal deficits. Stressful life events can trigger depressive episodes in vulnerable individuals, and depressive episodes compromise interpersonal functioning, making it difficult to manage stressful life events, and often triggering further negative life events (Bleiberg & Markowitz, 2007).

IPT was also built on the interpersonal theory of Adolph Meyer (1957) and Harry Stack Sullivan (1953), and on the attachment theory of John Bowlby (1973). The interpersonalists broadened the scope of psychiatry by emphasizing social, cultural, and interpersonal factors. Sullivan stressed the role of interpersonal relationships in the development of mental illness and the use of interpersonal relationships to understand, assess and treat mental illness. Sullivan also indicated that life events and relationships occurring *after* early childhood influenced psychopathology, in contradistinction to the then current focus on pre-Oedipal life events.

Bowlby (1973) posited that the disruption of secure attachments can contribute to the onset of depression, and that psychiatric disorders result from difficulties in forming and maintaining secure attachments. Indeed, social supports protect against depression. In psychiatry, the idea that mental illness was influenced by current life events and not (simply) due to early childhood experiences was novel in an era divided between psychoanalytic and biological approaches (Klerman, Weissman, Rounsaville, & Chevron, 1984).

PRINCIPLES OF IPT: THE IPT MODEL OF DEPRESSION

Two basic principles of IPT explain the patient's depression and situation. These principles are simple enough to grasp, even for a very depressed patient with poor concentration. First, the IPT therapist defines depression as a medical illness and explains that the patient has a common illness that comprises a discrete and predictable set of symptoms, thus making the symptoms seem less overwhelming and more manageable. The IPT therapist assumes that the etiology of depression is complex and multidetermined: The etiology may comprise biology, life experiences, and family history, among other factors. The IPT therapist emphasizes that *depression is a medical illness that is treatable and not the patient's fault*. Explaining that depression is treatable inspires in

patients the hope that they can feel better. Hopelessness, a potentially deadly depressive symptom, distorts the generally good prognosis of the illness. Depressed patients often see their symptoms and consequent difficulties in functioning as reflections of a personal failure, character flaw, or weakness.

Defining depression as a blameless illness helps to combat the depressed patient's guilt and self-criticism. The therapist diagnoses depression using DSM-IV or *International Classification of Diseases* (ICD-10; World Health Organization, 1992) criteria and assesses symptoms using rating scales such as the Hamilton Depression Rating Scale (HDRS; Hamilton, 1960) or the Beck Depression Inventory–II (BDI-II; Beck, Steer, & Brown, 1996). IPT's use of the medical model to define depression distinguishes it from other psychotherapies and makes it highly compatible with antidepressant medication in combination treatment.

The second principle of IPT is that the patient's depression is connected to a current or recent life event. Stressful life events can precipitate depressive episodes in vulnerable individuals and, conversely, depression can make it difficult for individuals to manage stressful life events. IPT focuses on solving an interpersonal problem in the patient's life, a problem area—complicated bereavement, a role dispute, a role transition, or interpersonal deficits—connected to the patient's current depressive episode. By solving an interpersonal crisis, the patient can improve his or her life situation and simultaneously relieve depressive symptoms.

CHARACTERISTICS OF IPT

Several characteristics define IPT, sometimes distinguishing it from other psychotherapies.

• *IPT is time-limited and focused.* Acute treatment is set at the start at 12 or 16 weekly sessions. Some studies have included continuation and maintenance phases, which involve biweekly and monthly sessions. IPT's time limit provides hope for patients that their symptoms and life situation can rapidly improve; the time limit encourages patients to stay focused in treatment. It also pressures both patient and therapist to work hard and efficiently within the therapeutic window of opportunity. Therapist and patient agree to focus on one, or at most two, problem areas at the beginning of treatment.

• *IPT is empirically grounded.* Because IPT has shown repeated efficacy in research studies, therapists can offer and deliver the treatment with confidence and optimism, and patients can feel hopeful about the treatment they are receiving.

• *IPT is diagnosis-targeted.* IPT focuses on a specific diagnosis, its symptoms, and how symptoms interfere and interact with social functioning. IPT is not intended for all patients, but it has been tested in a series of randomized controlled trials to determine its efficacy.

• *IPT has a "here-and-now" focus.* IPT focuses on the present and on improving the patient's situation for the future—not on what happened in the patient's past. The IPT therapist relates current symptoms and interpersonal difficulties to recent or current life events. Although past depressive episodes and relationships are reviewed and relationship patterns are identified, treatment focuses on current relationships—building social supports and resolving disputes—and social functioning.

• *IPT focuses on interpersonal problems.* The IPT therapist may recognize intrapsychic defenses but does not see the patient's current difficulties as a function of internal conflict. Instead, the therapist focuses on interpersonal relationships and functioning.

• *IPT focuses on the interrelationship between mood and current life events.* The IPT therapist emphasizes that stressful life events can trigger episodes of major depression and, reciprocally, depression compromises psychosocial functioning. This makes it difficult to manage life stressors, leading to further negative life events.

• *IPT emphasizes eliciting affect.* Depressed patients often have difficulty understanding, identifying, and articulating what they are feeling. Whereas patients with depression tend to report feeling "bad," they have often difficult identifying negative feelings more specifically, such as anger, hurt, shame, rejection, disappointment. Furthermore, depressed patients who do recognize such negative affects tend to feel ashamed of having such "bad" emotions. The IPT therapist helps the patient to better identify what she[1] is feeling, validates emotions such as anger and disappointment as normal and useful interpersonal signals, and helps the patient to use such emotion as a guide. Patients in IPT learn to manage their feelings better and

to use them to decide how to behave and what to say in interpersonal encounters.

IPT COMPARED WITH OTHER PSYCHOTHERAPIES

Although IPT has a distinct rationale and is distinguishable from other psychotherapies (Hill, O'Grady, & Elkin, 1992; Weissman, Markowitz, & Klerman, 2000), it is an eclectic psychotherapy that uses techniques seen in other treatment approaches. IPT also includes the so-called "common" factors of psychotherapy (Frank, 1971). IPT shares the "here and now," diagnostic focus and time limit, and active approach with cognitive-behavioral therapy (CBT). IPT and CBT both include role playing and skills building. However, IPT is much less structured and assigns no formal homework, although the IPT therapist does encourage activity between sessions to improve mood and as it relates to resolving the interpersonal problem area. Whereas the CBT therapist defines depression as a consequence of dysfunctional thought patterns and attributes the patient's difficulties to them, the IPT therapist emphasizes that depression is a medical illness and relates difficulties to feeling depressed and to recent life events. IPT emphasizes eliciting affect rather than ("hot," affectively charged) automatic thoughts. IPT addresses interpersonal issues in a manner similar to that in marital therapy. Much like a supportive therapist, IPT therapists provide support and encouragement (Bleiberg & Markowitz, 2007).

IPT has been termed a "psychodynamic" psychotherapy on occasion, but it is not (Markowitz, Svartberg, & Swartz, 1998). IPT employs the medical model of depressive illness, whereas psychodynamic psychotherapy uses a conflict-based approach. The IPT therapist does not address unconscious processes, or explore or interpret the transference, but instead focuses on current relationships outside of the treatment room. Childhood experiences are recognized but not emphasized. The IPT therapist relates current symptoms and interpersonal problems to recent life events, not to childhood experiences. IPT acknowledges the influence of past experiences on present difficulties, but only to identify patterns of interpersonal behavior and to empathize with the patient's struggle. Unlike psychodynamic treatment, the goal in IPT is to improve symptoms and social functioning, not to change character or personality. Like the psychodynamic psychotherapist, however, the IPT therapist emphasizes facilitating affect in the treatment room and helping patients become aware of feelings they may not have been aware of previously (Weissman et al., 2000).

THE IPT THERAPIST

The IPT therapist conducts treatment in an office in an academic, hospital, or private practice setting. The therapist typically does not consult with the patient's family or friends.

The IPT therapist takes a non-neutral, active stance, providing psychoeducation about depression, emphasizing the IPT rationale, teaching social skills, and instilling hope. A somewhat directive approach is essential for adhering to the time limit in IPT and keeping the treatment focused on the interpersonal problem area. Taking an active stance may be challenging for therapists with psychodynamic orientations who are used to taking a neutral stance and offering little guidance in the session.

On the other hand, the IPT therapist does not want to reinforce the passivity and dependency that are characteristic of depression. A therapist who solves all problems may reinforce the patient's sense of inadequacy. Hence, the IPT therapist encourages the patient to come up with ideas, explore options, and test them out between sessions. Hence, the patient deserves (and is given) credit for making the life changes that lead to improvement in treatment.

The IPT therapist needs to be supportive, enthusiastic, and optimistic to instill hope that the depression will improve and changes will be forthcoming, and to encourage and inspire the patient to make changes. The structure of the IPT manual (Weissman et al., 2000) and the empirical validation of IPT in randomized controlled studies help to bolster therapist confidence. The IPT therapist frequently congratulates the patient on her progress in treatment and efforts to make changes.

Given the emphasis on helping the patient to identify and express feelings, the IPT therapist needs to feel comfortable encouraging expression of affect and tolerating intense negative affects. The therapist can show by example that feelings are indeed potent, but they are only feelings, and can be understood in an interpersonal context and will pass, if tolerated.

THE IPT PATIENT

Research has demonstrated that a wide range of patients are good candidates for IPT for major depression. IPT has been validated with minor modifications as a treatment for adolescent, adult, and geriatric depression. The patient should ideally report some recent life stressor and have some social contacts. Patients with depression who report no recent life events and lack basic social skills tend to do least well in IPT. IPT is not intended for patients with delusional depression, which requires antidepressant and antipsychotic pharmacotherapy or electroconvulsive therapy. Patients with comorbid moderate or severe personality disorder may be less likely to respond to short-term psychotherapy (Weissman et al., 2000). Accordingly, the recent adaptation of IPT for borderline personality disorder allows up to 32 weeks of treatment (Markowitz et al., 2006).

THE FOUR INTERPERSONAL PROBLEM AREAS

Treatment with IPT focuses on solving one of the following four interpersonal problem areas related to the onset or maintenance of the patient's current depressive episode. The IPT therapist follows strategies specific to each problem area.

Grief

This problem area addresses a patient's complicated bereavement following the death of a significant other. The therapist facilitates the mourning process, encourages catharsis, and ultimately helps the patient to form new relationships and find new activities to compensate for the loss. The therapist explores the relationship and the associated feelings the patient had with the loved one. Patients with complicated bereavement often have had a conflicted relationship with the deceased, often reporting unresolved feelings about and anger toward the person, and feeling guilty or uncomfortable with such feelings. Patients may feel guilty about what they did or did not say to or do for the person who died. The therapist encourages exploration of these feelings, and validates and normalizes negative feelings, allowing the patient to let go of the guilt she experiences.

The release of negative affects in the therapy office can help to diminish the intensity of such feelings. The therapist also explores positive feelings the patient had for the person she lost and empathizes with her loss. Finally, the therapist helps the patient explore options for forming new relationships and finding new activities that help to substitute for the lost relationship and give the patient a new sense of direction. The loss may provide opportunities for the patient to meet people and engage in activities she might not otherwise have encountered.

Role Disputes

A role dispute is a conflict with a significant other: a spouse, friend, parent, relative, employer, coworker, or close friend. The therapist and patient explore the relationship, the nature of the dispute, and options to resolve it. Patients with depression tend to put other people's needs ahead of their own. They have difficulty asserting themselves, confronting others, or getting angry effectively, which makes it difficult for them to manage interpersonal conflicts. The therapist discusses these depressive tendencies with patients and explains: "It is not your fault. You can learn how to assert yourself."

The therapist validates the patient's feelings in the relationship: recognizing anger as a natural response to someone bothering the patient, for example. The next question is how to express such feelings. The therapist helps the patient to conceive ways to communicate thoughts and feelings more effectively and roleplays potential interactions with her. If, after exploring and attempting to implement options to resolve the dispute, the conflict has reached an impasse, the therapist helps the patient to consider ways to live with the impasse or end the relationship.

Role Transitions

A role transition is a change in life status, such as beginning or ending a relationship, starting a new job or losing one, a geographic move, graduation or retirement, becoming a parent,

or the diagnosis of a medical illness. The therapist helps the patient to mourn the loss of the old role, to explore positive and negative aspects of the new role, and to determine what positive aspects of the old role, if any, she can retain. Ultimately, the therapist helps the patient adjust to and gain a sense of mastery over the new role. Even if a new role is wanted or positive, the role may be accompanied by unanticipated loss. For example, getting married may involve having to spending less time with one's family of origin because of having to spend time with the spouse's family. Moving to a new, larger house in a new and better neighborhood may disrupt relationships with friends in the old neighborhood. If a new role is undesired, a patient may discover unseen benefits in therapy. A patient who has lost a job may come to see the loss as an opportunity to pursue a better job.

Interpersonal Deficits

Interpersonal deficits is the least developed of the four problem areas. It is used as the focus of IPT for major depression only when a patient reports no recent life events and, therefore, lacks any of the first three problem areas. Patients in this category tend to be socially isolated and to have few social supports and a history of difficulty forming and sustaining relationships or finding relationships unfulfilling. The goal of treatment in this problem area is to reduce the patient's isolation. Because the patient lacks current relationships, treatment focuses on patterns in past relationships and starting to form new ones. The therapist reviews past significant relationships, exploring positive and negative aspects and identifying recurrent problems. The therapist helps the patient to explore options for meeting people and participating in activities that she used to enjoy.

Unlike treatment for the other problem areas, treatment for interpersonal deficits also focuses on the relationship with the therapist. In the absence of other relationships, and with the understanding that the patient is likely to feel uncomfortable in the therapeutic situation, the therapist encourages the patient to discuss her feelings about the therapist and work on problems that arise in their relationship. Ideally, the relationship with the therapist can serve as model for the patient to form other relationships. Given that IPT usually focuses on a life event, it is not surprising that patients who lack such life events have been shown to respond least well to IPT. It is important to identify patients who have underlying dysthymic disorder, because such patients often describe few recent life events. There is an IPT protocol adapted to the treatment of dysthymic patients (Markowitz, 1998; Weissman et al., 2000).

THE PROCESS OF IPT TREATMENT

Acute IPT treatment for major depression comprises initial, middle, and termination phases. IPT techniques help the patient to pursue the goals of treatment for each interpersonal problem area. This section leads into a case example illustrating the implementation of these techniques.

The Initial Phase (Sessions 1–3)

Tasks of the initial sessions of IPT for major depression include eliciting the patient's chief complaint, reviewing her symptoms and establishing a diagnosis, determining the interpersonal context for the current depressive episode, forming a therapeutic alliance, and setting the frame of the treatment, including the treatment goals and strategies. Although these tasks are common to other psychotherapeutic interventions, the techniques and process for accomplishing them are unique to IPT.

Diagnosing Major Depression

To diagnosis MDD, the therapist reviews current symptoms of depression using either DSM-IV or ICD-10 criteria, inquiring about each symptom and about any past history of depression. The therapist may administer the HDRS (Hamilton, 1960) or the BDI-II (Beck et al., 1996) and repeat these instruments every few weeks to monitor the patient's progress. The therapist rules out other diagnoses, such as bipolar illness, depression due to general medical condition or substance, and other psychiatric disorders. If the patient meets criteria for MDD, the therapist tells her, describing explicitly each of the symptoms she reported. The therapist states:

"You have an illness called major depression. The symptoms you describe having had for the past couple of months—feeling down most of the time, having difficulty enjoying things, feeling like you have to push yourself to get things done, difficulty sleeping, loss of appetite, trouble concentrating, and feeling very self-critical and down on yourself and pessimistic about your future—are all symptoms of depression. Depression is a treatable illness. It is not your fault that you feel this way and have had difficulty functioning, any more than it would be your fault if you had asthma or high blood pressure, or any other medical problem. And although you're feeling hopeless, your prognosis with treatment is quite good. You can feel better."

In the initial phase and as needed throughout the treatment the therapist provides psychoeducation about depression and how it affects social functioning. The therapist helps the patient to identify and understand her depressive symptoms and how better to manage them, and to distinguish between the illness and premorbid strengths and capabilities. The therapist determines the need for medication based on symptom severity, past response to medications, and patient preference.

The "Sick Role"

The IPT therapist gives the patient the "sick role" (Parsons, 1951), a temporary role intended to help the patient to recognize that she suffers from an illness that comprises a distinct set of symptoms that compromise functioning. By assuming the sick role, the patient is relieved of self-blame and exempted from responsibilities that the depression compromises until she recovers. The therapist educates the patient about the way depression can impair social functioning and how to explain the illness to family and friends to gain support. The sick role also gives the patient the responsibility of working on improving her symptoms in treatment.

The Interpersonal Inventory

In IPT the psychiatric history includes the "interpersonal inventory," a thorough review of the patient's past and current social functioning, close relationships, relationship patterns, expectations of others within relationships, and the perceived expectations that others have of the patient. The interpersonal inventory should give the therapist a sense of how the patient interacts with other people. It should also illuminate how relationships may have contributed to the current depressive episode and, conversely, how depressive symptoms may be affecting current relationships. To glean this information, the IPT therapist asks detailed questions about the patient's past and current relationships. An inquiry about current relationships might include the following questions:

"Who is in your life currently? . . . Do you have a significant other? . . . Girlfriend/boyfriend? . . . What is your relationship like with him or her? . . . What do you like about him or her? . . . What don't you like? . . . Do you and your spouse argue? . . . What kinds of things to do you argue about? . . . What happens when you argue—what do you do/say? . . . What do you expect of him or her? . . . What do you think he or she expects of you?"

Identification of Interpersonal Problem Areas

The primary goal of the interpersonal inventory is to determine which interpersonal issues are most related to the patient's current depressive episode. The therapist should identify major interpersonal problem areas that will become the focus of the treatment. The therapist inquires about any changes in the patient's life that occurred around the onset of current depressive symptoms: "What was going on in your life when you became depressed?" The therapist also explores different areas in the patient's life: home, work, relationships with significant others, family members, and friends. The therapist should pick one, or at most two, problem areas on which to focus; too many treatment foci yield an unfocused treatment. The therapist relates the depression to a problem area and presents this to the patient in a formulation:

"It seems from what you have been telling me that the main problem has been your difficulty in getting along with your husband. Although the causes of depression are complex and not fully known, we do know that conflicts with significant others can be related to depression. Furthermore, depression can make it difficult to handle conflicts with

other people. I suggest that we meet for the next 12 weeks to figure out how you can better deal with the problems with your husband you've described. In IPT, we call that conflict a 'role dispute.' As you solve your role dispute, both your life and your depression should improve. Does this make sense to you?"

Only with the patient's explicit agreement to work on the chosen interpersonal problem area does the therapist proceed to the middle phase of treatment. The patient's agreement on the focus allows the therapist to bring her back to this theme thereafter, maintaining a thematic flow for the treatment.

Explanation of the Treatment Contract and the IPT Approach

In addition to agreeing on a treatment focus, the therapist and patient discuss and come to an understanding about other aspects of the treatment in the initial sessions. The therapist discusses practical aspects of the treatment, including the time limit, the specific length and frequency of sessions, termination date, appointment time, fee, and so forth. The therapist explains that IPT is one of several empirically supported treatments for depression and describes the basic IPT principles. The therapist emphasizes the "here and now," and the social and interpersonal focus of the treatment, explaining:

"We'll work together to try to understand how current stresses and relationships may be affecting your mood. We will work on helping you to better manage these stresses and the problems you may be having in relationships. We'll explore what you want and need in your relationships and help you figure out how to get what you want and need."

The therapist continues: "I'll be interested in hearing each week about what's going on in your relationships with other people, how those interactions make you feel, and also how your feelings influence what happens with other people." The therapist encourages the patient to bring up any discomforts she has about the sessions. "If anything bothers you, please bring it up. I do not intend to do anything to make you uncomfortable, but if you feel that way, please tell me, so that we can address the issue. It's just the sort of interpersonal tension that we need to focus on in your outside life as well."

The Middle Phase (Sessions 4–9)

Once the treatment contract has been made and an interpersonal problem area is chosen as the focus of treatment, the therapist can proceed to the middle phase of sessions, in which the goal is to work on resolving the focal problem area.

Each session begins with the question, "How have you been feeling since we last met?" This question elicits an interval history of mood, events, and interpersonal interactions that transpired between sessions. It also keeps the patient focused on current mood and situation. The patient is likely to respond by describing a mood ("I felt really down") or an event ("My husband and I had a huge fight"). After further inquiry, the therapist links the patient's mood to a recent event, or an event to her mood ("No wonder you felt depressed given the fight you had with your husband").

Inquiring about emotionally laden interpersonal interactions, the therapist uses *communication analysis*—the reconstruction and evaluation of affectively charged interactions—to help the patient understand how she felt in the situation and what she might have done to communicate more effectively. The therapist *explores the patient's wishes and options*, helping her to decide what she wants and exploring the options for achieving it.

"What did you want to happen in that situation? . . . What could you have done to get what you wanted in that situation?"

Depressed patients often have difficulty seeing that they have options, and their tendency to deem their needs less important than others' contributes to difficulty in being self-assertive. The therapist explains this to the patient and offers empathy, blaming the depressive syndrome for the patient's difficulties where appropriate. To help the patient choose which options to pursue, the therapist uses *decision analysis*. These techniques are elaborated in the case example presented later in this chapter.

The therapist *role-plays* potential interactions with the patient to prepare her for inter-

personal interactions in real life. Rather than supply words for the patient during role play, the therapist instead encourages her to come up with her own words. This empowers the patient, because it fosters her independence from the therapist. The therapist points out that the patient is able to figure out what to say and do in interpersonal interactions, but that depression can make her feel unable to do so. The therapist asks the patient how she felt during role play and how she imagines it will feel to say the words in reality. When a patient communicates effectively during role play—and, ultimately, in real life—the therapist reinforces the adaptive behavior with congratulations and encouragement. Real-life successes not only improve mood but also inspire patients to try to assert themselves in subsequent situations.

Depressed patients tend to withdraw socially and to lose interest in activities they previously found pleasurable. The therapist encourages the patient to resume social activity and to explore options for new activities and opportunities to form new relationships, if applicable. The therapist empathizes with how difficult it may be for the patient to push herself to engage with others, but stresses that, once engaged, she will likely feel better. Indeed, the IPT therapist asks the patient to take risks—both in asserting herself with others and in pushing herself to reengage in social activities. The therapist explicitly acknowledges that he or she is asking the patient to take risks, yet assures her that these risks will likely lead to improvement of her mood and life situation.

The Termination Phase (Sessions 10–12)

In the final sessions, the therapist reviews the patient's progress in symptom improvement, as well as the extent to which the patient has resolved the focal problem area. By reviewing why the patient is better, through the actions the patient has taken to resolve the interpersonal focus, the therapist reinforces the patient's growing self-esteem by pointing out that the patient's actions have led to her gains. The therapist congratulates the patient on her progress and hard work, and expresses optimism that the patient can maintain that progress independent of the therapist.

The therapist addresses nonresponse in patients whose moods and life situations do not improve, or only partially improve. The therapist should explain that is the *treatment* that failed—*not* the patient. The therapist gives the patient hope by emphasizing that depression is treatable and many other effective treatments exist, and by encouraging her to explore alternative treatments.

The therapist explores the patient's feelings about the treatment and termination. The therapist acknowledges not only his or her own sadness to be ending their relationship but also happiness about the patient's improvement and confidence that the patient will be able to maintain the progress she made in treatment. Should symptoms recur, the patient has gained tools to manage symptoms of depression on her own. Furthermore, the patient can return to IPT for "booster" sessions as needed.

Using the IPT medical model, the therapist provides psychoeducation about relapse and recurrence of major depression and prepares the patient about potential for relapse. Patients who have experienced one or more episodes of major depression are unfortunately vulnerable to future episodes. The therapist explains this and advises that given the link between stressful life events and mood, the patient can anticipate that she may have difficulty with future, stressful life events. Fortunately, the patient can use the coping skills she gained in treatment to ward off a worsening of symptoms. If the patient has improved in IPT but has either significant residual symptoms or a history of multiple episodes, therapist and patient may contract for continuation or maintenance IPT, which has also demonstrated efficacy in forestalling relapse.

CASE STUDY

The following case demonstrates how a clinician (K. L. B.) implemented IPT for major depression in a 12-week acute treatment and illustrates how one works with the problem area of grief. In IPT, grief (complicated bereavement) is considered as a focal problem area when the onset of depression is related to the death of a significant other and the patient is experiencing an abnormal grief reaction (Weissman et al., 2000). Although cases that focus on the grief problem area usually address complicated bereavement related to the death of a person who has actually lived, the following case involves complicated bereavement related to a stillbirth. Indeed, the IPT problem areas can apply to a wide range of cases. IPT

treatment goals and techniques specific to working with the grief problem area are demonstrated.

Background Information

Sara, a 35-year-old, married, childless woman, was referred for treatment of depression following the death of her baby girl *in utero* at 27 weeks' gestation. Her doctor explained that a bacterial infection was the most likely cause of the stillbirth. Sara's chief complaint was: "I feel like I should be over it."

At 27 weeks, after not feeling the baby move for at least several hours, Sara called her doctor, who told her to come to the hospital. The doctor was unable to find a heartbeat and told her that he needed to deliver the fetus. Sara recalled feeling shocked, numb, and unable to cry at first. She was given medication to induce labor and an epidural, and delivered the baby vaginally. Despite efforts to revive her, the baby was pronounced dead shortly after delivery. Sara said that she wanted to hold the baby and was given the baby to hold. She held the baby, who was swaddled in a white-and-pink blanket. She recalled that she and her husband cried uncontrollably while they took turns holding the baby and for a long time after giving the baby back to the doctor. She remembers that the baby was "very cute" and looked like her husband. She was given pictures of the baby and footprints to take home. Sara and her husband decided not to have a funeral or memorial service for the baby.

Sara reported that since the stillbirth 2 months earlier, she had been feeling sad and irritable most of day, nearly every day, and unable to enjoy things she used to enjoy, such as reading fiction, cooking, going to the movies, and exercise. She worked as a nurse on an inpatient medical floor in a New York City hospital, and prior to the stillbirth had very much enjoyed her work. She now felt unable to enjoy her work because of her mood, and she feared having to talk about her loss with coworkers who knew she had been pregnant. She was crying frequently, socially withdrawn, had low energy and difficulty concentrating, experienced decreased appetite, and felt very bad about herself. She denied ever having thoughts of suicide or feeling that life was not worth living.

Sara reported that she tried not to think about the baby's death, but she was frequently bothered by thoughts about the baby, often wondering what her life would have been like had she survived. Sara had returned to work 3 weeks after the stillbirth, hoping that it would serve as a distraction and help her "get over" her loss. She reported feeling very angry at and avoiding other pregnant women, including close friends and women with newborns, in addition to other reminders of her pregnancy. She felt angry at having had to go through pregnancy, labor, and delivery without gaining the pleasure of having a child.

Sara was plagued by inappropriate guilt. She felt guilty because she feared that she had done something to cause her loss, despite the doctor telling her that there was nothing she could have done to prevent it. He explained that when bacterial infections cause fetal death, they often cause no symptoms in the mother and go undiagnosed, until they cause serious complications. Nevertheless, Sara felt that she should have known about the infection, and she felt guilty about having waited until age 35 to try to conceive. She described feeling like a failure for having had a stillbirth. Sara felt guilty that she had disappointed and upset her husband by losing the baby, and she did not want to burden him with her feelings about the loss.

Sara had never sought treatment prior to her current evaluation. She described one prior episode of major depression in her late 20s lasting 4–6 weeks, precipitated by a breakup with a boyfriend of several years, but reported feeling much worse since losing the baby. She reported that her mother had been treated for depression with antidepressant medication with good results.

Sara was an attractive woman of average height and weight who looked her stated age. She was casually but neatly dressed in jeans and a large sweater. Sara's movements were slightly slowed; her speech was fluent. Her mood was depressed and her affect, congruent and tearful. She denied current or past suicidal ideation and any history of substance abuse or psychotic symptoms. She denied current or past medical conditions, including thyroid dysfunction. She reported no known prior pregnancies, pregnancy losses, or fertility issues prior to the stillbirth. In fact, she had conceived after just a couple of months of trying to get pregnant.

Sara was good candidate for IPT: She met criteria for major depression and had experienced a recent life event that could be easily linked to the onset of her symptoms. Furthermore, IPT could address the interpersonal problems she was experiencing related to the onset of her symptoms. Sara was also a potential candidate for CBT, pharmacotherapy, or (evidence-based antidepressant) psychotherapy combined with medication. She was uninterested in doing written homework and resistant to taking medication, because she was hoping to conceive again in the near future.

IPT Treatment with Sara

Acute Phase (Sessions 1–3)

Treatment with Sara followed the IPT format for acute treatment. In the first three sessions, the therapist obtained a thorough psychiatric history and set the treatment framework. In the first session, she obtained a chief complaint and a history of Sara's present illness. Using DSM-IV criteria, the therapist determined that Sara met criteria for major depression, recurrent. She administered the HDRS to assess the severity of Sara's symptoms.

The therapist offered Sara empathy for her pregnancy loss, saying: "I am *so* sorry. You've suffered a terrible loss. No wonder you have been feeling so badly and having such a difficult time." The therapist gave Sara her diagnosis of major depression, reviewed her specific symptoms, and gave her the "sick role."

"The symptoms you've described having in the past couple of months—depressed mood, not being able to enjoy things and your loss of interest in things, feeling very badly about yourself and guilty, your difficulty eating and sleeping, and difficulty concentrating—are all symptoms of major depression. Major depression is an *illness* that is *treatable*. It is *not* your fault that you have been feeling this way."

The therapist explained that Sara's HDRS score of 24 indicated moderately severe depression and that she would readminister the HDRS at regular intervals to monitor Sara's progress. Given the severity of Sara's symptoms, her willingness to participate in psychotherapy, and her reluctance to take medication in anticipation of trying to conceive again, the therapist did not think medication was needed.

The therapist described IPT and the treatment rationale:

THERAPIST: I am trained in a psychotherapy called interpersonal psychotherapy, which I think could be helpful to you. Interpersonal psychotherapy—often referred to as IPT—is a time-limited treatment that focuses on how recent life events and stresses—such as losing a baby—affect mood, and how mood symptoms make it difficult to current life events and stresses, particularly problems in relationships. Although we will take the first few sessions to review your history, our sessions will focus on the here and now, on your *current* difficulties and relationships, not on the past. Does this make sense to you?

SARA: Yes.

THERAPIST: Often, people respond to treatment with IPT in 12 weekly sessions. I propose that we meet once a week for a 50-minute session for the next 12 weeks. If it's helpful, at the end of the 12 sessions, we can discuss whether it might be useful to have additional sessions to work on issues and maintain your progress. How does that sound to you?

SARA: It sounds good. I hope I can feel better in 12 weeks.

THERAPIST: You *can* feel better in 12 weeks. IPT has been shown in numerous research studies to be effective in treating symptoms like the ones you have described.

After the first session Sara felt somewhat more hopeful but stated that she did not like the idea that she had a diagnosis of major depression. Although she could understand that there was relationship between her stillbirth and her mood, Sara still felt that she should be feeling better after 2 months and did not want to think of herself as depressed, like her mother, and in need of help. Sara stated that she was always the "strong one" and was used to functioning at a very high level. The therapist was not surprised by Sara's initial skepticism, because it can take time for patients to accept the medical model. Furthermore, patients with depression often feel uncomfortable about seeking help, because they fear burdening others. Nevertheless, therapist and patient agreed to work together for 12 weeks, then decide whether further sessions were needed.

In obtaining Sara's psychiatric history, the therapist conducted an *interpersonal inventory*, carefully reviewing Sara's past and current social functioning and close relationships. She started the inventory by asking about Sara's family.

"Where did you grow up? . . . Who was in your family? . . . How would you describe your relationship with your mother? . . . With your brother?"

Sara grew up in Canada with her father and mother, both in their early 60s, and her younger brother, age 33, all of whom still lived near Toronto where she had been raised. She reported that her father had worked a lot while she was growing up, and although she was fond of him, she did not feel so close to him. Sara felt closer to her mother and spoke with her weekly but was easily irritated by her. It bothered Sara that her mother was not assertive and was intermittently depressed. She spoke weekly with her brother, who lived in Canada with his wife and 2-year-old son. She described her relationship with her brother as fairly close. She reported speaking to her brother less often since the stillbirth, because she felt jealous that he had a child. When they did speak, Sara avoided asking about her nephew.

After exploring Sara's relationships with family members, the therapist asked about other important people in her life and asked her about the relationship with her husband. At age 33, Sara met her husband, Steve, who was 1 year her junior. She described Steve as warm and charming, and reported that he took great care of her. She felt she did not "deserve him," because he was "such a good guy." She described her previous boyfriends as less emotionally available and "not very nice." Both Sara and Steve were originally from Canada but met in New York City, when they were introduced by mutual friends. Sara had moved to New York in her early 20s, whereas her husband had moved there 2 years prior to their meeting.

Since the stillbirth, Sara felt distant from Steve and argued with him about "little things." She reported feeling guilty that she had let him down by losing the baby and feared that he blamed her for the baby's death. She did not want to burden him further by sharing her own distress about the loss. She also felt that Steve would not be able to understand her fears about trying to conceive again.

Sara reported having a few close girlfriends who lived in the tristate area and, until the pregnancy loss, spoke to them about once per week. She had several friends at work, with whom she chatted almost daily until the loss. She described herself as "independent," "outgoing," and "not one to lean on other people" prior to becoming depressed. She was the one to whom her friends turned when they had problems. Sara said that before the depression, her friends would describe her as hardworking and energetic. Sara reported that she rarely argued with friends because she felt "uncomfortable" with conflict. She avoided confronting friends and coworkers when she disagreed or felt angry with them.

The therapist asked Sara if there was anyone to whom she had turned for comfort after her loss, because it is important to have someone in whom to confide after such a terrible loss or any stressful experience. Sara replied that she had been avoiding her friends and family since the loss. She had felt uncomfortable talking to friends, family, and coworkers about her pregnancy when she was pregnant, because she did not like being the center of attention and felt guilty that she did not enjoy the first trimester of her pregnancy. She felt even more uncomfortable discussing her pregnancy loss. Her parents and in-laws came to see Sara and her husband after the loss, but she felt unable to talk with them about what had happened and how she was feeling. All of her coworkers knew that she had been pregnant, and Sara felt obligated to say something to them about what had happened. The therapist noted that it sounded like Sara could trust no one with her feelings about the stillbirth. Sara did not want to reach out to family or friends, or let them know how bad she felt; she explained: "I don't want to bother people with my problems. I don't want to be weak."

The therapist reframed Sara's difficulty in reaching out to others, using the medical model to explain how depression affects social functioning:

THERAPIST: You are not weak—you are *depressed*—and that's not your fault. People with depression tend to minimize their own needs and avoid seeking help from their friends, as you have been, because they fear being a burden. However, it is not only appropriate to seek support from others but it also can be *really* helpful to get support from others. In fact, support from others has been

shown to help in recovery from depression. I appreciate your dilemma. Your depression makes you feel uncomfortable seeking support, yet support from others has been shown to reduce depression and protect people from becoming depressed. Does this make sense to you?

SARA: Yes, but I also don't want to hear what they have to say. It just makes me more upset. They don't understand what I have been through.

THERAPIST: What kinds of things have people said to you?

Sara replied that it bothered her when people said things like "You'll get pregnant again" or "I know someone who also lost a baby." These statements made her feel angry. She felt that others could not understand what she had experienced. One close friend had recently given birth to her first child, and Sara had avoided calling and seeing her. She felt that it was unfair that her friend had a baby when she did not. A coworker had been pregnant at the same time but had a relatively easy pregnancy. Sara felt that her coworker was not sympathetic to her physical discomfort during pregnancy.

By the end of the first phase of treatment, the therapist had connected Sara's major depressive episode to her interpersonal situation in a *formulation* centered on an IPT focal problem area. Sara's chief complaint reflected that she was still grieving the loss of her baby and unable to resume her normal level of functioning. Her situation was a clear example of the grief problem area: Sara was suffering from complicated bereavement. While it is normal to grieve for months after losing a loved one, the severity of Sara's depressive symptoms—especially the excessive guilt, low self-esteem, and social isolation—and her avoidance of thoughts, feelings, and reminders of the baby and the baby's death, reflected an abnormal grief reaction. She had not sought emotional support after the stillbirth and had not really mourned the loss of her baby. In fact, people often develop complicated bereavement when they lack or have not used their social network to help them mourn the loss of their loved one.

The therapist presented this formulation to Sara:

THERAPIST: From what you are telling me, it's clear that the loss of your baby triggered your current depression. You have suffered a terrible loss and you are having trouble grieving. No wonder you are having such a hard time. This is not your fault. Furthermore, your loss and your depression have affected your relationships with people in your life, like your husband, your friends and coworkers, and you're having difficulty expressing your feelings to them. I suggest that we focus our sessions on handling your grief over this terrible event. Grief is one of the problem areas that IPT has been shown to treat. I suggest we work on helping you to mourn the loss and to improve your relationships that have been affected by your loss. How does this sound to you?

SARA: It sounds good.

With Sara's explicit agreement about the treatment focus, the therapist began the middle phase of treatment.

Middle Phase (Sessions 4–9)

During the middle phase, therapist and patient worked on resolving Sara's interpersonal problem area. In IPT, the strategy for working with grief is to help the patient to tolerate and manage the affect of loss, and to gather social support to help the patient through mourning. In addition, the therapist helps the patient to use existing social supports, to reestablish interests and relationships, and to form new relationships and explore new activities to compensate for the loss (Weissman et al., 2000).

The therapist continued providing psychoeducation about complicated bereavement and how depression affects social functioning, and repeatedly linked Sara's depression to the identified problem area. She began each session with the *opening question:* "How have things been since we last met?" This question elicited affect and a history of Sara's mood and events between sessions, and kept her focused on her current mood and life events.

To facilitate the mourning process, the therapist encouraged Sara to think about the loss. In fact, this process had begun during the initial phase, while the therapist took a history of the events related to the onset of Sara's depression. The therapist asked Sara to describe the events

prior, during, and after the baby's death—often a source of patient guilt—and explored Sara's feelings associated with these events. In helping a patient mourn the loss of a loved one, the IPT therapist asks the patient to describe her feelings about the death and about the person who died. The therapist explores what the patient and the deceased did together, what the patient liked and did not like about the person, and what the patient wished they had done together but did not have a chance to do. The therapist asks the patient to describe how the deceased died and how she learned about the death, and explores the patient's related feelings. Given that the Sara's baby died *in utero*, the therapist modified this inquiry somewhat by encouraging Sara to talk about her experience of being pregnant, about the baby, and what she imagined the baby would be like. The therapist asked Sara what she liked about carrying the baby, what she did not like, and what she had hoped to do with the baby.

Sara tearfully described having had mixed feelings about her pregnancy. She reported that she and Steve started trying to conceive 6 months after getting married and, to her surprise, she got pregnant after 2 months. When she discovered she was pregnant, Sara felt really happy, but scared about becoming a parent. She questioned whether she was "ready." Sara reported that she made a great effort to practice good prenatal care: She ate healthy, pregnancy-safe foods, took prenatal vitamins, and started prenatal yoga classes. Practicing good prenatal care made her feel good, "as if I was already a mom taking care of my baby."

Sara quickly began to experience terrible fatigue and unrelenting nausea, which lasted for the first 12 weeks of the pregnancy. She described feeling as if she had been "taken over" by the pregnancy. She complained that she loved to cook but did not want to cook, because she felt so sick. Despite the nausea, she ensured that she was getting the nutrients she needed for the baby. The fatigue and the nausea were so debilitating that Sara could no longer meet the physical demands of her job as a nurse. As a result, she was unable to hide her pregnancy from her coworkers; she told her supervisor, who was happy to accommodate Sara by giving her more administrative responsibilities in lieu of patient care, until she felt better. Sara resented having to give up clinical work with patients, which was the part of her job she enjoyed. She felt self-conscious about her symptoms and very guilty that her coworkers had to absorb her patient load, despite their being very supportive. It bothered her that others idealized pregnancy when she found it so unpleasant. At the same time, she felt guilty and selfish that she had complained about the pregnancy: Sara felt that she should have just been grateful she was pregnant.

The therapist empathized with Sara's discomfort during her first trimester and validated her need to complain:

THERAPIST: The first trimester of pregnancy can be really difficult and disruptive. Give yourself a break! It can be hard to appreciate being pregnant when you are feeling so terrible. It sounds like you did appreciate being pregnant—you made a great effort to take care of yourself. You watched your diet carefully and rearranged your work situation.

SARA: I don't know . . . I guess that is true.

When the exhaustion and nausea subsided in her second trimester, Sara began to feel more optimistic and excited about having a child. Seeing sonograms made the baby seem "more real" and helped Sara feel connected to the baby. At Week 16, Sara learned that the baby was a girl. She felt excited and immediately began considering names and envisioning what the baby would look like. Sara imagined that she would look like a combination of herself and her husband, with blue eyes and blond, curly hair. She thought the baby would be a kind person, like her husband. She imagined walking to the park with the baby in a stroller, and playing with her. At Week 20, Sara began to feel the baby move, which she very much enjoyed. When the baby moved, Sara would stop whatever she was doing to watch and feel her abdomen. She described feeling the movements as "some of the happiest moments in my life." Neither she nor her husband had thought of a name for the baby, but referred to her as "Sweetie" *in utero*.

For weeks after the stillbirth, Sara struggled with physical reminders of the baby. After delivering the baby, she had leaky breasts for a few days and vaginal bleeding for several weeks. She reported that she still looked pregnant for weeks after delivering the baby, as her uterus slowly returned to its prepregnancy size.

At the time of her initial evaluation, Sara reported that she still had to lose 5 pounds to return to her prepregnancy weight. Sara missed being pregnant and described feeling "empty" and "alone" without the baby inside her. She was eager and ready to be a parent, yet felt scared about conceiving again, because she feared losing another baby.

A couple of weeks after the stillbirth, Sara's doctor determined that an undetected bacterial infection caused the stillbirth. The doctor explained that there was nothing Sara or her husband could have done to prevent the loss, and that this kind of loss was very rare. Despite her doctor's explanation, Sara blamed herself for her baby's death and feared that her husband blamed her too, although he repeatedly denied this. The therapist explored Sara's guilt further:

THERAPIST: What could you have done to prevent your baby's death?

SARA: (*tearfully*) I don't know. . . . I should have been able to do something.

The therapist offered Sara empathy and support, and related her guilt to depression:

THERAPIST: It would be great if there was something you could have done to prevent this tragedy, but there is generally nothing parents can do to prevent a pregnancy loss. It sounds like you did everything you could— you took very good care of yourself. You are struggling with inappropriate and excessive guilt—a symptom of depression. You are blaming yourself for something you didn't do. Perhaps when you find yourself feeling guilty, you can try to label this as a symptom of depression.

SARA: Yes. I guess I can try.

Talking about the pregnancy, the baby, and the baby's death, and exploring related feelings enabled Sara to develop a more balanced and realistic perception of her relationship with the baby and her role in the baby's death. She realized that she had not taken her pregnancy for granted. In fact, she had done everything she could to manage a difficult first trimester and take care of her baby. In addition, her experience with the pregnancy and the baby made Sara realize that, despite her initial anxiety, she was ready and excited to become a parent. By the end of the first month of treatment, Sara's mood was somewhat improved and her HDRS score had fallen to 18. She was less self-critical and more hopeful.

An important part of treating grief is facilitating the expression of affect related to the loss of the loved one. The therapist explored Sara's feelings as she spoke about the baby and her loss, giving her time to articulate what she was feeling and to cry. Although IPT therapists generally take an active stance, when facilitating the expression of painful feelings, it is important to allow for silences. By listening silently, the therapist showed that she could tolerate Sara's painful feelings, and that catharsis was an important part of mourning her loss. Sara was able to express feelings that she not only had been avoiding but also feelings of which she had previously been unaware.

Sara had avoided looking at the pictures and footprints of the baby from the hospital, which had been stored in a box under her bed. She and the therapist explored what it would be like for her to look at these items. Sara feared it would be scary, and that she would feel really bad. The therapist gently encouraged Sara to take a risk and look, because it might make her feel better to experience the feelings she had been avoiding:

"Your feelings are not going to hurt you. You might actually feel better if you allow yourself to let out some of the feelings you have been trying to keep inside. I know I am asking you to take a risk, but you might be pleasantly surprised."

Between sessions, Sara looked at the pictures and the footprints. The therapist asked what it was like for her.

SARA: I cried a lot. She was so cute. It wasn't as hard as I thought it would be. It felt like a release. I was surprised that I felt a little better afterwards.

THERAPIST: I am *so* glad you took a risk and looked. It sounds like it made you feel better.

In fact, every few weeks before the end of treatment, Sara looked at the pictures and the footprints. She explained that the pictures were sort of comforting, because they made her feel a connection to her baby.

In addition to encouraging catharsis, the therapist encouraged Sara to work on her interpersonal interactions, to reconnect with the people in her life, and to consider opportunities to form new relationships and start new activities to compensate for the loss. The therapist explained that people with depression tend to isolate themselves and stop engaging in previously pleasurable activities, both of which can perpetuate depression. Sara reported not wanting to talk to people, because she feared that she would have to talk about the loss, or that things people said would make her feel worse. In fact, as Sara and the therapist discussed, *she could guide the conversation* in a way that made her feel comfortable. They explored and role-played options for maintaining control of such conversations. Furthermore, Sara could tell people what would be helpful to her. The therapist explained:

"People with depression often have difficulty asserting their needs. If you communicate your needs to others—like your husband, friends, coworkers, and your family—you might improve those relationships *and* your mood. The people in your life may not know what you need. If you tell them, you might not only get support from them, but you might enjoy their company again and feel better."

Using *communication analysis*, the therapist asked Sara to recount arguments and unpleasant interactions with others—what she was feeling during the interaction, what she said or did, and what the other person said or did. They explored what Sara wished other people would say or do, and what *options* she had for asking them to do these things, and *role-played* Sara asking for what she wanted. Sara reported that she hated running into people who knew she had been pregnant but did not know about the stillbirth. In fact, she avoided going places, because she feared having to answer questions about the stillbirth. Sara and the therapist explored these interactions and how Sara could handle them more effectively:

THERAPIST: What kinds of things have people asked, or what are you afraid they will ask?

SARA: People have asked "How's your baby?" or "Weren't you pregnant?"

THERAPIST: How does that make you feel?

SARA: Awful!

THERAPIST: How do you handle it?

SARA: I don't know. . . . Sometimes I say "It didn't work out" or "My baby died."

THERAPIST: That sounds good. How does it feel for you to say that?

SARA: It feels OK, but then they want to know what happened and say stupid things like "At least you know you can get pregnant" or "You can have another one."

THERAPIST: What would you like them to say or do?

SARA: I would like them to just say "I'm sorry," and not ask any questions. I don't want to talk about what happened.

THERAPIST: How could you convey that?

SARA: I guess I could say, "I'm sorry, but I'd rather not talk about it."

THERAPIST: How does that sound? How did it feel to say that?

SARA: It felt OK. Don't you think that is rude to say that?

THERAPIST: No. You said it politely and it is appropriate for you to assert your needs. It is an uncomfortable situation for both you and the person who asked the question. If you are polite and direct with people, they are likely to understand. But why not try it and see?

Sara reported that she had avoided returning calls from old friends. She explained that she did not feel comfortable seeing her friends who had babies, because it would remind her of the baby she had lost. Sara also did not want to have to talk about the loss. She did not want to tell them how she felt, because she feared hurting their feelings. Sara and the therapist role-played Sara telling her friends about her discomfort and explaining that she did not want to offend them. Role play helped Sara feel prepared and less anxious about going to work, walking around her neighborhood, and talking to old friends. As a result, she gradually starting going out more and began returning phone calls. She returned to the yoga studio, where she had taken prenatal yoga, and started taking regular yoga classes, which helped her mood and provided an opportunity to be among other people. By midtreatment Sara's HDRS had fallen to 13, consistent with mild depression.

Since the stillbirth, Sara had been bickering with her husband Steve "over stupid things" and felt "distant from him." The therapist asked her to describe a recent incident. Sara said that Steve came home from work and told her that his friend's wife had just had a baby. She felt it was insensitive for him to tell her about other people's positive pregnancy experiences. It bothered her that Steve did not seem as uncomfortable as she was with this information, and that he no longer seemed as upset as she about the loss. The interaction made her feel "alone." She had responded to him by saying, "That's nice," then leaving the room and ruminating for the rest of the evening about his insensitivity.

Sara reported that they often had similar interactions. The therapist once again related Sara's difficulty asserting herself with her husband to depression, and noted that keeping her feelings inside might actually be making Sara feel worse. They explored interpersonal options for handling this situation in a way that might make Sara feel better. The therapist also helped Sara to explore what her husband's intentions might have been in the situation she described. She wondered whether he was trying to make her feel better, because his friend's wife had experienced several miscarriages. They role-played Sara telling her husband how she felt. Subsequently, when Sara was able to express her feelings to him, she learned that Steve was, in fact, telling her these stories to give her hope. Furthermore, her husband revealed that he was still upset about the loss of their baby but did not want to upset *her* by sharing his feelings. Sara was relieved that she and Steve were "on the same page" and felt good that she was able to feel close to him again. They subsequently were able to share more of their mixed feelings about the pregnancy experience.

Termination Phase (Sessions 10–12)

During the final sessions the therapist and Sara reviewed the progress Sara had made. She reported that her mood was much improved. Her HDRS was now a 5, consistent with euthymia and remission. Sara's affect was brighter, and she was less preoccupied with the loss of her baby: "I still get upset when I think about my baby, but I don't get as upset. It doesn't ruin my entire day. I am actually able to enjoy things again." Furthermore, Sara no longer blamed herself for her baby's death. She felt good about her ability to communicate her feelings more effectively with her husband, friends, and others, and to enjoy socializing and other activities again.

The therapist congratulated Sara on her hard work and achievements, and told her how happy she was that Sara felt so much better. They discussed the potential for relapse and how Sara could maintain her progress. Given Sara's history of depression, the therapist explained that Sara was, unfortunately, vulnerable to future episodes; however, Sara could anticipate that she would be vulnerable in the setting of stressful life events—role disputes, role transitions, deaths—and use the coping skills she had learned during their work together. Sara anticipated starting treatments for her clotting disorder, trying to conceive again, and, she hoped, getting pregnant for a second time—all role transitions. The therapist and Sara explored ways Sara could take care of herself during this potentially stressful time. They discussed Sara's reaching out to others for support, communicating with her husband about how she was feeling, and forgiving herself if she found herself having a hard time.

In the final session, Sara told the therapist that she had reread her diary entries from the days before beginning treatment, and she could not believe how far she had come, that her pregnancy loss had forced her to seek treatment for depression that she now realized had been a lifelong problem; in retrospect, she had suffered numerous episodes of mild to moderate depression. Sara admitted that she was initially very resistant to the medical model. Defining depression as a medical illness ultimately relieved Sara of her shame and guilt about her difficulty in functioning. Furthermore, being able to see depression as a set of discrete symptoms made it seem more manageable. Sara reported that she was getting along better with her mother; now that she understood depression, she felt more sympathy for her mother's struggle with depression. She was grateful for the opportunity to learn coping skills that she felt confident about maintaining. In addition, Sara said that she would not hesitate to seek treatment in the future should she find herself becoming depressed again.

The therapist's frequent encouragement, the time limit, and the brief duration of IPT helped keep Sara motivated. Sara said that she appreciated the opportunity to talk about her feelings about her pregnancy, her baby, and her baby's death, and that she felt the therapist understood and supported her. She recognized that her feelings, while powerful, made sense in context and had subsided with discussion. Sara confessed that she appreciated the therapist's "pushing" her to reconnect with others. She had not thought she could handle being with others but was pleasantly surprised.

Although each patient is unique, Sara's therapy resembled other IPT treatments for major depression and is a good example of working with the problem area of grief. The exploration and normalization of affect, communication analysis, exploration of options, use of role play, encouragement to take social risks, and other techniques employed in Sara's treatment are characteristic of working with interpersonal difficulties related to any of the four IPT problem areas.

COMMON PROBLEMS THAT ARISE DURING TREATMENT

The problems that typically arise during IPT treatment for major depression are (1) those inherent to working with depressed patients and (2) those related to the therapeutic frame. Although these problems are not unique to IPT, how the therapist views and treats these issues distinguishes IPT from other psychotherapies. In keeping with important IPT themes, the therapist attributes problems to depression, and to the patient's difficulties handling interpersonal interactions and communicating effectively outside of the treatment. The therapist continues to maintain an optimistic, supportive, and nonjudgmental stance and avoids transference interpretations.

For example, patients with major depression superimposed on dysthymic disorder ("double depression") and their therapists are often discouraged by the chronicity of their depression. In these cases, the therapist should remain hopeful and optimistic. Some depressed patients feel that their depression is incurable despite reassurances from the therapist. In these cases, the IPT therapist employs the medical model, labeling the hopelessness as a symptom of depression, and emphasizes that patients need not feel hopeless since depression is treatable. Depressed patients often view seeking treatment as a personal failure. The IPT therapist frames seeking treatment as the appropriate and smart way to treat a medical illness, and a positive step toward gaining mastery over their problems (Weissman et al., 2000).

The most serious problem to arise in any treatment for depression is when a patient expresses suicidal ideation. In IPT, as in any treatment, the therapist determines whether hospitalization is necessary, based on the seriousness of the intent and the availability of the patient's social supports. The therapist is as available as possible to the patient and schedules extra sessions as needed. The therapist assesses the circumstances in which the suicidal ideation developed and what the patient hoped to accomplish by ending her life, and reviews how the patient imagines others would react to her suicide. The therapist helps the patient explore alternative ways of expressing what she intended to communicate by committing suicide. Furthermore, the therapist provides psychoeducation about suicide, explaining that it is the most deadly symptom of depression, and that therapist and patient have to work together to keep the patient alive long enough to get through successful treatment. Augmenting the therapy with medication treatment should be considered for severely suicidal patients. The therapist remains optimistic that the patient's depression will improve, and that she will no longer feel as if life is not worth living (Weissman et al., 2000).

Problems may arise in the relationship with the therapist. For example, a patient who has poor social supports may come to view the therapeutic relationship as a substitute for relationships outside of the therapy. Because IPT focuses on relationships *outside* of the treatment, the therapist gently refocuses the patient to outside relationships. Whereas the therapist notes that the patient's ability to connect within the treatment relationship reflects her ability to form intimate relationships, he or she clarifies that they are not friends or family and emphasizes the importance of the patient's life outside of the treatment. The therapist helps the patient explore options for connecting with others that are similar to the way she connected with the therapist (Weissman et al., 2000).

Missed and late sessions are also considered to be symptomatic of depression. The therapist calls attention and empathizes with the fact that the patient has missed or is late to a session, and notes that difficulty getting to sessions may reflect functioning that is characteristic of depression. It is likely that the patient is late to appointments outside of the therapy. The therapist can remind the patient of the time limit of IPT to motivate her to come to sessions. In the event that the patient misses or is late to sessions because she is uncomfortable with the material being discussed in session, or because she has some other negative feeling about the treatment or the therapist, the therapist empathizes with the patient's feelings and helps her to explore ways to express these feelings directly.

When a patient is silent to the extent that it seems she is refraining from sharing thoughts and feelings, or when she changes or avoids subjects, or has problems with self-disclosure, the therapist notes this behavior and explores the patient's feelings related to the behavior. These behaviors are particularly problematic in a time-limited, focused treatment such as IPT, because they make it difficult to work on the chosen problem area. The patient may feel uncomfortable and ashamed to share her thoughts and feelings with the therapist. The therapist assures the patient that there is little that can surprise him or her, and that the patient does not have to talk about everything.

PREDICTORS OF RESPONSE

Although there is repeated evidence that IPT is an efficacious treatment for major depression and other disorders, there are fewer data on factors that predict response to IPT. Data from comparative treatment studies involving IPT suggest some clinical predictors of response. In the multisite National Institute of Mental Health Treatment of Depression Collaborative Research Program (NIMH TDCRP; Elkin et al., 1989), 250 outpatients with major depression were randomly assigned to 16 weeks of imipramine (IMI), IPT, CBT, or placebo. The TDCRP dataset has been examined for predictors of response by several researchers. Sotsky and colleagues (1991) found that TDCRP subjects with low-baseline-level social dysfunction responded well to IPT, whereas those with interpersonal deficits responded less well. These findings support the discussion earlier in this chapter that IPT works least well for patients with few or no social contacts, who report no recent life events, and whose treatment, therefore, focuses on the IPT problem area of interpersonal deficits. High initial symptom severity and impaired functioning predicted superior response to IPT and to IMI compared to CBT (Sotsky et al., 1991; Weissman et al., 2000) In another analysis, TDCRP subjects with symptoms of atypical depression, such as mood reactivity and reversed neurovegetative symptoms, responded better to IPT and CBT than to IMI or to placebo (Stewart, Garfinkel, Nunes, Donovan, & Klein, 1998).

Barber and Muenz (1996) found that among patients who completed treatment in the TDCRP study, IPT was more efficacious than CBT for patients with obsessive–compulsive personality disorder, whereas CBT was better for patients with avoidant personality disorder, as measured by the HDRS. However, another study examining the relationship between personality traits and outcome in the same dataset found no significant differences among personality traits (Blatt, Quinlan, Pilkonis, & Shea, 1995; Weissman et al., 2000).

In another study, Thase and colleagues (1997) found that among 91 patients with depression, patients who had abnormal electroencephalographic (EEG) sleep profiles had significantly poorer response to IPT than did patients with normal profiles. In this study, unlike the Sotsky and colleagues (1991) study, symptom severity did not significantly predict response to IPT (Weissman et al., 2000).

Patients taking medication, or those who wish to augment their psychotherapy with medication, may respond well to IPT, which shares the medical model of depression with pharmacotherapy, although no research to date has supported this hypothesis. Additional potential predictors of response are noted in the section describing the IPT patient Sara earlier in this chapter.

CONCLUSION

In summary, IPT is a time-limited, diagnosis-targeted treatment with demonstrated efficacy for patients with major depression and other mood disorders. It has been adapted for the treatment of anxiety disorders, eating disorders, and, most recently, personality disorders. Although there is substantial evidence of IPT's efficacy for the treatment major depression and other mood and psychiatric disorders, further

evidence of predictors of response to IPT is warranted. This chapter has focused on the original IPT protocol: IPT as an individual treatment for major depression.

IPT employs the medical model and focuses on *current* or recent life events, interpersonal difficulties, and symptoms. IPT emphasizes the interrelationship between mood and life events: Negative or stressful life events affect mood and, conversely, mood symptoms affect how people manage negative or stressful life events. Treatment with IPT focuses on one of four interpersonal problem areas—grief, role disputes, role transitions, and interpersonal deficits. The therapist helps patients recover from depression by relieving depressive symptoms and by helping them to resolve the chosen interpersonal problem area. The IPT therapist takes an active, optimistic, and supportive stance.

The case of Sara clearly demonstrates the techniques used and the process of treatment with IPT. IPT is an eclectic treatment that uses techniques employed by other psychotherapies. The combination of IPT's main principles, techniques, strategies, therapist and patient characteristics, and its proven clinical efficacy distinguishes it from other antidepressant treatments.

For further information about IPT and its adaptations, readers should consult the *Comprehensive Guide to Interpersonal Psychotherapy* by Weissman and colleagues (2000).

NOTE

1. For stylistic simplicity, patients are referred to in the feminine. Indeed, most depressed patients are women.

REFERENCES

American Psychiatric Association. (2000) *Diagnostic and statistical manual of mental disorders* (4th ed., text rev.). Washington, DC: Author.

Barber, J. P., & Muenz, L. R. (1996). The role of avoidance and obsessiveness in matching patients to cognitive and interpersonal psychotherapy: Empirical findings from the Treatment for Depression Collaborative Research Program. *Journal of Consulting and Clinical Psychology, 64,* 951–958.

Beck, A. T., Steer, R. A., & Brown, G. K. (1996). *Beck Depression Inventory manual* (2nd ed.). San Antonio, TX: Psychological Corporation.

Blatt, S. J., Quinlan, D. M., Pilkonis, P. A., & Shea, M. T. (1995). Impact of perfectionism and need for approval on the brief treatment of depression: The National Institute of Mental Health Collaborative Research Program revisited. *Journal of Consulting and Clinical Psychology*, 63, 125–32.

Blazer, D. G., II. (2000). Mood disorders epidemiology. In B. J. Sadock & V. A. Sadock (Eds.), *Kaplan and Sadock's comprehensive textbook of psychiatry* (7th ed., Vol. 1, pp. 1298–1308). Philadelphia: Lippincott/Williams & Wilkins.

Bleiberg, K. L., & Markowitz, J. C. (2005). Interpersonal psychotherapy for posttraumatic stress disorder. *American Journal of Psychiatry*, 162, 181–183.

Bleiberg, K. L., & Markowitz, J. C. (2007). Interpersonal psychotherapy and depression. In C. Freeman & M. Power (Eds.), *Handbook of evidence-based psychotherapies: A guide for research and practice* (pp. 41–60). London: Oxford University Press.

Bowlby, J. (1973). *Attachment and loss*. New York: Basic Books.

Elkin, I., Shea, M. T., Watkins, J. T., Imber, S. D., Sotsky, S. M., Collins, J. F., et al. (1989). National Institute of Mental Health Treatment of Depression Collaborative Research Program: General effectiveness of treatments. *Archives of General of Psychiatry*, 46, 971–982.

Fairburn, C. G., Jones, R., Peveler, R. C., Hope, R. A., & O'Connor, M. (1993). Psychotherapy and bulimia nervosa: Longer-term effects of interpersonal psychotherapy, behavior therapy, and cognitive behavior therapy. *Archives of General Psychiatry*, 50, 419–428.

Fairburn, C. G., Norman, P. A., Welch, S. L., O'Connor, M. E., Doll, H. A., & Peveler, R. C. (1995). A prospective study of outcome in bulimia nervosa and the long-term effects of three psychological treatments. *Archives of General Psychiatry*, 52, 304–312.

Frank, E. (2005). *Treating bipolar disorder: A clinician's guide to interpersonal and social rhythm therapy*. New York: Guilford Press.

Frank, J. (1971). Therapeutic factors in psychotherapy. *American Journal of Psychotherapy*, 25, 350–361.

Hamilton, M. (1960). A rating scale for depression. *Journal of Neurology, Neurosurgery, and Psychiatry*, 2, 56–62.

Hill, C. E., O'Grady, K. E., & Elkin, I. (1992). Applying the Collaborative Study Psychotherapy Rating Scale to rate therapist adherence in cognitive-behavior therapy, interpersonal therapy, and clinical management. *Journal of Consulting and Clinical Psychology*, 60, 73–79.

Kessler, R. C., Berglund, P., Demler, O., Koretz, D., Merikangas, K. R., Rush, A. J., et al. (2003). The epidemiology of major depressive disorder: Results of the National Comorbidity Survey Replication (NCS-R). *Journal of the American Medical Association*, 289, 3095–3105.

Klerman, G. L., Weissman, M. M., Rounsaville, B. J., &

Chevron, E. S. (1984). *Interpersonal psychotherapy of depression*. New York: Basic Books.

Lipsitz, J. D., Fyer, A. J., Markowitz, J. C., & Cherry, S. (1999). An open trial of interpersonal psychotherapy for social phobia. *American Journal of Psychiatry*, 156, 1814–1816.

Markowitz, J. C. (1998). *Interpersonal psychotherapy for dysthymic disorder*. Washington, DC: American Psychiatric Press.

Markowitz, J. C., Klerman, G. L., Perry, S. W., Clougherty, K. F., & Mayers, A. (1992). Interpersonal therapy of depressed HIV-seropositive patients. *Hospital and Community Psychiatry*, 43, 885–890.

Markowitz, J. C., Kocsis, J. H., Fishman, B., Spielman, L. A., Jacobsberg, L. B., Frances, A. J., et al. (1998). Treatment of HIV-positive patients with depressive symptoms. *Archives of General Psychiatry*, 55, 452–457.

Markowitz, J. C., Skodol, A. E., & Bleiberg, K. (2006). Interpersonal psychotherapy for borderline personality disorder: Possible mechanisms of change. *Journal of Clinical Psychology*, 62, 431–444.

Markowitz, J. C., Svartberg, M., & Swartz, H. A. (1998). Is IPT time-limited psychodynamic psychotherapy? *Journal of Psychotherapy Practice and Research*, 7, 185–195.

Meyer, A. (1957). *Psychobiology: A science of man*. Springfield, IL: Thomas.

Mufson, L., Moreau, D., & Weissman, M. M. (1993). *Interpersonal psychotherapy for depressed adolescents*. New York: Guilford Press.

Mufson, L., Weissman, M. M., Moreau, D., & Garfinkel, R. (1999). Efficacy of interpersonal psychotherapy for depressed adolescents. *Archives of General Psychiatry*, 56, 573–579.

Murray, C. L., & Lopez, A. D. (1996). *The global burden of disease* (Vol. 1). Cambridge, MA: Harvard University Press.

O'Hara, M. W., Stuart, S., Gorman, L. L., & Wenzel, A. (2000). Efficacy of interpersonal psychotherapy for postpartum depression. *Archives of General Psychiatry*, 57, 1039–1045.

Parsons, T. (1951). Illness and the role of the physician: A sociological perspective. *American Journal of Orthopsychiatry*, 21, 452–460.

Sholomskas, A. J., Chevron, E. S., Prusoff, B. A., & Berry, C. (1983). Short-term interpersonal therapy (IPT) with the depressed elderly: Case reports and discussion. *American Journal of Psychotherapy*, 36, 552–566.

Sotsky, S. M., Glass, D. R., Shea, M. T., Pilkonis, P. A., Collins, J. F., Elkin, I., et al. (1991). Patient predictors of response to psychotherapy and pharmacotherapy: Findings in the NIMH treatment of depression collaborative research program. *American Journal of Psychiatry*, 148, 997–1008.

Spinelli, M., & Endicott, J. (2003). Controlled clinical trial of interpersonal psychotherapy versus parenting education program for depressed pregnant women. *American Journal of Psychiatry, 160,* 555–562.

Stewart, J. W., Garfinkel, R., Nunes, E. V., Donovan, S., & Klein, D. F. (1998). Atypical features and treatment response in the National Institute of Mental Health Treatment of Depression Collaborative Research Program. *Journal of Clinical Psychopharmacology, 18*(6), 429–434.

Sullivan, H. S. (1953). *The interpersonal theory of psychiatry.* New York: Norton.

Thase, M. E., Buysse, D. J., Frank, E., Cherry, C. R., Cornes, C. L., Mallinger, A. G., et al. (1997). Which depressed patients will respond to interpersonal psychotherapy?: The role of abnormal EEG profiles. *American Journal of Psychiatry, 154,* 502–509.

Weissman, M. M., Markowitz, J. C., & Klerman, G. L. (2000). *Comprehensive guide to interpersonal psychotherapy.* New York: Basic Books.

World Health Organization. (1992). *The ICD-10 classification of mental and behavioral disorders: Clinical descriptions and diagnostic guidelines.* Geneva, Switzerland: Author.

CHAPTER 8

Behavioral Activation
for Depression

SONA DIMIDJIAN
CHRISTOPHER R. MARTELL
MICHAEL E. ADDIS
RUTH HERMAN-DUNN

New to this edition, the behavioral activation (BA) approach to treating depression has received very strong empirical support in the past few years, with results as good or better than cognitive therapy and antidepressant medications, even for the most severe cases of depression. Seemingly counterintuitive at first blush, this treatment does not focus on the notion of "just do it" but takes a comprehensive look at contingent relationships in the patient's life across the full range of behavior, cognition, and affect that may be maintaining the depression. As such, this very idiographic approach does not prescribe a set number of sessions to accomplish certain goals but is very adaptable to the individual with depression. In the detailed and very human description of the treatment of "Mark," readers will also note a very up-to-date focus on the role of rumination in depression (or worry in anxiety) as a fundamentally avoidant technique. The illustration of creative therapeutic strategies for activating clients and overcoming rumination will be of interest to all therapists treating depression.—D. H. B.

Behavioral activation (BA) is a structured, brief psychosocial approach that aims to alleviate depression and prevent future relapse by focusing directly on behavior change. BA is based on the premise that problems in vulnerable individuals' lives, and their behavioral responses to such problems, reduce their ability to experience positive reward from their environment. The treatment aims to increase activation systematically in ways that help clients to experience greater contact with sources of reward in their lives and to solve life problems. The treatment procedures focus directly on activation, and on processes that inhibit activation, such as escape and avoidance behaviors and ruminative thinking, to increase experiences that are pleasurable or productive and improve life context. We believe that BA is an important new treatment for depression for two main reasons. First, its efficacy is supported by recent empirical research; second, it is based on simple and easily grasped underlying principles and utilizes a small set of straightforward procedures.

BEHAVIORAL MODELS OF DEPRESSION

Basic Concepts

The central premise in virtually all behavioral models is the assumption that depression is associated with particular behavior–environment relationships that evolve over time in a person's life. "Behavior" is a very broad construct in these models and includes everything from taking a walk to grieving over the loss of a loved one. Behaviors can be fairly circumscribed (e.g., lying on the couch watching television after dinner) or they can be part of a more general repertoire (e.g., avoiding asserting one's own needs and desires in conflictual interactions).

"Environment" is also a broad construct that can best be thought of as the settings in which behaviors currently occur, as well as those in which behaviors have evolved over time. The temporal nature of environments is crucial for understanding behavioral approaches to depression. Often, behavior that appears to serve no function in a person's current environment has served a very important function in the past. Thus, when practitioners wonder why a depressed person is engaging in a particular set of behaviors, such as remaining in a dead-end job, it is often necessary to consider how particular repertoires (e.g., avoiding potential losses) have evolved over time.

Finally, all behavioral models of depression emphasize the importance of contingent relationships between behaviors and the environments in which they occur. Contingent relationships are "if–then" relationships between human activities and their (often interpersonal) environmental consequences. For example, practitioners working within a behavioral framework are probably less interested in the *fact* that a depressed client stays in bed each morning worrying, for example, about the future of a troubled marriage, than they are about the consequences of this behavior. What happens as a result? Does the client become more or less depressed? By staying in bed, does the client avoid something aversive, such as confronting a spouse about an issue in the marriage, or going to work and facing a pile of uncompleted tasks? Understanding contingent relationships is a central feature of behavioral models of depression and a requisite skill of BA therapists.

Behavioral Roots of BA

These general behavioral concepts were developed and refined into specific conceptual frameworks and treatments for depression by both Ferster (1973, 1981) and Lewinsohn and colleagues (Lewinsohn, 1974; Lewinsohn, Antonuccio, Breckenridge, & Teri, 1984; Lewinsohn, Biglan, & Zeiss, 1976). Ferster's primary assumption was that depression is the result of a learning history in which the actions of the individual do not result in positive reward from the environment, or in which the actions are reinforced because they allow the individual to escape from an aversive condition. Over time, behavior that would typically produce positive consequences ceases to do so. For example, for a variety of different reasons, a person's efforts to form close relationships with others might gradually fade away, because they are not followed by positive reinforcement (e.g., reciprocal efforts from others).

Ferster reasoned that this decrease in response-contingent positive reinforcement produces two further consequences that facilitate depression. First, when people's efforts do not result in reward, they often become more focused on responding to their own deprivation than to potential sources of positive reinforcement in the environment. This is the classic "turning inward" that is often seen in depression, and that makes sense from a behavioral perspective; when individuals learn that their own behavior is an unreliable predictor of positive consequences in their environment, they naturally spend less time attending to contingencies in that environment.

The second consequence of decreased rates of positive reinforcement that Ferster observed was a narrowing of individuals' repertoire of adaptive behaviors. This makes logical sense as well, because fewer and fewer behaviors are being maintained by positive reinforcement. Individuals may adopt extremely passive repertoires (e.g., "doing nothing"), because they have learned that their active attempts to become engaged in life do not produce positive consequences.

Finally, Ferster observed that increases in aversive consequences following behavior typically lead depressed individuals to become preoccupied with escape and avoidance. In effect, more energy is expended attempting to avoid or escape from anticipated aversive consequences than in attempting to contact potential positive reinforcers in the environment.

Lewinsohn's (1974) early behavioral model of depression was very compatible with many of the ideas proposed by Ferster. Lewinsohn similarly emphasized the importance of response-contingent reinforcement and conceptualized that its rate was influenced by three factors: the number of potentially reinforcing events for an individual; the availability of reinforcement in the environment; and the instrumental behavior of the individual required to elicit the reinforcement. Lewinsohn also identified social avoidance as a core part of his model. Importantly, Lewinsohn, Sullivan, and Grosscup (1980) developed the first stand-alone behaviorally oriented treatment for depression. *The Coping with Depression Course* (Lewinsohn et al., 1984) is a structured group treatment for depression that includes both behavioral and cognitive components. The behavioral component consists of self-monitoring, and structuring and scheduling specific pleasant activities that are intended to reverse the decrease in positive behavior–environment transactions.

Beck, Rush, Shaw, and Emery (1979) also pioneered early work on BA. Incorporating BA strategies as a core component of cognitive therapy (CT) for depression, Beck and colleagues formalized and widely disseminated some of the principal BA strategies. Although these strategies were utilized within a larger model that emphasized the importance of cognition in the etiology and treatment of depression, the formalization and dissemination of BA within CT advanced work on behavioral strategies significantly.

Current Conceptualization

The current version of BA was influenced by Ferster, Lewinsohn, and Beck in important ways. With respect to a conceptual model of depression, the current conceptualization draws heavily on the work of Ferster and Lewinsohn in emphasizing the central importance of context and activity in understanding depression. While acknowledging that genetic, biological, and other, distal factors may be causally related to depression, the current behavioral conceptualization focuses on the aspects of a person's life context that may have triggered depression, and particular ways of responding to this context that may be maintaining depression. Specifically, the model assumes that one reason people get depressed is because changes in the context of their lives provide low levels of positive reinforcement and high levels of aversive control. Lives that are "less rewarding" can lead to feelings of sadness and depressed mood. And when people get depressed, they often pull away from the world in important ways, and the basic routines of their lives become easily disrupted. Both of these processes can increase depressed mood and make it difficult to solve problems effectively in one's life. In fact, these processes are conceptualized as "secondary problem behaviors," because they frequently (1) prevent people from connecting with aspects of their lives that may provide some improvement in mood and (2) prevent people from solving problems that may help to decrease stress and improve life context.

The BA approach to therapy addresses both of the factors that may be contributing to depression: those aspects of one's life that need to be changed to reduce depression and the ways withdrawal from the world may be maintaining or increasing depression. BA accomplishes these aims through guided activation, which refers to a series of behavior change strategies that the therapist and client develop together on the basis of a careful examination of what activities will be reinforcing for a given client and will help to disrupt the relationships that are maintaining the depression. The point of BA is not to engage in increased activation at random or activities that are "generally" thought to be pleasing or to improve mood (e.g., seeing a movie); in contrast, activation strategies are highly individualized and "custom tailored." The role of the BA therapist is to act as a "coach" as the client implements the activation strategies, providing expert help in setting achievable goals, breaking difficult tasks down into manageable units, troubleshooting problems that arise, and maintaining motivation during the process of change. The specific treatment strategies also draw heavily from the pioneering work of Lewinsohn and Beck. Moreover, in accordance with the primary emphasis of Ferster's work, avoidant behavioral repertoires are a primary clinical target in BA.

EMPIRICAL CONTEXT

The first study to revitalize interest in a purely behavioral approach to treating depression was conducted by Jacobson and colleagues (1996), who proposed a simple but provocative question: Could the behavioral component of CT account for the efficacy that CT has demonstrated in previous clinical trials? Adults with major depression were randomly assigned to one of three treatment conditions, including BA only, BA plus interventions designed to modify automatic thoughts, and the full CT package. Results suggested that BA was comparable to the full CT package in both acute efficacy (Jacobson et al., 1996) and prevention of relapse over a 2-year follow-up period (Gortner, Gollan, Dobson, & Jacobson, 1998).

On the basis of these findings, BA was developed into a more fully articulated behavioral intervention that included the behavioral aspects of CT and incorporated the early behavioral work of Ferster and Lewinsohn, as described earlier. This expanded BA model was articulated in published reports (Jacobson, Martell, & Dimidjian, 2001; Martell, Addis, & Jacobson, 2001) and in a patient-oriented self-help manual (Addis & Martell, 2004). BA was further tested in a large, randomized, placebo-controlled clinical trial that compared its acute and long-term efficacy to both CT and antidepressant medication (ADM).

Two hundred forty-one patients were randomly assigned to BA, CT, ADM, or pill-placebo, and severity was used as a stratification variable during randomization. The findings suggested that BA is a particularly promising treatment for depression (Dimidjian et al., 2006). Among more severely depressed patients, its performance was comparable to the current standard of care, ADM, and demonstrated better retention. Both BA and ADM were superior to CT among more severely depressed patients. Moreover, follow-up results indicate that BA appears to have promising enduring effects (Dobson et al., 2007). Finally, BA may demonstrate an important cost-effectiveness advantage compared to continuing patients on medication.

These results are consistent with a range of other studies suggesting that activation interventions are particularly important components of cognitive-behavioral treatments. In a classic study, Zeiss, Lewinsohn, and Munoz (1979) reported comparable outcomes for depressed patients who received treatment focused on interpersonal skills, pleasant activities, or cognitive change. In addition, in a study with depressed older adults, Scogin, Jamison, and Gochneaur (1989) found no differences in outcome between a cognitive bibliotherapy treatment and a behavioral bibliotherapy treatment among mildly and moderately depressed older adults. The importance of behavioral strategies has also been reported in other studies across multiple diagnostic categories (e.g., Borkovec, Newman, Pincus, & Lytle, 2002; Foa, Rothbaum, & Furr, 2003; Gloaguen, Cottraux, Cucherat, & Blackburn, 1998) and across other activation-oriented approaches with depressed clients (e.g., Blumenthal et al., 1999; Hopko, Lejuez, LePage, Hopko, & McNeil, 2003). Process-oriented research on CT has similarly emphasized the importance of the BA components of CT (Bennett-Levy et al., 2004) and has suggested the possibility of negative outcomes when therapists work on changing clients' thoughts about interpersonal relationships as opposed to changing actual interpersonal relationships (Hayes, Castonguay, & Goldfried, 1996).

In addition, Ferster's early focus on avoidance has also been underscored by contemporary behavior therapists. Specifically, Linehan (1993) incorporates the use of "opposite action" for sadness as a means to target depression in dialectical behavior therapy. And Hayes and colleagues (1996) have emphasized the role of experiential avoidance in the development of a wide range of psychopathologies and in the conceptualization of acceptance and commitment therapy (ACT; Hayes, Strosahl, & Wilson, 1999). A study on an early precursor to ACT found significant treatment benefits for depressed clients in comparison to standard CT (Zettle & Rains, 1989).

ASSESSING DIAGNOSTIC, CLINICAL, AND FUNCTIONAL DOMAINS

The application of BA is based on a comprehensive diagnostic, clinical, and functional assessment. Some of these assessment activities are completed as a precursor to the initiation of therapy, and others are ongoing throughout the course of therapy.

In our treatment outcome research, we used a number of structured diagnostic interview instruments to assess all five axes of *Diagnostic and Statistical Manual of Mental Disorders*, fourth edition (DSM-IV; American Psychiatric Association, 1994) diagnosis, including the Structured Clinical Interview for DSM-IV Axis I Disorders (SCID-I; First, Spitzer, Gibbon, & Williams, 1997), and the Structured Clinical Interview for DSM-IV Axis II Personality Disorders (SCID-II; First, Spitzer, Gibbons, Williams, & Benjamin, 1996). In addition, we used two measures to assess depressive severity: the clinician-administered Hamilton Depression Rating Scale (HDRS; Hamilton, 1960) and the client self-reported Beck Depression Inventory–II (BDI-II; Beck, Steer, & Brown, 1996). In routine clinical practice, we recommend conducting a baseline diagnostic interview (although it can be administered using a less structured format than a research-based interview), and the ongoing use of a measure to assess depressive severity is important. Typically, the most easily administered measure is the BDI-II (Beck et al., 1996).

Also, a number of self-report instruments currently under development will serve as useful assessment measures of patient activity level and of the reward available in a client's environment. The Behavioral Activation for Depression Scale (BADS; Kanter, Mulick, Busch, Berlin, & Martell, 2007) is a 29-item measure that assesses clients on four subscales: Activation, Avoidance/Rumination, Work/School Impairment, and Social Impairment. Initial psychometric studies on nonclinical samples have demonstrated good internal consistency and sufficient test–retest reliability and construct validity. A second measure, the Environmental Reward Observation Scale (EROS; Armento & Hopko, 2007), is a 10-item scale developed to measure the construct of response-contingent positive reinforcement. Whereas the BADS focuses on activities in which the individual did or did not engage, the EROS measures increased behavior and improvement in positive affect as a consequence of rewarding environmental experiences. Initial psychometric studies indicate that the EROS has strong internal consistency and good test–retest reliability. Clinicians who want a nomothetic measure of pleasurable activities to augment the idiographic behavioral assessment (described in more detail below) can use the Pleasant Events Schedule (Lewinsohn & Graf, 1973).

These measures may prove to be useful clinical tools that can be administered periodically throughout the course of treatment to assess change in activity and reward.

Because functional capacity is such a key component of BA treatment, it is important to gather detailed information about the impact of the client's depression on functional status across multiple life domains, including work, family, social, and so forth. These domains can be assessed using clinical interview or standard assessment instruments (e.g., the Social Adjustment Scale [Weissman & Bothwell, 1976] and the Medical Outcomes Study 36-Item Short Form Health Survey [Ware & Sherbourne, 1992]).

COURSE OF TREATMENT

BA is a theory-driven as opposed to a protocol-driven treatment and, as such, is highly idiographic in its application. Treatment does not follow a required session-by-session format; however, it does follow a general course over time. This general course comprises the following activities, which are described in greater detail below:

- Orienting to treatment
- Developing treatment goals
- Individualizing activation and engagement targets
- Repeatedly applying and troubleshooting activation and engagement strategies
- Reviewing and consolidating treatment gains

Orienting to Treatment

BA begins with orienting the client to the treatment, a process that is typically the focus of the first two sessions. The primary tasks to accomplish during this initial phase of treatment include discussing the BA model of depression and primary treatment strategies, and providing information about the structure of treatment, and the roles and responsibilities of the client and therapist.

The presentation of the treatment model includes describing the behavioral approach to depression and the process of change during treatment, discussing the specific ways the model fits with the client's experiences, and encouraging and responding to questions and concerns about the model. The model is presented both verbally during the first session and in a brief, written description that is given to the client at the end of the first session. A detailed transcript illustrating the presentation of the treatment rationale is included in the case study below, and the key points to address are summarized in Table 8.1.

During the second session, therapist and client again discuss the treatment model and the client's reactions. It is essential that the thera-

TABLE 8.1. Ten Key Points to Address When Presenting the Treatment Model

1. Behavioral activation (BA) is based on the idea that the events in your life and how you respond to such events influence how you feel.
2. BA assumes that one reason people get depressed is that their lives are providing too few rewards and too many problems.
3. Sometimes it is possible to identify easily stressors or problems; other times there are no clearly identifiable stressors, but there is still not adequate reward from the environment.
4. When life is less rewarding or stressful, people sometimes pull away from the world around them and find that basic routines in their lives become disrupted.
5. Pulling away from the world when feeling down is natural and understandable. The problem is that it also can increase depression and make it hard to solve life problems effectively.
6. In this treatment, we will work together to help you become more active and engaged in your life.
7. BA is not just about "doing more." If feeling better were that easy, you would already have done it. My expertise lies in figuring out what activities would be most helpful *and* what small and manageable steps you can take to get started. You can think of me as a coach or consultant to you in the process of change.
8. Each session will involve developing practical and doable steps to engage in activities that improve mood and to solve specific life problems.
9. Between sessions, you will work on homework assignments that we develop together; these assignments are an essential part of therapy and will focus on reconnecting or building parts of your life that increase feelings of pleasure or accomplishment and bring you closer to important life goals.
10. Activating and engaging in specific ways can help you experience more reward and effectively solve life problems. When you are active, engaged, and solving problems effectively, it is likely that you will be moving toward important life goals and feeling better.

pist obtain "buy in" from the client with the basic elements of the treatment model. Therapy works best if the client accepts and buys into the rationale for treatment and the case conceptualization (Addis & Carpenter, 2000). The therapist is advised to guard against moving too quickly if the client does not express agreement with the key tenets of the model. Thus, during the initial sessions, it is essential that the therapist encourage the client to ask questions and elicit the client's potential doubts and concerns.

For instance, some clients may find it difficult to accept the idea that changing behavior directly is an effective way to work with depression. Often, clients are strongly committed to a biological explanation for their depression. It is not advisable for therapists to debate this position; instead, therapists can explain that there are many sources of vulnerability to depression, and that one of the effective ways to change depression is by changing what one does. At times, clients may also think that the emphasis on behavioral change means that all they need to do is exercise more, go to a few more movies, or take a few more walks, and their depression will remit. If clients understand BA in this way, then it is not surprising when they feel that the treatment invalidates their degree of distress and the difficulty they face in overcoming depression. We often find it helpful to talk to clients about two points. First, behavior can have a powerful effect on our moods and people are often unaware of this link, particularly when they are depressed. For example, subtly shifting the way someone approaches interactions with family members may not rid that person of depression, but it can reduce the severity of depressed mood, thereby setting the stage for other changes that collectively help to reverse the depression. The second point is that behavior change is not easy; if it were, we would all behave exactly as we think we should all the time (and we know this is not the case!). Changing behavior requires knowing what to change, and this can take some serious and sustained "detective work" in therapy. The therapist can again emphasize his or her role as a coach in helping the client to figure out what to change and how to do it.

In addition to presenting and discussing the treatment model, it is also important to discuss thoroughly the structure of treatment and the roles of therapist and client. It is necessary to emphasize three key elements: between-session practice, collaboration, and the structure of sessions.

1. It is important early in treatment to highlight the active nature of BA and establish the importance of between-session practice. The therapist sets the tone of therapy and expectations by highlighting that BA is a very action-oriented and problem-focused treatment in which the majority of the "work" of therapy goes on between sessions, as the client implements plans that therapist and client devise in session. Subsequent sessions examine what the client has learned, highlight relevant consequences of activities, and identify barriers and troubleshoot to maximize the likelihood of success on future attempts. The assignment of homework begins in the very first session, when the therapist asks the client to read the brief pamphlet that reviews the key ideas of the BA approach (see Martell et al., 2001).

2. Therapists should explain that BA is a collaborative approach to therapy, in which therapist and client work together in the service of the client's goals.

3. Therapists should explain the structured nature of each treatment session. Although the specific foci of each session vary across clients and across time, each session nonetheless follows a similar general outline. Specifically, as in cognitive therapy for depression (Beck et al., 1979), each session begins with therapist and client setting an agenda in a collaborative fashion. The aim of the agenda is to organize the time effectively and to ensure that sessions address the client's most important topics and have maximal likelihood of helping the client reach key goals. Because the goal of treatment is activation, the more control given to the client in setting the agenda, the better. In addition, given the integral role of homework in BA, the majority of each session is devoted to reviewing homework from the previous session and assigning homework for the next session. The ending of each session includes asking the client to reiterate a "take-home message" from the session, verifying that the client has a clear understanding of the assigned homework, and reviewing the time for the next scheduled session and methods to reach the therapist in the interim.

In attending to each of these specific tasks, the therapist must also establish his or her credibility as an expert who can help the client.

Doing so requires conveying a sense of hope and establishing a strong foundation of collaboration in which the client and therapist work together toward the client's goals.

Developing Treatment Goals

The ultimate goal of BA is to help clients modify their behavior to increase contact with sources of positive reinforcement in their lives. Typically, this process involves first addressing basic avoidance patterns and areas of routine disruption and, second, addressing short- and long-term goals. A good deal of the therapist's time in BA is spent helping clients to increase awareness of their escape and avoidance repertoires and to replace them with active coping responses. Often, part of this process also involves changing basic routines (e.g., sleep, eating, and social contact). Thus, short-term goals are set to specify concrete accomplishments that can help clients shift their life situations in a less depressing direction. Common examples might include getting the house cleaned, spending time with friends and family, making headway on a large pile of paperwork on which the client has procrastinated, exercising more frequently, and so on. Often, behaviors necessary for progress on short-term goals can be scheduled and structured in such a way that they substitute for maladaptive secondary coping responses. A therapist works with a client to make progress on short-term goals *regardless of how the client is feeling*. In other words, one of the therapist's primary goals is to help the client change the pattern of having his or her behavior governed by mood. Rather, the objective is to make progress on goals regardless of how one feels at a particular point in time, under the assumption that progress on life goals is itself antidepressive. This is a crucial point, because clients often judge the success of a particular behavior change based on how it makes them feel in the moment. Thus, it is important for therapists to remain mindful of the consequence of different behaviors specifically with respect to whether they help clients move toward or achieve treatment goals.

Once the short-term goals relating to avoidance, withdrawal, and routine disruption have been addressed, clients are assisted in addressing larger life circumstances that may be related to depression. Larger life goals are those shifts that take time to accomplish but have the potential to alter a person's life situation in substantial ways. Common examples include finding a new job, getting out of a distressing relationship, starting a new relationship, or moving to a new city or town. BA can be helpful in teaching and encouraging clients to continue to make progress toward these goals even though their actual realization may take some time to accomplish. Essentially, in BA, clients learn basic change strategies that can be used to accomplish short-term and larger life goals.

Individualizing Activation and Engagement Targets

No two people are the same, and no person is exactly the same from situation to situation. In the context of treating depression, this means that the particular activation strategies that work for one person may not work for another person, and they may work for the same person sometimes, but not always. Consider the behaviors associated with a client meeting a friend for lunch, which might include getting in the car or walking to a restaurant, talking with a friend about current events, sharing details of his or her personal life with the friend, eating, worrying about what the friend thinks of him or her, and so on. Each of these different repertoires of activity can be associated with positive or negative shifts in mood depending on a person's particular history and the way events unfold in the present. Whether these activity–environment transactions shift someone's mood in a positive or negative direction is an empirical question, and one that requires careful attention and assessment to answer.

Much of the skill of doing competent BA relies on just this kind of careful examination. In BA, this process is referred to as "functional analysis," which is the key to individualizing activation targets and the heart of BA. Functional analysis involves identifying for each client the variables that maintain the depression and are most amenable to change. This understanding forms the basis of the case conceptualization and guides the idiographic application of specific activation strategies. In general, the therapist must engage the client in a detailed examination of the following:

- What is maintaining the depression?
- What is getting in the way of engaging in and enjoying life?
- What behaviors are good candidates for maximizing change?

This process sounds simple, yet in practice, it can be complicated given that we all frequently lack awareness of the contingencies that control our behavior. Given this reality, early in treatment, we talk explicitly about the goal (and the challenge!) of identifying these relationships.

A number of steps are involved in identifying the contingencies that control behavior. First, therapist and client must clearly and specifically define the behavior of interest; this includes defining the frequency, duration, intensity, and setting of the behavior. The behaviors of greatest interest are those most closely tied to changes in mood. Often, therapists are uncertain about how to sequence treatment targets; generally, we focus initially on behavior change that has the greatest likelihood of success, which may be based on ease of accomplishment or level of importance to client goals. For instance, for one client, difficulty completing basic household tasks was maintaining and exacerbating his experience of depression. It was important to specify the problems of (1) filling and closing bags of household trash, then leaving them in the pantry room rather than taking them to the dumpster behind the house for the past 6 weeks; and (2) receiving bills in the mail and placing them unopened in a file drawer for the past 4 months. Treatment with this client began with a series of graded tasks to accomplish the goal of taking out the trash. This was selected as an initial focus, because the therapist and client decided it was more easily accomplished than addressing the bills, which the client experienced as overwhelming. Next, the therapist and client worked to identify the antecedent and consequences of the behavior, with the goal of specifying the variables that elicited or reinforced the depression.

Understanding basic behavioral principles can often be of great value in identifying these contingent relationships. What does this mean in practical terms? For depressed clients, a number of contingent relationships are often observed. First, as we discussed earlier, negative reinforcement contingencies are often pervasive. Negative reinforcement means that the likelihood of a behavior occurring is increased by the removal of something from the environment, typically an aversive condition. Negative reinforcement contingencies can be a very adaptive part of human behavior. For instance, putting on a warm coat to avoid getting cold, stopping at stop signs to avoid getting in accidents, and being extra nice to a parent after crashing the car to avoid being punished are all examples of ways that negative reinforcement can serve one well. Unfortunately, however, when individuals become depressed, their behavioral repertoires can become dominated by escape and avoidance behaviors that temporarily allow a person to escape from painful feelings or difficult interpersonal situations. In this way, many avoidant and escape behaviors may be understood as secondary coping responses—efforts to cope with the experience of depression that, unfortunately, make it worse. For example, a person might attempt to escape from feelings of hopelessness and fatigue by taking a long nap in the middle of the afternoon. This might, as a consequence, temporarily remove the person from an aversive context, but it can also prevent him or her from taking the steps necessary to shift into a less depressive context overall (exercising, applying for jobs, cleaning the house, etc.). Substance abuse, excessive sleeping, watching too much television, and general inactivity are all common examples of secondary coping responses that can be maintained by negative reinforcement. These types of negative reinforcement contingencies are often central in preventing people from coming into contact with potentially reinforcing environments that contribute to leading a more adaptive and engaged life. Careful assessment is required to identify whether and how specific negative reinforcement contingencies are active in a client's life.

Second, positive reinforcement contingencies may also be problematic for clients. In these cases, the likelihood of a behavior is increased, because it is contingently associated with positive consequences. For instance, going to bed early may be positively reinforced by family members offering empathy and support. Some behaviors, such as overeating and substance abuse, can also provide immediate positive reinforcement but detract from long-term goals, thereby maintaining the depression.

How do we conduct functional analyses in BA? Activity monitoring is the heart of the process. Through detailed and ongoing activity monitoring that the client completes between sessions, therapist and client can work together to develop an understanding of the questions listed earlier. Given the role of activity monitoring, it is important early in treatment for the

therapist to set the stage to clearly explain how to do it, and carefully and skillfully review monitoring tasks to reinforce the client's efforts to begin developing activation and engagement assignments.

Therapists may elect to use a number of different formats for activity monitoring, the most basic form of which includes recording both an activity and a mood rating for each hour of the client's waking day. Time sampling procedures may also be used. In such a procedure, client and therapist agree on a specified number of hours when activities will be monitored during the week between sessions. Time sampling procedures need to include a variety of situations in which the client functions during the week. Therefore, times during the early morning, the work day, and the evening and weekend should be set aside for monitoring.

Therapists can provide clients with a simple weekly Activity Record for monitoring assignments (e.g., see Figure 8.1). However, as is often emphasized in BA, the function of the behavior is more important than its form; thus, clients may eschew monitoring on an Activity Record but be comfortable using personal calendars, personal digital assistants, or other idiosyncratic recording methods. Adapting the monitoring assignment to a form that is compatible with the client's normal daily routine is highly encouraged. For instance, some clients who spend a lot of time in their car may keep their records above the visor; others may find it helpful to keep it taped to the refrigerator or bathroom mirror; still others find it useful to carry it with them in a pocket, purse, backpack, or briefcase. In general, therapists will want to encourage clients to complete entries at regular intervals throughout the day and are advised to work with clients to develop plans for recording that take advantage of natural cues and rhythms in their lives to facilitate such regular recording.

When a client has completed an activity monitoring assignment, it is essential for the therapist to review it in detail. Failing to review activity monitoring records may mean missed opportunities to reinforce the client's behavior and to develop the case conceptualization. Much of competent BA lies in skillfully reviewing a completed Activity Record. What does the competent therapist attend to when reviewing the records? In general, the therapist will want to keep the case conceptualization ques-

Instructions: Record your activity for each hour of the day, and record a mood rating associated with each activity. Use the scale below with the anchors that you and your therapist develop to guide your mood rating. Aim to make entries on your Activity Record at least every 3–4 hours each day.

	Monday	Tuesday	Wednesday	Thursday	Friday	Saturday	Sunday
5–6							
6–7							
7–8							
8–9							
9–10							
10–11							
11–12							
12–1							
1–2							
2–3							
3–4							
4–5							
5–6							
6–7							
7–8							
8–9							
9–10							
10–11							
11–12							
12–1							
1–2							
2–3							
3–4							
4–5							

Mood Ratings: 0: Feeling really good; not depressed at all *(Examples of associated activities:* _____)

5: Intermediate *(Examples of associated activities:* _____)

10: Feeling the worst *(Examples of associated activities:* _____)

FIGURE 8.1. Activity Record (hourly).

tions listed earlier in the forefront of his or her mind when reviewing a completed activity log. The therapist reviews the Activity Record to understand the client's activities, routines, and life context, and to begin to identify patterns that may be maintaining or exacerbating depressed mood.

Specific questions that therapists can use to guide their review of activity schedules are listed below:

- What would the client be doing if he or she were not depressed (working, managing family responsibilities, exercising, socializing, engaging in leisure activities, eating, sleeping, etc.)?
- Is the client engaging in a wide variety of activities, or have his or her activities become narrow?
- What is the relationship between specific activities and mood?
- What is the relationship between specific life contexts/problems and mood?
- In what ways are avoidance and withdrawal maintaining or exacerbating depression? What does the client avoid or from what is he or she pulling away? In what specific ways? Are there routine disruptions?
- Where has contact with reinforcers been lost?
- Are there deficits in coping skills and strategies?

To answer these questions, it is essential to focus on the parts of the client's activity and context that change and the parts that are consistent over time. It is not uncommon for depressed clients to report that their mood is always low, no matter what they are doing or where they are doing it. They may describe that they simply feel "blah" all the time or that, perhaps, their mood changes, but such changes are minor or irrelevant. A central premise of BA, however, is that variability is everywhere, though sometimes it is difficult to detect. Moreover, the variability is not random. Instead, *variations in behavior and its settings have a direct effect on a person's mood* and, as such, provide critical information about central contingencies. When clients report that they feel depressed "all the time," it is either because they are inaccurately reporting on their mood retrospectively, their behavioral repertoires are extremely narrow (e.g., lying in bed all day long), or they have not learned to discriminate between subtle differences in mood. This last point is a critical one. One of the key tasks for therapists is to help clients understand that their moods are intimately linked to what they are doing, where they are doing it, and the resulting consequences. Treating depression requires making a series of strategic changes in each of these domains, all of which are based on understanding the basic contingent relationships.

Repeatedly Applying and Troubleshooting Activation and Engagement Strategies

Given the idiographic nature of BA, the course of treatment may look quite different across a range of clients. Despite this diversity, a few, straightforward behavioral methods are frequently used. These are discussed below.

Activity Scheduling and Self-Monitoring

The major work of therapy in BA occurs between treatment sessions. It is uncommon for clients to leave a session without some specific activities with which to experiment during the week. Thus, activity scheduling and monitoring of outcome are standard methods used throughout treatment. At the end of each session, the client should clearly understand the specific activity assignment and have a clear strategy for implementing it during the week.

Specifically scheduling the activity is a useful tool for having the client commit to times when he or she will do the homework. When the assignment is listed in writing on a particular day of the week, at a particular hour, the client has the benefit of an external aid to motivate behavior change (i.e., working from the "outside-in" as opposed to the "inside-out"). Activity scheduling is also used frequently for clients with significant routine disruptions. Schedules can be an aid in the effort to develop and follow regular routines for eating, working, sleeping, exercising, and maintaining social contact. Depending on the activity, the client may not specifically schedule the time, but may instead record its completion on a daily log.

A key part of scheduling activities frequently involves careful attention to contingency management. As social psychologists have long known, "The correlations between intention and behavior are modest . . . the weak intention–behavior relation is largely due to people having good intentions but failing to act on them" (Gollwitzer, 1999, p. 493). Given this reality, it is essential for BA therapists to consider ways they can help clients structure their environment so as to maximize success with treatment assignments and goals. One helpful method of contingency management is the use of public commitment to enhance the likelihood of completing assignments (Locke & Latham, 2002). Often, we explore whether friends, coworkers, or family members are available to be included in activation plans. For instance, one of our clients learned in treatment that when his depression was more severe, it was essential for him to tell his wife each morning the primary tasks he intended to complete that day. For him, "keeping his word" was an effective reinforcer that helped to increase his activation. In addition, we work with clients to structure their environments in ways that will enhance activation. Thus, for a client who works on an exercise plan during the week, putting on her exercise clothes before she leaves work at the end of the day is an essential part of the plan. Finally, clients may also experiment with the use of arbitrary reinforcers for specific behavior change tasks. Although the emphasis of BA is heavily on increasing contact with natural reinforcers in one's environment, the selective use of arbitrary reinforcers can at time be helpful. The client we noted earlier planned a special dinner with his wife at the end of a week of adherence with activation tasks; the client who was working on the exercise program bought a new shirt for exercising after she started her new program.

Occasionally, therapists may suggest the use of aversive contingencies to help promote behavior change; for instance, one client found it useful to agree to call his therapist if he was going to stay in bed and miss work for the day. We have described to other clients the method of writing donation checks to their least favored charities, which are then cashed if they do not complete scheduled activities (Watson & Tharp, 2002). Often, simply the suggestion of an aversive contingency is sufficient to motivate change. For instance, the client who agreed to call his therapist did, in fact, call early one Monday morning; when he was halfway through leaving a message, he stated, "This is ridiculous. Forget it, I am going to work."

When clients do activity scheduling, it is also essential to build in a monitoring component such that they record the context and consequences of activation. This provides both information about the specific activation assignment, and regular and ongoing practice in noticing contingent relationships between activity and mood. It is essential for the therapist to discuss what the client learned from the activation and self-monitoring tasks in each session. In addition, the therapist needs to provide regular feedback about progress and to highlight areas of improvement or

troubleshoot problems that may have arisen. It is essential for the therapist not to shy away from asking about homework that is incomplete or not done. Attending to these domains is exactly the job of the BA therapist. Repeated and persistent focus on a small set of activation tasks often occupies a great deal of the course of treatment. Asking about what prevented the completion of homework gives the therapist and client essential information about important barriers and possible examples of avoidance patterns. The purpose of such discussions is not to punish or shame the client, so it is important to approach homework review with a direct and nonjudgmental attitude. At the same time, discussing incomplete or partially completed homework may be experienced as aversive by the client, which may help to facilitate his or her doing the homework next time (i.e., through being negatively reinforced by escaping from the therapist's uncomfortable questioning). If this occurs naturally, it is not a problem and can in fact enhance treatment progress. However, the therapist should never use shame or criticism, however subtly, to enhance homework completion.

Graded Task Assignment

Graded task assignment, which is a core part of cognitive therapy for depression (Beck et al., 1979), is also a hallmark of BA and a key part of most activity scheduling efforts. Thus, it is important for therapists to help clients break down behaviors into specific, achievable units to facilitate successful behavior change. Knowing how to break down tasks and grade them appropriately in a stepwise progression from simple to complex requires therapists to use a broad array of basic self-management and problem-solving skills. Toward this end, it is also important for therapists to help clients learn the method of grading tasks during therapy, so that they can apply this skill to new contexts and tasks after therapy has ended. In explaining the tool of graded task assignment, it is often important to remind clients that the goal is not to accomplish all parts of the activity; rather, the goals are to get started on important tasks, increase activation, and disrupt avoidance. Therapists can also explain to clients that breaking tasks down helps to ensure success with subtasks, and such success experiences can in turn reinforce and motivate work on successive components of the larger task.

It is very important to break down tasks in such a way that early success is guaranteed. If clients experience difficulty with tasks, therapists may want to revisit explicitly whether the task was broken down and graded sufficiently. Clients also can be asked to envision the steps involved in a given task before attempting it outside of therapy, and to anticipate any obstacles that might arise. If this process suggests that certain components may be difficult to master, the therapist and client can grade that task into smaller and more achievable components.

Avoidance Modification and Problem Solving

This is perhaps one of the most rich and varied aspects of BA. As noted earlier, clients may be addressing avoidance of concrete tasks at work or home, avoidance of painful emotions such as grief or fear, avoidance of interpersonal conflict, and so forth. The specific methods used to address these areas are tied to the specific nature of the avoidance. For instance, a client who avoids the experience of grief over a lost relationship may be assisted in spending time each day reviewing photos of the former partner, reminiscing about times they shared, and so forth. A client who avoids tasks at work may be assisted in breaking down tasks, making specific to-do lists, asking others for help, and so forth. A client who avoids interpersonal conflict may be assisted in practicing assertive communication in role plays in sessions, experimenting with discussions with friends, bringing a family member to a therapy session, and so forth. That said, within this broad domain, a number of basic strategies may be helpful in planning treatment.

First, it is essential when addressing avoidance to start from a collaborative stance with the client. It is important to understand and communicate an understanding of the discomfort that a client may experience in a particular situation, which is then followed by some action on the part of the client to end the aversive experience. Therapists can emphasize the ways that avoidance may serve an adaptive function in the short term but be problematic in the long term. Given that many avoidant behaviors may

be under the control of immediate contingencies, it is often helpful to highlight repeatedly the long-term consequences of particular behaviors.

Second, basic problem-solving methods are frequently used to address avoidance. Although we rarely teach problem-solving steps in a structured and formal manner, addressing avoidance typically involves figuring out how to approach and solve problems. Thus, it is essential for therapists to maintain a problem-solving mindset with respect to avoidance and to work with clients to generate a range of options for possible alternative coping behaviors. Problem-solving strategies include defining and assessing the problem, generating alternative solutions, managing environmental contingencies, and trouble-shooting the solution when needed. It should also be noted that all of the other basic strategies are also frequently used in the service of avoidance modification and problem solving (e.g., activity scheduling and monitoring, graded task assignment, etc.).

Third, to help maintain a consistent focus on avoidance, clients may be assisted by several mnemonic devices. These devices help to organize a method of examining, "What is the function of a behavior; what are its consequences?" We have used the acronym ACTION to identify the general approach that we ask clients to take (Martell et al., 2001):

- Assess—Is this behavior approach or avoidance? Will it be likely to make me feel better or worse?
- Choose—Either choose to continue this behavior, even if it makes me feel worse, or try a new behavior.
- Try—Try the behavior chosen.
- Integrate—Any new behavior needs to be given a fair chance, so integrate new behaviors into a routine before assessing whether it has been helpful or not.
- Observe the Results—Pay close attention and monitor the effects of the new behavior.
- Never Give Up—Remembering that making changes can often require repeated efforts and attempts.

When clients demonstrate behavioral patterns characterized by avoidance behaviors, therapists may use the acronym of being in a TRAP (Martell et al., 2001):

- Trigger—usually something in the environment (e.g., criticized by employer)
- Response—usually an emotional reaction (e.g., feels shame and sadness)
- Avoidance Pattern—The avoidance behavior(s) used to cope with the emotional response (e.g., leaves work early, complains to partner about displeasure with job)

Therapists then ask the client to get out of the TRAP and back on TRAC; that is, under the same trigger and response conditions they are asked to experiment with "Alternative Coping" behaviors.

Engagement Strategies

Research has well documented the frequency and negative consequences of ruminative behavior among people with depression (Nolen-Hoeksema, 2000). The BA approach considers ruminating as a behavior that frequently prevents people from engaging fully with their activities and environments. BA therapists are on alert for client reports of ruminating and are also careful to assess whether ruminating is a problem when clients return to sessions reporting that an activation assignment "didn't work." If, for example, a client reports that she experienced little mood improvement while playing with her son in the park, the therapist will want to examine whether she was only partially engaged with the task of playing because her mind was focused on why her former partner did not want to continue their relationship, what that meant about her value as a woman, and so forth.

In addressing rumination in BA, we are less interested in the particular content of ruminative thoughts than in the context and consequences of rumination. For instance, in working with a client who frequently ruminated about a job that he regretted having declined, the BA therapist asked him to examine the following types of questions: What were you doing while you were thinking about the other job? How engaged were you with the activity of the moment and with your surroundings? What happened during and after your thinking about the other job? In examining these questions, the therapist and client identified that the client was more likely to ruminate when he was working on aversive tasks in his current job, about which he felt significant anxiety; thus,

ruminating was negatively reinforced by distracting the client from anxiety and decreasing his focus on the aversive tasks. BA therapists may ask clients who ruminate frequently to experiment with "attention to experience" practice, in which they deliberately focus their attention on their current activity and surroundings. For instance, they may be asked to bring their full awareness to physical sensations (colors, sounds, smells, tastes, physical movements, etc.). These strategies are akin to mindfulness practices (Segal, Williams, & Teasdale, 2001) and are also very consistent with the dialectical behavior strategy of "opposite action all the way" (Linehan, 1993).

Reviewing and Consolidating Treatment Gains

As the therapist and client agree that there has been sufficient improvement and termination seems indicated, remaining sessions should focus on relapse prevention, which largely involves reviewing and consolidating gains the client has made. Toward the end of therapy, it is often wise to focus on anticipating situations in the client's life that may trigger depressive feelings and behaviors, and to generate plans for coping with such situations. Upcoming life events that can be anticipated as challenges for the client (e.g., the death of a parent, a career change) should be discussed in detail, and the client can draft a self-help plan to activate in the face of the stressor. In addition, it is also very important to review the basic methods used in therapy to ensure that the client is leaving with a solid understanding of how to apply these as tools in the future. For instance, therapists will want to review how to approach mood from a behavioral perspective (e.g., identifying the pattern of antecedents and consequences), how to set specific and concrete goals, how to use graded task assignment, and how to identify and target primary avoidance patterns (noticing that one is ruminating more at work, noticing that one is starting to fail to return phone calls of friends, etc.).

The Therapy Setting

BA therapy has been most widely investigated in the context of outpatient individual psychotherapy settings. Treatment duration has ranged from 12- to 24-session formats over 16 weeks. In our research protocol, sessions were offered twice per week during the first 8 weeks of treatment and once per week for the remaining 8 weeks. This intensity of sessions accommodated comparisons with other treatments included in our research designs; however, limitations of client resources, insurance reimbursement, and other factors may make such a course of therapy impractical in many treatment settings. Twice-weekly appointments are always be recommended in the beginning of therapy with severely depressed clients. When doing BA in settings that are not compatible with this level of frequency, we often schedule brief phone contacts between sessions to reinforce the interpersonal connection to the therapist and the importance of completing the between-session assignments, and to provide an opportunity to address questions or problems with the between-session assignments. Although BA is an individual treatment modality, significant others in clients' lives are often included in sessions across the course of treatment. Decisions about whether to include significant others in treatment follow from the functional analysis; thus, they are determined on an idiographic basis. Conjoint sessions can be helpful in assessing patterns that may be maintaining the client's depression, providing information and education to the family member about the treatment rationale and approach, and providing opportunities for the client and family member to practice new interpersonal behaviors with the therapist's direct and immediate feedback.

BA has also been applied in a group format. Peter Lewinsohn and colleagues developed the Coping with Depression Course for adolescents (Lewinsohn et al., 1984). This treatment program includes activity scheduling, relaxation training, assertiveness and social skills training, and cognitive restructuring. Admittedly, the inclusion of cognitive restructuring in the Coping with Depression Course places this program in the broader area of CBT rather than specific BA, but the emphasis is on scheduling pleasant events.

Therapist Qualities

In our experience, a number of qualities are important for BA therapists to bring to their clinical work. All of the BA strategies require the basic skill of being a good problem solver. Therapists approach most matters that arise in treatment simply as problems to be solved.

Thus, therapists must be naturally curious about factors that maintain problems and be skilled at generating a range of more functional alternative behaviors. Toward this end, it is important to be comfortable being concrete, specific, and structured in one's approach to therapy. In addition, therapists also need to be comfortable with a direct, matter-of-fact, and nonjudgmental manner of communication. This is essential in reviewing homework assignments effectively and troubleshooting problems that may arise. It is important to be skilled in maintaining a persistent focus on activation assignments within and across sessions. Therapists must also balance a genuine sense of empathy and understanding for the suffering and struggles of their clients with an optimistic and dogged commitment to the possibility of change. Finally, understanding basic behavioral concepts and principles can help therapists conceptualize cases according to a behavioral model of depression and present a coherent framework to clients.

In our treatment outcome research, we have used ongoing clinical supervision and therapist consultation teams to assist therapists in adhering to and refining these important therapist qualities. Therapists typically meet together weekly for 1–2 hours. The teams help therapists increase skills with basic treatment strategies (conceptualizing treatment plans, doing functional analysis, effectively grading tasks, etc.). In the context of a focus on specific cases and strategies, the team also provides essential reinforcement for the therapist qualities of empathy, nonjudgment, problem-solving curiosity and persistence, and optimism about change. Although we have not tested this hypothesis empirically, we strongly suspect that it would be difficult for many therapists to maintain these qualities in their work with clients struggling in particular with severe, complicated, or chronic depression without the support of an effective consultation team.

Client Variables

Our treatment outcome research suggests that depressed adults can experience acute and enduring clinical benefit from a course of BA. Our current work explores what specific characteristics help to predict whether a client will respond to BA. Our clinical impressions are that engagement with the basic treatment rationale and willingness to complete homework assignments are both important predictors of outcome in BA. Moreover, it is important to note that we used a number of client characteristics as exclusionary criteria in our treatment research. For instance, if a client was acutely suicidal, such that his or her risk could not be managed on an outpatient basis, then we would refer him or her for more acute and intensive treatment. In addition, if a client had a comorbid diagnostic disorder that was more severe and prominent (more interfering and the primary focus of the client), and necessitated another evidence-based treatment (e.g., obsessive–compulsive disorder), then we would also refer him or her to a more specifically appropriate treatment. We also carefully evaluated any potential medical problems that may have contributed to depression and referred clients for appropriate concurrent medical treatment, if necessary.

CASE STUDY

Background Information

The following section presents the treatment of Mark, a 43-year-old man with a long history of depression, who sought treatment after the end of his second marriage. Mark was in treatment for 19 sessions across 4 months. The description here is presented to illustrate the implementation of core BA principles and strategies. Earlier sessions are described in greater detail to provide the reader with "how-to" information regarding the primary principles and strategies. Later sessions emphasize a thematic focus for which the same types of principles and strategies are applied. It is important to emphasize at the outset that this case description is not intended to communicate a prescriptive course of treatment, and readers are advised against following the sequence of strategies in a lockstep fashion. BA is a highly idiographic treatment in which the choice of specific activation strategies is driven by functional analysis; given this, the reader is encouraged to attend to the ways the therapist conceptualizes Mark's difficulties and implements treatment strategies over the course of therapy. It is our hope that this detailed illustration will inspire readers to apply the basic principles and core strategies in a flexible and idiographic manner.

Mark sought treatment at the urging of his primary care physician. His recent episode of depression had lasted without remission for 3 years. Mark also had a history of alcohol abuse. His early alcohol abuse had caused significant problems in Mark's first marriage, which ended in divorce when he was in his early 20s; however, problems with alcohol were not a cause of current concern. He had been in therapy previously, during his separation and divorce 4 years earlier. However, Mark described it as unstructured and unfocused, and reported that he stopped going after a few sessions. He lived alone, although he had joint custody of his twin adolescent daughters; he and his ex-wife alternated parenting every other week.

Mark reported that he had had periods of depression for "as long as I can remember." In particular, he recalled his first episode of depression at age 12, shortly after his father abruptly left and severed all contact with Mark and his family. Mark reported that he had believed that his parents were happily married and, at that time, blamed himself for his father's departure. Mark reported that his mother and older siblings never discussed his father. In describing his mood during adolescence and adulthood, he reported, "I have periods when I'm able to function OK. I go to work and all that, but I'm never really happy." Mark's primary depressive symptoms included depressed mood, loss of pleasure in nearly all activities, excessive guilt, fatigue, difficulty concentrating, and occasional passive thoughts of death.

Mark had had a social network that revolved primarily around his former marriage, but he had been withdrawn from that network since his separation and divorce. Currently, he spent most of his time alone, with the exception of caring for his daughters. Mark was college educated and worked as an accountant for a local manufacturing company. He also wrote children's stories and, prior to his most recent episode of depression, was working on a number of stories as a member of a local writer's group.

Case Conceptualization and Overview of Treatment

Mark's depression was conceptualized as being controlled by a pattern of interpersonal avoidance that was negatively reinforced by reductions in grief and anxiety. Specifically, Mark had trouble fully engaging in his significant relationships and, instead, avoided intimacy in various ways that included ruminating about mistakes he made in the past, and failing to express commitment to the relationship and what he thought or felt about various topics on a regular basis. Over the course of treatment, the therapist and Mark hypothesized that avoiding close interpersonal connections in his adult life kept Mark detached enough that he would not feel subsequent losses as acutely as those he felt as a child. However, these patterns of avoidance also maintained his depression by limiting Mark's experience of reward in many of his current contexts. Treatment focused initially on increasing activation and addressing many secondary problems and routine disruptions that had become established. Although Mark increased activation relatively quickly, his mood did not improve significantly. This led to a primary focus on Mark's rumination and the ways it functioned to avoid intimacy in his relationships, and experimentation with new behaviors designed to move Mark closer to his goal of having a close intimate relationship.

Session 1

Session 1 focused on reviewing the results from the assessment process, presenting the treatment model, encouraging questions and feedback, and tailoring the model to Mark's specific experiences. The review of the assessment process is typically brief; in this part of the session, the aim of the therapist is to ensure that he or she has a solid understanding of the client's presenting problems, relevant history, and previous experience with treatment, if any. The therapist also reviews the basic diagnostic formulation to ensure that the assessment outcome matches the client's subjective experience of his or her current problems. Discussion of the treatment typically forms the bulk of the early sessions. The following transcript provides an example of the therapist presenting the treatment model and responding to frequently asked questions about the etiology of depression. Specifically, the therapist puts forth the idea that depression is treated behaviorally, regardless of etiology.

THERAPIST: Let me tell you a little about the basic model that guides BA. The first idea is that there are often things that happen in people's lives that make it hard for them to connect with the kinds of experiences that would normally help them feel good. These shifts can be clear and easy to detect changes like major losses or disruptions in life. And they can also be smaller things, like the kind of things that just bug you a little but they keep happening, or you have a bunch of them happen all around the same period of time. The most important part is the idea that the effect of these events in your life is that it's harder to connect with the kinds of experiences that could give you a sense of pleasure or accomplishment in your life, and that could help you feel better.

MARK: I would say that is true for me. There isn't much that helps me feel better. Even things that I think should help me feel better don't do much.

THERAPIST: Yes, exactly. What we find often happens is that people can respond to these changes by pulling away from their lives even more. This pulling away can happen sometimes in obvious ways, like staying in bed or calling in sick to work, or canceling social engagements, and sometimes in more subtle ways, like being focused more on your thinking than on the activities you are engaged in. The problem with pulling away like this is that it tends to keep people stuck in feeling depressed, and the pulling away can become a problem in its own right. So, the ultimate goal of our work together is to figure out what sorts of experiences may potentially have a positive effect on your mood, and then help you activate and engage to connect with these experiences. And to figure out how to solve the problems that are creating stress or dissatisfaction in your life. How do you see this fitting with your experience? Do you have questions about what I've said? Parts that fit or don't fit?

MARK: I understand what you are saying, and I think some of it fits, but I guess I don't understand why I get so depressed. I mean, other people have stressful things in their lives and they seem to function. Other people get divorced or have crappy jobs, and they move on. I mean, come on, I've been divorced for 4 years now. I think depression runs in my family. My older brother has been depressed forever, and I sometimes wonder if my dad was depressed when he took off. Sometimes, I can't really identify anything that has happened in my life. I mean, I am never really happy and then, it's just like a switch goes in my brain and I'm back in that dark hole again. But how does that fit with what you are saying?

THERAPIST: That is an excellent question. What I mean as I talk about depression is that some people are more vulnerable than others. And, there are many ways that you may be vulnerable to depression—through genetics, biology, or experiences in your history. What this treatment emphasizes is that it's possible to change depression by making changes in what you do.

MARK: That makes sense to me. One part of what you said definitely fits for me—the part about pulling away more. I definitely do that. Sometimes I don't talk to another person or get out of bed all weekend. I know it makes it all worse. But I still do it. I guess I don't really understand that part either. It fits, but it doesn't make much sense to me.

As the therapist replies to these very common questions, she seeks to normalize avoidant responses to depression. It is essential for the client to experience the therapist as someone who understands and has sincere empathy for his or her struggle. The therapist must communicate that the client's behaviors make sense, even though they may not serve the client well in the long term. In this way, the client is more likely to experience the therapist as an ally in the change process as opposed to someone who oversimplifies or "doesn't get" the challenges of making changes. Additionally, the therapist also emphasizes to Mark the importance of guided activity, highlighting her role as an expert and the importance of careful assessment. She emphasizes the difference between assignments derived from a list of pleasurable activities and those that are guided by functional analysis, a key aspect of the treatment, to which the therapist will return many times.

THERAPIST: Those are great observations and are really on target with what I have noticed for a lot of people as well. What many people experience is that when they start to activate and engage, they can actually feel worse initially! The troubling fact about pulling away or avoiding is that it does provide some short-term relief. But in the long term, it sets up a downward spiral and can keep you trapped in depression.

MARK: That makes a ton of sense to me. I just don't want to do anything. Making a meal makes me tired. I feel irritated by the sound of silverware scratching on plates. It's kind of crazy, but I just want to crawl in a hole, to turn out a light in my head and make it all go away. Then, I end up feeling worse when I do stay in bed. I used to drink, too. I knew it would make it worse, and I don't do it much anymore, but it helped in the moment, even though I knew it didn't *really* help. I guess I felt better temporarily and that was enough.

THERAPIST: Yes, exactly. Avoidance is a perfectly natural response to depression. What unfortunately happens, though, is that you are not in touch with all those things that can give you pleasure and a sense of accomplishment, *and* you are not engaged in solving the problems that create stress in your life.

MARK: I know that would help, but it just all feels so overwhelming. Just the thought of it . . .

THERAPIST: Yes, I know. That is where I come in. It's important to emphasize that this treatment is not just about me saying you should "do more" in general. Sometimes I tell people that it's not the Nike approach to therapy, where I tell you each week to "just do it." You have probably received feedback like that from other people in your life, and you may even say something similar to yourself.

MARK: Yeah, guilty as charged.

THERAPIST: My assumption is that if this were easy to figure out, you would already have done it. The reason that you are here is that it's not so easy, and that is where my expertise comes in. A major part of this treatment is the idea of *guided activation*. This means that you and I will be working together to identify specific ways in which you can experiment with activation. My expertise lies in figuring out, first, where the places are that would be the most helpful in increasing your activation and engagement, *and* second, what small and manageable steps you can take to get started. You can think of me as a coach or consultant to you in the process of change. We will work together, in small steps, all along the way. How does that sound?

MARK: The idea of it sounds good. I guess it's worth trying.

THERAPIST: I'd like to ask you to read a short

pamphlet about this treatment, between now and the next time that we meet. It will provide you with more information. When we meet next time, we can talk more about how we will put the ideas into practice.

With this initial session, the therapist has begun to teach the client about the treatment model and is getting the client actively involved in and on board with the rationale. The therapist has oriented the client to their roles in treatment and has given the client his first homework assignment (reading the treatment rationale pamphlet). These critical tasks of the first session set the stage for additional discussion in Session 2.

Session 2

In Session 2, the therapist carefully follows up on a number of the key orienting tasks, including ensuring that Mark is on board with the basic treatment model and explaining the structure of the therapy. The therapist attends to these topics in the opening of the session:

THERAPIST: It's great to see you today, Mark.

MARK: Thanks. It's good to be back here.

THERAPIST: That's great. You know, when I was thinking about our session last time, I realized that there were a couple of points I wanted to emphasize more. One of the important ones is that this is a very collaborative approach to therapy, and one that is also fairly structured. So each time we meet, we will start out by setting an agenda for the session, and we will do this collaboratively. In fact, over time, you will set the agenda more and more, though I may have more to say about it in the beginning. The idea is that I'm the expert on how to get over depression, and you are the expert on yourself and your life, and what things help or don't help.

MARK: That sounds reasonable to me.

THERAPIST: Great. So in terms of the agenda for today, I have a couple of things. I'd like to talk more about the treatment approach and your reaction, and more about how we put some of the ideas into practice. Do you have items you want to be sure we address today?

MARK: No, that sounds good. I did read the pamphlet, and it really hit home. It was like

they wrote it about me, basically. I thought, "Thank goodness somebody has figured this out."

THERAPIST: That's great. I think one of the core ideas of the model is things happen that tend to trigger depressed mood, and then people tend to do things, or not do things, that make the depression worse. For you, my understanding is that the main trigger was your divorce.

MARK: Yeah, I've really pulled back on a lot, like not exercising and not doing things with other people or even with my girls. We used to cook these great dinners together and now it's like an effort to get organized to order pizza. It's kind of like that everywhere—at work, too. I'm just managing the minimum and, honestly, a lot of times I'm not even doing that.

THERAPIST: I know. It can be very hard to keep doing the sort of things that will keep you feeling well. And that is where this therapy comes in. From our session last time and from your reading, what is your understanding of what we are going to be doing in here, and how I am going to be helpful? If you were to tell a friend of yours what we were going to do in this therapy, what would you say?

MARK: I guess I would say that we are going to pinpoint the activities that give me some pleasure or help me feel like I'm handling things well. Then, we will figure out how to help me get into the position of being more involved in some of those things.

THERAPIST: Yes, that is a big part of it. Sometimes in people's lives something that is completely beyond their control triggers depression, and then what I call secondary problem behaviors get triggered or made worse. These are the behaviors that involve pulling away or avoiding, as you were saying, like stopping fun activities with your girls or withdrawing at work. And in those cases we work on the secondary problem behaviors, and that is the core of the therapy. Other times, we also need to address larger problems in your life that may be related to what makes you vulnerable to depression. In those cases, therapy can involve *both* directly addressing the secondary problem behaviors *and* working directly on the problems, after we have kind of cleared the path for doing some problem solving by getting you activated and engaged.

MARK: That sounds like it's probably the case for me, because I know I had a lot of problems relating to Diane that were part of our divorce, and those are not any better.

THERAPIST: Yes, we will talk more as we go along about what set off the depression for you. In a global sense, we know now that it was the divorce. But, as we start following your mood and activities day to day, we will see the ways that your mood has ups and downs. We will work together and look at that carefully, asking what set that off, how you responded to your mood hitting that point, and whether it would help if you tried something different.

The therapist has now stated twice that generally a contextual event triggers depression, while earlier acknowledging that several things can contribute to vulnerability. This is a subtle but important point, because clients sometimes believe their depression came "out of the blue" or that it is simply "biological" and not modifiable by behavioral means. By emphasizing an environmental antecedent (e.g., a loss of positive reinforcement), the therapist sets up the idea that rather than depression being completely beyond patients' control, their depressive response makes sense, and more importantly, it is possible to make behavioral changes to regain or establish new reinforcers in their lives. Moreover, the therapist has continued to emphasize the importance of carefully monitoring and assessing the relationships among mood, activity, and context as a key part of designing effective behavior change plans. The therapist then builds on this foundation as she moves into the other main focus of Session 2—the initiation of activity monitoring. Here, the therapist explains to Mark why activity monitoring is important, begins to teach him how to complete an Activity Record (see Figure 8.1), and links it directly to some of his recent experiences.

THERAPIST: One of the main tools that we use in this therapy is called an Activity Record. This is one example (*hands Mark the record*); as you can see, it has blocks for each hour of the day. I'd like you to use this to start recording your activity and your mood. It's basically a way to keep track of how you are spending your time during the day and how you are feeling. We want to learn what you are doing on an hour-by-hour and day-to-day basis. What things in your life help you feel better, and what things make you feel worse? You and I will review these very carefully together, focusing on how you are spending your time and how you feel. Sometimes the Activity Record tells us right away where changes need to be made, and other times we have to look at it over a couple of weeks.

MARK: OK.

THERAPIST: Is there anything you have been doing since you started to feel more depressed that is different from what you normally do?

MARK: Yes, exercising less, watching more TV, and just the amount of time I spend thinking about all this. It's just crazy.

THERAPIST: It's hard not to do that, but also it's not helping you very much. And it's very difficult, which is why you are here. We can start to figure this out together. It's great that you are already aware of those patterns, and those are good examples of looking concretely at what you are doing. This therapy is about increasing your awareness of how your mood is affected subtly from activity to activity and increasing those that tend to be more rewarding.

MARK: So, should I write all this down? Do you really want me to do this every hour?

THERAPIST: Here's the guideline that I use: I want people to record their activity frequently enough that they are not relying heavily on memory. The problem with memory when you are depressed is that your awareness can be dulled or biased by the depression. So you don't have to do it every hour. We have to be realistic about the rest of your life! But you may want to experiment with doing it every 3–4 hours. Sometimes, people like to do it at breakfast, lunch, dinner, and before bed.

MARK: That might work for me.

THERAPIST: Let's go over what to write down. You put your activity down for each hour block and then for each hour block you also assign a mood rating from 0 to 10. Let's look at today as an example. What were you doing in the hours before you came here?

MARK: I was at work.

THERAPIST: Okay, great. What were you doing at work?

MARK: I was teaching a new employee how to use our computer system. It was really frustrating because she wasn't picking it up and I didn't have much patience.

THERAPIST: That's great information to record. Why don't you write down "working–teaching new employee." Now, I also want you to record your mood on a 0- to 10-point scale of depression, so let's see if we can get some anchors here. What would be 0 mood for you? This would mean that you feel really good, absolutely no depression or feeling down at all. What would be 10? This would be when you feel your absolute worst, the worst you could possibly feel. It might be helpful to think of some activities that are a 5 or in between, when you're not feeling your best but you're not feeling particularly bad either. Which activities might be associated with each?

The therapist and Mark then worked together to identify activities that were associated with the low, middle, and high ends of the scale. This was completed to provide Mark with anchors to use when completing the monitoring at home. It should also be noted that therapists may ask clients to rate mastery and pleasure associated with activities (Beck et al., 1979). Mastery and pleasure may be rated instead of or in addition to mood. Often we begin by asking clients to record mood ratings given that this is an easier starting place for many clients because it requires less discrimination of subjective experience; moreover, the mood rating provides essential information about the relationships between specific activities and depression. For some clients, it is helpful to build on this by teaching them how to how to distinguish between mastery and pleasure, and the ways in which both can be helpful in regulating mood. In the case of rating mood or mastery–pleasure, it is important to review carefully the method and scale we want clients to use.

THERAPIST: Given this scale, what was your mood rating for the 2 hours of "working" today?

MARK: Probably a 5.

THERAPIST: That's exactly it. Now, sometimes what happens is that people don't fill it out because they think, "I wasn't doing anything." It's important to realize that even if you are not doing an activity, we want to know that, too.

MARK: What do you mean?

THERAPIST: Well, when people think "activities," they often think of things like "going to the store," "watching a movie," "picking up my child from school." But, we are conceptualizing activity more broadly. It might be driving by Diana's house, or having a significant phone conversation with someone, or even lying in bed, spending time thinking about Diana.

MARK: That would be true on a lot of days.

THERAPIST: Yes, and you can write that down. Those are some of the most important things. In some ways, the more detail, the better. We want to start noticing subtle changes. We want to build on those times that you feel just a little better, and we want to figure out what the problem is when you feel worse.

MARK: I think I got it.

THERAPIST: Great! People usually come away from this thinking that it sounds really simplistic. And it does. It sounds simple, but in practice it is not that simple. It can be difficult to do in the beginning, to really look at all your activities and figure out how your mood is related to them. It takes skill and hard work on both our parts.

The therapist ended the session by asking Mark to review his understanding of the homework assignment, encouraged him to make contact by phone if any questions arose, and offered encouragement about the likelihood that she could be helpful to him.

Session 3

As noted earlier, one of the necessary competencies of a BA therapist is the ability to review an Activity Record and glean information that will help to customize activation and engagement strategies. Session 3 focused heavily on reviewing Mark's Activity Record (see Figure 8.2) and using the information collected as a springboard for more detailed assessment of key problem behaviors. Again, the therapist's

Instructions: Record your activity for each hour of the day, and record a mood rating associated with each activity. Use the scale below with the anchors that you and your therapist develop to guide your mood rating. Aim to make entries on your Activity Record at least every 3–4 hours each day.

	Monday	Tuesday	Wednesday	Thursday	Friday	Saturday	Sunday
5-6							
6-7			Awake, thinking in bed (9)				
7-8							
8-9		At work (7)					
9-10			Getting ready for work (8)				
10-11			At work (7)				
11-12							
12-1							
1-2							
2-3							
3-4	Working/ teaching employee (5)	Home (7)					
4-5							
5-6							
6-7	Therapy (5)	Making Dinner (6)					
7-8		TV (9)	TV (9)				
8-9							
9-10							
10-11							
11-12							
12-1							
1-2							
2-3							
3-4							
4-5							

Mood Ratings: 0: Feeling really good; not depressed at all (*Examples of associated activities:* writing; playing with my kids   )

5: Intermediate (*Examples of associated activities:* doing a work task that is only moderately interesting but I'm focused and concentrating   )

10: Feeling the worst (*Examples of associated activities:* thinking about how I've screwed everything up   )

FIGURE 8.2. Sample completed Activity Record (hourly) (assigned on Monday and reviewed on Thursday).

focus in these early sessions is on increasing activation in areas that will improve Mark's mood; this work will set the foundation for later work on avoidance modification and problem solving.

THERAPIST: Shall we go over your Activity Record?

MARK: Okay. (*Hands the therapist the record.*)

THERAPIST: Why don't you walk me through it? (*Hands the record back to Mark.*)

MARK: I'm not sure if this is what you had in mind. I started the next day after our last session. I went to work that day, but I was feeling so lousy that I left early and came home. I was just kind of fiddling around the house until dinner. I felt really down all day up to that point; I rated my mood as a 7. I did make dinner, which was a little better for me. I used to love to cook for Diana and myself, and we would make these big feasts sometimes with the girls. Since the divorce, though, sometimes I just grab a bag of chips or something like that, or on a good night, I might order a pizza. When I was cooking, I felt a little better then, about a 5.

THERAPIST: This is terrific. You did a really great job with this. You completed the record exactly as we talked about—writing down your activities and also your mood rating—and all of this information is extremely useful. I want to ask you some more questions about specific parts of the day in a minute, but right now let me just get an overall sense of things.

Notice how the therapist is careful to reinforce her client's efforts early in the review process. Clients are often uncertain about how to complete the record, and it is not uncommon for them to return with partially or improperly completed records. In such cases, therapists must balance the need to provide corrective feedback and to reinforce the client's efforts. Frequent client errors include writing down activities very globally (e.g., "at work" for 6 hours), failing to record mood ratings, or failing to record anything because they did "nothing." In such cases, the therapist should address these problems in a straightforward and matter-of-fact manner.

THERAPIST: What happened after you made dinner?

MARK: Well, after dinner, I started watching TV, and everything kind of tanked from there. I sat and watched TV until 2:00 in the morning. I guess it helped in that it kept my mind off of worries about work and just feeling lousy about Diana, but I was really depressed the whole time. In fact, I rated my mood as a 9.

THERAPIST: That is really important information. I see that you were also up the next night watching TV until 1:00 A.M. Is this true of a lot of nights for you, or are these two more like exceptions?

MARK: I wish they were exceptions, but no, it's been more the rule. And then what happens is that I just can't get up in the morning. Well, I guess I do wake up, but I just lie there in bed. I've been getting to work pretty late, and some days I just call in sick.

THERAPIST: So we'll use this log to pick up themes of specific activities that can help you feel good and those that may be contributing to your depression. It seems like there are a few that might be important. I'm thinking that the watching TV and going to bed late is one big one, and the other two are cooking and how you are doing at work.

MARK: I think the TV is a really big one.

Notice here that the therapist identified a few broad areas that appear to be related to the maintenance of the client's depression. The BA therapist is also alert to disruptions in the client's normal routines; in Mark's case, both eating and sleeping routines appear to have been significantly altered. The therapist then works collaboratively with Mark to target a specific area for further assessment and problem solving (i.e., nighttime TV watching). At this point, the therapist begins the more explicit process of functional analysis.

THERAPIST: OK, why don't we start there? Let's get clear first about what the problem is, because it doesn't sound like it's watching TV in general.

MARK: That's true. Normally, I would watch some TV, like I might watch for an hour. But, actually, come to think of it, I was more involved in my writing then, too. So, normally, I might watch TV until about 9:00 P.M. and then turn off the TV and write for another hour. Or, if I had the girls, we might watch a show together and then turn off the TV and read or play a game, or just hang out together, or maybe I'd be on a phone call or something.

THERAPIST: So, this is different for you. The problem, then, is that you don't turn off the TV at 9:00 P.M. and instead watch it for an additional 4–5 hours.

MARK: Yes, that's the problem.

THERAPIST: Are you doing this every night of the week or just on work nights?

MARK: I hate to admit it, but it's pretty much all nights, not always so late, but pretty much always later than is good for me.

To this point, the therapist has worked successfully to define the problem in specific and behavioral terms. With a clear and mutual understanding of the problem, the therapist and client can begin to consider the contingencies that may be maintaining the problem and what may be amenable to change.

THERAPIST: We should probably look at what gets in the way of turning the TV off, since it does not seem to have a great effect on your mood. If you were to turn off the TV at 9:00 P.M. now, what do you think would happen?

MARK: I thought about turning it off last night, but I just didn't want to think about all of this stuff.

THERAPIST: By "all this stuff," do you mean the divorce and the pressures at work?

MARK: Yes, both of them.

THERAPIST: So, that is what you are actively avoiding. And the TV helps you to distract?

MARK: Yes, I just don't have the mental awareness now to start writing. I can't focus on it, and I'm just not interested.

THERAPIST: I think you have the right idea in terms of distraction, but the problem is that you are distracting yourself with something that doesn't give you much pleasure and not much accomplishment.

MARK: And meanwhile the house is a mess. I haven't paid my bills in months, and . . .

THERAPIST: I think it might be good to help you solve the problem of watching TV. It might

be simple to solve, but my guess is that there is more to understand about it.

Notice how easily the client can become overwhelmed and hopeless in response to the myriad problems in his life. The therapist is alert to this possibility during sessions and is careful to refocus the client on the problem at hand. In addition, the therapist also takes a keen interest in the "minutiae" of the client's day-to-day behavior, particularly if such behavior is related to mood. This detailed level of interest is critical. Its intent is twofold: First, such discussions guide the choice of activation targets and specific assignments; and second, it is the intent that such discussions will teach Mark to take a similar interest and begin to notice patterns that are more and less helpful in working his way out of depression.

THERAPIST: Let's understand better what happens with the TV. Does it come into your mind, the thought that you might be better off if you turned off the TV?

MARK: Typically, I think, "I should go to bed." But I know that if I go to bed, I'll just lie there awake anyway, thinking about what Diana is doing, thinking about how much I am going to hate being at work the next day. So, then I think I might as well watch TV and distract myself.

THERAPIST: Is that what happens in bed? You lie there and ruminate about Diana or things you have done or haven't done at work?

MARK: Pretty much exactly.

In this transcript, the therapist has effectively identified a number of key relationships. These include the following: (1) nighttime TV watching is associated with deteriorated mood; (2) nighttime TV watching is associated with poor performance at work; and (3) nighttime TV watching is potentially maintained via a process of negative reinforcement in which negative affect (specifically, grief and anxiety) are reduced when the client is watching TV. The therapist has done so in a collaborative and nonjudgmental manner, and the client is on board. At this point, the therapist explicitly examines her hypothesis with Mark about the relationship between TV and mood. On the basis of this understanding, they can then consider possible activation strategies.

THERAPIST: I'm wondering if part of what is happening is that watching TV is helpful in the short run, because it takes your mind away from these topics that are connected to a lot of potential sadness and also anxiety about the future.

MARK: Yeah, that's true.

THERAPIST: But the tough part is that while it works in the short run, it's that same vicious cycle in the long run, because watching TV gives you almost no pleasure and it keeps you from doing activities that you previously got a lot out of, and it sets you up for having problems at work.

MARK: Yes, exactly. It's crazy, I know, but it's such an easy way out when I'm just beaten by the day.

THERAPIST: Absolutely! So we have to take that into account when we think about making any changes here. I'm thinking that you could try going to bed in spite of that, and we could work on the ruminating. Or, if you are going to be up, you could do things that are better than the TV. Which do you lean toward?

The therapist attends to the function (distraction) of the problem behavior (TV watching), while engaging in problem solving in a very collaborative manner.

MARK: Probably finding other things, better than the TV. I used to go to a book group one night a week. It was made up of other writers and I liked a few of the people a lot, so when I was doing that, I was also doing reading in the evenings, too.

THERAPIST: OK, does reading seem more of a way you could start getting back into some of your writing, versus jumping in with writing itself?

MARK: Yes, there is no way I could write now. I would just be staring at a blank page, feeling like crap.

THERAPIST: OK, that makes sense. So what about starting with this? One option is that you could have a limit for yourself of 9:00 P.M. for TV and we could work on identifying a book that you could read instead.

MARK: It's a good idea. It's more a question of my doing it.

It is very important that the therapist not gloss over comments such as Mark's final statement. When clients express doubt about how or whether they will implement an activation strategy, it is essential to attend to this in detail. Additionally, it is helpful for the therapist to be attentive to statements such as "I'll just have to make myself do it," which generally indicate that the therapist and client have not sufficiently identified the contingencies that control the behavior. In our experience, use of sheer willpower is unlikely to meet with great success, and suggestions of such signal that further assessment is required, as the therapist illustrates.

THERAPIST: So we need to be sure we are getting at the real problem, instead of just saying, "Oh, you are going to do this," and leaving it at that. What kind of reader are you? Are you someone who can get really involved in a book?

MARK: I do get really involved. In fact, I'll think about the book a lot during the day, if I'm already into it.

THERAPIST: But getting yourself to do it is hard.

MARK: Yes, it's getting started on things.

THERAPIST: That is great to know. So, we have to somehow get you involved in the book so that when 9:00 P.M. rolls around, you are already involved, so it will be easier to turn off the TV.

MARK: That would make it easier.

THERAPIST: What if you were to buy a book on the way back from our session and begin reading it in the café of the bookstore.

MARK: Oh, yeah, that is right on the way back. I can do that.

THERAPIST: Mark, I think the trick with all of this is to figure out what is going to help you move toward the things that will be beneficial for your mood. And this is what is really hard—getting yourself to go back to the things that you used to enjoy, when you have no interest in them right now. When you feel good, you take it for granted that it's easy to do things like reading, spending time with friends or your girls, and even writing. When you don't feel good, you really notice it. The problem is that you're in this vicious cycle again. The longer you do not do things, the more badly you feel and the less you want to do. The trick for us is to figure out ways to help you start to do some of the things that will give you pleasure again.

The therapist acknowledges to the client that the new behavior will be hard to initiate because of mood, and that it is necessary to do so anyway. Many times, clients employ an "inside-out" or mood-dependent approach to their depression; that is, they passively wait for their mood to improve before making behavioral changes. BA therapists teach clients that when they feel down, they cannot afford to wait for a better mood to strike them. The goal is to get active when they feel bad (as hard as that is). Increasing activation will eventually improve mood, even if not immediately, and it will interrupt the pattern of secondary problems created by withdrawal and avoidance. Addressing mood-dependent behavior (or talking about an outside-in vs. inside-out approach) is a sensitive point in therapy, in which a *great* deal of empathy for the experience of feeling depressed is required. *The therapist must skillfully balance encouragement for action with validation of the difficulty of activating when depressed.* In addition, heavily reinforcing the client (frequently with the use of significant praise) for any steps taken is essential in supporting the process of change.

MARK: Yeah, I know. A lot of the time I might know what I need to do, but I have no idea how to get myself to do it. I've just dropped a lot of stuff, like anything social in the evenings. I don't try to make plans. And, like I said, for almost a year I was going to that writer's book group every Thursday. But then I said to myself, I'm not writing. This whole divorce is wiping me out. What is the point of going? I have nothing to add." But, it's true that when I went, I used to get a lot out of it. I'm just not interested now, though.

THERAPIST: Yes, exactly. That's where you and I will work together. I want to come back to the social connections and the routines around writing, but let's stick with the reading and nighttime TV for a bit longer first, if that's OK?

MARK: Yeah, that makes sense.

THERAPIST: Let's think through this book plan again. Is there anything that might come up

between here and the bookstore that would derail that plan?

At this point, the therapist and Mark spend the remainder of the session discussing particular books he could purchase that would maximize his engagement, and they discuss potential barriers that might arise to derail him from the intended plan. They also continued to review the Activity Record to identify other key problems, including ruminating at work, withdrawing from social networks, and experiencing disruptions in routines that previously brought him pleasure (e.g., cooking, exercise). In each case, the therapist uses a similar method that she used with the problem of TV watching: defining the problem, identifying the antecedent and consequences, and checking out hypotheses about how the activity is related to mood with client. In each case, the therapist also continues to emphasize that simply deciding to "make myself do it" is not likely to be an effective activation strategy for Mark, and that it is essential to tie the activation plan to a clear understanding of the function of the problem behaviors. The therapist employs a combination of gentle prompting, consistent validation of the difficulty of the tasks and understanding of the temptation of withdrawal and avoidance, and repeated discussion of potential barriers to activation plans. Importantly, the therapist also highlights for Mark that compliance with the homework assignments may not bring immediate relief.

"What will be really good this week is to see what effect these things have on your mood. Even if they have just a little bit of a positive effect, then we know that we are on the right track. And, Mark, they might not have an immediate positive effect on your mood. It might be that the act of getting yourself to do it is the success itself, and that you need to keep doing it for a while before you start to feel good again. But, it's my guess that some of this stuff will help your mood a little bit, even in the short run."

The session concluded with the therapist and Mark reviewing the homework assignments, which included purchasing a new book, starting to read it in the café, and turning off the TV every night at 9:00 P.M. and reading. In addition, they agreed that Mark would return a telephone call of an old friend, Mary, who lived in his neighborhood and had been trying to contact him recently.

Session 4

Mark returned to Session 4 with little improvement in the severity of his depression. He reported that he had increased his social contact, but that he was not feeling any better. Mark also had delayed the task of purchasing the new book and continued to watch TV late at night. The therapist addressed both of these problems in a direct, matter-of-fact way.

MARK: It was a really bad weekend. I did call Mary and ended up going to this kind of cocktail party at the community pool that she had organized. I was kind of shocked that I went, but I thought being outside would do me good. I was thinking about what we were talking about, and I thought about how much I used to love swimming. I was actually a lifeguard during summers in college. But I think I felt worse after I went. I suppose there were moments that were fun, but I was so frustrated by it all. I just spent the rest of the weekend holed up in my apartment.

THERAPIST: Would that be good to put on the agenda? Doing things that you used to enjoy and not enjoying them?

MARK: Sure.

THERAPIST: And I want to make sure we check in about how it went with the book versus the TV, too. Which do you want to talk about first—calling Mary and the party or the TV?

MARK: I guess we can do the TV first. I just bought the book today. On Friday, I was at that party, so I didn't get home and in bed until midnight.

THERAPIST: Did you watch TV then?

MARK: No, I do think I was more tired from being outside all night, so I just fell asleep when I got back.

THERAPIST: And what about Saturday and last night?

MARK: It was kind of par for the course. I stayed up late both nights.

Given the importance of attending consistently and regularly to the completion of home-

work, here the therapist assesses what interfered with Mark's full completion of the previous assignment.

THERAPIST: I'm glad you bought the book. What got in the way of getting it sooner? Am I recalling correctly that you were going to buy it on the way back from the session last week?

MARK: Yeah, I was, but when I left someone called me from work about needing to meet, so I didn't have as much time as I thought. But I thought I could do it after work, and then in the evening, I thought, "I'll get it on the weekend because I'll have more time." I don't know.

THERAPIST: If you go back to your leaving the session last time, when you got the phone call from work, was there anything else that derailed the plan?

MARK: No, that was really it. I was still pretty optimistic about getting the book. It was just that I didn't have as much time as I thought I would, and I had to get to work.

THERAPIST: OK, that is good to know. So your plan was to get the book on the weekend, and you just bought it today. On the weekend, did you think about getting it, or did it just come up again today?

MARK: I did, but I felt so bad after the party I just couldn't get myself to do it.

THERAPIST: It sounds like you were really down. Let's talk about the party in a bit. I'm curious how it was that you got yourself to get the book today. Are you feeling better, or is it something else?

MARK: I'm not feeling quite as bad, and given that I was already out, it was easier to go get the book. Plus I knew that we were going to meet and you were probably going to ask me about it.

THERAPIST: That is so great to know! So one thing we know is that I have got to keep following up about these things, because it helps you do them.

MARK: (*laughing a little*) True, not that I was enjoying imagining being called to task on it, but it did help, I guess.

THERAPIST: And getting yourself out of the house to buy a book this weekend was a lot harder then getting yourself out this morning, since you were already leaving to go to work. Being out already made it easier to accomplish your task.

MARK: Right. That sort of thing seems to happen a lot lately.

THERAPIST: So one solution would be to not wait for the weekend when you've got a specific task to do, because that seems to be a harder time for you to accomplish things. The other thing would be for us to set up a system of phone check-ins when you are feeling particularly down, since it seems to help to know that we will be following up on these tasks when we meet. The other issue, though, is to figure out what brought you down so much this weekend, and what to do about that.

MARK: I think that is the biggest thing.

THERAPIST: Shall we talk a bit about the party and the weekend in order to figure out what is going to help most? How does that sound? And we'll make sure to come back to the TV and reading plan.

MARK: OK. I would like not to feel as lousy as I was feeling.

THERAPIST: Why don't we take a look at your Activity Record? (*Reviews the record.*) It looks like your mood ratings were moderate on Thursday and Friday after we met. Then, Friday, at the party and for the rest of the weekend, they were high, 7's, 8's, and 9's, too.

MARK: I'm not sure this is for me, honestly. I think I gave it a fair shot, calling Mary, going to the party. I didn't want to do either, but I did. And I felt worse afterwards.

When clients report that they are increasing activation and their mood is not improving, it is important to assess a number of possible explanations. First, therapists may consider whether the activation assignments were too ambitious and did not incorporate successful grading. In such cases, it is important for therapists to acknowledge responsibility for this and recommend assignment based on smaller components of the task. Second, therapists want to consider whether the functional analysis was accurate. Is it possible that they are activating the client in a domain that is unlikely to yield improvements in mood? Third, therapists want to consider whether ruminative thinking is interfering with activation. In such cases, clients "physically" engage in the activation assign-

ments, whereas "mentally" they remain disengaged from their context and are less likely to have an opportunity to contact whatever reinforcement is available. Fourth, it is possible that although activation may not immediately improve mood, it may still be "on the right track," because clients are taking active steps toward solving problems and addressing important life goals.

In Mark's case, the therapist decided initially to pursue the possibility that rumination was interfering with activation, based on Mark's comments in earlier sessions about frequently ruminating about Diana and their divorce.

THERAPIST: I guess one thing we could explore together is what was on your mind during the party. When you were standing by the pool talking to other people, or even swimming in the water, what was on your mind?

MARK: You know, when I was diving into the water, I do remember that those were the pleasurable moments of the party. The sound of the water splashing, the coolness, the silence under the water, that was all great. That is what I used to love about swimming too. But the other part—I think I was mentally checking out. I was with a lot of people I really like. Mary is great, and her whole family was back visiting from the East Coast. I haven't seen them in years and I really enjoy all of them. They are great people. But, it didn't really matter. I just wasn't there.

THERAPIST: Were you thinking about Diana or yourself in relation to her?

MARK: Yeah, that was mainly it.

THERAPIST: Were the other folks there conversing with you?

MARK: Yes, and I was talking with them. I mean, I could hear the words coming out of my mouth, but I was just not there.

THERAPIST: So you have one rating on this record for the party, a 7. But, if we were to break these different pieces apart—the swimming, when you were fully engaged with the activity, and the talking, when your mind was elsewhere—what would you rate each?

MARK: The swimming . . . it was good. I guess that would be a 3, if 0 is feeling good; I mean it didn't take it all away. But the talking . . . that was terrible, a 9.

The therapist has successfully identified the problem that was interfering with the potential benefits of activation. She continues to assess the nature and scope of the problem.

THERAPIST: I'm trying to figure out if when you are actively engaged in an activity, which kind of requires some attention to it, are those the times that are more enjoyable?

MARK: Yeah, that's true.

THERAPIST: Is this a problem that also interferes with your mood and accomplishment of tasks at work?

MARK: Yes, exactly. I go into my office and it's like where does the time go? Hours go by and I haven't done a damn thing. I'm just wandering over and over things that happened with Diana, what I said, what I could have said. It's awful.

THERAPIST: OK, so we know this is an important problem to address. It's interfering with your enjoyment of times that have the potential to improve your mood, and it's interfering with managing your job well. Can we spend a little more time on what happened at the party?

MARK: OK.

THERAPIST: How would you normally be when talking with Mary's family, if you were not thinking about all these things? What would I see differently in those times than what I might have observed on Friday?

MARK: I'd be talking to everyone. I wouldn't be feeling so bad.

THERAPIST: Yes, that is exactly true. What I'm really curious about is, when you are not feeling so bad, what would you be doing differently? Would you be asking them more questions? Making more eye contact? Responding differently?

MARK: Yeah, all of those things. I'd be more active in the conversation.

THERAPIST: So you would be more engaged.

MARK: Yes, more engaged. Less of that heavy feeling; you know, that "this really sucks" feeling.

In the preceding portion of the session, the therapist has begun to define behaviorally what Mark does in interpersonal interactions when he is not depressed. Carefully specifying these behaviors is an important step in developing some possible plans for targeted change in how Mark approaches similar situations.

THERAPIST: Do you think that if you could practice talking, when you weren't feeling down, more like you normally would with these people that you might feel better?

MARK: I don't know.

THERAPIST: I think the key is to notice what you do in response to the ruminating and to see whether that is helping or not helping your mood, and then for us to begin to explore what you may need to do differently. It seems that at the party, what you were doing when your mood was better, was to be more engaged.

MARK: It's true. But, when I'm like this, I don't have much to say.

THERAPIST: Yes, when you are depressed, you are more quiet and withdrawn.

MARK: Yes, because it's painful. I see Mary's parents and I think, "They've been married for 30 years. I could have had that with Diana." Then, I start thinking that she is with someone else. It just goes downhill from there.

THERAPIST: You are absolutely right. There is a lot of pain there. And what's happened is that in response to that pain, you have narrowed activity in your life. So you not only feel the pain of being reminded of that loss, but also there is not a lot else going on in your life. And even when you are doing things, you are not as engaged, because you are feeling so much pain. I think we need to get you back to doing the things you did before you had the breakup, and before the two of you got together. We need to get you back to your baseline, and once we do that, we can figure out how to get you feeling even better than that.

MARK: It sounds good.

THERAPIST: I know you are thinking this is like pie in the sky, but we can figure out how to do this. The key is to figure out some concrete and manageable steps to help you engage more when you are doing some of these activities, like going to the party. You are right. It's worlds harder to do when you are not feeling well, but these behaviors are partly why you enjoyed those occasions more in the past. We know that you enjoyed

Mary and her family in the past, and we know that you got a lot of pleasure from swimming when your mind was fully present with the activity. So the trick is not only to call your friends, like you did so wonderfully with Mary, but also to go to the gathering, and to get yourself really to interact instead of just being there at the party. For times when you find yourself withdrawing into your thoughts, we need to develop specific strategies to help you do less of that. Can you think of anything that would help you do that?

MARK: I don't know. I just don't seem to have much to say these days.

THERAPIST: I know it's hard. There are a variety of things you could try, such as asking more questions, and then closely attending to the response. Or you could focus on something more specific, such as voice or facial expression, to keep your mind from wandering. Sometimes it works just to notice that you've drifted and to take a deep breath to refocus on your goal in that moment.

MARK: I suppose I could try it. My mind just seems to keep wandering.

THERAPIST: I know. So your job here would be to practice being more vigilant as to when that happens, because it will happen. The more you notice you're drifting, the more you can practice refocusing yourself back on your friend. Does your mind wander in here?

MARK: I guess a little.

THERAPIST: Why don't we try it in here? Let's pick something to focus on, and then you can practice here.

MARK: OK. What do I do?

THERAPIST: I'm going to time us for the next 5 minutes and, as we talk, I want you to practice fully engaging in our discussion. Your mind is going to wander, particularly if we are talking about something that reminds you of Diana, I would guess. So let's pick something you can focus on to bring your attention back to our conversation. How about the sound of my voice, like changes in tone, how I articulate words, the pace of my speech?

MARK: I can try.

THERAPIST: Great. So, let's talk about some options for social connections that you could make this weekend.

The therapist and Mark continued this discussion for the next few minutes, at which time, the therapist interrupted their conversation to ask Mark for feedback about his experience.

THERAPIST: What did you notice?

MARK: I don't know, maybe you are talking kind of softly.

THERAPIST: How engaged were you with our discussion? Why don't you give me a rating, with 0 being not engaged at all and 10 being totally engaged?

MARK: I guess maybe 7. It wasn't that hard here, because I was really focused. I guess I did start to think about Diana a little when we were talking about my calling Mary. I did remind myself to pay attention to your voice, and I guess you just sounded so interested. It made it harder for me to wander off in my thoughts when you seemed to be paying so much attention to what we were talking about.

THERAPIST: That was my impression, too, that your engagement was generally high, and that you did appear to refocus your attention a couple times. That is terrific!

MARK: Yeah, but it was a little strange. I mean, usually people aren't that focused when they are just talking about usual stuff.

THERAPIST: That is very true. I might have been paying closer attention to what you were doing and saying than other folks are in typical social interactions. And this may feel pretty artificial now in general. My guess, though, is that once you get more engaged in social interactions, it won't be necessary to concentrate so hard. It will just come automatically again.

MARK: That makes sense.

In this way, the therapist generates a strategy to block avoidance (rumination) by substituting a new behavior in the form of attending to direct and immediate experience. Although, in this case, Mark experimented with directing his attention to interpersonal stimuli, clients may also be directed to experiment with attention to other aspects of sensory stimuli, such as sights, smells, and so forth. The in-session behavioral rehearsal is very important in that it allows the client to practice and receive direct feedback from the therapist, both of which increase the likelihood of success outside of the session. The therapist then returns to the specific task of reviewing and developing behavioral assignments for the next session.

THERAPIST: Let's go back to your not getting out all weekend. Do you think going out to buy the book was too hard? Is there something easier you could've done to help you get a little more engaged this weekend?

MARK: I'm not sure. How hard is it to go out and buy a book?

THERAPIST: Very hard, when you're really down. Let's think about smaller steps. If you can do a smaller step and get a little reinforcement for it, then it becomes easier to move toward your goal.

The therapist and client continue along these lines with graded task assignment. Given that Mark has previously enjoyed socializing, he and the therapist came up with a plan that on the weekend, he would start by returning some phone calls from friends and inviting Mary for lunch. During lunch, he would focus specifically on attending to their conversation. The therapist also raised the possibility of swimming as an exercise activity. Mark reported that he thought his plate was full with the assignments they had already developed, and they decided to table further discussion of swimming. The therapist then uses the final moments of the session to review the homework, to instill hope in Mark, to validate the difficulty of change, and to reinforce the basic treatment model.

Session 5

At the outset of the session, Mark reports improvement in his mood and the therapist includes this as an item on the agenda. Their discussion allows the therapist to emphasize an important point about maintaining new behaviors in consistent and regular routines. In this session, the therapist continues to emphasize the pattern of social connections and to assess factors that increase Mark's vulnerability to exacerbated mood when alone.

THERAPIST: Let's understand in more detail how it is that you are feeling better?

MARK: I think the reading plan is helping. I finished the book.

THERAPIST: Great! So you probably need another book.

MARK: (*laughing*) I guess that's true. You don't think just the one cured the problem?

THERAPIST: (*laughing*) Oh, how I wish that were the case! Seriously, though, Mark, I think that is such an important question. There is a real temptation when you start feeling a little better to back off from some of the very things that are helping. It makes sense, because making these changes requires so much effort, I know. But maintaining the routines are so important.

MARK: It's true. I actually think I've been doing pretty well with that this week. I've been reaching out more to other people.

THERAPIST: This is fantastic.

MARK: And Mary called me again. So, I guess I didn't do what we talked about in terms of calling her, but I did ask her about lunch when she called. I didn't really want to, because I was feeling down when she called. I had just gotten a letter from the lawyer about some new money stuff with Diana. But, I did ask Mary, and I took the girls, too. I think they enjoyed it a lot. I did really focus on asking them all a lot of questions during lunch. I think that helped, too.

THERAPIST: Mark, you have definitely had more social contact in the last few days! You are doing a huge part of this treatment, which is acting in accordance with the goals and plans that we are setting here, as opposed to being directed by how you feel in the moment.

MARK: I tried.

THERAPIST: You did it! You talked about having lunch with your coworker. Did you do that?

MARK: I did do that.

THERAPIST: You did a lot! That's great. OK, I may be pushing our luck here, but what do you think about adding swimming to our agenda?

MARK: I knew you were going to ask about that again.

THERAPIST: (*laughing*) You know me too well. What's your thought about it?

MARK: It's probably a good idea. There is actually a swim lesson that the girls like to do on the weekends, and I could take them and do laps at the same time in the other pool.

THERAPIST: Fantastic! Do you have them with you this weekend? Could we schedule that for the weekend?

MARK: Yeah, I think that would help.

THERAPIST: Mark, do you think that reconnecting with people and some of these activities, like reading, are connected with your improved mood?

MARK: Yes, that definitely had a lot to do with it. I am still not sure that we are getting to the real problem with all of this, but you are right that it does help.

THERAPIST: So we should talk about that, too. Before we move to that, is there anything else that you think is contributing to your positive mood, or is it mostly having more social contact, which you find reinforcing?

MARK: It's the social contact and trying to distract myself with the reading.

THERAPIST: That is so great! Good reminder, too. Let's talk some about another book and how to keep up that schedule.

At this point, the therapist and Mark focus on developing a specific plan for selecting and purchasing a new book to continue the reading routine. Next, the therapist returns to Mark's comments about whether the interventions are addressing what is most important.

THERAPIST: What you mentioned before about the real problem . . . I'm curious what you meant.

MARK: I guess I'm still thinking about Diana a lot. I think that there is a part of me that has to let go, yet just isn't letting go. I am thinking, just asking myself, "Is there still a chance for us? What did I do to screw it all up so badly?" And then I start thinking, "Is this all I have now—having lunch with people, reading by myself at night?" You know, the kind of stuff we've been focusing on . . . I don't know. Is it really going to fix anything?

THERAPIST: Mark, I know it feels like this stuff isn't really getting at the real problem in terms of your thinking about Diana, and I agree that is really important to talk about. At the same time, I don't want us to lose sight of the fact that this other stuff makes a huge difference. It's important for you to re-connect with ways to buoy up your mood before you start to tackle some of the past problems and those that still come up with Diana. Also, I think we will find that there are some similar patterns, so maybe the ways you have tended to pull away from other people since you've been down might have some connections with what happened with Diana.

MARK: That's true. I guess they are not totally separate.

THERAPIST: Are you saying that it's time now to start focusing our time more directly on those topics?

MARK: I think so. Maybe I'm more aware of it because I'm feeling a little better. I guess I'm asking more often, "Is this all there is now?" It just seems like a damn lonely life to be leading, if this is it.

The therapist and Mark end the session by reviewing the assignments. In addition, they agree on a plan to return to Mark's important questions in the next session.

Sessions 6–9

In this next series of sessions, the therapist and Mark return to Mark's question from Session 5. In repeated sessions, he reports improvements in mood related to making progress on projects at home, exercising, and becoming more socially connected in casual and friendship circles. These areas of progress are reflected consistently on his Activity Record forms, which now specifically target the areas of social engagement, reading, and swimming (see Figure 8.3). (This version of the Activity Record can be considered when the activation targets are clear and well developed, and the detailed information gained via hour-by-hour monitoring is not as necessary. It can also be used for clients who have difficulty with the more detailed Activity Record.)

Even with clear areas of improved activation and mood, Mark also reports that his mood is vulnerable to his tendency to ruminate frequently about his ex-wife. The therapist and Mark begin to explore the potential function of rumination about his ex-wife. As they did with respect to both TV watching and rumination during social interactions, they develop some initial hypotheses about the consequences of Mark's ruminating about his ex-wife.

Task	Monday	Tuesday	Wednesday	Thursday	Friday	Saturday	Sunday
Reading	✓	✓	✓	✓			✓
Reaching out to other people	✓	✓	✓			✓	✓
Swimming						✓	✓
Mood	5	5	5	6	8	3	3

FIGURE 8.3. Sample completed Activity Record (daily).

THERAPIST: Is it possible that ruminating might be a form of avoidance itself? It's like your mind gets stuck in a broken record format. You keep replaying what you did wrong, what you could have done, and one of the effects is that you are actually avoiding the painful emotions about the loss of the relationship, and maybe also avoiding exploring new relationships?

MARK: It feels like I can't stand the loss of it. That's what I can't accept—that it is lost. I keep thinking maybe there is a way to recapture it, even though I know there simply is not. We can't even communicate about the kids' health care without a lawyer.

THERAPIST: So, in a way, ruminating may be a way to avoid dealing with grief and sadness. I wonder if part of this comes from what you learned about how to cope with major loss after your dad left. It seems like no one talked about that and you got pretty caught up in thinking about how you might have been responsible. I wonder if it's hard to know what to do emotionally right now.

MARK: It's certainly true about what happened when I was a kid.

THERAPIST: So one possibility we could experiment with is taking time specifically to experience the sadness and loss.

MARK: I don't know. Thinking about her and what I've lost seems overwhelming. I just want to be done with it and move on.

THERAPIST: I know. Exactly! The problem is that ruminating seems to have the effect of keeping you from moving on. Instead of moving onto other relationships or pursuits in your life, your mind keeps replaying what happened and didn't happen with Diana.

MARK: I just don't know if I'm ready for other relationships.

THERAPIST: So, if you weren't ruminating as much, do you think you might experience more fear?

MARK: When I think about getting into another relationship. . . . You know, I think that there is actually a person at work who is interested in dating, but that's been part of the reason that I've kind of held back from doing things with her. She's asked me to lunch a couple of times. I just don't want to be back in the same place again 2 years from now. I can't take this whole thing again, and I don't want to subject my kids to it either.

THERAPIST: So, it may be possible that ruminating has the effect of keeping at bay not only feelings of loss about Diana but also fears about future loss.

The therapist also emphasize the importance of continuing with activation plans developed in earlier sessions to maintain adaptive routines and improve mood. In particular, they highlight the need for consistent attention to social contact, exercise, and reading. In addition, the therapist and Mark begin to discuss his return to the writers' group in more detail, beginning to break down that larger task in manageable pieces. Work on these targets forms the majority of the middle of the course of treatment. As Mark begins to address feelings of loss more directly and continues his work on social connections, exercise, and limiting TV watching, he also begins to express interest in dating again.

Sessions 10–15

In this section of treatment, the therapist and Mark begin to address directly the prospect of his developing new intimate relationships in his life, specifically with a woman at work to whom he is attracted. They explore what is necessary to approach rather than avoid Mark's fear of starting a new relationship, and the therapist hypothesizes in particular that Mark's ruminative style may have functioned to avoid learning from patterns in past relationships. The therapist used the TRAP/TRAC acronym as a simple way to help Mark recognize the conditions under which he was likely to avoid (the TRAP), and to then engage in more adaptive coping behavior to get back on "TRAC." For example, Mark reported that he would see the woman at work (trigger) and begin to feel nervous (response) and either not talk with her or restrict his conversation to perfunctory work issues (the avoidance pattern). His alternative coping under the same conditions involved asking her if she would like to have coffee. Sessions then focus heavily on examining in detail what he might learn from his former marriage that would be instructive in future relationships. The following dialogue provides an example of the types of foci that these sessions target.

MARK: One of the things that happened a lot with Diana is I never felt like I was really present with her or the girls. It was like they were in this little world together and I was always on the outside somehow. I often thought that I should put myself more in the center, like say more of what I thought, but I just didn't. I never did.

THERAPIST: Did that cause conflict with her?

MARK: Yes, absolutely. It was one of things that she said when she ended things. Being on the outside is a big thing for me.

THERAPIST: What does being on the outside involve specifically? How would I know if you were doing that?

MARK: It's just not being willing to speak up about things. She always said it was like I wasn't really in or out on anything, just kind of on the fence the whole time.

THERAPIST: Can you think of a specific example when that was an issue?

MARK: Well, my mother and brothers never really liked Diana very much, but I didn't do much to stand up for her with them. I just kind of let things unfold. . . .

THERAPIST: So, that might have been a TRAP with her? Was it a trigger that you thought she wanted something from you in terms of your commitment?

MARK: Yes, it was, because I ended up feeling really overwhelmed by that.

THERAPIST: And the avoidance pattern was withdrawing.

MARK: I did. I just backed off, and she had to handle the whole scene with my family.

THERAPIST: So with your coworker, if you were to take a stand with her now, what would that look like? What would alternative coping be?

MARK: I have no idea.

THERAPIST: Do you think there is a similar trigger?

MARK: Maybe, because I think she is wondering what's up with me? Like am I interested or not?

THERAPIST: Have you been clear with her about being interested in dating her?

MARK: Not really. We talk often at work, but I can't say that I've really said much about it.

THERAPIST: Would you like to ask her out?

MARK: Yes, I guess I would.

THERAPIST: Why don't we think of some specific things you could say as alternatives to withdrawing and practice with some of them?

In these sessions, the therapist and Mark define, in very specific and concrete terms, the types of behaviors associated with decreased satisfaction and quality in his former marriage. For instance, the therapist's following question to Mark is a central question asked repeatedly over the course of BA: "What does being on the outside involve specifically? What does it look like? How would I know if you were doing that?" The therapist emphasizes identifying clear, specific, and observable behaviors when analyzing behaviors and defining goals. Then, the therapist and Mark work to identify specific strategies that he can use to practice alternative behaviors in pursuing a future relationship. They continue to use the TRAP/TRAC framework to examine situations that arise and Mark's response, and to guide him toward a more engaged approach to intimate interpersonal relationships. As Mark begins dating, they have ample opportunity to revise and refine strategies through activation assignments that target being direct and present in intimate interactions.

Sessions 16–19

By Session 16, the therapist and Mark agree that the bulk of the work of understanding and problem-solving Mark's depression in terms of his unique life context and avoidant response patterns that maintain his depression has been completed. Mark has been successfully activated both in terms of his secondary problem behaviors (e.g., increased reading, exercise, social contacts, and projects around the house; decreased TV watching). He has also been activated toward solving his primary problem (avoidance of intimacy) via initiating a new relationship.

Thus, the final sessions of treatment focused on reviewing and consolidating primary themes and methods used in therapy. Specifically, the therapist and Mark identified the importance of continuing to practice his new skills of blocking rumination by attending to immediate goals and to his direct and immediate experience, and being more direct and expressive with his new partner. In addition, the therapist carefully reviewed with Mark the ways he had learned to use the fundamentals of behavioral activation himself. Together they reviewed ways that Mark would know when he was starting to feel depressed or to engage in avoidance response patterns. They also reviewed specific steps he could take to begin self-monitoring his mood and activities, and to problem-solve alternative coping behaviors. They also specifically identified a number of alternative behaviors that were uniquely helpful in breaking the vicious cycle of depression, avoidance, and withdrawal. Mark reported that he felt well equipped with these tools and the opportunities he had had to practice them in therapy. He also reported feeling encouraged about the positive changes he had already made in his life. He ended treatment expressing optimism about his future and warmly thanked the therapist for all of their work together. Over time, Mark continued to maintain the gains he made in treatment. He established a

new relationship with a woman, and they became engaged over the course of the following year. He continued to practice many of the skills he had learned in therapy in the context of this new relationship, with his children, and with his coworkers and friends.

Case Summary

The course of treatment with Mark provides an example of many of the core principles and strategies of BA. The treatment followed from careful and ongoing functional analysis of key problems that Mark presented, which in turn allowed the therapist to develop the organizing case conceptualization. This work was completed in collaboration with Mark during sessions and was also a focus of the ongoing clinical consultation team meetings, of which Mark's therapist was a key member. During treatment, the therapist used a range of specific strategies, including goal setting, self-monitoring, graded task assignment, problem solving, behavioral rehearsal, and attention to experience. She also addressed a number of important treatment targets frequently observed in BA, including interpersonal avoidance, rumination, and routine disruption. Overall, the therapist worked as a coach throughout therapy, helping Mark to problem-solve specific steps to overcome patterns of avoidance and to engage in activities. She also taught Mark to understand the pattern of antecedents to depressed mood and how his responses contributed to either maintaining or improving his mood. She skillfully balanced acknowledging the difficulty of change when depressed with emphasizing the importance of action, even when mood is low. She maintained a matter-of-fact, nonjudgmental, problem-solving approach to difficulties that arose during the course of Mark's therapy, and returned regularly and persistently to the selected targets of change.

CONCLUSION

This chapter provides the conceptual basics and the how-to specifics that are required to use BA with depressed clients. Evolving from the seminal foundation established by the work of Ferster, Lewinsohn, and Beck, BA highlights the power of direct and sustained attention to behavior change. BA aims to help clients become active and engaged in their lives in ways that reduce current depression and help to prevent future episodes. BA therapists help depressed clients to increase activities that bring greater reward and to solve important problems. Clients are assisted in approaching important life goals and engaging directly and immediately with problematic aspects of their lives. Both outcome research and other converging lines of empirical inquiry suggest that BA holds promise as an efficacious treatment for depression. Future research will examine in greater detail the process of change in BA and the ease with which BA can be transported to applied community settings.

REFERENCES

Addis, M. E., & Carpenter, K. M. (2000). The treatment rationale in cognitive behavioral therapy: Psychological mechanisms and clinical guidelines. *Cognitive and Behavioral Practice, 7*(2), 147–156.

Addis, M. E., & Martell, C. R. (2004). *Overcoming depression one step at a time: The new behavioral activation approach to getting your life back.* Oakland, CA: New Harbinger.

American Psychiatric Association. (1994). *Diagnostic and statistical manual of mental disorders* (4th ed.). Washington, DC: Author.

Armento, M. E. A., & Hopko, D. R. (2007). The Environmental Reward Observation Scale (EROS): Development, validity, and reliability. *Behavior Therapy, 38*, 107–119.

Beck, A. T., Rush, A. J., Shaw, B. F., & Emery, G. (1979). *Cognitive therapy of depression.* New York: Guilford Press.

Beck, A. T., Steer, R. A., & Brown, G. K. (1996). *Manual for the BDI-II.* San Antonio, TX: Psychological Corporation.

Bennett-Levy, J., Butler, G., Fennell, M., Hackman, A., Mueller, M., & Westbrook, D. (2004). *Oxford guide to behavioural experiments in cognitive therapy.* Oxford, UK: Oxford University Press.

Blumenthal, J. A., Babyak, M. A., Moore, K. A., Craighead, W. E., Herman, S., Khatri, P., et al. (1999). Effects of exercise training on older patients with major depression. *Archives of Internal Medicine, 159*, 2349–2356.

Borkovec, T. D., Newman, M. G., Pincus, A. L., & Lytle, R. (2002). A component analysis of cognitive-behavioral therapy for generalized anxiety disorder and the role of interpersonal problems. *Journal of Consulting and Clinical Psychology, 70*, 288–298.

Dimidjian, S., Hollon, S. D., Dobson, K. S., Schmaling, K. B., Kohlenberg, R. J., Addis, M., et al. (2006). Randomized trial of behavioral activation, cognitive therapy, and antidepressant medication in the acute treatment of adults with major depression. *Journal of Consulting and Clinical Psychology, 74*, 658–670.

Dobson, K. S., Hollon, S. D., Dimidjian, S., Schmaling, K. B., Kohlenberg, R., Gallop, R., et al. (2007). *Behavioral activation therapy, cognitive therapy and pharmacotherapy for depression: Relapse prevention.* Manuscript under review.

Ferster, C. B. (1973). A functional analysis of depression. *American Psychologist, 28*, 857–870.

Ferster, C. B. (1981). A functional analysis of behavior therapy. In L. P. Rehm (Ed.), *Behavior therapy for depression: Present status and future directions* (pp. 181–196). New York: Academic Press.

First, M. B., Spitzer, R. L., Gibbon, M., & Williams, J. B. W. (1997). *User's guide for the Structured Clinical Interview for DSM-IV Axis I Disorders.* Washington, DC: American Psychiatric Press.

First, M. B., Spitzer, R. L., Gibbons, M., Williams, J. B. W., & Benjamin, L. (1996). *User's guide for the Structured Clinical Interview for DSM-IV Axis II Personality Disorders (SCID-II).* New York: Biometrics Research Department, New York State Psychiatric Institute.

Foa, E. B., Rothbaum, B. O., & Furr, J. M. (2003). Augmenting exposure therapy with other CBT procedures. *Psychiatric Annals, 33*, 47–53.

Gloaguen, V., Cottraux, J., Cucherat, M., & Blackburn, I. M. (1998). A meta-analysis of the effects of cognitive therapy in depressed patients. *Journal of Affective Disorders, 49*, 59–72.

Gollwitzer, P. M. (1999). Implementation intentions: Strong effects of simple plans. *American Psychologist, 54*, 493–503.

Gortner, E. T., Gollan, J. K., Dobson, K. S., & Jacobson, N. S. (1998). Cognitive-behavioral treatment for depression: Relapse prevention. *Journal of Consulting and Clinical Psychology, 66*, 377–384.

Hamilton, M. A. (1960). A rating scale for depression. *Journal of Neurology, Neurosurgery, and Psychiatry, 23*, 56–61.

Hayes, A. M., Castonguay, L. G., & Goldfried, M. R. (1996). Effectiveness of targeting the vulnerability factors of depression in cognitive therapy. *Journal of Consulting and Clinical Psychology, 64*(3), 623–627.

Hayes, S. C., Strosahl, K. D., & Wilson, K. G. (1999). *Acceptance and commitment therapy: An experiential approach to behavior change.* New York: Guilford Press.

Hopko, D. R., Lejuez, C. W., LePage, J. P., Hopko, S. D., & McNeil, D. W. (2003). A brief behavioral activation treatment for depression: A randomized pilot trial within an inpatient psychiatric hospital. *Behavior Modification, 27*, 458–469.

Jacobson, N. S., Dobson, K. S., Truax, P. A., Addis, M. E., Koerner, K., Gollan, J. K., et al. (1996). A component analysis of cognitive-behavioral treatment for depression. *Journal of Consulting and Clinical Psychology, 64*, 295–304.

Jacobson, N. S., Martell, C. R., & Dimidjian, S. (2001). Behavioral activation treatment for depression: Returning to contextual roots. *Clinical Psychology: Science and Practice, 8,* 255–270.

Kanter, J. W., Mulick, P. S., Busch, A. M., Berlin, K. S., & Martell, C. R. (2007). The Behavioral Activation for Depression Scale (BADS): Psychometric properties and factor structure. *Journal of Psychopathology and Behavioral Assessment, 29,* 191–202.

Lewinsohn, P. M. (1974). A behavioral approach to depression. In R. M. Friedman & M. M. Katz (Eds.), *The psychology of depression: Contemporary theory and research* (pp. 157–185). New York: Wiley.

Lewinsohn, P. M., Antonuccio, D. O., Steinmetz-Breckenridge, J., & Teri, L. (1984). *The coping with depression course: A psychoeducational intervention for unipolar depression.* Eugene, OR: Castalia.

Lewinsohn, P. M., Biglan, A., & Zeiss, A. S. (1976). Behavioral treatment of depression. In P. O. Davidson (Ed.), *The behavioral management of anxiety, depression and pain* (pp. 91–146). New York: Brunner/Mazel.

Lewinsohn, P. M., & Graf, M. (1973). Pleasant activities and depression. *Journal of Consulting and Clinical Psychology, 41,* 261–268.

Lewinsohn, P. M., Sullivan, J. M., & Grosscup, S. J. (1980). Changing reinforcing events: An approach to the treatment of depression. *Psychotherapy: Theory, Research, Practice, and Training, 17,* 322–334.

Linehan, M. M. (1993). *Cognitive-behavioral treatment of borderline personality disorder.* New York: Guilford Press.

Locke, E. A., & Latham, G. P. (2002). Building a practically useful theory of goal setting and task motivation: A 35-year odyssey. *American Psychologist, 57,* 705–717.

Martell, C. R., Addis, M. E., & Jacobson, N. S. (2001). *Depression in context: Strategies for guided action.* New York: Norton.

Nolen-Hoeksema, S. (2000). The role of rumination in depressive disorders and mixed anxiety/depressive symptoms. *Journal of Abnormal Psychology, 109,* 504–511.

Scogin, F., Jamison, C., & Gochneaur, K. (1989). Comparative efficacy of cognitive and behavioral bibliotherapy for mildly and moderately depressed older adults. *Journal of Consulting and Clinical Psychology, 57,* 403–407.

Segal, Z. V., Williams, J. M. G., & Teasdale, J. D. (2002). *Mindfulness-based cognitive therapy for depression.* New York: Guilford Press.

Ware, J. E., & Sherbourne, C. D. (1992). The MOS 36-Item Short-Form Health Survey (SF-36), I: Conceptual framework and item selection. *Medical Care, 30,* 473–483.

Watson, D. L., & Tharp, R. G. (2002). *Self directed behavior.* Belmont, CA: Wadsworth/Thomson Learning.

Weissman, M. M., & Bothwell, S. (1976). Assessment of social adjustment by patient self-report. *Archives of General Psychiatry, 33*(9), 1111–1115.

Zeiss, A. M., Lewinsohn, P. M., & Munoz, R. F. (1979). Nonspecific improvement effects in depression using interpersonal skills training, pleasant activity schedules, or cognitive training. *Journal of Consulting and Clinical Psychology, 47,* 427–439.

Zettle, R. D., & Rains, J. C. (1989). Group cognitive and contextual therapies in treatment of depression. *Journal of Clinical Psychology, 45*(3), 436–445.

CHAPTER 9

Dialectical Behavior Therapy for Borderline Personality Disorder

MARSHA M. LINEHAN
ELIZABETH T. DEXTER-MAZZA

This chapter presents one of the more remarkable developments in all of psychotherapy. Few therapists are willing to undertake the overwhelmingly difficult and wrenching task of treating individuals with "borderline" characteristics, yet these people are among the neediest encountered in any therapeutic setting. They also impose an enormous burden on the health care system. Over the past two decades, Linehan and her colleagues have developed a psychological treatment for individuals with borderline personality disorder (BPD). Importantly, data indicate that this treatment is effective when compared to alternative interventions. If results from the initial trials continue to hold up in future clinical trials, then this treatment will constitute one of the most substantial contributions to the armamentarium of the psychotherapist in recent times. What is even more interesting is that this approach blends emotion regulation, interpersonal systems, and cognitive-behavioral approaches into a coherent whole. To this mix Linehan adds her personal experience with Eastern philosophies and religions. Among the more intriguing strategies incorporated into this approach are "entering the paradox" and "extending," borrowed from *aikido*, a Japanese form of self-defense. Yet the authors remain true to the empirical foundations of their approach. The fascinating case study presented in this chapter illustrates Linehan's therapeutic expertise and strategic timing in a way that will be invaluable to all therapists who deal with personality disorders. The surprising and tragic outcome illustrates the enormous burden of clinical responsibility inherent in any treatment setting, as well as the practical issues that arise when treatment ultimately fails.—D. H. B.

Clinicians generally agree that clients with a diagnosis of borderline personality disorder (BPD) are challenging and difficult to treat. As a result, BPD has become a stigmatized disorder resulting in negative attitudes, trepidation, and concern with regard to providing treatment (Aviram, Brodsky, & Stanley, 2006; Lequesne & Hersh, 2004; Paris, 2005). Perhaps of greatest concern is the generally high incidence of suicidal behavior among this population. Approximately 75% of clients who meet criteria for BPD have a history of suicide attempts, with an average of 3.4 attempts per individual (Soloff, Lis, Kelly, Cornelius, & Ulrich, 1994). Suicide threats and crises are frequent, even among those who never engage in any suicidal or nonsuicidal self-injurious behavior (NSSI). Although much of this behavior is without lethal consequence, follow-up studies of individuals with BPD have found suicide rates of about 7–8%, and the percentage who eventually commit suicide is estimated at 10% (for a review, see Linehan, Rizvi, Shaw-Welch, & Page, 2000). Among all individuals who have committed suicide, from 7 to 38% meet criteria for BPD when personality disorders are assessed via a psychological autopsy, with the higher incidence occurring primarily among young adults with the disorder (Brent et al., 1994; Isometsa et al., 1994, 1997; Lesage et al., 1994; Rich & Runeson, 1992). Individuals with BPD also have difficulties with anger and anger expression. Not infrequently, intense anger is directed at their therapists. The frequent coexistence of BPD with both Axis I conditions (e.g., mood or anxiety disorders) and other personality disorders clearly complicates treatment further.

The criteria for BPD, as defined within the text revision of the fourth edition of the *Diagnostic and Statistical Manual of Mental Disorders* (DSM-IV-TR; American Psychiatric Association, 2000) and the Revised Diagnostic Interview for Borderlines (DIB-R; Zanarini, Gunderson, Frankenburg, & Chauncey, 1989), the most commonly used research assessment instrument, reflect a pervasive pattern of instability and dysregulation across all domains of functioning. Other assessment measures used to diagnose BPD include the International Personality Disorders Examination (IPDE; Loranger, 1995) and the Diagnostic Interview for DSM-IV Personality Disorders (DIPD-IV; Zanarini, Frankenburg, Sickel, & Yong, 1996). The Borderline Symptom List (BSL; Bohus et al., 2001) and the McLean Screening Instrument for Borderline Personality Disorder (MSI-BPD; Zanarini et al., 2003) are both screening measures for BPD.

Linehan (1993a) has reorganized and summarized the diagnostic criteria of BPD into five domains. First, individuals with BPD generally experience emotional dysregulation and instability. Emotional responses are reactive, and the individuals generally have difficulties with episodic depression, anxiety, and irritability, as well as problems with anger and anger expression. Second, individuals with BPD have patterns of behavioral dysregulation, as evidenced by extreme and problematic impulsive behavior. As noted earlier, an important characteristic of these individuals is their tendency to direct apparently destructive behaviors toward themselves. Attempts to injure, mutilate, or kill themselves, as well as actual suicides, occur frequently in this population. Third, individuals with BPD sometimes experience cognitive dysregulation. Brief, nonpsychotic forms of thought and sensory dysregulation, such as de-

personalization, dissociation, and delusions (including delusions about the self), are at times brought on by stressful situations and usually cease when the stress is ameliorated. Fourth, dysregulation of the sense of self is also common. Individuals with BPD frequently report that they have no sense of a self at all, feel empty, and do not "know" who they are. Finally, these individuals often experience interpersonal dysregulation. Their relationships may be chaotic, intense, and marked with difficulties. Even though their relationships are so difficult, individuals with BPD often find it extremely hard to relinquish relationships. Instead, they may engage in intense and frantic efforts to prevent significant individuals from leaving them. The polythetic format of the DSM-IV-TR definition allows for considerable heterogeneity in diagnosis (indeed, the requirement that five of nine criteria be met for the diagnosis yields 256 ways in which the BPD diagnosis may be met), and clinical experience with these clients confirms that this diagnostic category comprises a heterogeneous group.

This chapter focuses primarily on describing dialectical behavior therapy (DBT), a comparatively new approach to treatment of BPD (Linehan, 1993a, 1993b). It has the distinction of being one of the first psychosocial treatments demonstrated to be effective in a randomized clinical trial (Linehan, Armstrong, Suarez, Allmon, & Heard, 1991). Before describing DBT, we first review other treatments for BPD and provide information on their theoretical rationales and supporting data (when such data are available). This is followed by a more in-depth description of DBT—its philosophical roots, underlying theory, and treatment protocols.

OVERVIEW OF OTHER TREATMENT APPROACHES

Various approaches have been applied to the treatment of BPD. Although it is not our purpose to present a scholarly review of all the many treatments for BPD, we believe it helpful to review briefly the status of other, current treatments before presenting DBT in detail.

Psychodynamic

Psychodynamic approaches currently receiving the greatest attention include those of Kernberg

(1975, 1984; Clarkin et al., 2001; Kernberg, Selzer, Koenigsberg, Carr, & Appelbaum, 1989), Adler and Buie (1979; Adler, 1981, 1985, 1993; Buie & Adler, 1982), and Bateman and Fonagy (2004). Among these, Kernberg's (1975, 1984) theoretical contributions are clearly prominent. His object relations model is comprehensive as to theory and technique, and has had considerable influence on the psychoanalytic literature. His expressive psychotherapy for clients with "borderline personality organization" (BPO) or BPD, transference-focused therapy (TFT), emphasizes three primary factors: interpretation, maintenance of technical neutrality, and transference analysis. The focus of the therapy is on exposure and resolution of intrapsychic conflict. Treatment goals include increased impulse control and anxiety tolerance, ability to modulate affect, and development of stable interpersonal relationships. TFT also uses a target hierarchy approach to the first year of treatment. The targets are (1) containment of suicidal and self-destructive behaviors, (2) therapy-destroying behaviors, and (3) identification and recapitulation of dominant object relational patterns, as experienced in the transference relationship (Clarkin et al., 2001). Kernberg has also distinguished a supportive psychotherapy for more severely disturbed clients with BPO or BPD. Like expressive psychotherapy, supportive psychotherapy also places great emphasis on the importance of the interpersonal relationship in therapy (transference); however, interpretations are less likely to be made early in treatment, and only the negative responses to the therapist and to therapy (negative transference) are explored. Both expressive and supportive psychotherapy are expected to last several years, with primary foci on suicidal behaviors and therapy-interfering behaviors. The data supporting the use of TFT are not extensive. Clarkin and colleagues have published results from a preliminary study of TFT. Additionally, one completed randomized clinical trial has compared TFT to schema-focused therapy (SFT; Giesen-Bloo et al., 2006). The results of this study are described in the section on cognitive-behavioral treatments.

The preliminary study of TFT assessed pre- and posttreatment changes over the course of a 1-year treatment for adult women with BPD (N = 23). Of the 23 clients who were considered intent-to-treat (ITT), 17 completed the treatment. Both the ITT sample and the completer sample

were analyzed. There were no significant reductions in number of suicide attempts, number of NSSI behaviors (referred to as "parasuicide" in the article), medical risk of either type of self-injury, or physical condition after either type of self-injury in the ITT sample. However, significant decreases in medical risk and physical condition after NSSI behaviors occurred in the completer sample. Furthermore, the number of hospitalizations over the course of the treatment year compared to the year prior to treatment reduced significantly for both groups. Given the lack of a control group in this study and the small sample size, these findings should be reviewed with caution (Clarkin et al., 2001).

Mentalization therapy, developed by Bateman and Fonagy (2004), is an intensive therapy grounded in attachment theory (i.e., BPD is viewed as an attachment disorder), with a focus on relationship patterns and nonconscious factors inhibiting change. "Mentalization" refers to one's perception or interpretation of the actions of others and oneself as intentional. The treatment is based on the theory that individuals with BPD have an inadequate capacity for mentalization. Treatment, therefore, is focused on bringing the client's mental experiences to conscious awareness, facilitating a more complete, integrated sense of mental agency. The goal is to increase the client's capacity for recognizing the existence of the thoughts and feelings he or she is experiencing.

A randomized trial of mentalization therapy offered in a partial hospitalization setting provides additional supporting data for psychoanalytic treatment of BPD. This study by Bateman and Fonagy (1999) consisted of random assignment of clients to either standard psychiatric care constrained only by the requirement that individual psychotherapy was not allowed (control condition) or to partial hospitalization, a treatment program with the following goals of therapy: (1) psychoanalytically informed engagement of clients in treatment; (2) reduction of psychopathology, including depression and anxiety; (3) reduction of suicidal behavior; (4) improvement in social competence; and (5) reduction in lengthy hospitalizations. The experimental treatment group received once-weekly individual psychotherapy provided by psychiatric nurses, once-weekly psychodrama-based expressive therapy, thrice-weekly group therapy, a weekly community meeting, a monthly meeting with a case administrator, and a monthly medications review. At the end of the 18-month treatment, the group receiving mentalization therapy showed significant reductions in suicidal behavior (suicide attempts and self-mutilation), inpatient hospitalization stays, measures of psychopathology (including depression and anxiety), and social functioning relative to the control group. These gains were maintained and increased during an 18-month follow-up period consisting of twice-weekly group therapy (Bateman & Fonagy, 2001). The researchers note that their program contained three characteristics that they hypothesize to be related to treatment effectiveness: a consistent theoretical rationale for treatment, a relationship focus, and consistent treatment over time.

Psychopharmacological

Reviews of the literature regarding drug treatments for BPD highlight a dilemma for the prescribing pharmacotherapist: BPD involves dysregulation in too many domains for a single drug to serve as a panacea (Dimeff, McDavid, & Linehan, 1999; Lieb, Zanarini, Linehan, & Bohus, 2004; Nose, Cipriani, Biancosino, Grassi, & Barbui, 2006). In general, results indicate that several agents may be useful for improving global functioning, cognitive perceptual symptoms (e.g., suspiciousness, ideas of reference, transitory hallucinations), emotion dysregulation, or impulsive–behavioral dyscontrol (for reviews, see Lieb et al., 2004; Nose et al., 2006). Nose and colleagues (2006) conducted a meta-analysis of 22 randomized, placebo-controlled clinical trials, published between 1986 and 2006, examining the effects of pharmacotherapy for individuals with BPD. Organization of results was based on five primary outcome measures: affective instability and anger, impulsivity and aggression, interpersonal relationships, suicidality, and global functioning. First, no medication had a more positive effect than placebo on suicidality. Overall, across the studies, fluoxetine, an antidepressant, and topiramate and lamotrigine, mood stabilizers, showed more positive effects than placebo for affective instability and anger. Additionally, valproate, an anticonvulsant and mood stabilizer, has effectively treated behavioral dysregulation in clients with BPD, including those with aggressive and impulsive behavior (Stein, Simeon, Frenkel, Islam, & Hollander, 1995). As a class, antipsychotics were more effective than placebo for impulsivi-

ty, interpersonal relationships, and global functioning, and specifically, olanzapine was better than placebo relative to global functioning (Nose et al., 2006) and has been shown to decrease impulsive aggression and chronic dysphoria more effectively compared to fluoxetine (Zanarini, Frankenburg, & Parachini, 2004). In summary, although some drug treatments may be effective, caution is in order when considering pharmacotherapy for this particular client population. Clients with BPD are notoriously noncompliant with treatment regimens, may abuse the prescribed drugs or overdose, and may experience unintended effects of the drugs. With these caveats in mind, carefully monitored pharmacotherapy may be a useful and important adjunct to psychotherapy in the treatment of BPD.

Cognitive-Behavioral

Treatment of BPD has received increasing attention from cognitive theorists. The cognitive approach views the problems of the client with BPD as residing within both the content and the process of the individual's thoughts. Beck's approach to treating BPD (Beck & Freeman, 1990) is representative of cognitive psychotherapy generally, with the focus of treatment on restructuring thoughts and on developing a collaborative relationship through which more adaptive ways of viewing the world are developed. More specifically it focuses on decreasing negative and polarized beliefs that result in unstable affect and destructive behaviors (Brown, Newman, Charlesworth, Crits-Christoph, & Beck, 2004). In an open clinical trial of cognitive therapy for clients with BPD, Brown and colleagues found decreases in clients meeting BPD criteria, depression, hopelessness, and suicide ideation at the end of the 12-month treatment and 6-month follow-up posttreatment.

The cognitive-behavioral therapies of Young, Klosko, and Weishaar (Kellogg & Young, 2006; Young, 2000; Young, Klosko, & Weishaar, 2003; Pretzer, 1990); Blum and colleagues (Blum, Pfohl, St. John, Monahan, & Black, 2002) and Schmidt and Davidson (as cited in Weinberg, Gunderson, Hennen, & Cutter, 2006) attempt to address some of the difficulties experienced in applying traditional cognitive approaches to the treatment of BPD. Pretzer's (1990) approach emphasizes modifying standard cognitive therapy to address difficulties often encountered in treating clients with BPD, such as establishing a collaborative relationship between therapist and client, maintaining a directed treatment, and improving homework compliance. Blum and colleagues (2002) developed a twice-weekly outpatient group treatment that uses a psychoeducational approach to teaching skills to clients with BPD and to their support systems (e.g., family, friends, other care providers). The treatment focuses on destigmatization of BPD, emotional control, and behavioral control. At present, outcome data are limited for Pretzer's approach. A pilot study has shown potential for the group treatment developed by Blum and colleagues and a randomized control trial is currently being conducted (Van Wel et al., 2006).

Young's schema-focused therapy (SFT) (Young et al., 2003) postulates that stable patterns of thinking ("early maladaptive schemas") can develop during childhood and result in maladaptive behavior that reinforces the schemas. SFT includes a variety of interventions aimed at challenging and changing these early schemas through the identification of a set of dysfunctional schema modes that control the individual's thoughts, emotions, and behaviors (i.e., detached protector, punitive parent, abandoned/abused child, angry/impulsive child). Giesen-Bloo and colleagues (2006) completed the first randomized clinical trial of TFT and SFT. Transference focused therapy was compared to schema focused therapy in a study where 88 participants received three years of twice per week individual sessions of either schema focused therapy or transference based therapy. Study results indicated an overall decrease in BPD symptoms for both treatments, however, participants who received SFT had significantly greater improvements overall and a lower attrition rate. Suicide and NSSI behaviors were not assessed as an outcome measure in this study.

Weinberg and colleagues (2006) completed a randomized, controlled trial of Schmidt and Davidson's manual-assisted cognitive treatment (MACT) and treatment as usual (TAU). MACT is a brief cognitive-behavioral treatment that incorporates strategies from DBT, cognitive therapy, and bibliotherapy. The treatment targets NSSI behaviors occurring in individuals with BPD. MACT was provided as an adjunctive treatment to TAU for study participants ($N = 30$). Participants were 30 women diagnosed with BPD, with a history of NSSI be-

haviors and at least one in the last month; however, suicide was considered one of the exclusionary criteria for study participation. Participants were randomly assigned to MACT plus TAU or to TAU-alone conditions. Upon completion of the 6-week treatment and at the 6-month follow-up, individuals who received MACT had significantly fewer and less severe NSSI behaviors than those in the TAU-alone condition. The authors state that these results should be interpreted with caution due to small sample size and the use of self-report measures only in assessment of NSSI behaviors.

DIALECTICAL BEHAVIOR THERAPY

DBT evolved from standard cognitive-behavioral therapy as a treatment for BPD, particularly for recurrently suicidal, severely dysfunctional individuals. The theoretical orientation to treatment is a blend of three theoretical positions: behavioral science, dialectical philosophy, and Zen practice. Behavioral science, the principles of behavior change, is countered by acceptance of the client (with techniques drawn both from Zen and from Western contemplative practice); these poles are balanced within the dialectical framework. Although dialectics was first adopted as a description of this emphasis on balance, dialectics soon took on the status of guiding principles that have advanced the therapy in directions not originally anticipated. DBT is based within a consistent behaviorist theoretical position. However, the actual procedures and strategies overlap considerably with those of various alternative therapy orientations, including psychodynamic, client-centered, strategic, and cognitive therapies.

Efficacy

Although several treatments (Bateman & Fonagy, 1999, 2001; Giesen-Bloo et al., 2006; Marziali & Munroe-Blum, 1994) have shown efficacy in the treatment of individuals with BPD, DBT has the most empirical support at present and is generally considered the frontline treatment for the disorder. DBT has been evaluated in six randomized controlled trials (RCTs) conducted across three independent research teams (Koons et al., 2001; Linehan et al., 1991, 1999, 2002, 2006; Linehan, Heard, & Armstrong, 1993; Linehan,

Tutek, Heard, & Armstrong, 1994; Verheul et al., 2003). Two of the RCTs specifically recruited clients with suicidal behaviors (Linehan et al., 1991, 1993, 1994, 1999). The results in general have shown DBT to be an effective evidenced-based treatment for the disorder. In four of the six studies participants treated with DBT demonstrated significantly greater reductions in suicide attempts, intentional self-injury, and suicidal ideation (Koons et al., 2001; Linehan et al., 1991, 1999, 2002; Verheul et al., 2003). Treatment superiority was maintained when DBT was compared to only those control subjects who received stable individual psychotherapy during the treatment year, and even after researchers controlled for number of hours of psychotherapy and of telephone contacts. (Linehan & Heard, 1993; Linehan et al., 1999). Two studies with participants with substance dependence and BPD found DBT to be more effective than control treatments in reducing substance use, and increasing global and social adjustment (Linehan et al., 1999, 2002). In the original study of recurrently suicidal patients with BPD, participants treated with DBT were significantly less likely than TAU participants to attempt suicide or NSSI behaviors during the treatment year, had less medically severe NSSI behaviors, were less likely to drop out of treatment, had fewer inpatient psychiatric days per participant, and improved more on scores of both global and social adjustment. More specifically, Linehan and colleagues' (2006) study showed that participants treated with DBT were half as likely to engage in suicidal behaviors compared to participants in the treatment by community experts (TBCE) condition, further indicating that DBT is an effective treatment for reducing suicidal behavior. This study suggests that the efficacy of DBT is due to specific treatment factors, and not general factors or the expertise of the treating psychotherapists. In two studies to date, DBT has been shown to be effective in reducing substance use disorders (Linehan et al., 1999, 2002).

In addition to these studies of DBT for individuals with BPD, three studies have examined its effectiveness with other disorders. First, Lynch, Morse, Mendelson, and Robins (2003) found that a DBT skills group plus antidepressant medication showed greater reductions in depressive symptoms in older (over 60-years-old) depressed individuals compared to TAU plus antidepressant medication group at the 6-month follow-up time point in a 28-week treatment program. DBT has also been adapted for use with individuals without BPD who are diagnosed with binge-eating disorder (BED). Telch, Agras, and Linehan (2001) compared women diagnosed with BED receiving an adapted 20-week group DBT treatment to waiting-list controls. Participants in the DBT condition had significantly fewer days of binge-eating episodes compared to those in the wait-list control condition and were more likely to abstain from bingeing at follow-up. Additionally, those in the wait-list control group who were offered the DBT treatment after the study had similar results. DBT continues to be examined in a variety of settings and for a variety of different diagnoses. However, it is important to highlight that when DBT is adapted for use with different populations, it may not be as effective, given that many adaptations have not been rigorously tested. We recommend that until it is tested in an RCT, adaptations should not be made to DBT. If using DBT with different populations, then the most important change should be in the examples used when teaching, not in the content itself.

Philosophical Basis: Dialectics

The term "dialectics" as applied to behavior therapy refers both to a fundamental nature of reality and to a method of persuasive dialogue and relationship. (See Wells [1972, cited in Kegan, 1982] for documentation of a shift toward dialectical approaches across all the sciences during the last 150 years; more recently, Peng & Nisbett [1999] discuss both Western and Eastern dialectical thought.) As a worldview or philosophical position, dialectics guide the clinician in developing theoretical hypotheses relevant to the client's problems and to the treatment. Alternatively, as dialogue and relationship, dialectics refers to the treatment approach or strategies used by the therapist to effect change. Thus, central to DBT are a number of therapeutic dialectical strategies. These are described later in this chapter.

Dialectics as a Worldview

DBT is based on a dialectical worldview that emphasizes wholeness, interrelatedness, and process (change) as fundamental characteristics of reality. The first characteristic, the Principle of Interrelatedness and Wholeness, provides a perspective of viewing the system as a whole and how individuals relate to the system, rather than seeing individuals as if they exist in isolation. Similar to contextual and systems theories, a dialectical view argues that analysis of parts of any system is of limited value unless the analysis clearly relates the part to the whole. The second characteristic is the Principle of Polarity. Although dialectics focuses on the whole, it also emphasizes the complexity of any whole. Thus dialectics asserts that reality is nonreducible; that is, within each single thing or system, no matter how small, there is polarity. For example, physicists are unable to reduce even the smallest of molecules to one thing. Where there is matter there is antimatter; even every atom is made up of both protons and electrons: A polar opposite is always present. The opposing forces are referred to as the thesis and antithesis, present in all existence. Dialectics suggests that the thesis and antithesis move toward a synthesis, and inherent in the synthesis will be a new set of opposing forces. It is from these opposing forces that the third characteristic is developed. This characteristic of the dialectical perspective refers to the Principle of Continuous Change. Change is produced through the constant synthesis of the thesis and the antithesis, and because new opposing forces are present within the synthesis, change is ongoing. These dialectical principles are inherent in every aspect of DBT and allow for continuous movement throughout the therapy process. A very important dialectical idea is that all propositions contain within them their own oppositions. Or, as Goldberg (1980, pp. 295–296) put it, "I assume that truth is paradoxical, that each article of wisdom contains within it its own contradictions, that truths stand side by side. Contradictory truths do not necessarily cancel each other out or dominate each other, but stand side by side, inviting participation and experimentation." One way that the client and therapist address this in therapy is by repeatedly asking each other or oneself the question: "What is being left out?" This simple question can assist in finding a synthesis and letting go of an absolute truth, a nondialectical stance.

Dialectics as Persuasion

From the point of view of dialogue and relationship, dialectics refers to change by persuasion and by making use of the oppositions inherent in the therapeutic relationship rather than by formal impersonal logic. Through the therapeutic opposition of contradictory positions, both client and therapist can arrive at new meanings within old meanings, moving closer to the essence of the subject under consideration. The spirit of a dialectical point of view is never to accept a proposition as a final truth or an undisputable fact. Thus, the question addressed by both client and therapist is "What is being left out of our understanding?" Dialectics as persuasion is represented in the specific dialectical strategies described later in this chapter. As readers will see, when we discuss the consultation strategies, dialectical dialogue is also very important in therapist consultation meetings. Perhaps more than any other factor, attention to dialectics can reduce the chances of what psychodynamic therapists have labeled "staff splitting," that is, the frequent phenomenon of therapists' disagreeing or arguing (sometimes vehemently) about how to treat and interact with an individual client who has BPD. This "splitting" among staff members is often due to one or more factions within the staff deciding that they (and sometimes they alone) know the truth about a particular client or clinical problem.

Dialectical Case Conceptualization

Dialectical assumptions influence case conceptualization in DBT in a number of ways. First, dialectics suggests that a psychological disorder is best conceptualized as a systemic dysfunction characterized by (1) defining the disorder with respect to normal functioning, (2) assuming continuity between health and the disorder, and (3) assuming that the disorder results from multiple rather than single causes (Hollandsworth, 1990). Similarly, Linehan's biosocial theory of BPD, presented below, assumes that BPD represents a breakdown in normal functioning, and that this disorder is best conceptualized as a systemic dysfunction of the emotion regulation system. The theory proposes that the pathogenesis of BPD results from numerous factors: Some are genetic–biological predispositions that create individual differences in susceptibility to emotion dysregulation, known as emotion vulnerability; others result from the individual's interaction with the environment, referred to as the invalidating environment. Assuming a systemic view compels the theorist to integrate work from a variety of fields and disciplines.

A second dialectical assumption that underlies Linehan's biosocial theory of BPD is that the relationship between the individual and the environment is a process of reciprocal influence, and that the outcome at any given moment is due to the transaction between the person and the environment. Within social learning theory, this is the principle of "reciprocal determinism." Besides focusing on reciprocal influence, a transactional view also highlights the constant state of flux and change of the individual–environment system. Therefore, BPD can occur in multiple environments and families, including chaotic, perfect, and even ordinary families. Millon (1987) made much the same point in discussing the etiology of BPD and the futility of locating the "cause" of the disorder in any single event or time period.

Both transactional and interactive models, such as the diathesis–stress model of psychopathology, call attention to the role of dysfunctional environments in bringing about disorder in the vulnerable individual. A transactional model, however, highlights a number of points that are easy to overlook in an interactive diathesis–stress model. For example, a person (Person A) may act in a manner stressful to an individual (Person B) only because of the stress Person B is putting on Person A. Take the child who, due to an accident, requires most of the parents' free time just to meet survival needs. Or consider the client who, due to the need for constant suicide precautions, uses up much of the inpatient nursing resources. Both of these environments are stretched in their ability to respond well to further stress. Both may invalidate or temporarily blame the victim if any further demand on the system is made. Although the system (e.g., the family or the therapeutic milieu) may have been predisposed to respond dysfunctionally in any case, such responses may have been avoided in the absence of exposure to the stress of that particular individual. A transactional, or dialectical, account of psychopathology may allow greater compassion, because it is incompatible with the assignment of blame, by highlighting the reality of the situation rather than judgments about the individuals. This is particularly relevant with a label as stigmatized among mental health professionals as "borderline" (for examples of the misuse of the diagnosis, see Reiser & Levenson, 1984).

A final assumption in our discussion regards the definition of behavior and the implications of defining behavior broadly. Linehan's theory, and behaviorists in general, take "behavior" to mean anything an organism does involving action and responding to stimulation (*Merriam-Webster's New Universal Unabridged Dictionary*, 1983, p. 100). Conventionally, behaviorists categorize behavior as motor, cognitive/verbal, and physiological, all of which may be either public or private. There are several points to make here. First, dividing behavior into these three categories is arbitrary and is done for conceptual clarity rather than in response to evidence that these response modes actually are functionally separate systems. This point is especially relevant to understanding emotion regulation, given that basic research on emotions demonstrates that these response systems are sometimes overlapping, somewhat independent, but definitely not wholly independent, thus remaining consistent with the dialectical worldview. A related point here is that in contrast to biological and cognitive theories of BPD, biosocial theory suggests that there is no a priori reason for favoring explanations emphasizing one mode of behavior as intrinsically more important or compelling than others. Rather, from a biosocial perspective, the crucial questions are under what conditions a given behavior–behavior relationship or response system–response system relationship holds, and under what conditions these relationships enter causal pathways for the etiology and maintenance of BPD.

BIOSOCIAL THEORY

Emotion Dysregulation

Linehan's biosocial theory suggests that BPD is primarily a dysfunction of the emotion regulation system. Behavioral patterns in BPD are functionally related to or are unavoidable consequences of this fundamental dysregulation across several, perhaps all, emotions, including both positive and negative emotions. From Linehan's point of view, this dysfunction of the emotion regulation system is the core pathology; thus, it is neither simply symptomatic nor definitional. Emotion dysregulation is a product of the combination of emotional vulnerability and difficulties in modulating emotional reactions. Emotional vulnerability is conceptualized as high sensitivity to emotional stimuli, intense emotional responses, and a slow return to emotional baseline. Deficits in emotion modulation may be due to difficulties in (1) inhibiting mood-dependent behaviors; (2) organizing behavior in the service of goals, independently of current mood; (3) increasing or decreasing physiological arousal as needed; (4) distracting attention from emotionally evocative stimuli; and/or (5) experiencing emotion without either immediately withdrawing or producing an extreme secondary negative emotion (see Gottman & Katz, 1990, for a further discussion).

Conceptually, the deficit in the emotion regulation system leads to not only immense emotional suffering but also multiple behavioral problems in individuals with BPD. When clinician's ratings of characteristics associated with psychopathology are examined, tendencies toward being chronically anxious and unhappy, depressed, or despondent are the most highly descriptive of the BPD (Bradley, Zittel, & Westen, 2005). Dysfunction leads the individual to attempt to escape aversive emotions, often leading to further suffering. For example, a female client may be experiencing intense anger after a fight with her partner, and in an effort to escape the anger, she engages in cutting behaviors. She begins to feel relief from her anger for a short period of time. However, once her anger begins to subside, shame in response to the cutting behavior begins to increase and the cycle of emotion escape behavior continues. Although the mechanisms of the initial dysregulation remain unclear, it is likely that biological factors play a primary role. Siever and Davis (1991) hypothesized that deficits in emotion regulation for clients with BPD are related to both instability and hyperresponsiveness of catecholamine function. The etiology of this dysregulation may range from genetic influences to prenatal factors to traumatic childhood events affecting development of the brain and nervous system. Furthermore, adoption studies of monozygotic (MZ) twins (Davison & Neale, 1994) suggest a genetic vulnerability. However, researchers do not claim that genetic or biological factors accounted for all pathology. If pathology were solely determined by genetics, then 100% of the MZ twins would have been presumed to share the same pathology. Because this does not occur, we can explain the differences through the transactions between biology, as described earlier, and the environment.

Invalidating Environments

Most individuals with an initial temperamental vulnerability to emotion dysregulation do not develop BPD. Thus, the theory suggests further that particular developmental environments are necessary. The crucial developmental circumstance in Linehan's theory is the transaction between emotion vulnerability and the presence of the "invalidating environment" (Linehan, 1987a, 1987b, 1989, 1993a), which is defined by its tendency to negate, punish, and/or respond erratically and inappropriately to private experiences, independent of the validity of the actual behavior. Private experiences, and especially emotional experiences and interpretations of events, are not taken as valid responses to events by others; are punished, trivialized, dismissed, or disregarded; and/or are attributed to socially unacceptable characteristics, such as overreactivity, inability to see things realistically, lack of motivation, motivation to harm or manipulate, lack of discipline, or failure to adopt a positive (or, conversely, discriminating) attitude. The invalidating environment can be any part of an individual's social environment, including immediate or extended family, school, work, or community. Within each of these environments are even more specific idiosyncrasies that may impact the environment, such as birth order, years between siblings, teachers and peers, and/or coworkers. It is important to note that because two children grew up in the same home does not mean that they were raised in identical environments. Furthermore, individuals are often not aware of their invalidating behaviors and are not acting with a malicious intent.

There are three primary characteristics of the invalidating environment. First, the environment indiscriminately rejects communication of private experiences and self-generated behaviors. For example a person may be told, "You are so angry, but you won't admit it" or "You can't be hungry, you just ate." Second, the invalidating environment may punish emotional displays and intermittently reinforce emotional escalation. For example, a woman breaks up with her partner and is feeling depressed. Her friends and family begin telling her to "Get over it," "He wasn't worth it," "Don't feel sad." Over the course of the next week, she becomes more depressed and is beginning to withdraw from daily activities. Again, her environment responds in an invalidating manner. Finally after another 3 days of high emotional arousal she makes a suicide attempt. At that moment the environment jumps in and provides support by taking care of her. Unfortunately, this type of pattern often results in inadvertent reinforcement of extreme dysfunctional behavior. Finally, the invalidating environment may oversimplify the ease of problem solving and meeting goals for an individual.

The high incidence of childhood sexual abuse reported among individuals with BPD (Bryer, Nelson, Miller, & Krol, 1987; Herman, 1986; Herman, Perry, & van der Kolk, 1989; Wagner, Linehan, & Wasson, 1989) suggests that sexual abuse may be a prototypic invalidating experience for children. The relationship of early sexual abuse to BPD, however, is quite controversial and is open to many interpretations. On the one hand, Silk, Lee, Hill, and Lohr (1995) reported that the number of criterion BPD behaviors met was correlated with severity of childhood sexual abuse in a group of clients with BPD. On the other hand, a review by Fossati, Madeddu, and Maffei (1999) suggested that sexual abuse is not a major risk factor for BPD.

The overall results of this transactional pattern between the emotionally vulnerable individual and the invalidating environment are the emotional dysregulation and behavioral patterns exhibited by the borderline adult. Such an individual has never learned how to label and regulate emotional arousal, how to tolerate emotional distress, or when to trust his or her own emotional responses as reflections of valid interpretations of events resulting in self-invalidation (Linehan, 1993a). In more optimal environments, public validation of one's private, internal experiences results in the development of a stable identity. In the family of a person with BPD, however, private experiences may be responded to erratically and with insensitivity. Thus, the individual learns to mistrust his or her internal states, and instead scans the environment for cues about how to act, think, or feel. This general reliance on others results in the individual's failure to develop a coherent sense of self. Emotional dysfunction also interferes with the development and maintenance of stable interpersonal relationships, which depend on both a stable sense of self and a capacity to self-regulate emotions. The invalidating environment's tendency to trivialize or ignore the expression of negative emotion also shapes

an expressive style later seen in the adult with BPD—a style that vacillates from inhibition and suppression of emotional experience to extreme behavioral displays. Behaviors such as overdosing, cutting, and burning have important affect-regulating properties and are additionally quite effective in eliciting helping behaviors from an environment that otherwise ignores efforts to ameliorate intense emotional pain. From this perspective, the dysfunctional behaviors characteristic of BPD may be viewed as maladaptive solutions to overwhelming, intensely painful negative affect.

DIALECTICAL DILEMMAS

Linehan (1993a) describes "dialectical dilemmas" as behavioral patterns of the client that often interfere with therapy. These behavioral patterns, also referred to as "secondary targets" in treatment (compared to other targets that we describe later) represent six behaviors that are dichotomized into a set of three dimensions of behavior defined by their opposite poles (see Figure 9.1). At one end of each dimension is the behavior that theoretically is most directly influenced biologically via deficits in emotion regulation. At the other end is behavior that has been socially reinforced in the invalidating environment. These secondary targets are characteristics of individuals with BPD that often interfere with change, thus interfering with therapy.

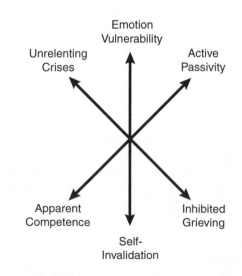

FIGURE 9.1. Dialectical dilemmas in DBT.

Emotion Vulnerability/Self-Invalidation

One dialectical dilemma is represented by biologically influenced emotional vulnerability on the one hand (e.g., the sense of being out of control or falling into the abyss) and by socially influenced self-invalidation on the other (e.g., hate and contempt directed toward the self, dismissal of one's accomplishments). Along this dimension of behavior, clients with BPD often vacillate between acute awareness of their own intense, unbearable, and uncontrollable emotional suffering on the one hand, and dismissal, judgment, and invalidation of their own suffering and helplessness on the other.

Emotion vulnerability here refers to the client's acute experience and communication of emotional vulnerability and excruciating emotional pain. "Vulnerability" here means the acute experience of vulnerability rather than the sensitivity to emotional cues that defines the term when discussing the emotion dysregulation difficulties of the BPD person. In the case here, vulnerability is experienced; in the latter case, the vulnerability may not be experienced. Three reactions to emotional vulnerability are common in BPD: (1) freezing or dissociating in the face of intense emotion; (2) rage, often directed at society in general or at individuals who are experienced as invalidating; and (3) intense despair. Suicide here can function to communicate to others the depth of one's suffering ("I'll show you") and/or as an escape from an unendurable life.

On the other side of this polarity is self-invalidation. What is invalidated, in essence, is one's own emotional experiencing and dysregulated responses. The most typical pattern here is a reaction to emotional pain with intense self-blame and self-hate. These individuals identify themselves as perpetrators, which results in intense levels of shame and contempt toward the self ("There is nothing wrong with me, I'm just a bad person"). Mood-dependent perfectionism is also common. Here, the individual belittles, ignores, or discounts the difficulty of his or her own life or may overestimate the ease of solving current problems. Unfortunately, this may initiate the start of a cycle that may eventually end in death. Extreme perfectionism often ultimately leads to failure, especially in individuals who overestimate their abilities; the failure then results in self-hatred, which cues suicidal behaviors in these individuals. Finally, self-invalidation can also be expressed through willful suppression, meaning that the individual actively denies the experience of all emotion. Often clients who come into our offices simply state, "I don't do emotions." As with emotion vulnerability, self-invalidation needs to be attended to actively and directly with individuals with BPD, due to the lethal consequences of these behaviors.

Active Passivity/Apparent Competence

A second dimension of behavior is a tendency toward active passivity versus the socially mediated behavior of apparent competence. Either pole of this dimension can lead to anger, guilt, or shame on the part of the client, and a tendency for the therapist to either under- or overestimate the client's capabilities.

"Active passivity" may be defined as passivity in solving one's own problems, while actively engaging others to solve one's problems. It can also be described as passivity that appears to be an active process of shutting down in the face of seeing problems coming in the future. In a sense, individuals with BPD do not appear to have the ability to regulate themselves internally, particularly when the regulation required is non-mood-dependent behaviors. Individuals with BPD appear to be "relational selves" rather than "autonomous selves"; that is, they are more highly regulated by their environment than by internal dialogues, choices and decisions. Their best form of self-regulation is to regulate their environment, such that it then provides the regulation they need. The problem here is that managing one's environment and getting the support one needs requires a good deal of emotional consistency and regulation, characteristics that ordinarily are difficult for individuals with BPD. Lorna Benjamin has described this characteristic as "My misery is your command" (1996, p. 192).

On the opposite side of the polarity is apparent competence. "Apparent competence" refers to the tendency of other individuals to overestimate the capabilities of the individual with BPD. Thus, this characteristic is defined by the behavior of the observer rather than the behavior of the individual with BPD. This failure to accurately perceive their difficulties and "disability" has serious effects on individuals with BPD. Not only do they not get the help they need, but also their emotional pain and difficulties may easily be invalidated, leading to a further sense of being misunderstood. A number of behavioral patterns can precipitate this overestimation of the competence of the individual with BPD. Often, a significant discrepancy between the individual's verbal and nonverbal presentations results in the individual with BPD believing that he or she has sufficiently communicated his or her level of distress, when in fact the observer interprets the individual as effectively managing a difficult situation. An example would be a woman speaking nonchalantly and without emotion about urges toward suicide after a fight with her husband. Individuals with BPD also frequently have difficulty generalizing behaviors across situations, especially in relationships. For example, the person may be able to cope well in the presence of one person, such as a therapist, but be unable to cope when he or she is alone or with someone other than the therapist. The therapist, understandably, may then fail to predict the dysregulation that occurs as the client walks away from the therapy session. Additionally, there may be a difficulty in generalizing coping behaviors across different moods. In one mood, a problem is solvable; in another, it is not. This may not be so difficult for the observer to figure out if mood changes are readily apparent to the observer, but often they are not. Thus, accurate estimates of the person's competence actually require the observer, such as the therapist, constantly to anticipate mood changes that might occur to be able to predict what a client might or might not do. It is this characteristic, more than any other, that leads so often to a client walking out of a session, with the therapist believing all is well, only to end up in the emergency department with a suicide attempt 2 hours later. At times, client failures are nothing more than failures of the therapist (and often the client, also) to predict future behavior accurately.

Unrelenting Crisis/Inhibited Grieving

The third dimension of behavior is the tendency of the client with BPD to experience life as a series of unrelenting crises as opposed to the behavior of "inhibited grieving" (i.e., an inability to experience emotions associated with significant trauma or loss). The client experiences each of these extremes in a way that facilitates movement to the other extreme; for example, attempting to inhibit emotional experiences related to current crises may result in problem behaviors that add to existing crises. As with all of these dialectical dilemmas, the solution is for therapist and client to work toward a more balanced position that represents a synthesis of the opposing poles.

Individuals with BPD who experience unrelenting crises have lives that are often characterized as chaotic and in crisis. "Crisis" is defined as the occurrence of problems that are extreme, with significant pressure to resolve them quickly. The consequence of the unrelenting crisis is that the individual with BPD, as well as the person's environmental resources, such as family, friends, coworkers, and even the therapist, slowly wear down. There are three typical scenarios that result in a pattern of unrelenting crisis. First, individuals with extreme impulsivity and emotion dysregulation engage in behaviors that result in crisis situations. Poor judgment is a key element to assess when analyzing the impulsive behaviors of individuals with BPD. Second, situations that do not start out as crises can quickly become critical due to the lack of resources available to many individuals with BPD. This may be due to socioeconomic status, or to lack of family or peer support. Finally, unrelenting crises can be due simply to fate or bad luck at a given moment, a phenomenon that is out of the person's control. For example, an unexpected disaster in a client's apartment due to the neighbors running the water in their sink for an extended period of time, might occur. The floors in the client's apartment are damaged by the water and he or she does not have the financial resources to pay for renter's insurance or to replace the carpet in the apartment. His or her apartment is now uninhabitable but he or she does not have any place else to stay. This problem is out of the person's control, but it is still that person's responsibility to solve.

At the other extreme, and often precipitated by a crisis, is the phenomenon of "inhibited grieving." In this context, "grief" refers to the process of grieving, including experiencing multiple painful emotions associated with loss, particularly traumatic loss, not just the one emotion of deep sadness or grief. Individuals with BPD may not be able to experience or process the grief related to the loss of the life they had expected for themselves, and ordinarily do not believe they will recover from the grief if they actually try to experience or to cope with it on their own.

As one client said to us, "I don't do sadness." Another said, "I feel sad, I die." Individuals with BPD may not recognize their own emotional avoidance and shutdown. Thus, it is crucial that the therapist attend to emotional avoidance, particularly of sadness and grief, and assist clients through the grief process. Areas that must be confronted, grieved, and finally accepted include an insurmountably painful childhood, a biological makeup that makes life harder rather than easier, inability to "fit in" in many environments, absence of loving people in the current environment, or loss of hope for a particular future for which one had ardently hoped. What must be confronted by the therapist is that egregious losses can be real and clients might be right: They really cannot get out of the abyss if they fall into it. Regardless of the situation to be grieved, avoidance of these situations may lead to increased shame. The shame is a result of believing that one is unloved, being alone, or fearing that one will not be able to cope in the face of emotional situations. Many of our clients believe that if they begin to address any of these areas, they will not be able to function in their lives, and often this is true. They do not have the skills or resources to assist them with the process of experiencing emotions. We often tell clients that managing grief or processing emotions requires going to the cemetery to pay tribute to what is lost, but building a house at the cemetery and living there is not a good idea. It is a place to visit, experience the sadness of the loss, and then leave. The use of this metaphor has helped many of our clients to experience emotion without falling into the abyss.

STAGES OF THERAPY AND TREATMENT GOALS

In theory, treatment of all clients with BPD can be organized and determined based on their levels of disorder, and is conceptualized as occurring in stages. "Level of disorder" is defined by the current severity, pervasiveness, complexity, disability, and imminent threat presented by the client. Clients can enter into five stages of treatment based on their current level of disorder. First, a pretreatment stage prepares the client for therapy and elicits a commitment to work toward the various treatment goals. Orientation to specific goals and treatment strategies, and commitment to work toward goals

addressed during this stage, are likely to be important throughout all stages of treatment. In Stage 1 of therapy, the primary focus is on stabilizing the client and achieving behavioral control. Out-of-control behaviors constitute those that are disordered due to the severity of the disorder (e.g., as seen in an actively psychotic client) or due to severity combined with complexity of multiple diagnoses (e.g., as seen in a suicidal client who has BPD with comorbid panic disorder and depression). Generally, the criteria for putting a client in Stage 1 are based on level of current functioning, together with the inability of the client to work on any other goals before behavior and functioning come under better control. As Mintz (1968) suggested in discussing treatment of the suicidal client, all forms of psychotherapy are ineffective with a dead client. In the subsequent stages (2–4), the treatment goals are to replace "quiet desperation" with nontraumatic emotional experiencing (Stage 2); to achieve "ordinary" happiness and unhappiness, and to reduce ongoing disorders and problems in living (Stage 3); and to resolve a sense of incompleteness and to achieve freedom (Stage 4). In summary, the orientation of the treatment is first to get action under control, then to help the client to feel better, to resolve problems in living and residual disorder, and to find freedom (and, for some, a sense of transcendence). All research to date has focused on the severely or multiply disordered clients who enter treatment at Stage 1. Understanding a client's severity of disorder and level of treatment through accurate and thorough assessment can assist a therapist in two ways. First, it aids in treatment planning and conceptualization with the client, and in identifying the appropriate level of care needed. Second, it can assist a therapist in determining whether to accept the client into care based on the level of severity. For example, if a therapist has multiple Stage 1 clients, he or she may not want to take on one more Stage 1 client, until treatment is either completed with the others or far enough along that the therapist does not have multiple clients in crisis at one time. Furthermore, some therapists may also use level of severity to determine that a client's condition is not severe enough for the type of treatment the therapist provides; for example, DBT may be too intensive a treatment for someone with a single diagnosis of major depressive disorder.

Pretreatment: Orienting and Commitment

Specific tasks of orientation are twofold. First, client and therapist must arrive at a mutually informed decision to work together. Typically, the first one to four sessions are presented to the client as opportunities for client and therapist to explore this possibility. Diagnostic interviewing, history taking, and formal behavioral analyses of high-priority, targeted behaviors can be woven into initial therapy sessions or be conducted separately. Second, client and therapist must negotiate a common set of expectancies to guide the initial steps of therapy. Agreements outlining specifically what the client and therapist can expect from each other are discussed and agreed to. When necessary, the therapist attempts to modify the client's dysfunctional beliefs regarding the process of therapy. Issues addressed include the rate and magnitude of change that can reasonably be expected, the goals of treatment and general treatment procedures, and various myths the client may have about the process of therapy in general. The dialectical/biosocial view of BPD is also presented. Orientation covers several additional points. First, DBT is presented as a supportive therapy requiring a strong collaborative relationship between client and therapist. DBT is not a suicide prevention program, but a life enhancement program in which client and therapist function as a team to create a life worth living. Second, DBT is described as a cognitive-behavioral therapy with a primary emphasis on analyzing problematic behaviors and replacing them with skillful behaviors, and on changing ineffective beliefs and rigid thinking patterns. Third, the client is told that DBT is a skills-oriented therapy, with special emphasis on behavioral skills training. The commitment and orienting strategies, balanced by validation strategies described later, are the most important strategies during this phase of treatment. The therapist places a strong effort into getting the client to commit to not engaging in suicidal or NSSI behaviors for some specified period of time before allowing the client to leave the session; it can be for 1 year, 6 months, until the next session, or until tomorrow.

Stage 1: Attaining Basic Capacities

The primary focus of the first stage of therapy is attaining behavioral control in order to build a life pattern that is reasonably functional and stable. Furthermore, DBT does not promote itself as a suicide prevention program; instead, it focuses on life improvement. Therefore, the primary treatment goal in DBT and in Stage 1 specifically is to assist clients in building a life worth living. DBT attains this goal by focusing the treatment on specific behavioral targets agreed upon by both therapist and client. Specific targets in order of importance are to reduce life-threatening behaviors (e.g., suicide attempts, increase in suicide ideation, NSSI behaviors, homicidal threats and behaviors), therapy-interfering behaviors (e.g., late to session, missing sessions, not following treatment plan, hostile attacks on the therapist), and quality-of-life–interfering behaviors (e.g., substance abuse, eating disorder, homelessness, serious Axis I disorders), and to increase behavioral skills. These targets are approached hierarchically and recursively as higher-priority behaviors reappear in each session. However, this does not mean that these behaviors must be addressed in this specific order during a session; it means that based on the hierarchy, all relevant behavior must be addressed at some point within the session. For example, if a client is 10 minutes late to session (therapy-interfering behavior) and has cut within the last week (life-threatening behavior), the therapist may choose to address the therapy-interfering behavior first, then move on to address the life-threatening behaviors.

With severely dysfunctional and suicidal clients, significant progress on first stage targets may take up to 1 year or more. In addition to these therapy targets, the goal of increasing dialectical behaviors is universal to all modes of treatment. Dialectical thinking encourages clients to see reality as complex and multifaceted, to hold contradictory thoughts simultaneously and learn to integrate them, and to be comfortable with inconsistency and contradictions. For individuals with BPD, who are extreme and dichotomous in their thinking and behavior, this is a formidable task indeed. A dialectical emphasis applies equally to a client's patterns of behavior, because the client is encouraged to integrate and balance emotional and overt behavioral responses. In particular, dialectical tensions arise in the areas of skills enhancement versus self-acceptance, problem solving versus problem acceptance, and affect regulation versus affect tolerance. Behavioral extremes, whether emotional, cognitive, or overt responses, are constantly confronted while more balanced responses are taught.

Life-Threatening Behaviors

Keeping a client alive must, of course, be the first priority in any psychotherapy. Thus, reducing suicide crisis behaviors (any behaviors that place the client at high and imminent risk for suicide or threaten to do so, including credible suicide threats, planning, preparations, obtaining lethal means, and high suicide intent) is the highest priority in DBT. The target and its priority are made explicit in DBT during orientation and throughout treatment, simply because suicidal behavior and the risk of suicide are of paramount concern for clients with BPD. Similarly, any acute, intentional NSSI behaviors share the top priority. The priority here is due both to the risk of suicidal and NSSI behavior as the single best predictor of subsequent suicide. Similarly, DBT also targets suicide ideation and client expectations about the value and long-term consequences of suicidal behavior, although these behaviors may not necessarily be targeted directly.

Therapy-Interfering Behaviors

Keeping clients and therapists working together collaboratively is the second explicitly targeted priority in DBT. The chronic nature of most problems among clients with BPD, including their high tendency to end therapy prematurely, and the likelihood of therapist burnout and iatrogenic behaviors when treating BPD require such explicit attention. Both client and therapist behaviors that threaten the relationship or therapeutic progress are addressed directly, immediately, consistently, and constantly—and most importantly, before rather than after either the therapist or the client no longer wants to continue. Interfering behaviors of the client, including those that actually interfere with receiving the therapy (e.g., lateness to sessions, missed sessions, lack of transportation to sessions, dissociating in sessions) or with other clients benefiting from therapy (in group or milieu settings; e.g., selling drugs to other clients in the program), and those that burn out or cross the personal limits of the therapist (e.g., repeated crisis calls at three in the morning, repeated verbal attacks on the therapist) are treated within therapy sessions. Behaviors of the therapist include any

that are iatrogenic (e.g., inadvertently reinforcing dysfunctional behaviors), as well as any that cause the client unnecessary distress or make progress difficult (e.g., therapist arriving late to sessions, missing sessions, not returning phone calls within a reasonable time frame). These behaviors are dealt with in therapy sessions, if brought up by either the client or the therapist, and are also discussed during the consultation/supervision meeting.

Quality-of-Life–Interfering Behaviors

The third target of Stage 1 addresses all other behaviors that interfere with the client having a reasonable quality of life. Typical behaviors in this category include serious substance abuse, severe major depressive episodes, severe eating disorders, high-risk and out-of-control sexual behaviors, extreme financial difficulties (uncontrollable spending or gambling, inability to handle finances), criminal behaviors that are likely to lead to incarceration, employment- or school-related dysfunctional behaviors (a pattern of quitting jobs or school prematurely, getting fired or failing in school, not engaging in any productive activities), housing-related dysfunctional behaviors (living with abusive people, not finding stable housing), mental health–related patterns (going in and out of hospitals, failure to take or abuse of necessary medications), and health-related problems (failure to treat serious medical disorders). The goal here is for the client to achieve a stable lifestyle that meets reasonable standards for safety and adequate functioning.

Behavioral Skills

The fourth target of Stage 1 is for the client to achieve a reasonable capacity for acquiring and applying skillful behaviors in the areas of distress tolerance, emotion regulation, interpersonal effectiveness, self-management, and the capacity to respond with awareness without being judgmental ("mindfulness" skills). In our outpatient program, the primary responsibility for skills training lies with the weekly DBT skills group. The individual therapist monitors the acquisition and use of skills over time, and aids the client in applying skills to specific problem situations in his or her own life. Additionally, it is the role of the individual therapist, not the skills group leader, to provide skills coaching to the client as needed when problems arise.

Stage 2: Posttraumatic Stress Reduction

Stage 1 of DBT takes a direct approach to managing dysfunctional behavioral and regulating emotional patterns. Although the connection between current behavior and previous traumatic events (including those from childhood) may be explored and noted, the focus of the treatment is distinctly on analyzing the relationship among current thoughts, feelings, and behaviors, and on accepting and changing current patterns. The aim of Stage 2 DBT is to reduce "quiet desperation," which can be defined as extreme emotional pain in the presence of control of action (Linehan et al., 1999). A wide range of emotional experiencing difficulties (e.g., avoidance of emotions and emotion-related cues) are targeted in this stage, with the goal of increasing the capacity for normative emotional experiencing (i.e., the ability to experience a full range of emotions without either severe emotional escalation or behavioral dyscontrol). Because many individuals with BPD have histories of severe and chronic traumatic experiences, these problems frequently take the form of posttraumatic stress disorder (PTSD) and related behaviors and are treated through exposure therapy (formal and informal). Stage 2 addresses four goals: remembering and accepting the facts of earlier traumatic events; reducing stigmatization and self-blame commonly associated with some types of trauma; reducing the oscillating denial and intrusive response syndromes common among individuals who have suffered severe trauma; and resolving dialectical tensions regarding placement of blame for the trauma.

Stage 3: Resolving Problems in Living and Increasing Respect for Self

In the third stage, DBT targets the client's unacceptable unhappiness and problems in living. At this stage, the client with BPD has either done the work necessary to resolve problems in the prior two stages or was never severely disordered enough to need it. Although problems at this stage may still be serious, the individual is functional in major domains of living. The goal here is for the client to achieve a level of ordinary happiness and unhappiness, as well as independent self-respect. To this end, the client is helped to value, believe in, trust, and validate him- or herself. The targets here are the abilities to evaluate one's own behavior nondefensively, to trust one's own responses, and to hold on to self-evaluations, independent of the opinions of others. Ultimately, the therapist must pull back and persistently reinforce the client's independent attempts at self-validation, self-care, and problem solving. Although the goal is not for clients to become independent of all people, it is important that they achieve sufficient self-reliance to relate to and depend on others without self-invalidating.

Stage 4: Attaining the Capacity for Freedom and Sustained Contentment

The final stage of treatment in DBT targets the resolution of a sense of incompleteness and the development of a capacity for sustained contentment. The focus on freedom encompasses the goal of freedom from the need to have one's wishes fulfilled, or one's current life or behavioral and emotional responses changed. Here the goals are expanded awareness, spiritual fulfillment, and the movement into experiencing flow. For individuals at Stage 4, long-term insight-oriented psychotherapy, spiritual direction or practices, or other organized experiential treatments and/or life experiences may be of most benefit.

STRUCTURING TREATMENT: FUNCTIONS AND MODES

Functions of Treatment

Treatment in DBT is structured around the five essential functions it serves. Treatment functions to (1) enhance behavioral capabilities by expanding the individual's repertoire of skillful behavioral patterns; (2) improve the client's motivation to change by reducing reinforcement for dysfunctional behaviors and high-probability responses (cognitions, emotions, actions) that interfere with effective behaviors; (3) ensure that new behaviors generalize from the therapeutic to the natural environment; (4) enhance the motivation and capabilities of the therapist so that effective treatment is rendered; and (5) structure the environment so that effective behaviors, rather than dysfunctional behaviors, are reinforced.

Modes of Treatment: Who Does What and When

Responsibility for performing functions and meeting target goals of treatment in DBT is spread across the various modes of treatment, with focus and attention varying according to the mode of therapy. The individual therapist (who is always the primary therapist in DBT) attends to one order of targets and is also, with the client, responsible for organizing the treatment so that all goals are met. In skills training, a different set of goals is targeted; during phone calls, yet another hierarchy of targets takes precedence. In the consultation/supervision mode, therapists' behaviors are the targets. Therapists engaging in more than one mode of therapy (e.g., individual, group, and telephone coaching) must stay cognizant of the functions and order of targets specific to each mode, and switch smoothly from one hierarchy to another as the modes of treatment change.

Individual Therapy

DBT assumes that effective treatment must attend both to client capabilities and behavioral skills deficits, and to motivational and behavioral performance issues that interfere with use of skillful responses (function 2). Although there are many ways to effect these principles, in DBT the individual therapist is responsible for the assessment and problem solving of skill deficits and motivational problems, and for organizing other modes to address problems in each area.

Individual outpatient therapy sessions are scheduled on a once-a-week basis for 50–90 minutes, although twice-weekly sessions may be held as needed during crisis periods or at the beginning of therapy. The priorities of specific targets within individual therapy are the same as the overall priorities of DBT discussed earlier. Therapeutic focus within individual therapy sessions is determined by the highest-priority treatment target relevant at the moment. This ordering does not change over the course of therapy; however, the relevance of a target does change. Relevance is determined by either the client's most recent, day-to-day behavior (since the last session) or by current behavior during the therapy session. If satisfactory progress on one target goal has been achieved or the behavior has never been a

problem, or if the behavior is currently not evident, then the therapist shifts attention to another treatment target according to the hierarchy. The consequence of this priority allocation is that when high-risk suicidal behaviors or intentional self-injury, therapy-interfering behaviors, or serious quality-of-life–interfering behaviors are occurring, at least part of the session agenda must be devoted to each of these topics. If these behaviors are not occurring at the moment, then the topics to be discussed during Stages 1, 3, and 4 are set by the client. The therapeutic focus (within any topic area discussed) depends on the stage of treatment, the skills targeted for improvement, and any secondary targets. During Stage 1, for example, any problem or topic area can be conceptualized in terms of interpersonal issues and skills needed, opportunities for emotion regulation, and/or a necessity for distress tolerance. During Stage 3, regardless of the topic, the therapist focuses on helping the client decrease problems in living and achieve independent self-respect, self-validation, and self-acceptance both within the session and within everyday life. (These are, of course, targets all through the treatment, but the therapist pulls back further during Stage 3 and does less work for the client than during the two preceding stages.) During Stage 2, the major focus is on reducing pervasive "quiet desperation," as well as changing the extreme emotions and psychological meanings associated with traumatizing cues.

For highly dysfunctional clients, it is likely that early treatment will necessarily focus on the upper part of the hierarchy. For example, if suicidal or NSSI behavior has occurred during the previous week, attention to it takes precedence over attention to therapy-interfering behavior. In turn, focusing on therapy-interfering behaviors takes precedence over working on quality-of-life–interfering behaviors. Although it is often possible to work on more than one target (including those generated by the client) in a given session, higher-priority targets always take precedence, but all relevant targets must be addressed adequately during the session. Again, targets do not need to be addressed in sequential order, they just have to be addressed during the session. Determining the relevance of targeted behaviors is assisted by the use of diary cards. These cards are filled out by the client during at least the first two stages of therapy and are brought to weekly sessions.

Failure to complete or to bring in a card is considered a therapy-interfering behavior and should be openly addressed as such. Diary cards record daily instances of suicidal and NSSI behavior, urges to self-harm or to engage in suicide behaviors (on a 0- to 5-point scale), "misery," use of substances (licit and illicit), and use of behavioral skills. Other targeted behaviors (bulimic episodes, daily productive activities, flashbacks, etc.) may also be recorded on the blank area of the card. The therapist doing DBT must develop the pattern of routinely reviewing the card at the beginning of each session. The card acts as a road map for each session; therefore, a session cannot begin until a diary card has been completed. If the card indicates that a life-threatening behavior has occurred, it is noted and discussed. If high suicide or self-harm urges are recorded, or there is a significant increase (e.g., an increase of 3 points or higher on the 0- to 5-point scale for urges) over the course of the week, they are assessed to determine whether the client is at risk for suicide. If a pattern of substance abuse or dependence appears, it is treated as a quality-of-life–interfering behavior.

Work on targeted behaviors involves a coordinated array of treatment strategies, described later in this chapter. Essentially, each session is a balance between structured, as well as unstructured, problem solving (including simple interpretive activities by the therapist) and unstructured validation. The amount of the therapist's time allocated to each—problem solving and validating—depends on (1) the urgency of the behaviors needing change or problems to be solved, and (2) the urgency of the client's needs for validation, understanding, and acceptance without any intimation of change being needed. However, there should be an overall balance in the session between change (problem solving) and acceptance (validation) strategies. Unbalanced attention to either side may result in a nondialectical session, in addition to impeding client progress.

Skills Training

The necessity of crisis intervention and attention to other primary targets makes skills acquisition within individual psychotherapy very difficult. Thus, a separate component of treatment directly targets the acquisition of behavioral skills (function 1). In DBT this usually takes the form of separate, weekly, 2- to 2½-hour group skills training sessions that clients must attend, ordinarily for a minimum of 6 months and preferably for a year. Skills training can also be done individually, although it is often more difficult to stay focused on teaching new skills in individual than in group therapy. After a client has gone through all skills modules twice (i.e., for 1 year), remaining in skills training is a matter of personal preference and need. Some DBT programs have developed graduate groups for individuals who have acquired the skills but still need weekly consultation in applying the skills effectively to everyday difficulties. It is important to note that there is no research to date on the effectiveness of graduate groups. In adolescent programs, family members are usually invited. Some programs include a separate friends and families skills training group as well.

Each group typically has a leader and a coleader. Whereas the primary role of the leader is to teach the skills, the coleader focuses on managing group process by keeping members both focused and attending to the material being taught, as well as processing the information (e.g., ensuring everyone is on the correct page, noticing when the leader's invalidation has led to a member shutting down, waking someone up, sitting next to a member who is crying during group). We have found that it is difficult to keep the group focused and the leader on schedule for teaching the skills if the leader attempts to manage both roles on his or her own. Oftentimes, the coleader role is the more difficult position to learn.

Skills training in DBT follows a psychoeducational format. In contrast to individual therapy, in which the agenda is determined primarily by the problem to be solved, the skills training agenda is set by the skill to be taught. As mentioned earlier, skills training also has a hierarchy of treatment targets that are used to keep the group focused: (1) therapy-destroying behaviors (e.g., using drugs on premises, which could lead to the clinic being shut down; property damage; threatening imminent suicide or homicidal behavior to a fellow group member or therapist); (2) increasing skills acquisition and strengthening; and (3) decreasing therapy-interfering behaviors (e.g., refusing to talk in a group setting, restless pacing in the middle of sessions, attacking the therapist and/or the therapy). However, therapy-interfering behaviors are not given the attention in skills training that they are given in the individual psychotherapy mode. If such behaviors were a primary focus, there would never be time for teaching behavioral skills. Generally, therapy-interfering behaviors are put on an extinction schedule, while a client is "dragged" through skills training and simultaneously soothed. In DBT, all skills training clients are required to be in concurrent individual psychotherapy. Throughout group or individual skills training, each client is urged to address other problematic behaviors with his or her primary therapist; if a serious risk of suicide develops, the skills training therapist refers the problem to the primary therapist.

Although all of the strategies described below are used in both individual psychotherapy and skills training, the mix is decidedly different. Skills acquisition, strengthening, and generalization strategies are the predominant change strategies in skills training. In addition, skills training is highly structured, much more so than the individual psychotherapy component. Half of each skills training session is devoted to reviewing homework practice of the skills currently being taught, and the other half is devoted to presenting and practicing new skills. Except when interpersonal process issues seriously threaten progress, the agenda and topics for discussion in skills training are usually set by the group leader.

Four skills modules are taught on a rotating basis over the course of 6 months. In standard DBT, mindfulness skills are taught in 2 consecutive weeks at the beginning of each of the subsequent modules. New members are able to join a group during either the 2 weeks of mindfulness or the first 2 weeks of the subsequent module. If a new member is not ready to join after this point, he or she must wait until the start of the next mindfulness module.

Mindfulness skills are viewed as central in DBT; thus, they are labeled the "core" skills. These skills represent a behavioral translation of meditation (including Zen and contemplative prayer) practice and include observing, describing, spontaneous participating, being nonjudgmental, focusing awareness, and focusing on effectiveness. Unlike standard behavior and cognitive therapies, which ordinarily focus on changing distressing emotions and events, a major emphasis of DBT is on learning to manage pain skillfully. Mindfulness skills reflect the ability to experience and to observe one's thoughts, emotions, and behaviors without evaluation, and without attempting to change

or control them. Distress tolerance skills comprise two types of skills. First, crisis survival skills are used to regulate behavior in order to manage painful situations without making them worse (e.g., without engaging in life-threatening behavior) until the problem can be solved. Second, accepting reality skills are used to tolerate the pain of problems that cannot be solved in either the short-term future or that may have occurred in the past and, therefore, cannot be changed ever. Emotion regulation skills target the reduction of emotional distress through exposure to the primary emotion in a nonjudgmental atmosphere. Emotion regulation skills include affect identification and labeling, mindfulness to the current emotions (i.e., experiencing nonjudgmentally), identifying obstacles to changing emotions, increasing positive emotional events, and behavioral expressiveness opposite to the emotion. Interpersonal effectiveness skills teach effective methods for deciding on objectives within conflict situations (either asking for something or saying "no" to a request) and teach strategies that maximize the chances of obtaining those objectives without harming the relationship or sacrificing self-respect. Self-management skills are taught in conjunction with the other behavioral skills; however, there is not a specific module allocated to these skills, because behavioral principles are inherent in all of DBT. Self-management skills include knowledge of the fundamental principles of learning and behavior change, and the ability to set realistic goals, to conduct one's own behavioral analysis, and to implement contingency management plans.

Telephone Consultation

Telephone calls between sessions (or other extratherapeutic contact when DBT is conducted in other settings, e.g., inpatient units) are an integral part of DBT. Telephone consultation calls also follow a target hierarchy: (1) to provide emergency crisis intervention and simultaneously break the link between suicidal behaviors and therapist attention; (2) to provide coaching in skills and promote skills generalization (function 3); and (3) to provide a context for repairing the therapeutic relationship, without requiring the client to wait until the next session. With respect to calls for skills coaching, the focus of a phone call varies depending on the complexity and severity of the problem to be solved and the amount of time the therapist is willing to spend on the phone. It is important to note that these calls are not considered therapy sessions and should not be used as such. Therapists must keep the function of the call in mind so that they do not begin conducting sessions over the phone; this behavior could easily lead to therapist burnout with the client. With easy or already clear situations, in which it is reasonably easy to determine what the client can or should do in the situation, the focus is on helping the client use behavioral skills (rather than dysfunctional behaviors) to address the problem. Alternatively, with complex problems, or with problems too severe for the client to resolve soon, the focus is on ameliorating and tolerating distress, and inhibiting dysfunctional problem-solving behaviors until the next therapy session. In the latter case, resolving the problem that set off the crisis is not the target of telephone coaching calls.

With the exception of taking necessary steps to protect the client's life when he or she has threatened suicide, all calls for help are handled as much alike as possible. This is done to break the contingency between suicidal and NSSI behaviors, and increased phone contact. To do this, the therapist can do one of two things: refuse to accept any calls (including suicide crisis calls), or insist that the client who calls during suicidal crises also call during other crises and problem situations. As Linehan (1993b) notes, experts on suicidal behaviors uniformly say that therapist availability is necessary with suicidal clients. Thus, DBT chooses the latter course and encourages (and at times insists) on calls during nonsuicidal crisis periods. In DBT, calling the therapist too infrequently, as well as too frequently, is considered therapy-interfering behavior. Through orientation to coaching calls during pretreatment the client learns what to expect during the calls. For example, a therapist may communicate to the client in session what the therapist will ask during the call, "What's the problem? What skills have you used? Where is your skills book? Go get it, and let's figure out what other skills you can use to get through this situation." It is important to highlight that clients and therapists can easily fall into the trap of considering the act of calling for phone consultation a skill. Although asking for help may be a current target of treatment, it is not considered a skill to be used when the client is in distress. Therapists want to reinforce the client for effectively reaching out; however, they do not want to reinforce the client who does not try using actual skills to manage the problem at hand prior to calling the therapist.

Additionally, the therapist is balancing the change-focused strategies with validation throughout the call. It is important that the therapist be aware of the contingency management principles that may be occurring during the phone calls to avoid inadvertently reinforcing crisis behaviors and to increase therapist–client contact between sessions.

A skills trainer uses phone calls for only one reason: to keep a client in the therapy (including, of course, when necessary, keeping the client alive). All other problems are handled by the primary therapist, and suicidal crises are turned over to the primary therapist as soon as possible. We have learned that this can be one of the most difficult distinctions for group leaders to uphold. Clients may call group leaders for a variety of reasons, and it is the role of the group leader consistently to refer the client back to the individual therapist. For example, a client may call a group leader to ask for assistance with the homework assigned the previous week. Although this may seem appropriate for the skills trainer to address, it should be referred back to the individual therapist. At most, the group leader may repeat what the assignment was but should not provide any coaching in how to complete the assignment.

The final priority for phone calls to individual therapists is relationship repair. Clients with BPD often experience delayed emotional reactions to interactions that have occurred during therapy sessions. From a DBT perspective, it is not reasonable to require clients to wait up to a whole week before dealing with these emotions, and it is appropriate for a client to call for a brief "heart-to-heart" talk. In these situations, the role of the therapist is to soothe and to reassure. In-depth analyses should wait until the next session.

Consultation Team

DBT assumes that effective treatment of BPD must pay as much attention to the therapist's behavior and experience in therapy as it does to the client's. Treating clients with BPD is enormously stressful, and staying within the DBT therapeutic frame can be tremendously difficult (function 4). Thus, an integral part of the therapy is the treatment of the therapist. Every therapist is required to be on a consultation team either with one other person or with a group. DBT consultation meetings are held weekly and are attended by therapists currently providing DBT to clients. At times, the clinical setting may require that the team be part of an administrative meeting due to time and space restraints. When this occurs, it is important to set a specific agenda and time limitations on each part of the meeting (administration, DBT) to ensure that therapist consultation issues are addressed. The roles of consultation are to hold the therapist within the therapeutic frame and to address problems that arise in the course of treatment delivery. Thus, the fundamental target is increasing adherence to DBT principles for each member of the consultation group. The DBT consultation team is viewed as an integral component of DBT; that is, it is considered peer group therapy for the therapists, in which each member is simultaneously a therapist to other members and a client. The focus is on applying DBT strategies to increase DBT-adherent behaviors and decrease non-DBT behaviors.

There are three primary functions of consultation to the therapist in DBT. First, a consultation team helps to keep each individual therapist in the therapeutic relationship. The role here is to cheerlead and to support the therapist. Second, the supervisor or consultation team balances the therapist in his or her interactions with the client. In providing balance, consultants may move close to the therapist, helping him/her maintain a strong position. Or consultants may move back from the therapist, requiring the therapist to move closer to the client to maintain balance. Third, within programmatic applications of DBT, the team provides the context for the treatment.

JOINING THE CONSULTATION TEAM

Each team comprises therapists who are currently treating a DBT client or are available to take on a DBT client. Prior to joining the team, it is important that the therapist be completely aware of his or her commitment. As with clients during the pretreatment phase of DBT, therapists must make a commitment to the team (see Table 9.1). A commitment session between the new member and either the team leader, a team member, or, in some cases, the entire team can be extraordinarily helpful here. The team member conducting the commitment session will use the same strategies and techniques used in a first

TABLE 9.1. DBT Consultation Team Commitment Session

1. To keep the agreements of the team, especially remaining compassionate, mindful, and dialectical.
2. To be available to see a client in whatever role one has joined the team for (e.g., individual therapist, group skills trainer, clinical supervisor, pharmacotherapist).
3. To function as a therapist in the group (to the group) and not just be a silent observer or a person that only speaks about his or her own problems.
4. To treat team meetings in the same way one treats any other group therapy session (i.e., attending the weekly meetings [not double scheduling other events or clients], on time, until the end, with pagers, PDAs, and phones out of sight and off or, if necessarily on, on silent).
5. To come to team meetings adequately prepared.
6. To be willing to give clinical advice to people who have more experience (especially when it's hard to imagine yourself as being able to offer anything useful).
7. To have the humility to admit your mistakes/difficulties and the willingness to have the group help you solve them.
8. To be nonjudgmental and compassionate of your fellow clinicians and clients. To ring the bell of nonjudgmentalness to remind yourself to not be judgmental or unmindful, but not to ring it as a proxy for criticizing someone. The bell is a reminder, not a censor.
9. To properly assess the problem before giving solutions (do unto others as you wish they would more often do unto you).
10. To call out "Elephant in the room" when others are ignoring or not seeing the elephant.
11. To be willing to go through a chain analysis even though you were only 31 seconds late and you would have been there on time if it were not for that traffic light that always takes all day to change.
12. To participate in team by sharing the roles of Leader, Observer, Note Taker or other tasks critical to team functioning.
13. If you feel that the consult team is not being useful or don't like the way it is being run, then say something about it rather than silently stewing in frustration.
14. To repair with the team in some way when team meetings are missed, because the team is only as strong as the weakest link. Therefore, the absence of any team member is felt.
15. To carry on even when feeling burnt out, frustrated, tired, overworked, underappreciated, hopeless, ineffective (easier committed to than done, of course).

session with a DBT client (e.g., devil's advocate, pros and cons, troubleshooting). In addition to the commitment items listed in Table 9.1, two fundamental commitments must be agreed to by each member of the team. First, as mentioned previously, the primary function of the team is to increase therapists' motivation and capability in providing DBT. Therefore, each member agrees to work actively toward increasing the team member's effectiveness and adherence when applying DBT principles and strategies to clients and to other team members. Second, the consultation team is a community of therapists treating a community of clients. Thus, each team member agrees to be responsible for treatment and outcomes of all clients treated by the team. For example, members of the team are agreeing that if a client being treated by any member of the team commits suicide, then all members will say "Yes" when asked if they have ever had a client commit suicide.

CONSULTATION MEETING FORMAT

There are multiple ways to run a DBT team meeting. The following is the way we conduct our meetings at the University of Washington (although it is important to note that even this format could change as needs of members change). Each of our DBT teams has an identified team leader. This person is typically the most experienced DBT therapist on the team, and his or her role is to articulate the DBT principles when necessary for overseeing the fidelity of the treatment provided. Additionally, a team may have an observer who rings a bell whenever team members make judgmental comments (in content or tone) about themselves, each other, or a client; stay polarized without seeking synthesis; fall out of mindfulness by doing two things at once; or jump in to solve a problem before assessing the problem. The point of these observations is not to lay blame, but to focus the team's awareness on the behavior and move past it.

A team may begin with a mindfulness practice. There are several functions of mindfulness on a team. First, it helps members transition into the team by participating fully and focusing on only one thing in the moment, using a DBT mindset. Second, it can provide an opportunity for team members to enhance their skills in leading and providing feedback about the practice with other team members. Consulta-

tion team agreements (see Table 9.2) have been developed to facilitate a DBT frame and help to create a supportive environment for managing client–therapist and therapist–therapist difficulties. Therefore, a team may elect to read one or all of the team agreements during the team meeting. Most importantly, an agenda is set by the team following the DBT hierarchy of targets, with a specific focus on the needs of the therapist rather than the problems of the clients. Our agenda at the University of Washington uses the following format; however, the following items can be prioritized differently based on the needs of an individual team: (1) the therapists' need for consultation around clients' suicidal crises or other life-threatening behaviors; (2) therapy-interfering behaviors (including client absences and dropouts, as well as therapist therapy-interfering behaviors); (3) therapist team-interfering behaviors and burnout; (4) severe or escalating deterioration in quality-of-life behaviors; (5) reportage of good news and therapists' effective behaviors; (6) a summary of the work of the previous skills group and graduate group by group leaders; and (7) discussion of administrative issues (requests to miss team or be out of town, new client contacts; changes in skills trainers or group time, format of consultation group, etc.). This agenda spans the 1-hour consultation meeting. Although the agenda may look impossibly long, therapists ordinarily manage the time by being explicit about their need for help and consultation from the team.

Ancillary Care

When problems in the client's environment interfere with the client's functioning or progress, the therapist moves to the case management strategies. Although not new, case management strategies direct the application of core strategies (discussed later) to case management problems. There are three case management strategies: the consultant-to-the-client strategy, environmental intervention, and the consultation/supervision team meeting (described above). Because DBT is grounded in dialectics and avoids becoming rigid, a therapist intervenes in the client's environment only under very specific conditions: (1) The client is unable to act on her own behalf and outcome is extremely important; (2) the environment will only speak with someone who is in high power

TABLE 9.2. DBT Consultation Team Agreements

1. *Dialectical agreement*: We agree to accept a dialectical philosophy: There is no absolute truth. When caught between two conflicting opinions, we agree to look for the truth in both positions and to search for a synthesis by asking questions such as "What is being left out?"

2. *Consultation to the client agreement*: We agree that the primary goal of this group is to improve our own skills as DBT therapists, and not serve as a go-between for clients to each other. We agree to not treat clients or each other as fragile. We agree to treat other group members with the belief that others can speak on their own behalf.

3. *Consistency agreement*: Because change is a natural life occurrence, we agree to accept diversity and change as they naturally come about. This means that we do not have to agree with each others' positions about how to respond to specific clients, nor do we have to tailor our own behavior to be consistent with everyone else's.

4. *Observing limits agreement*: We agree to observe our own limits. As therapists and group members, we agree to not judge or criticize other members for having different limits from our own (e.g., too broad, too narrow, "just right").

5. *Phenomenological empathy agreement*: All things being equal, we agree to search for nonpejorative or phenomenologically empathic interpretations of our clients', our own, and other members' behavior. We agree to assume that we and our clients are trying our best and want to improve. We agree to strive to see the world through our clients' eyes and through one another's eyes. We agree to practice a nonjudgmental stance with our clients and with one another.

6. *Fallibility agreement*: We agree ahead of time that we are each fallible and make mistakes. We agree that we have probably either done whatever problematic things we're being accused of, or some part of it, so that we can let go of assuming a defensive stance to prove our virtue or competence. Because we are fallible, it is agreed that we will inevitably violate all of these agreements, and when this is done, we will rely on each other to point out the polarity and move to a synthesis.

(e.g., the therapist instead of the client); (3) when the client's or others lives are in imminent danger; (4) when it is the humane thing to do and will cause no harm; and (5) when the client is a minor.

CONSULTATION TO THE CLIENT STRATEGY

The consultation-to-the-client strategy was developed with three objectives in mind. First, clients must learn how to manage their own lives and care for themselves by interacting effectively with other individuals in the environment, including health care professionals. The consultation-to-the-client strategy emphasizes clients' capacities and targets their ability to take care of themselves. Second, this strategy was designed to decrease instances of "splitting" between DBT therapists and other individuals interacting with clients. Splitting occurs when different individuals in a client's network hold differing opinions on how to treat the client. A fundamental tenet of this strategy is that therapists do not tell others, including other health care professionals, how to treat the client. The therapist may suggest, but may not demand. What this means in practice is that the therapist is not attached to others treating a client in a specific way. By remaining in the role of a consultant to the client, the therapist stays out of such arguments. Finally, the consultation-to-the-client strategy promotes respect for clients by imparting the message that they are credible and capable of performing interventions on their own behalf.

As mentioned previously, it is the responsibility of the individual DBT therapist to coordinate and organize care with ancillary treatment providers (function 5; e.g., case managers, pharmacotherapists). The consultation-to-the-client strategy balances the consultation-to-the-therapist strategy described earlier, primarily by providing direct consultation to the client in how to interact with other providers, rather than consulting with the environment on how to interact with the client. Except for special circumstances listed earlier, DBT therapists do not discuss clients with ancillary providers, or other individuals in the client's environment, without the client present. The therapist works with the client to problem-solve difficulties he or she has with his or her network, leaving the client to act as the intermediary between the therapist and other professionals.

ENVIRONMENTAL INTERVENTION

As outlined earlier, the bias in DBT is toward teaching the client how to interact effectively with his or her environment. The consultation-to-the-client strategy is thus the dominant case management strategy and is used whenever possible. There are times, however, when intervention by the therapist is needed. In general, the environmental intervention strategy is used over the consultation-to-the-client strategy when substantial harm may befall the client if the therapist does not intervene. The general rule for environmental intervention is that when clients lack abilities that they need to learn or that are impossible to obtain, or are not reasonable or necessary, the therapist may intervene.

Client Variables

DBT was developed to treat the multidiagnostic, difficult-to-treat individuals. Therefore, there are a number of requisite client characteristics for Stage 1 DBT. Of these, voluntary participation and a commitment to a specified time period (e.g., 16 weeks, 6 months to 1 year) are critical. The effective application of DBT requires a strong interpersonal relationship between therapist and client. The therapist must first work to become a major reinforcer in the life of the client, then use the relationship to promote change in the client. Continuing the relationship can only be used as a positive contingency when a client wants to be in treatment; thus, contingency management is seriously compromised with involuntary clients. Court-ordered treatment is acceptable, if clients agree to remain in therapy even if the order is rescinded. A client characteristic necessary for group therapy is the ability to control overtly aggressive behavior toward others. DBT was developed and evaluated with perhaps the most severely disturbed portion of the population with BPD; all clients accepted into treatment had histories of multiple suicidal and NSSI behaviors. However, the treatment has been designed flexibly and is likely to be effective with less severely disturbed individuals.

Therapist Variables

In comparison to other aspects of therapy, the therapist characteristics that facilitate DBT have received comparatively little attention. However, evidence supports the assumption that effective therapy for clients with BPD requires the proficient balancing of acceptance and change strategies (Shearin & Linehan, 1992). This research also found that therapists' nonpejorative perceptions of clients were associated with less suicidal behavior.

Linehan (1993b) describes requisite therapist characteristics in terms of three bipolar dimensions that must be balanced in the conduct of therapy. The first dimension represents the balance of an orientation of acceptance with an orientation of change. The therapist must be able to inhibit judgmental attitudes (often under very trying circumstances) and to practice acceptance of the client, of him- or herself, and of the therapeutic relationship and process exactly as these are in the current moment. Nevertheless, the therapist remains cognizant that the therapeutic relationship has originated in the necessity of change, and he or she assumes responsibility for directing the therapeutic influence. Second, the therapist must balance unwavering centeredness with compassionate flexibility. "Unwavering centeredness" is the quality of believing in oneself, the therapy, and the client. "Compassionate flexibility" is the ability to take in relevant information about the client and to modify one's position accordingly by letting go of a previously held position. In balancing these two dimensions, the therapist must be able to observe his or her own limits without becoming overly rigid, especially in the face of attempts by the client to control the therapist's behaviors. Finally, the DBT therapist must be able to balance a high degree of nurturing with benevolent demanding. "Nurturing" refers to teaching, coaching, assisting, and strengthening the client, whereas "benevolent demanding" requires the therapist to recognize existing capabilities, to reinforce adaptive behavior, and to refuse to "do" for the client when the client can "do" for him- or herself. Above all, the ability to demand requires a concomitant willingness to believe in the client's ability to change; the effective DBT therapist must see his or her client as empowered.

TREATMENT STRATEGIES

"Treatment strategies" in DBT refer to the role and focus of the therapist, as well as to a coordinated set of procedures that function to achieve specific treatment goals. Although DBT strategies usually consist of a number of steps, use of a strategy does not necessarily require the application of every step. It is considerably more important that the therapist apply the intent of the strategy than that he or she should inflexibly lead the client through a series of prescribed maneuvers.

DBT employs five sets of treatment strategies to achieve the previously described behavioral targets: (1) dialectical strategies, (2) core strategies, (3) stylistic strategies, (4) case management strategies (discussed earlier), and (5) integrated strategies. DBT strategies are illustrated in Figure 9.2. Within an individual session and with a given client, certain strategies may be used more than others, and all strategies may not be necessary or appropriate. An abbreviated discussion of the first three types of DBT treatment strategies follows. For greater detail, the reader is referred to the treatment manual (Linehan, 1993a).

Dialectical Strategies

Dialectical strategies permeate the entire therapy, and their use provides the rationale for adding the term "dialectical" to the title of the therapy. There are three types of dialectical strategies: those having to do with how the therapist structures interactions; those pertaining to how the therapist defines and teaches

skillful behaviors; and certain specific strategies used during the conduct of treatment.

Dialectics of the Relationship: Balancing Treatment Strategies

"Dialectical strategies" in the most general sense of the term have to do with how the therapist balances the dialectical tensions within the therapy relationship. As noted earlier, the fundamental dialectic within any psychotherapy, including that with a client who has BPD, is that between acceptance of what is and efforts to change what is. A dialectical therapeutic position is one of constant attention to combining acceptance and change, flexibility and stability, nurturing and challenging, and a focus on capabilities and a focus on limitations and deficits. The goals are to bring out the opposites, both in therapy and in the client's life, and to provide conditions for syntheses. The presumption is that change may be facilitated by emphasizing acceptance, and acceptance by emphasizing change. The emphasis upon opposites sometimes takes place over time (i.e., over the whole of an interaction), rather than simultaneously or in each part of an interaction. Although many, if not all, psychotherapies, including cognitive and behavioral treatments, attend to these issues of balance, placing the

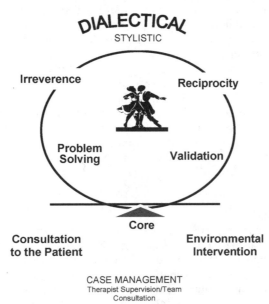

FIGURE 9.2. Treatment strategies in DBT. From Linehan (1993b). Copyright 1993 by The Guilford Press. Reprinted by permission.

concept of balance at the center of the treatment ensures that the therapist remains attentive to its importance.

Three primary characteristics are needed to maintain a dialectical stance in the therapeutic relationship: movement, speed, and flow. Movement refers to acting with certainty, strength, and total commitment on the part of the therapist. If the therapist only moves half-heartedly, the client will only move halfheartedly. Speed is of the essence and entails keeping the therapy moving, so that it does not become rigid or stuck. Finally, flow refers to being mindful to the moment-to-moment unfolding of a session and responding smoothly, and with apparent effortlessness.

Teaching Dialectical Behavior Patterns

Dialectical thinking is emphasized throughout the entire treatment. Not only does the therapist maintain a dialectical stance in his or her treatment of the client but he or she also focuses on teaching and modeling dialectical thinking to the client. The therapist helps the client move from an "either–or" position to a "both–and" position, without invalidating the first idea or its polarity when asserting the second. Behavioral extremes and rigidity— whether cognitive, emotional, or overtly behavioral —are signals that synthesis has not been achieved; thus, they can be considered nondialectical. Instead, a "middle path" similar to that advocated in Buddhism is advocated and modeled. The important thing in following the path to Enlightenment is to avoid being caught and entangled in any extreme and always follow the Middle Way (Kyokai, 1966). This emphasis on balance is similar to the approach advocated in relapse prevention models proposed by Marlatt and his colleagues (e.g., Marlatt & Gordon, 1985) for treating addictive behaviors.

Specific Dialectical Strategies

There are eight specific dialectical treatment strategies: (1) entering and using paradox, (2) using metaphor, (3) playing the devil's advocate, (4) extending, (5) activating the client's "wise mind," (6) making lemonade out of lemons (turning negatives into positives), (7) allowing natural change (and inconsistencies even within the therapeutic milieu), and (8) as-

sessing dialectically by always asking the question "What is being left out here?" Due to space limitations, a selection of these strategies is included in the following sections. For a complete review, the interested reader is referred to the DBT treatment manual (Linehan, 1993a).

ENTERING THE PARADOX

Entering the paradox is a powerful technique because it contains the element of surprise. The therapist presents the paradox without explaining it and highlights the paradoxical contradictions within the behavior, the therapeutic process, and reality in general. The essence of the strategy is the therapist's refusal to step in with rational explanation; the client's attempts at logic are met with silence, a question, or a story designed to shed a small amount of light on the puzzle to be solved. The client is pushed to achieve understanding, to move toward synthesis of the polarities, and to resolve the dilemma him- or herself. Linehan (1993b) has highlighted a number of typical paradoxes and their corresponding dialectical tensions encountered over the course of therapy. Clients are free to choose their own behavior but cannot stay in therapy if they do not work at changing their behavior. They are taught to achieve greater independence by becoming more skilled at asking for help from others. Clients have a right to kill themselves, but if they ever convince the therapist that suicide is imminent, they may be locked up. Clients are not responsible for being the way they are, but they are responsible for what they become. In highlighting these paradoxical realities, both client and therapist struggle with confronting and letting go of rigid patterns of thought, emotion, and behavior, so that more spontaneous and flexible patterns may emerge.

USING METAPHOR: PARABLE, MYTH, ANALOGY, AND STORYTELLING

The use of metaphor, stories, parables, and myth is extremely important in DBT and provides an alternative means of teaching dialectical thinking. Stories are usually more interesting, are easier to remember, and encourage the search for other meanings of events under scrutiny. Additionally, metaphors allow clients to distance themselves from the problem being discussed and can therefore be less threatening. In general, the idea of metaphor is to take something the client does understand and use it as an analogy for something the client does not understand. Used creatively, metaphors aid understanding, suggest solutions to problems, and reframe the problems of both clients and the therapeutic process. Furthermore, metaphors and stories can be developed by both therapist and client taking turns throughout a session or over the course of treatment. When the therapist and client relate to a metaphor, it can be a powerful tool to use throughout the treatment, reminding the client what he or she is working on. For example, changing behavior by learning new skills can be compared to building a new hiking trail in the woods. At first, the current trail is defined and easy to navigate; however, it always leads to a dead end (old dysfunctional behavior). To build a new trail (skillful behaviors), the hiker must repeatedly go through a new, undefined area until it becomes worn in. This takes time and the hiker moves slowly and deliberately clearing away the brush. Additionally, while the new path is developing, the old path is slowly becoming grown over. This story can be returned to throughout treatment, each time the client begins to struggle between trying new skills and returning to old dysfunctional behavior.

PLAYING DEVIL'S ADVOCATE

The devil's advocate technique is quite similar to the argumentative approach used in rational–emotive and cognitive restructuring therapies as a method of addressing a client's dysfunctional beliefs or problematic rules. With this strategy, the therapist presents a propositional statement that is an extreme version of one of the client's own dysfunctional beliefs, then plays the role of devil's advocate to counter the client's attempts to disprove the extreme statement or rule. For example, a client may state, "Because I'm overweight, I'd be better off dead." The therapist argues in favor of the dysfunctional belief, perhaps by suggesting that because this is true for the client, it must be true for others as well; hence, all overweight people would be better off dead. The therapist may continue along these lines: "And since the definition of what constitutes being overweight varies so much among individuals, there must be an awful lot of people who

would be considered overweight by someone. That must mean they'd all be better off dead!" Or "Gosh, I'm about 5 pounds overweight. I guess that means I'd be better off dead, too." Any reservations the client proposes can be countered by further exaggeration, until the self-defeating nature of the belief becomes apparent. The devil's advocate technique is often used in the first several sessions to elicit a strong commitment from the client and in commitment sessions with new therapists joining the DBT team. The therapist argues to the client that since the therapy will be painful and difficult, it is not clear how making such a commitment (and therefore being accepted into treatment) could possibly be a good idea. This usually has the effect of moving the client to take the opposite position in favor of therapeutic change. To employ this technique successfully, it is important that the therapist's argument seem reasonable enough to invite counterargument by the client, and that the delivery be made with a straight face, in a naive but offbeat manner.

EXTENDING

The term "extending" has been borrowed from *aikido*, a Japanese form of self-defense. In that context, extending occurs when the student of *aikido* waits for a challenger's movements to reach their natural completion, then extends a movement's endpoint slightly further than what would naturally occur, leaving the challenger vulnerable and off balance. In DBT, extending occurs when the therapist takes the severity or gravity of what the client is communicating more seriously than the client intends. This strategy is the emotional equivalent of the devil's advocate strategy. It is particularly effective when the client is threatening dire consequences of an event or problem to induce change in the environment. Take the interaction with the following client, who threatens suicide if an extra appointment time for the next day is not scheduled. The following interchange between therapist and client occurs after attempts to find a mutually acceptable time have failed.

CLIENT: I've got to see you tomorrow, or I'm sure I will end up killing myself. I just can't keep it together by myself any longer.

THERAPIST: Hmm, I didn't realize you were so

upset! We've got to do something immediately if you are so distressed that you might kill yourself. What about hospitalization? Maybe that is needed.

CLIENT: I'm not going to the hospital! Why won't you just give me an appointment?

THERAPIST: How can we discuss such a mundane topic as session scheduling when your life is in danger? How are you planning to kill yourself?

CLIENT: You know how. Why can't you cancel someone or move an appointment around? You could put an appointment with one of your students off until another time. I can't stand it any more!

THERAPIST: I'm really concerned about you. Do you think I should call an aid car?

The aspect of the communication that the therapist takes seriously (suicide as a possible consequence of not getting an appointment) is not the aspect (needing an extra appointment the next day) that the client wants taken seriously. The therapist takes the consequences seriously and extends the seriousness even further. The client wants the problem taken seriously, and indeed is extending the seriousness of the problem.

MAKING LEMONADE OUT OF LEMONS

Making lemonade out of lemons is similar to the notion in psychodynamic therapy of utilizing a client's resistances; therapeutic problems are seen as opportunities for the therapist to help the client. The strategy involves taking something that is apparently problematic and turning it into an asset. Problems become opportunities to practice skills; suffering allows others to express empathy; weaknesses become one's strengths. To be effective, this strategy requires a strong therapeutic relationship between therapist and client; the client must believe that the therapist has a deep compassion for his or her suffering. The danger in using this strategy is that it is easily confused with the invalidating refrain repeatedly heard by clients with BPD. The therapist should avoid the tendency to oversimplify a client's problems, and refrain from implying that the lemons in the client's life are really lemonade. While recognizing that the cloud is indeed black, the therapist assists the client in finding the positive characteristics of a situation—thus, the silver lining.

Core Strategies

Validation

Validation and problem-solving strategies, together with dialectical strategies, make up the core of DBT and form the heart of the treatment. Validation strategies are the most obvious acceptance strategies, whereas problem-solving strategies are the most obvious change strategies. Both validation and problem-solving strategies are used in every interaction with the client, although the relative frequency of each depends on the particular client, the current situation, and the vulnerabilities of that client. However, throughout an entire session, there should be an overall balance between the acceptance and change strategies. Many treatment impasses are due to an imbalance of one type of strategy over the other. We discuss validation strategies in this section and problem-solving strategies in the next.

Clients with BPD present themselves clinically as individuals in extreme emotional pain. They plead, and at times demand, that their therapists do something to change this state of affairs. It is very tempting to focus the energy of therapy on changing the client by modifying irrational thoughts, assumptions, or schemas; critiquing interpersonal behaviors or motives contributing to interpersonal problems; giving medication to change abnormal biology; reducing emotional overreactivity and intensity; and so on. In many respects, this focus recapitulates the invalidating environment by confirming the client's worst fears: The client is the problem and indeed cannot trust his or her own reactions to events. Mistrust and invalidation of how one responds to events, however, are extremely aversive and can elicit intense fear, anger, and shame, or a combination of all three. Thus, the entire focus of change-based therapy can be aversive, because the focus by necessity contributes to and elicits self-invalidation. However, an entire focus of acceptance-based therapy can also be invalidating when it appears to the client that the therapist does not take his or her problems seriously. Therefore, once again, a dialectical stance focuses on a balance between the two poles.

Validation (according to the *Oxford English Dictionary*; Simpson & Weiner, 1989) means "the action of validating or making valid . . . a strengthening, reinforcement, confirming; an establishing or ratifying." It also encompasses activities such as corroborating, substantiating, verifying, and authenticating. The act of validating is "to support or corroborate on a sound or authoritative basis . . . to attest to the truth or validity of something" (Merriam-Webster, Inc., 2006). To communicate that a response is valid is to say that it is "well-grounded or justifiable: being at once relevant and meaningful . . . logically correct . . . appropriate to the end in view [or effective] . . . having such force as to compel serious attention and [usually] acceptance" (*Webster's Dictionary*, 1991). Being "valid implies being supported by objective truth or generally accepted authority" (*Webster's Dictionary*, 1991); "being well-founded on fact, or established on sound principles, and thoroughly applicable to the case or circumstances," and "soundness and strength," "value or worth," and "efficacy" (Simpson & Weiner, 1989). These are precisely the meanings associated with the term when used in the context of psychotherapy in DBT:

> The essence of validation is this: The therapist communicates to the client that her [*sic*] responses make sense and are understandable within her [*sic*] *current* life context or situation. The therapist actively accepts the client and communicates this acceptance to the client. The therapist takes the client's responses seriously and does not discount or trivialize them. Validation strategies require the therapist to search for, recognize, and reflect to the client the validity inherent in her [*sic*] response to events. With unruly children, parents have to catch them while they're good in order to reinforce their behavior; similarly, the therapist has to uncover the validity within the client's response, sometimes amplify it, and then reinforce it. (Linehan, 1993b, pp. 222–223, original emphasis)

Two things are important to note here. First, validation means the acknowledgment of that which is valid. It does not mean "making" valid. Nor does it mean validating that which is invalid. The therapist observes, experiences, and affirms, but he or she does not create validity. Second, "valid" and "scientific" are not synonyms. Science may be one way to determine what is valid, logical, sound in principle, and/or generally accepted as authority or normative knowledge. However, an authentic experience or apprehension of private events (at least, when similar to the same experiences of others or when in accord with other, more observable events) is also a basis for claiming validity. Validation can be considered at any one

of six levels. Each level is correspondingly more complete than the previous one, and each level depends on one or more of the previous levels. They are definitional of DBT and are required in every interaction with the client. These levels are described most fully in Linehan (1997), and the following definitions are taken from her discussion.

LISTENING AND OBSERVING (V1)

Level 1 validation requires listening to and observing what the client is saying, feeling, and doing, as well as a corresponding active effort to understand what is being said and observed. The essence of this step is that the therapist is staying awake and interested in the client, paying attention to what the client says and does in the current moment. The therapist notices the nuances of response in the interaction. Validation at Level 1 communicates that the client per se, as well as the client's presence, words, and responses in the session have "such force as to compel serious attention and [usually] acceptance" (see earlier definitions of validation; pp. 360–361)

ACCURATE REFLECTION (V2)

The second level of validation is the accurate reflection back to the client of his or her own feelings, thoughts, assumptions, and behaviors. The therapist conveys an understanding of the client by hearing what the client has said and seeing what the client does, and how he or she responds. Validation at Level 2 sanctions, empowers, or authenticates that the individual is who he or she actually is (p. 362).

ARTICULATING THE UNVERBALIZED (V3)

In Level 3 of validation, the therapist communicates understanding of aspects of the client's experience and response to events that have not been communicated directly by the client. The therapist "mind-reads" the reason for the client's behavior and figures out how the client feels and what he or she is wishing for, thinking, or doing just by knowing what has happened to the client. The therapist can make the link between precipitating event and behavior without being given any information about the behavior itself. Emotions and meanings the client has not expressed are articulated by the therapist (p. 364).

VALIDATING IN TERMS OF PAST LEARNING OR BIOLOGICAL DYSFUNCTION (V4)

At Level 4, behavior is validated in terms of its causes. Validation here is based on the notion that all behavior is caused by events occurring in time; thus, in principle, it is understandable. The therapist justifies the client's behavior by showing that it is caused by past events. Even though information may not be available to determine all the relevant causes, the client's feelings, thoughts and actions make perfect sense in the context of the client's current experience, physiology, and life to date. At a minimum, what "is" can always be justified in terms of sufficient causes; that is, what is "should be," in that whatever was necessary for it to occur had to have happened (p. 367).

VALIDATION IN TERMS OF PRESENT CONTEXT OR NORMATIVE FUNCTIONING (V5)

At Level 5, the therapist communicates that behavior is justifiable, reasonable, well-grounded, meaningful, and/or efficacious in terms of current events, normative biological functioning, and/or the client's ultimate life goals. The therapist looks for and reflects the wisdom or validity of the client's response and communicates that the response is understandable. The therapist finds the relevant facts in the current environment that support the client's behavior. The therapist is not blinded by the dysfunctionality of some of the client's response patterns to those aspects of a response pattern that may be either reasonable or appropriate to the context. Thus, the therapist searches the client's responses for their inherent accuracy or appropriateness, or reasonableness (as well as commenting on the inherent dysfunctionality of much of the response, if necessary) (pp. 370–371).

RADICAL GENUINENESS (V6)

In Level 6, the task is to recognize the person as he or she is, seeing and responding to the strengths and capacities of the client, while keeping a firm empathic understanding of his or her actual difficulties and incapacities. The therapist believes in the client and his or her capacity to change and move toward ultimate life goals just as the therapist may believe in a friend or family member. The client is responded to as a person of equal status, due equal respect. Validation at the highest level is the validation of the individual as "is." The therapist sees more than the role, more than a "client" or "disorder." Level 6 validation is the opposite of treating the client in a condescending manner or as overly fragile. It is responding to the individual as capable of effective and reasonable behavior rather than assuming that he or she is an invalid. Whereas Levels 1–5 represent sequential steps in validation of a kind, Level 6 represents change in both level and kind (p. 377).

Cheerleading strategies constitute another form of validation and are the principal strategies for combating the active passivity and tendencies to hopelessness in clients with BPD. In cheerleading, therapists communicate the belief that clients are doing their best and validate clients' ability to eventually overcome their difficulties (a type of validation that, if not handled carefully, can simultaneously invalidate clients' perceptions of their helplessness). In addition, therapists express a belief in the therapy relationship, offer reassurance, and highlight any evidence of improvement. Within DBT, cheerleading is used in every therapeutic interaction. Although active cheerleading by therapists should be reduced as clients learn to trust and to validate themselves, cheerleading strategies always remain an essential ingredient of a strong therapeutic alliance.

Finally, functional validation, another form of validation that is used regularly in DBT, is a form of nonverbal or behavioral validation that at times may be more effective than verbal validation. For example, a therapist drops a 50-pound block on the client's foot. It would be considered invalidating for the therapist simply to respond verbally, saying, "Wow, I can see that really hurts! You must be in a lot of pain." Functional validation would entail the therapist removing the block from the client's foot.

Problem Solving

We have previously discussed how therapies with a primary focus on client change are typically experienced as invalidating by clients with BPD. However, therapies that focus exclusively on validation can prove equally problematic. Exhortations to accept one's current situation offer little solace to an individual who experiences life as painfully unendurable. Within DBT, problem-solving strategies are the core change strategies, designed to foster an active problem-solving style. For clients with BPD, however, the application of these strategies is fraught with difficulties. The therapist must keep in mind that with clients with BPD the process will be more difficult than with many other client populations. In work with clients who have BPD, the need for sympathetic understanding and interventions aimed at enhancing current positive mood can be extremely important. The validation strategies just described, as well as the irreverent communication strategy described later, can be tremendously useful here. Within DBT, problem solving is a two-stage process that concentrates first on understanding and accepting a selected problem, then generating alternative solutions. The first stage involves (1) behavioral analysis; (2) insight into recurrent behavioral context patterns; and (3) giving the client didactic information about principles of behaviors, norms, and so on. The second stage specifically targets change through (4) analysis of possible solutions to problems; (5) orienting the client to therapeutic procedures likely to bring about desired changes; and (6) strategies designed to elicit and strengthen commitment to these procedures. The following sections specifically address behavioral analysis, solution analysis, and problem-solving procedures.

Behavioral Analysis

Behavioral analysis is one of the most important strategies in DBT. It is also the most difficult. The purpose of a behavioral analysis is first to select a problem, then to determine empirically what is causing it, what is preventing its resolution, and what aids are available for solving it. Behavioral analysis addresses four primary questions:

1. Are ineffective behaviors being reinforced, are effective behaviors followed by aversive outcomes, or are rewarding outcomes delayed?
2. Does the client have the requisite behavioral skills to regulate his or her emotions, respond skillfully to conflict, and manage his or her own behavior?
3. Are there patterns of avoidance, or are effective behaviors inhibited by unwarranted fears or guilt?
4. Is the client unaware of the contingencies operating in his or her environment, or are effective behaviors inhibited by faulty beliefs or assumptions?

Answers to these questions guide the therapist in the selection of appropriate treatment procedures, such as contingency management, behavioral skills training, exposure, or cognitive modification. Thus, the value of an analysis lies in helping the therapist assess and understand a problem fully enough to guide effective therapeutic response. The first step in conducting a behavioral analysis is to help the client identify the problem to be analyzed and describe it in behavioral terms. Identifying the problem can be the most difficult task for the therapist, and if not done accurately and specifically, can lead the therapist and client down a path of solving only a related problem, without getting to the true heart of the problem behavior at hand. Problem definition usually evolves from a discussion of the previous week's events, often in the context of reviewing diary cards. The assumption of facts not in evidence is perhaps the most common mistake at this point. Defining the problem is followed by a chain analysis—an exhaustive, blow-by-blow description of the chain of events leading up to and following the behavior. In a chain analysis, the therapist constructs a general road map of how the client arrives at dysfunctional responses, including where the road actually starts (highlights vulnerability factors and prompting events), and notes possible alternative adaptive pathways or junctions along the way. Additional goals are to identify events that automatically elicit maladaptive behavior, behavioral deficits that are instrumental in maintaining problematic responses, and environmental and behavioral events that may be interfering with more appropriate behaviors. The overall goal is to determine the function of the behavior, or, from another perspective, the problem the behavior was instrumental in solving.

Chain analysis always begins with a specific environmental event. Pinpointing such an event may be difficult, because clients are frequently unable to identify anything in the environment that set off the problematic response. Nevertheless, it is important to obtain a description of the events co-occurring with the onset of the problem. The therapist then attempts to identify both environmental and behavioral events for each subsequent link in the chain. Here the therapist must play the part of a very keen observer, thinking in terms of very small chunks of behavior, and repeatedly identifying what the client was thinking, feeling, and doing, and what was occurring in the environment from moment to moment. The therapist asks the client, "What happened next?" or "How did you get from there to there?" Although, from the client's point of view, such links may be self-evident, the therapist must be careful not to make assumptions. For example, a client who had attempted suicide once stated that she decided to kill herself because her life was too painful for her to live any longer. From the client's point of view, this was an adequate explanation for her suicide attempt. For the therapist, however, taking one's life because life is too painful was only one solution. One could decide life is too painful, then decide to change one's life. Or one could believe that death might be even more painful and decide to tolerate life despite its pain. In this instance, careful questioning revealed that the client actually assumed she would be happier dead than alive. Challenging this assumption, then, became a key to ending her persistent suicide attempts. It is equally important to pinpoint exactly what consequences are maintaining the problematic response. Similarly, the therapist should also search for consequences that serve to weaken the problem behavior. As with antecedent events, the therapist probes for both environmental and behavioral consequences, obtaining detailed descriptions of the client's emotions, somatic sensations, actions, thoughts, and assumptions. A rudimentary knowledge of the rules of learning and principles of reinforcement is crucial.

The final step in behavioral analysis is to construct and test hypotheses about events that are relevant to generating and maintaining the problem behavior. The biosocial theory of BPD suggests several factors of primary importance. For example, DBT focuses most closely on intense or aversive emotional states; the amelioration of negative affect is always suspected as being among the primary motivational variables for dysfunctional behavior in BPD. The theory also suggests that typical behavioral patterns, such as deficits in dialectical thinking or behavioral skills, are likely to be instrumental in producing and maintaining problematic responses.

Solution Analysis

Once the problem has been identified and analyzed, problem solving proceeds with an active attempt at finding and identifying alternative solutions. DBT posits that there are five responses to any one problem: (1) Solve the problem; (2) change the emotional reaction to the problem; (3) tolerate the problem; or (4) stay miserable. An alert client suggested another response, which we have added: (5) Make things worse. These five options are presented to the client at pretreatment and throughout sessions prior to problem solving to ensure that therapist and client are working toward the same goal at any given point.

At times, solutions are discussed throughout the behavioral analysis, and pointing to these alternative solutions may be all that is required, rather than waiting until the behavioral analysis is completed. The therapist may ask, "What do you think you could have done differently here?" Throughout this process, the therapist is actively modeling effective problem solving and solution generation, with a heavier emphasis on modeling and guiding the client early on in treatment. At other times, a more complete solution analysis is necessary. Here the task is to "brainstorm" or generate as many alternative solutions as possible. Solutions should then be evaluated in terms of the various outcomes expected. The final step in solution analysis is to choose a solution that will somehow be effective. Throughout the evaluation, the therapist guides the client in choosing a particular behavioral solution. Here, it is preferable that the therapist pay particular attention to long-term over short-term gain, and that chosen solutions render maximum benefit to the client rather than benefit to others.

Problem-Solving Procedures

DBT employs four problem-solving procedures taken directly from the cognitive and behavioral treatment literature. These four—skills training, contingency procedures, exposure, and cognitive modification—are viewed as primary vehicles of change throughout DBT, since they influence the direction that client changes take from session to session. Although they are discussed as distinct procedures by Linehan (1993b), it is not clear that they can in fact be differentiated in every case in clinical practice. The same therapeutic sequence may be effective because it teaches the client new skills (skills training), provides a consequence that influences the probability of preceding client behaviors occurring again (contingency procedures), provides nonreinforced exposure to cues associated previously but not currently with threat (exposure procedures), or changes the client's dysfunctional assumptions or schematic processing of events (cognitive modification). In contrast to many cognitive and behavioral treatment programs in the literature, these procedures (with some exceptions noted below) are employed in an unstructured manner, interwoven throughout all therapeutic dialogue. Thus, the therapist must be well aware of the principles governing the effectiveness of each procedure in order to use each in immediate response to events unfolding in a particular session. The exceptions are in skills training, where skills training procedures predominate, and Stage 2, where exposure procedures predominate.

Skills Training

An emphasis on skills building is pervasive throughout DBT. In both individual and group therapy, the therapist insists at every opportunity that the client actively engage in the acquisition and practice of behavioral skills. The term "skills" is used synonymously with "ability" and includes, in its broadest sense, cognitive, emotional, and overt behavioral skills, as well as their integration, which is necessary for effective performance. Skills training is called for when a solution requires skills not currently in the individual's behavioral repertoire, or when the individual has the component behaviors but cannot integrate and use them effectively. Skills training in DBT incorporates three types of procedures: (1) skills acquisition (modeling, instructing, advising); (2) skills strengthening (encouraging *in vivo* and within-session practice, role playing, feedback); and (3) skills generalization (phone calls to work on applying skills; taping therapy sessions to listen to between sessions; homework assignments).

Contingency Procedures

Every response within an interpersonal interaction is potentially a reinforcement, a punishment, or a withholding or removal of reinforcement. Contingency management requires therapists to organize their behavior strategically so that client behaviors that represent progress are reinforced, while unskillful or maladaptive behaviors are extinguished or lead to aversive consequences. Natural consequences should be used over arbitrary consequences whenever possible. An important contingency for most clients with BPD is the therapist's interpersonal behavior with such clients. The ability of the therapist to influence the client's behavior is directly tied to the strength of the relationship between the two. Thus, contingency procedures based on the relationship are less useful in the very early stages of treatment (except, possibly, when the therapist is the "only game in town").

A first requirement for effective contingency management is that the therapist orient the client to the principles of contingency management and explain how learning takes place. The therapist must attend to the client's behaviors and use the principles of shaping to reinforce those behaviors that represent progress toward DBT targets. Equally important is that the therapist takes care not to reinforce behaviors targeted for extinction. In theory, this may seem obvious, but in practice, it can be quite difficult. The problematic behaviors of clients with BPD are often quite effective in obtaining reinforcing outcomes or in stopping painful events. Indeed, the very behaviors targeted for extinction have been intermittently reinforced by mental health professionals, family members, and friends. Contingency management at times requires the use of aversive consequences, similar to "setting limits" in other treatment modalities. Three guidelines are important when using aversive consequences. First, punishment should "fit the crime," and a client should have some way of terminating its application. For example, in DBT, a detailed behavioral analysis follows a suicidal or NSSI act; such an analysis is an aversive procedure for most clients. Once it has been completed, however, a client's ability to pursue other topics is restored. Second, it is crucial that therapists use punishment with great care, in low doses, and very briefly, and that a positive interpersonal atmosphere be restored following any client improvement. Third, punishment should be just strong enough to work. Although the ultimate punishment is termination of therapy, a preferable fallback strategy is putting clients on "vacations from therapy." This approach is considered when all other contingencies have failed, or when a situation is so serious that a therapist's therapeutic or personal limits have been crossed. When utilizing this strategy, the therapist clearly identifies what behaviors must be changed and clarifies that once the conditions have been met, the client can return. The therapist maintains intermittent contact by phone or letter, and provides a referral or backup while the client is on vacation. (In colloquial terms, the therapist kicks the client out, then pines for his or her return.) Observing limits constitutes a special case of contingency management involving the application of problem-solving strategies to client behaviors that threaten or cross a therapist's personal limits. Such behaviors interfere with the therapist's ability or willingness to conduct the therapy, thus constituting a special type of therapy-interfering behavior. Therapists must take responsibility for monitoring their own personal limits and clearly communicate to their clients which behaviors are tolerable and which are not. Therapists who do not do this eventually burn out, terminate therapy, or otherwise harm their clients. DBT favors natural over arbitrary limits. Thus, limits vary among therapists, and with the same therapist over time and circumstance. Limits should also be presented as for the good of the therapist, not for the good of the client. The effect of this is that although clients may argue about what is in their own best interests, they do not have ultimate say over what is good for their therapists.

Cognitive Modification

The fundamental message given to clients in DBT is that cognitive distortions are just as likely to be caused by emotional arousal as to be the cause of the arousal in the first place. The overall message is that, for the most part, the source of a client's distress is the extremely stressful events of his or her life rather than a distortion of events that are actually benign. Although direct cognitive restructuring procedures, such as those advocated by Beck and colleagues (Beck, Brown, Berchick, Stewart, & Steer, 1990; Beck, Rush, Shaw, & Emery, 1979) and by Ellis (1962, 1973), are used and taught as part of emotion regulation, they do not hold a dominant place in DBT. In contrast, contingency clarification strategies are used relentlessly, highlighting contingent relationships operating in the here and now. Emphasis is placed on highlighting immediate and long-term effects of clients' behavior (both on themselves and on others), clarifying the effects of certain situations on clients' own responses, and examining future contingencies that clients are likely to encounter. An example here is orienting a client to DBT as a whole and to treatment procedures as they are implemented.

Exposure

All of the change procedures in DBT can be reconceptualized as exposure strategies. Many of the principles of exposure as applied to DBT have been developed by researchers in exposure techniques (see Foa & Kozak, 1986; Foa, Steketee, & Grayson, 1985). These strategies work by reconditioning dysfunctional associations that develop between stimuli (e.g., an aversive stimulus, hospitalization, may become associated with a positive stimulus, nurturing in the hospital; a client may later work to be hospitalized) or between a response and a stimulus (e.g., an adaptive response, healthy expression of emotions, is met with an aversive consequent stimulus, rejection by a loved one; a client may then try to suppress emotions). As noted earlier, the DBT therapist conducts a chain analysis of the eliciting cue, the problem behavior (including emotions), and the consequences of the behavior. Working within a behavior therapy framework, the therapist operates according to three guidelines for exposure in DBT. First, exposure to the cue that precedes the problem behavior must be non-reinforced (e.g., if a client is fearful that discussing suicidal behavior will lead to his or her being rejected, the therapist must not reinforce the client's shame by ostracizing him/her). Second, dysfunctional responses are blocked in the order of the primary and secondary targets of treatment (e.g., suicidal or NSSI behavior related to shame is blocked by getting the client's cooperation in throwing away hoarded medications). Third, actions opposite to the dysfunctional behavior are reinforced (e.g., the therapist reinforces the client for talking about painful, shame-related suicidal behavior).

Therapeutic exposure procedures are used informally throughout the whole of therapy and formally during Stage 2, in which the client is systematically exposed to cues of previous traumatic events. Exposure procedures of the DBT therapist involve first orienting the client to the techniques and to the fact that exposure to cues is often experienced as painful or frightening. Thus, the therapist does not remove the cue to emotional arousal, and at the same time he or she blocks both the action tendencies (including escape responses) and the expressive tendencies associated with the problem emotion. In addition, the DBT therapist works to assist the client in achieving enhanced control over aversive events. A crucial step of exposure procedures is that the client be taught how to control the event. It is critical that the client have some means of titrating or ending exposure when emotions become unendurable. The therapist and client should collaborate in developing positive, adaptive ways for the client to end exposure voluntarily, preferably after some reduction in the problem emotion has occurred.

Stylistic Strategies

DBT balances two quite different styles of communication that refer to how the therapist executes other treatment strategies. The first, reciprocal communication, is similar to the communication style advocated in client-centered therapy. The second, irreverent communication, is quite similar to the style advocated by Whitaker (1975) in his writings on strategic therapy. Reciprocal communication strategies are designed to reduce a perceived power differential by making the therapist more vulnerable to the client. In addition, they serve as a model for appropriate but equal interactions within an important interpersonal relationship. Irreverent communication is usually riskier than reciprocity. However, it can facilitate problem solving or produce a breakthrough after long periods when progress has seemed thwarted. To be used effectively, irreverent communication must balance reciprocal communication, and the two must be woven into a single stylistic fabric. Without such balancing, neither strategy represents DBT.

Reciprocal Communication

Responsiveness, self-disclosure, warm engagement, and genuineness are the basic guidelines of reciprocal communication. Responsiveness requires attending to the client in a mindful (attentive) manner and taking the client's agenda and wishes seriously. However, this does not mean that the therapist gives priority to the client's agenda over the treatment hierarchy. It refers to the therapist validating the importance of the client's agenda openly. It is a friendly, affectionate style reflecting warmth and engagement in the therapeutic interaction. Both self-involving and personal self-disclosure, used in

the interests of the client, are encouraged to increase problem solving or to reinforce therapeutic activities. Self-involving self-disclosure is the therapist's immediate, personal reactions to the client and his or her behavior. This strategy is used frequently throughout DBT. For example, a therapist whose client complained about his coolness said, "When you demand warmth from me, it pushes me away and makes it harder to be warm." Similarly, when a client repeatedly failed to fill out diary cards but nevertheless pleaded with her therapist to help her, the therapist responded, "You keep asking me for help, but you won't do the things I believe are necessary to help you. I feel frustrated because I want to help you, but I feel that you won't let me." Such statements serve both to validate and to challenge. They constitute both an instance of contingency management, because therapist statements about the client are typically experienced as either reinforcing or punishing, and an instance of contingency clarification, because the client's attention is directed to the consequences of his or her interpersonal behavior. Self-disclosure of professional or personal information is used to validate and model coping and normative responses. The key point here is that a therapist should only use personal examples in which he or she has successfully mastered the problem at hand. This may seem like an obvious point, but it is very easy to fall into this pit by trying actively to validate the client's dilemma. For example, when working with a client whose goal is to wake up early each morning to exercise but who is having difficulty getting out of bed, the therapist may attempt to validate the behavior as normative by stating, "Yeah, I struggle with getting up every morning, too, even though I tell myself every night that I am going to exercise in the morning." However, this self-disclosure is only be useful to the client if the therapist continues by stating what skillful behavior he or she uses to get up each morning and exercise successfully.

Irreverent Communication

Irreverent communication is used to push the client "off balance," get the client's attention, present an alternative viewpoint, or shift affective response. It is a highly useful strategy when the client is immovable, or when therapist and client are "stuck." It has an "offbeat" flavor and uses logic to weave a web the client cannot escape. Although it is responsive to the client, irreverent communication is almost never the response the client expects. For irreverence to be effective it must be both genuine (vs. sarcastic or judgmental) and come from a place of compassion and warmth toward the client. Otherwise, the client may become even more rigid. When using irreverence the therapist highlights some unintended aspect of the client's communication or "reframes" it in an unorthodox manner. For example, if the client says, "I am going to kill myself," the therapist might say, "I thought you agreed not to drop out of therapy." Irreverent communication has a matter-of-fact, almost deadpan style that is in sharp contrast to the warm responsiveness of reciprocal communication. Humor, a certain naivete, and guilelessness are also characteristic of the style. A confrontational tone is also irreverent, communicating "bullshit" to responses other than the targeted adaptive response. For example, the therapist might say, "Are you out of your mind?" or "You weren't for a minute actually believing I would think that was a good idea, were you?" The irreverent therapist also calls the client's bluff. For the client who says, "I'm quitting therapy," the therapist might respond, "Would you like a referral?" The trick here is to time the bluff carefully, with the simultaneous provision of a safety net; it is important to leave the client a way out.

CASE STUDY

Background

At the initial meeting, "Cindy," a 30-year-old, white, married woman with no children, was living in a middle-class suburban area with her husband. She had a college education and had successfully completed almost 2 years of medical school. Cindy was referred to one of us (M. M. L.) by her psychiatrist of 1½ years, who was no longer willing to provide more than pharmacotherapy following a recent hospitalization for a near-lethal suicide attempt. In the 2 years prior to referral, Cindy had been hospitalized at least 10 times (once for 6 months) for psychiatric treatment of suicidal ideation; had engaged in numerous instances of both NSSI behavior and suicide attempts, including at least 10 instances of drinking Clorox bleach, multiple deep cuts, and burns; and had had three medically severe or nearly lethal suicide

attempts, including cutting an artery in her neck. At the time of referral, Cindy met DSM-III-R (American Psychiatric Association, 1987) as well as Gunderson's (1984) criteria for BPD. She was also taking a variety of psychotropic drugs. Until age 27, Cindy was able to function well in work and school settings, and her marriage was reasonably satisfactory to both partners, although her husband complained about Cindy's excessive anger. When Cindy was in the second year of medical school, a classmate she knew only slightly committed suicide. Cindy stated that when she heard about the suicide, she immediately decided to kill herself also, but had very little insight into what about the situation actually elicited her inclination to kill herself. Within weeks she left medical school and became severely depressed and actively suicidal. Although Cindy self-presented as a person with few psychological problems before the classmate's suicide, further questioning revealed a history of severe anorexia nervosa, bulimia nervosa, and alcohol and prescription medication abuse, originating at the age of 14 years. Indeed, she had met her husband at an Alcoholics Anonymous (AA) meeting while attending college. Nevertheless, until the student's suicide in medical school, Cindy had been successful at maintaining an overall appearance of relative competence.

Treatment

At the initial meeting, Cindy was accompanied by her husband, who stated that he and Cindy's family considered his wife too lethally suicidal to be out of a hospital setting. Consequently, he and Cindy's family were seriously contemplating the viability of finding long-term outpatient care. However, Cindy stated a strong preference for inpatient treatment, although no therapist in the local area other than M. M. L. appeared willing to take her into outpatient treatment. The therapist agreed to accept Cindy into therapy, contingent on the client's stated commitment to work toward behavioral change and to stay in treatment for at least 1 year. (It was later pointed out repeatedly that this also meant the client had agreed not to commit suicide.) Thus, the therapist began the crucial first step of establishing a strong therapeutic alliance by agreeing to accept the client despite the fact that no one else was willing to do so. She pointed out, however, that acceptance into therapy did not come without a cost.

In this manner, the therapist communicated acceptance of the client exactly as she was in the current moment, while concomitantly making clear that Cindy's commitment toward change was the foundation of the therapeutic alliance. At the fourth therapy session, Cindy reported that she felt she could no longer keep herself alive. When reminded of her previous commitment to stay alive for 1 year of therapy, Cindy replied that things had changed and she could not help herself. Subsequent to this session, almost every individual session for the next 6 months revolved around the topic of whether (and how) to stay alive versus committing suicide. Cindy began coming to sessions wearing mirrored sunglasses and would slump in her chair or ask to sit on the floor. Questions from the therapist were often met with a minimal comment or long silences. In response to the therapist's attempts to discuss prior self-injurious behavior, Cindy would become angry and withdraw (slowing down the pace of therapy considerably). The client also presented with marked dissociative reactions, which would often occur during therapy sessions. During these reactions, Cindy would appear unable to concentrate or hear much of what was being said. When queried by the therapist, Cindy would describe her experience as feeling "spacey" and distant. The client stated that she felt she could no longer engage in many activities, such as driving, working, or attending school. Overall, the client viewed herself as incompetent in all areas.

The use of diary cards, which Cindy filled out weekly (or at the beginning of the session, if she forgot), assisted the therapist in carefully monitoring Cindy's daily experiences of suicidal ideation, misery, and urges to harm herself, as well as actual suicide attempts and NSSI behaviors. Behavioral analyses that attempted to identify the sequence of events leading up to and following Cindy's suicidal behavior soon became an important focus of therapy. At every point the therapist presented self-injurious behavior as to be expected, given the strength of the urge (but considered it ultimately beatable), and pointed out repeatedly that if the client committed suicide, therapy would be over, so they had better work really hard now, while Cindy was alive.

Over the course of several months, the behavioral analyses began to identify a frequently recurring behavioral pattern that preceded suicidal behaviors. For Cindy, the chain of events would often begin with an interpersonal encounter (almost always with her husband), which culminated in her feeling threatened, criticized, or unloved. These feelings were often followed by urges either to self-mutilate or to kill herself, depending somewhat on the covarying levels of hopelessness, anger, and sadness. Decisions to self-mutilate and/or to attempt suicide were often accompanied by the thought, "I'll show you." At other times, hopelessness and a desire to end the pain permanently seemed predominant. Both are examples of emotional vulnerability. Following the conscious decision to self-mutilate or to attempt suicide, Cindy would then immediately dissociate and at some later point cut or burn herself, usually while in a state of "automatic pilot." Consequently, Cindy often had difficulty remembering specifics of the actual acts. At one point, Cindy burned her leg so badly (and then injected it with dirt to convince the doctor that he should give her more attention) that reconstructive surgery was required. Behavioral analyses also revealed that dissociation during sessions usually occurred following Cindy's perception of the therapist's disapproval or invalidation, especially when the therapist appeared to suggest that change was possible. The therapist targeted in-session dissociation by immediately addressing it as it occurred.

By several months into therapy, an apparently long-standing pattern of suicidal behaviors leading to inpatient admission was apparent. Cindy would report intense suicidal ideation, express doubts that she could resist the urge to kill herself, and request admission to her preferred hospital; or, without warning, she would cut or burn herself severely and require hospitalization for medical treatment. Attempts to induce Cindy to stay out of the hospital or to leave the hospital before she was ready typically resulted in an escalation of suicidality, followed by her pharmacotherapist's (a psychiatrist) insistence on her admission or the hospital's agreement to extend her stay. Observation of this behavioral pattern led the therapist to hypothesize that the hospitalization itself was reinforcing suicidal behavior; consequently, she attempted to change the contingencies for suicidal behaviors. Using didactic and contingency clarification strategies, the therapist attempted to help Cindy understand how hospitalization might be strengthening the very behavior they were working to eliminate. This issue became a focal point of disagreement within the therapy, with Cindy viewing the therapist's position as unsympathetic and lacking understanding of her phenomenal experience. In Cindy's opinion, the intensity of her emotional pain rendered the probability of suicide so high that hospitalization was necessary to guarantee her safety. She would buttress her position by citing frequently her difficulties with dissociative reactions, which she reported as extremely aversive and which, in her opinion, made her unable to function much of the time. From the therapist's perspective, the deleterious long-term risk of suicide created by repeated hospitalization in response to suicidal behavior was greater than the short-term risk of suicide if hospitalization stays were reduced. These differences in opinion led to frequent disagreements within sessions. It gradually became clear that Cindy viewed any explanations of her behavior as influenced by reinforcement as a direct attack; she implied that if hospitalization was reinforcing her suicidal behavior, then the therapist must believe that the purpose of her suicidality was for admission into the hospital. This was obviously not the case (at least some of the time), but all attempts to explain reinforcement theory in any other terms failed. The therapist compensated somewhat for insisting on the possibility that she (the therapist) was correct by doing three things. First, she repeatedly validated the client's experience of almost unendurable pain. Second, she made certain to address the client's dissociative behavior repeatedly, explaining it as an automatic reaction to intensely painful affect (or the threat of it). Third, she frequently addressed the quality of the relationship between Cindy and herself to strengthen the relationship and maintain Cindy in therapy, even though to do so was a source of even more emotional pain. By the fifth month, the therapist became concerned that the current treatment regimen was going to have the unintended consequence of killing the client (via suicide). At this point, the therapist's limits for effective treatment were crossed; therefore, she decided to employ the consultation-to-the-client strategy to address Cindy's hospitalizations. The first-choice strategy would have been to get Cindy to negotiate a new treatment plan with her preferred hospital and admitting psychiatrist. Cindy refused to go along, however, because she disagreed with the wisdom of changing her current unlimited access to the inpatient unit. The therapist was able to get her to agree to a consultation meeting with all of her treatment providers, and, with some tenacity, the therapist actually got Cindy to make all the calls to set up the meeting (including inviting her insurance monitor, who was coordinating payment for treatment).

At the case conference, the therapist presented her hypothesis that contingent hospitalization was reinforcing Cindy's suicidal behavior. She also assisted Cindy in making the case that she (the therapist) was wrong. Using reciprocal communication and contingency management, the therapist stated that she simply could not conduct a therapy she thought might kill the client (and she had to go along with what she thought was best even if she were wrong—"to do otherwise would be unethical"), and she requested that a new system of contingencies be agreed upon to disrupt the functional relationship between Cindy's suicidal behavior and hospitalization. Therefore, a plan was developed wherein the client was not required to be suicidal to gain hospital admittance. Under this new set of contingencies, Cindy could elect, at will, to enter the hospital for a stay of up to 3 days, at the end of which time she would always be discharged. If she convinced people that she was too suicidal for discharge, she would be transferred to her least-preferred hospital for safety. Suicidal and NSSI behaviors would no longer be grounds for admission except to a medical unit, when required. Although there was some disagreement as to the functional relationship between suicidal behavior and hospitalization, this system was agreed upon. Following this meeting, Cindy's husband announced that he was no longer able to live with or tolerate his wife's suicidal behavior, and that the constant threat of finding her dead had led to his decision to file for divorce. The focus of therapy then shifted to helping Cindy grieve over this event and find a suitable living arrangement. Cindy alternated between fury that her husband would desert her in her hour of need (or "illness," as she put it) and despair that she could ever cope alone. She decided that "getting her feelings out" was the only useful therapy. This led to many tearful sessions, with the therapist simultaneously validating the pain; focusing on Cindy's experiencing the affect in the moment, without escalating or blocking it; and cheerleading Cindy's ability to manage without going back into the hospital. Due to Cindy's high level of dysfunctionality, she and her therapist decided that she would enter a residential treatment facility for a 3-month period. The facility had a coping skills orientation and provided group but not individual therapy. Cindy saw her therapist once a week and talked to her several times a week during this period. With some coaching, Cindy looked for and found a roommate to live with and returned to her own home at the end of 3 months (the ninth month of therapy). Over the course of treatment, the therapist used a number of strategies to treat Cindy's suicidal, NSSI, and therapy-interfering behaviors. In-depth behavioral chain and solution analysis helped the therapist (and sometimes the client) gain insight into the factors influencing current suicidal behavior. For Cindy, as for most clients, performing these analyses was quite difficult, because the process usually generated intense feelings of shame, guilt, or anger. Thus, behavioral analysis also functioned as an exposure strategy, encouraging the client to observe and experience painful affect. It additionally served as a cognitive strategy in helping to change Cindy's expectancies concerning the advantages and disadvantages of suicidal behavior, especially as the therapist repeatedly made statements such as "How do you think you would feel if I got angry at you and then threatened suicide if you didn't change?" Finally, behavioral analysis served as contingency management, in that the client's ability to pursue topics of interest in therapy sessions was made contingent on the successful completion of chain and solution analysis.

Cindy presented early in therapy with exceedingly strong perceptions as to her needs and desires, and with a concomitant willingness to engage in extremely lethal suicidal behavior. As previously mentioned, several of these acts were serious attempts to end her life, whereas others functioned as attempts to gain attention and care from significant others. This client also presented with an extreme sensitivity to any attempts at obvious change procedures, which she typically interpreted as communicating a message about her incompetence and unworthiness. Although Cindy initially committed herself to attending weekly group skills training for the first year of therapy, her attendance at group meetings was quite erratic, and she generally tended either to miss entire sessions (but never more than three in a row) or to leave during the break. Cindy answered the therapist's attempts to address this issue by

stating that she could not drive at night due to night blindness. Although considered a therapy-interfering behavior and frequently addressed over the course of therapy, missing skills training was not a major focus of treatment, due to the continuing presence of higher-priority suicidal behavior. The therapist's efforts to engage the client in active skills acquisition during individual therapy sessions were also somewhat limited and were always preceded by obtaining Cindy's verbal commitment to problem solving. The stylistic strategy of irreverent communication was of value to the therapeutic process. The therapist's irreverence often served to "shake up" the client, resulting in a loosening of dichotomous thinking and maladaptive cognitions. The result of this was Cindy's increased willingness to explore new and adaptive behavioral solutions. Finally, relationship strategies were heavily employed as tools to strengthen the therapeutic alliance and to keep it noncontingent on suicidal and/or dissociative behaviors. Included here were between-session therapist-initiated telephone calls to see how Cindy was doing, the therapist routinely giving out phone numbers when she was traveling, and sending the client postcards when she was out of town.

By the 12th month of therapy, Cindy's suicidal and self-injurious behavior, as well as urges to engage in such behavior, receded. In addition, her hospital stays were reduced markedly, with none occurring after the eighth month. While living at home with a roommate, Cindy was readmitted to medical school. Part of the reason for returning to school was to turn her life around, so that she could try to regain her husband's love and attention, or at least his friendship. As the therapy continued to focus on changing the contingencies of suicidal behavior, reducing both emotional pain and inhibition, and tolerating distress, a further focus on maintaining sobriety and reasonable food intake was added. During the first months of living in her home without her husband, Cindy had several alcoholic binges, and her food intake dropped precipitously. These behaviors became immediate targets. The therapist's strong attention to these behaviors also communicated to Cindy that the therapist would take her problems seriously even if she were not suicidal. Therapy focused as well on expanding her social network. As with suicidal behaviors, attention to these targets served as a pathway to treating associated problems. As crisis situations decreased in frequency, much greater attention was paid to analyzing family patterns, including experiences of neglect and invalidation, that might have led to Cindy's problems in later life. Cindy did not report a history of sexual or physical abuse. Thus, the explicit goal of Stage 2 (which was being cautiously entered as an overlap to Stage 1) was to understand Cindy's history and its relationship to her current problems.

In other cases, especially when there has been sexual and/or physical abuse in childhood, movement to Stage 2 before Stage 1 targets have been mastered is likely to result in retrogression to previously problematic behaviors. For example, another client treated by the same therapist (M. M. L.), Terry, had been quite seriously abused physically by her mother throughout childhood and sexually abused by her father, beginning at age 5. The sexual advances were nonviolent at first but became physically abusive at approximately age 12. Prior to this therapy, Terry had not disclosed the incidents of abuse to anyone.

After successful negotiation of Stage 1 targets, the therapist proceeded to expose Terry to trauma-related cues by simply having her begin to disclose details of the abuse. These exposure sessions were intertwined with work on current problems in Terry's life. Following one exposure session focused on the sexual abuse, Terry reverted to some of her previously problematic behaviors, evidenced by withdrawal and silence in sessions, suicidal ideation, and medication noncompliance. The appearance of such behavior marked the necessity of stopping Stage 2 discussions of previous sexual abuse to address Stage 1 targets recursively. Three sessions were devoted to a behavioral analysis of Terry's current suicidal, therapy-interfering, and quality-of-life–interfering behaviors; these were eventually linked both to fears about how the therapist would view her childhood emotional responses to her father, and to holiday visits with her father that precipitated conflicts over how Terry should be feeling about him in the present. This two-steps-forward, one-step-back approach is common to therapy for clients with BPD, and in particular may mark the transition between Stage 1 and Stage 2.

As previously mentioned, Stage 3 targets the client's self-respect, regardless of the opinions of others. Betty, who was also in treatment with the same therapist (M. M. L.), had successfully negotiated Stages 1 and 2, and had become a highly competent nurse with training and supervisory responsibilities. Therapy with Betty was then focused on maintaining her self-esteem in the face of very powerful significant others (e.g., her supervisor) who constantly invalidated her. Components of the treatment included the therapist's noting and highlighting for Betty her tendency to modify her self-opinion in accordance with that of others, persistent attempts to extract from Betty self-validation and self-soothing, and imagery exercises wherein the client imagined and verbalized herself standing up to powerful others. Much of the therapy focus was on Betty's interpersonal behavior within the therapy session, with attention to relating this behavior to her interactions with other important people. Thus, treatment at that point was very similar to the functional-analytic psychotherapy regimen developed by Kohlenberg and Tsai (1991). Overall, this third stage of therapy involved the movement to a more egalitarian relationship between the client and the therapist, in which emphasis was placed on the client's standing up for her own opinions and defending her own actions. This approach required that the therapist both reinforce the client's assertions, and step back and refrain from validating and nurturing the client in the manner characteristic of Stages 1 and 2. In addition, therapy sessions were reduced to every other week, and issues surrounding eventual termination were periodically discussed.

Stage 4 of DBT targets the sense of incompleteness that can preclude the experience of joy and freedom. Sally started Stage 1 treatment with the same therapist (M. M. L.) 15 years ago. Stage 1 lasted 2 years; this was followed by a break of 1 year, after which treatment resumed for several years of bimonthly sessions leading to monthly sessions, and currently consists of four or five sessions a year. Sally has been married for 30 years to an irregularly employed husband who, though devoted and loyal, is quite invalidating of her. Although apparently brilliant, he is usually dismissed from jobs for his interpersonal insensitivity. She has been employed full-time at the same place for years, working with children. The son she felt closest to died in a plane accident 2 years ago; her mother died last year, and her father is very ill. Despite having a stable marriage, working in a stable and quite fulfilling job, having raised two well-adjusted sons, and still being athletic, life feels meaningless to Sally. In the past she was very active in spiritual activities; following meditation retreats or extended periods of daily meditation, she would report contentment and some sense of joy. Since her son died, Sally has let go of most of her spiritual activities. Following 2 years of focusing on grieving, she is now ready for Stage 4. Treatment planning focused on actively practicing and keeping track of progress in radical acceptance (or "letting go of ego," in Zen terminology), either alone or with group support.

TRANSCRIPTS

The following (composite) transcripts represent actual examples of the process of therapy occurring over several sessions with different clients. These particular dialogues between therapist and client have been chosen to provide the reader with comprehensive examples of the application of a wide range of DBT treatment strategies. The session targets in the following transcript were orienting and commitment. The strategies used were validation, problem solving (insight, orienting, and commitment), dialectical (devil's advocate), and integrated (relationship enhancement).

Obtaining the client's commitment is a crucial first step in beginning therapy with clients who have BPD. As illustrated in the following transcript, the dialectical technique of devil's advocate can be highly effective when used as a commitment strategy. In this first therapy session, the therapist's ultimate goal was to obtain the client's commitment to therapy, as well as a commitment to eliminate suicidal behavior. She began by orienting the client to the purpose of this initial session.

THERAPIST: So are you a little nervous about me?

CLIENT: Yeah, I guess I am.

THERAPIST: Well, that's understandable. For the next 50 minutes or so, we have this opportunity to get to know each other and see if we want to work together. So what I'd like to do is talk a little bit about the program and how you got here. So tell me, what do you want out of therapy with me, and what are you doing here?

CLIENT: I want to get better.

THERAPIST: Well, what's wrong with you?

CLIENT: I'm a mess. (*Laughs.*)

THERAPIST: How so?

CLIENT: Umm, I don't know. I just can't even cope with everyday life right now. And I can't even . . . I'm just a mess. I don't know how to deal with anything.

THERAPIST: So what does that mean exactly?

CLIENT: Umm, well, everything I try these days just seems overwhelming. I couldn't keep up on my job, and now I'm on medical leave. Plus everyone's sick of me being in the hospital so much. And I think my psychiatrist wants to send me away because of all my self-harming.

THERAPIST: How often do you self-harm?

CLIENT: Maybe once or twice a month. I use my lighter or cigarettes, sometimes a razor blade.

THERAPIST: Do you have scars all over?

CLIENT: (*Nods yes.*)

THERAPIST: Your psychiatrist tells me you've also drunk Clorox. Why didn't you mention that?

CLIENT: I guess it didn't enter my mind.

THERAPIST: Do things just not enter your mind very often?

CLIENT: I don't really know. Maybe.

THERAPIST: So maybe with you I'm going to have to be a very good guesser.

CLIENT: Hmm.

THERAPIST: Unfortunately, though, I'm not the greatest guesser. So we'll have to teach you how to have things come to mind. So what is it exactly that you want out of therapy with me? To quit harming yourself, quit trying to kill yourself, or both?

CLIENT: Both. I'm sick of it.

THERAPIST: And is there anything else you want help with?

CLIENT: Um, well, I don't know how to handle money, and I don't know how to handle relationships. I don't have friends; they don't connect with me very often. I'm a former alcoholic and a recovering anorexic/bulimic. I still have a tendency toward that.

THERAPIST: Do you think maybe some of what is going on with you is that you've replaced your alcoholic and anorexic behaviors with self-harm behaviors?

CLIENT: I don't know. I haven't thought about

it that way. I just feel that I don't know how to handle myself, and—you know, and I guess work through stuff, and that is obviously getting to me, because if it wasn't, I wouldn't be trying to kill myself.

THERAPIST: So from your perspective, one problem is that you don't know how to do things. A lot of things.

CLIENT: Yeah, and a lot of it is, I do know how, but for some reason I don't do it anyway.

THERAPIST: Um hmm.

CLIENT: You know, I mean I know I need to save money, and I know that I need to budget myself, and I do every single month, but every single month I get in debt. But, um, you know, it's really hard for me. You know, it's like sometimes I know it, or I know I shouldn't eat something and I do it anyway.

THERAPIST: So it sounds like part of the problem is you actually know how to do things; you just don't know how to get yourself to do the things you know how to do.

CLIENT: Exactly.

THERAPIST: Does it seem like maybe your emotions are in control—that you are a person who does things when you're in the mood?

CLIENT: Yes. Everything's done by the mood.

THERAPIST: So you're a moody person.

CLIENT: Yes. I won't clean the house for 2 months, and then I'll get in the mood to clean. Then I'll clean it immaculately and keep it that way for 3 weeks—I mean, just immaculate—and then when I'm in the mood I go back to being a mess again.

THERAPIST: So one of the tasks for you and me would be to figure out a way to get your behavior and what you do less hooked up with how you feel?

CLIENT: Right.

The therapist used insight to highlight for the client the observed interrelationship between the client's emotions and her behavior. She then began the process of shaping a commitment through the dialectical strategy of devil's advocate.

THERAPIST: That, of course, is going to be hell to do, don't you think? Why would you want to do that? It sounds so painful.

CLIENT: Well, I want to do it, because it's so in-

consistent. It's worse, you know, because when I'm . . . I know that, like with budgeting money or whatever, I know I need to do it, and then when I don't do it, it makes me even more upset.

THERAPIST: Why would you ever want to do something you're not in the mood for?

CLIENT: Because I've got to. Because I can't survive that way if I don't.

THERAPIST: Sounds like a pretty easy life to me.

CLIENT: Yeah, but I can't afford to live if I just spend my money on fun and stupid, frivolous things that I . . .

THERAPIST: Well, I guess maybe you should have some limits and not be too off the wall, but in general, I mean, why clean the house if you're not in the mood?

CLIENT: Because it pisses me off when it's a mess. And I can't find things, like I've lost bills before and then I end up not paying them. And now I've got collection agencies on my back. I can't deal with all this, and I end up self-harming and going into the hospital. And then I just want to end it all. But it still doesn't seem to matter, because if I'm not in the mood to clean it, I won't.

THERAPIST: So the fact that it makes horrible things happen in your life so far hasn't been enough of a motivation to get you to do things against your mood, right?

CLIENT: Well, obviously not (laughs), because it's not happening.

THERAPIST: Doesn't that tell you, though? This is going to be a big problem, don't you think? This isn't going to be something simple. It's not like you're going to walk in here and I'm going to say, "OK, magic wand," and then all of a sudden you're going to want to do things that you're not in the mood for.

CLIENT: Yeah.

THERAPIST: Yeah, so it seems to me that if you're not in the mood for things, if you're kind of mood-dependent, that's a very tough thing to crack. As a matter of fact, I think it's one of the hardest problems there is to deal with.

CLIENT: Yeah, great.

THERAPIST: I think we could deal with it, but I think it's going to be hell. The real question is whether you're willing to go through hell to get where you want to get or not. Now I figure that's the question.

CLIENT: Well, if it's going to make me happier, yeah.

THERAPIST: Are you sure?

CLIENT: Yeah, I've been going through this since I was 11 years old. I'm sick of this shit. I mean, excuse my language, but I really am, and I'm backed up against the wall. Either I need to do this or I need to die. Those are my two choices.

THERAPIST: Well, why not die?

CLIENT: Well, if it comes down to it, I will.

THERAPIST: Um hmm, but why not now?

CLIENT: Because, this is my last hope. Because if I've got one last hope left, why not take it?

THERAPIST: So, in other words, all things being equal, you'd rather live than die, if you can pull this off.

CLIENT: If I can pull it off, yeah.

THERAPIST: OK, that's good; that's going to be your strength. We're going to play to that. You're going to have to remember that when it gets tough. But now I want to tell you about this program and how I feel about you harming yourself, and then we'll see if you still want to do this.

As illustrated by the foregoing segment, the therapist's relentless use of the devil's advocate strategy successfully "got a foot in the door" and achieved an initial client commitment. The therapist then "upped the ante" with a brief explanation of the program and its goals.

THERAPIST: Now the most important thing to understand is that we are not a suicide prevention program; that's not our job. But we are a life enhancement program. The way we look at it, living a miserable life is no achievement. If we decide to work together, I'm going to help you try to improve your life, so that it's so good that you don't want to die or hurt yourself. You should also know that I look at suicidal behavior, including drinking Clorox, as problem-solving behavior. I think of alcoholism the same way. The only difference is that cutting, burning, unfortunately—it works. If it didn't work, nobody would do it more than once. But it only works in the short term, not the long term. So to quit cutting, trying to hurt your-

self, is going to be exactly like quitting alcohol. Do you think this is going to be hard?

CLIENT: Stopping drinking wasn't all that hard.

THERAPIST: Well, in my experience, giving up self-harm behavior is usually very hard. It will require both of us working, but you will have to work harder. And like I told you when we talked briefly, if you commit to this, it's for 1 year—individual therapy with me once a week, and group skills training once a week. So the question is, are you willing to commit for 1 year?

CLIENT: I said I'm sick of this stuff. That's why I'm here.

THERAPIST: So you've agreed to not drop out of therapy for a year, right?

CLIENT: Right.

THERAPIST: And do you realize that if you don't drop out for a year, that really does, if you think about it, rule out suicide for a year?

CLIENT: Logically, yeah.

THERAPIST: So we need to be absolutely clear about this, because this therapy won't work if you knock yourself off. The most fundamental mood-related goal we have to work on is that, no matter what your mood is, you won't kill yourself or try to.

CLIENT: All right.

THERAPIST: So that's what I see as number one priority—not our only one but number one—that we will work on that. And getting you to agree—meaningfully, of course—and actually follow through on staying alive and not harming yourself and not attempting suicide, no matter what your mood is. Now the question is whether you agree to that.

CLIENT: Yes, I agree to that.

The therapist, having successfully obtained the client's commitment to work on suicidal behavior again employed the strategy of devil's advocate to reinforce the strength of the commitment.

THERAPIST: Why would you agree to that?

CLIENT: I don't know. (*Laughs.*)

THERAPIST: I mean, wouldn't you rather be in a therapy where, if you wanted to kill yourself, you could?

CLIENT: I don't know. I mean, I never really thought about it that way.

THERAPIST: Hmm.

CLIENT: I don't want to . . . I want to be able to get to the point where I could feel like I'm not being forced into living.

THERAPIST: So are you agreeing with me because you're feeling forced into agreeing?

CLIENT: You keep asking me all these questions.

THERAPIST: What do you think?

CLIENT: I don't know what I think right now, honestly.

A necessary and important skill for the DBT therapist is the ability to sense when a client has been pushed to his or her limits, as well as the concomitant skill of being willing and able to step back and at least temporarily refrain from further pressuring the client. In these instances, continued pressure from the therapist is likely to boomerang and have the opposite effect of what the therapist intends. Here the therapist noticed the client's confusion and sensed that further pushing was likely to result in the client's reducing the strength of her commitment. Consequently, the therapist stepped back and moved in with validation.

THERAPIST: So you're feeling pushed up against the wall a little bit, by me?

CLIENT: No, not really. (*Starts to cry.*)

THERAPIST: What just happened just now?

CLIENT: (*pause*) I don't know. I mean, I don't think I really want to kill myself. I think I just feel like I have to. I don't think it's really even a mood thing. I just think it's when I feel like there's no other choice. I just say, "Well, you know there's no other choice, so do it." You know. And so right now, I don't see any ray of hope. I'm going to therapy, which I guess is good. I mean, I know it's good, but I don't see anything any better than it was the day I tried to kill myself.

THERAPIST: Well, that's probably true. Maybe it isn't any better. I mean, trying to kill yourself doesn't usually solve problems. Although it actually did do one thing for you.

CLIENT: It got me in therapy.

THERAPIST: Yeah. So my asking you all these questions makes you start to cry. You look like you must be feeling pretty bad.

CLIENT: Just overwhelmed, I guess the word is.

THERAPIST: That's part of the reason we're having this conversation, to try to structure our relationship so that it's very clear for both of us. And that way, at least, we'll try to cut down on how much you get overwhelmed by not knowing what's going on with me. OK?

CLIENT: Um hmm.

THERAPIST: And so I just want to be clear on what our number one goal is, and how hard this is, because if you want to back out, now's the time. Because I'm going to take you seriously if you say, "Yes, I want to do it."

CLIENT: I don't want to back out.

THERAPIST: OK. Good. Now I just want to say that this seems like a good idea right now. You're in kind of an energized mood today, getting started on a new program. But in 5 hours, it might not seem like such a good idea. It's kind of like it's easy to commit to a diet after a big meal, but it's much harder when you're hungry. But we're going to work on how to make it keep sounding like a good idea. It'll be hell, but I have confidence. I think we can be successful working together.

Note how the therapist ended the session by preparing the client for the difficulties she was likely to experience in keeping her commitment and working in therapy. Cheerleading and relationship enhancement laid the foundation for a strong therapeutic alliance. The following session occurred approximately 4 months into therapy. The session target was suicidal behavior. The therapist used validation, problem solving (contingency clarification, didactic information, behavioral analysis, and solution analysis), stylistic (irreverent communication), dialectical (metaphor, making lemonade out of lemons), and skills training (distress tolerance) strategies.

The therapist reviewed the client's diary card and noted a recent, intentional self-injury, in which the client opened up a previously self-inflicted wound following her physician's refusal to provide pain medication. The therapist began by proceeding with a behavioral analysis.

THERAPIST: OK. Now you were in here last week telling me you were never going to hurt yourself again because this was so ridiculous, you couldn't stand it, you couldn't hurt yourself any more. So let's figure out how that broke down on Sunday, so we can learn something from it. OK. So when did you start having urges to hurt yourself?

CLIENT: My foot began to hurt on Wednesday. I started to have a lot of pain.

THERAPIST: It hadn't hurt before that?

CLIENT: No.

THERAPIST: So the nerves were dead before that or something, huh? So you started having a lot of pain. Now when did you start having the pain, and when did the urge to harm yourself come?

CLIENT: At the same time.

THERAPIST: They just come at the identical moment?

CLIENT: Just about.

The specification of an initial prompting environmental event is always the first step in conducting a behavioral chain analysis. Here the therapist began by directly inquiring when the urges toward suicide and NSSI began. Note also the therapist's use of irreverent communication early in the session.

THERAPIST: So how is it that feeling pain sets off an urge to self-harm? Do you know how that goes? How you get from one to the other?

CLIENT: I don't know. Maybe it wasn't till Thursday, but I asked my nurse. I go, "Look, I'm in a lot of pain, you know. I'm throwing up my food because the pain is so bad." And the nurse tried. She called the doctor and told him I was in a lot of pain, and asked if he'd give me some painkillers. But no! So I kept asking, and the answer kept being no, and I got madder and madder and madder. So I felt like I had to show somebody that it hurt, because they didn't believe me.

THERAPIST: So let's figure this out. So is it that you're assuming that if someone believed it hurt as bad as you said it does, they would actually give you the painkillers?

CLIENT: Yes.

THERAPIST: OK. That's where the faulty thinking is. That's the problem. You see, it's entirely possible that people know how bad the pain is but still aren't giving you medication.

CLIENT: I believe firmly, and I even wrote it in my journal, that if I'd gotten pain medication when I really needed it, I wouldn't have even thought of self-harming.

The therapist proceeded by obtaining a description of the events co-occurring with the onset of the problem. Here it became apparent that maladaptive thinking was instrumental in the client's decision to self-harm. In the following segment, the therapist used the dialectical strategy of metaphor to highlight for the client her cognitive error.

THERAPIST: Now let me ask you something—you've got to imagine this, OK? Let's imagine that you and I are on a raft together out in the middle of the ocean. Our boat has sunk and we're on the raft. And when the boat sank, your leg got cut really badly. And together we've wrapped it up as well as we can. But we don't have any pain medicine. And we're on this raft together and your leg really hurts, and you ask me for pain medicine, and I say no. Do you think you would then have an urge to hurt yourself and make it worse?

CLIENT: No, it would be a different situation.

THERAPIST: OK, but if I did have the pain medication and I said no because we had to save it, what do you think?

CLIENT: If that were logical to me, I'd go along with it and wouldn't want to hurt myself.

THERAPIST: What if I said no because I didn't want you to be a drug addict?

CLIENT: I'd want to hurt myself.

THERAPIST: OK. So we've got this clear. The pain is not what's setting off the desire to self-harm. It's someone not giving you something to help, when you feel they could if they wanted to.

CLIENT: Yes.

The therapist used contingency clarification to point out the effects of others' responses on the client's own behavior. In the following segment, the therapist again employed contingency clarification in a continued effort to highlight for the client the communication function of NSSI.

THERAPIST: So, in other words, hurting yourself is communication behavior, OK? So what we have to do is figure out a way for the communication behavior to quit working.

CLIENT: Why?

THERAPIST: Because you're not going to stop doing it until it quits working. It's like trying to talk to someone; if there's no one in the room, you eventually quit trying to talk to them. It's like when a phone goes dead, you quit talking.

CLIENT: I tried three nights in a row in a perfectly assertive way and just clearly stated I was in a lot of pain.

THERAPIST: You know, I think I'll switch chairs with you. You're not hearing what I'm saying.

CLIENT: And they kept saying, "No," and then some little light came on in my head.

THERAPIST: I'm considering switching chairs with you.

CLIENT: And it was like, "Here, now can you tell that it hurts a lot?"

THERAPIST: I'm thinking of switching chairs with you.

CLIENT: Why?

THERAPIST: Because if you were sitting over here, I think you would see that no matter how bad the pain is, hurting yourself to get pain medication is not a reasonable response. The hospital staff may not have been reasonable either. It may be that they should have given you pain medicine. But we don't have to say they were wrong in order to say that hurting yourself was not the appropriate response.

CLIENT: No, I don't think it was the appropriate response.

THERAPIST: Good. So what we've got to do is figure out a way to get it so that the response doesn't come in, even if you don't get pain medicine. So far, it has worked very effectively as communication. And the only way to stop it is to get it to not work any more. And of course, it would be good to get other things to work. What you're arguing is "Well, OK, if I'm not going to get it this way, then I should be able to get it another way."

CLIENT: I tried this time!

THERAPIST: Yes, I know you did, I know you did.

CLIENT: A lady down the hallway from me was getting treatment for her diabetes, and it got real bad, and they gave her pain medication.

THERAPIST: Now we're not on the same wavelength in this conversation.

CLIENT: Yes, we are. What wavelength are you on?

THERAPIST: I'm on the wavelength that it may have been reasonable for you to get pain medicine, and I certainly understand your wanting it. But I'm also saying that no matter what's going on, hurting yourself is something we don't want to happen. You're functioning like if I agreed with you that you should get pain medication, I would think this was OK.

CLIENT: Hmm?

THERAPIST: You're talking about whether they should have given you pain medication or not. I'm not talking about that. Even if they should have, we've got to figure out how you could have gotten through without hurting yourself.

As illustrated by the foregoing exchange, a client with BPD often wants to remain focused on the crisis at hand. This poses a formidable challenge for the therapist, who must necessarily engage in a back-and-forth dance between validating the client's pain and pushing for behavioral change. This segment also illustrates how validation does not necessarily imply agreement. Although the therapist validated the client's perception that the nurse's refusal to provide pain medication may have been unreasonable, she remained steadfast in maintaining the inappropriateness of the client's response.

CLIENT: I tried some of those distress tolerance things and they didn't work.

THERAPIST: OK. Don't worry, we'll figure out a way. I want to know everything you tried. But first I want to be sure I have the picture clear. Did the urges start building after Wednesday and get worse over time?

CLIENT: Yeah. They started growing with the pain.

THERAPIST: With the pain. OK. But also they started growing with their continued refusal to give you pain medicine. So you were thinking that if you hurt yourself, they would somehow give you pain medicine?

CLIENT: Yeah. 'Cause if they wouldn't listen to me, then I could show them.

THERAPIST: OK, so you were thinking, "If they won't listen to me, I'll show them." And when did that idea first hit? Was that on Wednesday?

CLIENT: Yeah.

THERAPIST: OK. Well, we've got to figure out a way for you to tolerate bad things without harming yourself. So let's figure out all the things you tried, and then we have to figure out some other things, because those didn't work. So what was the first thing you tried?

At this juncture the behavioral analysis remained incomplete, and it would normally have been premature to move to the stage of solution analysis. However, in the therapist's judgment, it was more critical at this point to reinforce the client's attempts at distress tolerance by responding to the client's communication that she had attempted behavioral skills.

CLIENT: I thought that if I just continued to be assertive about it that the appropriate measures would be taken.

THERAPIST: OK, but that didn't work. So why didn't you harm yourself right then?

CLIENT: I didn't want to.

THERAPIST: Why didn't you want to?

CLIENT: I didn't want to make it worse.

THERAPIST: So you were thinking about pros and cons —that if I make it worse, I'll feel worse?

CLIENT: Yeah.

One aspect of DBT skills training stresses the usefulness of evaluating the pros and cons of tolerating distress as a crisis survival strategy. Here the therapist employed the dialectical strategy of turning lemons into lemonade by highlighting for the client how she did, in fact, use behavioral skills. Note in the following response how the therapist immediately reinforced the client's efforts with praise.

THERAPIST: That's good thinking. That's when you're thinking about the advantages and disadvantages of doing it. OK, so at that point the advantages of making it worse were outweighed by the disadvantages. OK.

So you keep up the good fight here. Now what else did you try?

CLIENT: I tried talking about it with other clients.

THERAPIST: And what did they have to say?

CLIENT: They said I should get pain medication.

THERAPIST: Right. But did they say you should cut yourself or hurt yourself if you didn't get it?

CLIENT: No. And I tried to get my mind off my pain by playing music and using mindfulness. I tried to read and do crossword puzzles.

THERAPIST: Um hmm. Did you ever try radical acceptance?

CLIENT: What's that?

THERAPIST: It's where you sort of let go and accept the fact that you're not going to get the pain medication. And you just give yourself up to that situation. You just accept that it ain't going to happen, that you're going to have to cope in some other way.

CLIENT: Which I did yesterday. I needed a little Ativan to get me there, but I got there.

THERAPIST: Yesterday?

CLIENT: Yeah. I took a nap. When I woke up I basically said, "Hey, they're not going to change, so you've just got to deal with this the best that you can."

THERAPIST: And did that acceptance help some?

CLIENT: I'm still quite angry about what I believe is discrimination against borderline personalities. I'm still very angry about that.

THERAPIST: OK. That's fine. Did it help, though, to accept?

CLIENT: Um hmm.

THERAPIST: That's good. That's great. That's a great skill, a great thing to practice. When push comes to shove, when you're really at the limit, when it's the worst it can be, radical acceptance is the skill to practice.

CLIENT: That's AA.

During a solution analysis, it is often necessary that the therapist facilitate the process by helping the client "brainstorm," or by making direct suggestions for handling future crises.

Here the therapist suggested a solution that is also taught in the DBT skills training module on distress tolerance. The notion of radical acceptance stresses the idea that acceptance of one's pain is a necessary prerequisite for ending emotional suffering.

THERAPIST: OK. Now let's go back to how you gave in to the urge. Because you really managed to battle all the way till then, right? OK. Usually, with you, we can assume that something else happened. So let's figure out Sunday and see if there wasn't an interpersonal situation that day that made you feel criticized, unloved, or unacceptable.

CLIENT: Well, on Saturday I was so pissed off and I went to an AA meeting. And it got on my brain how alcohol would steal away my pain. I went looking all around the neighborhood for an open store. I was going to go get drunk. That's how much my pain was influencing me. But I couldn't find a store that was open, so I went back to the hospital.

THERAPIST: So you got the idea of getting alcohol to cure it, and you couldn't find any, so you went back to the hospital. You were in a lot of pain, and then what happened?

CLIENT: I told the nurse, "I've been sober almost 10 years and this is the first urge I've had to drink; that's how bad my pain is." And that wasn't listened to.

THERAPIST: So you figured that should have done it?

CLIENT: Yeah.

THERAPIST: Yeah. 'Cause that's a high-level communication, that's like a suicide threat. Very good, though. I want you to know, that's better than a suicide threat, because that means you had reduced the severity of your threats.

The response above was very irreverent, in that most clients would not expect their therapists to view making a threat as a sign of therapeutic progress. The therapeutic utility of irreverence often lies in its "shock" value, which may temporarily loosen a client's maladaptive beliefs and assumptions, and open the client up to the possibility of other response solutions.

CLIENT: And I just told her how I was feeling about it, and I thought that would do it. And the doctor still wouldn't budge.

THERAPIST: So what did she do? Did she say she would call?

CLIENT: She called.

THERAPIST: OK. And then what happened?

CLIENT: She came back. She was really sweet, and she just said, "I'm really sorry, but the doctor said no."

THERAPIST: Then did you feel anger?

CLIENT: I don't know if I was really angry, but I was hurt.

THERAPIST: Oh, really? Oh, that's pretty interesting. OK. So you were hurt . . .

CLIENT: Because I ended up hugging my teddy bear and just crying for a while.

THERAPIST: Before or after you decided to hurt yourself?

CLIENT: Before.

THERAPIST: OK. So you didn't decide right away to hurt yourself. You were thinking about it. But when did you decide to do it?

CLIENT: Later on Saturday.

THERAPIST: When?

CLIENT: After I got sick of crying.

THERAPIST: So you laid in bed and cried, feeling uncared about and hurt, abandoned probably, and unlovable, like you weren't worth helping?

CLIENT: Yes.

THERAPIST: That's a really adaptive response. That's what I'm going to try to teach you. Except that you've already done it without my teaching it to you. So how did you get from crying, feeling unloved and not cared about, and you cry and sob—how did you get from there to deciding to hurt yourself, instead of like going to sleep?

CLIENT: Because then I got angry. And I said, "Fuck this shit, I'll show him."

THERAPIST: Now did you quit crying before you got angry, or did getting angry make you stop crying?

CLIENT: I think getting angry made me stop crying.

THERAPIST: So you kind of got more energized. So you must have been ruminating while you were lying there, thinking. What were you thinking about?

CLIENT: For a long time I was just wanting somebody to come care about me.

THERAPIST: Um hmm. Perfectly reasonable feelings. Makes complete sense. Now maybe there you could have done something different. What would have happened if you had asked the nurse to come in and talk to you, hold your hand?

An overall goal of behavioral analysis is the construction of a general road map of how the client arrives at dysfunctional responses, with notation of possible alternative pathways. Here the therapist was searching for junctures in the map where possible alternative responses were available to the client.

CLIENT: They don't have time to do that.

THERAPIST: They don't? Do you think that would have helped?

CLIENT: I don't know. She couldn't help me.

THERAPIST: She could have made you feel cared about. That would have been a caring thing to do.

CLIENT: Yeah, but I don't think it would have helped.

THERAPIST: What would have helped?

CLIENT: Getting pain medication.

THERAPIST: I thought you'd say that. You have a one-track mind. Now listen, we've got to figure out something else to help you, because it can't be that nothing else can help. That can't be the way the world works for you. There's got to be more than one way to get everywhere, because we all run into boulders on the path. Life is like walking on a path, you know, and we all run into boulders. It's got to be that there are other paths to places. And for you, it really isn't the pain in your ankle that's the problem; it's the feeling of not being cared about. And probably a feeling that has something to do with anger, or a feeling that other people don't respect you—a feeling of being invalidated.

CLIENT: Yes.

THERAPIST: So I think it's not actually the pain in your ankle that's the problem. Because if you were out on that raft with me, you would have been able to handle the pain if I hadn't had any medicine, right? So it's really not the pain; it's the sense of being invalidated and the sense of not being cared about. That's my guess. Do you think that's correct?

CLIENT: Yes.

THERAPIST: See, the question is, is there any other way for you to feel validated and cared about, other than them giving it to you?

CLIENT: No.

THERAPIST: Now is this a definite, like "I'm not going to let there be any other way," or is it more open, like "I can't think of another way, but I'm open to the possibility?"

CLIENT: I don't think there's another way.

THERAPIST: Does that mean you're not even open to learning another way?

CLIENT: Like what?

THERAPIST: I don't know. We have to figure it out. See, what I think is happening is that when you're in a lot of pain and you feel either not cared about or not taken seriously, invalidated, that's what sets you up to hurt yourself, and also to want to die. The problem that we have to solve is how to be in a situation that you feel is unjust without having to harm yourself to solve it. Are you open to that?

CLIENT: Yeah.

As illustrated here, behavioral analysis is often an excruciating and laborious process for client and therapist alike. The therapist often feels demoralized and is tempted to abandon the effort, which may be likened to trying to find a pair of footprints hidden beneath layers of fallen leaves; the footprints are there, but it may take much raking and gathering of leaves before they are uncovered. With repeated analyses, however, the client learns that the therapist will not "back down." Such persistence on the part of the therapist eventually extinguishes a client's refusal to attempt new and adaptive problem-solving behaviors. As clients increasingly acquire new behavioral skills, more adaptive attempts at problem resolution eventually become discernible.

In the following session (approximately 10 months into therapy), the client arrived wearing mirrored sunglasses (again) and was angry because collection agencies were persistent in pressuring her for payment on delinquent accounts. In addition, her therapist had been out of town for a week. The session targets were emotion regulation and interpersonal effectiveness. Dialectical (metaphor), validation (cheerleading), problem solving (contingency clarification, contingency management), stylistic (reciprocal communication, irreverent communication), and integrated (relationship enhancement) strategies were used. In this first segment, the therapist used cheerleading, contingency clarification, and the contingency management strategy of shaping to get the client to remove her sunglasses and work on expressing her anger.

THERAPIST: It's not a catastrophe that the collector did this to you, and it's not a catastrophe to be mad at the collector. It's made your life a lot harder, but you can handle this. You can cope with this. This is not more than you can cope with. You're a really strong woman; you've got it inside you. But you've got to do it. You've got to use it. I'm willing to help you, but I can't do it alone. You have to work with me.

CLIENT: How?

THERAPIST: Well, by taking off your sunglasses, for starters.

The therapist began the exchange by attempting to normalize the issue ("It's not a catastrophe"), validating the client ("It's made your life a lot harder"), and cheerleading ("You can handle this. You can cope. . . . You're a really strong woman"). The therapist then moved to contingency clarification by pointing out that provision of the therapist's assistance was contingent on the client's willingness to work. She immediately followed this by requesting a response well within the client's behavioral repertoire.

CLIENT: I knew you'd say that.

THERAPIST: And I knew you knew I'd say that.

CLIENT: Sunglasses are your biggest bitch, I think.

THERAPIST: Well, how would you like to look at yourself talking to someone else? (long pause) They make it difficult for me. And I figure they make it harder for you. I think you do better when you're not wearing those sunglasses. It's like a step; you always do better when you go forward. And when you do, you feel better. I've noticed that. (long pause) So that's what you should do; you should take off your sunglasses, and then we should problem-solve on how to cope when you can't get angry. There's nothing freakish about that. Something has happened in your life that has made it so that you're afraid to

be angry, and we just have to deal with that, you and me. It's just a problem to be solved. It's not a catastrophe; it's not the worst thing anyone ever did. It's just a problem that you have, and that's what you and I do. We solve problems; we're a problem-solving team. (pause)

CLIENT: (Removes sunglasses.) All right.

THERAPIST: Thank you. That's a big step, I know, for you.

The therapist's use of reciprocal communication informed the client of her feelings regarding the sunglasses. Note the matter-of-fact attitude taken by the therapist and her continued attempt to normalize the issue (i.e., "There's nothing freakish about that . . . it's not the worst thing anyone ever did"). Also note the framing of the issue as a problem to be solved, as well as the therapist's use of the relationship strategy to enhance the therapeutic alliance. The therapist also made a point of validating the client by letting her know that she realized this was difficult.

THERAPIST: Now, c'mon, I want you to find it inside yourself. I know you've got it; I know you can do it. You can't give up. You can't let your feet slip. Keep going. Just express directly to me how you feel. That you're angry at yourself, that you're angry at the collection agency, and that you're damn angry with me. (long pause)

CLIENT: (barely audible) I'm angry at you, at myself, and the collection agency.

The therapist continued to rely on cheerleading and praise as she continued the shaping process in an attempt to get the client to express her anger directly.

THERAPIST: Good, did that kill you? (long pause) That's great. Is that hard? (long pause) It was, wasn't it? Now say it with a little vigor. Can't you say it with a little energy?

CLIENT: (Shakes her head no.)

THERAPIST: Yes, you can. I know you've got it in you. I have a good feel for what your strengths are. I don't know how I've got this good feel, but I do. And I know you can do it and you need to do it, and you need to say it with some energy. Express how angry you are. You don't have to yell and scream or throw things. Just say it aloud—"I'm angry!" (*long pause*) You can scream, of course, if you want; you can say, "I'm angry!"

CLIENT: That's it. That's all I can do.

THERAPIST: Listen, you have to take the risk. You're not going to get past this or through this. You have to take the risk. You are like a person mountain climbing and we've come to this crevasse and it's very deep, but we can't go back because there's an avalanche, and the only way to go forward is for you to jump over this crevasse. You've got to do it. Tell me how mad you are, in a way that I can understand how you really feel.

CLIENT: (*long pause*) I can't do any of it.

THERAPIST: That is bullshit.

CLIENT: You want me to get angry at you, don't you?

THERAPIST: I don't care who you get angry at. I think you already are angry. I just want you to express it. I'm not going to ask you to do anything more today, by the way. I figure the only thing today you have to do is say "I'm angry," in a voice that sounds angry, and I figure you're capable of that. And I might be angry if you don't do it. I don't think I will be, but I might. That's OK. I can be angry, you can be angry, we can be angry sometimes, and it isn't going to kill either one of us.

Cheerleading and metaphor were unsuccessful in moving the client to express her anger more forcefully. Consequently, the therapist switched to irreverent communication in an attempt to get the client to "jump track." Also note how the therapist communicated to the client the potential negative consequences of her continued refusal to express her anger (i.e., ". . . I might be angry . . ."). In this manner, the therapist used the relationship as a contingency in order to promote change in the client.

THERAPIST: OK, so how angry are you? On a scale of 1 to 100, how angry would you say you are? At 100, you're ready to kill. You're so enraged, you'd go to war if you could.

CLIENT: (*barely audible*) Maybe 100.

THERAPIST: Really?

CLIENT: They know my situation.

THERAPIST: Um hmm.

CLIENT: They're persistent.

THERAPIST: Um hmm. (*pause*) Who's the safest to be angry at? Yourself, me, or the collection agency?

CLIENT: Collection agency.

THERAPIST: OK, then, tell me how angry you are. You don't have to make it sound like 100. Try to make it sound like 50.

CLIENT: They really pissed me off! (*said in a loud, angry voice*)

THERAPIST: Well, damn right. They piss me off, too.

As illustrated by the foregoing exchange, a primary difficulty in working with clients who have BPD is their not uncommon tendency to refuse to engage in behavioral work. Thus, it is absolutely necessary that the therapist maintain persistence and not give up in the face of a client's "I can't" statements. In situations like these, the use of irreverent communication often succeeds in producing a breakthrough and gaining client compliance.

POSTVENTION

After completing the writing of Cindy's case history for publication in this *Handbook*, 14 months into therapy, Cindy died of a prescription drug overdose plus alcohol. We considered dropping the case history and replacing it with a more successful case. However, in Cindy's honor, and because we think much can be learned from both failed and successful therapy, we decided to leave the case in. The immediate precipitant for Cindy's overdose was a call to her estranged husband, during which she discovered that another woman was living with him. As Cindy told her therapist during a phone call the next morning, her unverbalized hope that they might someday get back together, or at least be close friends, had been shattered. She phoned again that evening in tears, stating that she had just drunk half a fifth of liquor. Such drinking incidents had occurred several times before, and the phone call was spent "remoralizing" Cindy, offering hope, problem-solving how she could indeed live without her husband, and using crisis intervention techniques to get her through the evening, until her appointment the following day.

Cindy's roommate was home and agreed to talk with her, watch a TV movie together, and go to bed (plans on which the roommate did follow through). Cindy stated that although she felt suicidal, she would stop drinking and would not do anything self-destructive before her appointment. She was instructed to call the therapist back later that evening if she wanted to talk again. The next day, when Cindy did not arrive for her appointment, the therapist called her home, just as her roommate discovered Cindy dead, still in bed from the night before. At this point, the therapist was faced with a number of tasks. The therapist called to inform other therapists who had been treating the client, and she spoke with a legal consultant to review the limits of confidentiality when a client has died. Once the family (Cindy's parents and estranged husband) were alerted, the therapist called each to offer her condolences. The next day, the therapist (who was the senior therapist and supervisor on the treatment team) called a meeting of the treatment team to discuss and process the suicide. It was especially important to notify the individual therapists of the remaining three members of Cindy's skills training group. Group members were notified of the suicide by their individual psychotherapists. Within minutes of the beginning of the next group session, however, two members became seriously suicidal, and one of them had to be briefly hospitalized. (By the third week following the suicide, however, both had regained their forward momentum.) A third group member took this occasion to quit DBT and switch to another therapy, saying that this proved the treatment did not work. In the days and weeks following the suicide, the therapist attended the funeral and met with Cindy's roommate and with her parents.

What can we learn from this suicide? First, it is important to note that even when a treatment protocol is followed almost to the letter, it may not save a client. Even an effective treatment can fail in the end. In this case, DBT failed. This does not mean that the progress made was unimportant or not real. Had this "slippery spot over the abyss" been negotiated safely, perhaps the client would have been able to develop, finally, a life of quality. Risk is not eliminated, however, just because an individual makes substantial progress. In this case, the therapist did not believe during the last phone call that the client was at higher than ordinary risk for imminent suicide. In contrast to many previous phone calls and therapy sessions in

which the client had cried that she might not be able to hold on, during the last call the client made plans for the evening, agreed to stop drinking and not to do anything suicidal or self-destructive, and seemed to the therapist (and the roommate) to be in better spirits following the phone call. Her roommate was home and available. Thus, the therapist did not take extraordinary measures that evening to prevent suicide. Indeed, the problem behavior focused on during the call was the drinking. The topic of suicide was brought up by the therapist, in the course of conducting a risk assessment.

Could the therapist have known? Only (perhaps) if she had paid more attention to the precipitant and less to the affect expressed at the end of the phone call. In reviewing notes about the client, the therapist saw that each previous near-lethal attempt was a result of the client's believing that the relationship with her husband had irrevocably ended. Although the client could tolerate losing her husband, she could not tolerate losing all hope for a reconciliation at some point, even many years hence. Had the therapist linked these two ideas (complete loss of hope and suicide attempt), she might have been able to work out a better plan with the client for a reemergence of the crisis later in the evening. The value of both conducting thorough behavioral assessments and organizing them into a coherent pattern is highlighted in this case. Second, when all is said and done, an individual with BPD must ultimately be able and willing to tolerate the almost unimaginable pain of his or her life until the therapy has a chance to make a permanent difference. Ultimately, the therapist cannot save the client; only the client can do that. Even if mistakes are made, the client must nonetheless persevere. In this case, the DBT protocol of "no lethal drugs for lethal people" was violated, even though the client had a past history of near-lethal overdoses. Why was the protocol not enforced? There were two primary reasons. First, the client came into therapy with a strong belief that the host of medications she was on were essential to her survival. Any attempt on the therapist's part to manage her medications would have been met by very strong resistance. Although the drugs were dispensed in small doses, the only safe alternative would have been to have the person living with her (her husband at first, then her roommate) manage her medications, which the client also resisted. In addition, the "no lethal drugs" protocol of

DBT is regularly criticized by some mental health professionals, who believe that psychoactive medications are a treatment of choice for suicidal individuals. In the face of professional and client resistance to the policy in this case the therapist relented. The second reason was that the lethal behavior of the client during therapy consisted of cutting and slashing; thus, her using drugs to commit suicide did not seem likely, and the therapist allowed herself a false sense of safety with respect to them. Third, a group member's suicide is extraordinarily stressful for clients with BPD who are in group therapy. Although it is easy to believe that alliances are not strong in a psychoeducational behavioral skills group, this has universally not been our experience. The suicide of one member is a catastrophic event and can lead to contagious suicide and NSSI behavior, and therapy dropouts. Thus, extreme care is needed in the conduct of group meetings for some time following a suicide. Similar care is needed with the treatment team, where the thread of hope that maintains therapists in the face of a daunting task is also strained. It is important that the personal reactions of therapists, as well as a period of mourning and grieving, be shared and accepted. Fears of legal responsibility, never far from the surface, must be confronted directly; legal counsel must be sought as necessary; and, in time, a careful review of the case and the therapy must be conducted, if only to improve treatment in the future.

ACKNOWLEDGMENTS

The writing of this chapter was supported by National Institute of Mental Health Grant No. MH34486 to Marsha M. Linehan. Parts of this chapter are drawn from Linehan (1993b), Linehan and Koerner (1992), Koerner and Linehan (1992), and Linehan (1997). The quotations from Linehan (1997) in the section on validation are reprinted with the permission of the American Psychological Association. Finally, this chapter is a revision of the same chapter in the previous edition of this book. Many contributions to this chapter were made by previous authors Bryan M. Cochran and Constance A. Kehrer.

REFERENCES

Adler, G. (1981). The borderline–narcissistic personality disorder continuum. *American Journal of Psychiatry*, *138*, 46–50.

Adler, G. (1985). *Borderline psychopathology and its treatment*. New York: Aronson.

Adler, G. (1993). The psychotherapy of core borderline psychopathology. *American Journal of Psychotherapy*, *47*, 194–206.

Adler, G., & Buie, D. H. (1979). Aloneness and borderline psychopathology: The possible relevance of child development issues. *International Journal of Psychoanalytic Psychotherapy*, *60*, 83–96.

American Psychiatric Association. (1987). *Diagnostic and statistical manual of mental disorders*. (3rd ed., rev.). Washington, DC: Author.

American Psychiatric Association. (2000). *Diagnostic and statistical manual of mental disorders* (4th ed., text rev.). Washington, DC: Author.

Aviram, R. B., Brodsky, B. S., & Stanley, B. (2006). Borderline personality disorder, stigma, and treatment implications. *Harvard Review of Psychiatry*, *14*, 249–256.

Bateman, A., & Fonagy, P. (1999). Effectiveness of partial hospitalization in the treatment of borderline personality disorder: A randomized controlled trial. *American Journal of Psychiatry*, *156*, 1563–1569.

Bateman, A., & Fonagy, P. (2001). Treatment of borderline personality disorder with psychoanalytically oriented partial hospitalization: An 18-month follow-up. *American Journal of Psychiatry*, *158*, 36–42.

Bateman, A. W., & Fonagy, P. (2004). Mentalization-based treatment of BPD. *Journal of Personality Disorders*, *18*, 36–51.

Beck, A. T., Brown, G., Berchick, R. J., Stewart, B. L., & Steer, R. A. (1990). Relationship between hopelessness and ultimate suicide: A replication with psychiatric outpatients. *American Journal of Psychiatry*, *147*, 190–195.

Beck, A. T., & Freeman, A. (1990). *Cognitive therapy of personality disorders*. New York: Guilford Press.

Beck, A. T., Rush, A. J., Shaw, B. F., & Emery, G. (1979). *Cognitive therapy of depression*. New York: Guilford Press.

Benjamin, L. S. (1996). *Interpersonal diagnosis and treatment of personality disorders* (2nd ed.). New York: Guilford Press.

Blum, N., Pfohl, B., St. John, D., Monahan, P., & Black, D. W. (2002). STEPPS: A cognitive-behavioral systems-based group treatment for outpatients with borderline personality disorder—a preliminary report. *Comprehensive Psychiatry*, *43*, 301–310.

Bohus, M., Limberger, M. F., Frank, U., Sender, I., Gratwohl, T., & Stieglitz, R. D. (2001). [Development of the borderline symptom list]. *Psychotherapies, Psychosomatik, Medizinische Psychologie*, *51*, 201–211.

Bradley, R., Zittel, C. C., & Westen, D. (2005). The borderline personality diagnosis in adolescents: Gender differences and subtypes. *Journal of Child Psychology and Psychiatry*, *46*, 1006–1019.

Brent, D. A., Johnson, B. A., Perper, J., Connolly, J., Bridge, J., Bartle, S., et al. (1994). Personality disorder, personality traits, impulsive violence, and completed suicide in adolescents. *Journal of the American Academy of Child and Adolescent Psychiatry*, *33*, 1080–1086.

Brown, G. K., Newman, C. F., Charlesworth, S. E., Crits-Christoph, P., & Beck, A. T. (2004). An open clinical trial of cognitive therapy for borderline personality disorder. *Journal of Personality Disorders*, 18, 257–271.

Bryer, J. B., Nelson, B. A., Miller, J. B., & Krol, P. A. (1987). Childhood sexual and physical abuse as factors in adult psychiatric illness. *American Journal of Psychiatry*, 144, 1426–1430.

Buie, D. H., & Adler, G. (1982). Definitive treatment of the borderline personality. *International Journal of Psychoanalytic Psychotherapy*, 9, 51–87.

Clarkin, J. F., Foelsch, P. A., Levy, K. N., Hull, J. W., Delaney, J. C., & Kernberg, O. F. (2001). The development of a psychodynamic treatment for patients with borderline personality disorder: A preliminary study of behavioral change. *Journal of Personality Disorders*, 15, 487–495.

Davison, G. C., & Neale, J. M. (1994). *Abnormal psychology* (6th ed.). New York: Wiley.

Dimeff, L. A., McDavid, J., & Linehan, M. M. (1999). Pharmacotherapy for borderline personality disorder: A review of the literature and recommendations for treatment. *Journal of Clinical Psychology in Medical Settings*, 6, 113–138.

Ellis, A. (1962). *Reason and emotion in psychotherapy*. New York: Lyle Stuart.

Ellis, A. (1973). *Humanistic psychotherapy: The rational–emotive approach*. New York: Julian Press.

Foa, E. B., & Kozak, M. J. (1986). Emotional processing of fear: Exposure to corrective information. *Psychological Bulletin*, 99, 20–35.

Foa, E. B., Steketee, G., & Grayson, J. B. (1985). Imaginal and *in vivo* exposure: A comparison with obsessive–compulsive checkers. *Behavior Therapy*, 16, 292–302.

Fossati, A., Madeddu, F., & Maffei, C. (1999). Borderline personality disorder and childhood sexual abuse: A meta-analytic study. *Journal of Personality Disorders*, 13, 268–280.

Giesen-Bloo, J., Van Dyck, R., Spinhoven, P., van Tilburg, W., Dirksen, C., van Asselt, T., et al. (2006). Outpatient psychotherapy for borderline personality disorder: Randomized trial of schema-focused therapy vs transference-focused psychotherapy. *Archives of General Psychiatry*, 63, 649–658.

Goldberg, C. (1980). The utilization and limitations of paradoxical intervention in group psychotherapy. *International Journal of Group Psychotherapy*, 30, 287–297.

Gottman, J. M., & Katz, L. F. (1990). Effects of marital discord on young children's peer interaction and health. *Developmental Psychology*, 25, 373–381.

Gunderson, J. G. (1984). *Borderline personality disorder*. Washington, DC: American Psychiatric Press.

Herman, J. L. (1986). Histories of violence in an outpatient population: An exploratory study. *American Journal of Orthopsychiatry*, 56, 137–141.

Herman, J. L., Perry, J. C., & van der Kolk, B. A. (1989).

Childhood trauma in borderline personality disorder. *American Journal of Psychiatry*, 146, 490–495.

Hollandsworth, J. G. (1990). *The physiology of psychological disorders*. New York: Plenum Press.

Isometsa, E., Heikkinen, M., Henriksson, M., Marttunen, M., Aro, H., & Lonnqvist, J. (1997). Differences between urban and rural suicides. *Acta Psychiatrica Scandinavica*, 95, 297–305.

Isometsa, E. T., Henriksson, M. M., Aro, H. M., Heikkinen, M. E., Kuoppasalmi, K. I., & Lonnqvist, J. K. (1994). Suicide in major depression. *American Journal of Psychiatry*, 151, 530–536.

Kegan, R. (1982). *The evolving self: Problem and process in human development*. Cambridge, MA: Harvard University Press.

Kellogg, S. H., & Young, J. E. (2006). Schema therapy for borderline personality disorder. *Journal of Clinical Psychology*, 62, 445–458.

Kernberg, O. F. (1975). *Borderline conditions and pathological narcissism*. New York: Aronson.

Kernberg, O. F. (1984). *Severe personality disorders: Psychotherapeutic strategies*. New Haven, CT: Yale University Press.

Kernberg, O. F., Selzer, M. A., Koenigsberg, H. W., Carr, A. C., & Appelbaum, A. H. (1989). *Psychodynamic psychotherapy of borderline patients*. New York: Basic Books.

Koerner, K., & Linehan, M. M. (1992). Integrative therapy for borderline personality disorder: Dialectical behavior therapy. In J. C. Norcross & M. R. Goldfried (Eds.), *Handbook of psychotherapy integration* (pp. 433–459). New York: Basic Books.

Kohlenberg, R. J., & Tsai, M. (1991). *Functioned analytic psychotherapy: Creating intense and curative therapeutic relationships*. New York: Plenum Press.

Koons, C. R., Robins, C. J., Tweed, J. L., Lynch, T. R., Gonzalez, A. M., Morse, J. Q., et al. (2001). Efficacy of dialectical behavior therapy in women veterans with borderline personality disorder. *Behavior Therapy*, 32, 371–390.

Kyokai, B. D. (1966). *The teachings of Buddha*. Japan: Bukkyo Dendo Kyokai.

Lequesne, E. R., & Hersh, R. G. (2004). Disclosure of a diagnosis of borderline personality disorder. *Journal of Psychiatric Practice*, 10, 170–176.

Lesage, A. D., Boyer, R., Grunberg, F., Vanier, C., Morissette, R., Menard-Buteau, C., et al. (1994). Suicide and mental disorders: A case–control study of young men. *American Journal of Psychiatry*, 151, 1063–1068.

Lieb, K., Zanarini, M., Linehan, M. M., & Bohus, M. (2004). Seminar section: Borderline personality disorder. *Lancet*, 364, 453–461.

Linehan, M. M. (1987a). Dialectical behavior therapy for borderline personality disorder: Theory and method. *Bulletin of the Menninger Clinic*, 51, 261–276.

Linehan, M. M. (1987b). Dialectical behavioral therapy: A cognitive behavioral approach to parasuicide. *Journal of Personality Disorders*, 1, 328–333.

Linehan, M. M. (1989). Cognitive and behavior therapy

for borderline personality disorder. In A. Tasman, R. E. Hales, & A. J. Frances (Eds.), *Review of psychiatry, Volume 8* (pp. 84–102). Washington DC: American Psychiatric Press.

Linehan, M. M. (1993a). *Cognitive-behavioral treatment of borderline personality disorder.* New York: Guilford Press.

Linehan, M. M. (1993b). *Skills training manual for treating borderline personality disorder.* New York: Guilford Press.

Linehan, M. M. (1997). Validation and psychotherapy. In A. Bohank & L. Greenberg (Eds.), *Empathy reconsidered: New directions in psychotherapy* (pp. 353–392). Washington, DC: American Psychological Association.

Linehan, M. M., Armstrong, H. E., Suarez, A., Allmon, D., & Heard, H. L. (1991). Cognitive-behavioral treatment of chronically parasuicidal borderline patients. *Archives of General Psychiatry, 48,* 1060–1064.

Linehan, M. M., Comtois, K. A., Murray, A., Brown, M. Z., Gallop, R. J., Heard, H. L., et al. (2006). Two-year randomized trial + follow-up of dialectical behavior therapy vs. therapy by experts for suicidal behaviors and borderline personality disorder. *Archives of General Psychiatry, 63,* 757–766.

Linehan, M. M., Dimeff, L. A., Reynolds, S. K., Comtois, K., Shaw-Welch, S., Heagerty, P., et al. (2002). Dialectical behavior therapy versus comprehensive validation plus 12-step for the treatment of opioid dependent women meeting criteria for borderline personality disorder. *Drug and Alcohol Dependence, 67,* 13–26.

Linehan, M. M., & Heard, H. L. (1993). Impact of treatment accessibility on clinical course of parasuicidal patients: In reply to R. E. Hoffman [Letter to the editor]. *Archives of General Psychiatry, 50,* 157–158.

Linehan, M. M., Heard, H. L., & Armstrong, H. E. (1993). Naturalistic follow-up of a behavioral treatment for chronically parasuicidal borderline patients. *Archives of General Psychiatry, 50,* 971–974.

Linehan, M. M., & Koerner, K. (1992). A behavioral theory of borderline personality disorder. In J. Paris (Ed.), *Borderline personality disorder: Etiology and treatment* (pp. 103–121). Washington, DC: American Psychiatric Association.

Linehan, M. M., Rizvi, S. L., Shaw-Welch, S., & Page, B. (2000). Psychiatric aspects of suicidal behaviour: Personality disorders. In K. Hawton & K. van Heeringen (Eds.), *International handbook of suicide and attempted suicide* (pp. 147–178). Sussex, UK: Wiley.

Linehan, M. M., Schmidt, H., III, Dimeff, L. A., Craft, J. C., Kanter, J., & Comtois, K. A. (1999). Dialectical behavior therapy for patients with borderline personality disorder and drug-dependence. *American Journal of Addiction, 8,* 279–292.

Linehan, M. M., Tutek, D. A., Heard, H. L., & Armstrong, H. E. (1994). Interpersonal outcome of cognitive behavioral treatment for chronically suicidal borderline patients. *American Journal of Psychiatry, 151,* 1771–1776.

Loranger, A. W. (1995). *International Personality Disorder Examination (IPDE) manual.* White Plains, NY: Cornell Medical Center.

Lynch, T. R., Morse, J. Q., Mendelson, T., & Robins, C. J. (2003). Dialectical behavior therapy for depressed older adults: A randomized pilot study. *American Journal of Geriatric Psychiatry, 11,* 33–45.

Marlatt, G. A., & Gordon, J. R. (1985). *Relapse prevention: Maintenance strategies in the treatment of addictive behaviors.* New York: Guilford Press.

Marziali, E., & Munroe-Blum, H. (1994). *Interpersonal group psychotherapy for borderline personality disorder.* New York: Basic Books.

Merriam-Webster's New Universal Unabridged Dictionary. (1983). Cleveland, OH: Dorset & Baber.

Merriam-Webster, Inc. (2006). Merriam-Webster Online Dictionary. Available online at *www.m-w.com*

Millon, T. (1987). On the genisis and prevalence of the borderline personality disorder: A social learning thesis. *Journal of Personality Disorders, 1,* 354–372.

Mintz, R. S. (1968). Psychotherapy of the suicidal patient. In H. L. P. Resnick (Ed.), *Suicidal behaviors: Diagnoses and management* (pp. 271–296). Boston: Little, Brown.

Nose, M., Cipriani, A., Biancosino, B., Grassi, L., & Barbui, C. (2006). Efficacy of pharmacotherapy against core traits of borderline personality disorder: Meta-analysis of randomized controlled trials. *International Clinical Psychopharmacology, 21,* 345–353.

Paris, J. (2005). Borderline personality disorder. *Canadian Medical Association Journal, 172,* 1579–1583.

Peng, K., & Nisbett, R. E. (1999). Culture, dialectics, and reasoning about contradiction. *American Psychologist, 54,* 741–754.

Pretzer, J. (1990). Borderline personality disorder. In A. Freeman, L. Pretzer, B. Fleming, & K. M. Simon (Eds.), *Clinical applications of cognitive therapy* (pp. 181–202). New York: Plenum Press.

Reiser, D. E., & Levenson, H. (1984). Abuses of the borderline diagnosis: A clinical problem with teaching opportunities. *American Journal of Psychiatry, 141,* 1528–1532.

Rich, C. L., & Runeson, B. S. (1992). Similarities in diagnostic comorbidity between suicide among young people in Sweden and the United States. *Acta Psychiatrica Scandinavica, 86,* 335–339.

Shearin, E. N., & Linehan, M. M. (1992). Patient–therapist ratings and relationship to progress in dialectical behavior therapy for borderline personality disorder. *Behavior Therapy, 23,* 730–741.

Siever, L. J., & Davis, K. L. (1991). A psychobiological perspective on the personality disorders. *American Journal of Psychiatry, 148,* 1647–1658.

Silk, K. R., Lee, S., Hill, E. M., & Lohr, N. E. (1995). Borderline personality disorder symptoms and severity of sexual abuse. *American Journal of Psychiatry, 152,* 1059–1064.

Simpson, J. A., & Weiner, E. S. (1989). *Oxford English*

Dictionary (2nd ed.) [Online]. Retrieved December 17, 2000, from *www.oed.com*

Soloff, P. H., Lis, J. A., Kelly, T., Cornelius, J., & Ulrich, R. (1994). Risk factors for suicidal behavior in borderline personality disorder. *American Journal of Psychiatry, 151*, 1316–1323.

Stein, D. J., Simeon, D., Frenkel, M., Islam, M. N., & Hollander, E. (1995). An open trial of valproate in borderline personality disorder. *Journal of Clinical Psychiatry, 56*, 506–510.

Telch, C. F., Agras, W. S., & Linehan, M. M. (2001). Dialectical behavior therapy for binge eating disorder: A promising new treatment. *Journal of Consulting and Clinical Psychology, 69*, 1061–1065.

Van Wel, B., Kockmann, I., Blum, N., Pfohl, B., Black, D. W., & Heesterman, W. (2006). STEPPS group treatment for borderline personality disorder in The Netherlands. *Annals of Clinical Psychiatry, 18*, 63–67.

Verheul, R., van den Bosch, L. M. C., Koeter, M. W. J., de Ridder, M. A. J., Stijnen, T., & van den Brink, W. (2003). Dialectical behaviour therapy for women with borderline personality disorder: 12-month, randomised clinical trial in The Netherlands. *British Journal of Psychiatry, 182*, 135–140.

Wagner, A. W., Linehan, M. M., & Wasson, E. J. (1989). *Parasuicide: Characteristics and relationships to childhood sexual abuse.* Unpublished work, University of Washington, Seattle.

Weinberg, I., Gunderson, J. G., Hennen, J., & Cutter, C. J., Jr. (2006). Manual assisted cognitive treatment for deliberate self-harm in borderline personality disorder patients. *Journal of Personality Disorders, 20*, 482–492.

Wells, H. K. (1972). Alienation and dialectical logic. *Kansas Journal of Sociology, 3*, 7–32.

Whitaker, C. A. (1975). Psychotherapy of the absurd: With a special emphasis on the psychotherapy of aggression. *Family Process, 14*, 1–16.

Young, J. E. (2000). *Schema therapy for borderline personality disorder: Detailed treatment model.* New York: Cognitive Therapy Center of New York.

Young, J. E., Klosko, J. S., & Weishaar, M. E. (2003). *Schema therapy: A practitioner's guide.* New York: Guilford Press.

Zanarini, M. C., Frankenburg, F. R., & Parachini, E. A. (2004). A preliminary, randomized trial of fluoxetine, olanzapine, and the olanzapine–fluoxetine combination in women with borderline personality disorder. *Journal of Clinical Psychiatry, 65*, 903–907.

Zanarini, M. C., Frankenburg, F. R., Sickel, A. E., & Yong, L. (1996). *The Diagnostic Interview for DSM-IV Personality Disorders.* Belmont, MA: McLean Hospital, Laboratory for the Study of Adult Development.

Zanarini, M. C., Gunderson, J. G., Frankenburg, F. R., & Chauncey, D. L. (1989). The Revised Diagnostic Interview for Borderlines: Discriminating borderline personality disorder from other Axis II disorders. *Journal of Personality Disorders, 3*, 10–18.

Zanarini, M. C., Vujanovic, A. A., Parachini, E. A., Boulanger, J. L., Frankenburg, F. R., & Hennen, J. (2003). A screening measure for BPD: The McLean Screening Instrument for Borderline Personality Disorder (MSI-BPD). *Journal of Personality Disorders, 17*, 568–573.

CHAPTER 10

Bipolar Disorder

DAVID J. MIKLOWITZ

Our goal in this book is to present creative and important psychological treatments with empirical support. This chapter on bipolar disorder by David J. Miklowitz was new to the previous edition but existing evidence for the efficacy of this approach continues to grow. Based on years of systematic research on psychological factors contributing to the onset and maintenance of bipolar disorder, this sophisticated family therapy approach targets the most important psychosocial factors linked to the disorder and associated with poor outcome (e.g., disruptions in circadian rhythms and certain specific styles of interpersonal interactions). This chapter, and especially the very useful case study, also illustrate an essential linkage between psychological and pharmacological approaches to this very severe form of psychopathology.—D. H. B.

Bipolar disorder is one of the oldest and most reliably recognized psychiatric disorders. Our thinking about this disorder has evolved over this century, but the original descriptions (Kraepelin, 1921) of "manic–depressive insanity" greatly resemble our current conceptualizations. This chapter begins with a review of basic information about the disorder, its diagnosis, its longitudinal course, and drug treatment. This information about the illness is interesting in its own right, but it also provides the rationale for using psychosocial treatment as an adjunct to pharmacotherapy. The majority of the chapter describes a focused, time-limited, outpatient psychosocial treatment—family-focused treatment (FFT)—

that comprises three interrelated modules: psychoed- ucation, communication enhancement training (CET), and problem-solving skills training (Miklowitz & Goldstein, 1997). It is designed for patients who have had a recent episode of mania or depression.

THE DIAGNOSIS OF BIPOLAR DISORDER

DSM-IV Criteria

The core characteristic of bipolar disorder is extreme affective dysregulation, or mood states that swing from extremely low (depression) to extremely high (mania). Patients in a manic episode have euphoric, elevated mood or irritable mood; behavioral activation (e.g., increased goal-directed activity, excessive involvement in high-risk activities, decreased need for sleep, increased talkativeness or pressure of speech); and altered cognitive functioning (grandiose delusions or inflated self-worth, flight of ideas or racing thoughts, distractibility)—typically for more than 1 week. For the diagnosis of a manic episode, there must be evidence that the person's psychosocial functioning (marital, occupational, or social) is disrupted; that hospitalization is required; or that psychotic features (e.g., grandiose delusions) are present (see the fourth edition of the *Diagnostic and Statistical Manual of Mental Disorders* [DSM-IV; American Psychiatric Association, 1994a]).

A patient in a hypomanic episode shows many of the same symptoms, but the duration is typically shorter (i.e., 4 days or more). Hypomanic symptoms also do not bring about severe impairment in social or occupational functioning and are not associated with the need for hospitalization or with psychosis. However, the symptoms must reflect a real change in a person's ordinary behavior—one that is observable by others. The distinction between mania and hypomania, which is really one of degree rather than type of illness, is difficult for clinicians to make reliably. Often the degree to which the behavioral activation affects a patient's functioning is underestimated by the patient, who can see nothing but good in his or her behavior. A theme of this chapter is the value of including significant others (i.e., parents, spouses/partners, and siblings) in patients' assessment and treatment.

Some patients with bipolar disorder (40% or more; Calabrese, Fatemi, Kujawa, & Woyshville, 1996) experience mixed episodes, in which the criteria for a major depressive episode and a manic episode are met nearly every day for a minimum duration of 1 week. The symptoms of both poles of the illness are experienced simultaneously. The boundaries between "pure" mania and mixed mania are not entirely clear, because depression often lurks beneath the manic exterior and is easily evoked by situational factors (Young & Harrow, 1994). Children and adolescents with the disorder are particularly prone to mixed states (Geller et al., 2002).

DSM-IV proceeds with the diagnosis of bipolar disorder somewhat differently than past DSM systems have done. First, the diagnostician determines whether the patient satisfies the cross-sectional criteria for a manic or mixed episode. If he or she does meet these criteria, the diagnosis of bipolar I disorder is applied. If the patient currently meets DSM-IV criteria for a major depressive episode, he or she is diagnosed as having bipolar disorder only if there is a past history of manic, mixed, or hypomanic episodes; otherwise, the diagnosis is likely to be major depressive disorder (single episode or recurrent) or another mood disorder. If the patient presents in remission, there must be evidence of prior manic or mixed episodes. One implication of this rather complicated set of diagnostic rules is that a single manic or mixed episode, even in the absence of documentable depression, is enough to warrant the bipolar I diagnosis. The key word here is "documentable," because patients often underreport their depression histories and reveal them only upon careful questioning.

How Has the Diagnosis of Bipolar Disorder Changed?

Every version of the DSM has brought changes in the way we think about bipolar disorder, and modifications are likely to continue as new editions are published. For example, DSM-V will probably contain separate criteria for diagnosing the disorder in children and adolescents. Currently, DSM-IV uses the same criteria to diagnose mania in adults and children, despite the clear developmental differences in presentation (Leibenluft, Charney, Towbin, Bhangoo, & Pine, 2003).

DSM-IV distinguishes between bipolar I and bipolar II disorders. In the former, patients have fully syndromal manic or mixed episodes. In bipolar II illness, patients only have hypomanic episodes. Unlike bipolar I disorder, a major depressive episode must have occurred for a diagnosis of bipolar II disorder. (In this chapter, the term "bipolar disorder" refers either to bipolar I or bipolar II disorder as defined in DSM-IV, unless otherwise specified). DSM-IV also includes a course descriptor, "rapid cycling," which appears to characterize between 13 and 20% of patients (Calabrese et al., 1996), and more often females (Coryell, Endicott, & Keller, 1992; Schneck et al., 2004). This much misunderstood course subtype is often confused with mixed episodes. A mixed episode refers to the presentation of mania and major depression within a single episode, whereas in rapid cycling a patient has had four or more discrete major depressive, manic, mixed, or hypomanic episodes in a single year. The confusion in applying this course descriptor lies in the fact that it is difficult to tell when one episode has ended and another begins: If a patient quickly switches from mania to depression in a 48-hour period (what some refer to as "ultrarapid cycling"), is this truly a new episode or just a different presentation of the same episode? Rapid cycling appears to be a transient state of the disorder and not a lifelong phenomenon (Coryell et al., 1992).

Finally, DSM-IV deals with the thorny problem of patients with depression who develop manic, mixed, or hypomanic episodes that are brought on by antidepressants or other activating drugs. Because of the effects of antidepressants on the serotonin, norepinephrine, and dopamine systems, there is the potential for these drugs to induce activation, particularly in a patient who is already biologically vulnerable to mood swings. If a patient has never had a manic episode but then develops one after taking an antidepressant, the likely diagnosis is substance-induced mood disorder. The diagnosis of bipolar disorder is only then considered if the symptoms of mania preceded the antidepressant (a difficult historical distinction), or if the mania symptoms continue for at least a month after the antidepressant is withdrawn. Similar diagnostic considerations apply to patients who abuse drugs (e.g., cocaine, amphetamine) that are "psychotomimetics" and can induce manic-like states.

Comorbidity and Differential Diagnosis

Bipolar disorder, in its various forms, affects 3.9% of the population (Kessler, Berglund, Demler, Jin, & Walters, 2005). It is often comorbid with other conditions. When 1-year prevalence rates were considered within a community epidemiological sample, the highest correlations were observed between mania/hypomania and attention-deficit/hyperactivity disorder, followed by oppositional defiant disorder, agoraphobia, panic disorder, generalized anxiety disorder, alcohol dependence, and drug abuse (Kessler, Chiu, Demler, & Walters, 2005). The disorders with which bipolar disorder is comorbid have the common underpinning of affective dysregulation. In the Epidemiologic Catchment Area study (Regier et al., 1990), 46% of patients with bipolar disorder, as defined by DSM-III (American Psychiatric Association, 1980), also met DSM-III criteria for lifetime alcohol abuse (15%) or dependence (31%); 41% met the criteria for other substance abuse (13%) or dependence (28%). A total of 61% met criteria for any substance abuse or dependence.

The distinction between bipolar disorder and Axis II disorders is especially difficult. Notably, the hallmark of borderline personality disorder is affective instability. Akiskal (1996) has argued that what is commonly seen by clinicians as Axis II pathology is actually undertreated subsyndromal mood disorder. When studies of the overlap of bipolar disorder and Axis II disorders are done carefully, the estimates of Axis II comorbidity are actually quite conservative. For example, studies by Carpenter, Clarkin, Glick, and Wilner (1995) and George, Miklowitz, Richards, Simoneau, and Taylor (2003) estimate that only about 22–28% of patients with bipolar disorder meet the diagnostic criteria for Axis II disorders when patients are evaluated during a period of remission. Furthermore, the comorbid Axis II diagnosis is not always borderline personality disorder; it is often a disorder from cluster C (e.g., avoidant or dependent personality disorder).

The boundaries between bipolar and unipolar illness are sometimes difficult to draw. Depressions in bipolar and unipolar disorders may look quite similar. There is some evidence that bipolar depressions are more likely to be characterized by greater psychomotor retardation but less agitation, anxiety, and somatization than unipolar depressions (Beigel & Murphy, 1971; Goodwin & Jamison, 1990; Katz, Robins, Croughan, Secunda, & Swann, 1982). Other evidence indicates that bipolar depressions are shorter than unipolar depressions and are more often characterized by mood lability, diurnal variation, feeling worse in the morning, and derealization (Goldberg & Kocsis, 1999; Mitchell et al., 1992). Even more complicated is the distinction between agitated depression of the unipolar type and mixed mania of the bipolar type; both are characterized by sadness and a highly anxious, restless, activated state. Goldberg and Kocsis (1999) recommend that clinicians attempting to make these distinctions place emphasis on attributes such as goal-drivenness and undiminished energy (despite lack of sleep), both of which tip the scales toward bipolar disorder rather than unipolar depressive illness.

The distinction between bipolar disorder and schizophrenia is also a difficult judgment call. When a patient who has schizophrenia presents with a psychotic episode, he or she can appear acutely activated, grandiose in thinking and actions, and elated or depressed. In a highly influential paper published prior to the appearance of DSM-III, Pope and Lipinski (1978) argued strongly that patients with traditionally schizophrenic "Schneiderian first-rank symptoms" (e.g., thought broadcasting, delusions of control) often have bipolar or even unipolar depressions.

In part to deal with these diagnostic ambiguities, DSM-IV makes a distinction between schizoaffective disorder and major mood disorders with psychotic features. In schizoaffective disorder, delusions and hallucinations have been present for at least 2 weeks, even when there have been no prominent affective symptoms. In major mood disorders, psychotic symptoms occur only during periods of significant mood disturbance. Importantly, psychotic symptoms, particularly "mood-incongruent" features (delusions or hallucinations that have no clear content related to sadness or elation, such as the belief that thoughts are being inserted into one's head), are a poor prognostic sign in bipolar and unipolar disorders (Brockington, Hillier, Francis, Helzer, & Wainwright, 1983; Coryell, Keller, Lavori, & Endicott, 1990; Grossman, Harrow, Fudula, & Meltzer, 1984; Grossman, Harrow, Goldberg, & Fichtner, 1991; Kendler, 1991; Miklowitz, 1992; Tohen, Waternaux, & Tsuang, 1990).

DSM-IV also describes a subsyndromal or subaffective condition: cyclothymic disorder. Patients with cyclothymic disorder alternate between periods of hypomanic symptoms and brief periods of depression that fall short of the criteria for major depressive illness. As soon as the person develops a full manic, mixed, or depressive episode, the diagnosis of bipolar I or II disorder is substituted. Again, these distinctions really concern the degree and duration of symptoms rather than their form. In my own experience, clinicians are prone to "push" patients with cyclothymia into the bipolar II category, especially if they feel that the patients are not reliable in their historical reporting. Sometimes it is better to observe the mood lability of a patient over time than to attempt to distinguish cyclothymic disorder and bipolar disorder cross-sectionally.

The accuracy of patients' reporting is increased by self-report records kept over periods of a year or more. Examples are "life charts" that show, prospectively, the duration, severity, polarity, and functional impairment associated with mood disorder fluctuations (Leverich & Post, 1998).

DRUG TREATMENT AND THE COURSE OF BIPOLAR DISORDER

Standard Pharmacotherapy

The course of bipolar illness (its pattern of relapsing and remitting over time) is best considered with reference to the drug treatments that help stabilize patients and allow most to function in the community. In the prepharmacological era (i.e., prior to 1960), patients were hospitalized for years at a time (Cutler & Post, 1982). Nowadays, the availability of mood stabilizers such as lithium carbonate, the anticonvulsants (e.g., divalproex sodium [Depakote], lamotrigine [Lamictal], and other agents), and the atypical antipsychotics (e.g., olanzapine [Zyprexa], quetiapine [Seroquel], and risperidone [Risperdal], Ziprasidone [Geodon] or aripiprazole [Abilify]) has done much to ameliorate the course of bipolar illness (Goldberg, 2004). Some of these drugs not only control the acute episodes of the illness but also have "prophylactic value," meaning that they help prevent future episodes or minimize the duration or severity of episodes that do occur.

Most psychiatrists describe three phases of drug treatment: an acute phase, in which the goal is to control the most severe symptoms of the manic, mixed, or depressive disorder; a stabilization phase, in which the goal is to help the patient recover fully from the acute phase, which often means treating residual symptoms (e.g., mild depression) or levels of social–occupational impairment; and a maintenance phase, in which the goal is to prevent recurrences and continue to treat residual symptoms. The drugs recommended for bipolar disorder vary according to the phase of treatment. During the acute and stabilization phases, an antipsychotic medication may accompany a mood stabilizer. An antidepressant may be recommended after a manic episode has stabilized if a patient has ongoing, residual depression symptoms. These phases of treatment are also relevant to the psychosocial–psychotherapeutic treatment of bipolar disorder, as discussed later.

Symptomatic Outcome

If drug treatment is so effective, then why do we need psychosocial treatment? The problem that consistently arises in the drug treatment of bipolar disorder is "breakthrough episodes." With lithium or anticonvulsant treatment, rates of relapse over 1 year vary between 37 (Gitlin, Swendsen, Heller, & Hammen, 1995) and 67% (Shapiro, Quitkin, & Fleiss, 1989). Gelenberg and colleagues (1989) found that the 2-year "survival rate" (i.e., the proportion of patients not relapsing) for bipolar disorder was 40% on typical lithium regimens. Gitlin and colleagues (1995) found that the 5-year survival rate was only 27%.

In a representative longitudinal study, Keck and colleagues (1998) examined the 12-month course of bipolar disorder among 134 patients who began in an acute manic or mixed episode. The majority of the patients (N = 104) were treated with mood stabilizers, with or without accompanying antipsychotics or antidepressants. The investigators made a distinction among "syndromic recovery," in which patients no longer met the DSM-III-R (American Psychiatric Association, 1987) criteria for a manic, mixed, or depressive episode for at least 8 weeks; "symptomatic recovery," a tougher criterion by which patients had to have minimal or no mood disorder symptoms for 8 weeks; and "functional recovery," which required that patients regain their premorbid (preillness) level of employment, friendships, interests, and independent living status. Of the 106 patients who completed the study, 51 (48%) achieved syndromic recovery by 12-month follow-up. Only 28 (26%) achieved symptomatic recovery, and 25 (24%) reached functional recovery at follow-up. Predictors of poor outcome included low socioeconomic status, medication noncompliance, and longer duration of illness.

Even more problematic are the residual symptoms between episodes. In a 13-year study, subsyndromal symptoms, particularly depression, were present during approximately half of the weeks of follow-up (Judd et al., 2002). Patients generally take longer to recover from depressive episodes than from manic episodes (Kupfer et al., 2000).

Social–Occupational Functioning

The problems patients with bipolar disorder experience in social–occupational recovery are substantial, even when they are given mood-stabilizing medications. Dion, Tohen, Anthony, and Waternaux (1989) found that about one in every three patients with mania could not work in the 6 months following a manic episode, and only about one in five worked at their expected level. Coryell and colleagues (1993) found that social–occupational dysfunction—including high rates of marital separations and divorces—could be observed up to 5 years after a mood episode. Goldberg, Harrow, and Grossman (1995), in a 4½-year follow-up of patients with major mood disorders, found that patients with bipolar illness had lower work functioning scores than patients with unipolar illness. Furthermore, only 41% were rated as having a "good overall outcome" at follow-up. Patients in this study were usually taking lithium alone or lithium with antipsychotic medications.

A study of 253 bipolar I and II patients revealed that only about 33% of the patients worked full time and only 9% worked part time outside of the home (Suppes et al., 2001); 57% of patients reported being unable to work or able to work only in protected settings.

What predicts social–occupational functioning? In our 9-month follow-up of lithium- or anticonvulsant-treated young adults with bipolar disorder, family conflict, as measured by negative parent-to-patient verbal interactions during a family problem-solving task, predicted levels of social functioning at follow-up (Miklowitz, Goldstein, Nuechterlein, Snyder, & Mintz, 1988). Patient gender also appears to be important: Harrow, Goldberg, Grossman, and Meltzer (1990) found that women with mania had better work functioning at follow-up than did men with mania.

Not surprisingly, patients with higher socioeconomic status have more favorable functional outcomes than patients with lower socioeconomic status (Harrow et al., 1990; Keck et al., 1998). It appears that social functioning and symptomatic outcome are two correlated but separate domains of outcome in bipolar disorder, or "open-linked systems" (Strauss & Carpenter, 1972). Whereas many assume that severe symptoms predispose patients to worse functional outcomes, at least one study (Gitlin et al., 1995) found the reverse: Poor social functioning, especially job functioning, predicted a shorter time to relapse in a 4⅓-year follow-up.

Medication Nonadherence

Part of the reason why patients with bipolar disorder have breakthrough episodes is drug nonadherence. In the Keck and colleagues (1998) study, only 47% of the patients were fully adherent with their medications at follow-up. Miklowitz and colleagues (1988) found that only about 30% of young patients with recent-onset mania took their medications on a routinely scheduled basis during a 9-month follow-up. Whereas rates vary with the methods and criteria for measuring adherence, it is clearly a significant risk factor in this disorder. Jamison and colleagues (Jamison & Akiskal, 1983; Jamison, Gerner, & Goodwin, 1979) identified the following factors as predictors of nonadherence: negative feelings about having one's moods controlled by a medication; missing high or euphoric periods; and side effects, which for lithium can include weight gain, thirst, and tremor of the hands.

Why Psychotherapy?

What is the role of psychosocial treatment in a disorder with such a heavy biological and genetic basis? There is little doubt that medication is the first-line treatment for bipolar disorder. The evidence that lithium and the anticonvulsants reduce relapse rates and improve functioning is substantial. But can we do better? An optimal and perhaps overly optimistic view of the outcome of patients with bipolar disorder would include symptom stability for extended periods, minimal disruptions in social role functioning after episodes, and becoming consistent contributors to society. One role of psychotherapy as an adjunct to medication is to teach skills for symptom management, to augment social and occupational role functioning, and to keep patients adherent to their drug regimens. Implicit in this objective is that the physiology and psychology of major psychiatric disorders are not fully separable. We know that changes in brain function (as revealed in positron emission tomography scans) in obsessive–compulsive disorder can be detected before and after treatment among responders to behavior therapy and responders to fluoxetine (Prozac) (Baxter et al., 1992). The

time has come to think about psychotherapy and medication as working synergistically in the major mood disorders.

The strongest argument for including psychotherapy in an outpatient treatment program is to help patients to cope with stress triggers. As noted in the next section, certain forms of life events and family tensions are risk factors in the course of the disorder. Psychotherapy can target these factors and teach patients adaptive coping mechanisms, which can then be brought to bear during periods of wellness to help stave off the likelihood of a future relapse.

A VULNERABILITY–STRESS MODEL OF RECURRENCES

Implicit in the notion that psychotherapy would be helpful to a patient with bipolar disorder is the notion that stress plays a role in eliciting symptoms of mood disorder. What is the evidence for this view? What are the targets for psychosocial intervention? Figure 10.1 summarizes a model that takes into account the background of biochemical (e.g., serotonin, dopamine, norepinephrine, or gamma-aminobutyric acid [GABA]) imbalances, genetic vulnerability, and the two types of stress targeted in FFT: life events and disturbances in family functioning (see Goodwin & Jamison, 1990; Miklowitz & Frank, 1999; Miklowitz & Goldstein, 1997).

Life Events Stress

In this model, life events affect the onset of bipolar mood symptoms through the avenue of disrupting daily routines and sleep–wake cycles ("social rhythms"). The social rhythm stability hypothesis (Ehlers, Kupfer, Frank, & Monk, 1993) states that major life events can disrupt daily rhythms in mood disorders via one of two avenues. They can act as *zeitstorers*, which disrupt established social and circadian rhythms (e.g., the production of neuroendocrines as a function of the time of day). For example, a previously unemployed patient who gets a job with constantly shifting work hours is forced to adopt a new pattern of daily routines, which may include changes in sleep–wake habits. Major events can also result in the loss of *zeitgebers*, which maintain the stability of rhythms. For example, a spouse or partner

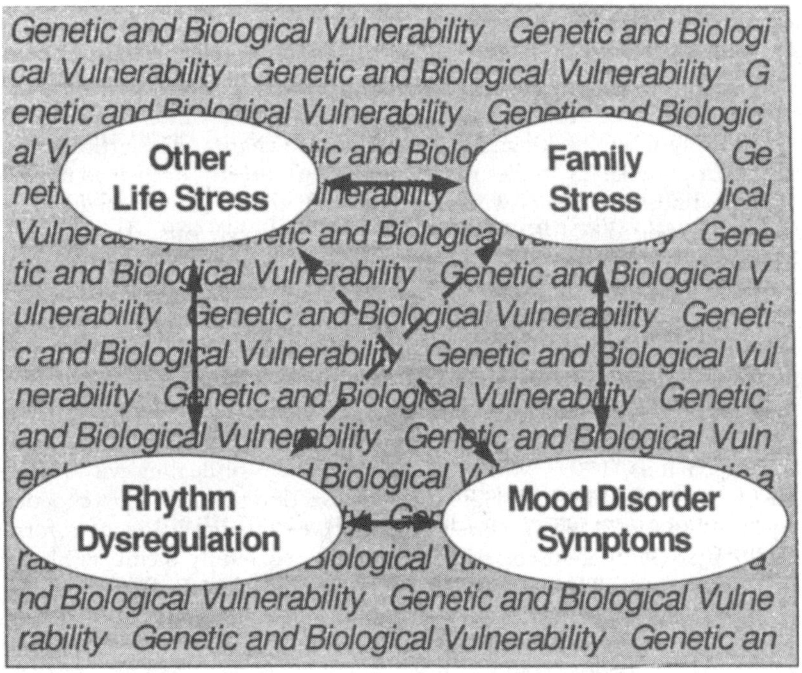

FIGURE 10.1. A vulnerability–stress "instability" model of mood episodes in bipolar disorder. From Miklowitz and Goldstein (1997). Copyright 1997 by The Guilford Press. Reprinted by permission.

helps maintain a person on predictable social and sleep schedules. A relationship separation, in addition to being a significant emotional event, results in the loss of this human time-keeper.

Patients with bipolar disorder are exquisitely sensitive to even minor changes in sleep–wake habits. A study by Malkoff-Schwartz and colleagues (1998) found that manic episodes were often precipitated by life events that changed sleep–wake habits (e.g., changing time zones due to air travel). However, depressive episodes were not differentially associated with rhythm-disruptive life events. Similar findings emerged from a second study (Malkoff-Schwartz et al., 2000).

One of the clinical implications of these findings is that if patients can be taught to regularize their social rhythms, especially in the face of life events that normally disrupt those rhythms, then the outcome of bipolar disorder should be improved. Thus, variability in the sleep–wake cycle is a target for treatment. This is a central tenet of interpersonal and social rhythm therapy, an individual psychotherapy discussed below (Frank, 2005).

Family Stress

Family conflicts may also become a breeding ground for increased cycling of bipolar disorder (see Figure 10.1). One method of measuring family stress is to evaluate a family's level of "expressed emotion" (EE). In this procedure, a researcher administers the Camberwell Family Interview (Vaughn & Leff, 1976) to a family member (parent, spouse/partner, or sibling) for approximately 1 hour to assess the relative's reactions to the patient's psychiatric disorder, with particular emphasis on a recent illness episode. Later, a trained judge evaluates tapes of these interviews on three primary dimensions: "critical comments" (e.g., "When I talk to him, I get upset that he just shuts down. It's like there's no one there!"); "hostility," or personal, generalized criticism of the patient (e.g., "I like nothing about him"); and "emotional over-involvement," or the tendency to be over-concerned, overprotective, or to use inordinately self-sacrificing behaviors in the patient's care (e.g., "I don't invite people to the house because Allen [son] doesn't like it"). Family members who score high on one or more of these dimensions are called "high-EE"; those who do not are called "low-EE."

EE is a well-established predictor of the course of schizophrenia. In Butzlaff and Hooley's (1998) meta-analysis of 28 longitudinal studies of EE in schizophrenia, 23 studies replicated the same core finding: Patients who return after an illness episode to high-EE families are two to three times more likely to relapse in 9-month to 1-year prospective follow-ups than those returning to low-EE families. Several studies have also documented a link between high EE in families and relapse among patients with bipolar disorder followed either prospectively or retrospectively (Honig, Hofman, Rozendaal, & Dingemanns, 1997; Miklowitz et al., 1988; O'Connell, Mayo, Flatow, Cuthbertson, & O'Brien, 1991; Priebe, Wildgrube, & Muller-Oerlinghausen, 1989; Yan, Hammen, Cohen, Daley, & Henry, 2004). A 2-year study of EE and bipolar adolescents undergoing family treatment also replicated this longitudinal association (Miklowitz, Biuckians, & Richards, 2006).

On first examination, one might conclude that patients with bipolar disorder are sensitive to stress in the family milieu, and that levels of EE elicit an underlying biological vulnerability. But the relationship is far from simple. First, it appears that the high-EE relatives of patients with bipolar illness, unipolar illness, or schizophrenia are more likely than low-EE relatives to interpret the patients' negative problem behaviors as controllable by the patients (see, e.g., Brewin, MacCarthy, Duda, & Vaughn, 1991; Hooley, 1987; Hooley & Licht, 1997; Weisman, Lopez, Karno, & Jenkins, 1993; Wendel, Miklowitz, Richards, & George, 2000). Second, relatives and patients coping with bipolar disorder are often locked into verbally aggressive, negative cycles of face-to-face interaction. We (Simoneau, Miklowitz, & Saleem, 1998) found that high-EE relatives of patients with bipolar disorder were more negative than low-EE relatives during face-to-face problem-solving interactions. The relatives and patients in high-EE families were also more likely to engage in counterproductive "attack–counterattack" cycles. Often the patients were provocateurs in these interchanges; they were not the "victims" of verbally aggressive or punitive relatives (Miklowitz, Wendel, & Simoneau, 1998; Simoneau et al., 1998).

Clearly, a psychosocial treatment program should consider aspects of the family's affective environment—such as high-EE attitudes in relatives or the negative interchanges that characterize relative–patient communication—to be targets for intervention. But does one attempt to change these attitudes and interaction patterns directly, or instead make an "end run" around them? Family members coping with a spouse/partner, offspring, or sibling who has bipolar disorder are understandably quite angry, and it makes little sense to tell them they should not be. Others feel that their overprotective behavior is more than warranted by the situation.

In developing FFT, we (Miklowitz & Goldstein, 1997) concluded that at least one component of dealing with these attitudes and transaction patterns is psychoeducation, which involves the provision of information to patients and family members about the disorder and its manifestations. As discussed earlier, relatives (parents, spouses, or siblings) need to realize that at least some proportion of the patient's aversive behaviors (e.g., irritability, aggression, inability to work, or low productivity) can be attributed to a biochemically driven illness state. This may seem obvious to us as clinicians, but to family members who deal with the patient on a day-to-day basis, it is easy to attribute aversive behaviors to personality factors or laziness, or to believe that "He or she is doing this to hurt me." In parallel, patients need to become more cognizant of the way they provoke anger and resentment in family members.

Negative face-to-face interactions cannot be eradicated, but they can be made more productive through the techniques of communication and problem-solving skills training. Thus, families or couples can be taught to stick with one problem topic rather than trying to solve many at a time, or to use listening skills to avoid counterproductive attack–counterattack cycles. Later in this chapter, these methods are explained with reference to a difficult treatment case.

TREATMENT OUTCOME STUDIES

Controlled psychotherapy outcome studies are relatively new to the field of bipolar disorder and certainly have not kept pace with the research on drug treatment. This section describes several randomized controlled trials of individual and family/marital interventions.

More thorough reviews of the studies in this area are available (Miklowitz, 2006; Miklowitz & Otto, 2006).

Individual Therapy

Two controlled trials of individual therapy deserve special emphasis here. Each focused on a specific risk factor in the course of bipolar disorder: medication noncompliance (Cochran, 1984) and disruptions in social rhythms (Frank et al., 1999, 2005). These therapy models are to be distinguished from earlier, psychoanalytically oriented models whose aim was to restructure personality or deal with early childhood conflicts (e.g., Cohen, Baker, Cohen, Fromm-Reichmann, & Weigert, 1954).

In Cochran's (1984) study, 28 lithium-treated outpatients with bipolar disorder were randomly assigned to lithium carbonate with six sessions of individual cognitive therapy or to a lithium-only group. The cognitive therapy was oriented toward restructuring cognitions associated with noncompliance. At a 6-month follow-up, patients who received the cognitive intervention had significantly better medication adherence, fewer hospitalizations, and fewer mood episodes precipitated by drug nonadherence.

Lam, Hayward, Watkins, Wright, and Sham (2005; Lam et al., 2003) examined a 6-month, 12- to 18-session cognitive-behavioral therapy (CBT) model with drug treatment versus drug treatment alone (N = 103). Patients had been in remission for at least 6 months but had had at least three episodes in the past 5 years. At a 1-year follow-up, 44% of patients in CBT had relapsed compared with 75% of the patients who received drug treatment alone. Twelve to 30 months after treatment, CBT did not prevent relapse relative to drug treatment alone, but it did continue to show a positive influence on mood and days spent in episodes.

A recent multicenter effectiveness trial of CBT in the United Kingdom (N = 253) indicated that not all subpopulations of bipolar patients are equally likely to benefit from CBT (Scott et al., 2006). The study compared 22 sessions of CBT plus pharmacotherapy to treatment as usual (TAU) plus pharmacotherapy. The patients had been in a variety of symptomatic states before study entry. No effects were found for CBT on time to recurrence. A post hoc analysis revealed that patients with less than 12 prior episodes had fewer recurrences in CBT than in TAU. However, patients with 12 or more episodes were more likely to have recurrences in CBT than in TAU. Possibly, CBT is most applicable to patients in the early stages of their disorder or in those whose course is less recurrent.

Frank and colleagues (2005) investigated the efficacy of an interpersonal psychotherapy for bipolar disorder—one that included not only the core elements of Klerman, Weissman, Rounsaville, and Chevron's (1984) model of interpersonal psychotherapy for depression but also a component in which patients self-regulated their daily routines and sleep–wake cycles. Patients with a recent mood episode were randomly assigned either to 45-minute interpersonal and social rhythm therapy (IPSRT) sessions and mood-stabilizing medications or to an active clinical management intervention, also with medications. The latter consisted of 20-minute sessions with a psychotherapist who focused on drug side effects and symptom management. Session frequencies were identical across the two groups. Randomization was done first during an acute phase of treatment, with sessions held weekly, and again at the beginning of a preventive, maintenance phase of treatment, with sessions held biweekly or monthly for up to 2 years. IPSRT in the acute phase was associated with more time before recurrences in the maintenance phase than in the clinical management condition. IPSRT was most effective in delaying recurrences in the maintenance phase, when patients succeeded in stabilizing their daily routines and sleep–wake cycles during the acute phase. Thus, consistency of routines may protect against a worsening course of the disorder (Frank et al., 2005).

Family and Marital Therapy

There are now several studies of family interventions as adjuncts to medications for patients with bipolar disorder. The first, by a group at the Cornell University Medical College (Clarkin et al., 1990; Glick, Clarkin, Haas, Spencer, & Chen, 1991) randomly assigned 186 inpatients with psychotic or mood disorders to either a brief family intervention or to standard hospital care. The family intervention averaged nine weekly or twice-weekly sessions, and focused on helping patients and family members to cope with the hospital experience and make plans for a positive posthospital adjustment. At 6- and 18-month follow-ups, female patients who had received the family intervention had less severe symptoms and higher global functioning than those who had originally received standard hospital care. Interestingly, among female patients from both the mood disorder and psychotic disorder groups, family treatment led to improvements at 6 and at 18 months in relatives' emotional attitudes (e.g., less rejecting feelings toward the patients). In the small subsample of patients with bipolar disorder ($N = 21$), the effects of family intervention were only seen among 14 female patients, so the findings cannot be considered conclusive.

Another randomized controlled trial by the Cornell group (Clarkin, Carpenter, Hull, Wilner, & Glick, 1998) compared a psychoeducational marital intervention and pharmacotherapy with pharmacological care alone. The sample size ($N = 33$) was small, but patients who received the marital treatment had better drug adherence and better global functioning scores over 11 months of treatment than those in the comparison group. No effect was observed for marital intervention on the symptomatic outcome of patients.

Three randomized trials have been completed on FFT, one at the University of California, Los Angeles (UCLA—Goldstein, Rea, & Miklowitz, 1996; Rea et al., 2003;) one at the University of Colorado (Miklowitz et al., 2000; Miklowitz, George, Richards, Simoneau, & Suddath, 2003), and one in the context of the Systematic Treatment Enhancement Program for Bipolar Disorder (STEP-BD; Miklowitz et al., 2007). These studies are examined in detail below.

The UCLA and Colorado Studies

The UCLA and Colorado studies each examined a 9-month, 21-session FFT intervention that comprised psychoeducation, communication enhancement training, and problem-solving training. Participants were patients and their parents or spouses. Patients were recruited during an index episode of bipolar disorder and maintained on mood-stabilizing medications, with or without antipsychotic or antidepressive agents. However, the studies differed in an important respect: At Colorado, the comparison "crisis management" group received two sessions of family education and individual crisis sessions, as needed, over 9 months. In the UCLA study, patients in the

comparison group received an individual case management and problem-solving intervention that was of similar intensity (21 sessions) to the FFT intervention.

Despite these design differences, the results that emerged from the Colorado and UCLA studies were quite similar. In the Colorado study (Miklowitz et al., 2000, 2003), FFT and medication led to lower frequencies of relapses and longer delays prior to relapses over a 2-year period than did crisis management and medication. FFT was also associated with more improvement in depression and mania symptoms—effects that did not appear until the 9- and 12-month follow-ups, but continued for the full 24 months of follow-up. In the UCLA study (Goldstein et al., 1996; Rea et al., 2003), the effects of FFT were seen on hospitalization rates over a 2-year follow-up. The effects of FFT on time to relapse were not seen in the first year but did appear in the second year. Notably, rates of rehospitalization in the 1- to 2-year period following the 9-month treatment were 12% in the FFT group and 60% in the individual therapy group; for relapse, the rates were 28% and 60%, respectively. Both studies suggested that there may be a delayed effect of FFT: Patients and family members may need to "absorb" the treatment and incorporate the education and skills training into their day-to-day lives before it has ameliorative effects on the illness.

This latter point was clarified further by Simoneau, Miklowitz, Richards, Saleem, and George (1999), who examined family interaction transcripts obtained in the Colorado study before and after FFT or crisis management treatment. Families (patients with their parents or spouses) participated in interactional assessments that comprised 10-minute problem-solving discussions, which were transcribed and coded via the Category System for Coding Partner Interactions (Hahlweg et al., 1989). Forty-four families returned at 1 year for the same assessment, after the FFT or crisis management protocol had been completed. Interestingly, at the posttreatment (1 year) interactional assessments, patients in FFT and those in crisis management could not be distinguished on the basis of frequency of negative interactional behaviors (e.g., criticisms). But there were clear differences at posttreatment in positive interactional behaviors, particularly in the nonverbal sphere. After FFT, patients and relatives were more likely to smile at each other, nod when others were speaking, and lean toward each other when speaking. Moreover, the degree to which patients improved in their nonverbal interactional behavior over the course of psychosocial treatment was correlated with their degree of symptom improvement over the year of treatment.

FFT appeared to have ameliorated certain tensions within the family environments. Future studies using multiple, time-lagged assessments of family interaction and patients' symptoms would help to disentangle the directional relationship between improvements in family communication and patients' symptomatic outcomes.

The STEP-BD Study

STEP-BD examined the effectiveness of treatment with mood stabilizers in combination with psychosocial treatments in 15 participating sites in the United States (Miklowitz et al., 2007). Bipolar patients in a depressive episode (N = 293) were randomly assigned to mood-stabilizing medications—with or without antidepressants—and 30 sessions of FFT, interpersonal and social rhythm therapy, cognitive-behavioral therapy, or collaborative care (CC), a three-session psychoeducational treatment. Patients assigned to any intensive psychotherapy had higher recovery rates over 1 year and recovered an average of 110 days faster than patients in CC. Patients in intensive therapy were also more likely to remain stable in mood over the year-long study. In FFT, 77% of the patients recovered by 1 year; in interpersonal therapy, 65%; and in CBT, 60%. In the CC condition, 52% recovered. The differences between the intensive modalities did not reach statistical significance.

The findings of STEP-BD, one of the largest randomized treatment studies for bipolar disorder, suggests that psychotherapy is an essential component of the effort to stabilize bipolar patients in a depressive episode. The common ingredients of intensive treatments—such as teaching strategies to manage mood, identifying and intervening early with prodromal symptoms, enhancing patients' compliance with medications, and working toward resolution of key interpersonal or family problems— contributed to more rapid recoveries. FFT proved to be a particularly potent treatment in this study, although its limitations also became apparent: only 54% of the patients assessed for the study had families who were accessible and willing to participate in treatment.

Family Psychoeducation in Early-Onset Bipolar Disorder

More recent applications of family psychoeducation have focused on patients with juvenile-onset bipolar disorder, who most frequently live with or are strongly connected with their families of origin. A revision of FFT for adolescents has been developed (Miklowitz et al., 2004), using the same 21-session structure adapted to the developmental needs of this age group (e.g., the occurrence of more frequent, briefer episodes, typically with a mixed presentation). A 2-year open trial of 20 adolescent patients revealed significant improvements over time in manic symptoms, depressive symptoms, and parent-rated problem behaviors (Miklowitz et al., 2006). A second open trial found positive benefits for the combination of FFT and CBT for school-age children with bipolar disorder (Pavuluri et al., 2004). A two-site pilot randomized trial of FFT and pharmacotherapy versus brief psychoeducation and pharmacotherapy (N = 58) is nearing completion (Miklowitz et al., 2006).

Fristad, Gavazzi, and Mackinaw-Koons (2003) have developed a multifamily psychoeducation group for school-age bipolar and unipolar depressed children. Children with mood disorders who were assigned to multifamily groups showed greater mood stability over 6 months than children on a waiting list. Improvements extended to parents as well: Parents who participated in the groups reported a greater understanding of depression and bipolar disorder, more positively toned family interactions, and increased use of psychosocial and medical services than did waiting-list parents.

Summary

The addition of psychosocial treatment— family, group, or individual—to pharmacotherapy leads to more positive outcomes of bipolar disorder than can be achieved with pharmacotherapy alone. In drawing conclusions from this small literature, we must keep in mind the different domains of outcome that have been targeted. For some, the targeted outcomes have been relapse rates or symptom severity. For others, outcomes have been levels of global functioning or medication compliance.

Few of these studies have examined social, occupational, or school functioning, or the domain cited as the most important to patients: quality of life.

The remainder of this chapter is devoted to the specifics of delivering FFT. For whom is it intended? How does it proceed? How are families educated about bipolar disorder, and how do they learn new styles of communicating or solving problems? In reviewing these methods, the reader may wish to reflect on the various targets of family intervention (i.e., family attitudes or expectations, interpersonal conflict, medication nonadherence) and the various domains of outcome that are presumed to be influenced by family interventions via their impact on these targets.

CONTEXT OF THERAPY

Treatment Objectives and Structure

FFT has six objectives, all of which concern coping with an episode of bipolar disorder. These are summarized in Table 10.1. Some of these pertain to dealing with the current episode; others are more focused on anticipating episodes in the future, and the stress triggers for these episodes. A strong case is made for the protective effects of medication and a stable, nonstressful family environment.

FFT is delivered in 21 outpatient sessions lasting 1 hour each. Sessions are given weekly for 3 months, biweekly for 3 months, and monthly for 3 months. This structure was originally proposed by Falloon, Boyd, and McGill (1984) for the behavioral treatment of families

TABLE 10.1. The Six Objectives
of Family-Focused Treatment

Assist the patient and relatives in the following:

- Integrating the experiences associated with mood episodes in bipolar disorder
- Accepting the notion of a vulnerability to future episodes
- Accepting dependency on mood-stabilizing medication for symptom control
- Distinguishing between the patient's personality and his or her bipolar disorder
- Recognizing and learning to cope with stressful life events that trigger recurrences of bipolar disorder
- Reestablishing functional relationships after a mood episode

of patients with schizophrenia. The session-by-session plan is more a guide for the clinician than a requirement, because some families require less intensive contact at the beginning, others require more intensive contact later, and still others simply do not need this much treatment. The treatment is designed to parallel stages of recovery from a mood episode. During the stabilization phase, about seven sessions are devoted to psychoeducation, in which patients and their relatives become acquainted with the nature, course, and treatment of bipolar disorder. At this stage, patients are often still symptomatic and are usually functioning socially or occupationally at a level lower than their preepisode capabilities (see Keck et al., 1998; Strakowski et al., 1998). Psychoeducation is an attempt to hasten clinical stabilization by reducing the family tensions that often accompany the stabilization phase. This is done through helping a patient and his or her family members make sense of the different events that have precipitated the acute episode, come to a common understanding of the causes and the treatment of the illness, develop plans for how the family will act if there are signs of a developing recurrence, and modulate expectations for the patient's and family's functioning in the recovery period.

Once the family has begun the communication training module (7–10 sessions), the patient is usually fully stabilized from the acute episode, although he or she may still have residual mood symptoms. At this point, the patient is usually able to tolerate exercises oriented toward resolving family conflict and promoting behavior change. For example, he or she can practice listening while another family member speaks, and family members can do the same for him or her. These exercises can be difficult when a patient's emotions are still dysregulated, but the structure introduced by communication training can help the patient modulate how he or she expresses emotions.

During the final phase, problem-solving training (four to five sessions), the mood episode is largely remitted and the patient has moved into the maintenance phase of drug treatment. At this stage, and sometimes even earlier, the patient and family are motivated to identify and address quality-of-life issues that have been disrupted by the illness (e.g., how a married/cohabiting patient can find work; how parents can help a young adult offspring move out of the home and gradually become more independent). The last few sessions of FFT, held monthly, help to consolidate gains made during the 9-month treatment.

Setting

Our laboratory, the Colorado Family Project, was established in 1989 at the University of Colorado at Boulder's Department of Psychology. The staff members are psychology postdoctoral fellows, psychology graduate students, and psychiatrists from the community with whom we have developed collaborative relations. Since 1989, we have involved over 200 adults and adolescents with bipolar disorder in various forms of psychosocial care and research follow-up. We identify patients for our programs through inpatient screening or through referral from outpatient psychiatrists when patients have acute episodes.

In the Colorado study of FFT, we recruited 82 patients from hospital settings and 19 from outpatient clinics. It is worth noting that as the effects of managed care cost containment have taken hold, fewer and fewer of our patients are recruited from hospital wards. The initial diagnostic evaluation (see below) is done in the hospital (for inpatients) or in our outpatient research clinic at the Department of Psychology. A pretreatment family assessment (see below) is also done in this laboratory setting. Treatment and research follow-up interviews are typically done in this same laboratory, although some of our earlier work (Miklowitz et al., 2003) involved family sessions in patients' homes. The UCLA FFT study was entirely outpatient clinic–based. Home-based treatment can enhance the generalization of skills training (Falloon et al., 1984), and may also allow clinicians to treat patients of lower socioeconomic status, who ordinarily would not have the resources to travel to a university clinic. However, meeting at families' homes raises many logistical and financial problems for therapists. Thus, we have moved almost entirely to an outpatient clinic–based model, unless home-based treatment would greatly enhance compliance or treatment success.

Client Variables

FFT is usually administered to adult patients with bipolar disorder who live with (or in close proximity to) their parents, siblings, or spouses/partners. Patients can be of any age, including adolescents or preteen children. Although there is no contraindication for offering FFT to patients with remitted bipolar disorder, in our experience they and their family members are less motivated for treatment than those who have recently coped with a mood episode.

Patients with bipolar disorder can present as manic, mixed, hypomanic, depressed, or rapid-cycling. The polarity of the most recent episode, however, is a moving target—it may change before the patient is seen next. Patients who are manic or hypomanic, particularly those who are elated and grandiose, are often in denial about whether they are really ill, and may believe that the disorder and its treatment are simply ways for others to control them. Depressed patients may be more motivated for psychosocial treatment but may have cognitive difficulty assimilating the educational content of sessions. Patients with a mixed episode or rapid-cycling bipolar disorder are candidates for FFT, but their illness often follows a more pernicious course (Keller et al., 1986; McElroy et al., 1992; Post et al., 1989).

Patients with comorbid alcohol or other substance use disorders pose special problems. These patients are usually resistant to psychosocial treatment and medication. They are also difficult to diagnose; the effects of drugs or alcohol can mimic the cycling of a mood disorder. Generally, patients with active substance use disorders are more successfully treated if they are "dry" before FFT commences. If not, it is usually necessary to supplement FFT with chemical dependency programs (e.g., dual-diagnosis Alcoholics Anonymous groups).

Concurrent Drug Treatment

We require that our patients be seen simultaneously by a psychiatrist, who monitors the patient's medications. Typically, a regimen includes a primary mood stabilizer, usually lithium carbonate or divalproex sodium (Depakote), or newer agents, such as lamotrigine (Lamictal). The choice of these mood stabilizers is at least in part a function of whether the patient presents with clear-cut episodes of mania or depression, in which case lithium is often recommended. If there is evidence of mixed states or rapid cycling, the anticonvulsants are often recommended (Goldberg, 2004). More and more, we are seeing patients treated with atypical antipsychotics (e.g., olanazapine [Zyprexa], risperidone [Risperdal], quetiapine

[Seroquel], or clozapine [Clozaril]), either as adjuncts to traditional mood stabilizers or as substitutes for them. There is evidence that these agents are highly effective in controlling mania, and some (notably, olanzapine and quetiapine) have antidepressant properties as well (Goldberg, 2004; Kowatch et al., 2005; Kowatch & DelBello, 2003). These agents are particularly valuable if the patient is highly agitated or psychotic. Antidepressants (e.g., paroxetine [Paxil], venlafaxine [Effexor], bupropion [Wellbutrin]) are still recommended as adjuncts to mood stabilizers or atypical antipsychotics if the patient's depression does not remit, but they are given sparingly, because there is a risk of switching from depression into manic, mixed, or rapid-cycling states (Altshuler et al., 1995). In children, there is concern about a slightly increased risk of suicidal ideation or behaviors (Vitiello & Swedo, 2004). Very few of our patients (i.e., fewer than 5%) receive electroconvulsive therapy in addition to drug treatment.

A core principle of FFT is that the family therapist must have regular contact with the patient's psychiatrist. This contact is established early in treatment. A close affiliation between the psychosocial and pharmacological treatment team enhances the likelihood of the patient's remaining compliant with his or her medications; it also decreases the likelihood of "splitting," or the tendency for a patient (or even family members) to have a "good doctor" and a "bad doctor." For example, patients frequently complain about their physicians and say to their FFT clinicians, "I wish you could just monitor my medications." An FFT clinician who has a regular dialogue with a patient's physician can avoid the trap that is being set by encouraging the patient to bring up these problems with the physician directly.

Some patients who refuse all medications assume that coming to therapy will be a substitute for drug treatment. These patients often have had bad experiences with pharmacotherapy and psychiatrists, and may also believe that they are not ill, or that the illness they do have can be treated using "alternative medicine." We have generally taken a hard line with these patients and do not accept them into FFT unless they commit to standard pharmacotherapy (usually lithium, anticonvulsants, and/ or atypical antipsychotics). Patients with bipolar disorder who are unmedicated are highly likely to have relapses, and it is not in their best interests for the clinician to imply that their illness can be managed with psychosocial treatment alone.

Therapist Variables

In the Colorado Treatment Outcome Study of adults (Miklowitz et al., 2003), therapist age varied from 23 to 46 years and from 1 to 14 years of clinical experience. The majority were graduate students in clinical psychology or clinicians with recent doctorates. Few had extensive background in family therapy before learning FFT. The 15-site Systematic Treatment Enhancement Program for Bipolar Disorder (STEP-BD; Miklowitz et al., 2007) involved therapists with doctorates or social workers who varied considerably in treatment experience. In other words, there are no requirements that an FFT therapist have a certain degree or amount of clinical training at the outset.

There are no studies of therapist variables as predictors of the course of family psychoeducational treatments. Our own clinical sense has been that there are two predictors of success in learning FFT. The first positive predictor is the ability to think of a family or couple as a system in which members are interdependent and mutually influence other members' behaviors. Therapists who have trouble with FFT often have difficulty making the transition to this systemic way of thinking. They tend, for example, to conduct family sessions as if they were individual sessions, with one patient and several observers. Some of these same problems arise in learning other forms of family therapy.

The second positive predictor is the willingness to think biopsychosocially—that is, to see bipolar disorder as a biologically based illness that requires medication treatment, even if its symptoms are partially evoked by concurrent stressors. Thus, a therapist often must argue for the patient's drug adherence even when psychosocial issues are more interesting and seem more pressing.

We have found that the following training protocol works well for learning FFT. First, clinicians attend group supervision sessions in which trained FFT therapists discuss their cases. They read the published treatment manual (Miklowitz & Goldstein, 1997) and an updated manual for adolescents (Miklowitz & George, 2004), and watch sample FFT videotapes. Then they serve as cotherapists to trained FFT therapists. After treating two cases with close supervision, they are usually ready to see families or couples independently, or to take on trainees themselves.

The cotherapy model has advantages separate from training. It has a long history in the family therapy literature (see, e.g., Napier & Whitaker, 1978). Cotherapists have a way of keeping their fellow therapists on track. Also, if one member of the family appears to be feeling "ganged up on" by one clinician and other family members, the other therapist can bridge the gap by allying him- or herself with this family member. In-session dialogue between the clinicians can also provide effective modeling of communication skills for members of a family or couple.

PRETREATMENT ASSESSMENTS

Diagnostic Evaluation

Bipolar disorder is becoming an increasingly common diagnosis in inpatient and outpatient community settings. Although this is a positive development given its underidentification in the past, there is also an element of sloppiness in modern diagnostic evaluations. Nowhere is this more obvious than in the diagnosis of children and adolescents, who are now being called "bipolar" with little supporting evidence (McClellan, 2005). The inadequacy of community diagnostic evaluations derives in part from inadequate insurance reimbursement for the evaluation phases of a patients' treatment. Some of the patients referred to us have been more aptly diagnosed as having cyclothymic disorder, borderline personality disorder, or even major depressive disorder, recurrent. Many adolescents are referred with "rage attacks." Our colleagues in community practice have often noted the same problems when patients who presumably have bipolar disorder are referred to them.

Upon seeing a new patient, a clinician often finds it useful to do a formal assessment using all or part of a structured diagnostic interview to determine the reliability of the diagnosis. Within our research protocols, we have used the Structured Clinical Interview for DSM-IV—Patient Version (SCID; First, Spitzer, Gibbon, & Williams, 1995) as the diagnostic assessment device. The SCID is well described elsewhere (Spitzer, Williams, Gibbon, & First, 1992). When the patient is under age 18, we use the Schedule for Affective Disorders and Schizophrenia for School-Age Children—Present and Lifetime Version (K-SADS-PL; Chambers et al., 1985; Kaufman et al., 1997), which requires separate interviews with the child and at least one parent, and then a consensus rating.

Some of the factors that can affect the reliability of the data obtained from the SCID or K-SADS-PL include whether the patient is acutely ill or stable; acutely ill patients are less reliable in their symptom reports. Typically, patients in a manic state minimize their symptoms, whereas depressed patients may do the reverse. Patients with bipolar disorder also have trouble with retrospective reporting: "I've had over 1,000 episodes" and "I've been constantly manic–depressed since I was an infant" are common responses to diagnostic interviews.

Whether one uses the structured or an open-ended clinical interview, it is often difficult to determine whether a patient's mood dysregulations and associated changes in activity are at the subsyndromal or syndromal levels. Some patients report brief periods of hypomania or irritability that alternate with more severe depressions. These brief, activated periods do not always reach the DSM-IV duration threshold for hypomania (4 days or more), especially among children and teens. In some cases, the patient is "one symptom short." Some of these patients are better labeled as having cyclothymic disorder or major depressive disorder. For children with manic symptoms who do not meet the duration or symptom count criteria, the diagnosis of "bipolar disorder, not otherwise specified" is often given (Birmaher et al., 2006).

Hagop Akiskal (1996; Akiskal & Akiskal, 1992) has encouraged clinicians to consider a broader bipolar spectrum that includes core temperamental disturbances. In addition to cyclothymia, Akiskal describes a "bipolar III" or "pseudounipolar" subtype, in which patients have recurrent major depressions, with an underlying temperament marked by hyperthymia (exuberance, overoptimism, grandiosity, stimulus seeking, physical intrusiveness with others), and/or a family history of bipolar disorder. He also describes a subgroup of patients with "subbipolar dysthymia," marked by mild depressions with hypomanias evoked by antidepressant treatment. Akiskal argues that these "soft-spectrum" patients respond to the same medications as traditional patients with bipolar I disorder and have similar family histories.

In FFT, the broadening of the bipolar spectrum to include these patients introduces a quandary: Does the clinician proceed with such patients in the same way as with patients with bipolar I or bipolar II disorder? How does the clinician educate the patient and family about the factors that bring about manic or depressive episodes if discrete episodes cannot be identified? If a patient has never had a true manic episode in the absence of antidepressants, then should the treatment proceed under the assumption that eventually he or she will develop mania spontaneously? Do we tell the family of a child with bipolar disorder, not otherwise specified, that he or she is at risk for developing the full syndrome, or are we on shaky ground in doing so? Do the same self-management techniques (e.g., using problem solving to minimize family conflict) apply?

For our research, we have opted to include only patients with bipolar I or II disorder as defined by DSM-IV criteria. Our general impression has been that patients who do not go through clear-cut cycles of mood episodes are a different population of patients. However, we see value in further research on Akiskal's conceptualization of the soft spectrum of bipolar disorder, and particularly research that evaluates whether psychosocial interventions should play the same or a different—perhaps even a more intensive—role in the treatment of such patients.

Mood Chart

Clarity on the diagnosis, as well as the patient's progress in treatment, is aided by asking the patient to keep a daily mood record. One such instrument is the Social Rhythm Metric (Monk, Flaherty, Frank, Hoskinson, & Kupfer, 1990; Monk, Kupfer, Frank, & Ritenour, 1991), which asks the patient to document daily mood on a −5 (*Depressed*) to +5 (*Euphoric/activated*) scale, along with social routines that may influence these moods (e.g., sleep–wake times, times when the patient socializes, the intensity of this social stimulation, the patient's exercise habits, and other factors).

Leverich and Post (1998) have developed a self-rated "life chart" that requires the patient to keep track of daily mood variations, medications, life stressors, and sleep. Data from mood/activity charts help the clinician and patient to evaluate collaboratively the type of cycling the patient experiences and the degree to which social stressors contribute to mood fluctuations. Figure 10.2 is an example of a mood chart; note the cycling of the disorder in relation to specific social stressors and sleep patterns reported by the patient. In this example, a stressor (a pet's illness) is associated with sleep disruption and the appearance of mixed mood symptoms at the subsyndromal level.

Family Assessments

Psychoeducational approaches usually begin with a thorough assessment of family attitudes

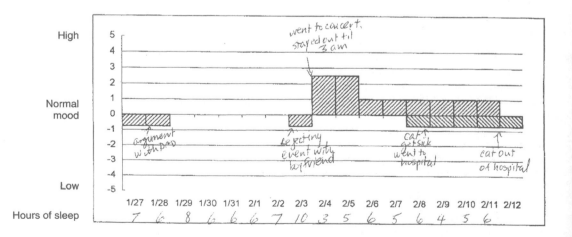

FIGURE 10.2. Example of a self-rated mood chart.

and behaviors to identify the targets of intervention. In our research studies, we have begun with the Camberwell Family Interview, the instrument for rating EE discussed earlier. This interview, usually done when the patient is acutely symptomatic, focuses on the prior 3-month period, which usually includes the prodromal phases of symptom buildup. For the purposes of clinical planning over research, the interview yields answers to the following questions: What is the current level of tension in the household and in the relative/patient relationship? Which of the patient's behaviors are eliciting stimuli for family arguments or hostility? Do family members understand that the patient has bipolar disorder, or are they likely to attribute the patient's negative behaviors to internal or controllable factors?

A problem with the EE/Camberwell Family Interview method is its lack of easy exportability to community care settings. Interviews with two parents can total 3 hours, and the coding of interview tapes can add an additional 6 person-hours per family. If a clinician's purpose is treatment planning rather than research, he or she may be able to substitute a self-report measure such as the Perceived Criticism Scale (Hooley & Teasdale, 1989). This measure simply asks the patient to rate, on a 1–10 scale, the degree to which close relatives express critical comments toward him or her, and the degree to which he or she expresses critical comments toward relatives. In one prospective study, self-reported scores on this instrument were just as strong in predicting depressive relapse among patients with recurrent major depression as were EE scores from the Camberwell Family Interview method (Hooley & Teasdale, 1989). Evaluation of this scale as a predictor of the course of adult bipolar disorder was recently accomplished in the multicenter STEP-BD study ($N = 360$; Miklowitz, Wisniewski, Miyahara, Otto, & Sachs, 2005). In that study, the degree to which patients reported being upset or distressed by criticism from relatives was a strong predictor of their levels of depression over a 1-year prospective period. Interestingly, the *amount* of criticism they perceived from relatives was not prognostically significant.

In our research protocols, we typically bring the family in for an interactional assessment once the patient has achieved some degree of remission. First, each member of the family, including the patient, is interviewed individually and asked to identify two family problem topics. Then each participant is asked to verbalize the nature of this problem as if the family member to whom the problem statement is directed were sitting across from him/her (e.g., a mother states, "Ralph, you never tell me when something is wrong, even though I know it is"). A tape recording of this problem statement is then played for the opposing family member, who is asked to respond on tape contiguously (e.g., "Mom, I don't talk to you because when I do, it makes things worse"). Two simulated "conversations" are obtained from each family member, and the clinician or experimenter chooses one from the patient and one from a relative as stimuli for family discussions.

Next, the family is brought into a meeting room with videotaping capability. The first of these two problem cue–response sequences is played, and the family members are asked to discuss the problem for 10 minutes; to tell each other why they said what they did on the tape, and how they each feel about the issue; and to try to reach a resolution. The clinician then exits the room, and the discussion ensues. Then he or she reenters the room and plays the second cue–response sequence, and a second 10-minute discussion ensues. Transcripts of these 10-minute problem-solving discussions can then be coded, using the Category System for Coding Partner Interactions (discussed earlier) or a similar interactional coding system. Unfortunately, obtaining this information from transcripts is very labor-intensive and cannot usually be carried out before the treatment begins.

The clinician can also rely on simple observations of the family's communication and problem-solving behavior to inform the skills training modules of FFT. To quote Yogi Berra, "You can observe a lot by watching." First, many family members or patients are unable to focus on a single problem, and instead begin to "cross-complain" or to accuse other family members to counteract the accusations directed at them. Some engage in attack–counterattack cycles, which may include negative verbal or nonverbal behaviors. For any particular family, the clinician must first identify the form these interchanges take, which dyadic or triadic relationships they involve; the content areas that trigger the interchanges (e.g., medication-taking habits, independence, boundaries within the family), and whether members of the family are able to stop these cycles before they spiral out of control. Who criticizes whom, and how often? How does the target person respond? Does the original problem ever get solved?

During these unsupervised family interactions, some family members combine negative affect with unclear or fragmented communication, which has been called "communication deviance" in the schizophrenia literature (Wynne, Singer, Bartko, & Toohey, 1977). We have found that the relatives of patients with bipolar disorder and the relatives of patients with schizophrenia do not differ in levels of communication deviance (Miklowitz et al., 1991). Patients with bipolar disorder and their relatives often speak in a hurried, driven manner, and often jumble phrases, get words out of order, or express fragments of ideas. The extent to which these communication styles reflect situational stress or enduring patterns of relating in the family is not clear. Nonetheless, FFT can include exercises that focus on communication clarity, as well as affective balance.

PROCESS OF TREATMENT

Psychoeducation

The initiation of the psychoeducation module of FFT requires three conditions. First, the patient must be seeing a psychiatrist and have begun a medication regimen. Second, he or she must have achieved some degree of clinical stability, although there is no requirement that the acute episode be fully remitted. Third, the family should have undergone an assessment of attitudes and interactional behaviors, even if not as formalized as described for the research protocols. Table 10.2 summarizes the topical domains that are covered in the first module of FFT, psychoeducation. In the seven or more weekly sessions that comprise this module, participants (patients and their close relatives) become acquainted with the symptoms of bipolar disorder; the way episodes develop; the roles of genetics, biology, and stress; pharmacological treatments; and the role of stress management strategies.

The Initial Sessions: Providing a Rationale

As in most other forms of therapy, the clinicians begin by explaining the rationale for the FFT program. Many participants ask why family or couple sessions should accompany medication for a patient adjusting to a recent

TABLE 10.2. Issues in Psychoeducation

The symptoms and course of the disorder
- The signs and symptoms of bipolar disorder
- The development of the most recent episode
- The recent life events survey
- Discussing the hospitalization experience
- Variations in prognosis: The course of the disorder

The etiology of bipolar disorder
- The vulnerability–stress model
- The roles of stress and life events
- Genetic and biological predispositions
- Risk and protective factors

Intervening within the vulnerability–stress model
- Types of medication and what they do
- Psychosocial treatments
- How the family can help
- The self-management of the disorder
- The relapse drill

Note. From Miklowitz and Goldstein (1997). Copyright 1997 by The Guilford Press. Reprinted with permission.

episode of bipolar disorder. Particularly helpful in orienting participants is the "reentry model":

> "An episode of mood disorder can be quite traumatic to all members of the family. . . . In bipolar disorder, when the person returns home and begins to recover, there is a 'getting reacquainted' period in which everyone has to get to know everyone else again, and when everyone tries to make sense of what happened. This is a tough time for any family, and part of our purpose here is to make this 'reacquaintance period' less disturbing to all of you. We'd like during this year to get you, as a family, back to where you were before _____ became ill. We want to give you some tools to deal with this recovery period." (Miklowitz & Goldstein, 1997, p. 93)

There are two purposes for this introduction. First, it communicates to the family members that their emotional reactions to the patient's illness—even if quite negative—are normal and expectable. Second, it implies that the therapy will include exploration and clarification of participants' emotional reactions to information about the disorder. This feature of the therapy can be made even more explicit:

> "If feelings come up for you when we're discussing this material, please bring them up. We're interested in knowing how this material applies to

you and your own experiences. You may or may not agree with some of the material we present here. . . . The purpose of focusing on this material is to put your experiences into a context that will make sense." (Miklowitz & Goldstein, 1997, p. 99)

Next, the treatment is previewed:

"We're going to work with you on two different levels. One is on encouraging _____'s ongoing work with his/her psychiatrist so that he or she can get himself/herself stabilized on the medications. The second is on how you as a family can minimize stress. . . . We think there are several ways to do this, including acquainting you with the facts about bipolar disorder, and working with you on improving your communication and problem solving with each other. These strategies should increase _____'s chances of making a good recovery and help you as a family cope with the disorder. How does this sound to you?" (Miklowitz & Goldstein, 1997, p. 94)

The Symptoms of Bipolar Disorder

FFT proceeds with a series of handouts that are used as stimuli for generating family or couple discussions. The first of these is a list of symptoms of manic, hypomanic, depressive, and psychotic episodes. The purpose of this handout is not for the participants to memorize the DSM-IV criteria. Rather, it is a starting point for destigmatizing the illness and breaking family taboos against talking about it. The patient is asked to scan the list and describe to his or her family members the way it feels when one is euphoric, irritable, unable to sleep, or activated by racing thoughts or grandiose plans. Likewise, family members describe the behaviors they observe when the patient cycles into mania or hypomania. A similar dialogue is undertaken for depression symptoms. Consider the following dialogue among a patient, mother, father, and therapist.

PATIENT: Well, the thing is, there's the manic and then there's the hypomanic. When I'm manic, I really should be hospitalized. I control the weather; I'm famous. When I'm hypomanic, well, I just can get into that from having too much stress, too much caffeine, and being all revved up . . .

MOTHER: I can tell when she's high, because I start getting real mad at her. She provokes me.

FATHER: And she gets this look in her eyes. And she says we're not listening to her . . .

PATIENT: But you're not! That's when you're most likely to tune me out!

THERAPIST: Let's hold on that for now, about listening. It's very important, and certainly something we'll want to focus on as we go along, but what else do you notice when you get manic or hypomanic? [Redirects the focus.]

PATIENT: I get sort of, well, reactive . . . I experience everything so intensely, but see, they know this as who I am.

Note the themes that arise in this discussion of symptoms, and how these relate to the six objectives of FFT outlined in Table 10.1. The patient's vulnerability to recurrences is made explicit by the family's identification of the prodromal signs of her episodes. The patient points to the role of disturbed family communication. She alludes to questions about whether some of her symptoms are really just personality traits (i.e., intensity and reactivity). There is a beginning discussion of stress factors that may play a role in triggering her episodes.

The Vulnerability–Stress Model and the Life Events Survey

Early in psychoeducation, the family clinicians make a strong argument for the conjoint influences of stress, biological imbalances of the brain, and genetic vulnerability in the course of bipolar illness. A handout illustrating these vulnerability–stress interactions is provided, and various risk and protective factors are reviewed. For example, the patient and family members are warned of the impact of "poor sleep hygiene" (i.e., keeping irregular hours, having unpredictable bedtimes); alcohol and drug use; stressful family interchanges; and provocative, overstimulating interpersonal interactions. They are encouraged to make use of available protective factors (e.g., social supports), and to help the patient maintain adherence to his or her pharmacotherapy regimen. The purposes of the patient's various medications are given, and the role of blood level monitoring is reviewed. In outlining protective factors, a special emphasis is placed on keeping the family environment low in conflict and on relatives' maintaining reasonable performance expectations of the patient during the recovery period. In the following vignette, the clinician reminds the patient and his mother that depression is not the same as lack of effort, and that a period of recovery prior to regaining one's premorbid occupational status is to be expected.

THERAPIST: (*to Gary, the patient*) I think you can't expect too much just yet. You're still recovering from your episode. It may take some time to get back on track.

MOTHER: How long? He's been like this now for a while.

THERAPIST: I'm sure that's frustrating, but you have to think of this as a convalescent period. When someone has a bad flu, he may need an extra day or two in bed to recover completely. For bipolar disorder, this period of time can average 3 to 6 months. But, Gary, with your medication treatments and our family sessions, I have every expectation that you'll recover and be able to get back to work.

The clinician here offers hope but does not paint a rosy picture of the future. Often the family has been through these episodes before, and a clinician who offers an excessively optimistic view of the future will be dismissed as unrealistic.

Describing the biology and genetics of the disorder is critical to justifying the role of medications. However, it is not necessary for the clinician to go into detail about the neurophysiology of the disorder. Instead, the clinician begins by asking the participants to review their family pedigree and discuss any other persons in the family who have had episodes of bipolar disorder. In reviewing this history, the family is told that the vulnerability to bipolar disorder may take many forms, including major depression without mania, alcoholism, suicide, and dysthymia. Next, the clinician explains the notion of biochemical imbalances:

"Sometimes the cells may have too much activity and communicate messages a little too quickly, at least when a person is getting manic. When a person gets depressed, the messages may not get through fast enough. These imbalances of brain chemicals can't be controlled by you through conscious effort, but the medications you take can go a long way toward balancing the activity in your nervous system."

When family members begin to attribute the patient's aversive behaviors to willfulness (the "fundamental attributional error"), the clinician can remind them of the existence of biochemical imbalances. But the family and patient should also be discouraged from overemphasizing the biological nature of the disorder, to the point of neglecting stress factors such as longstanding family conflicts. In other words, the patient is not entirely taken off of the hook: He or she is encouraged to self-monitor when getting into arguments with family members, and to determine whether his or her reactions to these conflicts reflect an unresolved symptom state or a reemergence of conflicts that would have been troublesome even before he or she became ill.

Clarifying the development and triggers for the most recent episode is aided by a Life Events Survey, which lists over 100 life changes that could have occurred during the interval in which the episode was developing. Some of these events are quite severe and negative (e.g., death of a parent); others are quite mild but may have provoked changes in sleep–wake cycles (e.g., taking a vacation). The clinician passes out the life events list and engages the family or couple in a discussion about important triggers that may have provoked the current episode. The clinician individualizes this discussion as much as possible: The triggers for one patient's mania are not the same as those for another's, and triggers for mania and depression within the same patient can be quite different.

The Relapse Drill

Toward the end of psychoeducation, the family and patient are given their first exposure to problem solving. The task is to review the prodromal signs of a developing episode and go through the steps that are necessary to prevent a full relapse. Participants are asked to generate alternative courses of action should the patient relapse into mania or depression, which can include arranging emergency psychiatric services (e.g., calling the patient's psychiatrist, arranging for a serum lithium level to be taken) or less intensive strategies such as behavioral activation (e.g., helping the depressed patient schedule positive events during the day). Each family member is asked to perform a function in the relapse prevention plan. For example, in some families it may make sense for a parent to undertake contact with the physician. In others, the patient may want the first opportunity to do so. The family or couple is encouraged to leave phone numbers of emergency contact people, including the family clinicians, in an easily accessible place.

Dealing with Resistance to the Illness Concept

Patients with bipolar disorder have strong reactions to the psychoeducational materials, as do their family members. These materials require that the participants recognize bipolar disorder as an illness that will eventually recur. Younger patients are particularly likely to reject the notion of a recurrent illness, particularly if they are still hypomanic; they feel powerful and in control, and the idea of having an illness feels like shackles. Moreover, they are particularly attuned to the stigma associated with bipolar disorder or any other psychiatric diagnosis, and fear that their behavior will now be labeled as that of a crazy person. Resistance can also originate with family members. Relatives of depressed patients are apt to see the disorder as willfully caused and not the product of biochemical imbalances. Resistance that originates from the patient or his or her relatives is often associated with family conflict.

Accepting a psychiatric disorder is a painful process for patients and relatives. Often the psychoeducational materials raise questions, such as "Why me? Why now? What kind of life will I have? Will people treat me like I'm mentally ill from now on? Will I ever get back to normal?" Relatives ask themselves similar painful questions, such as "Will I always have to take care of him or her? Are my dreams and hopes for him or her gone?" Spouses/partners may ask, "Should I leave him or her?" When asking themselves these questions, some patients respond by "underidentifying," or denying the reality of the disorder, or by acknowledging the illness superficially but living their lives as if it were not real.

Others "overidentify" and unnecessarily limit themselves (e.g., one woman avoided romantic relationships, because "No one will ever be able to get close to me because of my mood swings"). Likewise, family members can deny the realities of the disorder or, in contrast, overmonitor the patient's health status and try to limit his or her behavior unnecessarily. Family conflict reaches a maximum when there is a mismatch between coping styles, such as when patients underidentify and relatives overidentify, or the reverse.

FFT clinicians proceed with a sensitivity to the painful emotional issues underlying these reactions to psychoeducation. One method for dealing with these reactions is to predict that denial will occur, and to reframe it as a sign of health. For example, consider a young man with hypomania who has accepted taking medications but denies being ill, and whose parents overcontrol and overmonitor his behavior. To this young man, the clinician might say:

"Although I appreciate that you're taking medication and going along with the treatment plan, I'm going to guess that you're not always going to want to do this. You probably have some questions about whether this diagnosis is right for you or whether you'll have more symptoms. I can understand why you'd have these questions. Coming to terms with having bipolar disorder—or really any illness—is a very painful process that can be hard to accept. This is a normal and a healthy struggle. So, as we're going through our material, you may find yourself reacting to it and feeling that it can't be relevant to you. But I'd like for you to agree that if you have these reactions, you'll bring them up so we can discuss them."

Note that this intervention has a paradoxical flavor. Paradoxical interventions have a long history in family systems therapy (see, e.g., Haley, 1963). However, note that the clinician stops short of actually encouraging the patient to remain resistant or to increase his level of disagreement with the diagnosis. Instead, the clinician reframes this denial as healthy and expectable, and connects it with an underlying emotional struggle.

A second way to intervene is through "spreading the affliction." Being labeled as mentally ill can put a person in a one-down position vis-à-vis other family members, including siblings with whom he or she may already feel competitive. A possible side effect of psychoeducation is the exaggeration of these structural family problems. The clinician can avoid this trap by encouraging other members of the family to discuss their own experiences with depression, anxiety, or other problems. This process can normalize and destigmatize psychiatric problems and take the patient "off the hot seat."

The following vignette involves Josh, a 25-year-old with a recent manic episode. He reacted strongly, because he thought everyone was telling him he was "whacked out." According to Josh, all he had done was "party too much." During one of the psychoeducation sessions, his father admitted to having had a depressive episode in college.

THERAPIST: Josh, you seem like you're reacting to something I just said about bipolar disorder. Were you offended?

JOSH: I dunno. It wasn't anything you said; just I get tired of being the only one in the family who has problems.

THERAPIST: Is that really true? Has anyone else in the family ever had any problems with depression? Or what I've called mania?

FATHER: (*pause*) I did, and I've told Josh about this. Remember what I told you about college?

JOSH: (*sullen*) I don't know. Why don't you clue us in?

FATHER: I had that long period when I couldn't sleep and eat, and I couldn't study. I dropped out for a semester.

The session then focused on the father and his own history of depression. He revealed a history of psychosis involving delusional thinking. The patient became more cooperative in the discussions that followed, and more willing to talk about how the illness label made him feel stigmatized.

A third method of dealing with resistance involves making analogies to medical disorders. The illness feels less humiliating if the patient can see it within the continuum of other kinds of chronic physical illness. It is equally important for family members to hear these analogies. Diabetes and hypertension are often good comparisons, particularly because the influence of stress can also be brought to bear:

"Bipolar disorder involves biological imbalances much like hypertension does, and it's affected by stress in much the same way. Most people have changes in blood pressure when something stressful happens. But people with hypertension have a vulnerability to extreme shifts in their blood pressure. In the same way, most people have mood changes when something important happens, but people with bipolar disorder operate at greater extremes."

In making these analogies, the clinician validates the patient's feelings about stigma:

"Although there are some similarities with illnesses like hypertension, bipolar disorder can be tougher to live with because other people tend to be afraid of it and don't know what it means. They can think you're doing it on purpose. You have to take the time to educate other people—particularly those people who are most important to you—and explain it in a way that they won't be freaked out by it."

Communication Enhancement Training

The second module of FFT, CET, begins at approximately Session 8 and lasts for about seven or eight sessions (five weekly sessions, followed by two or three biweekly sessions). CET is guided by two assumptions. First, aversive family communication is a common sequel to an episode of a psychiatric illness and to a large extent reflects distress within the family or couple in members' attempts to deal with the disorder. Second, the frequency of aversive communication can be reduced through skills training.

CET uses a role-playing format to teach patients and their relatives four communication skills: expressing positive feelings, active listening, making positive requests for changes in others' behaviors, and giving negative feedback. These skills are central to the behavioral family management approach to schizophrenia of Falloon and colleagues (1984) and Liberman, Wallace, Falloon, and Vaughn (1981). The degree to which each of these skills dominates the role-play exercises varies according to the family assessments conducted earlier. Treatment of a family with much heated conflict and high-EE attitudes might focus on adaptive ways in which participants could ask for changes in each other's behaviors. Treatment of an emotionally disengaged couple might focus on positive feedback and listening skills to coax the partners into experimenting with a more interdependent relationship.

The module begins with an explication of the CET method for the family:

"A person can be at risk for another relapse of bipolar disorder if the home environment is tense. . . . Good communication and problem solving can be among those 'protective factors' against stress that we talked about before. For a close relative, learning effective communication skills can be a way of decreasing tension and improving family relationships. . . . We want to help you communicate in the most clear and the least stressful way possible . . . we'll be asking you to turn your chairs to each other and practice new ways of talking among yourselves." (Miklowitz & Goldstein, 1997, pp. 191–193)

Note that CET is linked with two of the six objectives of the larger treatment program: helping participants to cope with stress triggers, and restoring functional family relationships after an illness episode. The first two skills, positive feedback and active listening, generally foster a feeling of collaboration between members of the couple or family. In contrast, making positive requests for change and giving negative feedback are more conflict-oriented, and are only introduced once participants are used to the role-playing and behavioral rehearsal format.

For each skill, the clinician gives participants a handout that lists its components (e.g., for active listening: make good eye contact, nod your head, ask clarifying questions, paraphrase/check out what you have heard). Then the clinician models the skill for the family. For example, the clinician might compliment one member of the family for his or her cooperativeness with the treatment, or model effective listening while another member of the family talks about a problem. If a cotherapist is available, the therapist can model these skills with him or her. After the skill is introduced and modeled, participants are asked to practice the skill with each other, with coaching and shaping by the clinician. Typically the therapist coaches one participant at a time on appropriate ways to use a given skill. The feedback of other family members is actively solicited. The speaker or listener is then asked to try the skill again, until he or she has reasonably approximated its use. A homework assignment, in which participants keep a written log of their efforts in using the skills between sessions, facilitates generalization of the learning process to the home and work settings.

Many times, the skills are harder than they look. Consider Jessie, a 38-year-old woman with bipolar disorder who had had several episodes of psychotic mania, and who also had a borderline level of mental retardation. She worked part time as a gift wrapper in a department store. Jessie was trying to move into her own apartment, and required help finding a moving van. She was instructed to learn to make positive requests of her father, with whom she and her sister lived.

THERAPIST: Maybe that's a good topic to ask your dad about. Can you look at this "Positive Requests" handout and use these steps to ask your dad to help you move?

FATHER: It won't help. There won't be anything for them to move, because she still hasn't packed a single box! (*Laughs.*)

JESSIE: Well, get me the damn boxes and I'll do it.

THERAPIST: (*derailing this interchange*) Do you think you could ask your dad for something specific, like helping you find a moving company?

JESSIE: (*Looks at father, smirking.*) Dad, will you help me find a moving company? (*Giggles.*)

FATHER: (*more serious*) You're not . . . you're not looking at this (*indicates handout*). You're supposed to say, "I'd appreciate it if you would . . ."

JESSIE: (*Shrugs.*) All right, I'd appreciate it if you would! Get me a phone number. Please.

THERAPIST: (*after pause*) Well, you got part of it that time, Jessie. Dad, what did you like about what she just said to you?

FATHER: (*sarcastically*) Gee, all the sincerity.

JESSIE: (*Laughs nervously.*)

THERAPIST: Well, if you didn't care for it, can you say how she might say it to you?

FATHER: How about something like "I'd appreciate it if you'd get me those phone numbers. It'd make it a lot more comfortable for me to plan my move."

THERAPIST: Nice job, Dad. Jessie, what did your dad do that you liked or didn't like?

JESSIE: He followed the sheet. He did all the things you said.

THERAPIST: True, but you don't have to say it exactly the way he did. You can put your own spin on it. Do you feel you could try doing it one more time?

JESSIE: (*Gasps, giggles.*)

THERAPIST: I know it's hard being in the hot seat. But you're doing fine. Keep trying.

JESSIE: Dad, could you get me those phone numbers of the movers? I'd appreciate it. That way I could be . . . I wouldn't have to worry about the move, and, well, just thank you for your help.

THERAPIST: That was very good, Jessie. Dad, how did you like it that time?

FATHER: (*a little tentative*) That was better. It made a lot more sense.

These kinds of skills are most difficult to learn if the patient is highly symptomatic and/or cognitively impaired, or if the level of conflict in the family is so severe that productive conversations cannot ensue. This patient was moderately hypomanic and also had limited intellectual resources. Clearly, the skills training taxed her and made her nervous. However, with patience and practice, Jessie was able to adopt some of the communication skills, and her relationship with her father gradually improved. Her father, who was often quite critical, became more and more convinced that her limited functioning was a result of her bipolar disorder rather than lack of effort, as he had believed previously.

In the FFT manual (Miklowitz & Goldstein, 1997), we have described "short-fuse" families. These families begin with apparently innocuous discussions, which quickly escalate into angry, back-and-forth volleys of criticism or hostility. Our research indicates that these are usually high-EE families or couples, but not invariably (Simoneau et al., 1998). We have been surprised that relatives who on the surface appear benign and supportive of the patient during the EE/Camberwell Family Interview become quite aggressive and confrontational when facing the patient in a one-to-one interaction. Not surprisingly, the likelihood that this will occur is greatly augmented if the patient is hypomanic and irritable. A short-fuse family typically has difficulty with communication training, because the participants' emotions quickly get out of hand (see the case study presented later). But much can be accomplished by modifying CET to adapt to this dynamic. For example, the therapist can encourage the participants to use active listening skills during arguments. After a negative, back-and-forth interchange involving a couple, a clinician said:

"I think this is an important discussion. You're a couple that really likes to get things out in the open. But I'm afraid that you're missing out on each other's viewpoints. So let's see if we can make it more productive. I want you each to paraphrase each other's statements before making your next argument, like we did in the active listening exercises. Also, why don't you turn your chairs to each other so that you can more easily keep eye contact?"

Note again the use of reframing. It is better to cast a couple's or family's ongoing dynamics (unless clearly abusive or threatening) as an adaptive way of coping that needs modification than to label these dynamics as "bad" or "dysfunctional."

A short-fuse family may also make good use of positive requests for change or negative feedback exercises, in which the partners make constructive suggestions about specific aspects of each other's behavior (e.g., "I don't like it when you talk down to me about my cleaning habits") and offer suggestions as to ways these behaviors could be improved (e.g., "Could you be more aware of your tone of voice?"). These exercises often set the stage for problem solving, the final module of FFT.

Problem-Solving Skills Training

Families of patients with bipolar disorder, whether these be couples (see, e.g., Hoover & Fitzgerald, 1981) or parental families of bipolar adults (Miklowitz, Goldstein, & Nuechterlein, 1987; Simoneau et al., 1998), have difficulty with problem solving, especially if the patient has recently been ill. Family problems in adjusting to the postepisode phases of bipolar disorder appear to fall into one of four categories: medication nonadherence, difficulty resuming prior work and social roles, repairing the financial and social damage done during manic episodes ("life trashing"), and relationship/living situation conflicts.

Problem solving is one of the oldest and most validated methods of family intervention (for a review, see Clarkin & Miklowitz, 1997). Its purposes in FFT are threefold: (1) to open a dialogue among family members about difficult conflict topics; (2) allow them a context to share their emotional reactions to these problems; and (3) to help them develop a framework for defining, generating, evaluating, and implementing effective solutions to problems. This module occupies the final four to five sessions of FFT, and usually begins by the 4th or 5th month, when sessions have been tapered to biweekly. Problem solving is positioned last in FFT, because the patient is usually in remission by this point and is more able, both cognitively and emotionally, to experiment with new ways of behaving. Furthermore, if the psychoeducation and CET have gone well, family members are more ready to see their own role in generating or maintaining family conflicts.

In problem solving, families are taught to break broad problems down into smaller units that are more amenable to solution. Family members are given a problem-solving worksheet in which they are asked to take the following steps: define the problem (with each participant's input); "brainstorm" all possible solutions without evaluating them; consider each solution individually and weigh its advantages and disadvantages; choose a best solution or combination of solutions; and plan and implement the chosen solutions. Once they have had at least a moderately successful experience in solving a relatively minor problem, participants are given a homework task in which they record their attempts to solve a new, larger problem. Assignments are sometimes quite modest; some families are simply given the task of defining one or more problems to work on in the upcoming session.

The rationale for problem solving is presented as follows:

"Up until now, we've been talking mainly about how you communicate with each other. Now we'd like to deal with some of the concrete problems of living you've all been alluding to. But rather than our just giving you suggestions about what to do about these—which probably wouldn't work that well anyway—we'd like to teach you a way of solving problems cooperatively, as a family." (Miklowitz & Goldstein, 1997, p. 240)

This rationale is then followed by a review of the steps for solving problems and familiarizing the family or couple with a problem-solving worksheet. The clinician also reviews some of the problems the members raised during earlier phases of treatment.

Consider this case example of the problem-solving method. Karla, age 35, moved in with her new boyfriend, Taki, shortly after her divorce. She was in poor shape financially; she had a tendency to "spend to improve my self-esteem." In fact, most of her spending sprees occurred during hypomanic periods, and Karla had become hypomanic shortly after meeting Taki, who was quite well off. Perhaps due to his eagerness to make the relationship work, he gave Karla access to his credit cards. During their first months together, his bills increased hugely. Karla's own employment was inconsistent. She had had trouble for years keeping to a budget and maintaining a checking account. They had begun to fight heavily about this problem. Karla argued that money was his way of controlling women, and Taki argued that she was taking advantage of him and being inconsiderate.

First, the clinician returned to the communication enhancement exercises. He encouraged the couple to expand on these broader issues before zeroing in on the more specific problem of spending. Karla voiced her opinion about what she felt was the "meat of the problem," while Taki listened. Then Taki described his take on the underlying issues, while Karla listened and paraphrased. The structure imposed by problem solving eventually helped them define the issue more specifically: Karla spent more on clothing and "comfort items" than either of them thought she should, but it was unrealistic for her to try to support herself given her unresolved symptomatic state. Various options were then considered: Taki doing most of the buying, Karla being assigned her own account with an upper limit negotiated each month, and the two of them simply separating their finances. Each of these and other options were evaluated as to their advantages and disadvantages. Finally, they agreed on a somewhat complicated but clever solution: Karla was to obtain three bank debit cards assigned to each of three accounts. Each card was labeled with an expense item (e.g., "doctor bills") and had a spending limit posted on it. They were to meet weekly to determine whether the solution was working, and to practice listening skills with each other when they began to disagree.

In this example, the problem was to some degree generated by the patient's residual symptoms. There were also underlying relationship dynamics: Karla tended to become overly dependent on men and then to devalue them, and Taki tended to rescue women and then become angry about being in the rescuer role. The clinician decided to let them first "ventilate" about these larger relationship themes. Allowing a certain amount of emotional expression about loaded issues often reduces a family's or couple's resistance to dealing with more specific problems (in this case, disagreements about spending).

When taking families or couples through their first problem-solving exercises, FFT clinicians monitor the participants' reactions to the method. Reactions can vary from "This is just what we need" to "Gee, how superficial." Patients with bipolar disorder and their family members seem to crave spontaneity and enjoy fast-paced, unpredictable interchanges. They get bored easily. The communication and problem-solving exercises impose structure, which, although encouraging the family to maintain goal-directedness, sometimes generates resistance. This can take the form of changing the subject, "cross-complaining," or being unwilling to cooperate with the homework tasks.

When addressing resistances, a clinician reiterates the rationale for problem solving (e.g., "Sometimes you have to gain confidence from solving minor problems before you move on to bigger ones"). But often he or she must determine whether it is really the problem-solving method that family members object to or whether there are certain costs or painful consequences associated with attempting to solve a problem (e.g., a mother's fear that her son with bipolar disorder will be unable to handle agreed-upon tasks that require greater independence). Families who fear the consequences of solving a problem often approach solutions, then quickly abandon the problem-solving process, arguing that "this is not really the issue." The therapist has a number of options available. One is to take responsibility for the unsolved problem. For example, he or she can say, "Perhaps it was wrong of me to encourage you to solve this problem. Maybe you have other things you want to deal with first. Would you like to table it for now?" Alternatively, the clinician may proceed more paradoxically, framing the family's difficulty as due to "healthy avoidance":

"Solving a problem as a family involves some cost–benefit thinking. There are certainly some benefits to solving this problem, but there may be some hidden costs as well. I think if the costs of solving this problem outweigh the benefits, it's certainly understandable that you'd want to avoid putting a solution in place. Is that what's happening here?"

Both of these interventions give the family members "permission" to leave the problem untouched. Later, when the pressure is off, they may be able to return to the problem and have more success the second time around.

Terminating FFT

FFT is usually terminated after 9 months. As the termination of treatment approaches, a therapist reviews with the family members the six goals for treatment (discussed earlier) and the degree to which those goals were or were not realized. The status of the patient's bipolar disorder is evaluated relative to the beginning of treatment. In some cases, maintenance or "tune-up" FFT sessions are recommended.

Referrals for subsequent treatment for both the patient and other family members are discussed. For example, some patients follow up FFT with individual therapy or mutual support groups involving other persons with bipolar disorder. Family members may choose to attend support groups of the Depressive and Bipolar Support Alliance (*www.ndmda.org*) or the National Alliance for the Mentally Ill (*www.nami.org*). In our experience, it is unusual for families to request additional family or couple therapy after FFT, but referrals are made, if requested.

The clinicians reiterates the importance of continued medication compliance and incorporation of communication and problem-solving skills into the family's day-to-day life. Finally, a review of the relapse drill (see the earlier "Psychoeducation" section) is conducted: The patient's prodromal signs are reviewed, and the steps the patient and family can take to avert a relapse are reiterated.

CASE STUDY

Debra, a 36-year-old European American woman, lived with her husband Barry, age 46, and their 8-year-old daughter Jill. She had completed 2 years of college and worked part time as a sales clerk in a luggage shop. She had been married previously. Debra was referred for FFT by a university clinic, where she had been diagnosed with bipolar II disorder. The initial SCID confirmed this diagnosis. Her depression was marked by loss of interests and "being bummed" for several weeks at a time. She also complained of loss of appetite, waking several times each night, fatigue, guilt, and loss of concentration. She denied having suicidal thoughts. She recounted that her current depression was "a really big one" and had lasted on and off for a full year. Debra also said, "I've had tons of small ones." She dated the first onset of her depression to approximately 8 years earlier, following her divorce.

Debra also admitted to having had hypomania in the previous month, including about 5 days of elevated and irritable mood. She explained, "My confidence level was up." She admitted to racing thoughts, increased activity and talkativeness, and becoming involved in many different projects. She had trouble dating the onset and offset of these periods, noting, "I've been this way all my life." She did admit that Barry had commented on these mood phases. Debra complained, "He now tells me I'm getting manic every time we get in an argument. . . . It's his newest weapon against me." She denied having delusions or hallucinations.

Debra had been treated previously with sertraline (Zoloft) and bupropion (Wellbutrin). Her psychiatrist had recently started her on divalproex sodium (Depakote) at 1,500 mg/day, a medication that she said had made a difference in stabilizing her mood.

Barry, an attorney, presented as a "nononsense" type of man. He responded to the clinicians in a very businesslike manner and insisted that he had no problems of his own to discuss "except those that relate to Debra's care." He denied any psychiatric history himself. He preferred to talk about FFT as an educational course and became defensive if his wife referred to it as "therapy." The clinicians did not dissuade him from labeling the treatment this way, believing that they would need to work on building a rapport with him before addressing his defensive style.

Family Assessment

Based on the Camberwell Family Interview, a staff member of the Colorado Family Project determined that Barry met the criteria for a high level of EE. He voiced nine criticisms during his 1-hour interview. He tended to complain at length about Debra's memory, work habits, and disorganization (e.g., "She never remembers about parent–teacher meetings," "She forgets to turn in her time sheet at work"). He admitted that he still loved her but found her very frustrating. He was convinced that she had attention-deficit/hyperactivity disorder, as well as bipolar disorder.

Debra and Barry came in for the family interactional assessment well dressed and smiling. The research staff interviewed them individually, and arrived at an important problem topic for them to discuss: Barry's claim that Debra lied to him. Her response was to apologize for her past misdeeds and to argue, "I'm not lying or withholding . . . those are usually things I've forgotten or just don't think are important." Upon discussing this issue, the couple's dynamics became apparent, with Barry speaking in an accusatory, scolding mode and Debra apologizing for and justifying her behavior. As Barry became more accusatory, Debra looked more and more depressed.

BARRY: Lying is a way of life for you. You twist the truth and say you don't remember things.

DEBRA: But I really don't. I've been trying to tell you everything. Sometimes I just forget. (*Starts rocking chair.*)

BARRY: (*holding her chair still*) Why do you think it's OK to lie to me?

DEBRA: I don't. I'm being up front with you. Maybe you want to believe there's more, but there's not.

BARRY: I think you'll always do this. It's your bag. How would you like it if I lied to you? How would it make you feel? Would you want to stay married to me?

DEBRA: (*sullen*) No, probably not. But I'm trying to be open with my feelings, kinda with you as a practice case. (*Smiles awkwardly.*)

BARRY: You're doing that little smile again. The one you do when you're trying to get away with something.

DEBRA: (*defensive*) Oh, give me a break.

BARRY: Is it because we're talking so directly? I don't know if it's your personality or if it's the bipolar stuff acting up, but you have no tolerance for anything these days, especially people.

The therapists who viewed this assessment were struck by Barry's level of criticism, paired with Debra's tendency to take a one-down position. They also learned during the assessment that Barry doled out Debra's medications and made her doctor appointments for her, and also usually attended them with her. An initial appointment for FFT was set with two project clinicians, a man and a woman.

Psychoeducation (Sessions 1–7)

During the initial session, the clinicians (Therapist 1 and Therapist 2 in the dialogues below) described the FFT program to Barry and Debra, with particular emphasis on the psychoeducational component. They previewed the communication enhancement and problem-solving modules. The couple listened politely but expressed skepticism.

BARRY: We've been in and out of therapy for years. I haven't been impressed.

THERAPIST 1: When you say "We," do you mean you as a couple?

BARRY: As a couple, and she's had her own therapy.

DEBRA: I thought Dr. Walker was good.

BARRY: Yeah, but you hadn't had the bipolar diagnosis yet. She was just treating you for depression. And she got into that whole "You were probably abused as a child" thing.

THERAPIST 1: What was your couple therapy like?

BARRY: A lot of digging into our childhoods and getting in touch with our feelings.

THERAPIST 1: Debra?

DEBRA: It wasn't that bad. I thought it was pretty useful.

THERAPIST 1: Well, it sounds like you've got different opinions on how helpful those things were. Let me tell you how this will be different. Our treatment is going to be focused mainly on the present, and we'll be working with you on how you as a couple are coping with bipolar disorder. Barry, you're going to be affected by the cycling of Debra's mood disorder, but Debra, you're also going to be affected by the way Barry responds to your symptoms. I'm not saying your past will be irrelevant, but it's just not our focus.

BARRY: I need help dealing with all of this. The more information I get, the better.

THERAPIST 1: I'm sure that's true. But we won't just throw a lot of information at you—we want to individualize it to your situation. I think you'll have a much easier time if you come to a common understanding of the disorder as a couple and learn to communicate about it.

In this dialogue, the therapist made a distinction between FFT and more generic forms of couple therapy. At this point, the clinicians already suspected that there would be resistance from Barry, especially around tasks in which he was asked to look at his own behavior and its contribution to Debra's mood problems.

The psychoeducation itself began in the second session and continued through the seventh. The first task was to encourage the couple to come to a shared definition of bipolar disorder. During the assessments, both had mentioned the term "cycling," but without apparent agreement on what it meant.

THERAPIST 1: I want to be sure we're all on the same page when we discuss the meaning of the term "bipolar." Let's start by reviewing your symptoms, Debra. (*Passes around a handout describing the symptoms of mania and depression.*) Barry, which of these have you observed when Debra gets hypomanic?

BARRY: (*surveying the handout*) Well, all of these except appetite disturbance. . . . I guess you could say she has grandioseness—she thinks one day she'll be wealthy. (*Laughs.*)

THERAPIST 2: When was the last time you think she was like that?

BARRY: Last time I was working on a case—she always gets like that when I'm working on a case.

DEBRA: I agree, but I think it's because I have a lot more to do when he's working all the time. . . . he thinks it's some "abandonment" thing, but I think he forgets the realities I face when he's gone. (*Looks at list.*) I get more energy, I feel uncomfortable in my own body, I jump outta my skin . . . probably a good day to go shopping! (*Giggles.*) I probably get crankier, don't have much tolerance for people in general.

BARRY: Especially me. (*Smiles.*)

This was the first time that Debra had defended herself, by commenting on how relationship problems fed into her mood swings. Interestingly, her assertive stance cut through some of her husband's negativity. The therapists soon realized that Barry and Debra lacked a consensus about what really constituted a bipolar episode. This is a critical point in FFT: The members of a couple or family need to come to a shared perception of when the patient is getting ill, so that they can institute procedures to keep the patient's episodes from spiraling (e.g., visits to the physician, reduction in the patient's workload, learning to deescalate negative verbal exchanges). But it was not yet clear that Debra had discrete episodes.

THERAPIST 2: Do you think you have what we're calling "episodes"? Like a couple of days of being wired?

DEBRA: There can be, like 2 or 3 days when I can do a lot of stuff, my memory gets better, and then 2 or 3 days when it's just not gonna work. I can . . .

BARRY: (*Interrupts.*) It's that household project thing. She starts redoing Jill's room over and over. She'll sponge-paint it purple and then wipe it out that same evening, put in new closets.

DEBRA: I can filter all my energy into housework instead of killing somebody. (*They both chuckle.*)

THERAPIST 1: Maybe I'm a little slow today, but I'm trying to figure out whether you both agree when these high and low periods are. Debra, have you ever kept a mood chart?

The therapist then produced a written assignment in which Debra and Barry were asked to track independently, on a daily basis, the ups and downs of Debra's mood states, so that agreements and disagreements about what constituted the symptoms of the disorder (as opposed to personality traits) could be tracked.

The dynamics of this couple became more evident in Sessions 3–5. Debra was inconsistent about keeping her mood chart, and Barry felt that his conscientiousness in charting her mood was not being rewarded. "She won't take responsibility for her illness," he argued. Nonetheless, Debra had good recall of her mood swings, even though she had not written them

down. The therapists offered the couple much praise for their somewhat halfhearted attempt to complete this assignment. Interestingly, Barry noted small changes in mood that he called "mania," which Debra argued were just her reactions to everyday annoyances.

BARRY: You were manic as hell on Saturday morning.

THERAPIST 2: What do you mean, Barry?

BARRY: I went to tell her that Jill needed to get to soccer, and she practically bit my head off!

DEBRA: Because you had told me eight times already. I wasn't manic, I was just getting annoyed. Even Jill said something about you overdoing it.

This became a theme throughout the treatment: Barry tended to overlabel Debra's mood swings, to the extent that he often called her "manic" when the real issue appeared to be her transient irritability. He also called her "depressed," whereas Debra claimed she was just "relaxing . . . bored . . . trying to unwind and keep to myself for a while." The therapists were careful not to attribute blame or to tell either of them that he or she was right. One therapist said:

"I think this is a very hard distinction to make. I wish I could give you a simple rule for determining when Debra is in and out of an episode. But as you've seen, it's not always so clear. I usually suggest that people go back to that symptom list and ask, 'Is there more than one of these symptoms? Does irritability go with more sleep disturbance? Racing thoughts?' Just being annoyed is not enough to be called 'manic,' unless it's ongoing, it cuts across different situations, or it goes along with some of these other symptoms and impairment in getting through your day."

The therapists outlined a vulnerability–stress model for understanding Debra's episodes. Debra recounted a family history of depression in her mother and alcohol abuse in her father: "My mom was probably bipolar, but we just didn't call it that back then." They also discussed stress triggers that may have contributed to Debra's prior depressions. Barry became very vocal when discussing her risk factors: He noted that crowded places (e.g., shopping malls) made her hypomanic, and that alcohol, even in small amounts, contributed to her sleep disturbance, which in turn contributed to her hypomanias. The therapists offered a handout on risk factors (e.g., substance abuse, sleep irregularity, unpredictable daily routines, family conflict, and provocative interpersonal situations) and protective factors (e.g., regular medications, good family communication, making use of treatment resources). Next, the therapists helped Barry and Debra devise a relapse prevention plan:

THERAPIST 1: The clients we've worked with who've done best with this illness have been able to rely on their spouses and other close family members at times of crisis. It's a fine line you have to walk between being able to turn to your spouse and say, "I think I'm getting sick again," and to take some of their advice without giving up control altogether. (to Debra) When your moods are going up and down, you are going to want more control. Barry, maybe you sometimes feel like you're walking a fine line as well: You want to say "Yes, you are getting sick, and I'd like to help you," without rubbing it in, to be able to give suggestions without taking over.

BARRY: That's one thing we have in common. We're both control freaks. I guess likes attract.

THERAPIST 1: Well, maybe the fact that you both like to be in control of your own fate was part of what attracted the two of you in the first place [reframing]. But like many things that attract people initially, something like not wanting to give up control can become a problem in the relationship later.

The couple came to some agreements about what the prodromal signs of Debra's hypomania looked like (e.g., increased interest in household projects, getting up extraordinarily early, irritability that occurred in multiple situations) and some of her triggers (e.g., alcohol). They conjointly developed a relapse prevention plan that involved keeping emergency phone numbers handy, avoiding alcohol, and avoiding high-stress, provocative interpersonal situations (e.g., conflicts between Debra and her mother). Barry and Debra also discussed how they could communicate if her symptoms started to escalate. Barry admitted that he "had

to learn not to lash out" at such times, and not to "just blurt out everything I think." Interestingly, both showed resistance to the suggestion that Debra try to maintain a regular sleep–wake cycle, even on weekends, when she had her worst mood swings. Barry scoffed, "Maybe we should just join the Army," and both emphasized that they were not about to give up their love of late-night partying.

The psychoeducation module ended with a discussion of the effects of the "illness" label on Debra's self-esteem. She had been alluding throughout the first six sessions to her discomfort with the diagnosis of bipolar II disorder.

THERAPIST 1: Sometimes when we go through our symptom lists and talk about the causes of bipolar disorder, people can feel labeled or picked apart. Debra, have you ever felt that way in here?

DEBRA: When I first came in here, I felt picked on. I felt like it was "blame Debbie time," and now there was this real biological reason to pin all our problems on.

THERAPIST 1: I hope you don't think we're saying that all of your problems as a couple stem from your bipolar disorder.

DEBRA: No, I think you guys have been fair about that. It was hard for me to talk about, and sometimes I think Barry is just objecting to me, as a person.

THERAPIST 1: In other words, the line between your personality and your disorder gets blurred.

DEBRA: Yes, and to me they're very different.

THERAPIST 1: I'm glad you're bringing this up. I think that's very important, to be very clear on when we're just talking about you, your styles of relating to people. . . . Not everything you do has to be reduced to this illness.

BARRY: And I probably do bring it up [the illness] too much.

DEBRA: (becoming activated) Yes, and you bring it up in front of other people. . . . That can be a real problem for me. We used to have such great conversations! I get tired of talking with you about my bipolar disorder all the time. That's all you seem to wanna talk about.

BARRY: (startled) Why haven't you told me this?

DEBRA: I probably do need to tell you. . . . I just

want more of a happy medium, between talking about it and not.

BARRY: So what do you want?

DEBRA: I'm not sure.

THERAPIST 1: I think it's understandable that you wouldn't know. . . . You're not always sure how much help you need from Barry. Maybe you're trying to find a good balance. That may take some time. I hope you don't feel that all *we're* interested in is your bipolar disorder, and not in you as a person [examines apparent resistance to the psychoeducational material].

DEBRA: I usually don't feel that way, except when I try to do that mood chart [acknowledges emotional pain underlying resistance to the therapeutic tasks]. I just want to have conversations with Barry like I have with my girlfriends. I'd like to talk about things other than my illness and my doctors.

Communication Enhancement Training (Sessions 8–14)

During Session 8, the therapists introduced CET to the couple. Barry and Debra both described a "demand–withdrawal" pattern in their communication. Barry would become intrusive in trying to understand Debra's mood state, and Debra would withdraw and become noncooperative. Debra admitted that she had a difficult time acknowledging being depressed and talking about it, because "you just didn't do that in my family." She grew up in a Southern family, where "you didn't air your dirty laundry." In contrast, Barry was from Los Angeles, where "you might spill your guts to whoever was stuck in traffic next to you."

The therapists began by exploring the demand–withdrawal pattern:

THERAPIST 1: This is one of the dynamics we've seen in couples dealing with bipolar disorder. People with the disorder can get irritable with their spouses, and then their spouses react because they feel under attack, and when they react, the arguments can really spiral. The person with the disorder feels there's something he or she is legitimately angry about, and the husband or wife sees the anger as evidence of the bipolar illness.

BARRY: Well, my problem is that Debra's not aware of her symptoms.

DEBRA: I'm aware of them, but I wanna be left alone. You finish my sentences . . .

BARRY: And then you walk out of the room. You don't want to have anything to do with normal communication. It's just like it was with your parents . . .

DEBRA: When I'm in that state [depression], the last thing I want is a serious conversation or to have someone question what I want to do or why.

THERAPIST 2: Let's talk about what happens between the two of you [draws couple back to relationship focus]. When you try to talk about something, what happens? One of you just won't talk? You do talk, but it doesn't go well?

BARRY: She procrastinates, she won't deal with things; then I yell; then she won't be around me and she withdraws; and then I start thinking about how long I can live like this.

THERAPIST 2: Debra, how would you describe it?

DEBRA: Barry gets frustrated when I don't give him the answers he's looking for, and then I feel bad that I frustrated him, and he feels bad that he got upset at me, and then I feel bad that I made him feel bad about upsetting me.

THERAPIST 2: Is that something you'd like to work on—your communication as a couple?

BARRY: Yes. There's been no communication because of the bipolar disorder. I don't know if we'd have these problems if she weren't bipolar. She gets depressed, her thoughts don't get communicated, she never even tries . . . and that reminds me of what I was gonna ask you: Do you think she might have attention deficit disorder as well as being bipolar?

DEBRA: Oh, no, here we go . . .

THERAPIST 1: Barry, no one can tell for sure, but regardless of what the cause is, it sounds like you're ready for us to start focusing more on your relationship [redirects discussion but doesn't directly challenge Barry's definition of the problem]. At least part of what you're describing sounds like the habits you have communicating with each other as a couple. We'll be teaching you some fairly straightforward skills for talking to each other, like how to praise each other for things done well, how to listen, and how to ask for changes in each others' behavior.

This will help you during these cycles, whether they be real mood cycles or just rocky periods in your relationship [provides rationale for upcoming communication module].

DEBRA: Yeah, I need to learn how to argue. He's a lawyer; he's a much better arguer than me.

BARRY: (*still angry*) But you see, no one ever said a damn thing in your family; no one was ever really there. So of course you're going to react to me because I'm passionate, and then when I get really pissed off, you finally take stock and listen. It's the only way I can get through to you.

THERAPIST 1: I think there's a lot for us to work with here. I'd like to take you (*to Debra*) off the "bipolar hook" for a while, and let's work on how you act and react with each other. We don't have to work on your communication just about bipolar disorder—maybe also how you talk about finances, friends . . .

BARRY: But that's all about doing it in here. . . . How are you gonna know how we communicate at home?

THERAPIST 1: We're gonna bug your house. (*All laugh.*) We'll do some exercises in here that involve role playing new ways of talking, but you'll have to practice these new ways in between sessions at home. I personally think this will benefit you a great deal, if you have the time to do it [expresses optimism].

The therapists now had a better understanding of this couple's communication patterns. The demand–withdrawal pattern in part derived from their different family histories, but it was equally true that Barry was rewarded for being critical; it got results, even if these results were accompanied by Debra's resentment. They disagreed on the extent to which these communication patterns were driven by her bipolar disorder. Barry assumed that most or all of their problems could be attributed to the disorder, but Debra saw this assumption as just an attempt to blame her for everything. The therapists' take was that the marital dynamics existed independently of Debra's mood swings but became magnified by her hypomanic and depressive episodes. During hypomanic episodes she was more touchy and reactive, and when depressed she was more likely to withdraw.

In Session 9, the therapists began the skills training. FFT begins with positive communication skills to increase the likelihood that members of a couple or family will collaborate when dealing with more difficult issues. One therapist began by introducing a handout entitled Expressing Positive Feelings, in which each partner is directed simply to praise the other for some specific behavior the other has performed, and to tell the partner how this behavior makes him/her feel. The therapists first modeled the skill. One of them praised Barry, saying, "I appreciate you taking the long drive up here [to the clinic] and making an adjustment to your schedule to make this possible. . . . It makes me feel like you value what we do here." Barry expressed appreciation for the compliment. The therapist then asked Barry and Debra to turn their chairs toward each other and select a behavior to praise in each other. Interestingly, neither had trouble selecting a topic. The problem was in staying with positive emotions and not letting negative ones leak in.

BARRY: I appreciated your taking Jill to soccer on Wednesday. It made me feel like you . . . like you knew I was overwhelmed that day, and that, you know, I'm usually the one doing all the parenting while you . . .

THERAPIST 2: (*interrupting*) Barry, I'd like to stop you before we get into that. Debra, can you tell me what you liked so far about how Barry said that? Did he follow the instructions on this sheet?

DEBRA: Well, like you said, he was starting to get into it, but I liked the first part. I'm glad he feels that way.

BARRY: Do you feel I give you enough positive feedback?

DEBRA: (*pause*) You have your days.

THERAPIST 2: Barry, I thought you did that pretty well. Could you try it without the tail at the end?

BARRY: (*Chuckles.*) There you go, stealing my thunder. OK, um, Deb, thanks again for taking Jill to soccer. It made me feel like you . . . like my schedule is important to you, and that you're thinking of me.

THERAPIST 2: Good. Debra, what'd you think?

DEBRA: Much better.

BARRY: Sometimes I think I was put on this earth to learn tact.

Sessions 10 and 11 of CET focused on active listening skills. One member of the couple listened while the other spoke, first about issues outside of the marriage (i.e., work relationships), then about couple-related matters. Both Barry and Debra required restructuring of their listening skills. Specifically, Debra tended to "space out" when Barry spoke, and required prompting to stay with the issues. She acknowledged that she sometimes felt she was being tested by Barry when he talked to her, to determine whether she could come up with thoughtful, intuitive replies. Her "checking out" was a way of coping with the performance anxiety that she experienced when listening to him.

Not surprisingly, Barry's difficulty with listening centered on withholding his natural tendency to give advice. When Debra began to talk, he would listen reflectively for a minute or two, but then he would begin to ask questions such as "Well, when are you gonna call that person?" or "Last time we talked you said you were going to finish that resumé. Why haven't you?" Repeated practice within sessions— supplemented by homework assignments to practice these skills—led Barry to become more aware of what he was doing. During a particularly poignant moment, he admitted, "I don't like the way I react to her. . . . I don't like the person I'm becoming."

As FFT passed the 3-month point and the frequency changed to biweekly, the clinicians introduced potentially more heated forms of communication, such as making requests for changes in each other's behaviors and expressing negative feelings (Sessions 12–14). At this point, Debra was not as depressed as she had been during the assessment phase, although Barry continued to complain about her low functioning. He argued that she had become unable to tell him what she had and had not accomplished during the day, and that she often made it appear that she had done things that, in reality, she had not. He labeled this her "lack of follow-through" problem. In contrast, Debra became increasingly assertive about his "micromanagement" of her behavior.

THERAPIST 1: One of the things we'd like to work on with you is how you ask each other to change in some way. What's an appropriate way to ask someone to help you? (*Gives Barry and Debra the handout titled Making a Positive Request.*) Try looking directly at each other; tell each other what you would like to see done differently, and how it would make you feel. Debra, a minute ago you were talking about how Barry micromanages you. Can you turn this into a positive—ask him what you would like him to do? Phrase it in a way that he can help you? How can he ask you to follow through without nagging you?

DEBRA: Uh, Barry, it would really make me happy if you . . . in situations where there's a dilemma, if you'd give me a little more freedom.

BARRY: For example? Do you mean you want us to do things at your pace?

THERAPIST 1: Barry, let it come from her.

DEBRA: Um, like, if there's some shopping to do, it would help me out if I could just say, "Yes, this is on my list and I'll do it . . . if you could wait for me to get it done in my own time." That would help ease the tension.

THERAPIST 2: Barry, how did you feel about how Debra asked you? Did she follow this sheet?

BARRY: I think she asked me just fine, but my question is, will she then do the shopping?

DEBRA: I think it would really help me to have some plan—like agreeing that if I do this part of the shopping, you'll do that part. Maybe that would stop me from saying, "I'll show him. He's not gonna run my life; I'm not gonna do it his way."

THERAPIST 1: A person who feels one-down often reacts by refusing to go along with the plan, even though going along with it might be of help to them personally. Debra, do you get into that sometimes?

The therapists were encouraging assertiveness in Debra, and at the same time gently confronting what Barry had earlier called her "passive–aggressiveness." They then moved on to Barry and asked him to make a positive request of Debra.

THERAPIST 2: Barry, can you think of something you could ask Debra to do, to change her behavior?

BARRY: (*looking at clinicians*) OK, Deb, it's very important to me . . .

THERAPIST 2: Can you tell this to her?

BARRY: (*turns toward Debra*) OK, it's very important to me that you not just walk away when we have discussions. That you don't just withdraw. Especially when we talk about Jill and our differences about her. That really irritates me.

The therapists at this point again observed Debra withdraw in reaction to Barry's "high-EE" behavior. They addressed this by commenting on her reactions.

THERAPIST 1: Debra, what's happening now? You seem like you're checking out.

DEBRA: (*Snaps back, smiles.*) Yeah, I guess I am. What were we talking about?

BARRY: You see, I think that's part of her attention deficit disorder. Do you think she needs Ritalin [medication for this condition]?

THERAPIST 1: Barry, in this case, I don't think so. I think that what happened, Debra, if I can speak for you for a moment, is that you withdrew because you felt you were under attack.

DEBRA: That's probably true. He got into his "You do this, you do that."

BARRY: (*frustrated*) Well, you just asked me to change something! Am I supposed to do all the work here?

THERAPIST 1: Barry, I'm going to encourage you to try again. Only this time, I'd like you to be more aware of how you phrase things. Notice you said what you didn't want her to do—withdraw when you were talking to her. That's quite important. But what would you like her to do instead?

BARRY: I want her to engage with me! To talk it out!

THERAPIST 1: Can you try again, only this time tell her what you want her to do?

BARRY: (*Sighs.*) Deb, when we talk, I'd really like . . . I'd really appreciate it if you'd hang in there and finish talking to me, especially about Jill. That would make me feel, I don't know, like we're partners.

THERAPIST 2: Barry, that was much better, and I'll bet it was easier to hear. Debra?

DEBRA: Yeah, I liked it . . . that's easier. We need to do more of this.

Much emphasis was placed throughout CET on between-session homework assignments. The couple was strongly encouraged to hold weekly meetings and to record efforts on homework sheets. Both spouses reported a reduction in tension in the relationship by the time problem solving was initiated.

Problem Solving (Sessions 15–18)

FFT sessions were held less frequently (biweekly) in the 4th, 5th, and 6th months. At Session 15, problem solving was introduced. After explaining the rationale, the therapists asked the couple to identify several specific problems for discussion, then reviewed the problem-solving steps with them.

The first issue chosen by the couple seemed superficial at first. They had two cats, one of which belonged to Debra (and had come with her from a previous marriage) and the other of which Barry had bought. They disagreed on how much the cats should be fed: Debra "wanted mine to be fat" and fed it frequently, whereas Barry wanted his to be thin. As a result, Barry's cat was waking them up in the middle of the night, needing to be fed. The resulting changes in Debra's sleep–wake cycles had resulted in her becoming irritable, restless, and possibly hypomanic. Despite a conscientious literature search, the therapists were unable to find any research on the influence of cat diets on the cycling of bipolar disorder.

The couple considered various alternatives: feeding the cats equal amounts, keeping Barry's cat in the garage, giving away Barry's cat, and feeding both cats before the couple went to bed. They eventually settled on the last of these. The problem itself generated humor and playfulness between them, and they derived some satisfaction from being able to deal with it collaboratively.

A second and potentially more serious source of conflict concerned their night life. Both liked going to parties, but Barry liked to stay longer than Debra. Debra, who that parties contributed to her mood cycling. She tended to become overstimulated by the interactions with many people and would quickly become fatigued. They considered these alternatives: going to the parties in separate cars, Barry agreeing to leave earlier, Debra going to the car and sleeping when she felt tired, and Debra taking a cab home. They eventually decided to discuss and agree upon a departure time before going to a party.

The couple was able to apply the problem-solving method successfully to other issues, such as paying the bills and helping Jill get to her afterschool activities. They continued to have trouble breaking problems down into smaller chunks, and tended to "cross-complain" or bring up larger problems in the middle of trying to solve smaller ones. Barry often complained, "We aren't dealing with the source of these problems, which is her bipolar disorder. We wouldn't have these problems if she weren't bipolar." Again, the therapists did not challenge his definition of the problem, but they continued to offer the message that regardless of whether the source of the problems lay in Debra, the couple still needed to work collaboratively to generate acceptable compromises.

Termination (Sessions 19–21)

By 7 months, Debra, whose depression had largely remitted, had obtained a new job working in sales at a clothing store. The therapists began the termination phase of treatment, which focused on reviewing what the couple had taken away from the psychoeducation, CET, and problem-solving skills training modules. Both reported that their relationship had improved, and that they "occasionally" used the communication skills at home. The therapists commented on how far they had come and encouraged them to pick a time each week to keep rehearsing one or more of the skills.

Barry was not entirely convinced of Debra's clinical improvement, however. In one of the final sessions, he returned to the issue of Debra's symptoms and her "unwillingness" to follow through on tasks such as cooking, depositing her paycheck, cleaning Jill's clothes, and doing other tasks they had agreed she would perform. The following interchange ensued:

BARRY: (*Laughs.*) I had this dream the other night that I was getting married, and I knew that I was marrying Debra, but I couldn't see her face, and I wasn't sure it was really her. And I wasn't sure if I should be there.

THERAPIST 1: And you were standing in front of everyone wearing your pajamas as well.

BARRY: (*Laughs.*) Yeah, and I was about to take the exam that I hadn't studied for. But really, sometimes I feel like she's not the same person, especially when she doesn't want to follow through on things we've talked about.

THERAPIST 1: Let me give you some perspective on this. I think a dilemma many spouses face is "Should I stick it out with my husband or my wife, or should I leave and take care of me?" There are certainly people who do that, who leave, and then there are many others who hang out and wait for things to get better, which in fact they often do.

BARRY: And I think things have gotten better.

DEBRA: I think so. I don't know why you're being so negative.

BARRY: Well, if you . . .

THERAPIST 1: (*Interrupts.*) Let me finish this thought. Barry, I think it's critical for you to make a distinction in your own mind between what Debra can and can't control. That's sometimes vague between the two of you. When you say she doesn't want to follow through, that certainly sounds like an intentional behavior—something she's doing to hurt you or annoy you. Debra, do the problems with following through ever feel like they're about problems with your concentration? Your attention or your memory?

DEBRA: (*nodding emphatically*) Absolutely! If you could get him to realize that, we'd be a lot farther along.

BARRY: That memory stuff—is that her bipolar disorder or her attention deficit disorder?

THERAPIST 1: I'm not sure that's really the question. That's just a diagnostic distinction, and I'm not sure my answering one way or the other will help you. Maybe what you're really wondering is whether these problems are controllable by her or not. If I were in your position, the things that would really anger me would be those things I thought she was doing intentionally.

BARRY: Yeah, and I don't always think about that.

THERAPIST 1: If I thought what she was doing was due to a biochemical imbalance, I might be more patient, more sympathetic—in the same way that if someone had a broken leg and had trouble walking up stairs, I might have more sympathy than if I thought she was deliberately trying to hold me up.

In this segment, the therapist was addressing directly what he felt was a major source of Barry's critical attitudes toward Debra: the belief that many of her negative behaviors were controllable and intentional (see Hooley & Licht, 1997; Miklowitz et al., 1998). In some instances, Barry may have been right about Debra's motivations. But questioning the controllability of her symptoms forced him to consider a different set of causal explanations for her behavior. The distinction between controllable and uncontrollable behavior is a key point in the psychoeducational treatment of families of patients with bipolar disorder.

Barry and Debra's Progress

After completing FFT, Debra continued to have mild periods of depression despite her adherence to medication. Her depressions were unpleasant but not so severe that she was unable to keep her job or attend to her parenting duties. Her brief hypomanic periods sometimes caused arguments between Debra and Barry but were not debilitating. Barry and Debra were communicating better, and both agreed that Barry was more patient and less critical of her. But Debra frequently found herself reacting with the line from the now famous movie, "What if this is as good as it gets?" Although she was functional, she expressed chagrin that she could not have the life she had wanted—a successful career, a more intimate relationship with her husband, more friendships, an easier relationship with her daughter, and more financial success. The reality of her disorder and its psychosocial effects were difficult for her to accept. However, Debra felt that FFT had been helpful, as was her medication, which she showed no inclination to discontinue. The therapists offered her a referral for individual or group therapy, but Debra decided to forgo further psychosocial treatment for the time being.

CONCLUSIONS

Family psychoeducational treatment appears to be a useful adjunct to pharmacotherapy. However, not all patients with bipolar disorder have families, and individual approaches such as those of Frank and colleagues (2005) are im-

portant alternatives to consider. The finding that mood-stabilizing medications are more powerful in alleviating manic than depressive symptoms, whereas the reverse appears true for psychotherapy, is an argument for combining medical and psychosocial interventions in the outpatient maintenance of bipolar disorder.

There is limited research on which families are the best candidates for FFT. Our exploratory analyses from one trial (Miklowitz et al., 2000) suggested that patients in high-EE families showed greater reductions in depression severity scores over 1 year than those in low-EE families. But reductions in bipolar relapses were observed in patients from both high- and low-EE families treated with FFT. Patients who are most symptomatic at the time of random assignment often benefit more from FFT than do those who are less symptomatic.

Our clinical observations also suggest that there are subgroups of patients who do not respond well to FFT. Specifically, patients who are unusually resistant to accepting the diagnosis of bipolar disorder often resent the educational focus of FFT. These patients usually see their troubles as having external origins (i.e., being mistreated by others) and resist interventions that require them to take more responsibility for their behavior. These same patients may also reject pharmacotherapy. Sadly, we have seen many patients require several hospitalizations before the reality of their disorder sets in.

A different kind of resistance originates from viewing the disorder as biologically based. Some patients prefer to limit their mental health contacts to visits with a psychiatrist for medication, and regard psychotherapy as irrelevant. We see nothing wrong with this position; a subset of patients does function well on medication only. Future research needs to determine whether this self-selected group is indeed different from patients who need psychotherapy, in terms of symptomatic, course-of-illness, or family/genetic variables.

Family members are sometimes a major source of resistance. Their reasons can include a desire to distance themselves from the patient (whom they may have tried to help for years without reward), time or distance constraints, or the discomfort of talking about family or couple issues in front of a stranger. More subtle is the fear of being blamed for the disorder (Hatfield, Spaniol, & Zipple, 1987). The family therapy movement has come a long way, but it still has its roots in a culture that faulted parents for causing mental illness. The theoretical model underlying FFT does not in any way link poor parenting to the onset of bipolar disorder. Nonetheless, a clinician often needs to make clear early in treatment that he or she does not adhere to this antiquated position.

FUTURE DIRECTIONS

Important future research will include effectiveness studies, which examine the clinical impact of psychotherapy as delivered to patients in "real-world" (typically community mental health) settings, by the clinicians who work in these settings and the time constraints within which they work. As explained earlier, FFT was found to be effective in stabilizing depression and maintaining wellness in the large-scale STEP-BD study of community effectiveness, which included therapists working in 15 outpatient sites (Miklowitz et al., 2007). It remains to be seen whether FFT, along with other treatments whose evidence-base includes STEP-BD (cognitive-behavioral therapy, interpersonal and social rhythm therapy), will be taken up by practicing clinicians.

A related problem is determining the proper structure of FFT. In many community settings, insurance companies only pay for six to eight sessions. FFT is rather time-intensive, and research is needed to determine which of its components predict the greatest proportion of variance in the outcome of participants. For example, it is possible that some families will benefit from just the psychoeducation module or just the communication module. Perhaps these modules could be streamlined without a great loss in treatment effect size. Ideally, decisions to modify treatments such as FFT will be based on clinical outcomes research rather than solely on the desire for cost containment.

A final research direction is the applicability of FFT and other psychotherapy treatments to child and adolescent patients with bipolar disorder, or even children who are genetically at risk for bipolar disorder and showing early prodromal signs. The fact that bipolar disorder even exists in these age groups is just now being recognized (Pavuluri, Birmaher, & Naylor, 2005); although there have been important developments, there are no currently accepted methods of psychosocial treatment (Kowatch et al., 2005). Whether the same diagnostic criteria that are applied to adults can be applied to children is a topic of some debate (Leibenluft et al., 2003; McClellan, 2005). If unrecognized, childhood-onset bipolar disorder can progress into the more severe forms of adult bipolar disorder (Leibenluft, Cohen, Gorrindo, Brook, & Pine, 2006; Sachs & Lafer, 1998). The addition of FFT to medication regimens in the early stages of the disorder may serve a protective function in the disorder's long-term course. Possibly the negative symptomatic and psychosocial outcomes of adult bipolar disorder can be mitigated through early detection and carefully planned preventive interventions.

ACKNOWLEDGMENTS

Preparation of this chapter was supported in part by National Institute of Mental Health Grant Nos. MH43931, MH55101, MH42556, MH62555, MH073871, and MH077856; a Distinguished Investigator Award from the National Association for Research on Schizophrenia and Depression; and a Faculty Fellowship from the University of Colorado's Council on Research and Creative Work.

REFERENCES

Akiskal, H. S. (1996). The prevalent clinical spectrum of bipolar disorders: Beyond DSM-IV. *Journal of Clinical Psychopharmacology, 16*(Suppl. 1), 4–14.

Akiskal, H. S., & Akiskal, K. (1992). Cyclothymic, hyperthymic, and depressive temperaments as subaffective variants of mood disorders. In A. Tasman & M. B. Riba (Eds.), *American Psychiatric Press review of psychiatry* (Vol. 11, pp. 43–62). Washington, DC: American Psychiatric Press.

Altshuler, L. L., Post, R. M., Leverich, G. S., Mikalauskas, K., Rosoff, A., & Ackerman, L. (1995). Antidepressant- induced mania and cycle acceleration: A controversy revisited. *American Journal of Psychiatry, 152*, 1130–1138.

American Psychiatric Association. (1980). *Diagnostic and statistical manual of mental disorders* (3rd ed.).Washington, DC: Author.

American Psychiatric Association. (1987). *Diagnostic and statistical manual of mental disorders* (3rd ed., rev.). Washington, DC: Author.

American Psychiatric Association. (1994a). *Diagnostic and statistical manual of mental disorders* (4th ed.). Washington, DC: Author.

American Psychiatric Association. (1994b). Practice guideline for the treatment of patients with bipolar disorder. *American Journal of Psychiatry, 12*(Suppl.), 1–36.

Baxter, L. R., Schwartz, J. M., Bergman, K. S., Szuba,

M. P., Guze, B. H. Mazziotta, J. C., et al. (1992). Caudate glucose metabolic rate changes with both drug and behavior therapy for obsessive–compulsive disorder. *Archives of General Psychiatry, 49,* 681–689.

Beigel, A., & Murphy, D. L. (1971). Differences in clinical characteristics accompanying depression in unipolar and bipolar affective illness. *Archives of General Psychiatry, 24,* 215–220.

Birmaher, B., Axelson, D., Strober, M., Gill, M. K., Valeri, S., Chiappetta, L., et al. (2006). Clinical course of children and adolescents with bipolar spectrum disorders. *Archives of General Psychiatry, 63*(2), 175–183.

Brewin, C. R., MacCarthy, B., Duda, K., & Vaughn, C. E. (1991). Attribution and expressed emotion in the relatives of patients with schizophrenia. *Journal of Abnormal Psychology, 100,* 546–554.

Brockington, I. F., Hillier, V. F., Francis, A. F., Helzer, J. E., & Wainwright, S. (1983). Definitions of mania: Concordance and prediction of outcome. *American Journal of Psychiatry, 140,* 435–439.

Butzlaff, R. L., & Hooley, J. M. (1998). Expressed emotion and psychiatric relapse: A meta-analysis. *Archives of General Psychiatry, 55,* 547–552.

Calabrese, J. R., Fatemi, S. H., Kujawa, M., & Woyshville, M. J. (1996). Predictors of response to mood stabilizers. *Journal of Clinical Psychopharmacology, 16*(Suppl. 1), 24–31.

Carpenter, D., Clarkin, J. F., Glick, I. D., & Wilner, P. J. (1995). Personality pathology among married adults with bipolar disorder. *Journal of Affective Disorders, 34,* 269–274.

Chambers, W. J., Puig-Antich, J., Hirsch, M., Paez, P., Ambrosini, P. J., Tabrizi, M. A., et al. (1985). The assessment of affective disorders in children and adolescents by semi-structured interview: Test–retest reliability. *Archives of General Psychiatry, 42,* 696–702.

Clarkin, J. F., Carpenter, D., Hull, J., Wilner, P., & Glick, I. (1998). Effects of psychoeducational intervention for married patients with bipolar disorder and their spouses. *Psychiatric Services, 49,* 531–533.

Clarkin, J. F., Glick, I. D., Haas, G. L., Spencer, J. H., Lewis, A. B., Peyser, J., et al. (1990). A randomized clinical trial of inpatient family intervention: V. Results for affective disorders. *Journal of Affective Disorders, 18,* 17–28.

Clarkin, J. F., & Miklowitz, D. J. (1997). Marital and family communication difficulties. In T. A. Widiger, A. J. Frances, H. A. Pincus, R. Ross, M. B. First, & W. Davis (Eds.), *DSM-IV sourcebook* (Vol. 3, pp. 631–672). Washington, DC: American Psychiatric Association.

Cochran, S. D. (1984). Preventing medical noncompliance in the outpatient treatment of bipolar affective disorders. *Journal of Consulting and Clinical Psychology, 52,* 873–878.

Cohen, M., Baker, G., Cohen, R. A., Fromm-Reichmann, F., & Weigert, V. (1954). An intensive study of 12 cases of manic–depressive psychosis. *Psychiatry, 17,* 103–137.

Coryell, W., Endicott, J., & Keller, M. (1992). Rapidly cycling affective disorder: Demographics, diagnosis, family history, and course. *Archives of General Psychiatry, 49,* 126–131.

Coryell, W., Keller, M., Lavori, P., & Endicott, J. (1990). Affective syndromes, psychotic features, and prognosis: II. Mania. *Archives of General Psychiatry, 47,* 658–662.

Coryell, W., Scheftner, W., Keller, M., Endicott, J., Maser, J., & Klerman, G. L. (1993). The enduring psychosocial consequences of mania and depression. *American Journal of Psychiatry, 150,* 720–727.

Cutler, N. R., & Post, R. M. (1982). Life course of illness in untreated manic–depressive patients. *Comprehensive Psychiatry, 23,* 101–115.

Dion, G., Tohen, M., Anthony, W., & Waternaux, C. (1989). Symptoms and functioning of patients with bipolar disorder six months after hospitalization. *Hospital and Community Psychiatry, 39,* 652–656.

Ehlers, C. L., Kupfer, D. J., Frank, E., & Monk, T. H. (1993). Biological rhythms and depression: The role of *zeitgebers* and *zeitstorers. Depression, 1,* 285–293.

Falloon, I. R. H., Boyd, J. L., & McGill, C. W. (1984). *Family care of schizophrenia: A problem-solving approach to the treatment of mental illness.* New York: Guilford Press.

First, M. B., Spitzer, R. L., Gibbon, M., & Williams, J. B. W. (1995). *Structured Clinical Interview for DSM-IV Axis I disorders.* New York: Biometrics Research Department, New York State Psychiatric Institute.

Frank, E. (2005). *Treating bipolar disorder: A clinician's guide to interpersonal and social rhythm therapy.* New York: Guilford Press.

Frank, E., Kupfer, D. J., Thase, M. E., Mallinger, A. G., Swartz, H. A., Fagiolini, A. M., et al. (2005). Two-year outcomes for interpersonal and social rhythm therapy in individuals with bipolar I disorder. *Archives of General Psychiatry, 62*(9), 996–1004.

Frank, E., Swartz, H. A., Mallinger, A. G., Thase, M. E., Weaver, E. V., & Kupfer, D. J. (1999). Adjunctive psychotherapy for bipolar disorder: Effects of changing treatment modality. *Journal of Abnormal Psychology, 108,* 579–587.

Fristad, M. A., Gavazzi, S. M., & Mackinaw-Koons, B. (2003). Family psychoeducation: An adjunctive intervention for children with bipolar disorder. *Biological Psychiatry, 53,* 1000–1009.

Gelenberg, A. J., Kane, J. N., Keller, M. B., Lavori, P., Rosenbaum, J. F., Cole, K., et al. (1989). Comparison of standard and low serum levels of lithium for maintenance treatment of bipolar disorders. *New England Journal of Medicine, 321,* 1489–1493.

Geller, B., Zimerman, B., Williams, M., Bolhofner, K., Craney, J. L., Frazier, J., et al. (2002). DSM-IV mania symptoms in a prepubertal and early adolescent bipolar disorder phenotype compared to attention deficit hyperactive and normal controls. *Journal of the American Academy of Child and Adolescent Psychopharmacology, 12,* 11–25.

George, E. L., Miklowitz, D. J., Richards, J. A., Simoneau, T. L., & Taylor, D. O. (2003). The comorbidity of bipolar disorder and Axis II personality disorders: Prevalence and clinical correlates. *Bipolar Disorders, 5,* 115–122.

Gitlin, M. J., Swendsen, J., Heller, T. L., & Hammen, C. (1995). Relapse and impairment in bipolar disorder. *American Journal of Psychiatry, 152*(11), 1635–1640.

Glick, I. D., Clarkin, J. F., Haas, G. L., Spencer, J. H., & Chen, C. L. (1991). A randomized clinical trial of inpatient family intervention: VI. Mediating variables and outcome. *Family Process, 30,* 85–99.

Goldberg, J. F. (2004). The changing landscape of psychopharmacology. In S. L. Johnson & R. L. Leahy (Eds.), *Psychological treatment of bipolar disorder* (pp. 109–138). New York: Guilford Press.

Goldberg, J. F., Harrow, M., & Grossman, L. S. (1995). Course and outcome in bipolar affective disorder: A longitudinal follow-up study. *American Journal of Psychiatry, 152,* 379–385.

Goldberg, J. F., & Kocsis, J. H. (1999). Depression in the course of bipolar disorder. In J. F. Goldberg & M. Harrow (Eds.), *Bipolar disorders: Clinical course and outcome* (pp. 129–147). Washington, DC: American Psychiatric Press.

Goldstein, M. J., Rea, M. M., & Miklowitz, D. J. (1996). Family factors related to the course and outcome of bipolar disorder. In C. Mundt, M. Goldstein, K. Hahlweg, & P. Fiedler (Eds.), *Interpersonal factors in the origin and course of affective disorders* (pp. 193–203). London: Gaskell Press.

Goodwin, F. K., & Jamison, K. R. (1990). *Manic–depressive illness.* New York: Oxford University Press.

Grossman, L. S., Harrow, M., Fudula, J., & Meltzer, H. Y. (1984). The longitudinal course of schizoaffective disorders: A prospective follow-up study. *Journal of Nervous and Mental Disease, 172,* 140–149.

Grossman, L. S., Harrow, M., Goldberg, J. F., & Fichtner, C. G. (1991). Outcome of schizoaffective disorder at two long-term follow-ups: Comparisons with outcome of schizophrenia and affective disorders. *American Journal of Psychiatry, 148,* 1359–1365.

Hahlweg, K., Goldstein, M. J., Nuechterlein, K. H., Magana, A. B., Mintz, J., Doane, J. A., et al. (1989). Expressed emotion and patient–relative interaction in families of recent-onset schizophrenics. *Journal of Consulting and Clinical Psychology, 57,* 11–18.

Haley, J. (1963). *Strategies of psychotherapy.* New York: Grune & Stratton.

Harrow, M., Goldberg, J. F., Grossman, L. S., & Meltzer, H. Y. (1990). Outcome in manic disorders: A naturalistic follow-up study. *Archives of General Psychiatry, 47,* 665–671.

Hatfield, A. B., Spaniol, L., & Zipple, A. M. (1987). Expressed emotion: A family perspective. *Schizophrenia Bulletin, 13,* 221–226.

Honig, A., Hofman, A., Rozendaal, N., & Dingemanns, P. (1997). Psychoeducation in bipolar disorder: Effect on expressed emotion. *Psychiatry Research, 72,* 17–22.

Hooley, J. M. (1987). The nature and origins of expressed emotion. In K. Hahlweg & M. J. Goldstein (Eds.), *Understanding major mental disorder: The contribution of family interaction research* (pp. 176–194). New York: Family Process Press.

Hooley, J. M., & Licht, D. M. (1997). Expressed emotion and causal attributions in the spouses of depressed patients. *Journal of Abnormal Psychology, 106,* 298–306.

Hooley, J. M., & Teasdale, J. D. (1989). Predictors of relapse in unipolar depressives: Expressed emotion, marital distress, and perceived criticism. *Journal of Abnormal Psychology, 98,* 229–235.

Hoover, C. F., & Fitzgerald, R. G. (1981). Marital conflict of manic–depressive patients. *Archives of General Psychiatry, 38,* 65–67.

Jamison, K. R., & Akiskal, H. S. (1983). Medication compliance in patients with bipolar disorders. *Psychiatric Clinics of North America, 6,* 175–192.

Jamison, K. R., Gerner, R. H., & Goodwin, F. K. (1979). Patient and physician attitudes toward lithium: Relationship to compliance. *Archives of General Psychiatry, 36,* 866–869.

Judd, L. L., Akiskal, H. S., Schettler, P. J., Endicott, J., Maser, J., Solomon, D. A., et al. (2002). The long-term natural history of the weekly symptomatic status of bipolar I disorder. *Archives of General Psychiatry, 59,* 530–537.

Katz, M. M., Robins, E., Croughan, J., Secunda, S., & Swann, A. (1982). Behavioral measurement and drug response characteristics of unipolar and bipolar depression. *Psychological Medicine, 12,* 25–36.

Kaufman, J., Birmaher, B., Brent, D., Rao, U., Flynn, C., Moreci, P., et al. (1997). Schedule for Affective Disorders and Schizophrenia for School-Age Children—Present and Lifetime version (K-SADS-PL): Initial reliability and validity data. *Journal of the American Academy of Child and Adolescent Psychiatry, , 36,* 980–988.

Keck, P. E., McElroy, S. L., Strakowski, S. M., West, S. A., Sax, K. W., Hawkins, J. M., et al. (1998). 12-month outcome of patients with bipolar disorder following hospitalization for a manic or mixed episode. *American Journal of Psychiatry, 155,* 646–652.

Keller, M. B., Lavori, P. W., Coryell, W., Andreasen, N. C., Endicott, J., Clayton, P. J., et al. (1986). Differential outcome of pure manic, mixed/cycling, and pure depressive episodes in patients with bipolar illness. *Journal of the American Medical Association, 255,* 3138–3142.

Kendler, K. S. (1991). Mood-incongruent psychotic affective illness: A historical and empirical review. *Archives of General Psychiatry*, 48, 362–369.

Kessler, R. C., Berglund, P., Demler, O., Jin, R., & Walters, E. E. (2005). Lifetime prevalence and age-of-onset distributions of DSM-IV disorders in the National Comorbidity Survey replication. *Archives of General Psychiatry*, 62, 593–602.

Kessler, R. C., Chiu, W. T., Demler, O., & Walters, E. E. (2005). Prevalence, severity, and comorbidity of 12-month DSM-IV disorders in the National Comorbidity Survey Replication. *Archives of General Psychiatry*, 62, 617–627.

Klerman, G. L., Weissman, M. M., Rounsaville, B. J., & Chevron, R. S. (1984). *Interpersonal psychotherapy of depression*. New York: Basic Books.

Kowatch, R., & DelBello, M. P. (2003). The use of mood stabilizers and atypical antipsychotics in children and adolescents with bipolar disorders. *CNS Spectrums*, 8, 273–280.

Kowatch, R. A., Fristad, M., Birmaher, B., Wagner, K. D., Findling, R. L., Hellander, M., et al. (2005). Treatment guidelines for children and adolescents with bipolar disorder. *Journal of the American Academy of Child and Adolescent Psychiatry*, 44(3), 213–235.

Kraepelin, É. (1921). *Manic–depressive insanity and paranoia*. Edinburgh: Livingstone.

Kupfer, D. J., Frank, E., Grochocinski, V. J., Luther, J. F., Houck, P. R., Swartz, H. A., et al. (2000). Stabilization in the treatment of mania, depression, and mixed states. *Acta Neuropsychiatrica*, 12, 110–114.

Lam, D. H., Hayward, P., Watkins, E. R., Wright, K., & Sham, P. (2005). Relapse prevention in patients with bipolar disorder: Cognitive therapy outcome after 2 years. *American Journal of Psychiatry*, 162, 324–329.

Lam, D. H., Watkins, E. R., Hayward, P., Bright, J., Wright, K., Kerr, N., et al. (2003). A randomized controlled study of cognitive therapy of relapse prevention for bipolar affective disorder: Outcome of the first year. *Archives of General Psychiatry*, 60, 145–152.

Leibenluft, E., Charney, D. S., Towbin, K. E., Bhangoo, R. K., & Pine, D. S. (2003). Defining clinical phenotypes of juvenile mania. *American Journal of Psychiatry*, 160, 430–437.

Leibenluft, E., Cohen, P., Gorrindo, T., Brook, J. S., & Pine, D. S. (2006). Chronic vs. episodic irritability in youth: A community-based, longitudinal study of clinical and diagnostic associations. *Journal of Child and Adolescent Psychopharmacology*, 16, 456–466.

Leverich, G. S., & Post, R. M. (1998). Life charting of affective disorders. *CNS Spectrums*, 3, 21–37.

Liberman, R. P., Wallace, C. J., Falloon, I. R. H., & Vaughn, C. E. (1981). Interpersonal problem solving therapy for schizophrenics and their families. *Comprehensive Psychiatry*, 22, 627–629.

Malkoff-Schwartz, S., Frank, E., Anderson, B. P., Hlastala, S. A., Luther, J. F., Sherrill, J. T., et al. (2000). Social rhythm disruption and stressful life events in the onset of bipolar and unipolar episodes. *Psychological Medicine*, 30, 1005–1016.

Malkoff-Schwartz, S., Frank, E., Anderson, B., Sherrill, J. T., Siegel, L., Patterson, D., et al. (1998). Stressful life events and social rhythm disruption in the onset of manic and depressive bipolar episodes: A preliminary investigation. *Archives of General Psychiatry*, 55, 702–707.

McClellan, J. (2005). Commentary: Treatment guidelines for child and adolescent bipolar disorder. *Journal of the American Academy of Child and Adolescent Psychiatry*, 44, 236–239.

McElroy, S. L., Keck, P. E., Pope, H. G., Hudson, J. I., Faedda, G. L., & Swann, A. O. (1992). Clinical and research implications of the diagnosis of dysphoric or mixed mania or hypomania. *American Journal of Psychiatry*, 149, 1633–1644.

Miklowitz, D. J. (1992). Longitudinal outcome and medication noncompliance among manic patients with and without mood-incongruent psychotic features. *Journal of Nervous and Mental Disease*, 180, 703–711.

Miklowitz, D. J. (2006). A review of evidence-based psychosocial interventions for bipolar disorder. *Journal of Clinical Psychiatry*, 67(Suppl. 11), 28–33.

Miklowitz, D. J., Biuckians, A., & Richards, J. A. (2006). Early-onset bipolar disorder: A family treatment perspective. *Development and Psychopathology*, 18, 1247–1265.

Miklowitz, D. J., & Frank, E. (1999). New psychotherapies for bipolar disorder. In J. F. Goldberg & M. Harrow (Eds.), *Bipolar disorders: Clinical course and outcome* (pp. 57–84). Washington, DC: American Psychiatric Press.

Miklowitz, D. J., & George, E. L. (2004). *Treatment manual for the family-focused treatment of adolescents with bipolar disorder*. Unpublished manual, University of Colorado, Boulder.

Miklowitz, D. J., George, E. L., Axelson, D. A., Kim, E. Y., Birmaher, B., Schneck, C., et al. (2004). Family-focused treatment for adolescents with bipolar disorder. *Journal of Affective Disorders*, 82(Suppl. 1), 113–128.

Miklowitz, D. J., George, E. L., Richards, J. A., Simoneau, T. L., & Suddath, R. L. (2003). A randomized study of family-focused psychoeducation and pharmacotherapy in the outpatient management of bipolar disorder. *Archives of General Psychiatry*, 60, 904–912.

Miklowitz, D. J., & Goldstein, M. J. (1997). *Bipolar disorder: A family-focused treatment approach*. New York: Guilford Press.

Miklowitz, D. J., Goldstein, M. J., & Nuechterlein, K. H. (1987). The family and the course of recent-onset mania. In K. Hahlweg & M. J. Goldstein (Eds.), *Understanding major mental disorder: The contribution of family interaction research* (pp. 195–211). New York: Family Process Press.

Miklowitz, D. J., Goldstein, M. J., Nuechterlein, K. H., Snyder, K. S., & Mintz, J. (1988). Family factors and the course of bipolar affective disorder. *Archives of General Psychiatry, 45,* 225–231.

Miklowitz, D. J., & Otto, M. W. (2006). New psychosocial interventions for bipolar disorder: A review of literature and introduction of the Systematic Treatment Enhancement Program. *Journal of Cognitive Psychotherapy, 20*(2), 215–230.

Miklowitz, D. J., Otto, M. W., Frank, E., Reilly-Harrington, N. A., Wisniewski, S. R., Kogan, J. N., et al. (2007). Psychosocial treatments for bipolar depression: A 1-year randomized trial from the Systematic Treatment Enhancement Program. *Archives of General Psychiatry, 64,* 419–427.

Miklowitz, D. J., Simoneau, T. L., George, E. A., Richards, J. A., Kalbag, A., Sachs-Ericsson, N., et al. (2000). Family-focused treatment of bipolar disorder: One-year effects of a psychoeducational program in conjunction with pharmacotherapy. *Biological Psychiatry, 48,* 582–592.

Miklowitz, D. J., Velligan, D. I., Goldstein, M. J., Nuechterlein, K. H., Gitlin, M. J., Ranlett, G., et al. (1991). Communication deviance in families of schizophrenic and manic patients. *Journal of Abnormal Psychology, 100,* 163–173.

Miklowitz, D. J., Wendel, J. S., & Simoneau, T. L. (1998). Targeting dysfunctional family interactions and high expressed emotion in the psychosocial treatment of bipolar disorder. *In Session: Psychotherapy in Practice, 4,* 25–38.

Miklowitz, D. J., Wisniewski, S. R., Miyahara, S., Otto, M. W., & Sachs, G. S. (2005). Perceived criticism from family members as a predictor of the 1-year course of bipolar disorder. *Psychiatry Research, 136*(2–3), 101–111.

Mitchell, P., Parker, G., Jamieson, K., Wilhelm, K., Hickie, I., Brodaty, H., et al. (1992). Are there any differences between bipolar and unipolar melancholia? *Journal of Affective Disorders, 25,* 97–106.

Monk, T. H., Flaherty, J. F., Frank, E., Hoskinson, K., & Kupfer, D. J. (1990). The Social Rhythm Metric: An instrument to quantify daily rhythms of life. *Journal of Nervous and Mental Disease, 178,* 120–126.

Monk, T. H., Kupfer, D. J., Frank, E., & Ritenour, A. M. (1991). The Social Rhythm Metric (SRM): Measuring daily social rhythms over 12 weeks. *Psychiatry Research, 36,* 195–207.

Napier, A. Y., & Whitaker, C. A. (1978). *The family crucible.* New York: Harper & Row.

O'Connell, R. A., Mayo, J. A., Flatow, L., Cuthbertson, B., & O'Brien, B. E. (1991). Outcome of bipolar disorder on long-term treatment with lithium. *British Journal of Psychiatry, 159,* 132–129.

Pavuluri, M. N., Birmaher, B., & Naylor, M. W. (2005). Pediatric bipolar disorder: A review of the past 10 years. *Journal of the American Academy of Child and Adolescent Psychiatry, 44*(9), 846–871.

Pavuluri, M. N., Graczyk, P. A., Henry, D. B., Carbray, J. A., Heidenreich, J., & Miklowitz, D. J. (2004). Child and family-focused cognitive behavioral therapy for pediatric bipolar disorder: Development and

preliminary results. *Journal of the American Academy of Child and Adolescent Psychiatry, 43,* 528–537.

Pope, H. G., & Lipinski, J. F. (1978). Diagnosis in schizophrenia and manic–depressive illness: A reassessment of the specificity of "schizophrenic" symptoms in the light of current research. *Archives of General Psychiatry, 35,* 811–828.

Post, R. M., Rubinow, D. R., Uhde, T. W., Roy-Byrne, P. P., Linnoila, M., Rosoff, A., et al. (1989). Dysphoric mania: Clinical and biological correlates. *Archives of General Psychiatry, 46,* 353–358.

Priebe, S., Wildgrube, C., & Muller-Oerlinghausen, B. (1989). Lithium prophylaxis and expressed emotion. *British Journal of Psychiatry, 154,* 396–399.

Rea, M. M., Tompson, M., Miklowitz, D. J., Goldstein, M. J., Hwang, S., & Mintz, J. (2003). Family focused treatment vs. individual treatment for bipolar disorder: Results of a randomized clinical trial. *Journal of Consulting and Clinical Psychology, 71,* 482–492.

Regier, D. A., Farmer, M. E., Rae, D. S., Locke, B. Z., Keith, S. J., Judd, L. L., et al. (1990). Comorbidity of mental disorders with alcohol and other drug abuse: Results from the Epidemiologic Catchment Area (ECA) study. *Journal of the American Medical Association, 264,* 2511–2518.

Sachs, G. S., & Lafer, B. (1998). Child and adolescent mania. In P. J. Goodnick (Ed.), *Mania: Clinical and research perspectives* (pp. 37–62). Washington, DC: American Psychiatric Press.

Sachs, G. S., Thase, M. E., Otto, M. W., Bauer, M., Miklowitz, D., Wisniewski, S. R., et al. (2003). Rationale, design, and methods of the systematic treatment enhancement program for bipolar disorder (STEP-BD). *Biological Psychiatry, 53,* 1028–1042.

Schneck, C. D., Miklowitz, D. J., Calabrese, J. R., Allen, M. H., Thomas, M. R., Wisniewski, S. R., et al. (2004). Phenomenology of rapid cycling bipolar disorder: Data from the first 500 participants in the Systematic Treatment Enhancement Program for Bipolar Disorder. *American Journal of Psychiatry, 161,* 1902–1908.

Scott, J., Paykel, E., Morriss, R., Bentall, R., Kinderman, P., Johnson, T., et al. (2006). Cognitive behaviour therapy for severe and recurrent bipolar disorders: A randomised controlled trial. *British Journal of Psychiatry, 188,* 313–320.

Shapiro, D. R., Quitkin, F. M., & Fleiss, J. L. (1989). Response to maintenance therapy in bipolar illness. *Archives of General Psychiatry, 46,* 401–405.

Simoneau, T. L., Miklowitz, D. J., Richards, J. A., Saleem, R., & George, E. L. (1999). Bipolar disorder and family communication: Effects of a psychoeducational treatment program. *Journal of Abnormal Psychology, 108,* 588–597.

Simoneau, T. L., Miklowitz, D. J., & Saleem, R. (1998). Expressed emotion and interactional patterns in the families of bipolar patients. *Journal of Abnormal Psychology, 107,* 497–507.

Spitzer, R. L., Williams, J. B., Gibbon, M., & First, M.

B. (1992). The Structured Clinical Interview for DSM-III-R (SCID): I. History, rationale, and description. *Archives of General Psychiatry, 49*(8), 624–629.

Strakowski, S. M., Keck, P. E., McElroy, S. L., West, S. A., Sax, K. W., Hawkins, J. M., et al. (1998). Twelve-month outcome after a first hospitalization for affective psychosis. *Archives of General Psychiatry, 55,* 49–55.

Strauss, J. S., & Carpenter, W. T. (1972). The prediction of outcome in schizophrenia. *Archives of General Psychiatry, 27,* 739–746.

Suppes, T., Leverich, G. S., Keck, P. E., Nolen, W. A., Denicoff, K. D., Altshuler, L. L., et al. (2001). The Stanley Foundation Bipolar Treatment Outcome Network: II. Demographics and illness characteristics of the first 261 patients. *Journal of Affective Disorders, 67,* 45–59.

Tohen, M., Waternaux, C. M., & Tsuang, M. T. (1990). Outcome in mania: A 4-year prospective followup of 75 patients utilizing survival analysis. *Archives of General Psychiatry, 47,* 1106–1111.

Vaughn, C. E., & Leff, J. P. (1976). The influence of family and social factors on the course of psychiatric illness: A comparison of schizophrenia and depressed neurotic patients. *British Journal of Psychiatry, 129,* 125–137.

Vitiello, B., & Swedo, S. (2004). Antidepressant medications in children. *New England Journal of Medicine, 350,* 1489–1491.

Weisman, A., Lopez, S. R., Karno, M., & Jenkins, J. (1993). An attributional analysis of expressed emotion in Mexican-American families with schizophrenia. *Journal of Abnormal Psychology, 102,* 601–606.

Wendel, J. S., Miklowitz, D. J., Richards, J. A., & George, E. L. (2000). Expressed emotion and attributions in the relatives of bipolar patients: An analysis of problem-solving interactions. *Journal of Abnormal Psychology, 109,* 792–796.

Wynne, L. C., Singer, M., Bartko, J., & Toohey, M. (1977). Schizophrenics and their families: Recent research on parental communication. In J. M. Tanner (Ed.), *Developments in psychiatric research* (pp. 254–286). London: Hodder & Stoughton.

Yan, L. J., Hammen, C., Cohen, A. N., Daley, S. E., & Henry, R. M. (2004). Expressed emotion versus relationship quality variables in the prediction of recurrence in bipolar patients. *Journal of Affective Disorders, 83,* 199–206.

Young, M. A., & Harrow, M. (1994). Bipolar disorders. In A. S. Bellack & M. Hersen (Eds.), *Psychopathology in adulthood* (pp. 234–248). Boston: Allyn & Bacon.

Schizophrenia and Other Psychotic Disorders

Nicholas Tarrier

Among the most remarkable advances in the last decade is the direct treatment of "positive" symptoms of schizophrenia with psychological treatments. Almost all of these advances emanate from the United Kingdom, where a group of senior investigators working in the context of the National Health Service have developed and evaluated these approaches. Nick Tarrier has been at the forefront of this group during this period. In the context of case management and antipsychotic medication, this very creative mix of treatment components has been proven effective for chronic patients who did not fully respond to medication, as well as for patients in an acute stage of the disorder. More recently, promising evidence is beginning to appear in the possibility of preventing the onset of the disorder for those at risk. The thrusts and parries of these techniques are illustrated in the case of "Jim," who had developed an intricate web of delusions reminiscent of Russell Crowe's character in *A Beautiful Mind*, concerning complex schemes by others, including friends and family, to take advantage of him and steal his money and his girlfriend. The therapist's skill in carrying out these new approaches is never better illustrated than in this chapter. These new, empirically supported psychological treatments represent the front line of our therapeutic work with these severely disturbed patients and hold promise of further alleviating to some degree the tragedy that is schizophrenia.—D. H. B.

Schizophrenia is a serious mental illness that is characterized by positive symptoms of hallucinations, delusions, and disorders of thought. Typically hallucinations are auditory, in the form of hearing voices that often talk about the person and in the third person, although hallucinations can occur in other senses. Delusions are frequently bizarre, are held with strong conviction, and often involve a misinterpretation of perception or experience. The content of delusions may include a variety of themes, including alien control, persecution, reference, and somatic, religious, or grandiose ideas. Dis-

orders of thought are inferred from disruption, and disorganization in language. Hallucinations and delusions, and sometimes thought disorders, are referred to as positive symptoms and reflect an excess or distortion of normal functioning. Negative symptoms are also frequently present and reflect a decrease in or loss of normal functioning. These include restrictions in the range and intensity of emotions, in the fluency and productivity of thought and language, and in the initiation of behavior. The consequences of these symptoms can be dysfunction in personal, social, occupational, and vocational functioning. Comorbid disorders, especially depression and anxiety, are frequently present and further impair functioning. Suicide risk is high. Aspects of description, diagnosis, and classification of schizophrenia and psychotic disorders have stimulated much debate and controversy over the decades, and details can be found in most psychiatry textbooks. They do not concern us here except to say that there can be considerable variation in clinical presentation between patients and in the same patient over time. Furthermore, the focus of cognitive-behavioral therapy for psychosis (CBTp) in recent years has mainly been on the reduction of positive symptoms, and that is the major concern of most of this chapter. The standard treatments for schizophrenia remain antipsychotic medication and some type of case management, and CBTp described in this chapter is assumed to be in addition to this.

DEVELOPMENT OF COGNITIVE-BEHAVIORAL THERAPY FOR SCHIZOPHRENIA

CBTp for schizophrenia, although following a common theme and set of principles, has developed in a number of centers, mostly in the United Kingdom, and has been informed by a number of theoretical and conceptual perspectives. A dramatic expansion in the use of cognitive-behavioral therapy (CBT) in the 1980s and 1990s in the treatment of anxiety and affective disorders influenced clinical psychologists working in the field of schizophrenia, who were trying to understand and treat schizophrenia from a psychological perspective. This was especially true in the United Kingdom, where clinical psychologists treated a range of disorders in adult mental health services and were able to transfer their treatment methods across diagnostic groups. The structure and function of a system of universal health care in the United Kingdom, the National Health Service (NHS), facilitated such skills transfer and multidisciplinary work. Furthermore, funding of the professional training of health professionals, especially clinical psychologists, has aided awareness and dissemination of CBT for patients in general and for psychotic patients in particular. However, dissemination of treatments

into the health service and the universal availability of CBTp has been slow and not without its problems (Brooker & Brabban, 2006; Tarrier, Barrowclough, Haddock, & McGovern, 1999)

RESEARCH EVIDENCE

Clinical, ethical, and economic considerations have encouraged clinical practice to be guided by an evidence base produced from evaluations of treatments. The evidence develops from uncontrolled studies and small-scale projects to controlled studies and then to large randomized controlled trials (RCTs) of efficacy and effectiveness. In spite of recent criticisms of the appropriateness of RCTs in mental health (Richardson, Baker, Burns, Lilford, & Muijen, 2000; Slade & Priebe, 2001), they remain the "gold standard" by which all treatments are judged (Doll, 1998; Pocock, 1996; Salkovskis, 2002; Tarrier & Wykes, 2004). Once a database of controlled trials has been established, then meta-analysis can provide a measure of the average level of therapeutic effect for that treatment. For CBTp with schizophrenia, a number of published meta-analyses indicate that CBTp is effective in treating positive psychotic symptoms in psychotic patients (e.g., Gould, Mueser, Bolton, Mays, & Goff, 2001; Pilling et al., 2002; Rector & Beck, 2001; Tarrier & Wykes, 2004; Zimmermann, Favrod, Trieu, & Pomini, 2005). For example, out of 20 controlled trials of CBT for schizophrenia identified by Tarrier and Wykes (2004), data were available from 19 studies on the effects of CBT on positive symptoms. These studies have a mean effect size of 0.37 ($SD = 0.39$, median = 0.32), with a range between -0.49 and 0.99. Using Cohen's (1988) convention for categorizing effect sizes, 14 (74%) studies achieved at least a small effect size, 6 (32%) at least a moderate effect size, and 3 (16%) achieved a large effect size. Overall these studies indicate a modest effect size in improving positive symptoms compared to standard psychiatric care (treatment as usual, or TAU), which is probably not surprising given the nature and severity of the disorder. An updated meta-analysis and review indicated that effect sizes were 0.476 for CBTp on positive symptoms from 30 trials, 0.474 for negative symptoms from 14 trials, 0.477 for social functioning from 11 studies, and 0.424 for depression from 11 studies (Wykes, Everitt, Steele, & Tarrier, 2007).

Symptom Management in Chronic Schizophrenia

In spite of maintenance medication, a considerable percentage of patients with schizophrenia continue to have persistent hallucinations and delusions that do not respond further to medication. The majority of the CBTp studies have been carried out with patients who have chronic illnesses. These studies, for which data were available for 16, have a mean effect size of 0.4 (SD = 0.32, median = 0.33), with a range from −0.32 to 0.99 (Tarrier & Wykes, 2004).

Symptom Recovery in Acute Schizophrenia

Three studies have investigated the use of CBTp in the treatment of acutely ill patients hospitalized for an acute psychotic episode. Because the participants are acutely ill and may well be suspicious, agitated, and unstable, the therapy is often implemented as a *therapy envelope*, which consists of a range of duration of therapy that can be delivered in a flexible manner. These three studies have produced effect sizes of −0.49, 0.12, and 0.93, indicating considerable variance in this small number of studies. The Socrates study (Lewis et al., 2002) which is by far the largest and methodologically rigorous study, recruited 309 patients with early-onset schizophrenia and produced an effect size of 0.12. The other two studies were considerably smaller.

Relapse Prevention

A number of studies have investigated relapse prevention, or the ability of CBTp to prevent or delay future acute episodes. Relapse is an important outcome because of the disruption, distress, and economic costs that symptom exacerbation brings. Studies of CBTp interventions in which relapse prevention was just one of a series of components achieved little success with four studies, showing a mean reduction in relapse of only 1.4% compared to control treatments. Whereas CBTp focused on and dedicated to relapse prevention resulted in some success, with two studies showing a mean relapse reduction 21% (Tarrier & Wykes, 2004).

Early Intervention

In addition to the effect on individuals with more established psychoses, there has recently been a growing interest in diverting the course in schizophrenia at an early stage. Morrison and colleagues (2004) reported a study using CBT techniques in this early group to attempt to avert or postpone the first acute episode of the disorder by intervening during a prodromal period. Their technique focused not on frank positive symptoms, but on problem-solving difficulties. The results of this first RCT appear promising. CBTp proved more beneficial than TAU in preventing progression into psychosis, preventing the prescription of antipsychotic medication, and reducing symptoms.

Summary of Evidence

The evidence for CBTp reducing positive symptoms in chronic, partially remitted patients with schizophrenia is good. Evidence that CBTp speeds recovery in acutely ill patients to the level of achieving a significant clinical benefit is more equivocal. Reductions in relapse rates are achieved when the intervention focuses on and is dedicated to relapse reduction, but they are disappointing for standard CBTp. There are promising, although as yet unreplicated, results that full psychosis can be prevented in vulnerable individuals.

THEORETICAL ADVANCES

There has been considerable debate about the theoretical understanding of schizophrenia, with biological explanations being dominant. However, psychological and social factors have been consistently shown to be influential, certainly in affecting the course of schizophrenia, and have been incorporated into stress–vulnerability models that have emphasized the importance of these psychosocial factors in precipitating and maintaining psychotic episodes (Nuechterlein, 1987). More recently cognitive models have been developed in tandem with advances in cognitive-behavioral treatments (Garety, Kuipers, Fowler, Freeman, & Bebbington, 2001). It is expected that as these cognitive models develop and are subjected to empirical tests, further refinements of CBTp treatment will develop. For example, CBTp appears to have little significant effect in reducing suicide risk (Tarrier et al., 2006); however, with a greater conceptual understanding of the psychological mechanisms underlying such risk, more focused intervention to reduce risk will arise (Bolton, Gooding, Kapur, Barrowclough, & Tarrier, 2007; Johnson, Gooding, & Tarrier, 2008).

BASIC CLINICAL PRINCIPLES

A number of common clinical strategies underlie all variants of CBTp for schizophrenia: engagement and establishment of a therapeutic relationship; assessment based on an individualized case formulation that identifies psychotic experience (symptoms) and establishes associations between the patient's cognition, behavior, and affect within the environmental context in response to this experience; and an intervention strategy based on this formulation that uses cognitive and behavioral methods to reduce psychotic symptoms and associated emotional distress. Patients are taught to be aware of their symptoms and to learn methods to control them (e.g., learning to control auditory hallucinations by switching their attention away from them, or by thinking about alternative explanations for their experiences).

Patients can acquire coping strategies that are broken down into elements, learned individually, then aggregated into an overall strategy. To ensure that these coping strategies can be implemented, patients overlearn them during the therapy session. Learning such control techniques allows patients to challenge beliefs they may have had about voices, such as "The voices are uncontrollable," "The voices are all powerful," and "I must obey the voices." Thus, by learning to control basic psychological processes such as attention, through attention switching and distraction, patients also learn to challenge their beliefs about their experiences and symptoms. Behavioral experiments and reality tests may also be used to disprove delusional and inappropriate beliefs. Particular attention is paid to identifying avoidance and safety behaviors that reinforce inappropriate beliefs. Changing these behaviors is a powerful method of changing beliefs and delusions. Patients may be assisted in their attempts at behavior change by means of self-instruction and coping strategies that decrease arousal (e.g., breathing exercises; quick relaxation;

guided imagery; and encouraging positive task-oriented internal dialogue). In some refractory cases, patients are convinced and unshakable in the belief that their delusions are true, and they are unwilling to examine the veracity of this subjective experience. In these cases, the clinician must negotiate treatment goals aimed at reducing distress rather than the symptoms themselves. A failure to do this will probably result in the patient disengaging and refusing treatment.

It is frequently the case that the patient's delusional beliefs persist in spite of evidence to contradict them, including both evidence that occurs naturally and evidence that is manufactured by the therapist through behavioral experiments and reality testing. To weaken these delusional explanations, the therapist should use all available opportunities, through guided discovery and Socratic questioning, to reappraise the evidence for the patient's explanation of events, thus weakening the delusions. Pointing out the contradictory evidence in a quizzical and puzzled manner, often known as the "Columbo technique," is advised, so the patient has to account for contradictions and review his or her explanation in light of this new and contradictory evidence. When delusions are strongly held, this can be a slow process, but the weakening of delusional beliefs can occur, or, as happens in some cases, the delusional interpretations remain or return, but their importance and distressing nature are greatly reduced. For example, one older adult female patient I treated experienced auditory hallucinations that were of a blasphemous and obscene nature. She believed that her brain acted as a transmitter and broadcast her thoughts, so that other people in the vicinity could hear her blasphemous and obscene thoughts. Her main social contact was with her local church and associated social club. One Sunday, during the church service, she heard the voices and became convinced that her own thoughts about the voices were broadcast aloud to the congregation. She was mortified and so ashamed that she left the church and was unable to return or to have any contact with her friends. She was convinced that she had become ostracized by the church congregation. On being asked about the evidence for this, she replied that she had since met other members of the church congregation in town and they had totally ignored her, which had further reinforced her sense of exclusion, shame, and self-disgust. On further questioning, she revealed that she had been walking on the pavement and had seen her friends drive by some distance away. There was a high probability that they had not seen her. Thus, her evidence for being ostracized was challenged. We agreed upon a treatment goal that would test her interpretation of the situation. If the fear that the church congregation would shun her if she returned was real, then she should expect a negative reaction when she returned to church. If the fear was irrational, there would be no negative reaction; in fact, the others should be pleased to see her return. She experienced considerable anxiety at the thought of returning to church but managed the return using methods she had learned to cope with both the experience of auditory hallucinations and anxiety. To her surprise, far from being shunned or ostracized, she was greeted with warmth and concern. This experience considerably weakened her beliefs that others could hear her thoughts, and her delusions were rated as minimal. On being asked about the events some months later at follow-up, she said that she believed others could hear her thoughts, but because it did not appear to bother them, she was no longer concerned about it either! In this case, her delusional explanation of past events had returned but no longer caused her any distress or disrupted her social functioning.

Emphasis has also been placed upon improving the patient's self-esteem and feelings of self-worth. This more recent addition to the treatment has been found to be effective and well received by patients (Hall & Tarrier, 2003). In this chapter I have placed these methods after the treatment of symptoms, indicating a progression from symptom reduction to improved self-esteem. However, there is no reason why improvements in self-esteem cannot be initiated at the beginning of treatment, and in some cases this may be desirable.

BACKGROUND AND ASSOCIATED FACTORS

Phases of the Disorder and Relationship to Aims of Treatment

Schizophrenia, a complex disorder that may well be lifelong, passes through a number of phases. For example, the prodromal phase that occurs before a full-blown psychotic episode is characterized by nonspecific symptoms and symptoms of anxiety, depression, irritability, insomnia, and quasi-psychotic experience (e.g., magical thinking, feelings of paranoia). The prodromal phase develops into a psychotic episode, during which the most florid psychotic symptoms are present and seriously interfere with functioning. A psychotic episode usually requires acute management, frequently including hospitalization. Recovery from an acute episode of psychosis is followed by a period of remission or partial remission with maintenance doses of antipsychotic medication. It is not uncommon for residual symptoms to remain during the recovery and remission phase, and in some cases, there is little recovery at all. Treatment aims and strategies for CBTp vary depending on the phase of the disorder. For example, during the prodromal phase, the aim is to prevent transition into a full psychotic episode; during an acute episode, the aim is to speed recovery; during partial remission, the aim is to reduce residual symptoms and to prevent further relapse; and in full remission, the aim is to keep the patient well. The specifics of CBTp may vary depending on these aims and the phase of the disorder in which they are applied. For example, during an acute admission for a psychotic episode, the patient is often disturbed, distressed, and agitated. Thus, therapy sessions are often brief and frequent, whereas in chronically ill patients living within the community, therapy sessions follow the normal outpatient format. In all cases, therapy is tailored to the tolerance of the patient. In all but the most exceptional cases, CBTp is used in addition to appropriate antipsychotic medication. The various phases of the disorder and appropriate treatment strategies are outlined in Table 11.1.

Associated Features and Disability

It is important that the clinician attend to associated features and complicating factors, as well as the symptoms of the disorder. These vary from the effects of the disorder on basic psychological processes, such as attention, to clinical issues, such as suicide risk, to social issues, such as social deprivation and poor employment opportunities. These associated features are outlined in Table 11.2.

The crucial point is that the clinician be aware that these problems can arise. Some of them can be dealt with by keeping the message simple and brief, but with plenty of repetition

TABLE 11.1. Treatment Aims and Methods in Different Phases
of the Schizophrenic Illness

Phase	Aim	Treatment method
Preillness prodrome	Prevention of translation into full psychosis	CBT for early signs and prevention of symptom escalation
Acute episode	Speed recovery	CBT and coping training
Partially remitted residual symptoms	Symptom reduction	CBT, coping training, self-esteem enhancement
Remission	Relapse prevention	CBT for staying well and family intervention
Relapse prodrome	Abort relapse	Early signs identification and relapse prevention

TABLE 11.2. Associated Features of Schizophrenia: Features That Need to Be Assessed
and Considered as Potential Difficulties in the Psychological Treatment of Schizophrenia

Psychological

- Disrupted or slowed thought processes
- Difficulty discriminating signal from noise
- Restricted attention
- Hypersensitivity to social interactions
- Difficulty in processing social signals
- Flat and restricted affect
- Elevated arousal and dysfunctional arousal regulation
- Hypersensitivity to stress and life events
- High risk of depression and hopelessness
- Effects of trauma
- Stigmatization
- Low self-esteem and self-worth
- High risk of substance and alcohol abuse
- High risk of suicide and self-harm
- Interference of normal adolescent and early adult development due to onset of illness

Psychosocial

- Hypersensitivity to family and interpersonal environment (including that created by professional staff)
- Risk of perpetrating or being the victim of violence

Social

- Conditions of social deprivation
- Poor housing
- Downward social drift
- Unemployment and difficulty in competing in the job market
- Restricted social network
- Psychiatric career interfering with utilization of other social resources

(i.e., using overlearning in the teaching of coping strategies). Writing down simple points for the patient as a memory aid can also be helpful, as can creating a small "workbook," so that the patient has a continuous record of these points. This is usually more effective than providing handouts that are rarely read and frequently lost. It is important to balance the nature and duration of sessions against the patient's level of tolerance. Initially, it might be best to keep sessions brief or allow the patient to leave when he or she has had enough. The one-to-one nature of therapy is highly stressful, so initial sessions may serve merely to provide habituation to the social stress of being with the clinician. Teaching the patient simple strategies to deal with tension and anxiety (e.g., brief relaxation) may be helpful in habituating to the therapy situation and also provides a concrete task on which to focus attention. Simple attention-focusing tasks, such as focusing on some item in the room for a short period, may be helpful in reducing the effect of irrelevant stimuli on the patient's conscious awareness. It is also important to recognize that the verbal and nonverbal cues that the therapist might expect to indicate severe distress, depression, or suicidality may not be expressed by someone with schizophrenia. Affect may be flat or inappropriate, which may result in the therapist missing important signs of risk. This can be avoided, in part, by knowing the person and how he or she reacts, by never making assumptions about mental state, and by having the patient agree from the outset that he or she will inform the therapist of important changes in his or her life or mood.

Unfortunately, some issues, such as social conditions, are often beyond the therapist's power to change but may well impact upon the treatment process. However, there is nothing wrong in assuming an advocacy role or in helping patients to empower themselves by aiding their attempts to improve their own circumstances. Finally, it is important that therapists adopt a noncritical approach and learn to accommodate their own frustrations if therapy is progressing more slowly than they had hoped. Aspects of schizophrenia can make some patients difficult to deal with, and the therapist needs to be aware of this and develop a tolerant approach. The lack of a positive relationship between case managers and patients has been shown to be associated with poorer prognosis (Tattan & Tarrier, 2000).

THE CONTEXT OF THERAPY

It is highly probable that by the time a referral is made for CBT the patient will be under the care of a multidisciplinary mental health team, and be receiving antipsychotic medication and some type of case management. People who develop a psychotic illness are usually diagnosed by a general practitioner or primary care team, or in an accident and emergency department, and referred on to the mental health services. Mental health services are organized in different ways in different countries depending on health care philosophies and structures, but what is delivered in terms of therapy content may be independent of how that service is organized. Thus, the therapeutic procedures described in this chapter can be utilized in different types of service structure and organization. We have provided CBT to patients on closed and open wards, in hospital and health center outpatient facilities, in community facilities, and in the patients' own homes. It is probable that the more flexible the system, the more likely the patient will be engaged and attend. To this end we often deliver treatment in the patient's home, which is a common procedure in the United Kingdom.

Evidence from research trials indicates that cognitive-behavioral treatments are delivered over about 20 treatment sessions. These can be intensive over 3 months or less intensive over 9 months. Clinical impressions indicate that some patients benefit from continued although less intensive treatment, whereas others benefit from booster sessions. The clinician should always be led by the clinical need of the patient rather than adhering to a rigid "one size fits all" protocol. It should be remembered that CBT does not "cure" schizophrenia, but it does help the patient cope with a chronic illness.

The presence of possible associated factors, as outlined earlier, signifies that patients may present with a number of clinical difficulties, as well as psychotic symptoms. The clinician needs to be aware that this may be the case and be prepared to address or treat these presenting problems before moving on to treat the psychotic symptoms. It may be necessary to tackle clinical problems such as high levels of anxiety, depression, hopelessness, and suicidal behavior and risk not only because they are clinical priorities but also because there may be important interactions between these other disorders and the psychosis.

The treatment described here is for individual CBT. It is possible to deliver treatment in a group format. Groups are well received by some patients and are advantageous, in that patients can learn from each other. The results suggest clinical benefits in terms of enhanced self-esteem, but reductions in symptoms are modest compared to those in individual treatments (e.g., Barrowclough et al., 2006).

Other psychosocial treatments may also be available, such as family interventions. There is a considerable literature on family interventions, which have been shown to reduce relapse rates in at-risk individuals. Details of family intervention are beyond the scope of this chapter (for the clinical application of family interventions, see Barrowclough & Tarrier, 1992/1997; Mueser & Glynn, 1995; see also Miklowitz, Chapter 10, this volume). We have combined individual CBT and family intervention with some success (e.g., Barrowclough et al., 2001) and suggest that therapists consider whether this strategy would be clinically beneficial. Concomitant family intervention may reduce stressful home environments and help to sustain improvement. Many patients live alone or are estranged from their relatives, so family intervention may not be an option.

Patient Variables

Patients with schizophrenia represent a heterogeneous group of whom 20–45% may be resistant to medication treatment (Kane, 1999) and 5–10% show no benefit from antipsychotic medication (Pantelis & Barns, 1996). Although there is confusion among the terms "treatment-resistant," "incomplete recovery," and "treatment intolerance," it is clear that conventional treatment with antipsychotic medication is ineffective in a significant number of patients in spite of well publicized advances in antipsychotic medication. It is important, therefore, in tailoring and refining treatments to understand what factors predict a good response to psychological treatment and perhaps the converse, which patients do not derive benefit. Unfortunately, little is known in any great detail about which patients will or will not benefit from cognitive-behavioral treatments (Tarrier &

Wykes, 2004). Factors that have been associated with poor outcome include negative symptoms of affective flattening and alogia (cognitive impoverishment) (Tarrier, 1996). Factors associated with better outcome include a shorter duration of illness, less severe symptoms at pretreatment (Tarrier, Yusupoff, Kinney, et al., 1998), and receptiveness to hypothetical contradiction (Garety et al., 1997). These results suggest that those patients with less severe illness and fewer severe cognitive deficits may respond better, but no hard-and-fast rules are currently supported by evidence. Treatment dropout is a further issue of importance. There is some evidence that patients who dropout of treatment tend to be male, unemployed and unskilled, and single, with a low level of educational attainment and a low premorbid IQ. They have a long duration of illness but at the time of discontinuation are not necessarily severely ill and can function at a reasonable level. Dropouts suffer from both hallucinations and delusions, are paranoid, although not necessarily suspicious of the treating clinician, and depressed and moderately hopeless. The majority cannot see the point of psychological treatment or think that they will not personally benefit from treatment (Tarrier, Yusupoff, McCarthy, Kinney, & Wittkowski, 1998).

Therapist Variables

Therapist variables encompass a number of factors, including training, experience, competency, and personal style. There is a tendency for health care planners to expect, mainly on economic grounds, that these complex therapies will be delivered by minimally qualified clinicians. This may well be a mistake (Tarrier et al., 1999). Psychological treatment of someone with a psychosis is complex, and besides having the skills and experience to treat the psychotic disorder itself, as outlined in this chapter, the clinician may well need to be able to treat a range of comorbid disorders, including anxiety, posttraumatic stress, depression, and addictive disorders. It seems reasonable that to treat successfully someone with a severe mental illness and very possibly a range of comorbid disorders, the clinician should be experienced and sufficiently well trained in CBT to be able to react to various clinical demands and levels of complexity. In my opinion the treatment of psychotic disorders does not lend itself well to merely following a highly prescriptive manual. As indicated in the previous section on associated features and disabilities, the clinician needs to be competent in recognizing and prioritizing a range of presenting clinical problems for treatment. Similarly, the clinician needs to have personal qualities that engage the patient, who may well be difficult to manage or disturbed, and to tailor the treatment to that individual. Previous research suggests that the absence of a positive relationship is associated with a poorer outcome (Tattan & Tarrier, 2000), so the clinician needs the experience and patience to develop that relationship and maintain engagement.

THE PROCEDURE OF CBT: THE MANCHESTER MODEL

A Clinical Model: The Coping–Recovery Model

The model I developed and describe bears many similarities to other models and has benefited from my contact and discussion with other clinical researchers in the field. The basic tenet is the recovery model, in which patients are coping with a potentially persistent illness that may well change many aspects of their lives, affect their hopes and aspirations, and be associated with comorbid disorders such as depression and anxiety disorders. The therapist aids the patient in facilitating, as much as possible, the process of recovery. The coping model strongly resembles and uses many methods of other CBT approaches but emphasizes coping with symptoms rather than curing them, and intervenes to modify cognitive processes (e.g., attention), as well as cognitive content and behavior.

The clinical model that guides treatment is presented in Figure 11.1. It assumes that the experience of psychotic symptoms, hallucinations, and delusions is a dynamic interaction between internal and external factors. Internal factors may be either biological or psychological and can be either inherited or acquired. For example, genetic factors may influence both the biochemical functioning of the brain and cognitive capacity. Alternatively, biological and psychological dysfunction may be acquired, for example, in deficits in cognitive flexibility and in the development of maladaptive attitudes. Such internal factors increase individuals' vulnerability to psychosis, and their risk is further increased through exposure to environmental stress, such as certain interpersonal or excessively demanding environments. The interaction between internal and external factors is important both in the origins of the disorder and in maintaining symptoms. A dysfunction in the processing of information, such as source monitoring in hallucinations (i.e., a belief about where the voice is coming from) and probabilistic reasoning in delusions, in combination with dysfunctions in the arousal system and its regulation, result in disturbances of perception and thought that are characteristic of psychosis. The individual is reactive to these experiences, and there is a process of primary and secondary appraisal in which the individual attempts to interpret these experiences and give them meaning, then react to their consequences. Often patients' appraisal of experience results in feelings of threat to their physical integrity or social standing and concomitant emotional reactions, and avoidant and safety behavior. The immediate reaction to the psychotic experience is multidimensional, including emotional, behavioral, and cognitive elements. Secondary effects, such as depressed mood, anxiety in social situations, and the effect of trauma may further compound the situation.

The important aspect of the model is that appraisal (including beliefs about experience) and reaction to the psychotic experience feed back through a number of possible routes and increase the probability of the maintenance or recurrence of the psychotic experience. For example, the emotional reaction to hearing threatening voices or experiencing strong feelings of paranoia may well be anxiety or anger. Both these emotions include elevated levels of autonomic arousal that act either directly, through sustained increased levels of arousal, or indirectly, through further disrupting information processing, to increase the likelihood of psychotic symptoms. Similarly, behavioral responses to psychotic symptoms may increase exposure to environmental stress or increase risk of trauma (e.g., becoming involved in violence or indulging in dangerous behavior) that maintains or aggravates psychotic symptoms. For example, paranoid thoughts may result in interpersonal conflict or, alternatively, social avoidance and withdrawal. Both situations are likely to increase the probability of symptoms occurring. Interpersonal conflict is likely to be interpreted as evidence for persecution, whereas withdrawal and isolation probably re-sult in confirmatory rumination and resent-ment, with a lack of opportunity to disconfirm these paranoid beliefs. The appraisal of the content of voices or delusional thoughts as valid and true may result in behavior consistent with these beliefs and a confirmatory bias to collecting and evaluating evidence on which to base future judgments of reality.

Psychotic experiences can lead to dysfunc-tional beliefs that are then acted upon in a way that leads to their confirmation or a failure to disconfirm. This can be termed the experience–belief–action–confirmation cycle, or EBAC cy-cle. It is suggested that such cycles maintain psychotic experience through reinforcement of maladaptive beliefs and behavior. The generic model indicated in Figure 11.1 provides an overarching picture of how the patient's prob-lems arise and are maintained. Embedded with-in this model are the microelements of specific, time-linked events such as the EBAC cycle (see Figure 11.2).

Assessment

The clinician needs to be able to assess and de-velop a formulation of the determinants of the patient's psychotic symptoms. Clinicians may find the use of standardized assessment instru-

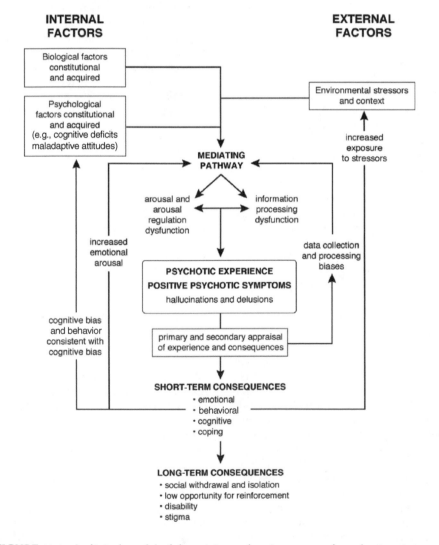

FIGURE 11.1. A clinical model of the origins and maintenance of psychotic symptoms.

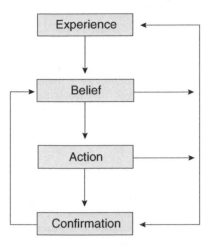

FIGURE 11.2. The experience–belief–action–confirmation (EBAC) cycle.

ments helpful (there are many of these, and they assess a range of functions; see Barnes & Nelson, 1994, for a detailed description and review of assessments). We recommend the Psychotic Symptom Rating Scales (PSYRATS; Haddock, McCarron, Tarrier, & Faragher, 1999) as an effective method of assessing the multidimensional nature of positive psychotic symptoms. The clinician needs to understand the individual variation in psychotic symptoms. This can be achieved by the use of a semistructured interview (the Antecedent and Coping Interview [ACI]; for more details, see Tarrier, 2002, 2006) that covers the nature and variation of positive psychotic symptoms experienced by the patient, including beliefs about psychotic symptoms, emotional reactions that accompany each symptom, antecedent stimuli and context in which each symptom occurs, consequences resulting from the symptoms and how the patient's behavior and beliefs are affected, and methods the patient uses to cope and manage his or her experiences. This allows the clinician to build up a comprehensive picture of how the patient experiences the psychosis on a daily basis and how his or her affect, behavior, and beliefs are changed. The clinician should be careful to identify avoidance and safety behaviors that occur because of psychotic symptoms, and examples in which the patient fails to disconfirm irrational or delusional beliefs. The clinician should use the clinical models shown in Figures 11.1 and 11.2 as a guide.

Intervention

Coping Strategies

When the clinician has constructed a comprehensive picture of the patient's psychotic experience, he or she can discuss this with the patient and present the rationale for CBTp. There may well be patients who are completely convinced of their delusional thoughts and will not accept any alternative view, in which case coping with distress should be advanced as a suitable goal.

The characteristics of CBTp and coping training are that it

- Is based on an individualized assessment or formulation.
- Emphasizes a normal and general process of dealing with adversity.
- Emphasizes that this is part of the recovery process.
- Is carried out systematically through overlearning, simulation, and role play.
- Is additive in that different strategies can be added together in a sequence that progresses to *in vivo* implementation.
- Is based on providing a new response set that will be a method of coping with an ongoing problem rather than being curative.
- The learning of cognitive coping skills is through a process of external verbalization that is slowly diminished until the required procedure is internalized as thought under internal control.
- Enhances executive function.
- Develops the learning of cognitive and behavioral coping skills through a process of graded practice or rehearsal.
- Provides opportunities for reappraisal and reattributions.

These coping methods include changes in cognitive processes, cognitive content, and behavior such as the following.

ATTENTION SWITCHING

A process whereby patients actively change the focus of their attention from one subject or experience to another. This involves inhibiting an ongoing response and initiating an alternative. Patients are trained within the session to switch attention on cue through rehearsal. This can be to external stimuli (e.g., an aspect of their environment, like describing a picture or being aware of background traffic noise) or to internal stimuli often to a set of positive images. For example, one patient who was asked to choose a positive scene to which to attend chose a restaurant in Blackpool, where he had had an enjoyable meal. He was trained to be able to elicit a visual image of the restaurant by describing the scene, furniture, decorations, and such in great detail. He was then asked to remember the experience of the meal in all his senses: the visual memory of the food; its smell and taste; the feel of holding the knife and fork in his hands; the experience of eating; and so on. He continually rehearsed the memory of the meal in the restaurant until he was able to elicit it at will. He then rehearsed switching his attention away from delusional thoughts to images of the meal. He was taught to use the onset of a delusion as a cue for attention switching (see "Awareness Training" below).

ATTENTION NARROWING

A process whereby patients restrict the range and content of their attention. Many patients talked about "blanking" their mind or focusing their attention as a method of coping. Evidence suggests that one problem faced by patients with schizophrenia is an inability to filter information input adequately, to distinguish signal from noise. Training patients to focus their attention and improve attentional control may assist them in overcoming this difficulty by narrowing and regulating their attention.

MODIFIED SELF-STATEMENTS AND INTERNAL DIALOGUE

That patients' use of self-statements can be incorporated successfully into intervention has been known for some years. The use of self-statements and internal dialogue may take on a number of functions in emotion control, such as teaching patients to overcome negative emotions associated with their voices; in cueing goal-directed behavior; and in cueing and directing reality testing. In each case the patient is taught statements that direct the appropriate response, such as "I don't need to be afraid," "I need to keep going and get on the bus," or "Why do I think that man is looking at me when I've never seen him before?" Within the session, the patient is first asked to repeat the set of statements or questions out loud when given the appropriate cue. The verbalized statements are then gradually reduced in loudness until they are internalized. The patient then practices these in simulated situations within the session. Learning such questioning statements is a useful stage in generating and evaluating alternative explanations for experience.

REATTRIBUTION

Patients are asked to generate an alternative explanation for an experience, then practice reattribution statements when that experience occurs. Initially, when we started coping training, we used reattributions that were illness related, such as "It's not a real voice, it's my illness," We have since abandoned this as unhelpful. We now try to use other, alternative explanations: "It may seem like a real voice, but it's just my own thoughts" and "It may seem as though people are looking at me, but they have to look somewhere." If patients do make changes that increase their control over their symptoms or circumstances, or challenge the omnipotence or infallibility of their voices, then these changes can be evidence for a reattribution concerning the nature of their symptoms or their ability to exert control—for example, "How can the voice be all powerful if it talks rubbish?" "I don't have to believe it if it isn't true."

AWARENESS TRAINING

Patients are taught to be aware of and monitor their positive symptoms, especially their onset. Patients not only become aware of their experiences but they also try to accept these experiences but not react to them. Patients are aware of their voices but do not react to them or become captured by their content. One function of awareness training is to make patients aware of the form and characteristics of their thoughts and perceptions rather than the content—for example, to monitor the physical onset of a voice, then use attention switching reduces the emotional impact of the content. The aim is twofold: to assist patients in becoming *mentally disengaged* from their symptoms, especially the content, and to use symptoms as a cue to alternative action.

DEAROUSING TECHNIQUES

Because high levels of arousal have been implicated in the psychopathology of schizophrenia and frequently occur as both antecedents and responses to psychotic experience, teaching patients to cope with these is important. These coping strategies may be simple passive behaviors to avoid agitation, such as sitting quietly instead of pacing up and down, or they may be more active methods of arousal control, such as breathing exercises or quick relaxation. We have not favored lengthy relaxation training, such as traditional progressive relaxation exercises, because these are time-consuming and off the point. What is functional here is a quick, usable skill.

INCREASED ACTIVITY LEVELS

Many patients are vulnerable to delusional thought or hallucinations during periods of inactivity, a problem to which patients with schizophrenia appear particularly prone. Many patients report that finding something to do is helpful. Thus, simple activity scheduling can be a powerful coping strategy, especially if implemented at the onset of the symptom, thus creating a dual task competing for attentional resources. Besides increasing purposeful activity this also reduces exposure to conditions under which symptoms are aggravated.

SOCIAL ENGAGEMENT AND DISENGAGEMENT

Although many patients tolerate social interactions poorly, surprisingly, many also find social engagement a useful method of coping. Possibly this may occur because social interaction serves as a dual task and source of distraction, and because it may help patients rationalize maladaptive thinking. It is beneficial to be able to titrate the amount of social stimulation involved in any interaction with the tolerance level of a particular patient, and to teach the patient that levels of social disengagement may be used to help develop tolerance of social stimulation. Social withdrawal and avoidance are common responses to experiencing overstimulation as a result of social interaction. However, patients can learn less drastic methods of disengagement, such as leaving the room for a short period and then returning, temporarily moving away from the social group, and practicing *functional disengagement* by not conversing for short periods or lowering their gaze. By using these methods, patients can control and tolerate social stimulation. Patients may also initiate social interaction more confi-

dently as a method to reduce the impact of their symptoms, if they feel they have some control over the intensity of those interactions. Simple training in specific skills for interaction and role plays can facilitate this.

BELIEF MODIFICATION

Patients can learn to examine their beliefs and to challenge them if they are inappropriate by examining the evidence and generating alternative explanations. Many patients do this to some extent already, but the level of arousal experienced, or the level of isolation and avoidance, can make these attempts unsuccessful. These methods are very similar to those used in traditional cognitive therapy except that the patient may need more prompting and the goal is to incorporate the skills of belief modification into a self-regulatory process. Patients can be encouraged to question their beliefs as they occur: "What would be the purpose of someone spying on me; how much effort and cost would it take; how would this be resourced and organized; and for what gain?" Similarly, patients can be encouraged to look for inconsistencies and to use these to challenge their beliefs. For example, the patient who was involved in a fight 15 years earlier, and still avoids young men because he fears that the same group is out to get revenge, may be asked to reflect on the fact that because the members of the gang are now in their middle to late 30s, he has been vigilant for the wrong age group. This can be used to challenge his fear that he needs to be vigilant to stay safe. In effect, his safety behaviors have not protected him from the source of danger. Patients can also learn to examine evidence to challenge their beliefs about the voices they hear. When patients perceive their voices as omnipotent and truthful, clinicians can investigate to see whether they have been wrong or incorrect. For example, the patient whose voices told him he was going to be murdered because he was a spy, concluded that the voices must be true and that he must deserve this fate. However, the voices also told him that he was soon to be married, and because he could find no supporting evidence for this, he decided it was untrue. However, he had never thought to challenge the voices' veracity concerning the threat of murder. Realizing that he was unlikely to be married in the near future, as the voices had asserted, helped him to challenge the idea that he was to be murdered by doubting the truthfulness of the voices and to look for further supporting, objective evidence of the spy ring, which was not forthcoming.

REALITY TESTING
AND BEHAVIORAL EXPERIMENTS

Probably the strongest way to test beliefs is to test them out in reality by some type of action; behavior change is probably the best way to produce cognitive change. Patients sometimes do this naturally, although a tendency toward biased interpretation and hypothesis protection may lead them to erroneous conclusions. Patients can learn to identify specific beliefs and to generate competing predictions that can be tested. The failure to do this in real life usually leads to patterns of avoidance, which can be reversed to challenge the beliefs that they underpin.

Enhancing Coping Strategies

Coping methods develop over time and vary in their complexity, from simple and direct attempts to control cognitive processes, such as attention, to more complex, self-directed methods that modify cognitive content and inference. Frequently, combinations of different coping strategies are built up, for example, the use of attention switching and dearousing techniques helps to dull the strength of a delusion, so that reality testing can be implemented. Without these initial coping methods the patient would not be able to undergo reality testing. Furthermore, the initial coping strategies can be used to challenge the strength of the delusion of the omnipotence of the voices and provide an increase in self-efficacy. The patient may ask questions, such as "You've used these attention-switching methods to cope effectively with your voices. What does that tell you about them being in total control and you being helpless?" The patient may well make statements that indicate the voices have been demonstrated to be fallible and he or she has some control over the situation, which can then be used as self-statements or a modified internal dialogue to further enhance self-efficacy and coping.

Modification of Behavior or Cognition

Changes in behavior and cognition complement each other, and one is not necessarily

better than the other. Changes in behavior should always be used to examine and potentially challenge maladaptive thoughts and beliefs or as learning experiences. Similarly, changes in cognition should be used as opportunities to change behavior and to establish new behaviors. The therapist should always look for opportunities to prompt patients to reappraise their beliefs. This can be carried out as part of formal behavioral experiments, naturally occurring changes, and frequent reflections on what has been achieved in treatment. In assessment and during formulation the therapist should always be alert to patients' avoidance or safety behaviors, or when patients do not behave in a way that could disconfirm their fears, delusions, or maladaptive cognitions. These can be used very early on in treatment as behavioral experiments to test out patients' beliefs or to provide opportunities for quick improvements to challenge despondent or hopelessness beliefs, such as "Nothing is worth it if I cannot change" or "I have no control over my life or circumstances." The belief of "no control" is often present and can be refuted by many small behavioral changes that may be repeated and referred to frequently. Finally, it is often helpful at the beginning of treatment to obtain some changes, however, although often small, in behavior and increase activity that may have a number of associated benefits and provide the opportunity for reappraisal.

Modification of Cognitive Content or Cognitive Process

Therapists frequently face the choice of whether to try to modify the content of hallucinations or delusions, or the attentional processes that these phenomena have captured. Traditionally, in cognitive therapy the content of cognition is the main focus. In the coping model intervention, this is broadened to modification of cognitive processes, because modifying cognitive processes provides greater clinical flexibility, and because deficits of the regulation of attention and executive function are often present in psychotic disorders. In practice, these tactics can work together. Initial modification of attentional processes through attention switching, for example, can decrease the emotional impact of the experience. A similar effect can be produced by attending to the physical characteristics of a hallucination rather than what the voice is actually saying.

This can provide not only an opening to challenge the truth of the content of the voice or delusional thought but also a sense of control over these experiences. Take, for example, a young man who is experiencing voices that accuse him of having committed a murder and that also say he is Russian. Initially, he can be taught to turn his attention away from the voices in a systematic way to reduce their emotional impact. This technique can be used to weaken the emotional strength of the experience, to elicit a sense of control, and to challenge the belief that the voices are all-powerful. With increased self-efficacy and a greater sense of power, the patient can later challenge the content of the voices that accuse him of murder by investigating the objective evidence that a murder has been committed. Furthermore, the untruthfulness of the voices in saying he is Russian can be used to challenge the veracity of the murder accusation; if the voices had been wrong about one issue, then they could be wrong about the other. Modification of cognitive process and content provides the therapist with two basic routes to intervention and the flexibility to move from one tactic to the other.

CASE STUDY

The following case example gives some indication of how CBTp works.

History

Jim, a 28-year-old man, developed a psychotic illness when he was 22. During his first episode, Jim became increasingly paranoid and accused people, including his friends, of stealing his money. He said that he could feel people taking money and his wallet from his pockets when he was socializing in his local pub and also when he was traveling by bus. The feeling that "something was wrong" had been with him for a few months, and Jim then began to hear voices warning him that people were against him and scheming to "do me down." These voices talked to Jim, warning him against "the schemes" and telling him who was involved and to be on his guard. These voices were especially insistent that those closest to Jim were the people most against Jim and the "worst schemers." The voices also told Jim that his girlfriend was unfaithful, and he experienced "visions," sent by the voices, of his girl-friend having sex with other men. He did not actually believe that his girlfriend was unfaithful, but he became very angry that the voices should make these accusations. On some occasions Jim did lose control and confronted some male friends about having affairs with his girlfriend. Usually he accepted their denials.

Jim also heard voices talking about him. These different voices were usually "scheming" and making insulting and accusatory comments. Sometimes these voices would laugh at Jim because his girlfriend was cheating on him, and make remarks about his sexual inadequacy, to which they attributed her infidelity.

Jim's friends and family noticed that he began to withdraw and became increasingly disheveled. He was often found muttering to himself or making sarcastic comments to family members about how they were "growing rich on my hard work." The voices also told him to "look for signs that the scheming is coming to a head." Jim began to write down an account of everyday events, such as the time certain buses arrived near his house and the type of advertisements on their sides. His parents, who would find these writings left around the house with various passages heavily underlined, increasingly worried about him and were also concerned that he was drinking considerable amounts of alcohol. Jim's friends began to avoid him and he was increasingly isolated. He broke up with his girlfriend, who could no longer deal with his accusations of infidelity.

The situation deteriorated very rapidly during the summer months, and Jim was hospitalized one evening and detained under the Mental Health Act. He had gone out early to his local pub. A number of his friends were there, but he kept away from them, drinking alone in a corner. Suddenly Jim got out of his seat and began shouting at his friends, accusing them of stealing his money, undermining his confidence, and spreading rumors about him. He took some loose change from his pockets and threw it at his friends. They tried to ignore him, but Jim became increasingly agitated and aggressive, and finally physically attacked one of them. A number of people became involved, and the situation became confused as a fight broke out. The police were called and Jim was arrested. He had suffered minor physical injuries, so he was taken to the accident and emergency department of the local hospital, and from there he was admitted to the psychiatric ward. He spent about 5 weeks in the hospital, during which time he was treated with antipsychotic medication. His health care plan included counseling, and his family received psychoeducation, in that they were given information about his diagnosis of schizophrenia and general advice on how to manage him at home. Jim's symptoms remitted during his hospital stay, and he was discharged with frequent outpatient appointments with his psychiatrist and home treatment with the assertive outreach team.

Over the intervening years Jim had five further relapses, during which a similar pattern would follow. He would become paranoid, hear voices and become isolated, and have increasing difficulty in caring for himself. Each relapse was followed by a short period of hospitalization with increased medication. However, residual symptoms became common following an episode, and in spite of increased medication and changes to atypical antipsychotics, Jim continued to experience auditory hallucinations, paranoid delusions, and delusions of reference. He often avoided going out or contacting people because of his paranoia. He was able to initiate and maintain a relationship, although the voices continued to send him "visions" and to question his girlfriend's faithfulness.

As a result of the increasing awareness of mental health service personnel to the potential benefits of psychological treatments, Jim was referred for CBT to treat his persistent positive psychotic symptoms as part of a multidisciplinary approach to his care and to promote recovery.

Current Situation

Jim now lived in his own apartment. He had good relations with his parents, who lived quite close by and whom he saw every few weeks. He was unemployed and received disability benefits. Jim attended a day center for people with mental health problems 2 or 3 days a week. He had attended a local college to study computers but had recently discontinued schooling because he found the social contact too stressful. Jim had a steady girlfriend, Sue, whom he saw regularly. He had lost contact with the friends he had had before he became ill, and although he occasionally saw them, he avoided them and places he thought they might go. He received antipsychotic medication, attended monthly outpatient appointments with a psychiatrist, and was visited at home once a week by a community psychiatric nurse who provided counseling and support, and monitored his mental state.

Mental State at Referral

Jim experienced auditory hallucinations in the form of a variety of voices talking to and about him. He described these as "helpful" voices and "evil" voices. The "helpful" voices warned him of the "schemes" of others and told him about dangerous situations and times when he was under threat. They warned him to avoid "dodgy people" who might attack or assault him. Jim thought their warnings were very helpful and was convinced that acting upon these warnings kept him from harm. The "evil" voices generally spoke about him, saying that he was "stupid, useless, and no good," "not up to it sexually," and other personally defamatory statements.

There were voices that told Jim that his girlfriend Sue was unfaithful and cheating on him. He was unsure whether these voices were "helpful" or "evil." These voices also sent him pictures of Sue being unfaithful and simultaneously told Jim that he was stupid and useless to put up with it. He described these pictures as "visions" that he found extremely distressing. Although Jim said he did not believe that Sue was unfaithful, the voices became increasingly more intense and compelling and he was unable to resist shouting back at them. Sue was able to reassure Jim that his fears were groundless.

Engagement

Initially Jim was resistant to contact with the clinician (in this case, Jim had been referred to a clinical psychologist for CBT). At the time of referral he was quite paranoid, and when he was visited at his home for the first appointment, having failed to attend his clinic appointment, Jim refused to open the door. (It is common practice for mental health professionals in the United Kingdom to do home visits.) A short conversation through the letter box ensued, ending with the clinician's statement that he would return at a more convenient time. Two further visits resulted in Jim refusing to open the door. The strategy here was just to make contact to reassure Jim that his views were perfectly valid and that another visit would be made at a later date to see how he felt about things then. In situations where the initial engagement is problematic, the best strategy is to "roll with resistance" and try to defuse the situation and reduce any agitation, maintain contact, and return at another time.

On the next occasion Jim was more relaxed and allowed the clinician into his flat. Given Jim's paranoia it was important for the clinician just to establish a positive interaction and relationship at this point and not to introduce the topic of symptoms or psychological treatment until Jim was completely comfortable with him. So, in Jim's case, the first couple of sessions were kept brief and covered his general well-being and topics of interest for him. The clinician's primary focus was to keep Jim engaged and to develop the beginnings of a therapeutic relationship. It is not always the case that assessment and treatment cannot be embarked upon more quickly, but maintaining engagement is essential.

The fourth session was longer and the clinician introduced the possibility of psychological treatment. This necessitated a discussion of Jim's symptoms, along the following lines:

CLINICIAN: I understand you have been hearing voices when no one is there? What do you make of this? Have you any idea what these voices are? Are the voices a difficulty for you? Would you want to try and do something about these voices?

These questions not only raise the topic of the psychotic experience and the suggestion of treatment but also attempt to obtain an idea of the patient's beliefs about the voices and whether they are perceived as real or not.

Similarly, the clinician can ask questions about the paranoid delusions:

"It is true that you are having difficulties with people?"
"Are you feeling that some people are against you? What do you make of these thoughts and feelings? Why do you think it is happening?"
"Are they a difficulty for you?"
"Would you want to try and do something about these thoughts and worries?"

Again, the clinician attempts to assess quickly how strongly Jim holds these delusions and whether he would consider treatment.

Jim was not enthusiastic about treatment. He thought that his fears were real, as were the voices, and that psychological treatment was not appropriate in his case. This reaction is often encountered in patients with residual and persistent psychotic symptoms. A number of important points should be considered:

• What needs to be done to maintain engagement?
• How can a clinically relevant problem be identified and mutually agreed upon?
• How can treatment be framed so that the patient sees it as achieving a positive and desired benefit?

First, it is important to validate the experience, but it is not necessary to agree on the cause. For example, in this case, it was important to agree that *Jim did hear voices*, and that he *believed that some people were against him*. This can be done without agreeing that the voices come from a real entity or that people are actually against him. This helps to separate *Jim's belief* about what is happening to him from the experience; that is, that Jim has the belief is not the same as that belief being true. Similarly, that Jim hears voices is not the same as believing these voices exist as an independent and real entity. It may not necessarily be possible to agree on these points at this time, but the clinician can return to these issues. At the moment, engagement is more important.

Next, it is often helpful to investigate the consequences of the experience. Some of the voices cause Jim distress, and his paranoid ideas cause him to be fearful. Thus, distress and fear are more likely to be problems that Jim will be willing to address. This can be introduced as follows:

"You have told me that the voices sometimes make you feel very upset. Perhaps that upset is something I can help you with and that you would like to work on?"

"The thoughts that some people out there are against you and want to harm you make you very frightened. Perhaps that fear is something we can work on together, so you feel less afraid? Maybe if you were less afraid you could cope better with dealing with people. Would that be helpful to you?"

So in cases when patients are very deluded or lack insight into their symptoms, trying to persuade them that eliminating their symptoms, the experiences that they believe to be real, can be counterproductive and jeopardize engagement. However, trying to reduce distress may be a viable alternative for a collaborative goal. There is also an assumption from the model that reducing emotional reactions to symptoms may well weaken the symptoms themselves.

However, Jim remained unenthusiastic about this treatment goal as well. His view was that being fearful about people was a reasonable reaction given that there were people who would harm him, and this emotion kept him on his "edge," so that he was more vigilant for threat and danger. His belief was that such vigilance actually kept him safe from harm, so there was little motivation to change and put himself in harm's way.

To protect engagement it is important not to dispute or argue with the patient, and most definitely not at this early stage, when the patient is not convinced that there is any benefit to be gained from treatment. The next strategy the clinician used to engage Jim was to ask him about his goals in life.

CLINICIAN: Jim, what sort of goals do you have? Is there anything you would like to achieve personally? Is there anything you would like to do that you haven't been able to do, for whatever reason?

JIM: Yes, lots of things. I'd like to get a job that's well paid. I'd like to go back to college. That would help me get a good job.

CLINICIAN: Going to college would help you get a good job. That is a very good idea. Would you like to go back to college?

JIM: I would but when I went before I had problems.

CLINICIAN: What sort of problems were they?

JIM: Well, I got scared of the people there. I thought some of them were scary, dodgy, money grubbers. The voices told me not to go. I have to do what the voices tell me.

CLINICIAN: So one of your important goals is to get to college so as to help you get a good job, but being scared of the people there and the voices is stopping you from going to college and achieving your goals. Is that about it?

JIM: Yes, I suppose you are right.

In this way Jim has realized that his important goals are being impeded by his psychosis, and he and the clinician are able to agree on a problem that needs to be addressed. Thus, Jim can see a benefit to receiving treatment.

As well as maintaining engagement, the clinician has learned quite a lot about Jim and his problems. The voices warn Jim about certain situations, and he listens to them and takes avoidant action; thus, he has developed a number of safety behaviors that protect him from perceived harm. Opportunities to test out or refute these threat cognitions by dropping safety behavior are not taken up. However, there are situations that lend themselves to reality testing. Jim experiences command hallucinations (voices that give him a direct order) to which he responds. The likelihood that Jim thinks the voices are powerful, and that he has little or no control over them, provides future opportunity to refute these attributions. Jim experiences some feelings of dissonance, in that he is now aware that his valued goals are impeded.

Case Formulation

Treatment naturally follows from an accurate assessment of the patient's problems and it is important to establish details of the antecedents and consequences of psychotic symptoms (see Tarrier & Calam, 2002, for a discussion of case formulation in general). In this case, Jim has many psychotic symptoms, and it is probably best to deal with them in stages.

Paranoid Delusions

Jim has paranoid delusions that occur in a number of situations. When alone in his flat, Jim worries that his old friends and family have stolen all his money and are scheming against him. This is reinforced by the voices telling Jim he needs to be on his guard. Jim also becomes very paranoid when he goes out. For example, in the street he scans the crowds for signs of his old friends, so that he can make good his escape if he sees them or "scary people" who might assault him. He is also paranoid at the day center, just as he was at college. The voices tell him the situation is dangerous, that there are dangerous people about, and that he must take care. Jim knows the voices will warn him of danger, so he listens out for them and is attentive to them when they occur. At the day center Jim becomes more agitated the longer he is there, and he usually goes home after a short time. In doing so he feels reassured that the voices have helped him and kept him from harm. Jim also wonders why the voices help him and concludes that it must be because he is special in some way. This puzzles him, because the "evil" voices are unpleasant and nasty to him. Jim concludes that because he is special, he is being tested by the "evil" voices to see whether he is worthy of their help. Only special people would be helped and be tested. In thinking this way, Jim has resolved the dissonance posed by experiencing both "helpful" and "evil" voices.

The clinician and Jim decide jointly to focus on the difficult situation at the day center:

CLINICIAN: OK, Jim, I'd like you to talk me through what happens at the day center. The reason I ask this is because you remember that attending college was an important goal you wanted to achieve but couldn't, because you felt suspicious of people there. Well, the situation at the day center is a lot like that at college, so we might learn how you can cope with returning to college if we examine the day center situation. Does that sound OK to you?

JIM: OK. Well one of the things that happens is that I know the voices know I'm vulnerable, because they can tell when I'm like that, which is when they attack me, but they also want to help me, so they warn me about the scary people there.

CLINICIAN: How do the voices know you are vulnerable?

JIM: They can tell, because they know how I feel.

CLINICIAN: How do you feel when you are vulnerable?

JIM: All shaky and on edge.

CLINICIAN: Is that like a feeling of being anxious or stressed?

JIM: Yes, a bit like that.

It appears that Jim becomes anxious in anticipation of going to the day center. There may be a range of reasons for this, such as anticipatory and situational anxiety, social anxiety, fear of being attacked, or general elevated levels of arousal. One hypothesis is that Jim picks up on this feeling of anxiety and misattributes it to being "vulnerable" to the voices. This is because his increased anxiety is associated with an increased probability of experiencing auditory hallucinations, but Jim attributes meaning to this association. Voices are imbued with attributes of power and intent.

CLINICIAN: OK, Jim, so you're feeling anxious and vulnerable. What happens next?

JIM: Well usually the voices will start. They can say a lot of things, but they will warn me about danger. I know that the voices will attack me, but I want to keep safe, and they will warn me so I listen out for them.

Here Jim is indicating that not only do the voices occur in this situation but also his attention is focused on listening out for them, which may indicate that the threshold for detecting them is being lowered. This suggests that a redirection of attention may be a helpful method of coping with this situation. The clinician does not suggest this method at this stage, but he may call upon it later.

CLINICIAN: When they warn you, how does it happen?

JIM: The voices will see someone that is dangerous and they will say, "See him? He's going to get you, he'll attack you. You better get out of here." When they say that, I can see this guy looks vicious and he's going to have a go at me, so I get out of there as fast as I can.

CLINICIAN: Then what happens?

JIM: I get out of there, and I feel real relieved that I've escaped. I feel real lucky that I've got the voices to keep me safe. Otherwise, I'd be in for it, I'd be in terrible trouble. The more I think about it, the more lucky and special I feel. They keep me safe.

It appears that Jim attributes both personal meaning to his voices and power to keep him safe. In fact he has developed a type of safety behavior that reduces his anxiety and helps him escape a feared consequence. His avoidant behavior also reinforces his feeling of being special.

This establishes a useful behavior cycle that the clinician may utilize to help Jim abandon his safety behaviors and to disprove his catastrophic predictions that he will be attacked. First, it is helpful to establish a little more detail.

CLINICIAN: You said that the voices warn you about danger at the day center most of the time. Does this always happen?

JIM: No, not every time. I always listen out very carefully for the voices, but sometimes they aren't there.

CLINICIAN: So when the voices aren't there, what happens?

JIM: Sometimes I still feel vulnerable, but I just get on with it.

CLINICIAN: Do you mean you don't leave, you stay there?

JIM: Yes, sometimes I get bored and go home, but usually I stay and have a chat and a cup of tea.

CLINICIAN: Tell me, Jim, is it pretty much the same people there whether you hear the voices or not?

JIM: Yes that's it, pretty much the same people all the time.

CLINICIAN: So sometimes the voices tell you someone is dangerous and you get out pretty quick, and feel relieved you weren't attacked, and at other times the voices aren't there, but you stay with the same people, those that you thought were dangerous before, and nothing happens. Doesn't that mean that at times they are dangerous and other times they're not dangerous? Isn't that strange?

JIM: Yes, I suppose it is. I'd not thought about that before.

Here, the clinician is looking for inconsistencies in situations that can be used to refute Jim's beliefs. The clinician highlights the inconsistency in the logical presence of threat and feeds it back to the patient, who is asked what he makes of it. The clinician pursues the point about the inconsistency of the occurrence of the voices.

CLINICIAN: Sometimes the voices aren't there. Why is that?

JIM: I don't know that either. Maybe they have to look after someone else on that day. Yes, that must be it. There must be other special people that they have to look after and they are helping them. Just goes to show how important the voices are if they have lots of special people to look after. Means I'm really special too, one of the real special people.

At this point Jim appears to be confabulating and absorbing this new information into his delusional thought network. New information is processed in a way that protects rather than challenges the delusional system. This is useful, because an alternative explanation—that the voices occur when Jim attends to them and feels stressed and are less likely to occur if he is more relaxed and engaged—can be advanced and tested as an alternative belief.

The clinician now needs to motivate Jim to test out some of his beliefs. He compares the day center situation with college and the achievement of an important goal to motivate Jim to attempt to cope better at the day center. Furthermore, it is established that generally Jim enjoys going, although ambivalence is maintained by his fear of attack. Being taught how to manage his fear and be more relaxed in the situation is also a motivating factor.

Jim needs to have a plausible set of alternative explanations of what is going on, so that he may process any new information differently and not reinforce his delusions. In the past Jim has been told that he is paranoid because he has a mental illness involving an imbalance of biochemicals in his brain. This is not a particularly attractive explanation to Jim. It does not reflect his actual experience, and it is stigmatizing. Jim needs to be presented with an alternative model of his experiences that allows him to collaborate in his psychological treatment.

The clinician might suggest that paranoia is a result of misunderstanding or misinterpreting situations, and that if Jim feels stressed and anxious, as he does at the day center, then he may misattribute this physical state to a "vulnerability." He is more likely to experience the voices when he is anxious, but this does not mean that the voices know he is vulnerable. The clinician might also suggest that Jim ignore the voices when they tell him he is about to be attacked and just get on with what he is doing at the day center. Because the same people are there, and they do not attack him when the voices are absent, it is unlikely that he will be attacked when the voices are present. Thus, a behavior experiment can be established to test out whether the voices keep Jim safe. This may help challenge Jim's belief that the voices are both truthful and helpful, and that they are powerful and all knowing.

When Jim did enter these situations, he was acutely aware that his voices might occur, so that he developed an internal focus to monitor for feeling "vulnerable" and an external attention scan for hearing the voices. The former meant that he was more likely to amplify any internal sensations. The latter meant that he was more likely to verbalize what the voices usually said to him as a match and also, paradoxically, to focus his attention internally. This process of internal focus and attention scanning was more likely to trigger the voices. Intervention here involved persuading Jim to use other attentional strategies when he entered these situations. These strategies were rehearsed in the sessions and prompted with appropriate internal dialogue.

Jim also made a number of attributions about the voices. He believed that the voices warned him of threat because he "might be special," and he thought they might be able to do this through telepathy, and that he had little control over this process. Jim was troubled because the voices were often unpleasant, and he could not understand why they would be so if they were helping him to avoid danger. But Jim concluded that because he was special, he needed to "be tested" by the voices, which in turn confirmed his belief that he was special. Of course, much of this explanation had been built up on the incorrect premise that the voices were actually warning him of a real danger, which could be challenged. An alternative explanation of his experience could be based on a normalization of this experience. Everyone has self-referent or bizarre thoughts at times, and in Jim's case these are perceived as external voices rather than being identified as part of the self and merely thoughts. Jim found this explanation plausible, although he was not entirely accepting of it. This is not unusual; however, it did seed doubt in his mind and could be constantly referred to, further weakening his delusional explanations.

Two difficulties arose with Jim. He did not have an alternative explanation for the voices other than they represented some, albeit vague and poorly defined, powerful entity or beings (delusional), or that they were the manifestation of a biochemical imbalance in his brain (disease). The clinician suggested to Jim that his voices might be his own thoughts or a leakage from memory into consciousness that was not identified as being part of his self. This was why the voices often reflected Jim's fears or concerns, or aspects of his past.

The voices warned Jim when he was in danger. He believed that the voices helped and protected him in these situations. For example, on one occasion when Jim was walking down a road, the voices told him that a man coming from the other direction was going to attack him. Jim crossed the road to avoid the man and believed that in doing so he had avoided being attacked. He also noticed that the man looked "suspicious," which further confirmed his belief that the voices had saved him from danger. Here is an example of an EBAC cycle to which I referred earlier in the chapter.

- Experience—Voices tell him of a suspicious person approaching.
- Belief—He is in imminent danger.
- Action—He crosses the road.
- Confirmation—He has avoided being attacked.

This can be used as another therapeutic example:

CLINICIAN: You've told me that when the man approached you in the street, he was looking at you and the voices told you you were in danger. What happened next?

JIM: Well, I knew he would go for me, so I crossed the street and got away.

CLINICIAN: When you crossed the street, did the man look at you or follow you, or say anything?

JIM: No I don't think so.

CLINICIAN: Isn't that strange, if he was out to attack you?

JIM: Yes, I suppose so. I'd not thought about that before, I was so glad to get away.

CLINICIAN: Tell me, Jim, when you walk down the street, where do you look?

JIM: Well, where I'm going, of course. That's a daft question!

CLINICIAN: Well, it may seem so, but think where was the man going when you thought he was looking at you to attack you.

JIM: Well, he was walking toward me, and he was looking in that direction.

The clinician continues his questioning, so that Jim keeps returning to the conclusion that the man happened to be looking at him because Jim was in his line of vision, nothing more. There was no evidence of an intent to attack, and once Jim was out of his line of vision, the man paid no further attention to him. Experiments can be constructed to further emphasize this point. Sometimes Jim may be drawing attention to himself by his own actions, which make people look at him (the self-fulfilling prophecy). Again, this can be drawn out by a similar line of questioning and tested. A similar approach can be taken with other examples of Jim's paranoid behavior, and his behavior with friends and family. The clinician always comes back to these past examples of successful belief and behavior change, and asks Jim how he feels about them and whether he can identify any common factors between these past successes and current problems.

"Visions" Sent by the Voices

Jim was very upset with the "visions" he experienced of his girlfriend having sex with other people. He thought these visions were sent by the voices, also by a process of telepathy. Jim did not believe his girlfriend was unfaithful, but he became very upset and angry when the voices told him this. He tried to push the images out of his mind but when this strategy failed, he became further convinced that the images were sent via telepathy. The more angry and upset Jim became, the more difficult he found it to resist the belief and to view the experience of the visions as collateral evidence. An alternative explanation was that the visions were mental images that had become very vivid and occurred in response to his catastrophic thoughts about his girlfriend's infidelity and persisted because Jim attempted to suppress them. The voices were his own thoughts, which again posed questions about his girlfriend's fidelity, because his constant ruminations on the topic had made him feel insecure about his relationship. This alternative explanation, in conjunction with a review of the objective evidence regarding the security of his relationship, significantly weakened Jim's delusional beliefs about infidelity, telepathy, and the reality of the voices. The clinician introduced thought suppression exercises to demonstrate the rebound effect of Jim pushing the images out of his mind. Exposure to the "visions" were also useful in this case (although they might not be in all cases), demonstrating that images held in attention fade with time, along with the distress they cause, which was further evidence of an internal phenomena and not external telepathy. Jim was also taught to identify the onset of the voices and to switch his attention to alternative stimuli as a way to reduce their impact and to demonstrate that these experiences were more likely internally generated rather than coming from an external entity. The clinician compared these experiences with anxiety disorders in which catastrophic beliefs and images serve to fuel irrational and threatening beliefs, pointing out that vivid imagery of "what might happen" or an imagined "catastrophe" would produce a sudden cascade of intense emotions. These experiences could then be relabeled as unpleasant but highly improbable situations rather than reality.

Any slight reduction in the strength of a delusional belief was also used to challenge Jim's general beliefs about control, threat, and veracity.

LOW SELF-ESTEEM: A COMMON PROBLEM

Patients with schizophrenia frequently have a poor perception of themselves and low self-esteem. These global concepts can be hypothesized to be manifest in terms of a negative self-schema. This is postulated as being a consequence of severe mental illness and all that goes with this. This can involve suffering the stigma of a mental illness and even harassment and exclusion, the effects of social rejection and negative interpersonal environments, and the projected sense of being valueless and devalued. Patients with depression and suicidal ideation may feel increased feelings of low self-worth because of their depressed mood. Furthermore, an attribution process can make them think that if they feel they want to kill themselves, then they must be worthless and deserve to die.

The factors that potentially impact upon and maintain negative self-schemas are represented in Figure 11.3. As can be seen, the factors that influence and maintain negative self-schema are strong, multiple, and relentless. The consequence of having a severe mental illness is the formation of such negative self-schemas, which then serve to bias the way information is assimilated, so that these negative schemas are maintained and strengthened rather than being challenged and modified.

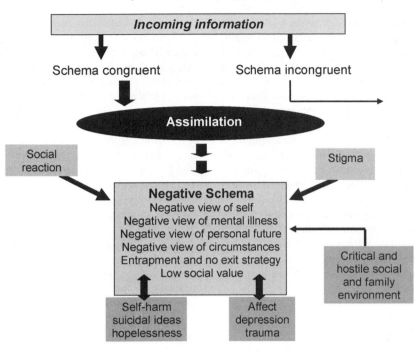

FIGURE 11.3. Maintenances of negative schemas.

Feelings of low self-worth can both inhibit the effective use of coping strategies and increase the risk of depression and self-harm.

Improving the Patient's Self-Esteem

The aim of this set of techniques is to produce generalizations of positive attributes, challenge negative self-schemas, improve global self-esteem, and elicit positive emotional reactions. This method can be carried out in two stages. The first stage elicits positive cognitions about the self, and the second elicits a positive emotional response. Alternatively, the two stages can be combined, so that the processes of cognitive and emotional responding occur together. The procedure for the two-stage process is described for convenience as follows:

Stage 1. Cognitive Responding

• Ask the patient to produce up to 10 positive qualities about him- or herself (the number can be varied dependent on the patient's capabilities; it is important that the patient not fail in generating the required number).

• Once the patient has produced a list of these qualities, ask him or her to rate each on how much he or she really believes it to be true on a 0- to 100-point scale (where 0 = *Not at all* and 100 = *Completely*).

• Ask the patient to produce specific examples of evidence of each quality; prompt specifically for actions that have occurred recently and can be time linked, such as "last week"; also use your knowledge of the patient to elicit examples. Prompt and list as many examples as possible.

• Ask the patient to rehearse the list of examples for each quality, which may be done through verbal description and mental imagery of the event, then to rerate his or her belief that he or she possesses this quality. (Usually the belief rating changes to show an increase; it should be emphasized to the patient that his or her belief can change depending on the evidence on which he or she focuses attention.)

• The patient is given a homework exercise to monitor his or her behavior over the next week and to record specific evidence to support the contention that he or she has these qualities. The aim is to produce generalization and experiential learning of a number of positive attributes.

• At the next session, provide feedback on examples and prompt further examples. Again, ask the patient to rerate his or her belief that he or she actually has these qualities, and further point out any changes in these beliefs.

• Ask the patient to reflect on the effect that eliciting and focusing on specific behaviors and evidence has on beliefs and qualities about him- or herself and how this could affect the general opinion of him- or herself. Reinforce all positive attributes and the process whereby the patient comes to a more positive view of him- or herself.

• Continue to repeat this procedure. Continually emphasize that the patient's beliefs about him- or herself vary depending on what is the focus of attention, and that self-esteem can be greatly affected by belief and is thus amenable to change.

The case of "Dave" illustrates implementation of this procedure. Dave had very successfully learned to cope with his symptoms, which had been markedly reduced, and he had significantly improved his level of functioning. Dave produced a number of attributes that he thought he might have: "helpful," which he gave a belief rating of 60 out of 100; "friendly," which he rated 50; and "a good father," which he rated as 30. He was then asked to suggest concrete and specific evidence to support all of these. For "helpful," he cited having lent money to a friend some months before, opening a door to someone the previous week, and helping his father in the garden that week. He rerated this belief as 90.

For "friendly," Dave cited that he had had many friends of 10 to 20 years' standing; his friends contacted him regularly and enjoyed his company; he could talk comfortably to people in pubs or on buses. He got on well with the friends of his parents. He thought he got on well with the therapist and enjoyed speaking to him, and that he could talk to different types of people from different backgrounds without difficulty or reserve. He rerated this belief as 100.

For being a "good father," Dave said that he enjoyed taking his son and daughter out every week (he was divorced from their mother, who had custody). He was upset when he did not see them. He liked to buy them presents. He was happy for them to decide on activities rather than doing things purely for convenience, and this in itself gave him pleasure. Dave rerated this belief as 60. However, at this point he introduced some negative evaluations. He felt that he could not be a good father, because he did not live with his children. He did not get on with their mother. He said that it was always easier for absent fathers, who saw their children for short periods of time and tended to spoil them. This was not responsible parenting in his view. At this point it was helpful for the clinician to go through the model of how negative views such as this are maintained (see Figure 11.3), and to discuss these thoughts as being negative schema–congruent and indicate that the statements were overgeneralizations, a process by which negatives are maximized and positives minimized. Furthermore, these thoughts and beliefs had a depressing effect on his mood, and maintained Dave's negative beliefs about himself, but did not accurately reflect circumstances. To challenge Dave's views of himself as a bad father, various exercises where undertaken: He was asked to define a "bad father" in explicit terms, then objectively compare his behavior to this definition. He was asked to compare his behavior with that of others in similar circumstances. Last, he was asked to give a realistic and objective appraisal of his performance and circumstances. While carrying out these exercises, the clinician emphasized the potential for negatively biased self-appraisals, along with strategies for coping with this in the future.

Stage 2: Affective Responding

Dave was also asked to explain why these qualities were important and the potential benefits of possessing them. The clinician used guided discovery and imagery during this process to ensure that the qualities selected were meaningful and important to Dave. Dave was then asked to generate practical examples of each quality. Particular emphasis was placed on describing specific behaviors associated with the quality and the context in which they were carried out. Attention was directed to Dave's emotional experiences when displaying that quality, thus generating the positive affect associated with that experience. Dave was asked to imagine the positive emotional reaction that another person would experience in interaction with him as he displayed a positive quality, and to vividly imagine the other person's experience and describe how he or she would feel and attempt to mimic this experience. Dave was then asked to describe how he himself felt when he had evoked the positive emotion in the other person.

For example, in displaying generosity by helping out a friend, Dave was asked to imagine through guided imagery how that friend felt when assisted by Dave. He was asked to intensify and sustain this positive emotion. Then, through a similar process, Dave was asked to imagine and describe how he himself felt when he realized how positive his friend had felt in being helped out. Again Dave was asked to intensify and sustain this emotion. A similar process should be carried out for all positive characteristics and scenarios.

PREVENTION OF RELAPSE

Relapses rarely occur without any forewarning. They are usually preceded by a period of prodromal symptoms that can last for days, or more usually weeks, and in some cases, months; the average prodrome is, however, about 4 weeks (Birchwood, MacMillan, & Smith, 1994). Common prodromal signs and symptoms include nonpsychotic symptoms, such as mild depression or dysphoria, anxiety, insomnia, irritability, mood fluctuations and interpersonal sensitivity, and low-level psychotic symptoms such as suspiciousness, magical thinking, ideas of reference, feelings that "something is strange or wrong" and that the individual does not "fit in" with others around him. During the prodromal phase, patients display behavior change, such as becoming more withdrawn, avoiding social contact, abandoning hobbies or interests, appearing more preoccupied, and being unable to continue with work or other routine or demanding activities. As the prodrome progresses, these signs and symptoms intensify and patients may exhibit strange and bizarre behavior, such as being unable to care for themselves, becoming socially or sexually inappropriate, making accusations against others, muttering to themselves, and disconnecting the television or telephone.

Patients may be asked to recall prodromal signs and symptoms that preceded previous episodes and relapses. This can be based on the onset of the episode or admission to the hospital, then identifying when changes were first noticed, what changes occurred, and how they progressed and in what sequence. Each sign or symptom may be written on a card, and the patient may be asked to arrange them in temporal

order of occurrence. In this way the patient's *relapse signature*, that is, the individual set of signs and symptoms that characterized the patient's prodrome and its time course leading to relapse, can be identified. Family members or professional mental health staff, if available, can help identify prodromal changes and their sequence. Clinicians may find the use of standardized assessments of prodromal symptoms helpful, such as the Early Signs Scale (Birchwood et al., 1989). Such instruments can also help the clinician cue or inquire about possible prodromal symptoms not spontaneously recalled by the patients. The patient needs to be able to discriminate between an actual relapse prodrome and normal mood fluctuations that do not signal a relapse. This is done through a process of discrimination training, whereby the patient monitors mood and experiences over a number of weeks, with a goal of learning to distinguish a real prodrome from the "false alarm" of a normal fluctuation in affect.

The next stage is to formulate a "game plan" to deal with a prodrome should one occur. Coping strategies can be formulated and rehearsed, the help of others can be elicited, and the assistance of psychiatric services can be requested, which may include an increase or change in medication. With an understanding of the time course of patients' prodromes, the clinician can identify different actions for different phases of the prodrome and the "window of opportunity" to intervene. An important part of the treatment approach is to plan for the future, especially for potentially stressful events that may occur and how to be aware of emerging symptoms and relapse. Patients can be monitored by returning to the clinician postcards indicating that they are well or that a prodrome may have started. The advent of new technology such as mobile phones and e-mail may provide new, innovative methods for clinicians to monitor patients and maintain contact, to identify early signs of relapse, and to intervene at the optimal time.

CLINICAL PROBLEMS AND DIFFICULTIES

Thought Disorder

Thought disorder, typically characterized by disruption to language, makes it difficult to comprehend the meaning that the patient is imparting. However, with experience and patience, it is often possible to follow some internal logic in the patient's speech. This can be accomplished by asking the patient to explain the meaning, or by reflecting back one's own understanding, which is then rephrased in more coherent language. Progressing through these organized steps in a calm manner can help prevent the patient from feeling overloaded with the emotional content of the discussion, which can occur, especially when the material being discussed is emotionally salient.

Intractable Psychotic Symptoms

Regrettably, there are cases in which the therapist's best efforts and optimum medication produce little improvement in the patient's symptoms. A number of options are available in such intractable cases. First, it is necessary to ensure that appropriate support services are in place, so that the patient's quality of life is maximized. Second, there should be regular reviews of treatment, especially of medication and of environmental circumstances, so that excessive stresses are avoided. Last, it is always worth continuing with a few simple and direct cognitive-behavioral strategies, because, over a long period of time, these may begin to have an effect.

Risk of Suicide and Self-Harm

The risk of suicide in patients with schizophrenia is significant. Risk factors include being young and male, and having a chronic illness with numerous exacerbations, high levels of symptomatology and functional impairment, feelings of hopelessness in association with depression, fear of further mental deterioration, and excessive dependence on treatment or loss of faith in treatment. In one study two paths to suicide risk, both of which were mediated by hopelessness, were also identified: (1) increased social isolation, to which longer illness duration, more positive symptoms, older age, and being unemployed contributed, and (2) greater negative views of the self, higher frequency of criticism from relatives, and more negative symptoms, to which being male, unmarried, and unemployed significantly contributed (Tarrier, Barrowclough, Andrews, & Gregg, 2004).

It is important for therapists to be aware that suicide attempts are a very real possibility while treating someone with schizophrenia. Unfortunately, patients with schizophrenia often commit suicide impulsively and use lethal methods, such as jumping from heights, immolation, or firearms. The presence of suicidal ideation needs to be assessed, and the patient needs to be asked whether he or she has made any specific plans or taken any actions, and whether the normal barriers to self-harm and suicide have broken down. It is necessary to be aware of factors that can elevate risk, including erosion of self-esteem; increased sense of hopelessness and despair, especially related to the patient's perception of the illness and recovery; disruptive family or social relationships; and any changes in social circumstances or loss of supportive relationships (e.g., changes in mental health staff, staff holidays, or leave). Furthermore, the occurrence of major life events, loss, or shameful experiences can lead to despondency.

Some factors that can increase risk for suicide are quite unique to the psychotic disorders, such as the experience of command hallucinations telling patients to self-harm. Other examples are more idiosyncratic. I had a patient who experienced strange physical sensations that he interpreted as the Queen of England entering his body. As a loyal subject, he thought he should vacate his body to give her sole possession, and he attempted to kill himself by slashing his wrists. This was not the result of a will to die, but was more driven by some sense of social protocol toward royalty. Fortunately, the attempt was unsuccessful.

Many clinicians hypothesize that psychotic symptoms have a protective aspect in masking the harsh realities of the burden of serious mental illness. Improvement in insight and symptomatology can bring with it an increased exposure to this burden, thus increasing the probability of potential escape through suicide. The clinician needs to be aware of all these factors, to know his or her patients well, and to monitor changes in their circumstances or mood that may be problematic. It is important to be aware of predictable changes and plan for them, to establish good communication with other mental health workers, and to address depressed mood and hopelessness in an open manner. Assessing acute suicide risk is further complicated by patients' flat or incongruous affect, so that the cues that a clinician would look for in a depressed patient may not be exhibited by a patient with schizophrenia. When risk is high, emergency psychiatric services should be called.

Dual Diagnosis: Comorbidity of Alcohol and Substance Use

Comorbid substance use disorders are an escalating problem in patients with schizophrenia. Dual-diagnosis patients tend to do worse than patients with schizophrenia alone on a range of outcomes. They tend to be more persistently symptomatic, to have more frequent and earlier relapse and readmission, to be more likely to present to the emergency services, to have higher levels of aggression and violence, and greater risk of suicide and self-harm.

Motivational interviewing has been used effectively to enhance motivation to change substance use behavior in nonpsychotic patients (Barrowclough et al., 2001; Haddock et al., 2003). Motivational interviewing has been termed a "style" rather than a specific intervention, and can be incorporated into a CBT approach to increase the patient's motivation to change substance or alcohol use behavior while concurrently addressing the psychosis. It is postulated that an important interaction between alcohol or substance use and psychotic symptoms requires this dual-treatment approach. Many patients do not consider their alcohol or substance use a problem, and perceive the positive benefits, such as self-medication, peer identification, or enjoyment, as outweighing any negative consequences. The aim during the initial sessions is to elicit change or motivational statements from the patient. The therapist uses the motivational interviewing skills of reflective listening, acceptance, and selective reinforcement to elicit such statements. Once the patient identifies substance or alcohol use as a problem and expresses a desire to change, therapy can then progress to practical ways to achieve this goal.

CONCLUSION

CBTp for psychosis does have significant benefits for patients with schizophrenia and psychosis. It should be carried out as part of a comprehensive care plan. It is unlikely to "cure" patients, but it may assist them in coping with and recovering from their illness. Intervention is based on a detailed assessment and formulation. It does require considerable skill, experience, and knowledge of CBT and psychosis, and it does not lend itself easily to a simple protocol format. Further research on theoretical aspects of understanding psychosis from a psychological perspective is important to further inform and develop CBT procedures. Research into dissemination and how new psychological treatments penetrate into mental health services and become accessible to patients is required.

REFERENCES

Barnes, T. R. E., & Nelson, H. E. (1994) *The assessment of psychoses: A practical handbook*. London: Chapman & Hall.

Barrowclough, C., Haddock, G., Lobban, F., Jones, S., Siddle, R., Roberts, C., et al. (2006). Group cognitive behaviour therapy for schizophrenia: randomized controlled trial. *British Journal of Psychiatry, 189*, 527–532.

Barrowclough, C., Haddock, G., Tarrier, N., Lewis, S., Moring, J., O'Brian, R., et al. (2001). Randomised controlled trial of motivational interviewing and cognitive behavioural intervention for schizophrenia patients with associated drug or alcohol misuse. *American Journal of Psychiatry, 158*, 1706–1713.

Barrowclough C., & Tarrier N. (1992). *Families of schizophrenic patients: A cognitive-behavioural intervention*. London: Chapman & Hall.

Birchwood, M., MacMillan, F., & Smith, J. (1994). Early intervention. In M. Birchwood & N. Tarrier (Eds.), *Psychological management of schizophrenia* (pp. 77–108). Chichester, UK: Wiley.

Birchwood, M., Smith, J., MacMillan, F., Hogg, B., Prasad, R., Harvey, C., et al. (1989). Predicting relapse in schizophrenia: The development and implementation of an early signs monitoring system using patients and families as observers. *Psychological Medicine, 19*, 649–656.

Bolton, C., Gooding, P., Kapur, N., Barrowclough, C., & Tarrier, N. (2007). Developing psychological perspectives of suicidal behaviour and risk in people with a diagnosis of schizophrenia: We know they kill themselves but do we understand why? *Clinical Psychology Review, 27*, 511–536.

Brooker, C., & Brabban, A. (2006). *Measured success: A scoping review of evaluated psychosocial interventions training for work with people with serious mental health problems*. London: National Health Service, National Institute for Mental Health in England.

Cohen, J. (1988). *Statistical power analysis for the behavioral sciences* (2nd ed.). Hillsdale, NJ: Erlbaum.

Doll, R. (1998). Controlled trials: The 1948 watershed. *British Medical Journal, 317,* 1217–1220.

Garety, P., Kuipers, E., Fowler, D., Freeman, D., & Bebbington, P. E. (2001). A cognitive model of the positive symptoms of psychosis. *Psychological Medicine, 31,* 189–195.

Garety, P. A., Fowler, D., Kuipers, E., Freeman, D., Dunn, G., Bebbington, P., et al. (1997). London–East Anglia randomised controlled trial of cognitive-behavioural therapy for psychosis: II. Predictors of outcome. *British Journal of Psychiatry, 171,* 420–426.

Gould, R. A., Mueser, K. T., Bolton, E., Mays, V., & Goff, D. (2001). Cognitive therapy for psychosis in schizophrenia: An effect size analysis. *Schizophrenia Research, 48,* 335–342.

Haddock, G., Barrowclough, C., Tarrier, N., Moring, J., O'Brien, R., Schofield, N., et al. (2003). Randomised controlled trial of cognitive-behavior therapy and motivational intervention for schizophrenia and substance use: 18 month, carer and economic outcomes. *British Journal of Psychiatry, 183,* 418–426.

Haddock, G., McCarron, J., Tarrier, N., & Faragher, B. (1999). Scales to measure dimensions of hallucinations and delusions: The Psychotic Symptom Rating Scales (PSYRATS). *Psychological Medicine, 29,* 879–890.

Hall, P. H., & Tarrier, N. (2003). The cognitive-behavioural treatment of low self-esteem in psychotic patients: A pilot study. *Behaviour Research and Therapy, 41,* 317–332.

Johnson, J., Gooding, P., & Tarrier, N. (in press). Suicide risk in schizophrenia: Explanatory models and clinical implications. *Psychology and Psychotherapy.*

Kane, J. M. (1999). Management strategies for the treatment of schizophrenia. *Journal of Clinical Psychiatry, 60*(Suppl. 12), 13–17.

Lewis, S. W., Tarrier, N., Haddock, G., Bentall, R., Kinderman, P., Kingdon, D., et al. (2002). Randomised controlled trial of cognitive-behaviour therapy in early schizophrenia: Acute phase outcomes. *British Journal of Psychiatry, 181*(Suppl. 43), 91–97.

Morrison, A. P., French, P., Walford, L., Lewis, S., Kilcommons, A., Green, J., et al. (2004). A randomised controlled trial of cognitive therapy for the prevention of psychosis in people at ultra-high risk. *British Journal of Psychiatry, 185,* 291–297.

Mueser, K., & Glynn, S. M. (1995). *Behavioral family therapy for psychiatric disorders.* Needham Heights, MA: Allyn & Bacon.

Nuechterlein, K. H. (1987) Vulnerability models for schizophrenia: State of the art. In H. Hafner, W. F. Gattaz, & W. Janzarik (Eds.), *Search for the cause of schizophrenia* (pp. 297–316). Heidelberg: Springer-Verlag.

Pantelis, C., & Barns, T. R. E. (1996). Drug strategies in treatment resistant schizophrenia. *Australian and New Zealand Journal of Psychiatry, 30,* 20–37.

Pilling, S., Bebbington, P., Kuipers, E., Garety, P., Geddes, J., Orbach, G., et al. (2002). Psychological treatments in schizophrenia: I. Meta-analysis of family interventions and cognitive behaviour therapy. *Psychological Medicine, 32,* 763–782.

Pocock, S. J. (1996). *Clinical trials: A practical approach.* Chichester, UK: Wiley.

Rector, N. A., & Beck, A. T. (2001). Cognitive behavioral therapy for schizophrenia: An empirical review. *Journal of Nervous and Mental Disease, 189,* 278–287.

Richardson, A., Baker, M., Burns, T., Lilford, R. J., & Muijen, M. (2000). Reflections on methodological issues in mental health research. *Journal of Mental Health, 9,* 463–470.

Salkovskis, P. M. (2002). Empirically grounded clinical interventions: Cognitive behaviour therapy progresses through a multi-dimensional approach to clinical science. *Behavioural and Cognitive Psychotherapy, 30,* 3–10.

Slade, M., & Priebe, S. (2001). Are randomised controlled trials the only gold that glitters? *British Journal of Psychiatry, 179,* 286–287.

Tarrier, N. (1996). A psychological approach to the management of schizophrenia. In M. Moscarelli & N. Sartorius (Eds.), *The economics of schizophrenia* (pp. 271–286). Chichester, UK: Wiley.

Tarrier, N. (2002). The use of coping strategies and self-regulation in the treatment of psychosis. In A. Morrison (Ed.), *A casebook of cognitive therapy for psychosis* (pp. 79–107). Cambridge, UK: Cambridge University Press.

Tarrier, N. (2006). A cognitive-behavioural case formulation approach to the treatment of schizophrenia. In N. Tarrier (Ed.), *Case formulation in cognitive behaviour therapy: The treatment of challenging and complex clinical cases* (pp. 167–187). London: Routledge.

Tarrier, N., Barrowclough, C., Andrews, B., & Gregg, L. (2004). Suicide risk in recent onset schizophrenia: The influence of clinical, social, self-esteem and demographic factors. *Social Psychiatry and Psychiatric Epidemiology, 39,* 927–937.

Tarrier, N., Barrowclough, C., Haddock, G., & McGovern, J. (1999). The dissemination of innovative cognitive-behavioural treatments for schizophrenia. *Journal of Mental Health, 8,* 569–582.

Tarrier, N., & Calam, R. (2002). New developments in cognitive-behavioural case formulation: Epidemiological, systemic and social context: An integrative approach. *Cognitive and Behavioural Psychotherapy, 30,* 311–328

Tarrier, N., Haddock, G., Lewis, S., Drake, R., Gregg, L., & the Socrates Trial Group. (2006). Suicide behaviour over 18 months in recent onset schizophrenic patients: The effects of CBT. *Schizophrenia Research, 83,* 15–27.

Tarrier, N., & Wykes, T. (2004). Is there evidence that

cognitive behaviour therapy is an effective treatment for schizophrenia: A cautious or cautionary tale? (Invited essay). *Behaviour Research and Therapy, 42,* 1377–1401.

Tarrier, N., Yusupoff, L., Kinney, C., McCarthy, E., Gledhill, A., Haddock, G., et al. (1998). A randomised controlled trial of intensive cognitive behaviour therapy for chronic schizophrenia. *British Medical Journal, 317,* 303–307.

Tarrier, N., Yusupoff, L., McCarthy, E., Kinney, C., & Wittkowski, A. (1998). Some reason why patients suffering from chronic schizophrenia fail to continue in psychological treatment. *Behavioural and Cognitive Psychotherapy, 26,* 177–181.

Tattan, T., & Tarrier, N. (2000). The expressed emotion of case managers of the seriously mentally ill: The influence of EE and the quality of the relationship on clinical outcomes. *Psychological Medicine, 30,* 195–204.

Wykes, T., Everitt, B., Steele, C., & Tarrier, N. (in press). Cognitive behaviour therapy for schizophrenia: Effect sizes, range of outcomes, clinical models and methodological rigor. *Schizophrenia Bulletin.*

Zimmermann, G., Favrod, J., Trieu, V. H., & Pomini, V. (2005). The effect of cognitive behavioural treatment on the positive symptoms of schizophrenia spectrum disorders: A meta-analysis. *Schizophrenia Research, 77,* 1–9.

CHAPTER 12

Alcohol Use Disorders

Barbara S. McCrady

Clinicians working with individuals with alcohol use problems, as well as clinicians in training, have found this chapter to be an extraordinarily useful resource in guiding their treatment approaches. In this thoroughly updated and edited revision, the author begins by describing how recent societal trends and legislative initiatives have altered the nature of the clientele who come for treatment with drinking problems. After briefly reviewing the available empirical evidence on treatment approaches that range from Alcoholics Anonymous to brief interventions to intensive inpatient treatment, the author describes the myriad factors that every clinician must consider in choosing and carrying out appropriate interventions for individuals with drinking problems. Using a variety of illuminating case vignettes, Barbara McCrady illustrates important therapeutic strategies, including methods for motivating these patients to begin treatment. In a manner that emphasizes the humanity of the couple and makes the partners come to life, the extended case study in this chapter illustrates the all-too-frequent tragic consequences of excessive drinking. In the context of this case description, the author describes in great detail what clinicians will not find in books that simply lay out various treatment procedures—that is, the thrusts and parries of a superb and experienced clinician in overcoming the roadblocks that inevitably emerge during treatment.—D. H. B.

Alcohol use disorders are a heterogeneous group of problems ranging in severity from the heavy-drinking college student who occasionally misses classes to the person with severe and chronic alcoholism who experiences serious medical and social consequences of drinking. Although the prevalence of alcohol use disorders is higher in males than in females and in younger than in older adults, these problems affect individuals from any sociodemographic, racial/ethnic, or occupational background. In mental health and medical settings, at least 25% of clients are likely to have an alcohol use disorder as part of their presenting problems,

so clinicians in health and mental health professions need to be competent to identify, assess, and plan an effective course of treatment for these clients. This chapter describes the social context of drinking and drinking problems, provides an integrative model for conceptualizing and treating alcohol use problems, and presents both a series of case vignettes and an extended case study to illustrate the clinical model.

The clinician functioning in the 21st century must provide treatment within a complex and contradictory treatment network; must have formal and systematic training in the treatment of alcohol and other drug use disorders; must have tools to work with involuntary and voluntary clients, those who adhere passionately to a traditional recovery perspective, and those who are offended by it; and may work either to promote major and enduring changes in alcohol use or to decrease the harm that individuals and groups may experience from their use.

Given this rather complex picture, and given the notorious reputation of persons with alcohol use disorders for being difficult and frustrating to treat, many clinicians might ask, "Why bother?" The answers to this question must, on one level, be as individual as each clinician's motives for doing therapy. This chapter, however, assumes that the clinician who has useful and effective tools for working with persons with drinking problems, and who has a bit of success with these tools, will find positive reasons to see these clients. Persons with drinking problems *are* treatable; they are both challenging and rewarding to treat; and when they change successfully, the clinician has the rare opportunity to participate in helping people make major and satisfying changes in their lives.

DEFINITIONS AND DIAGNOSIS OF ALCOHOL PROBLEMS

Diagnosis

Contemporary approaches to the diagnosis of alcohol problems are based on a hypothetical construct, the "alcohol dependence syndrome" (Edwards & Gross, 1976), a constellation of behavior patterns and problems that result from drinking and are hypothesized to constitute a diagnostic entity. The diagnosis of alcohol problems in the *Diagnostic and Statistical Manual of Mental Disorders*, fourth edition, text revision (DSM-IV-TR; American Psychiatric Association, 2000) is based on the alcohol dependence syndrome. The two primary DSM-IV-TR alcohol use disorder diagnoses are alcohol dependence and alcohol abuse. To be diagnosed as having alcohol dependence, an individual must meet at least three of seven criteria that relate to impaired control (a persistent desire or attempts to cut down or stop; using larger amounts or over longer periods of time than intended), physical tolerance, physical withdrawal, neglect of other activities, increased time spent using alcohol, and contin-

ued use despite knowledge of recurrent physical or psychological problems related to use. Alcohol dependence is diagnosed "with physiological dependence," if either the tolerance or the withdrawal criterion is met, or "without physiological dependence," if the individual has neither tolerance nor withdrawal. Alcohol dependence also may be classified as being in "partial remission" or in "full remission"; remission may be "early" (at least 1 month) or "sustained" (1 year or more). Alcohol abuse is diagnosed based on problems in at least one of four areas, including failure to fulfill major social role obligations at work, home, or school; drinking repeatedly in a manner that creates the potential for harm (e.g., drinking and driving); incurring repeated alcohol-related legal consequences; or continuing to drink despite known social or interpersonal problems because of drinking. If an individual has ever met criteria for alcohol dependence, he or she can no longer receive a diagnosis of alcohol abuse.

Researchers have been examining the reliability and validity of DSM-IV diagnostic criteria, and further changes are likely in DSM-V (e.g., one of the more interesting and radical proposals has been to restrict the diagnosis of alcohol dependence to those with signs of alcohol withdrawal) (Langenbucher et al., 2000). Such a shift would result in more individuals diagnosed with alcohol abuse than with alcohol dependence. Other suggestions for changes in diagnostic criteria have focused on elements of the alcohol abuse diagnosis. In particular, it appears that those who meet abuse criteria because of repeated drinking and driving may differ from others who meet abuse criteria (Hasin, Paykin, Endicott, & Grant, 1999). Such findings suggest that diagnostic criteria for alcohol use disorders will continue to evolve in future versions of the DSM.

Alternative Definitions

In contrast to the formal psychiatric diagnosis of alcohol abuse or dependence, behavioral researchers and clinicians have suggested that alcohol problems represent one part of a continuum of alcohol use, ranging from abstinence through nonproblem use to different types and degrees of problem use. From this perspective, problems may be exhibited in a variety of forms—some that are consistent with a formal diagnosis, and others that are milder or more intermittent. By using an alcohol problems perspective, the clinician can focus more clearly on the pattern of drinking, negative consequences that the individual has accumulated, his or her behavioral excesses and deficits across various areas of life functioning, and the client's particular strengths. A deemphasis on diagnosis forces the clinician to consider clients from a more individual perspective. Therefore, although formal diagnosis is useful for identifying and defining the severity of a client's problems and is necessary for formal record keeping, the approach to clinical assessment emphasized in this chapter attends less to diagnostic issues and more to problem identification.

This chapter views alcohol use problems as a multivariate set of problems, with alcohol consumption as a common defining characteristic. These problems vary in severity from severe alcohol dependence to mild and circumscribed problems. For some, alcohol consumption itself is a major presenting problem; for others, the consequences of alcohol use—such as disruption of a relationship, occupational problems, or health problems—are the major reason for seeking treatment. In viewing alcohol problems as multivariate, this chapter also assumes the existence of multiple etiologies for these problems, with genetic, psychological, and environmental determinants contributing in differing degrees for different clients.

Complicating Problems

Drinking problems are complicated by a variety of concomitant problems. Of significance is the comorbidity of alcohol use disorders with other psychiatric diagnoses. A high percentage of those diagnosed with alcohol abuse or dependence also experience other psychological problems, which may be antecedent to, concurrent with, or consequent to their drinking (Rosenthal & Westreich, 1999). The most common Axis I disorders are other psychoactive substance use disorders, depression, and anxiety disorders, occurring in up to 60% of males in treatment. The most common Axis II disorder comorbid with alcoholism in males is antisocial personality disorder, with rates ranging from 15 to 50%. Females more often present with depressive disorders; 25 to 33% of women with alcoholism experience depression prior to the onset of their alcoholism.

Alcohol problems also are complicated by problems with cognition, physical health, inter-personal relationships, the criminal justice system, the employment setting, and the environment. Many people with alcoholism have subtle cognitive deficits, particularly in the areas of abstract reasoning, memory, and problem solving (for a review of this literature, see Bates, Bowden, & Barry, 2002). Because verbal functioning is usually unimpaired, these cognitive problems are not immediately apparent. Heavy drinking also causes a variety of medical problems and can affect any organ system in the body. Heavy drinking may cause conditions such as cardiomyopathy, liver diseases, gastritis, ulcers, pancreatitis, and peripheral neuropathies. Even when obvious medical conditions are not present, the effects of heavy drinking can be insidious and debilitating. Many people eat poorly when drinking, which results in nutritional deficits, poor energy, or vague and diffuse physical discomfort. Mortality rates among persons of all ages are elevated with alcohol dependence, and are higher among women than among men.

Interpersonal relationships also may be disrupted. The rates of separation and divorce range up to seven times those of the general population (Paolino, McCrady, & Diamond, 1978); spousal violence is higher among both men and women with alcohol use disorders (Drapkin, McCrady, Swingle, & Epstein, 2005); and emotional and behavioral problems are more common among their spouses/partners and children (Moos & Billings, 1982; Moos, Finney, & Gamble, 1982). Health care utilization is elevated among the spouses and children of actively drinking individuals with alcohol use disorders (Spear & Mason, 1991).

Persons presenting for treatment of a drinking problem may be involved with the legal system because of charges related to driving while intoxicated (DWI), other alcohol-related offenses such as assault, or involvement with the child welfare system. Drug-related charges also may bring a client to treatment. Clients vary in the degree to which they recognize that their drinking is creating problems, and in their degree of motivation to change their drinking patterns.

In conclusion, the client presenting for treatment may be drinking in a manner that creates concern, be formally diagnosed as having alcohol dependence or alcohol abuse, and also meet criteria for one or more Axis I or Axis II disorders. The person also may have other major problems, such as cognitive impairment, physical health problems, interpersonal or occupational problems, and/or legal problems. Problem recognition and motivation to change may be low. How does the clinician develop a rational approach to conceptualizing and treating this rather complicated clinical picture?

THEORETICAL MODEL

This model assumes that treatment planning must be multidimensional and that there is more than one effective treatment for alcohol problems. Unlike certain disorders for which one treatment approach has demonstrable superiority over others, in the alcohol field there are a number of legitimate and empirically supported approaches to treatment. These treatments are based in different conceptualizations of the etiology, course, treatment goals, and length of treatment for alcohol problems. Among the treatments with the best support are brief and motivationally focused interventions, cognitive-behavioral treatment, 12-step facilitation treatment, behavioral couple therapy, cue exposure treatment, and the community reinforcement approach. A number of factors seem to be common to effective treatments. These are summarized in Table 12.1. A key therapist responsibility is to help a client find a treatment approach and treatment setting that is effective for him or her, rather than slavishly adhering to a particular treatment model or setting. A second and equally important therapist responsibility is to enhance the client's motivation to continue to try, even if the initial treatment setting is not effective. This treatment model takes into account seven major considerations: (1) problem severity, (2) concomitant life problems, (3) client expectations, (4) motivation and the therapeutic relationship, (5) variables maintaining the current drinking pattern, (6) social support systems, and (7) maintenance of change.

Problem Severity

Problem severity is relatively atheoretical, and is most important in decision making about the types of treatments to be offered, the intensity of the treatment, and the initial treatment setting. Severe alcohol dependence can best be conceptualized as a chronic, relapsing disorder (McLellan, Lewis, O'Brien, & Kleber, 2000), with relapses occurring even after extended periods of abstinence. As with other chronic disorders, such as diabetes, cardiovascular disease, or rheumatoid arthritis, the clinician necessarily takes a long-term perspective, and maximizing periods of positive functioning and minimizing periods of problem use should be the primary goals. In contrast, other individuals have alcohol-related problems that may be circumscribed and not progressive (Finney, Moos, & Timko, 1999). Epidemiological data suggest that for the majority of those with alcohol-related problems, the problems will resolve or remit without any need for formal treatment or intervention. The clinician encountering individuals at the mild end of the severity spectrum should plan a brief, motivationally enhancing intervention to complement the natural recovery process and inspire these individuals to make changes in their drinking.

Concomitant Life Problems

Clients with alcohol use disorders often have problems in multiple areas of life functioning—physical, psychological/psychiatric, familial, social/interpersonal, occupational, legal, child care, housing, transportation. Assessment of multiple areas of life functioning is crucial for the planning and delivery of effective treatment. Research suggests that targeting client problem areas can be successful in making appreciable changes in these problems, even with clients who are severely alcohol dependent and homeless (Cox et al., 1998). Furthermore, providing treatment directed at multiple problem areas enhances positive alcohol and drug use outcomes as well (McLellan et al., 1997; Morgenstern et al., in press).

Client Expectations

Clinicians should provide clients with accurate expectations about the intensity of their treatment and the probable course of their problems. To date, no research has examined ways to affect such client expectations, so the recommendations provided here derive from empirical findings about the course and treatment of alcohol use disorders, and remain to be tested.

The clinician can inform clients with circumscribed, less severe problems that treatment will be short in duration, that they are likely to be successful in reducing their drinking, and that the long-term prognosis is good. Such cli-

TABLE 12.1. Principles for Treatment of Substance Use Disorders

1. *Structure and organization of the treatment setting*
   - Clear and well organized
   - Actively involve the clients in the program
   - Provide a supportive and emotionally expressive environment
   - Emphasize self-direction, work, and social skills development
   - Expect clients to take responsibility for their treatment and follow through
2. *Type of provider and what the provider does*
   - Treatment by addictions specialists or mental health clinicians
   - Development of an effective therapeutic alliance is crucial
     - Accurate empathy
     - Respect for the experience of clients in therapy
     - Avoidance of confrontational struggles
   - Provide goal direction for the clients
   - Provide a moderate level of structure for the therapy
   - Handle ambivalence about changing or being in treatment:
     - Titrate level of confrontation to the level of clients' reactance
     - Avoid arguing with angry clients
     - Avoid pushing clients hard to accept their diagnosis or the need to change
3. *Level of care, continuity of care, and elements of treatment*
   - Pay attention to retaining clients in treatment
   - Determine the intensity and length of treatment partly by considering the severity of the substance use disorder.
     - For heavy drinkers with low alcohol dependence, less intense, briefer treatments are appropriate and intensive inpatient therapy yields poorer outcomes.
     - Clients with severe alcohol dependence have better outcomes with more intensive initial treatment, and respond most positively to treatment that focuses on 12-step counseling and involvement with 12-step groups.
   - Assess and arrange for attention to clients' other social service and medical care needs
4. *Contextual factors*
   - Involve a significant other
   - Help clients restructure their social environments to include persons that support change and abstinence.
   - With clients who have little commitment to remain in treatment or change their substance use, involve the family or other member of the social support system in the treatment to foster retention in treatment
   - In the treatment of adolescents with substance use disorders, use approaches that involve multiple systems, including the family, peers, and others
5. *Client characteristics*
   - Greater client readiness to change is associated with greater treatment success
   - Greater severity of the substance use disorder is associated with a poorer response to treatment
6. *Specific therapeutic elements*
   - Focus on client motivation
   - Help clients develop awareness of repetitive patterns of thinking and behavior that perpetuate their alcohol or drug use
   - Attend to the affective experiences of clients
   - Consider the role of conditioning in the development and maintenance of substance use disorders. Clinicians should carefully assess for indicators of specific conditioned responses to alcohol or drugs, and develop ways to change these conditioned responses
   - Enhance positive outcome expectancies
7. *Client–treatment matching*
   - Assess for comorbid disorders and use empirically supported treatments for additional presenting problems
   - Use female-specific treatment with women clients

Note. From Haaga, McCrady, and LeBow (2006). Copyright 2006 by Wiley Interscience. Reprinted by permission.

ents also can be told that now or at some point in the future they may decide to stop drinking completely (Miller, Leckman, Delaney, & Tinkcom, 1992), or that they may continue to drink in a moderated fashion.

Clients with more severe and chronic dependence, however, should be given a different set of expectations about treatment and the likely course of their problems. It is fair to tell them that about one-third of middle-class clients maintain sustained abstinence over extended periods of time (e.g., 4 years; Pettinati, Sugerman, DiDonato, & Maurer, 1982), and that more than half (57%) will sustain long-term remission (abstinence or drinking without problems) (Finney & Moos, 1991). The challenge for such clients is to learn skills to manage their drinking in a way that makes it minimally disruptive to their lives. Chronic illness metaphors may be helpful. For example, like a patient with diabetes, a client with severe alcohol dependence needs to make and maintain significant lifestyle changes to support healthy functioning. Like the patient with diabetes, the client with severe alcohol dependence needs to know warning signs that he or she may be getting into trouble and know what to do. And neither individual can afford to forget or ignore his or her chronic problem.

Motivation and the Therapeutic Relationship

Clients vary in the degree to which they recognize their drinking is problematic and in their readiness to change. Motivational models suggest that individuals initiate change when the perceived costs of the behavior outweigh the perceived benefits, and when they can anticipate some benefits from behavior change (Cunningham, Sobell, Sobell, & Gaskin, 1994). Prochaska and DiClemente (2005) have proposed a continuum of stages of readiness for change. The continuum includes the stages of "precontemplation," in which a person does not recognize a behavior as problematic; "contemplation," in which the person considers that a behavior pattern might be problematic; "determination" or "preparation," in which the individual resolves to change; and "action," in which a person initiates active behaviors to deal with the problem. Following "action" is "maintenance" if the behavior change is successful, or "relapse" if the person returns

to the problem behavior. Miller and Rollnick (2002) suggested that several factors influence a person's readiness to change, including awareness of problem severity, awareness of positive consequences for changing the behavior, and the perception of choice in making changes. Clients' apparent stage of change and their self-perception of their problems should guide a clinician's initial approach to treatment and treatment planning.

Contemporary models view motivation as a state that can be influenced by therapeutic behaviors and the client's life experiences. Therapeutic approaches to enhance motivation are associated with less client resistance to treatment and with more positive drinking outcomes (Miller, Benefield, & Tonigan, 1993). Motivationally enhancing approaches appear to be particularly effective with clients who enter treatment very angry and hostile (Project MATCH Research Group, 1997b). Miller and Rollnick (1991) described six common elements to enhance motivation, summarized in the acronym FRAMES: personalized feedback (F) to the client about his or her status; an emphasis on the personal responsibility (R) of the client for change; provision of clear advice (A) about the need for change, given in a supportive manner; providing the client with a menu (M) of options for how to go about changing, rather than insisting upon one treatment or treatment goal; providing treatment in a warm, empathic (E), and supportive style; and enhancing the client's perceived self-efficacy (S) for change.

Factors Maintaining the Current Drinking Pattern

Case conceptualization for treatment planning focuses on factors maintaining the problematic drinking pattern. Different treatment models use different frameworks for conceptualizing current factors that maintain drinking. Presented here is a cognitive-behavioral approach to case conceptualization. The cognitive-behavioral case formulation assumes that drinking can best be treated by examining current factors maintaining drinking rather than historical factors. Factors maintaining drinking may be individual, or related to environmental circumstances or interpersonal relationships. The model assumes external antecedents to drinking that have a lawful relationship to drinking through repeated pairings with positive or negative reinforcement or through the anticipation of reinforcement. The model assumes that cognitions and affective states mediate the relationship between external antecedents and drinking behavior, and that expectancies about the reinforcing value of alcohol play an important role in determining subsequent drinking behavior. Finally, the model assumes that drinking is maintained by its consequences, and that the sources of these consequences may be physiological, psychological, or interpersonal.

To integrate these assumptions about drinking, my colleagues and I use a functional analytic framework, in which the drinking response (R) is elicited by environmental stimuli (S) that occur antecedent to drinking; that the relationship between the stimulus and response is mediated by cognitive, affective, and physiological, or organismic (O) factors; and that the response is maintained by positive or the avoidance of negative consequences (C) as a result drinking. Various individual, familial, and other interpersonal factors are associated with drinking. At the individual level, environmental antecedents may be associated with specific drinking situations, times of the day, or the mere sight or smell of alcohol. Organismic variables may include craving for alcohol; withdrawal symptoms; negative affects such as anger, anxiety, or depression; negative self-evaluations or irrational beliefs; or positive expectancies about the effects of alcohol in particular situations. Individual reinforcers may include decreased craving or withdrawal symptoms, decreases in negative affect or increases in positive affect, decreased negative self-evaluations, or decreased focus on problems and concerns.

At the familial level, various antecedents to drinking occur. Alcohol may be a usual part of family celebrations or daily rituals. Family members may attempt to influence the problematic drinking behavior by nagging the person to stop or by attempting to control the drinking through control of the finances or liquor supply. These actions may become antecedents to further drinking. Families in which a member is drinking heavily may develop poor communication and problem-solving skills, as well as marital/couple, sexual, financial, and child-rearing problems that then cue further drinking. The person with the drinking problem may have a variety of reactions to these familial antecedents,

experiencing negative affect, low self-efficacy for coping with problems, and/or retaliatory thoughts. Family behaviors may serve to reinforce the drinking. The family may shield the person from negative consequences of drinking by taking care of the drinker when intoxicated or assuming his or her responsibilities. A number of investigators have observed positive changes in marital/couple interactions associated with drinking, such as increases in intimate exchanges or increased assertiveness by the drinker, suggesting that these positive behaviors may reinforce the drinking (e.g., Frankenstein, Hay, & Nathan, 1985).

There also are other interpersonal antecedents to drinking. These may include social pressures to drink; work-related drinking situations; friendships in which alcohol consumption plays a major role; or interpersonal conflicts with work associates, friends, or acquaintances. The person may react to interpersonal antecedents to drinking with craving, positive expectancies for alcohol use, social discomfort, or negative self-evaluations for not drinking. Positive interpersonal consequences of drinking may include decreased craving or social anxiety, an enhanced sense of social connectedness or fun, or increased social comfort or assertiveness.

Social Support

The behaviors of family and other members of the client's social network are integral to the case conceptualization. The availability of general social support, as well as social support for abstinence or moderate drinking, is crucial to successful treatment. Clients in a social network that is strongly supportive of drinking may need to take deliberate steps to detach from that social network and access new social networks that support abstinence or moderate drinking. Some data suggest that involvement with Alcoholics Anonymous (AA) can serve such a function (Longabaugh, Wirtz, Zweben, & Stout, 1998), and data on natural recovery from alcohol problems suggest that finding a new love relationship or involvement in religious activities also may be viable avenues for change (Vaillant & Milofsky, 1982).

Maintenance of Change

Implicit in much of the preceding discussion is a view that individuals with severe alcohol use disorders have a high probability of relapse, an ever-present consideration, both because long-term, ingrained habits are difficult to change, and because of the permanent physiological and metabolic changes stimulated by heavy drinking (Moak & Anton, 1999). Several models have been proposed to conceptualize the maintenance or relapse process, with associated treatments. The most prominent maintenance models include Marlatt and Gordon's (1985) relapse prevention (RP) model, and the disease model, best exemplified by the practices common to AA. The RP model is an extension of the functional-analytic model described earlier, and focuses on the interplay among environment, coping skills, and cognitive and affective responses in maintaining successful change. In the RP model, relapse occurs in response to a high-risk situation for which the client either lacks or does not apply effective coping skills. Low self-efficacy for coping with the situation may contribute to the difficulties. If the client does not cope effectively, use of alcohol is likely. Following initial drinking, Marlatt and Gordon suggested that a cognitive factor, the "abstinence violation effect" (AVE), is activated. The AVE represents all-or-nothing thinking; after drinking, the client makes a cognitive shift to viewing him- or herself as "drinking"; therefore, he or she continues to drink. RP treatment focuses on several points of intervention common to cognitive-behavioral treatment, such as identification of high-risk situation and acquisition of coping skills, as well as cognitive restructuring to help the client view a drinking episode as a "lapse" from which the client can learn and return to abstinence rather than a "relapse" into previous drinking patterns. RP also focuses on lifestyle changes to decrease the presence of high-risk situations, and encourages development of a balance between pleasures and desires, and obligations and responsibilities (a "want–should" balance) in the client's life. In his more recent work, Marlatt (Marlatt & Donovan, 2005; Witkiewitz & Marlatt, 2004) has described relapse as "multidimensional and dynamic" (Marlatt & Donovan, 2005, p. 21), and considers the influence of longer-term risk factors such as family history and social supports, and well as more proximal influences on relapse. He also suggests that there are reciprocal interactions among cognitions, coping skills, affect, and drinking.

Disease model perspectives view alcoholism as a chronic, progressive disease that can be arrested but not cured. Treatment then focuses on helping the client recognize that he or she has this disease, that abstinence and a lifelong program of recovery are the only means to arrest the disease, and that involvement in AA or other 12-step groups is essential to successful maintenance of change.

The model presented in this chapter is most closely allied with the RP model, but clinicians should be knowledgeable about the disease model underlying AA and recognize that some clients are drawn to it because they find the model and the program helpful and relevant to them.

CLINICAL APPLICATION OF THE THEORETICAL MODEL

Overview

The major elements of the treatment model have direct implications for facilitating problem recognition and entry into treatment, and for the planning and delivery of treatment. If an individual has not entered treatment, there are techniques to help that individual recognize his or her drinking as problematic and in need of change. For a client seeking alcohol treatment, the therapist must make decisions about the most appropriate setting in which to provide treatment and select the therapeutic modalities most appropriate to the client. Therapeutic techniques must be tailored to the client's needs related to drinking and other life problems. The therapist also must consider the social context in which drinking occurs, as well as the social context for change. He or she must be cognizant of the subtle and nonspecific aspects of providing treatment to clients with drinking problems and utilize a therapeutic stance that enhances the client's motivation to continue to engage in the change process. The therapist must attend to the client's own views about treatment and change, and provide the client with accurate long-term expectations about drinking outcomes. Core components of the treatment model are listed in Table 12.2.

Case Identification and Entry into Treatment

Before I discuss applications of the model to active treatment, it is important to consider how to help clients enter the treatment system.

TABLE 12.2. Steps in Treatment

1. Case identification and motivation to enter treatment
2. Assessment
3. Selection of treatment setting
4. Selection of treatment modalities
5. Enhancing and maintaining motivation to change
6. Selection of drinking goals
7. Initiation of abstinence
8. Developing a functional analysis
9. Early sobriety strategies
10. Coping strategies
11. Partner/family involvement
12. Long-term maintenance
13. Managing complicating conditions
14. Self-help groups

Case Identification and Screening

Many individuals do not think they have problems related to drinking. They may be unaware of the high-risk nature of their drinking pattern, or unaware of the negative consequences that are occurring. Feeling ashamed or guilty, they may be reluctant to tell others about their problems; or may perceive health care professionals as uninterested or unconcerned about drinking. Routine queries about drinking and its consequences in both medical and mental health care settings can obviate some of these difficulties. Given the high prevalence of drinking problems among individuals seeking health

and mental health services, questions about drinking should be part of all clinicians' intake interview.

Many screening interviews and questionnaires have been developed to identify clients with alcohol problems. At a minimum, all clients should be asked whether they drink, and drinkers should be asked follow-up questions about the quantity and frequency of their drinking. Drinking should be considered as heavy or high-risk if a man drinks more than 28 standard drinks in a week, or a woman drinks more than 21 standard drinks in a week.[1] Concern should also be heightened if a client reports heavy drinking (five drinks for men, four for women) twice or more than per month. Follow-up questions may be used to inquire about subjective and objective consequences of drinking. The CAGE (Mayfield, McLeod, & Hall, 1974; see Table 12.3) and the Alcohol Use Disorders Identification Test (AUDIT; Saunders, Aasland, Babor, de la Fuente, & Grant, 1993) are two useful screening interviews. Two affirmative responses to the CAGE suggest a high probability of an alcohol use disorder, but even one positive response warrants further clinical inquiry. The AUDIT includes both direct and subtle approaches to alcohol screening; therefore, it may be useful with clients who are reluctant to self-identify drinking problems. Suggested screening questions are summarized in Table 12.3.

Motivating a Drinker to Enter Treatment

The initial challenge for a clinician is to stimulate the client to initiate any change. Methods for motivating clients to enter treatment vary; a

TABLE 12.3. Questions to Screen for Alcohol Use and Problems

Type of question	Question
Quantity–frequency	1. Do you drink alcohol (including beer, wine, or hard liquor)? 2. How often do you drink? 3. When you drink, about how much do you usually drink? 4. What is the most you ever drink in a day? 5. How often do you drink your top amount?
Screening	CAGE[a]: 1. Have you ever felt you should cut (C) down on your drinking? 2. Have people annoyed (A) you by commenting on your drinking? 3. Have you ever felt bad or guilty (G) about your drinking? 4. Have you ever had a drink first thing in the morning (eye-opener [E])?

[a] From Mayfield, McLeod, and Hall (1974).

clinician may draw upon motivational interviewing techniques (Miller & Rollnick, 2002), may involve family and concerned others in either client-centered work (Miller, Meyers, & Tonigan, 1999), or may use confrontational approaches (Liepman, 1993). Implementation of motivational principles and techniques in ongoing clinical practice, however, presents creative challenges to the clinician. Three examples illustrate the application of different approaches to motivating clients to enter treatment.

Bill was a retired chemist with a long history of heavy drinking, multiple phobias, and bipolar disorder. I was initially contacted by his wife Diana, who told me that her husband had a 20-year drinking history, that his drinking had increased since his retirement, and that she did not know what to do: The children were angry and threatening to break off contact with him; she and he were arguing frequently; and she was beginning to feel increasingly anxious and depressed herself. Diana had consulted with a certified addictions counselor, who told her that they should set up an "intervention" —a meeting in which Diana and the children would confront Bill about his drinking, insist that he get treatment, then take him directly to an inpatient treatment facility. When Diana was hesitant, the counselor told her she was codependent and enabling him. She left the counselor's office discouraged, certain that she did not want to initiate an intervention, but also certain that something should be done. I tried the most minimal intervention first. Over the telephone, I suggested that Diana speak with Bill one morning (before he had begun drinking) and say, "Bill, I am concerned about your drinking. I have spoken with a psychologist who specializes in alcohol treatment, and she said that she would be happy to see you for an evaluation. At the end of the evaluation, she'll give us feedback about what we could do." I told her not to elaborate on this statement, but simply to respond to Bill's questions. If he refused, she was to get back in touch with me.

I next heard from Diana a month later. Bill had refused her request, and she wondered what else she could do. I suggested an individual consultation with me to discuss how to change her own actions to motivate Bill toward change. Diana came in, and after some further assessment of both Bill's drinking history and her current functioning, I suggested three basic behavioral strategies, which I drew from Thomas's unilateral family therapy (Thomas, Yoshioka, & Ager, 1996) and the community reinforcement and family training (CRAFT) model (Miller et al., 1999). First, I instructed Diana to leave Bill to his drinking as much as possible, to let negative consequences occur naturally. Second, I encouraged her to give him factual feedback about negative behaviors related to his drinking, but only at times when he was sober. The structure of the feedback was as follows: "Bill, I am concerned that X happened last night when you were drinking." Third, I encouraged her to spend time with him in positive pursuits when he was not drinking. Given that they were going to Florida for the winter, I suggested that just before they returned to New Jersey, she should repeat her request that he come to see me for an evaluation.

I next heard from Diana in the spring, when she called me to make an appointment for the two of them to come in for an evaluation. They both attended. What follows is our initial discussion.[2] (In this and other dialogues in this chapter, I am the therapist.)

THERAPIST: I'm so glad to get to meet you. As you know, Diana first spoke with me a few months ago, so I feel as though I know you a bit. I understand that you were initially reluctant to come in, and I'm pleased that you decided to come. How did that come about?

BILL: Well, Diana asked me, and I know she's been concerned, so I agreed. But I only agreed to come today—I'm not making any kind of commitment here.

THERAPIST: I understand that and certainly won't try to push you to do anything you're not comfortable with. What I'd like to do today is to get a better understanding about your drinking and the kinds of problems it might be causing. At the end of our time together, I'll give you some feedback and we can discuss some options for you, if you decide you want to make any changes. If I ask you anything that you're not comfortable answering, just let me know. OK?

Bill was visibly uncomfortable, and pushed his chair as far back into the corner of my office as possible. He sat with his body turned away from Diana and often looked up at the ceiling or sighed when she was speaking. Despite his visible discomfort, he gave a clear account of his drinking. He had been drinking heavily for the past 25 years, and at one point had been drinking a pint of Jack Daniels whiskey each evening. He was diagnosed with colon cancer in his early 60s and treated surgically. Since the surgery, he had been concerned about his health and had attempted to reduce his drinking. His current pattern was almost daily drinking, in the evenings, ranging from two to four bottles of Grolsch beer to an occasional (approximately twice per month) pint of Jack Daniels. He reported no withdrawal symptoms on days when he did not drink, and no apparent medical sequelae of his drinking. He said that he did not feel that he had control over his drinking, and expressed sadness that Diana was so upset. His love for her, apparent in his speech and demeanor, was clearly the primary reason he had come to see me.

Given Bill's discomfort, I did not try to complete any standardized assessment instruments or even to structure the initial interview as much as I might with other clients. Instead, I followed his lead, made frequent comments reflecting the emotions he was expressing, and at times asked Diana not to interrupt, so that Bill could express himself. In the last 15 minutes of the 1-hour interview, we shifted to feedback and discussion:

THERAPIST: I'd like to stop asking you so many questions now, and see if we can talk about possible options. I am glad that you came in and appreciate that this was not easy for you. From what you and Diana have told me, it does seem that it makes sense to be concerned about your drinking. The amount you're drinking is above the recommended levels for safe and healthy drinking; you are concerned by your own feelings of lack of control; and your drinking has been upsetting to your family, which is painful to you. What do you think?

BILL: I guess talking about all of this at once makes it clearer that I'm drinking too much. I don't want to stop, though—I appreciate good beer, and look forward to having a bottle or two in the evening. I just don't want to overdo it to the point of hurting Diana.

THERAPIST: So you are concerned and think that some kind of change makes sense, but you're not sure exactly what those changes should be?

BILL: Exactly.

THERAPIST: I think you have a number of options. Making some kind of change makes sense given the problems we've discussed. Probably your safest choice is to stop drinking—you can't create future health problems from drinking if you don't drink, and in some ways it might be easiest given that you're in a pretty daily routine of drinking now. But if you don't want to stop, we could also work toward your reducing your drinking to a level that is safer and healthier, and one that Diana and your children are comfortable with. I'd be willing to work with you to try to reach that goal. I don't think that you need intensive treatment in a hospital program right now, but you would probably benefit from some help to make changes. What do you think?

BILL: I'm surprised that you think I could reduce my drinking. I have to think about this. I'll have Diana get back to you.

The discussion continued with input from Diana as well, and the session ended with a commitment only to think about our discussion. Several days later, Diana called to indicate that Bill wanted to begin treatment with me, and we scheduled an appointment.

Dorothy, a 78-year-old, widowed, retired schoolteacher, was hospitalized at a local medical center after a fall in her apartment. Her blood alcohol level (BAL) on admission was 185 mg%, and she had extensive evidence of old bruises, as well as a dislocated shoulder and broken wrist from the fall. She was immediately started on medication for alcohol withdrawal, and our addictions consultation team was called in to see her on the second day of her hospitalization. Dorothy's son John was in the room when I came to see her. With his assistance, I was able to obtain a lengthy history of alcohol consumption that dated back to her early 40s. Although Dorothy had wanted to stop drinking, she had never been successful for more than a few days at a time, and had never received any form of alcohol treatment. Since her husband's death 2 years earlier, she had been consuming a pint bottle of blackberry brandy each day. She had completely withdrawn from her previous social activities with friends, her hygiene had deteriorated, and she had had multiple accidents in her house. Dorothy provided this information tearfully, expressing a great sense of shame about her behavior. John described her home as "a mess" and said that he was angry and disgusted with her. Dorothy's family history revealed many family members with alcohol dependence, including her father, two brothers, and a maternal uncle. Despite the medication, she showed visible signs of alcohol withdrawal during the interview. Dorothy was tearful and stated repeatedly that she was a "sinful, bad" person. My interviewing style with her was empathic: I asked her about her concerns, inquired how she felt, and reflected back her obvious distress with her current situation. I then told her that there were treatments available to help people with problems like hers. Her immediate and strong reaction was to say that she was too bad, and that her drinking was a sin. Although not usually a strong proponent of labeling alcohol dependence as a disease, I decided that this framework might in fact be acceptable and supportive to her. Given her long history of alcohol dependence with physiological dependence, and her heavy family history of alcohol dependence, such a framework seemed plausible and appropriate.

"Dorothy, it is clear to me that you are very, very upset by your drinking and by all the problems it has caused for you and your family. I understand that you blame yourself and seem to think your drinking shows that you are a bad person. There is another way of thinking about your drinking that I'd like to tell you about. You may or may not agree with me, but I hope you'll think about what I say. Some people say that alcoholism is a disease. In your case, I think that is true. You probably have genes that made you very vulnerable to alcohol—your father, your uncle, and your brothers all seem to have the same disease. We know that the vulnerability to alcoholism can be inherited, and I would guess that you inherited it. Over time, your body has become adapted to your drinking—it is more comfortable with alcohol than without it. If you try to stop, your body reacts badly. The shaking and nausea that you're experiencing now are signs that your body has become hooked on alcohol.

"What does all this mean? It means that your body reacts differently to alcohol than other people's, and probably has from the beginning of your drinking. It is no more your fault that you have a drinking problem than it is the fault of a diabetic that her body

can't make insulin. People are not responsible for the diseases they develop. But they *are* responsible for making the decision to take care of their disease, for getting help, and for following the advice of the people who give them that help. Except for the problems your drinking has caused, you're healthy, and you obviously have people who care about you. If you can get help, you have a good chance of getting better."

Dorothy initially was skeptical of this reframing of her problems. Without my prompting, when her son left the hospital that day he picked up some brochures about alcoholism as a disease, and brought them back for his mother to read. When I came to see her the next day, she had many questions about this disease notion and about treatment, which I answered as factually as possible, still maintaining a motivational interviewing stance—not trying to push her into treatment, but reflecting her interest and concern. By my third visit, she agreed to enter a treatment program. She entered a short-term residential rehabilitation program, followed by longer-term outpatient group therapy. She began to volunteer at the hospital where I first saw her, and she remained sober and an active volunteer for several years, until advancing age required that she retire.

Dennis was a 41-year-old dentist with a history of abuse of alcohol, prescription opiates, and benzodiazepines. Dennis's case illustrates the need for a full armamentarium of clinical techniques to motivate individuals to enter treatment. At the time that I saw Dennis, the Rutgers Center of Alcohol Studies had a contract with the New Jersey Dental Association to provide assessment, motivational, referral, and monitoring services for dentists with alcohol and drug problems. I was called about Dennis on a Friday afternoon by an emergency room physician. Dennis had taken an overdose of medications and had been rushed to the emergency room by his office staff. His condition had been stabilized, and he was now insisting that he leave the hospital. The physician wanted our program to "do something." In rapid succession, I received calls from the office staff, from Dennis's wife, and from another dentist, who had been serving as his AA sponsor. By telephone, they provided me with a horrific history of abuse of multiple substances, domestic violence, canceled afternoons of appointments with patients, extraction of the wrong tooth from a patient, and repeated failures in AA and outpatient treatment. Each caller described Dennis as intractable, and all were desperately concerned that he would kill himself. I asked them all to meet me at the hospital, and left my office to join them there. I informed the emergency room physician that I would be coming to the hospital, and asked him to hold Dennis there until I arrived.

When I arrived at the hospital, I first spoke with Dennis individually. He was alert, oriented, belligerent and angry, and utterly unwilling to speak with me at any length or to agree to any kind of plan of care. My best motivational interviewing skills failed completely with him. Given the crisis nature of the situation and the extremely severe substance use disorder, I decided to utilize a more confrontational technique—the intervention (Liepman, 1993). Interventions are designed to confront the resistant client and create a forced plan of action. Research suggests that two-thirds of families will not follow through with an intervention (as was the case with Diana and Bill), but that if an intervention is implemented, the probability of the client's entering treatment is very high (Miller et al., 1999). I gathered the office staff, Dennis's wife, and his AA sponsor together and asked them whether they would be willing to sit down with Dennis to talk with him about his problems. They were relieved and eager to do so. We spent about 30 minutes together, during which time I outlined the basic requirements for the intervention: (1) Each person's feedback should begin with an expression of caring or concern; (2) each person should provide concrete, behavioral feedback related to Dennis's drinking and drug use (e.g., mentioning his canceling appointments rather than saying he was irresponsible); (3) at the end of each person's feedback, he or she should repeat the expression of concern and request that Dennis get help. We then sat down with Dennis, and each person spoke. Dennis began to cry and after a lengthy period of time agreed that he needed help and would follow my recommendations for treatment.

Assessment

Once a client has entered treatment, the therapist should begin with an initial assessment of drinking, other drug use, and problems in other areas of life functioning. Assessment of motivation, as well as resources that the client brings to the treatment, is important. If the therapist provides cognitive-behavioral treatment, assessment for a functional analysis of drinking is necessary. If the client's spouse/partner or other family members are involved in the treatment, their role in the drinking, as well as overall relationship functioning, should be assessed.

Drinking Assessment

The clinical interview is used to assess drinking history and client perceptions of his or her current drinking. Major topics to cover in the clinical interview are outlined in Table 12.4. Typically, we use a handheld breath alcohol tester at the beginning of each session to assess current BAL. In addition to the clinical interview, two structured interviews—the Timeline Follow-Back Interview (TLFB; Sobell, Maisto, Sobell, Cooper, & Saunders, 1980), designed to assess drinking and drug use behavior each day in a set window of time before treatment; and the alcohol and drug sections of the Structured Clinical Interview for DSM-IV (SCID; Spitzer, Williams, Gibbon, & First, 1996)—provide standardized information about quantity, frequency, pattern of drinking, and other information needed to establish a formal diagnosis. Alternative structured interviews, such as the FORM-90 (Tonigan, Miller, & Brown, 1997), may be used to obtain information about drinking history, patterns, and consequences of use. Self-report measures may be used to assess severity of alcohol dependence (the Alcohol Dependence Scale [ADS]; Skinner & Allen, 1982) and negative consequences of drinking (the Drinker Inventory of Consequences or the Short Inventory of Problems; Miller, Tonigan, & Longabaugh, 1995).

Assessment of Other Problem Areas

The clinician can draw from a wide variety of measures to assess other life problems. Assessment may range from unstructured interviews to the use of simple problem checklists to formal interviewing techniques. The Addiction Severity Index (ASI; McLellan et al., 1992) is a widely used measure of client functioning across multiple domains; subscales include Medical, Psychological, Family/Social, Legal, Employment, Alcohol, and Drug. The ASI is in

TABLE 12.4. Topics to Cover in Initial Clinical Interview (Both Partners Present)

1. Initial orientation
   a. Introductions
   b. Breathalyzer reading
   c. Brief questionnaires
2. Initial assessment
   a. Presenting problems
   b. Role of drinking/drug use in presenting problems
   c. Other concerns
   d. How the drinking has affected the partner
   e. How the drinking has affected the relationship
3. Drinking/drug use assessment
   a. Identified patient
      i. Quantity, frequency, pattern of drinking
      ii. Last drink/drug use
      iii. Length of drinking/drug problem
      iv. Negative consequences of drinking/drug use
      v. DSM-IV-TR symptoms
      vi. Assessment of need for detoxification
   b. Partner
      i. Quantity, frequency, pattern of drinking
      ii. Last drink/drug use
      iii. Length of drinking/drug problem
      iv. Negative consequences of drinking/drug use
      v. DSM-IV-TR symptoms
      vi. Assessment of need for detoxification
2. Assessment of other problems
   a. Psychotic symptoms
   b. Depression
   c. Anxiety
   d. Cognitive impairment
   e. Health status
3. Assessment of domestic violence
   a. This assessment is done privately with each partner alone
   b. Review of Conflict Tactics Scale
      i. Identification of episodes of physical aggression
      ii. Determination of level of harm/injury from aggression
      iii. Assessment of individual's sense of safety in couple therapy

the public domain, and the instrument, instructions, and scoring programs can be downloaded from *www.tresearch.org/asi.htm*. The ASI can be administered as an interview in about 45 minutes, and computer-assisted interview versions are available. The ASI, however, does not provide diagnostic information for any psychological disorders, and the cautious clinician should use formal diagnostic screening questions to assess for the possible presence of other psychological disorders (Zimmerman, 1994).

Assessment of Motivation

Assessment of motivation should consider (1) reasons why the client is seeking treatment, with careful attention to external factors involved with help seeking; (2) the client's treatment goals; (3) the client's stage of readiness of change; and (4) the degree to which the client sees negative consequences of his or her current drinking pattern and envisions positive consequences of change. Clinical interviewing provides information about reasons for seeking treatment, and drinking goals may be assessed either by asking the client directly or by using a simple goal choice form (see Figure 12.1). The University of Rhode Island Change Assessment Scale (McConnaughy, Prochaska, & Velicer, 1983), the Readiness to Change Questionnaire (Rollnick, Heather, Gold, & Hall, 1992), and the Stages of Change Readiness and Treatment Eagerness Scale (SOCRATES; Miller & Tonigan, 1996) all measure stage of change. Perception of negative consequences of drinking and positive consequences of change also may be assessed through the clinical interview, or by developing a Decisional Balance Sheet (Marlatt & Gordon, 1985) with the client (see Figure 12.2).

Functional Analysis

Two assessment techniques may be used to identify antecedents to drinking. A self-report questionnaire, the Drinking Patterns Questionnaire (DPQ; Zitter & McCrady, 1979), lists potential environmental, cognitive, affective, interpersonal, and intrapersonal antecedents to drinking or drinking urges. The Inventory of Drinking Situations (Annis, 1982), a shorter measure that assesses situations in which a client drinks heavily, also is available. Daily self-

We would like to know the **one GOAL** you have chosen for yourself about drinking at this time. Please read the goals listed below and choose the **ONE** goal that best represents your goal at this time by checking the box next to the goal and by filling in any blanks as indicated for that goal.

☐ I have decided not to change my pattern of drinking.

☐ I have decided to cut down on my drinking and drink in a more controlled manner—to be in control of how often I drink and how much I drink. I would like to limit myself to no more than _____ drinks (upper limit amount) per _____ (time period).

☐ I have decided to stop drinking completely for a period of time, after which I will make a new decision about whether I will drink again. For me, the period of time I want to stop drinking is for _____ (time).

☐ I have decided to stop drinking regularly, but would like to have an occasional drink when I really have the urge.

☐ I have decided to quit drinking once and for all, even though I realize I may slip up and drink once in a while.

☐ I have decided to quite drinking once and for all, to be totally abstinent, and to never drink alcohol ever again for the rest of my life.

☐ None of this applies exactly to me. My own goal is _____

FIGURE 12.1. Goal choice questionnaire.

recording cards (Figure 12.3) are used throughout the treatment to record drinks and drinking urges. Discussing events associated with drinking or drinking urges can help the client and clinician to develop a clearer picture of drinking antecedents and consequences. Self-recording cards also allow the clinician to track progress in terms of quantity and frequency of drinking, as well as frequency and intensity of urges to drink.

Partner Assessment

Questionnaires and self-recording cards can be used to assess how the client's partner has coped with the drinking. Each day, the partner who is involved with treatment records his or her perceptions of the drinker's drinking and drinking urges on a Likert scale (*None, Light, Moderate,* or *Heavy*; Figure 12.4). In addition, the partner may complete the Coping Questionnaire (Orford, Templeton, Velleman, & Copello, 2005) to describe the variety of ways the partner has tried to cope with drinking. These include engaged, tolerant–inactive, and withdrawal coping. It also is important to assess other aspects of the couple's relationship, if both partners are to be involved in treatment. The Areas of Change Questionnaire (ACQ; Margolin, Talovic, & Weinstein, 1983) and the Dyadic Adjustment Scale (DAS; Spanier, 1976) are excellent self-report measures of relation-

	Not Drinking	Drinking
Pros		
Cons		

FIGURE 12.2. Decisional Balance Sheet.

Urges			Drinks/Drugs				
Time	Strength (1–7)	Trigger?	Time	Type	Amount	% Alcohol	Trigger?

Relationship
satisfaction:
    1 2 3 4 5 6 7

    Worst   Greatest
    ever   ever

FIGURE 12.3. Sample client self-recording card.

ship problems and satisfaction. The Revised Conflict Tactics Scale (Strauss, Hamby, Boney-McCoy, & Sugerman, 1996) provides a succinct measure of relationship conflict, including physical violence.

Selection of Treatment Setting

Information from the assessment of drinking, concomitant problem areas, and motivation is used to determine the appropriate setting in which to initiate treatment. As with other areas of health and mental health care, the principle of least restrictive level of care should apply to alcohol and drug treatment. Residential rehabilitation of fixed length (usually 28–30 days) historically was seen as the treatment of choice. However, studies comparing the effectiveness of different levels of care (e.g., see Fink et al., 1985; Longabaugh et al., 1983; McCrady et al., 1986) have found that most clients can be treated effectively in an ambulatory treatment setting. Intensive outpatient programs of fixed duration and standard outpatient care now are the most common settings for treatment (National Advisory Council on Alcohol Abuse and Alcoholism, 1996).

Both the Institute of Medicine (1990) and Sobell and Sobell (2000) have proposed stepped-care models for making decisions about level of care. The stepped-care model proposes brief interventions as the modal initial approach to treatment, with treatment "stepped up" to more intensive or extensive treatment based on the client's response to the initial treatment. Such models are economically

Day	Date	Drinking	Drug use	Urge intensity	Relationship satisfaction
		No L M H	No L M H	0 1 2 3 4 5 6 7	0 1 2 3 4 5 6 7
		No L M H	No L M H	0 1 2 3 4 5 6 7	0 1 2 3 4 5 6 7
		No L M H	No L M H	0 1 2 3 4 5 6 7	0 1 2 3 4 5 6 7
		No L M H	No L M H	0 1 2 3 4 5 6 7	0 1 2 3 4 5 6 7
		No L M H	No L M H	0 1 2 3 4 5 6 7	0 1 2 3 4 5 6 7
		No L M H	No L M H	0 1 2 3 4 5 6 7	0 1 2 3 4 5 6 7

Note. Use the reverse side of the card to track behaviors you are learning to change.

FIGURE 12.4. Sample spouse self-recording card.

conservative and maintain the principle of least restrictive level of care. However, some clients with more severe problems might not be served well by very brief treatment (e.g., Rychtarik et al., 2000), and studies using the American Society of Addiction Medicine (ASAM) criteria suggest that patients have poorer outcomes if they receive less intensive treatment than suggested by these criteria (Magura et al., 2003).

Proposed decision-making models to determine level of care have been implemented in many states. The ASAM (1996) has proposed a multidimensional decision-making model for selecting initial level of care. ASAM criteria consider need for supervised withdrawal, medical conditions that might require monitoring, comorbid psychiatric conditions, motivation for change and degree of treatment acceptance or resistance, relapse potential, and nature of the individual's social environment in recommending an initial level of care. These criteria are mapped onto four major levels of care, including outpatient, intensive outpatient, medically monitored intensive inpatient, and medically managed intensive inpatient treatment. Table 12.5 summarizes the way that the major

criteria are applied to level of care determinations. Studies of the ASAM criteria suggest a number of barriers to using the criteria in clinical practice. For example, among homeless individuals, treatment facilities may be inaccessible because of lack of insurance or money to pay. Also, such individuals often are placed on waiting lists because programs are full. Some programs also may lack adjunctive services needed by a homeless population, such as assistance with pragmatic issues (food stamps, housing, unemployment, medical care, mental health care, or family treatment) (O'Toole et al., 2004). Among other patients seeking alcohol treatment, some may receive treatment that is more intensive than that suggested by ASAM criteria, because their insurance or Medicaid only covered inpatient treatment, there may have been pressure from the family to go with inpatient treatment, or a specific level of care was mandated by an external agency (e.g., Employee Assistance Program). Patients also may receive treatment that is less intensive than that suggested by ASAM criteria, because of their work schedule or reluctance to commit to more (Kosanke, Magura, Staines, Foote, & DeLuca,

TABLE 12.5. American Society of Addiction Medicine General Guidelines for Selection of Treatment Settings

Level of care	Criteria
Level I. Outpatient treatment	No serious risk for major withdrawal or withdrawal seizures No acute or chronic medical or psychiatric problems that could interfere with treatment Some openness to change Some ability to maintain change Reasonable environmental support for change
Level II. Intensive outpatient treatment	No serious risk for major withdrawal or withdrawal seizures No acute or chronic medical or psychiatric problems that could be managed with intensive supervision *and* Some reluctance to change *or* Limited ability to maintain change *or* Limited environmental supports for change
Level III. Medically monitored intensive inpatient treatment	At least two: Risk for withdrawal Some level of acute or chronic medical or psychiatric problems that could be managed with intensive supervision Reluctance to change Limited ability to maintain change Limited environmental supports for change
Level IV. Medically managed intensive inpatient treatment	Serious risk for major withdrawal or withdrawal seizures *or* Acute or chronic medical *or* psychiatric problems that could interfere with treatment

2002). Additional considerations in determining initial level of care are discussed below.

Need for Detoxification

If a client is physically dependent on alcohol, then he or she will experience alcohol withdrawal symptoms when drinking is decreased or stopped. A number of signs suggest that a client may be physically dependent on alcohol, including daily drinking, drinking regularly or intermittently throughout the day, and morning drinking. Awakening during the night with fears, trembling, or nausea, or experiencing such symptoms upon first awakening also suggests dependence. Cessation or a substantial decrease in drinking will result in the appearance of minor withdrawal symptoms, such as tremulousness, nausea, vomiting, difficulty sleeping, irritability, anxiety, and elevations in pulse rate, blood pressure, and temperature. Such symptoms usually begin within 5–12 hours. More severe withdrawal symptoms (e.g., seizures, delirium, or hallucinations) may also occur, usually within 24–72 hours of the cessation of drinking. If a client has not consumed alcohol for several days prior to initial clinical contact, concerns about alcohol withdrawal are not relevant. If the client has stopped drinking within the last 3 days, the clinician needs to inquire about and observe the client for signs of withdrawal. If the client currently is drinking, the clinician must rely on drinking history, pattern, and the results of previous attempts to stop drinking to determine whether detoxification will be necessary.

If the client needs detoxification, four alternatives are available: inpatient or partial hospital medical detoxification, inpatient nonmedical detoxification, or outpatient medical detoxification. Inpatient, medically assisted detoxification is essential if the client has a history of disorientation, delirium, hallucinations, or seizures during alcohol withdrawal, or is showing current signs of disorientation, delirium, or hallucinations. If the client does not believe that he or she can stop drinking without being physically removed from alcohol, but does not show any major withdrawal signs, is in good health, and does not abuse other drugs, a social setting detoxification may be appropriate. If the client has some social supports, then detoxification can be initiated on a partial hospital or outpatient basis. The choice between these two latter settings is determined by how much support the person will need during withdrawal, and whether a structured program will be needed after detoxification. If the client needs a fairly structured program, then the partial hospital is the preferred setting for detoxification.

Medical Problems

The clinician who is considering the best setting for detoxification should take into account the presence of other medical problems. A cautious approach dictates that every client should have both a thorough physical examination, and blood and urine studies at the beginning of treatment. The clinician should routinely include questions about physical health in the first contact with a client, and if significant physical complaints are noted, the client should receive immediate medical attention. Some clients have medical problems that require hospitalization; if so, the hospitalization should initiate the treatment.

Treatment History

After physical health issues have been considered, the clinician should examine the client's previous treatment history. Questions to consider include the following:

1. Has the client attempted outpatient treatment in the past, and been able to stop or decrease drinking successfully? If so, then another attempt at outpatient treatment may be indicated.
2. Has the client dropped out of outpatient treatment in the past? If so, and there is no indication that any variables have changed in the interim, then a more intensive partial hospital or inpatient program should be considered.
3. Has the client dropped out of, or drunk repeatedly, while in a partial hospital program? If so, then inpatient treatment may be indicated.
4. Did the client relapse immediately after discharge from an inpatient program? If so, then a partial hospital or outpatient setting may be appropriate, because relapse may have been associated with problems in generalization from the inpatient to the natural environment. Alternatively, a halfway house may be considered to provide a longer-term structured environment.

Previous Quit Attempts

Many clients have successfully decreased or stopped drinking on their own at some time. Outpatient treatment is more likely to be successful for a client with a history of stopping successfully on his or her own than a client without any history of successful change.

Social Support Systems

Social support systems are a critical variable to consider in determining the appropriate setting for initial treatment. If a client has support from another person, *and* that person is perceived as an important source of support and reinforcement, *and* is willing to provide support and reinforcement, then the client is a good candidate for ambulatory treatment. If the client is lacking in social support, or is in an environment that supports heavy drinking, then inpatient or partial hospital treatment may be advisable. Alternatively, a halfway house may provide a good setting for treatment for persons who do not have current social supports and have not been successful at developing them in the past, even during periods of abstinence.

Personal Resources

The next area to consider encompasses the client's personal psychological resources. Has he or she been successful in other areas of life in setting goals, changing behavior, and completing tasks? If so, outpatient treatment is more feasible. Another aspect of personal resources is cognitive functioning. If the client shows significant cognitive deficits in memory, attention, abstraction, or problem solving, a higher level of care may be considered. Otherwise, the client may have difficulty with retaining information presented in treatment or generating successful ways to avoid drinking.

Other Psychological Problems

As noted earlier in the chapter, persons with drinking problems often have other, significant psychological problems. The clinician must not only assess these problems but also determine level of care based on the appropriate setting for treatment of these other problems. A client who presents with serious depression must be assessed for suicidality and appropriate precautions should be taken.

Attitudes about Treatment

Although difficult areas to assess, the client's commitment to treatment and desire to change are important factors in selecting level of care. The client who is ambivalent but willing to come to treatment may respond better to a more intensive program that provides higher density reinforcement for attending treatment and making changes. However, sometimes ambivalence makes it impossible to provide treatment in a more intensive setting, because the client is unwilling to disrupt his or her life to the extent required for such a program.

Practical Concerns

There are a number of practical concerns that the clinician must consider. Although in certain therapeutic approaches these issues might be considered evidence of client "denial," my colleagues and I view practical matters as real barriers to treatment and work with the client to overcome these barriers. Some practical barriers revolve around employment—whether the client can get time off from work, whether the job is in jeopardy, whether the employer is willing to support treatment, or whether missing any more work would result in termination of employment.

A second concern is the client's financial condition. Can the client afford to take time off from work and experience a reduction in income while he or she collects temporary disability (if sick time is not available)? If not, outpatient treatment, or a partial hospital program that allows the person to work, is appropriate. Another financial concern is the client's ability to pay for treatment.

Other practical concerns revolve around transportation and child care. Can the client get to outpatient appointments? Does he or she have a driver's license, and if not, is other transportation available? Is child care available if the person has to be hospitalized? If not, a day treatment setting may be preferred. The clinician must consider a range of pragmatic barriers to treatment.

Personal Preferences

Finally, the client's own preferences about the treatment must be considered carefully. If the client feels strongly about wanting to be in a hospital or residential treatment program, the clinician should listen carefully to this request, even if the initial assessment suggests that outpatient treatment may be feasible. Similarly, if the client wants outpatient treatment, the clinician should perhaps attempt it, even if he or she believes that a more intensive treatment is preferable.

General Considerations

In general, the selection of the initial treatment setting must be seen as a tentative decision. Often an initial contract must be established that includes the client's preferred setting, but with specification of the circumstances that will dictate a different level of care. For example, if the clinician believes that the client will find it extremely difficult to discontinue drinking on an outpatient basis, but this is the client's desire, then an initial contract may involve a plan for reducing or stopping drinking, learning skills to support that plan, and a time limit. If the person is unsuccessful within the specified time frame, then the contract is reviewed and alternative settings are considered. Thus, although the initial setting decision is important, continuing to consider and discuss other treatment settings is an important early step in the treatment process.

Selection of Treatment Modalities

If a client is referred to inpatient, residential, or intensive outpatient treatment, a mixture of treatment modalities is included in the treatment. Six major treatment modalities are available for the provision of alcoholism treatment: self-help groups, individual therapy, group therapy, couple therapy, family therapy, and intensive treatment programs. In the ambulatory setting, the clinician has more flexibility in selecting among these treatment modalities.

Self-Help Groups

AA is the most commonly utilized self-help group. With groups in all 50 states, as well as more than 150 countries throughout the world,

AA is widely available. It offers a specific approach to recovery, rooted in the view that alcoholism is a physical, emotional, and spiritual disease that can be arrested but not cured. Recovery is viewed as a lifelong process that involves working the 12 Steps of AA and abstaining from the use of alcohol (for a detailed description of AA, see McCrady, Horvath, & Delaney, 2003). The only requirement for membership in AA is a desire to stop drinking, and members do not have to pay dues or join the organization. Persons who become involved with AA usually attend different meetings; have a relationship with an AA sponsor that helps them with their recovery; and become involved with other AA-related activities, ranging from making the coffee before meetings to going on "commitments," where members of one AA group speak at another group. More active involvement is correlated with more successful change (Emrick, Tonigan, Montgomery, & Little, 1993).

Research suggests that persons most likely to affiliate with AA have a history of using social supports as a way to cope with problems, experience loss of control over their drinking, drink more per occasion than persons who do not affiliate, experience more anxiety about their drinking, believe that alcohol enhances their mental functioning, and are more religious or spiritual (Emrick et al., 1993). Outpatient treatment to facilitate involvement with AA (12-step facilitation) has been found to be as effective as other forms of outpatient therapy in controlled trials, and some evidence suggests that clients receiving 12-step facilitation are more likely to maintain total abstinence from alcohol than clients receiving more behaviorally oriented treatments (Project MATCH Research Group, 1997a). Twelve-step facilitation treatment appears to be particularly successful for individuals with social systems that support them in drinking heavily (Longabaugh et al., 1998).

Alternative self-help groups have developed in recent years. Self-Management and Recovery Training (SMART) is a self-help approach based largely on cognitive-behavioral principles. SMART offers several steps to recovery, emphasizing awareness of irrational beliefs, self-perceptions, and expectancies as core to successful change. SMART suggests abstinence as a preferred drinking goal, but emphasizes personal choice. Secular Organizations for Sobriety/Save Ourselves (SOS) was developed largely in response to the spiritual aspects of AA and does not invoke a Higher Power as a part of the change process. Women for Sobriety, a self-help approach for women, emphasizes women's issues such as assertiveness, self-confidence, and autonomy as a part of the change process. Moderation Management (2006) draws upon behavioral principles to accomplish moderate drinking outcomes. All of these alternative approaches are more compatible with behavioral approaches than is AA, but none are as widely available to clients.

Individual Treatment

Individual therapy is offered widely on an outpatient basis. Few data are available to guide the choice of individual versus group therapy. The literature on women with alcoholism is replete with suggestions that women respond better to individual than to group therapy, but empirical support for that assertion is lacking. Similar assertions apply to the treatment of older persons who have alcoholism, with a similar lack of empirical support.

Group Therapy

There is a strong belief in the alcohol field that group therapy is preferable to individual therapy (although see the previous comments in regard to women and older adults). Group therapy is more economical to provide, and interaction among group members provides opportunities for modeling, feedback, and behavioral rehearsal that are less available in the individual setting. Behavioral models for providing group therapy (Monti, Kadden, Rohsenow, Cooney, & Abrams, 2002) are well documented. Clients who are able to function in a group setting and do not require intensive individual attention because of other psychological problems can be assigned to group therapy.

Couple Therapy

A number of studies have suggested that involving the spouse/partner in alcoholism treatment increases the probability of a positive treatment outcome (reviewed in Epstein & McCrady, 2002). Despite the empirical evidence, traditional alcoholism counselors prefer individual or group therapy over couple therapy, emphasizing the importance of a focus on personal change before relationship change. Models for treatments that integrate individual and relationship treatment are available (Epstein & McCrady, 2002). Couple therapy is most appropriate for clients who have a stable relationship, in which the partner is willing to be involved in treatment and can function in a supportive manner in the early phases of treatment. Couples who have experienced severe domestic violence, or in which one partner's commitment to the relationship is highly ambivalent, are less appropriate for couple therapy.

Techniques also have been developed to provide treatment to partners of people with alcohol use disorders when the drinker will not seek help. Behavioral groups that emphasize personal decision making, communication, and limit setting around drinking are effective in motivating individuals to seek treatment or to decrease drinking (Miller et al., 1999; Sisson & Azrin, 1986; Thomas, Santa, Bronson, & Oyserman, 1987). Al-Anon offers a self-help approach to partners and other family members affected by alcoholism.

Family Therapy

Despite a strong interest in alcoholism in the family therapy field, models for working with whole families in which alcoholism is present are scarce. Within the self-help area, Alateen is available for teens affected by a family member's alcoholism, and Alatot is available for younger family members.

Intensive Treatment Programs

Although technically a treatment setting rather than a modality, intensive treatment programs have such a specific and defined role in alcohol treatment that they can be considered a treatment modality. The "Minnesota model" (Sheehan & Owen, 1999) is an intensive treatment approach that includes group therapy, education, self-help group involvement, and some individual counseling. Programs based on the Minnesota model emphasize confrontation of denial, acceptance that one is an alcoholic who is powerless over alcohol, development of caring and interdependent relationships, and commitment to AA involvement. Over time,

Minnesota model programs have incorporated many behavioral strategies and techniques, including social skills and relaxation training, as well as RP techniques. Minnesota model programs have been marketed as the most effective approach to alcoholism treatment, but data are lacking to support these claims. Most research on these programs has involved the evaluation of a single treatment program, and all the evaluations have been of private treatment centers. The evaluations suggest substantial levels of abstinence among persons receiving treatment (see, e.g., Filstead, 1991; Stinchfield & Owen, 1998), but the subjects in these studies tend to be good-prognosis patients, and without appropriate controls, conclusions cannot be drawn about the relative efficacy of these treatments compared to other approaches. Their wide visibility has made them the choice of many individuals with alcoholism and their families.

Enhancing and Maintaining Motivation to Change

Once a decision has been made about the level of care and the client has entered treatment, the clinician needs to continue to focus on motivation to be in treatment and to change. Techniques to enhance motivation include feedback, use of motivational interviewing techniques, mutual goal setting and decision making, treatment contracting, and the instillation of hope. Three clinical examples illustrate some of these techniques.

Bill (described earlier in this chapter) began treatment quite tentatively. He was willing to complete a standardized assessment of his drinking, so we completed a 1-month TLFB (Sobell et al., 1980), the Rutgers Consequences of Use Questionnaire (RCU; Rhines, McCrady, Morgan, & Hirsch, 1997), and a Decisional Balance Sheet (Marlatt & Gordon, 1985; see Figure 12.2). Based on this information, I provided him with a standardized feedback sheet (Figure 12.5) about his drinking. The sheet provided data about how his drinking compared to national norms (Miller, Zweben, DiClemente, & Rychtarik, 1995), as well as information about his peak BAL, usual BAL, and negative consequences of his drinking. Bill found the feedback interesting and asked questions about alcohol metabolism, epidemiological surveys, and alcohol and health effects.

Although his wife Diana was somewhat impatient with this conversation, I thought that Bill's interest in learning more about alcohol and its effects was a positive sign.

We discussed drinking goals, and I suggested the MM drinking guidelines for men (Moderation Management, 2000) of no more than 14 drinks in a week, no more than 4 days' drinking per week, and no more than four drinks per occasion. Bill indicated that he wanted to continue with daily drinking, but with a limit of three drinks per day. Diana was agreeable, saying that if he kept to this limit she would be "thrilled." Although his selected goal was higher than I would have liked, I agreed in order to engage him further in treatment. I then gave him his first "homework" assignment—to initiate self-recording of his drinking (see Figure 12.3). The assignment of homework serves as a useful behavioral probe for level of motivation, and I was pleased when Bill returned to the next session with completed self-recording cards.

Suzanne was a 39-year-old computer programmer whom I treated in outpatient therapy as part of a treatment research project. Suzanne drank daily, typically consuming three glasses of wine per day. She had made a number of unsuccessful attempts to stop drinking and felt that she had completely lost control over her drinking. She was concerned about her ability to be alert and available to her children in the evenings when she was drinking, particularly since her husband traveled frequently for his business. Suzanne sought treatment voluntarily and wanted to abstain from drinking completely. Despite her self-referral to treatment and her self-defined need for abstinence, Suzanne reacted to the same structured feedback quite differently than Bill did. She had provided information for the TLFB and completed the RCU, but when I gave her feedback that she had been drinking an average of 21.5 drinks per week, she told me that this figure was too high and that our measure was not very accurate. She also indicated that she was participating in a research study, not in therapy, which was why she thought it important that we have accurate data. I did not argue with her perspective, agreeing that she was in a research study, but that I hoped that the study would helpful to her. She continued with treatment, and several weeks later commented spontaneously, "You know, I know that I'm in treatment, and I really

For the Drinker:

1. Based on the information I obtained during the assessment, I calculated the number of "standard drinks" you consumed in a typical week, during the last month:

    Total number of standard drinks per week   _____

    Average number of standard drinks per day   _____

2. When we look at everyone who drinks in the United States, you have been drinking more than approximately ___ percent of the population of women/men in the country.

3. I also estimated your highest and average blood alcohol level (BAL) in the past month. Your BAL is based on how many standard drinks you consume, the length of time over which you drink that much, whether you are a man or a woman, and how much you weight. So,

    Your estimated peak BAL in an average week was   _____

    Your estimated average BAL in an average week was   _____

    This is a measure of how intoxicated you typically become. In New Jersey, the legal intoxication limit is 80 mg% or higher.

4. You have experienced many negative consequences from drinking. Here are some of the most important:

    _____   _____

    _____   _____

    _____   _____

For the Partner

1. You have been trying many ways to cope with your wife/husband's drinking. The things you have tried the most include:

    _____   _____

    _____   _____

    _____   _____

For the Couple:

1. You have a number of areas of your relationship that you are concerned about. Some are concerns for both of you:

    _____   _____

    _____   _____

    _____   _____

2. Some concerns are mostly concerns for the husband:

    _____   _____

    _____   _____

3. Some concerns are mostly concerns for the wife:

    _____   _____

    _____   _____

FIGURE 12.5. Drinking feedback sheet for a couple.

need it. I think I was just protecting my ego at the beginning by focusing on the research part so much."

Anne, a 32-year-old, married, college graduate working as a cocktail waitress, was the mother of a 20-month-old daughter, Breanne. Her husband Charlie was working full time and enrolled in a doctoral program in mechanical engineering. She entered treatment as part of our women's treatment research program. She was a daily drinker with a varying pattern of consumption. During the evenings, when her husband was at school, she drank one or two bottles of wine. When he was home, her typical consumption was one glass of wine with dinner. She also drank at the end of her shift at work, consuming four to six beers on those evenings. When I gave her the feedback about her alcohol consumption, indicating that her level of consumption placed her in the 99th percentile of women, her eyes filled with tears and she looked visibly distraught, saying repeatedly, "I knew it was bad, but I never knew it was this bad." As treatment progressed, Anne made few changes in her drinking. She canceled or changed appointments, and said on several occasions, "If I didn't like you, I'd probably just quit the whole thing." She continued:

ANNE: I really like to drink. When Charlie is at school, I make myself a nice dinner—a lamb chop, a salad—and have an excellent bottle of wine. No one bothers me, and I enjoy myself. But I know I should stop because of Breanne.

THERAPIST: [As part of the treatment protocol, we had completed a decisional matrix, and I suggest that we return to that form.] Anne, let's look at your decisional matrix again. We did this a few weeks ago. When you look at it now, what strikes you?

ANNE: Everything on it is still true. I'm not being a good mother with all this drinking. I'm out of it at night, and I have no energy during the day. I just plop her in front of the television, and she watches *Teletubbies*. I keep thinking about when she gets older. Do I want her to have a drunken mother?

THERAPIST: It seems as though those feelings are very strong right now, but it's hard for you to keep them in the front of your mind each day. I wonder if you could review this sheet every day at some point. Would that help?

ANNE: I think so. I can look at it while Breanne is eating her breakfast. My motivation would be sitting right in front of me then. I'll try that.

Anne began reviewing her decisional matrix every day. The task seemed helpful for about a month, and she began to decrease her drinking, joined a gym, and came to treatment regularly. However, these changes were short-lived, and she fairly quickly reverted to her pattern of erratic treatment attendance and heavy drinking.

Selection of Drinking Goals

The final major area to consider in treatment planning is the selection of drinking goals. Traditional approaches to alcoholism treatment view abstinence as the only appropriate drinking goal, because these approaches view alcoholism as a progressive disease that can only be arrested with abstinence. Behavioral clinicians have examined alternatives to abstinence and have developed a number of strategies to teach clients how to drink moderately. Although better accepted as a goal for individuals with alcohol abuse (rather than dependence), moderation training continues to be controversial, and the clinician who elects to provide such treatment may be vulnerable to criticism from the traditional, mainstream alcoholism treatment community. A number of studies suggest that the long-term outcomes of alcoholism include reduced drinking (e.g., Helzer et al., 1985; Vaillant, 1983), but data about the success of moderation training are more mixed. Two European studies have found that giving clients the opportunity to select treatment goals increases compliance with treatment and may improve treatment outcome (Ojehegan & Berglund, 1989; Orford & Keddie, 1986). I have argued in favor of abstinence as a preferred treatment goal (see, e.g., McCrady, 1992; Nathan & McCrady, 1987), and continue to view it as the preferred treatment goal. Abstinence is clearly defined and is in accord with usual clinical practice in the United States. Also, agreeing readily to a goal of controlled drinking may reinforce a client's distorted view that alcohol is important and necessary to his or her daily functioning.

Under certain circumstances, however, the use of a reduced drinking goal is appropriate. Moderation may be used as a provisional goal to engage a client in treatment, or may be used when the client will not agree to abstinence but does want assistance to change (as with Bill). A moderate drinking goal also is more appropriate if a client shows few signs of alcohol dependence or withdrawal, has a history of being able to drink in moderation, does not have medical or psychological problems that would be exacerbated by continued drinking, is younger, and does not have a family history of alcoholism (Rosenberg, 1993). If the clinician and client select a moderation goal, a period of initial abstinence usually makes it easier for the client to drink moderately. In selecting a moderation goal, the clinician should be careful to help the client recognize the current and potential negative consequences of excessive drinking, and make an informed and thoughtful choice in selecting a treatment goal. The clinician should view any initial drinking goal (abstinence or moderation) as tentative, to be reevaluated as therapy progresses.

Initiating Abstinence

For clients with goals of abstinence, the clinician has a variety of alternatives to help a client initiate abstinence. With a client whose goal is moderation, the most conservative approach is to initiate a period of abstinence, then gradually reintroduce alcohol. As noted earlier, several detoxification alternative strategies are available, including inpatient detoxification, ambulatory detoxification, "cold turkey" detoxification (in which the client simply stops drinking abruptly), or a graduated program of reduction of drinking over a period of weeks until the client reaches abstinence. A case example illustrates a graduated program of reduction of drinking.

Steve, a 48-year-old, homeless, unemployed man with a long history of heroin, cocaine, and alcohol dependence, entered treatment after heroin detoxification but was still drinking an average of eight drinks per day (usually a half-pint of hard liquor plus one to two beers). He was healthy and had no history of alcohol withdrawal symptoms. No inpatient detoxification facility was available to him given his homeless and economically destitute state. Initial treatment focused on helping him achieve a stable housing situation and obtaining temporary General Assistance (welfare). Following these social interventions, the therapist (one of our practicum students) began to focus on his

drinking. Steve expressed a strong preference for a program of graduated reduction in drinking. He was evaluated by a physician at the local free clinic and cleared medically. We had him record his drinking for 1 week to establish a clear baseline. We then set a program to reduce his drinking by 15% per week, or eight drinks per week. We discussed specific strategies to achieve this goal each week, and Steve continued to monitor his drinking. During the alcohol reduction period, Steve reestablished contact with a former long-term girlfriend who had terminated their relationship when he relapsed to alcohol and heroin use. She had heard that he was off heroin and expressed interest in being involved with him again. Her presence provided a strong incentive for him to follow the alcohol reduction program, because she was unaware that he had been drinking. The program progressed smoothly, and he stopped drinking after 7 weeks.

Developing a Functional Analysis

As described earlier, completing a behavioral assessment of the factors associated with a client's drinking includes both a structured and a qualitative dimension, and incorporates clinical interviewing, questionnaires, and self-recording of drinking and drinking urges. Suzanne, described briefly earlier, provides an excellent illustration of the complexity and results of the behavioral assessment process.

Suzanne came from a large Jewish family, many members of whom made demands on her. She had three daughters, ages 10, 8, and 4 years old. Her drinking had increased 5 years prior to treatment after a car accident that took the life of her fraternal twin brother. They had gone out to a Bruce Springsteen concert together, and her brother had had several drinks at the concert. An autopsy after the accident revealed that he had also been using cocaine, but Suzanne was completely unaware of his drug use. She blamed herself for allowing him to drive and for not insisting that he stop when he began to drive in a reckless manner. She began to drink immediately after the accident and quickly established a pattern of daily consumption of a half-bottle of wine per day.

Although the amount was not that great, she reported that the alcohol was very important, because it helped her avoid her overwhelming sadness about her brother's death, especially at the end of the day. The results of the behavioral assessment revealed a more complex pattern of drinking antecedents. On the DPQ, Suzanne rated emotional antecedents as most important, endorsing feelings of sadness, hurt, and frustration. She also indicated that certain environments were triggers for drinking, such as specific restaurants, times of the day (evening), and activities (particularly watching television). Other major triggers emerged from Suzanne's self-recording cards—her interactions with extended family members, interactions with friends, and situations related to her children. Her parents were highly critical of how she was raising her children. Suzanne and her husband Josh were attending a conservative temple, kept kosher in their home, did not allow violent video games, and expected each daughter to participate in a fine arts activity (music, dance, or painting). Her parents believed that their grandchildren's upbringing and Suzanne and Josh's standards were too strict and conservative, and were vocal in their criticisms. Other familial stressors included her interactions with a sister who was getting divorced and a cousin who was in economic straits. Each contacted Suzanne on a regular basis, demanding either her attention or her money. Suzanne's functional analysis is provided in Figure 12.6.

Early Sobriety Strategies

Early sobriety strategies help the client maintain abstinence from alcohol. Cognitive-behavioral techniques vary with the individual but may include stimulus control strategies to avoid or rearrange high-risk situations, development of skills to deal with urges to drink, learning to think differently about drinking and not drinking, identification of behaviors alternative to drinking in high-risk situations, developing alternative ways to obtain the reinforcers previously obtained from alcohol, and learning to refuse drinks.

Stimulus Control

Stimulus control strategies are designed to alter environmental cues for drinking by avoiding the cue, rearranging it, or implementing different responses in the same environment. Stimulus control strategies are compatible with the AA suggestion to be attuned to "people, places,

and things." Work with Suzanne illustrates stimulus control strategies.

With Suzanne, stimulus control strategies served a major function early in treatment. She developed specific strategies to deal with a number of the environmental high-risk situations identified in her functional analysis. Her first approach was to avoid such situations whenever possible. She suggested to Josh that they eat only at restaurants without liquor licenses, and asked that they decline several social invitations to places where alcohol would be the main focus of the evening (such as cocktail parties). The one situation that she could not avoid was the end of the day, after the children had gone to bed. Her usual routine had been to complete the dinner dishes while Josh helped the girls get ready for bed, then to sit down in the den with her wine and the television after reading the children a story. She decided that she needed to disrupt this pattern, and thought that if she got ready for bed herself, then curled up on the couch with a book and a cup of herbal tea, she would experience less urge to drink. It took her 3 weeks to get to a bookstore to buy some light novels, but once she had the books, Suzanne was able to implement this plan with success, except when she was upset.

Dealing with Urges

As individuals decrease their drinking or initiate abstinence, they may experience urges or cravings for alcohol. It is helpful to provide the client with a framework for understanding that urges are learned responses to drinking situations, and that urges abate if unfulfilled. Marlatt and Gordon (1985) suggest the use of imagery to help cope with urges, and describe either acceptance-oriented imagery (e.g., surfing with the urge) or action-oriented imagery (e.g., attacking the urge with a samurai sword).

Suzanne struggled with urges to drink, particularly when anything reminded her of her twin brother's death. During therapy, we focused on a variety of aspects of her feelings about her brother's death and also addressed the urges more directly. Suzanne initially reacted to the imagery techniques negatively, saying that she was not a person who imagined things much. She clearly needed some way to cope with these rather strong urges, so I pushed her a bit to try:

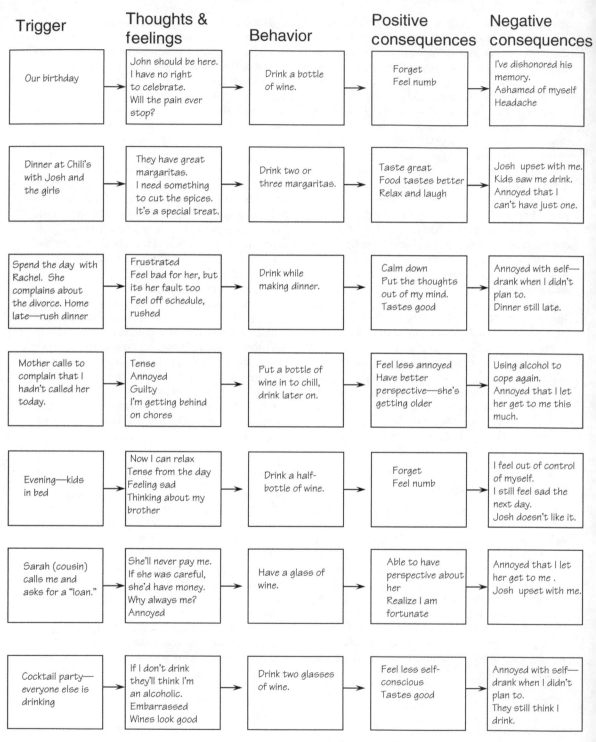

FIGURE 12.6. Suzanne's functional analysis.

THERAPIST: I appreciate that you don't think of yourself as imaginative, but maybe I can help you out. Just humor me for a minute, and let's see if we can come up with an image that grabs you. It doesn't matter what the image is—you could imagine climbing a mountain and coming down the other side, or spraying the urge with a fire extinguisher.

SUZANNE: (*smiling*) I know what I can imagine—I could picture you jumping out of the bottle and shaking your head at me.

THERAPIST: OK. Should I look mean?

SUZANNE: No, just having you there would help me deal with it.

THERAPIST: All right, I can live with that.

SUZANNE: In fact, I could picture a row of wine bottles—with you coming out of the first one, then showing me all the disgusting things in the other one.

THERAPIST: So what would be disgusting? Ticks?

SUZANNE: Ticks would be good, and maybe cockroaches, too.

THERAPIST: Let's try this out.

At that point, I had her practice using the imagery in an imagined urge situation. Remarkably, she used the imagery frequently and found it helpful.

A second technique for coping with urges is to enlist the assistance of a family member or friend. Persons involved with AA are told to call someone in the AA program when they feel the urge to drink, and they usually receive telephone numbers from several members. Clients not involved with AA can seek other sources of support. Suzanne, for example, asked her husband to help her when she had the urge to drink. She asked Josh to remind her of why she had stopped drinking and to say, "Of course, it has to be your decision."

Addressing Cognitive Distortions about Alcohol

People who drink heavily hold stronger positive expectancies about the effects of alcohol than do people who drink more lightly (Brown, Goldman, & Christiansen, 1985). Clients may believe that drinking facilitates social interactions, enhances sexual responsiveness, allows them to forget painful events or feelings, or makes them more capable. These beliefs often

are deeply held and difficult to challenge, particularly if a client continues to drink. Several cognitive strategies may help. First, effecting a period of abstinence allows the client to experience many situations without alcohol—an experience that often leads to reevaluation, with little input from the therapist. At some point, many clients are impressed with the vacuous nature of drunken conversation; the undesirable physical appearance, behaviors, and odors that accompany high BALs; and the shallow nature of drinking relationships. The wise therapist watches carefully for these observations and underscores their importance and self-relevance. If a client does not have such experiences spontaneously, the therapist facilitates new views of drunken comportment by developing a relatively safe way for the client to observe intoxicated behavior—through either movies or videotapes, or visits to a local bar (accompanied by someone who is aware of and supports the client's abstinence).

A second strategy reported in the self-change literature (Ludwig, 1985) is the ability to think past anticipated positive benefits of drinking to the clear, though often delayed, negative consequences of drinking. The therapist and client can generate a list of negative consequences of drinking, and use imaginal rehearsal in the session to help the client pair positive thoughts with the list of negatives. Continued rehearsal in the natural environment is then important. Third, some clients develop a set of erroneous beliefs about their drinking that set them up for drinking. Common beliefs include "I've been doing so well, I can just drink tonight," or "I'll have just one." Although moderate drinking is possible for some clients, others have histories of drinking until they lose control, which is in direct opposition to a belief in control, and need to learn how to counter these beliefs.

Work with Steve provides a simple illustration of cognitive strategies to address positive expectations about drinking. Steve had a long history of loss-of-control drinking. After a period of abstinence, he began to think, "I could have just one beer, and that would be fine." His therapist questioned the accuracy of that belief. Steve readily acknowledged that he had never been able to control his drinking in the past, that if his girlfriend found out she'd be very upset and probably leave him, and that relapses to heavy drinking usually led him to use of heroin. Steve and his therapist developed a simple cognitive formula to use when he thought about drinking: "1 = 32 = 10," meaning that for him, one drink would lead to a quart of liquor (32 ounces), which would lead to heroin use (10 bags a day).

Alternative/Distracting Behaviors

Drinking is a time-occupying activity, and clients may see few alternatives to help them through times when they previously would drink. Discussion of specific behavioral alternatives to drinking that are both time-occupying and mentally or physically absorbing is another helpful strategy early in treatment.

Steve's experiences provide a particularly powerful example of the alternatives that highly motivated clients may find. After Steve found a room in a rooming house and had begun the detoxification process, he was faced with the daunting prospect of filling his completely unstructured days. Some of his time was occupied with the time-consuming work of being poor—getting back and forth to the soup kitchen, waiting at the free clinic for medical services, getting an appropriate identification card so that he was eligible for other charitable programs, such as clothing distribution. But even with these necessary activities, Steve had hours and hours of free time. Steve began to address this challenge by creating his own activities. He obtained a library card and scheduled times for himself at the library. Instead of reading randomly or recreationally, he decided to read about the Crusades, which sparked an interest for him in medieval Christianity. A lapsed Catholic, he decided to attend Mass again, and began to attend daily. His daily attendance led to involvement in a Bible study group, and he became a thoughtful and passionate participant. A creative man, Steve then began to write short stories with religious themes.

Identifying Alternative Ways to Obtain Reinforcers

Among the more compelling aspects of alcohol and drug use are the psychoactive properties of the substances. In the short term, large quantities of alcohol effectively deaden negative affect, decrease obsessional thoughts, and decrease muscle tension, although these effects do not endure over the long term. Alcoholic beverages also have distinctive and desirable tastes that cannot be replaced with other beverages.

An important aspect of the functional analysis is articulating the client's perception of positive consequences of drinking. The clinician can address the power of these perceived reinforcers in several ways: helping the client develop alternative means of obtaining the same types of reinforcement; challenging the client's belief that the desirable consequences will occur (e.g., questioning whether the client is in fact more socially adept and appealing after consuming a quart of vodka); helping the client reevaluate the importance of these reinforcers; and/or helping the client identify other classes of reinforcers that might be valued more highly in the long run (e.g., valuing spirituality more highly than hedonism).

Drink Refusal Skills

Some drinkers find the interpersonal aspects of abstinence difficult. For them, identification of interpersonal situations as high risk for drinking, development of effective responses, and rehearsal of these responses all form an important component of treatment. Early research (Chaney, O'Leary, & Marlatt, 1978) suggested that giving a quick response is strongly associated with successful change. Suggested components of an effective way to refuse drinks include indicating clearly that the one does not want an alcoholic beverage, requesting an alternative beverage, communicating confidence and comfort with the request, and being persistent in the face of social pressure (Foy, Miller, Eisler, & O'Toole, 1976). In addition, clients who face excessive social pressure may be advised to consider avoiding certain social situations or persons.

Although the guidelines for refusing drinks appear simple, client beliefs and expectations often make the drink refusal process difficult. Common cognitions include "Everyone will think I'm an alcoholic," "My host will be offended if I don't drink," or "People will think I'm too good for them if I don't drink." As with other distorted beliefs, the clinician can provide alternative frameworks for thinking about drink refusal situations, suggesting that most people really are uninterested in others' drinking, or that hosts are most concerned that guests are enjoying themselves. Many clients also experience ambivalence about not drinking and find that the most difficult part of the drink refusal process is internal rather than interpersonal. Another complicated aspect of drink refusal is how much personal information the client wishes to divulge. Most people share different levels of personal information, depending on the closeness of the relationship and their knowledge of the other person's behavior and attitudes. For persons to whom a client does not want to disclose his or her drinking problem, we encourage use of a simple "No, thank you," or, if pressed, a simple response that would discourage pushing without being revealing, such as "I'm watching my weight and can't afford the calories," "I'm on medication that doesn't allow me to drink," or "My stomach's been acting up—I better pass." None of these replies protect the client against future offers, but each is effective in the moment. For closer relationships, the client makes a decision about when, where, and how much to reveal. Two clinical examples illustrate these points.

Steve was living in a boarding house and had friendly, sociable neighbors who liked to drink on the front porch. These neighbors were from the Portuguese Azores and spoke virtually no English. After accepting a beer from them one day, he insisted to his therapist that he could not refuse because he did not speak Portuguese. The therapist suggested that perhaps the word "No," spoken with a smile and a hand gesture, might be understood even in Portuguese. Steve acknowledged that his difficulty with refusing the drink came from his desire to drink, and that a friendly "No" would certainly work.

Suzanne did not want anyone to know that she had a drinking problem, or that she was abstaining. This stance posed problems for an upcoming cocktail party. Strategizing, Suzanne decided ahead that she would drink seltzer water during the evening, and that she would attempt to forestall offers of drinks by keeping a glass of seltzer in her hand at all times. If offered a drink, she decided to tell people that she had had some health problems that might be made worse by her drinking, so she was sticking to seltzer. Although she was concerned that one of her friends (a social worker) might surmise that she had an alcohol problem, the evening progressed uneventfully.

Coping Strategies

Clients face challenges beyond those directly related to their drinking. As do clients without drinking problems, clients with such problems face common life difficulties stemming from dysfunctional thoughts, negative affect, and interpersonal conflicts. As clients develop a greater ability to maintain abstinence or moderated drinking, the clinician may devote increasing attention to other problems clients are facing. Clinical techniques to deal with dysfunctional thoughts or social skills deficits can be used readily with clients with drinking problems.

Dealing with Negative Affect

There are multiple sources of negative affect in persons with alcohol abuse or dependence. As noted earlier in the chapter, comorbidity with other psychiatric disorders is high (e.g., mood and anxiety disorders are quite common). Rates of sexual and physical abuse are also elevated among those with alcohol use disorders (Stewart, 1996), and the sequelae of these problems often include a strongly negative affective component. In addition, persons who have used alcohol to cope with negative affect over an extended period of time may simply have limited experience, and limited skills, to cope with the pain that is a part of everyday life.

In focusing on negative affect, a careful assessment of the causes is essential. Intense negative affect associated with another disorder should be treated in accord with the appropriate approach for that disorder. Dealing with negative affect that is not necessarily disorder-based presents different challenges. Full behavioral mood management programs (e.g., Monti et al., 1990) have been developed, although a description of these is beyond the scope of the chapter. However, certain common principles are of value. When clients first reduce or stop drinking, they may experience all emotions as unfamiliar and intense. Cognitive reframing to help clients view these intense emotions as a natural part of the change process may be useful. For clients pursuing a moderation goal, avoidance of drinking at times of intense negative affect provides the opportunity to learn alternative coping strategies. Coping strategies may vary with the type of negative emotion, and may include relaxation, prayer or meditation, increasing the experience of pleasurable events to decrease depression, or use of anger management and assertiveness skills to cope with angry feelings.

Work with Suzanne illustrates several of these principles. Most difficult for Suzanne were any situations that reminded her of the death of her twin. Their birthday, the anniversary of his death, the celebration of Father's and Mother's Days, holiday celebrations, and special celebratory events for her children in which he would have been importantly involved with (such as a bat mitzvah) all elicited intense negative affect and a strong desire to drink. Given that Suzanne had begun drinking heavily right after her twin's death, she had spent little time experiencing grief or even discussing his death and her feelings about it. My initial approach in therapy was to give her opportunities to be exposed to these negative feelings by simply talking about him in the therapy session. The second approach was to discuss and identify ways to approach events that reminded her of him. I saw her over a 6-month period, during which a number of these situations arose naturally. For example, in the week prior to the anniversary of his death, we discussed ways that she could focus on his death and memories. Suzanne took one of her children to his gravesite, and they cleaned it up and planted flowers together. On the Saturday of the anniversary of his death, she went to temple with her family, then cooked what had been her twin's favorite dinner. The day was sorrowful and Suzanne cried several times, but it was the first anniversary that she felt she had honored him rather than shaming his memory by getting drunk. We also addressed her repetitive, self-blaming thoughts about his death by using cognitive restructuring techniques. She found it difficult not to blame herself for his death, and few cognitive strategies had much impact on the self-blame. Suzanne finally was able to begin to think, "I cannot torture myself forever with this blame. If I don't let go of it, I won't be a good mother. He'd be disappointed with me if I let my children down."

Lifestyle Balance and Pleasurable Activities

Marlatt and Donovan (2005) suggest that long-term success is supported by lifestyle changes that enhance positive experiences and allow for a balance between responsibilities and pleasure. Although some studies of successful self-changers (e.g., Vaillant & Milofsky, 1982) have revealed that development of an "alternate dependency" (e.g., obsessive involvement with work or exercise) is associated with successful long-term abstinence, we typically work toward a more balanced approach. As they begin to change, some of our clients believe that they need to make up for their previous lack of responsibility with a very high level of responsibility to family, job, and home. Taking on major redecorating or remodeling projects, trying to spend every free moment with their children, or cleaning out 10 years' worth of messy drawers and cabinets is not uncommon. This zeal for responsibility can be a double-edged sword for both client and family. Unrelenting attention to responsibilities may be simultaneously satisfying, and exhausting and unrewarding, and may lead the client to question the value of not drinking. Family members may be thrilled that the client is taking on responsibility but leery of the stability of the change and unwilling to give up responsibilities they have assumed for the client. They also may experience the client's enthusiasm as an intrusion on their own independent lives and schedules. Clients should be prepared for such reactions, and the clinician can help reframe the family's response as understandable. With most clients, it is important for the clinician to suggest the importance of leisure time, pleasurable activities, and self-reinforcement for positive changes made.

Helping Suzanne identify a half-hour per day during which she could relax, read, or exercise was a challenge. She believed that she should devote herself to her daughters—a belief that resulted in her being with them virtually all the time they were home. When they were at school, she focused on housecleaning, cooking, errands, paying bills, and other chores. She was exhausted and tense at the end of the day, and commented that alcohol had been a good way to "come down." We finally agreed on a half-hour block before lunch, during which she would use her exercise bike, read a book of daily meditations, or take a walk. She was only partially successful in these efforts, often citing other responsibilities that took precedence.

Partner/Family Involvement and the Social Context of Treatment

The literature on the treatment of alcohol use disorders suggests that the involvement of some significant social system is associated with positive treatment results. Because of these findings, the clinician's first inclination should be to involve the client's spouse/partner or some significant other in the treatment. There are a number of ways to involve significant others: using them as sources of information, having them provide differential reinforcement for drinking and abstinence, helping them to provide emotional or practical support, involving them in relationship-focused treatment, providing treatment to them without the person who drinks, and/or helping them access new social systems.

Information

Folklore suggests that persons with alcoholism minimize or lie about their drinking and its consequences. The empirical literature suggests that such individuals provide relatively accurate data when sober, and when there are no strong negative consequences for telling the truth (e.g., Sobell & Sobell, 2003). Despite these results, a number of clinical considerations suggest that obtaining information from a family member may be useful in the assessment phase of treatment.

Clients who are referred to or coerced into treatment may be reluctant to provide full information about their drinking. Collecting data from the referring agent helps both the client and clinician understand the reasons for the referral. Even with self-referred clients, significant others can provide information that may be unavailable to the clients because of problems with memory or recall. In addition, an intimate significant other usually has observed the drinker over a long period of time and in multiple environments, and may have valuable observations to contribute to the conceptualization of antecedents to drinking.

Responses to Drinking and Abstinence

A different type of social system involvement is the establishment of a network that provides differential reinforcement for abstinence and applies negative consequences for drinking. Such reinforcement may be relatively simple, such as positive comments and encouragement from friends and family, or it can involve the negotiation of detailed contracts that specify the consequences of drinking and abstinence. The "community reinforcement approach" (CRA; Meyers & Smith, 1995) helps clients access potential reinforcers (jobs, families, social clubs), teaches clients and partners behavioral

coping skills, and may involve development of contingency contracts to make access to reinforcers contingent on sobriety. In addition, clients may take Antabuse or Revia (naltrexone), and compliance may be monitored by a significant other. Evaluations of the CRA approach suggest that clients are significantly more successful than controls in maintaining abstinence and employment, avoiding hospitalizations or jail, and maintaining a stable residence. In addition to formal treatments that focus on manipulation of environmental contingencies, the therapist also may teach spouses/partners and other family members how to allow the client to experience the naturally occurring negative consequences of drinking. Many spouses/partners protect the drinker from these consequences by covering at work, doing their chores, or lying to friends and family about the drinking (e.g., Orford et al., 1975). Experience of these negative consequences may increase the client's awareness of the extent and severity of his or her drinking problem, and provide further motivation for change.

Decreasing Cues for Drinking

Significant others also may engage in behaviors that cue further drinking. A wife who wants her husband to stop drinking may nag him repeatedly about the problems his drinking is causing, hoping that her concerns will motivate him to change. Or a husband may try to get his wife to stop drinking by limiting her access to alcohol or tightly controlling their money. Such behaviors may have an unintended and negative effect, eliciting anger or defensiveness from the person with the drinking problem, and leading to further drinking. Helping spouses/partners learn to identify such behaviors, recognize the results of these actions, and find alternative ways to discuss concerns about drinking may be helpful.

Support for Abstinence

Significant others can provide many kinds of support to clients. Support may involve helping a client to implement behavior change, discussing urges to drink, supporting a client's plan to avoid high-risk situations for drinking, or (upon the request of the client) assisting in the implementation of other coping skills that support sobriety.

Relationship Change

For many clients, interactions with their spouses/partners, children, parents, or close friends cue drinking. Thus, treatment that focuses on changing those interpersonal relationships is another way that significant others may become involved. These interventions may include couple or family therapy, or parent skills training. Data (McCrady, Stout, Noel, Abrams, & Nelson, 1991) suggest that a focus on changing the couple relationship during conjoint alcoholism treatment results in greater stability of drinking outcomes, fewer separations, and greater couple satisfaction.

Accessing New Social Systems

Some clients have either no social support system or one that strongly supports heavy drinking. For such clients, it is important to access new systems that either reinforce abstinence or are incompatible with heavy drinking. Self-help groups are one potential source of such support. Because many religious groups are against the use of alcohol, serious involvement in such a group also may support abstinence. Many group activities are incompatible with drinking: Running, hiking, or cycling groups are examples. Unfortunately, alcohol can be involved in almost any activity, and therapist and client need to look carefully at activity groups to determine whether the group norm includes drinking.

In summary, decisions about the social context of alcoholism treatment are complicated. The initial assessment should involve at least one significant other. The results of the assessment should reveal persons who are most available for treatment, and who might be sources of support and reinforcement. For some clients with no readily accessible supports, new support systems need to be developed.

Long-Term Maintenance

Relapse Prevention

Marlatt and Gordon's (1985) RP model and Witkiewitz and Marlatt's (2004) revised RP model are comprehensive treatment models. Many elements of RP treatment model already have been described—identifying high-risk situations for drinking, developing alternative strategies to cope with high-risk situations, enhancing self-efficacy for coping, dealing with positive expectancies about the use of alcohol, and facilitating the development of a balanced lifestyle. An additional and important part of the RP model is addressing the possibility of relapse and developing preventive and responsive strategies related to relapse.

Clients are told that use of alcohol after treatment is not uncommon, and treatment addresses this possibility. Two basic strategies are used. First, a client is helped to develop a list of signs of an impending relapse, including behavioral, cognitive, interpersonal, and affective signs. If a client's spouse/partner is also involved with the treatment, he or she contributes to the list. After this list is developed, we develop a set of possible responses, should these signs arise. Most important is for the client to recognize that these warning signs should trigger action, rather than inaction and fatalistic cognitions about the inevitability of relapse. A second set of strategies involves response to drinking or heavy drinking. We attempt to address the possibility of the AVE (Marlatt & Gordon, 1985) by calling attention to the possibility that a client may have catastrophic thoughts if he or she drinks and helping him or her rehearse alternative thoughts. Marlatt and Gordon also suggested a series of behavioral steps: Introduce a behavioral delay (1–2 hours) between an initial drink and any subsequent drinks, get out of the immediate drinking situation, conduct a functional analysis of the drinking situation during that time, review possible negative consequences of drinking, and call someone who might be helpful. Some research evidence supports the use of such RP approaches. For example, we found in our own research (McCrady, Epstein, & Hirsch, 1999) that including RP procedures as part of conjoint alcoholism treatment was successful in reducing the length of relapse episodes compared to conjoint CBT without RP. O'Farrell, Choquette, and Cutter (1998), who incorporated RP techniques into their couple therapy treatment by providing additional therapy sessions over the 12 months after initial treatment, reported less frequent drinking among couples who received the additional therapy.

Maintaining Contact with Clients

Time-limited treatment is appropriate and effective for many clients, and there is good evidence of long-term, sustained improvement following a course of outpatient treatment (Project MATCH Research Group, 1998). However, periods of relapse are common. The clinical strategies I have described for RP are intended to minimize periods of problem use and to maximize positive outcomes. For some clients, however, alcohol dependence must be viewed as chronic, relapsing disorder (McLellan et al., 2000). As with other chronic health problems such as diabetes or rheumatoid arthritis, acute care models that treat individuals and send them on their way may be inappropriate and ineffective. An alternative strategy provides longer-term, low-intensity contact over an extended time interval (Stout, Rubin, Zwick, Zwyiak, & Bellino, 1999).

During the initial treatment of a client with a history of severe alcohol dependence, multiple treatment episodes, and difficulty maintaining successful change, the clinician may elect to set a different expectancy with that client—that some form of contact will be ongoing and long-term.

Lee, a 54-year-old married man, came to treatment with problems with alcohol dependence and agoraphobia. Treatment focused on both disorders, and he was successful both in becoming abstinent from alcohol and in gradually increasing the distances that he could drive by himself. Lee's home was an hour's drive from my office, and treatment had gone on for almost 12 months before he could drive to my office without his wife accompanying him. By the end of the year, we were meeting every 2 to 3 weeks. Given that Lee had been abstinent for a year and was functioning well, we discussed the possibility of termination. His response was instructive:

LEE: Doctor, I've been drinking a long, long time. One year is just a drop in the bucket in comparison. I think that I need to keep seeing you.

THERAPIST: Lee, I understand your concerns, but you've been doing well for quite a long time now. Maybe we should just cut down more on how often you come in. How about an appointment in a month, and making it a bit shorter—a half-hour instead of an hour?

LEE: I think that's a good idea. Let's try it.

I gradually tapered the frequency and length of my sessions with Lee, and saw him twice per year, 15 minutes per session, for the last 3½

years of his 5-year course of treatment. He described the importance of the sessions: "I just know I'll have to see you and tell you what I've been doing. It keeps me honest."

Managing Complicating Conditions

As I described earlier in the chapter, clients with alcohol use disorders may present with a myriad of other, complicating conditions. The clinician must assess and develop a treatment plan for the multiple needs of such clients. At a minimum, clinicians should consider possible problems related to housing, transportation, income, occupation/employment, the legal system, the family, child care, medical conditions, and comorbid psychological disorders. Knowledge of services and agencies in the local community, and the development of working relationships with a range of agencies, are essential to the treatment of complicated clients. Rose, Zweben, and Stoffel (1999) provide a comprehensive framework for interfacing with other health and social systems.

The Role of Self-Help Groups

Types of self-help groups were described in an earlier section of this chapter. Various therapeutic strategies may facilitate involvement in a self-help group, when appropriate. The clinician should first assess whether a client may be a good candidate for self-help group involvement. Clients with very high social anxiety or social phobia, clients who believe that a person should take care of problems alone, and clients with a history of negative experiences with self-help groups may be poorer candidates. Conversely, affiliative clients, those who are used to solving problems with assistance from others, those who are particularly anxious and concerned about their drinking, those whose social support systems strongly support continued heavy drinking, and those with more severe alcohol dependence are particularly good candidates for AA. Persons who are interested in the social support aspects of self-help but explicitly reject some of the constructs associated with AA (e.g., powerlessness or spirituality) may be best served by referral to an alternative self-help group.

As with all aspects of the therapy, the clinician should use a client-centered approach to the introduction of AA or other self-help groups. Such an approach suggests a dialogue between client and therapist, acknowledgment and discussion of the client's perceptions and concerns, and development of a mutually agreed-upon plan. Because many clients have misconceptions about AA and are unfamiliar with some of the alternative organizations, the clinician should be prepared to describe the organizations and answer questions. It also is helpful for the clinician to have some basic publications from each group available in the office. At times, I may encourage a reluctant client to try a few meetings to sample firsthand what actually occurs. We negotiate a very short-term agreement for a specified number of meetings in a specified length of time (such as six meetings in 3 weeks); we agree that if the client continues to be negative or reluctant after trying the groups, then we will abandon this idea; and we discuss the client's experiences and perceptions of the self-help group meeting in each therapy session. I use behavioral sampling with other aspects of therapy as well—clients often cannot visualize how a strategy might work without trying it—be it a relaxation technique, an AA meeting, or an assertive response—and I encourage clients to be open to new strategies. In AA, newcomers may be told, "Your best thinking got you here," suggesting that their own coping strategies have been ineffective. Behavioral sampling is based on this same construct.

Therapist Variables

As with any form of therapy, the therapist's relationship with the client and the therapeutic stance he or she assumes are important. Empathy, active listening, instillation of hope, flexible application of therapeutic principles and techniques, and establishing a sense that the therapist and client are working toward mutually agreed-upon goals are essential. Research suggests that in contrast to a confrontational style, an empathic, motivational style is associated with better treatment outcomes, and that confrontational behaviors by the therapist tend to elicit defensive and counteraggressive behaviors by the client (Miller et al., 1993). Such responses are hardly conducive to a constructive therapeutic alliance.

Working with a client with an alcohol use disorder often is difficult, both because of the client's behavior during treatment and because of his or her history of drinking-related behaviors that the therapist may find repugnant or upsetting. The client may lie about or minimize drinking during treatment. If the spouse/partner is also involved in the treatment, the therapeutic relationship becomes even more complicated.

By treating a client with a drinking problem along with a spouse/partner who wants that client to stop or decrease drinking, the therapist is allied de facto with the spouse/partner. That individual may attempt to enhance his or her alliance with the therapist by echoing the therapist's comments, expressing anger at the client's behavior, being confrontational, or, alternatively, being submissive and allowing the client to be verbally aggressive or dominant.

Certain therapist attitudes and behaviors appear to be conducive to successful treatment. First is a sense of empathy with the client. The therapist must develop some understanding of the client's subjective experience of entering therapy and the difficulty of admitting behaviors that are personally embarrassing and often not socially sanctioned. In addition, the therapist needs to have some appreciation of the incredible difficulties involved with long-term change in drinking behavior. The therapist may develop this appreciation by attempting to change a deeply ingrained behavior pattern of his or her own, by attending meetings of some self-help group (AA, SMART, SOS), and by listening carefully to clients.

A second important therapist skill is the ability to distinguish between the person and the drinking-related behavior. The client needs to be able to describe drinking-related actions not only without feeling that the therapist is repulsed, but also without feeling that the therapist condones or accepts such behaviors. This is a delicate balance to achieve, especially when a client describes drinking episodes in a joking manner that may hide embarrassment or disgust with the behavior. The client's motivation to change may be enhanced by discussing negative, drinking-related behaviors and experiencing the negative affect associated with thinking about those actions. The therapist also should communicate a sense of hope to the client by anticipating positive changes that might be associated with changes in drinking, and by emphasizing that it is possible to change. Thus, the implied message to the client is as follows:

"You have done many things when drinking that are distressing to you and to the people around you. The fact that you are in treatment is a statement that you want to change.

It is important to talk about things you have done when drinking, because being aware of them will strengthen your desire to stop drinking and to stop doing these things. Making changes will take time and a lot of work on your part, but I believe that you will be successful if you stick with treatment."

In other words, the therapist's message is positive about change, but negative about drinking-related behavior.

A third important therapist quality is integrity. Both because of their discomfort and their reinforcement history, it is difficult for some clients to report drinking episodes honestly, failed homework assignments, or their feelings and attitudes about being in treatment. The therapist can acknowledge how difficult it is to be honest given that lying was probably adaptive in the past, but he or she must make it clear that part of therapy involves learning how to be honest. The therapist also must provide a positive model of integrity. He or she should not ignore the smell of alcohol on a client's breath and should review the homework assigned each week. Attending to the client's behavior teaches the client the importance of following through on commitments and increases the chances that therapist and client will be able to identify problems and blocks to progress in treatment.

The therapist also must set clear expectations about both the client's and his or her own responsibilities to the therapy, and must be able to set appropriate limits. The therapist should set clear expectations for the client: coming to scheduled sessions on time, calling if unable to attend, paying the bill for therapy, coming in sober, and completing assigned homework. The therapist also should make his or her own commitment to therapy clear, by being at sessions on time, being reasonably available by telephone, providing coverage when away, and providing treatments with the best empirical support for their effectiveness. Being clear about expectations for the client's behavior during therapy emphasizes the therapist's commitment to therapy as a serious process.

Client Variables

Only a few client characteristics are consistent predictors of treatment outcome (Haaga, McCrady, & Lebow, 2006). Clients who have positive expectancies about the outcomes of treatment tend to have better outcomes. Additionally, clients with greater readiness to change have more positive outcomes. Finally, clients with more severe problems have poorer outcomes. Both treatment expectancies and readiness to change can be influenced by the therapist.

The clinician must be aware of and sensitive to a number of issues that persons with drinking problems bring to treatment. The emotional experience of the client, his or her beliefs and attitudes, physical state (described in the section on treatment settings), and the social context of drinking (described in the section on the social context of drinking) are all important aspects of the therapeutic plan.

A person has a variety of reactions to the initial realization that his or her drinking is causing problems. Most commonly, as negative consequences accumulate, an individual begins to feel out of control and ashamed of the behavior. The person's actions may be unacceptable to his or her self-definition. Thus, financial or work irresponsibility, neglecting family members, engaging in physical violence, or verbal abuse all may be actions about which the individual feels intense guilt and self-blame. The prospect of admitting these actions to a stranger is frightening and embarrassing, making it difficult for a client to discuss drinking-associated problems. Because many clients ascribe their problems to weakness or lack of willpower, and believe that if they were only "stronger" these events would not occur, they blame themselves. Thus, clients are unusually sensitive to implied criticisms from the therapist. The therapist can attenuate this difficulty by making empathic comments while asking questions, letting clients know that their actions are common among people who drink heavily, and listening to clients' descriptions of drinking-related actions in an accepting manner. Clients also hold a number of beliefs and attitudes about alcohol and their ability to change that make change difficult. People with alcohol use disorders have positive expectancies about the effects of alcohol on feelings and behavior, and they hold these more strongly than do people without drinking problems. They may attribute their drinking to reasons external to themselves and believe that they are not personally responsible for either drinking or changing. They may have low self-efficacy about their ability to change their drinking or to handle alcohol-related situations without drinking, or they may have unrealistically high self-efficacy that is not grounded in actuality. Finally, if people stop drinking and then consume alcohol again, cognitive dissonance may occur; they may experience the AVE (Marlatt & Gordon, 1985), characterized by an excessively negative reaction to initial alcohol consumption, and a self-perception that they have "blown" their abstinence and will inevitably relapse to the previous drinking pattern.

CASE STUDY

In the preceding sections, I have presented case examples to illustrate the application of parts of our treatment model. In this section, I present a complete outpatient therapy case to illustrate a number of the issues described earlier in the context of ongoing treatment. The couple was part of a research project evaluating different approaches to the maintenance of change following conjoint behavioral alcoholism treatment (McCrady et al., 1999).

Couples in the study had to have been married or cohabitating for at least 6 months; neither partner could have a primary problem with the use of illicit drugs or show evidence of gross cognitive impairment or psychosis; and only the male partner could show evidence of alcohol abuse or dependence. All couples were seen by a therapist for 15–17 sessions of weekly outpatient treatment, and agreed to a baseline assessment and 18 months of post-treatment follow-up.

Carl and Maria were married, and both were 32 years old. They came to treatment because of Carl's drinking. Maria was of average height, had long black, wavy hair and was heavy. Carl was also of average height, had blond hair, and was slim, but showed the beginnings of a "beer belly." Both were neat and attractive. The couple had been married 5 years and had known each other for 12 years. They had two boys, ages 2 and 3. Both came from intact families, although Carl's father had died a number of years previously. Carl's family was primarily Polish; Maria's was Italian.

At the time of treatment, Carl and Maria had been separated for 5 months. He was living with his mother in her home; Maria was renting a one-bedroom apartment in a poor community, where she lived with the two boys. Maria was a trained hairdresser; Carl was a carpenter who worked out of the union hall.

Carl was not working at the time, because he did not want to establish a pattern of support for Maria or the children in case she filed for divorce. In addition, if he did not work for a certain period of time, Carl would be able to withdraw his money from the union's pension plan, and he thought that would be an easy way to obtain money. Maria was not working because she had decided that Carl would have to babysit while she worked, and she did not think that he would be reliable about coming to her apartment to care for the children. She was supported by welfare; Carl worked odd jobs "under the table." Both were high school graduates.

The couple came to treatment at Maria's urging. She was very concerned about Carl's drinking and cited it as the primary reason for their marital separation.

Behavioral Assessment and Case Conceptualization

Carl and Maria were assessed using several approaches. Their assessment was somewhat more extensive than is usual in clinical practice because of their involvement with the treatment research project. However, the main elements of the assessment are applicable to clinical practice as well.

Drinking Assessment

To assess his drinking, we used a clinical interview to ask Carl about his drinking history and perceptions of his current drinking. A handheld Breathalyzer was used at the beginning of each session to assess his current BAL. In addition, we used two structured interviews, the TLFB (Sobell et al., 1980) and the Alcohol section of the Composite International Diagnostic Interview—Substance Abuse Module (CIDI-SAM; Robins et al., 1988), to obtain a more complete picture of his drinking. Maria was present for all interviews and contributed additional information.

The TLFB inquires about drinking behavior on each day in a set window of time before treatment. For this study, we asked about Carl's drinking in the prior 6 months, cueing his recall of drinking by noting other salient events in his and Maria's lives, such as social events, medical appointments, holidays, and other celebrations. The TLFB revealed that Carl had drunk alcohol virtually every day of the previous 6 months. His only abstinent day was when he and some friends were arrested for attempted breaking and entering. His preferred beverages were beer and vodka, and he reported that the most he drank any one day was about 32 drinks. His usual consumption was in the range of 10–12 drinks daily. Carl met criteria for a diagnosis of alcohol dependence with physiological dependence. He had been drinking since high school and reported having his first problems as a result of alcohol at the age of 25. Carl had experienced a variety of problem consequences of his use: three arrests for DWI, one arrest for breaking and entering, warnings from job supervisors for intoxication on the job, problems in his relationship with his wife, and the feeling that he had neglected his responsibilities to his wife and sons. He had experienced numerous blackouts and reported many signs of physical dependence, including morning drinking, a sense of "panic" when he thought he would not be able to obtain a drink when he wanted one, and drinking throughout the day. However, he said that he had never experienced any of the physical symptoms of alcohol withdrawal. He also reported no health or emotional problems associated with his drinking. When asked about his goals for treatment, he indicated that his own preference was to cut down and to drink moderately, but that his wife insisted on abstinence, and he was willing to work toward that goal.

We used two assessment techniques to identify antecedents to Carl's drinking, the DPQ (Zitter & McCrady, 1979) and self-recording cards. The DPQ was used to assess Carl's and Maria's perceptions of drinking antecedents. Carl completed the DPQ by checking off all antecedents that applied to his drinking in the previous 6 months, and Maria completed the measure as well, to indicate her views of his drinking. They also were asked to indicate what they thought were the most influential antecedents. Both perceived environmental influences as being most important to Carl's drinking, citing as most salient settings such as bars and his home, afternoons when he was not working, any celebratory occasions, and being around others who were drinking.

The second most important set of drinking cues pertained to their relationship, with Carl citing arguments, anger, feeling nagged, or having a good time together as antecedents. The third area of concern that both Carl and Maria cited was physiological antecedents, primarily restlessness and fatigue.

Carl used daily self-recording cards throughout the treatment to record drinks and drinking urges. Reviewing the information he recorded and discussing events associated with drinking or drinking urges made it clear that being with heavy-drinking friends was an important component of Carl's drinking. The self-recording cards also clarified factors associated with his feelings of "restlessness." When he and Maria were together and the children were being active, if he wanted to leave or go somewhere, then he would get restless and irritable, and want to drink to "take the edge off." Finally, it was apparent that Carl felt like drinking whenever Maria reminded him of a commitment that he had made (even something simple, such as bringing a book to her apartment), when she tried to get him to commit to any responsible course of action, or when he felt "trapped."

We used questionnaires and self-recording cards to assess how Maria coped with Carl's drinking. She recorded her perceptions of his drinking each day on a Likert scale (None, Light, Moderate, or Heavy) and recorded her daily marital satisfaction as well. Her responses antecedent to and consequent to drinking episodes were discussed in the therapy sessions. In addition, both partners completed a modified version of the Coping Questionnaire (Orford et al., 2005).

Data from these assessment sources made it apparent that Maria often questioned Carl about his actions, threatened him, or pleaded with him not to drink. She had reacted to his drinking in a number of negative ways—by separating from him, calling the police, and refusing to have sex with him. At the same time, she had made serious efforts to support him and encourage his abstinence by doing positive things with Carl when he did not drink, doing nice things for him, or talking about positive things they could do together if he did not drink.

Marital Relationship

We assessed the couple's relationship by administering the ACQ (Margolin et al., 1983) and the DAS (Spanier, 1976), and by viewing a videotape of the couple discussing a problem in their relationship. Maria had a number of major concerns about their relationship. In addition to Carl's drinking, she was concerned about his apparent lack of responsibility, citing his unwillingness to work, to care for the children, or to be independent of his mother. In general, Maria felt that Carl could not be relied upon for concrete or emotional support. A second concern that she expressed was their role definitions. She felt that Carl dictated her role to her, and that she allowed him to do so. She often felt angry and resentful as a result. Finally, she cited Carl's mother as a problem, describing her as an "enabler" who rescued Carl from his problems and made no demands upon him. She stated that when she and Carl first dated they liked to drink, stay out late, ride motorcycles, and have a good time, but she felt that it was now time to "move forward" with their lives and "get somewhere."

Carl had fewer marital concerns. He disliked Maria's "nagging" him or discussing his drinking, stating at one point, "If I had a different wife, I wouldn't have a drinking problem." He also disliked her "persistence" in wanting to discuss topics at length and her "attitude change" when he drank.

A videotape of their interactions revealed several communication problems. Carl and Maria interrupted each other frequently and did not listen to each other's comments. Each made frequent sarcastic and biting comments about the other, usually stating these with a smile and a funny comment. Maria complained about her excessive responsibilities, and Carl criticized her for not fulfilling her responsibilities but refused to acknowledge any responsibilities of his own.

Despite these considerable marital problems, they enjoyed each other's company, shared many activities and pleasures (e.g., fishing, going to parks with the children), and had a very positive sexual relationship. Maria said of their relationship, "We get along great when I don't demand anything."

Behavioral Formulation

Carl's drinking appeared to have developed in a social context, with virtually all his drinking occurring within social groups with similar drinking patterns. The pattern was reinforced by these positive social interactions, both with friends and (early in their relationship) with Maria. He had developed significant tolerance for alcohol, so that he could consume increasingly large amounts, resulting in a pattern of daily drinking with some signs of physical dependence on alcohol. For Carl, alcohol provided a number of positive consequences: He enjoyed the tastes and sensations associated with drinking, the social context of drinking, and the feelings of relaxation that drinking engendered. Although he had accumulated a number of significant negative consequences of drinking, none had affected his internal perceptions of himself or of alcohol. From his perspective, negative consequences were imposed on him by others—the police, job supervisors, and his wife. In addition, Carl had been able to avoid responsibility for his actions in many areas of his life. When he did not work, he was able to live with his mother, who shielded him from the negative consequences of not working by providing shelter and food for him. When his wife made demands on him that he experienced as aversive, he avoided or ignored her. To some degree, his problems with alcohol were accentuated by their different developmental stages: Maria was ready to move to a more adult stage of life, with increased responsibilities and long-term goals; Carl, in contrast, wanted to maintain the lifestyle and behavior patterns of his early 20s.

Despite Carl's externalizing attributions for his problems and his tendency to avoid negative consequences and responsibility, his wife and children were important to him, and he did not want to lose them from his life. Therefore, he came to treatment to maintain these desired reinforcers, but not necessarily to make the behavior changes his wife saw as necessary for them to have a successful long-term marriage.

As treatment progressed (see below), Carl engaged in a variety of maneuvers to maintain the relationship but avoid behavior change, and his wife, and at times the therapist, reinforced these behaviors. Maria had a limited repertoire of effective ways to obtain positive reinforcers for herself. She appeared to expect most positive feelings to come from external sources, and nagging and criticizing were the only verbal behaviors she used to try to get what she wanted. She reinforced Carl's drinking by continuing to have contact with him but engaged in aversive negative verbal behavior at the same time. She placed responsibility for her happiness with Carl, stating that she could not work (something she enjoyed a great deal) until he stopped drinking and was more responsible, and that she could not lose weight until he stopped drinking and she was less upset.

As a couple, Carl and Maria lacked the verbal skills to discuss these very major problems. Aversive control, avoidance of responsibility, and lack of empathic communication characterized their interactions.

Preparing the Client for Change

Carl and Maria were seen together for all phases of the evaluation. In the initial evaluation, both spouses were asked to describe their perceptions of Carl's drinking, their relationship, and how each had attempted to cope with Carl's drinking. By seeing the couple together, I communicated my view that the drinking was intimately connected to their relationship, and that both spouses would need to examine their own behavior to effect positive changes. At the end of the evaluation, I provided them with feedback about the main difficulties that I perceived (as summarized earlier), and oriented them to the plan for treatment. In discussing the treatment plan, I covered the following:

"We have asked you to come to treatment as a couple. This is because drinking affects many areas of your life, including your marriage and your family. I know from what you have said, Maria, that you have tried many different ways to cope with Carl's drinking, and that you have been angry and frustrated at times. It is clear that you have tried to help, but it seems, Carl, that you mostly have resented it when Maria has said anything about your drinking. During treatment we will look at your drinking, how you have tried to cope with it, and how the two of you are getting along as a couple. Right now the two of you are separated, and you have a lot of concerns about your relationship. As we go along in the therapy, I will help you improve your communication, and I will ask you to try new ways to spend time together and discuss problems. The therapy will focus on three main topics—your drinking (Carl), how you (Maria) have coped with it, and how to cope in ways that work better for both of you, and for your relationship with each other."

In addition to this overall orientation, which both Carl and Maria felt captured their goals for the treatment; we discussed Carl's drinking goals in more detail and made plans for how to achieve those goals. As indicated earlier, Carl's preferred drinking goal was moderate drinking. However, Maria felt strongly that she wanted him to abstain, and he had agreed to

that goal prior to coming to treatment. Since he had been drinking daily and showed evidence of tolerance to alcohol, I was concerned that he would not be able to stop drinking without assistance. I therefore discussed with him the possibility of being detoxified under medical supervision:

"I am concerned, Carl, that it will be difficult for you to stop drinking on your own. You drink every day and have been drinking a lot. On the questionnaires, you indicated that you 'panic' if you think that you will not be able to get any alcohol, and you typically drink throughout the day. All of these things suggest to me that you may be 'hooked' on alcohol, and that your body will have a strong reaction to going without any alcohol at all. The easiest way to get through the first few days without drinking is to check into a hospital detoxification program, and I would like you to consider it."

Carl had a very negative reaction to the thought of being hospitalized. He was afraid of being "locked up," and said, "I know that I would go crazy. I can't stand being confined. After 24 hours I would just have to leave. It's not a good idea." I was most interested in engaging Carl in treatment, so I thought it inappropriate to try to force Carl to enter a detoxification center. I was certain that if I made brief hospitalization a prerequisite to further treatment, he would leave treatment completely. Therefore, we developed a plan to achieve abstinence. The plan had two major components: (1) Carl was to come to therapy sessions sober, and his BAL would be verified by breath alcohol test reading; and (2) Carl would set goals to reduce his drinking gradually, with a target date for abstinence 6 weeks hence. If he was not able to achieve either goal, then we would reevaluate the need for supervised detoxification. He was amenable to this agreement, as was Maria.

Process of Treatment

The course of treatment is described sequentially to provide the reader with the clearest picture of the progress and pitfalls of a fairly typical therapy case. The treatment covered several major areas: (1) helping Carl to reduce then stop his drinking; (2) teaching Carl skills to maintain abstinence; (3) enhancing Carl's perception of his drinking as problematic; (4) teaching Maria more constructive coping strategies; (5) teaching the couple how to engage in positive interactions; and (6) teaching the couple mutual problem-solving techniques. In addition, as treatment progressed, we focused on some other areas of individual behavioral change for Maria.

Intake and Sessions 1–2

At the initial intake session, Carl had a BAL of greater than 400 mg%. Although he did not show gross signs of intoxication, he was belligerent, and the clinician doing the intake did not feel that he could conduct a reasonable intake interview. He suggested that Carl receive medical attention because his BAL was so high, but Carl refused, and the clinician rescheduled the intake. At the rescheduled appointment, Carl was sober and able to provide information, to give informed consent for the research aspects of the program, and to schedule the baseline data collection session.

At the first treatment session, however, Carl again had an elevated BAL (120 mg%). He acknowledged only having had "a couple of beers" and insisted that he was fine. We briefly discussed Carl's and Maria's concerns and goals, but I suggested that we would not be able to have a very productive session with Carl's BAL so high. (My general policy is to reschedule a treatment session if the client's BAL is greater than 50 mg%.) Carl agreed to come to the next session sober and to have no more than four drinks per day. I gave Carl and Maria self-recording cards, on which I asked them to record drinks, drinking urges, and marital satisfaction on a daily basis. Carl was given one card for each day and was asked to record each drink he actually consumed, to note urges to drink not followed by drinking, and to note on the back of the card the situations in which he drank or had urges to drink (see Figure 12.3).

Maria received one card to use for the entire week. I asked her to write on the card a daily estimate of Carl's drinking (*None*, *Light*, *Moderate*, or *Heavy*) and also to record her estimate of the strength of his urges to drink that day. She also made a daily rating of her marital satisfaction (see Figure 12.4).

When Carl and Maria came to the second session, his BAL was again elevated, at 60 mg%. He reported drinking about four beers during the day. We continued the discussion

of detoxification, and Carl said that he felt he was addicted to alcohol. He said that he would consider detoxification, and we scheduled a phone conversation to discuss detoxification further. After we spoke twice by phone, Carl again decided that he did not want to be hospitalized. He did not use the self-recording cards during these first 2 weeks, although Maria completed his cards for him while they drove to the treatment session. I did not feel that I had a clear picture of Carl's drinking, but it was clear that he was continuing to drink daily.

Sessions 3–5

Carl came to the third session with a BAL of 0. He again reiterated his desire to stop drinking without hospitalization, and we worked out a plan for him to reduce his drinking gradually to zero over a 6-week time period. In addition to setting drinking goals, we began to discuss a behavioral-analytic view of drinking. To introduce the couple to a behavioral way of thinking about their drinking, I said:

"Together we are going to observe carefully and analyze all the factors that seem to be part of your drinking. I think that we can look at your drinking and figure out what kinds of situations lead you to feel like drinking. If we can figure this out, then we can work together to come up with *alternatives* for these situations. We will be using these sheets, called 'triggers' sheets, to analyze your drinking. Let's go through one of these together."

I then asked Carl to identify a recent drinking situation. He indicated that he liked to drink when he went fishing. As we spoke, I completed the boxes on the "triggers" sheet, illustrated in Figure 12.7. Carl had a fairly nonpsychological view of his drinking. He described his thoughts as "I want to get some beer" and his feelings as "happy." He viewed drinking when fishing as having positive consequences—"I have a blast." He felt that the only negative consequences came from Maria, who would be angry when he came home.

Carl and Maria grasped the behavioral analysis quickly and found it a comfortable way to conceptualize his drinking. As homework, I then asked both of them to complete the DPQ and bring it to the next treatment session. I

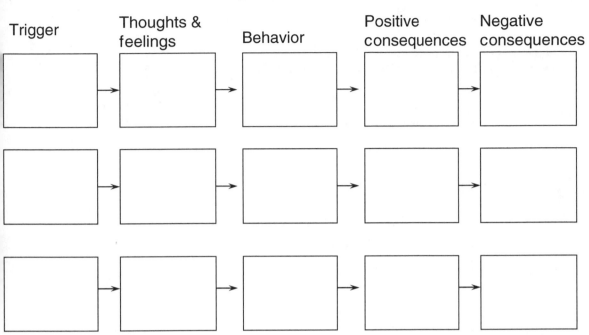

FIGURE 12.7. "Triggers" sheet.

gave them additional self-recording cards to use for the week.

Carl also came to the fourth session sober but reported heavy drinking over the weekend. The graph of his weekly alcohol consumption during treatment is reproduced in Figure 12.8. Carl's and Maria's average weekly marital satisfaction ratings are reproduced in Figure 12.9. Carl expressed no concern about his continued heavy drinking, and showed no evidence that he was trying to cut down.

"I am glad that you have come to the last two sessions sober—I know that's not easy for you, and it does show that you want treatment to succeed. However, I am concerned that you have not cut down at all between sessions. If anything, your drinking seems a

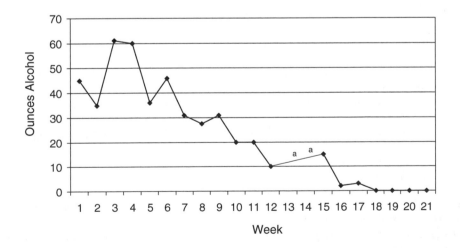

FIGURE 12.8. Carl's weekly alcohol consumption. Areas marked "a" represent missing self-recording data.

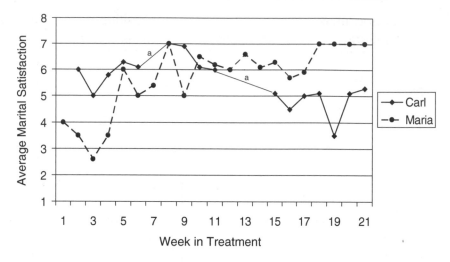

FIGURE 12.9. Carl and Maria's weekly marital satisfaction. Areas marked "a" represent missing self-recording data.

bit heavier. It's not clear to me whether you don't really want to cut down, or whether you just don't know how."

Carl said that it was hard to cut down, but that he was committed to stop drinking because he wanted to have Maria and the boys back again. We then discussed a number of potential strategies to help him avoid drinking, such as sleeping (his suggestion) or having alternative beverages available in the house (my suggestion), or going back to work (Maria's suggestion). He was reluctant to commit to any plans, and Maria challenged whether he was really willing to stop drinking.

To respond to Carl's ambivalence, I suggested that we examine other consequences of his drinking than Maria's disapproval and the couple's arguments about his drinking. Carl was unable to think of any other adverse consequences. I asked him about his legal problems from the DWIs and the arrest for breaking and entering, but he said that he did not believe that alcohol had anything to do with the latter charge, and that DWI laws were "ridiculous." He also indicated that he was still driving, even though he did not have a driver's license, and that he would continue to drive even if his license was revoked for 10 years (a real possibility, given that he had had three DWIs in less than 10 years, with two in the same month). Carl expressed a similar lack of concern about any other aspects of his drinking but again said that he was willing to stop because of his com-

mitment to the marriage and his children. I made a list of the negative consequences that he or Maria had reported at various times and asked him to review the list at least twice daily, and to think about which of these consequences were of concern to him. Carl reported looking at the list "once or twice" between sessions, but he was relatively indifferent to the content.

Despite my concern about Carl's relative lack of motivation to change, I decided to proceed with a behavioral analysis of his drinking. I thought that if we could identify a discrete set of antecedents to drinking, and if Carl could successfully avoid drinking in some of these situations some of the time, his motivation to change might increase as his self-efficacy increased. We discussed two other drinking situations in the session, and as homework, I had him complete two behavioral chains at home. A complete summary of the behavioral analysis of his drinking is provided in Figure 12.10.

Carl came to the next treatment session with a BAL of 118 mg% and reported drinking heavily for the last several days prior to the treatment session. After a lengthy discussion, he agreed to go for detoxification. Carl said he was afraid of the hospitalization and concerned that he would not be able to be abstinent after detoxification. I tried to emphasize that the detoxification was only the first step in treatment, and that we would be working together to help him learn ways of coping without drinking.

Trigger	Thoughts & feelings	Behavior	Positive consequences	Negative consequences
Going fishing	Get some beer and fish. Happy time	Drink beer	Have a blast	Come home to Maria, argue
Argument with Maria	She's angry because I had a drink. Angry Gotta get away	Leave house Drink	None	Feel like shit
Steve comes over, asks me to go out.	Sounds good, I'll go.	Go to a bar and drink	Have a blast	Get home late Maria's upset
Scott comes over with a 12-pack. No one else is home.	Glad to see him— like to talk to him. Like to see beer. It'll be fun to sit and rap.	Sit on patio Drink and talk Listen to radio	Feels good to talk— get things off my chest. Relaxed Takes the edge off	Maria comes home and gets mad. Scott leaves. I feel like shit. No sex
Get up at Maria's— kids get up, lots of action	Edgy A beer will take the edge off.	Have a morning beer	Takes the edge off	Maria unhappy Keeps the addiction going
Noontime at work	Time for a beer It'll be good to relax.	Split a six-pack	Relax Talk with other guys Tastes great when I'm thirsty	Boss doesn't like us to drink. Feel tired
Kids acting up, Maria's not handling it. I yell, but nothing happens.	Angry Tense Frustrated Don't know what to do	Leave house and drink.	Get away from it Calm down	Kids get away with acting up. Feel like a bad father
Maria reminds me about a responsibility.	Guilty Annoyed Where does she get off telling me what to do?	Leave house and drink; talk to guys at bar.	They agree with me that she's a nag. Feel better	Feel guilty when I sober up

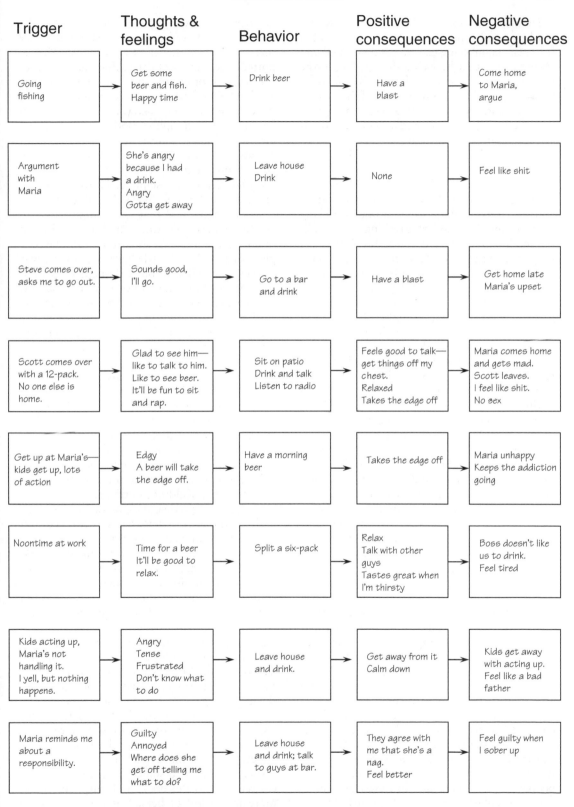

FIGURE 12.10. Sample behavioral analysis of Carl's drinking.

He also expressed his belief that life would not be fun if he did not drink. Maria oscillated between encouraging Carl to get detoxified and saying to me that he was only agreeing to the detoxification to get out of my office. Because he was so concerned, I had him call the detoxification center from my office to ask any questions he had. He did so, and scheduled himself for admission the next day.

Sessions 6–8

Carl did not admit himself for detoxification and stated again that he could not face being "locked up." He was still drinking daily, making minimal efforts to decrease his drinking. I suggested outpatient detoxification and gave him the phone number of a physician colleague who supervised outpatient detoxification, but I had little expectation that he would follow through with that referral either. Carl continued to express willingness to be in treatment and to change his drinking, and I decided to continue despite my doubts about whether he had sufficient incentives to change. We completed the behavioral analysis of his drinking during the sixth session, and identified several of Maria's actions that were antecedents to his drinking, including reminding him about responsibilities, her slow pace when they had an appointment and there was a lot to do to get themselves and their children ready to go out, and her comments about his drinking.

At one point during Session 6, Carl said, "You know, Maria has a real temper. You should ask her what she did to me at the beach." Maria responded immediately by saying, "Show Barbara your arms." Carl rolled up his sleeves, revealing a number of scratches and bruises covering his lower forearms. Maria then explained that she had been intensely frustrated with Carl because of his drinking, and often grabbed him, scratched him, or tried to hit him in the chest or abdomen when she was angry. The behavior had started in the last 4 months, and she found it very upsetting. She also indicated her concern that she might become abusive toward her children and admitted that she sometimes used physical punishment when she was angry at them. Although Maria's anger and frustration were not surprising and are common reactions of partners of people with alcoholism, the physical aggression, particularly in the absence of any physical abuse from Carl, was less usual. We discussed

her behavior toward the children in great detail, because I was concerned about whether there was any evidence of child abuse. She reported, and Carl confirmed, that she had never bruised, cut, or injured the children in any way, and that they had never had to take either of the children to a physician or emergency room because of her discipline. Both reported the belief that physical punishment, in the form of "swats on the bum" or physically removing the child from a dangerous situation, was an appropriate form of discipline. However, Maria felt that she did not always discipline the children rationally, and that she would occasionally hit them on the arm, or pull too hard when removing them from a situation. From the couple's reports, I did not believe that Maria was abusing the children, but I thought it was important to address her concerns in the therapy. I instructed Maria to use the self-recording cards to write down any times in the next 2 weeks when she felt that she was reacting too strongly to the children or when she was physically aggressive toward Carl.

Over the next two sessions, Carl began to decrease his drinking substantially and was abstinent for each treatment session. Carl and Maria had begun to spend more time together, and they reported that their time together was more positive. They had a family barbecue and went fishing at the beach with the children.

Maria had been faithful in recording her reactions to her children, noting two times each week when she either slapped one of the children on the arm or felt that she grabbed him too hard. We discussed the antecedents to these incidents and identified several salient aspects: Maria was tired, the child was tired, and she attempted to tell him to do something when she could not enforce it (she was across the room or had her hands full). In each situation, she repeated her verbal instructions to the boy several times to no avail, then felt angry and stomped across the room and grabbed him. We discussed alternative strategies, and I emphasized the importance of being able to follow through on a verbal instruction immediately rather than allowing herself to get frustrated. She quickly picked up on my suggestions and also expressed relief at being able to discuss her concerns. After the 2-week period, Maria reported no further instances of excessive physical reaction to the boys, and reported feeling more in control of herself as a parent again. Carl's observations confirmed her reports.

At the same time that we discussed Maria's problems with disciplining the children, we began to implement some self-management planning techniques for Carl. I suggested to Carl that it would be easier not to drink if he had ideas about how to handle certain triggers without alcohol. He could avoid situations or rearrange them to minimize the importance of alcohol in the situation. We used a self-management planning sheet to assist in the process (see Figure 12.11).

We selected fishing as a topic for self-management planning, because it was a high frequency, high-drinking activity for him. Carl had a number of ideas about how to fish without alcohol. These included taking his older son, taking his wife, or inviting an older friend who was an excellent fisherman and did not drink at all. In addition, he thought if he bought soft drinks the night before he went fishing and filled his cooler with the sodas before he left the house, he would be less tempted to stop by the liquor store at the end of his block. For homework, I asked Carl to implement this plan, and to develop another self-management plan for getting together with a friend without drinking.

Carl implemented the fishing plan successfully and also planned to ask his friend Scott to play tennis, then go to a fast-food restaurant to eat, because alcohol would not be available there. Although Carl saw no obstacles to implementing this plan, he never used it, and could provide no reasons for not following it up. He did, however, tell Scott that he was trying not to drink, and his friend reacted positively and supportively.

The other major topic of these several sessions was reinforcement for changes in Carl's drinking. Because Carl was so ambivalent about changing his drinking, I thought it particularly important that he experience some positive consequences for decreased drinking and for abstinence. I also wanted to give Maria some positive rather than coercive ways to interact with Carl about his drinking. In introducing this topic, I suggested that they both should think about ways to make abstinence and reduced drinking more positive. I first suggested that Maria might give him positive feedback when he was not drinking, but Carl reacted quite negatively to this suggestion, saying, "I would just think it was another one of her sneaky ways to try to pressure me to stop. I don't want her to say anything." In continuing with this discussion, I asked whether there was anything that Maria could *do* that would make abstinence worthwhile to him, and Carl suggested that she could refrain from talking about alcohol and spend time with him without being "picky." They decided on several mutually enjoyable activities to share when he was not drinking, such as sharing a shrimp dinner, and Maria telling Carl when she was enjoying their time together. They were able to implement these plans successfully, and although Carl drank while they were together, the amount was substantially less on these occasions.

Sessions 9–11

By this point in the treatment, Carl had reduced his drinking to approximately three to six drinks per day, but he had not abstained from drinking at all. His reports of urges to drink had also begun to decrease. Maria re-

	Trigger	Plan	Pluses	Minuses	How Hard
1.					
2.					

FIGURE 12.11. Sample self-management planning sheet.

ported high marital satisfaction almost every day (ratings of 7 on a 1- to 7-point scale), and they were spending most of their free time either at her apartment or at the home of Carl's mother. However, in the therapy sessions they began to argue more frequently, with their conflict revolving around two major topics— Maria's desire to move to North Carolina and her feeling that Carl was not emotionally supportive of her. I began to implement some structured communication training with them, teaching them skills that included allowing the other to finish before speaking, reflective listening, and making specific positive requests. These sessions were supplemented with handouts about communication. After reading the first handout, which covered basic topics, such as the value of being polite and respectful of your spouse, and some of the sources of bad communication, they came into the session absolutely surprised at the notion that calling each other names (e.g., "idiot," "asshole," or "shithead") could have any negative impact on their relationship. They had begun to use positive rather than negative communication at home and were pleased with the impact it had on their conversations.

Although we were making progress in the treatment, I was concerned that Carl was still drinking every day, and I relayed this concern to him. Carl stated that he believed that he could now stop, and he agreed to be abstinent for 2 days in the following week. The first week that he agreed to this contract, Carl did not want to discuss strategies for abstinence, and he was unsuccessful. The second week we discussed very specific plans for how he would abstain. He planned to be with Maria and the children for part of each day, and he decided not to buy more beer to have in his mother's house those days. In addition, he would stock up on soft drinks and plan to go to bed early. I also suggested that he might use Maria as a support in his attempts to abstain. I often encourage a client to find someone with whom to discuss urges, and the partner can be a good source of support. He again was resistant to involving Maria, saying, "I wouldn't tell her that I wanted to drink—all I'd get is a lecture." I suggested that he usually disliked her comments because they were unsolicited, but in this situation, he would be in charge, because he would be the person concerned about his drinking. He responded positively to this

reframing. I then asked him whether there was anything Maria could say that would be helpful to him, and he suggested that she tell him it was his choice. Maria indicated that it would be difficult not to lecture, but she agreed to a role play. They imagined that they were driving to the beach, and Carl said, "I want to stop to pick up a six-pack on the way down." Maria answered, "It's your choice if you want to, but we could stop to get some sodas instead, if you want." Carl was amazed at how much he liked her response, and although Maria acknowledged that it was very difficult to be that neutral, she liked feeling that it was not her responsibility to prevent him from drinking. They agreed to try out such a discussion once during the coming week.

Carl was not successful in maintaining any abstinent days, although he did implement most of the rest of the plans and drank only one beer on each of the 2 target days. However, he did not tell Maria about any of his urges to drink. He again expressed little concern about not meeting his goals. During the session, Carl and Maria announced that they were going to North Carolina for a 2-week trip. Carl knew a contractor who had offered him work there, and Maria was intrigued with the possibility of moving to an area with a lower cost of living and more rural environment in which to raise the children. She stated that she would not move while Carl was still drinking, but they both decided that a trip to explore the possibilities was appealing.

Sessions 12–15

Carl and Maria returned from their 2-week trip very enthusiastic about North Carolina. They believed that work was available, the cost of living was clearly lower, and both of them liked the area they had visited. Maria said again that she would not move unless Carl had been abstinent for a considerable length of time, because she did not want to leave her family if she could not depend on Carl. He again said that he would stop drinking. I had taken advantage of the break in the therapy to review all of my progress notes and to think about the couple with a bit more detachment. It was clear to me that although Carl had agreed to abstinence because of Maria's pressure, he wanted instead to reduce his drinking. However, he had dealt with this conflict by providing verbal reassurances that his behavior would change, without accompanying behavior changes. He had implemented only a few of the behavioral plans that we had developed, and I did not think that the lack of implementation reflected a skills deficit. I had decided to point out Carl's behavioral inconsistencies at this treatment session.

To initiate this discussion, I told Carl and Maria that I wanted to discuss their progress so far. I emphasized the positive changes that they had made so far: Carl had decreased his drinking substantially; he had developed some skills to assist him in drinking less; their communication had begun to improve; they were spending time together that was mutually enjoyable; and they had begun to consider possible long-term plans together. I noted, however, that Carl had made a series of promises about his drinking on which he had not followed through. I read them several passages from my progress notes, noting Carl's initial target date for abstinence, and his broken agreements about detoxification and abstinent days. I suggested two alternative explanations to them: Either Carl did not want to stop drinking completely but felt that he had to agree to abstinence to keep Maria happy or he really could not stop drinking and needed further assistance to do so. By framing my explanations this way, I tried to avoid labeling Carl as dishonest or unmotivated to change. I also suggested that Maria had helped Carl to keep drinking by reporting high marital satisfaction even though he was still drinking, and that perhaps reduced drinking really was acceptable to her as well. Both reacted quite strongly to my feedback. Carl said, "At first I didn't want to stop, but now it doesn't seem that bad. I'm not drinking enough now for it to mean anything, so I'll just quit. It's no big deal, and I don't want to disappoint you." Maria said, "I always feel like Carl is just saying whatever he has to say to get me or you off his back. But I have been so much happier since he cut down that I kind of lost sight of that fact that he's still drinking. I am afraid to move anywhere with him while he's still drinking at all. It was so bad before, I don't want to go back to that."

After this conversation, Carl denied that he preferred moderate drinking and announced that he was going to "quit for good." Over the next 2 weeks, Carl had one drinking day each week—one beer the first week and two beers the second week. Although we dis-

cussed a variety of behavioral coping strategies, such as developing behavioral alternatives for drinking situations, rehearsing strategies for refusing drinks, and using various strategies for coping with urges, Carl deemphasized their importance. Instead, he focused on cognitive coping strategies: When he had urges to drink, he would think about reasons not to drink ("It's not worth it—Maria and the kids are more important"). Or he would use delay tactics ("I won't have anything right now—if I still feel like drinking at 5:00 [or some other, later time during the day], then I'll have a beer"). Or he would deemphasize the positive aspects of alcohol ("One or two beers won't do anything for me, and I don't want to get blasted").

Carl and Maria also began to discuss their long-term goals. I asked them to write down how they would like their lives to be in 5 years. Carl wrote down the following[3]:

Comfortable place to live for Maria and this kids. Good schools, backyard. Get finances in order; save money, consolidate bills, improve credit. Maintain stable income ie. steady construction work or other. Obtain a loving relationship with Maria. Self improvement: manage money better, listen to Maria more objectivly, secure steadier employment. Maria: better self discipline, controll temper, improve self confidence, weight loss, less pessimistic in dialy matters. ie. scared of bugs, traffic, mishaps, ect.

Maria wrote down remarkably similar 5-year goals:

Five years from now—37 years old; Jonathan 8 years, Marc 7 years. We are living in North Carolina in a rented house. I'm working, Carls working the boys are in school. We have two cars. Carl is 5 yrs sober. I'm 4 years thin. We are two yrs away from getting credit back from filing bankruptcy. Some nights we will be together as a family to relax or to go to a baseball or soccer game of Jonathan's or Marc's. Other nights I will be out to socialize or run errands. Other nights Carl will do the same. We will be somewhat financialy comfortable. Three things I want out of life:

Maria	Carl:
calmness, thinness, responsability	*motivation, sobriety, contentness*
to feel secure, a car, money, independence, control over my life	

Because Carl and Maria's goals were so similar, I asked them if I could read them aloud. Both were amenable to this suggestion, and I did so. They reacted quite positively and felt encouraged; because their long-term goals were so similar, they could work together to achieve these goals. I began to teach them skills related to assertiveness and problem solving, discussing ways to implement these skills both in their relationship and in other interpersonal situations.

Sessions 16–18

Carl abstained from drinking from Session 15 to the end of the treatment. He reported a few urges to drink, but these soon decreased. However, he discussed very strong reactions to not drinking. He felt sad, saying that he missed drinking and felt that he had lost something important to him. He also said that it was frustrating, because he always had been able to drink when he felt bad, but now he could not do so. I tried to reframe his feelings for him, noting that his ability to recognize that he missed alcohol was an important step toward being able to reorganize his life without it, and that his reaction suggested that he was serious about his intentions not to drink. Carl seemed to find the reframing helpful, but he continued to find abstinence uncomfortable.

As Carl remained abstinent, his marital satisfaction ratings decreased. Previously he had reported fairly high marital satisfaction, but as Carl stopped drinking he became increasingly unhappy. When I asked him about his ratings, he said that he felt they were "going nowhere" in terms of reconciling. We had begun assertion and problem-solving training, and I suggested that Carl could use these skills to express his feelings to Maria more directly. They had a positive discussion during the session about his feelings and about wanting to reconcile, and her concerns about how difficult that would be, with each using some of the positive skills we had worked on. Both agreed that they now wanted to live together again, but it would be difficult to develop a plan to do so. We used structured problem-solving techniques over two treatment sessions to develop a plan. The major impediment to reconciliation was financial. Maria was receiving welfare, but if either she or Carl began to work, they would receive less public assistance. However, to be able to live together, they would have to save sufficient

money for a security deposit and first month's rent. They finally decided that Maria would begin to work a few hours a week as a hairdresser, working "under the table," and that Carl would care for the children while she worked. If that worked well, then Carl would begin to look for work again; once both were working, they would move in with his mother for a limited period of time to save money for the deposits and rent, then either obtain an apartment together in New Jersey or find a trailer to rent in North Carolina and move. They also used problem-solving techniques to develop a plan to deal with their other debts.

Termination

Because Carl and Maria were part of a clinical research study, we had to terminate treatment after 18 sessions (including the sessions when he was intoxicated). They had made significant progress during treatment: Carl had been abstinent for more than a month; Maria had learned more effective ways to discipline the children and no longer reported concerns about being overly punitive to them; the couple's relationship was significantly improved; and they had a constructive plan for reconciliation. I was concerned that Carl was still uncomfortable with abstinence, and I thought that he had acquired only a few effective coping strategies to deal with triggers for drinking. We had not worked directly on Carl's responsibility-avoiding style except by following through on his commitment to abstinence and on long-term goal setting. Whether Carl would implement his part of these agreements was relatively untested. The couple was fairly comfortable with termination but asked about possible follow-up treatment, inquiring specifically about AA or other support groups that focused on couples or on behavioral approaches to change. I referred them to SMART, and to a couples AA group. The constraints of the clinical research protocol precluded any longer-term treatment with me, even though I thought continued treatment would be beneficial.

Comment

Carl and Maria were a fairly typical couple. Carl's ambivalence about change, his entry into treatment solely because of an external agent, and his resistance to many behavioral interventions are fairly representative. I believe that he began to engage in treatment when he stopped feeling that he was the sole focus of the treatment, after Maria began to discuss her aggressive behavior and feelings. The second critical point in treatment was addressing his continued drinking. I was willing to allow them to renegotiate for a goal of moderate drinking, but I did not think it therapeutic for Carl to feel that he could verbally agree to abstinence, then avoid the agreement. Confronting Carl's behavior forced him either to be assertive and renegotiate treatment goals or to follow through on his commitment.

The role of behavioral skills training in facilitating Carl's abstinence was less important than with some clients. He tried various skills introduced during the treatment, but relied primarily on cognitive coping strategies. The role of reinforcement was probably more important in understanding his changed drinking behavior. Carl's marital relationship was important to him at the beginning of treatment, and focusing in the therapy on ways to improve that relationship increased its reinforcement value to him. Maria's consistency in saying that they could only reconcile if he were abstinent, in discussing long-term goals for the relationship, and in seeing the possible positive life they could live in North Carolina all contributed.

Finally, my relationship with the couple probably contributed to the positive changes they made. I found them a likable, appealing couple despite their difficulties. At times, I would tease or cajole Carl into compliance, and he commented at the end of the treatment, "At first I didn't know if I liked you or not, but then I decided you were kind of cute, and then I realized that you weren't going to let up on me, so I decided that I'd give it a try." I tried to reinforce Maria's ability to take care of herself, and I suspect that she saw me as a female role model in some ways. She often asked me personal questions (whether I was married, how old my son was), and gave me a desk calendar as a thank-you gift at termination. Our research has suggested that our more experienced therapists are more successful at keeping clients in treatment (Epstein, McCrady, Miller, & Steinberg, 1994; Raytek, McCrady, Epstein, & Hirsch, 1999), and I suspect that being able to deal with these complex relationships is one skill that our more experienced therapists have acquired more fully.

Typical Problems

The problems presented in this case are fairly typical—coming to treatment sessions intoxicated, continued drinking during treatment, ambivalence about change, noncompliance with assignments, and discovering new and major problems as the therapy progresses. Lying and failing to come to scheduled treatment sessions are other typical obstacles that clients with drinking problems sometimes present. By working with Carl and Maria together, I was able to minimize these particular difficulties, because Maria was highly motivated for treatment and very responsible about keeping scheduled appointments. Also, by having them both record Carl's drinking and drinking urges, I had a clearer picture of his drinking and was able to maintain a clear idea of our progress (or lack thereof).

CLINICAL PREDICTORS OF SUCCESS OR FAILURE

A number of factors predict the success or failure of therapy. However, before I address these factors, it is important to discuss definitions of "success." In any treatment, a minority of clients maintain successful change (abstinence or nonproblem drinking) for extended periods of time. The proportion varies with the demographic characteristics of the population, and persons who are married, have stable employment, a stable residence, and no comorbid psychopathology have the best treatment outcomes. In addition, a person's posttreatment environment plays an important role (Moos, Finney, & Cronkite, 1990) in determining long-term outcomes. Observations of the long-term instability of drinking outcomes have led many to consider alcoholism as a chronic, relapsing disorder, and to reconceptualize "success" as a process rather than a static outcome; that is, the client who learns not only effective skills to avoid drinking or heavy drinking but also ways to cope with relapses by minimizing their length and severity should be considered "successful" as well. In treatment outcome studies, investigators look at percentage of abstinent or moderate drinking days and length of periods of abstinence compared to periods of heavy drinking as ways to assess relative rather than absolute "success." From the individual clinician's perspective, certain client characteristics and behaviors bode well for the course of treatment. The client who has important incentives to change (either internal or external) and some recognition of a relationship between his or her drinking and life problems is easier to treat. Complying with early homework assignments, coming to sessions sober, and being honest about behavior outside of the treatment are also positive indicators. However, clinician behavior is another important predictor of success. Various studies have pointed to different aspects of clinician behavior —empathy, specific goal setting and treatment planning, developing drinking goals with the client rather than imposing goals, and providing the client with options for treatment—as all being associated with better compliance with treatment.

CONCLUSION

Providing treatment to persons with drinking problems is a complex and continuously fascinating process. The clinician is faced with decisions about matching each client to the appropriate level of care, setting for treatment, treatment modalities, and techniques. Diagnostic skills to identify concomitant medical, psychological, psychiatric, and cognitive problems are challenged by these clients. Therapy requires knowledge of a range of treatment techniques, an ability to be able to form a positive therapeutic relationship with sometimes frustrating and difficult clients, and the ability to "think on your feet."

From the briefest, one-session treatments to motivate heavy drinkers to reduce their drinking to the complex and longer treatment provided to individuals with chronic alcohol dependence, treatment is never dull or routine. The clinician has a large body of empirical literature to guide the selection of treatments and a significant clinical literature as well to illustrate clinical techniques and problems. And although many persons with drinking problems change successfully on their own or with minimal assistance, treatment also can provide an effective means for persons to change a major life problem.

So this chapter concludes as it began—as a "sales pitch" for clinicians to be knowledgeable about and receptive to providing thoughtful, informed treatment to persons with drinking problems.

ACKNOWLEDGMENT

Preparation of this chapter was supported in part by Grant No. R37 AA07070 from the National Institute on Alcohol Abuse and Alcoholism.

NOTES

1. A standard drink is equal to one 12-ounce beer, one 5-ounce glass of wine, or a 1.5-ounce shot of 86-proof liquor.
2. All dialogue in this chapter is paraphrasing of actual therapist or client comments.
3. These verbatim transcripts include the clients' spelling of all words.

REFERENCES

American Psychiatric Association. (2000). *Diagnostic and statistical manual of mental disorders* (4th ed., text rev.). Washington, DC: Author.

American Society of Addiction Medicine (ASAM). (1996). *Patient placement criteria for the treatment of psychoactive substance use disorders*. Chevy Chase, MD: Author.

Annis, H. M. (1982). *Inventory of Drinking Situations (IDS-100)*. Toronto: Addiction Research Foundation of Toronto.

Bates, M. E., Bowden, S. C., & Barry, D. (2002). Neurocognitive impairment associated with alcohol use disorders: Implications for treatment. *Experimental and Clinical Psychopharmacology, 10,* 193–212.

Brown, S. A., Goldman, M. S., & Christiansen, B. A. (1985). Do alcohol expectancies mediate drinking patterns of adults? *Journal of Consulting and Clinical Psychology, 53,* 512–519.

Chaney, E. F., O'Leary, M. R., & Marlatt, G. A. (1978). Skills training with alcoholics. *Journal of Consulting and Clinical Psychology, 46,* 1092–1104.

Cox, G. B., Walker, R. D., Freng, S. A., Short, B. A., Meijer, L., & Gilchrist, L. (1998). Outcome of a controlled trial of the effectiveness of intensive case management for chronic public inebriates. *Journal of Studies on Alcohol, 59,* 523–532.

Cunningham, J. A., Sobell, L. C., Sobell, M. B., & Gaskin, J. (1994). Alcohol and drug abusers' reasons for seeking treatment. *Addictive Behaviors, 19,* 691–696.

Drapkin, M. L., McCrady, B. S., Swingle, J. M., & Epstein, E. E. (2005). Exploring bidirectional couple violence in a clinical sample of female alcoholics. *Journal of Studies on Alcohol, 66,* 213–219.

Edwards, G., & Gross, M. M. (1976). Alcohol dependence: Provisional description of a clinical syndrome. *British Medical Journal, 1,* 1058–1061.

Emrick, C., Tonigan, J. S., Montgomery, H., & Little, L. (1993). Alcoholics Anonymous: What is currently known? In B. S. McCrady & W. R. Miller (Eds.), *Research on Alcoholics Anonymous: Opportunities and alternatives* (pp. 41–78). New Brunswick, NJ: Alcohol Research Documentation, Rutgers University.

Epstein, E. E., & McCrady, B. S. (2002). Couple therapy in the treatment of alcohol problems. In A. S. Gurman & N. A. Jacobson (Eds.), *Clinical handbook of couple therapy* (3rd ed., pp. 597–628). New York: Guilford Press.

Epstein, E. E., McCrady, B. S., Miller, K. J., & Steinberg, M. L. (1994). Attrition from conjoint alcoholism treatment: Do dropouts differ from completers? *Journal of Substance Abuse, 6,* 249–265.

Filstead, W. (1991). *Two-year treatment outcome: An evaluation of substance abuse services for adults and youths.* Park Ridge, IL: Parkside Medical Services.

Fink, E. B., Longabaugh, R., McCrady, B. S., Stout, R. L., Beattie, M., Ruggieri-Authelet, A., et al. (1985). Effectiveness of alcoholism treatment in partial versus inpatient settings: Twenty-four month outcomes. *Addictive Behaviors, 10,* 235–248.

Finney, J. W., & Moos, R. H. (1991). The long-term course of treated alcoholism: I. Mortality, relapse and remission rates and comparisons with community controls. *Journal of Studies on Alcohol, 52,* 44–54.

Finney, J. W., Moos, R. H., & Timko, C. (1999). The course of treated and untreated substance use disorders: Remission and resolution, relapse and mortality. In B. S. McCrady & E. E. Epstein (Eds.), *Addictions: A comprehensive guidebook* (pp. 30–49). New York: Oxford University Press.

Foy, D. W., Miller, P. M., Fisler, R. M., & O'Toole, D. H. (1976). Social skills training to teach alcoholics to refuse drinks effectively. *Journal of Studies on Alcohol, 37,* 1340–1345.

Frankenstein, W., Hay, W. M., & Nathan, P. E. (1985). Effects of intoxication on alcoholics' marital communication and problem solving. *Journal of Studies on Alcohol, 46,* 1–6.

Haaga, D. A. F., McCrady, B., & Lebow, J. (2006). Integrative principles for treating substance use disorders. *Journal of Clinical Psychology, 62,* 675–684.

Hasin, D., Paykin, A., Endicott, J., & Grant, G. (1999). The validity of DSM-IV alcohol abuse: Drunk drivers versus all others. *Journal of Studies on Alcohol, 60,* 746–755.

Helzer, J. E., Robins, L. N., Taylor, J. R., Carey, K., Miller, R. H., Combs-Orme, T., et al. (1985). The extent of long-term moderate drinking among alcoholics discharged from medical and psychiatric treatment facilities. *New England Journal of Medicine, 312,* 1678–1682.

Institute of Medicine. (1990). *Broadening the base of treatment for alcohol problems.* Washington, DC: National Academy Press.

Kosanke, N., Magura, S., Staines, G., Foote, J., & DeLuca, A. (2002). Feasibility of matching alcohol patients to ASAM levels of care. *American Journal on Addictions, 11,* 124–134.

Langenbucher, J., Martin, C., Labouvie, E., Sanjuan, P.

M., Bavly, L., & Pollock, N. (2000). Toward the DSM-V: The withdrawal-gate model vs. the DSM-IV in the diagnosis of alcohol abuse and dependence. *Journal of Consulting and Clinical Psychology, 68,* 799–809.

Liepman, M. R. (1993). Using family influence to motivate alcoholics to enter treatment: The Johnson Institute Intervention approach. In T. J. O'Farrell (Ed.), *Treating alcohol problems: Marital and family interventions* (pp. 54–77). New York: Guilford Press.

Longabaugh, R., McCrady, B., Fink, E., Stout, R., McAuley, T., & McNeill, D. (1983). Cost-effectiveness of alcoholism treatment in inpatient versus partial hospital settings: Six- month outcomes. *Journal of Studies on Alcohol, 44,* 1049–1071.

Longabaugh, R., Wirtz, P. W., Zweben, A., & Stout, R. L. (1998). Network support for drinking, Alcoholics Anonymous and long-term matching effects. *Addiction, 93,* 1313–1333.

Ludwig, A. M. (1985). Cognitive processes associated with "spontaneous" recovery from alcoholism. *Journal of Studies on Alcohol, 46,* 53–58.

Magura, S., Staines, G., Kosanke, N., Rosenblum, A., Foote, J., DeLuca, A., et al. (2003). Predictive validity of the ASAM Patient Placement Criteria for naturalistically matched vs. mismatched alcoholism patients. *American Journal on Addictions, 12,* 386–397.

Margolin, G., Talovic, S., & Weinstein, C. D. (1983). Areas of Change Questionnaire: A practical approach to marital assessment. *Journal of Consulting and Clinical Psychology, 51,* 921–931.

Marlatt, G. A., & Donovan, D. M. (Eds.). (2005). *Relapse prevention, second edition: Maintenance strategies in the treatment of addictive behavior.* New York: Guilford Press.

Marlatt, G. A., & Gordon, J. R. (Eds.). (1985). *Relapse prevention: Maintenance strategies in the treatment of addictive behaviors.* New York: Guilford Press.

Mayfield, D., McLeod, G., & Hall, P. (1974). The CAGE questionnaire: Validation of a new alcoholism instrument. *American Journal of Psychiatry, 131,* 1121–1123.

McConnaughy, E. A., Prochaska, J. O., & Velicer, W. F. (1983). Stages of change in psychotherapy: Measurement and sample profiles. *Psychotherapy: Theory, Research, and Practice, 20,* 243–250.

McCrady, B. S. (1992). A reply to Peele: Is this how you treat your friends? *Addictive Behaviors, 17,* 67–72.

McCrady, B. S., & Epstein, E. E. (Eds.). (1999). *Addictions: A comprehensive guidebook.* New York: Oxford University Press.

McCrady, B. S., Epstein, E. E., & Hirsch, L. (1999). Maintaining change after conjoint behavioral alcohol treatment for men: Outcomes at six months. *Addiction, 94,* 1381–1396.

McCrady, B. S., Horvath, A. T., & Delaney, S. I. (2003). Self-help groups. In R. K. Hester & W. R. Miller (Eds.), *Handbook of alcoholism treatment approaches. Effective alternatives, third edition* (pp. 165–187). Boston: Allyn & Bacon.

McCrady, B. S., Longabaugh, R. L., Fink, E., Stout, R., Beattie, M., Ruggieri-Authelet, A., et al. (1986). Cost effectiveness of alcoholism treatment in partial hospital versus inpatient settings after brief inpatient treatment: Twelve month outcomes. *Journal of Consulting and Clinical Psychology, 54*, 708–713.

McCrady, B. S., Stout, R., Noel, N., Abrams, D., & Nelson, H. F. (1991). Effectiveness of three types of spouse-involved behavioral alcoholism treatment. *British Journal of Addiction, 86*, 1415–1424.

McLellan, A. T., Grissom, G. R., Zanis, D., Randall, M., Brill, P., & O'Brien, C. P. (1997). Problem–service "matching" in addiction treatment: A prospective study in four programs. *Archives of General Psychiatry, 54*, 730–735.

McLellan, A. T., Kushner, H., Metzger, D., Peters, R., Smith, I., Grissom, G., et al. (1992). The fifth edition of the Addiction Severity Index. *Journal of Substance Abuse Treatment, 9*, 199–213.

McLellan, A. T., Lewis, D. C., O'Brien, C. P., & Kleber, H. D. (2000). Drug dependence, a chronic medical illness: Implications for treatment, insurance, and outcomes evaluation. *Journal of the American Medical Association, 284*, 1689–1695.

Meyers, R. J., & Smith, J. E. (1995). *Clinical guide to alcohol treatment: The community reinforcement approach.* New York: Guilford Press.

Miller, W. R., Benefield, R. G., & Tonigan, J. S. (1993). Enhancing motivation for change in problem drinking: A controlled comparison of two therapist styles. *Journal of Consulting and Clinical Psychology, 61*, 455–461.

Miller, W. R., Leckman, A. L., Delaney, H. D., & Tinkcom, M. (1992). Long-term follow-up of behavioral self-control training. *Journal of Studies on Alcohol, 53*, 249–261.

Miller, W. R., Meyers, R. J., & Tonigan, J. S. (1999). Engaging the unmotivated in treatment for alcohol problems: A comparison of three strategies for intervention through family members. *Journal of Consulting and Clinical Psychology, 67*, 688–697.

Miller, W. R., & Rollnick, S. (1991). *Motivational interviewing: Preparing people to change addictive behavior.* New York: Guilford Press.

Miller, W. R., & Rollnick, S. (2002). *Motivational interviewing, Preparing people for change* (2nd ed.). New York: Guilford Press.

Miller, W. R., & Tonigan, J. S. (1996). Assessing drinkers' motivations for change: The Stages of Change Readiness and Treatment Eagerness Scale (SOCRATES). *Psychology of Addictive Behaviors, 10*, 81–89.

Miller, W. R., Tonigan, J. S., & Longabaugh, R. (1995). *The Drinker Inventory of Consequences (DrInC): An instrument for assessing adverse consequences of alcohol abuse.* Rockville, MD: National Institute on Alcohol Abuse and Alcoholism.

Miller, W. R., Zweben, A., DiClemente, C. C., & Rychtarik, R. G. (1995). *Motivational enhancement therapy manual.* Rockville, MD: National Institute on Alcohol Abuse and Alcoholism.

Moak, D. H., & Anton, R. F. (1999). Alcohol. In B. S. McCrady & E. E. Epstein (Eds.), *Addictions: A comprehensive guidebook* (pp. 75–94). New York: Oxford University Press.

Moderation Management. (2006). *The MM limits* [Online]. Retrieved on September 21, 2006, from *www.moderation.org/readings.shtml#mmlimits*

Monti, P. M., Abrams, D. B., Binkoff, J. A., Zwick, W. R., Liepman, M. R., Nirenberg, T. D., et al. (1990). Communication skills training, communication skills training with family and cognitive behavioral mood management training for alcoholics. *Journal of Studies on Alcohol, 51*, 263–270.

Monti, P. M., Kadden, R. M., Rohsenow, D. J., Cooney, N. L., & Abrams, D. B. (2002). *Treating alcohol dependence: A coping skills training guide* (2nd ed.). New York: Guilford Press.

Moos, R. H., & Billings, A. (1982). Children of alcoholics during the recovery process: Alcoholic and matched control families. *Addictive Behaviors, 7*, 155–163.

Moos, R. H., Finney, J. W., & Cronkite, R. (1990). *Alcoholism treatment: Context, process, and outcome.* New York: Oxford University Press.

Moos, R. H., Finney, J. W., & Gamble, W. (1982). The process of recovery from alcoholism: II. Comparing spouses of alcoholic patients and matched community controls. *Journal of Studies on Alcohol, 43*, 888–909.

Morgenstern, J., Blanchard, K. A., McCrady, B. S., McVeigh, K. H., Morgan, T. J., & Pandina, R. J. (in press). A randomized field trial examining the effectiveness of intensive case management for substance dependent women receiving temporary assistance for needy families (TANF). *American Journal of Public Health.*

Nathan, P. E., & McCrady, B. S. (1987). Bases for the use of abstinence as a goal in the behavioral treatment of alcohol abusers. *Drugs and Society, 1*, 109–132.

National Advisory Council on Alcohol Abuse and Alcoholism, Subcommittee on Health Services Research. (1996). *Final report: Panel on financing and organization.* Washington, DC: U.S. Department of Health and Human Services.

O'Farrell, T. J., Choquette, K. A., & Cutter, H. S. G. (1998). Couples relapse prevention sessions after behavioral marital therapy for male alcoholics: Outcomes during the three years after starting treatment. *Journal of Studies on Alcohol, 59*, 357–370.

Ojehegan, A., & Berglund, M. (1989). Changes in drinking goals in a two-year outpatient alcoholic treatment program. *Addictive Behaviors, 14*, 1–10.

Orford, J., Guthrie, S., Nicholls, P., Oppenheimer, E., Egert, S., & Hensman, C. (1975). Self-reported coping behavior of wives of alcoholics and its association with drinking outcome. *Journal of Studies on Alcohol, 36*, 1254–1267.

Orford, J., & Keddie, A. (1986). Abstinence or controlled drinking in clinical practice: A test of the dependence and persuasion hypotheses. *British Journal of Addiction, 81,* 495–504.

Orford, J., Templeton, L., Velleman, R., & Copello, A. (2005). Family members of relatives with alcohol, drug and gambling problems: A set of standardized questionnaires for assessing stress, coping and strain. *Addiction, 100,* 1611–1624.

O'Toole, T. P., Freyder, P. J., Gibbon, J. L., Hanusa, B. J., Seltzer, D., & Fine, M. J. (2004). ASAM Patient Placement Criteria treatment levels: Do they correspond to care actually received by homeless substance abusing adults? *Journal of Addictive Diseases, 23,* 1–15.

Paolino, T. J., Jr., McCrady, B. S., & Diamond, S. (1978). Some alcoholic marriage statistics: An overview. *International Journal of the Addictions, 13,* 1252–1257.

Pettinati, H. M., Sugerman, A. A., DiDonato, N., & Maurer, H. S. (1982). The natural history of alcoholism over four years after treatment. *Journal of Studies on Alcohol, 43,* 201–215.

Prochaska, J. O., & DiClemente, C. C. (2005). The transtheoretical approach. In J. C. Norcross & M. R. Goldfried (Eds.), *Handbook of psychotherapy integration* (2nd ed., pp. 147–171). New York: Oxford University Press.

Project MATCH Research Group. (1997a). Matching alcoholism treatments to client heterogeneity: Project MATCH posttreatment drinking outcomes. *Journal of Studies on Alcohol, 58,* 7–29.

Project MATCH Research Group. (1997b). Project MATCH secondary a priori hypotheses. *Addiction, 92,* 1671–1698.

Project MATCH Research Group. (1998). Matching alcoholism treatments to client heterogeneity: Project MATCH three-year drinking outcomes. *Alcoholism: Clinical and Experimental Research, 22,* 1300–1311.

Raytek, H. S., McCrady, B. S., Epstein, E. E., & Hirsch, L. S. (1999). Therapeutic alliance and the retention of couples in conjoint alcoholism treatment. *Addictive Behaviors, 24,* 317–330.

Rhines, K. C., McCrady, B. S., Morgan, T. J., & Hirsch, L. S. (1997). Integrated assessment of alcohol and drug use: The Rutgers Consequences of Use Questionnaire [Abstract No. 544]. *Alcoholism: Clinical and Experimental Research, 21,* 94A.

Robins, L. N., Wing, J., Wittchen, H. U., Helzer, J. E., Babor, T. F., Burke, J., et al. (1988). The prevalence of psychiatric disorders in patients with alcohol and other drug problems. *Archives of General Psychiatry, 45,* 1023–1031.

Rollnick, S., Heather, N., Gold, R., & Hall, W. (1992). Development of a short "Readiness to Change" Questionnaire for use in brief opportunistic interventions. *British Journal of Addictions, 87,* 743–754.

Rose, S. J., Zweben, A., & Stoffel, V. (1999). Interfaces between substance abuse treatment and other health and social systems. In B. S. McCrady & E. E. Epstein (Eds.), *Addictions: A comprehensive guidebook* (pp. 421–438). New York: Oxford University Press.

Rosenberg, H. (1993). Prediction of controlled drinking by alcoholics and problem drinkers. *Psychological Bulletin, 113,* 129–139.

Rosenthal, R. N., & Westreich, L. (1999). Treatment of persons with dual diagnoses of substance use disorder and other psychological problems. In B. S. McCrady & E. E. Epstein (Eds.), *Addictions: A comprehensive guidebook* (pp. 439–476). New York: Oxford University Press.

Rychtarik, R. G., Connors, G. J., Whitney, R. B., McGillicuddy, N. B., Fitterling, J. M., & Wirtz, P. W. (2000). Treatment settings for persons with alcoholism: Evidence for matching clients to inpatient versus outpatient care. *Journal of Consulting and Clinical Psychology, 68,* 277–289.

Saunders, J. B., Aasland, O. G., Babor, T. F., de la Fuente, J. R., & Grant, M. (1993). Development of the Alcohol Use Disorders Screening Test (AUDIT): WHO collaborative project on early detection of persons with harmful alcohol consumption-II. *Addiction, 88,* 791–804.

Sheehan, T., & Owen, P. (1999). The disease model. In B. S. McCrady & E. E. Epstein (Eds.), *Addictions: A comprehensive guidebook* (pp. 268–286). New York: Oxford University Press.

Sisson, R. W., & Azrin, N. (1986). Family-member involvement to initiate and promote treatment of problem drinkers. *Journal of Behavior Therapy and Experimental Psychiatry, 17,* 15–21.

Skinner, H., & Allen, B. A. (1982). Alcohol dependence syndrome: Measurement and validation. *Journal of Abnormal Psychology, 91,* 199–209.

Sobell, L. C., & Sobell, M. B. (2003). Alcohol consumption measures. In J. P. Allen & V. B. Wilson (Eds.), *Assessing alcohol problems: A guide for clinicians and researchers, second edition* (pp. 75–99), Bethesda, MD: National Institute on Alcohol Abuse and Alcoholism.

Sobell, M. B., Maisto, S. A., Sobell, L. C., Cooper, T., & Saunders, B. (1980). Developing a prototype for evaluating alcohol treatment effectiveness. In L. C. Sobell, M. B. Sobell, & E. Ward (Eds.), *Evaluating alcohol treatment effectiveness: Recent advances* (pp. 129–150). New York: Pergamon Press.

Sobell, M. B., & Sobell, L. C. (2000). Stepped care as a heuristic approach to the treatment of alcohol problems. *Journal of Consulting and Clinical Psychology, 68,* 573–579.

Spanier, G. (1976). Measuring dyadic adjustment: New scales for assessing the quality of marriage and similar dyads. *Journal of Marriage and the Family, 38,* 15–28.

Spear, S. F., & Mason, M. (1991). Impact of chemical dependency on family health status. *International Journal of the Addictions, 26,* 179–187.

Spitzer, R. L., Williams, J. B. W., Gibbon, M., & First, M. B. (1996). *Structured Clinical Interview for DSM-IV: Patient Edition (with Psychotic Screen—Version 1.0).* Washington, DC: American Psychiatric Press.

Stewart, S. H. (1996). Alcohol abuse in individuals exposed to trauma: A critical review. *Psychological Bulletin, 120,* 83–112.

Stinchfield, R., & Owen, P. (1998). Hazelden's model of treatment and its outcome. *Addictive Behaviors, 23,* 669–683.

Stout, R. L., Rubin, A., Zwick, W., Zywiak, W., & Bellino, L. (1999). Optimizing the cost-effectiveness of alcohol treatment: A rationale for extended case monitoring. *Addictive Behaviors, 24,* 17–35.

Strauss, M., Hamby, S. L., Boney-McCoy, S., & Sugerman, D. B. (1996). The Revised Conflict Tactics Scale (CTS-2): Development and preliminary psychometric data. *Journal of Family Issues, 17,* 283–316.

Thomas, E. J., Santa, C., Bronson, D., & Oyserman, D. (1987). Unilateral family therapy with the spouses of alcoholics. *Journal of Social Service Research, 10,* 145–162.

Thomas, E. J., Yoshioka, M., & Ager, R. D. (1996). Spouse enabling of alcohol abuse: Conception, assessment, and modification. *Journal of Substance Abuse, 8,* 61–80.

Tonigan, J. S., Miller, W. R., & Brown, J. M. (1997). The reliability of FORM 90: An instrument for assessing alcohol treatment outcome. *Journal of Studies on Alcohol, 58,* 358–364.

Vaillant, G. (1983). *The natural history of alcoholism.* Cambridge, MA: Harvard University Press.

Vaillant, G., & Milofsky, E. S. (1982). Natural history of male alcoholism: 4. Paths to recovery. *Archives of General Psychiatry, 39,* 127–133.

Witkiewitz, K., & Marlatt, G. A. (2004). Relapse prevention for alcohol and drug problems: That was zen, this is tao. *American Psychologist, 59,* 224–235.

Zimmerman, M. (1994). *Interview guide for evaluating DSM-IV psychiatric disorders and the Mental Status Examination.* East Greenwich, RI: Psych Products Press.

Zitter, R. E., & McCrady, B. S. (1979). *The Drinking Patterns Questionnaire.* Unpublished manuscript, Butler Hospital, Providence, RI.

CHAPTER 13

Drug Abuse and Dependence

STEPHEN T. HIGGINS
STACEY C. SIGMON
SARAH H. HEIL

In this chapter we follow the case of "Bill," a 24-year-old individual with cocaine dependence who would ordinarily be considered to be among the most difficult types of patients for someone administering psychological interventions. As is typical with this population, Bill presented with not only cocaine dependence but also alcohol dependence; problems with anger management; heavy use of cigarettes and marijuana; suicidal ideation; and major interpersonal, social, and occupational problems (including a prohibition from visiting his 5-year-old daughter). The fact that Stephen T. Higgins and his team of close associates have been able to create a treatment protocol for individuals such as Bill—a protocol with strong empirical support—is in itself a remarkable achievement. But only those most familiar with this approach have a good idea of the multifaceted nature of this brief semistructured strategy, which includes attention to the full range of addictive behaviors, as well as mood disturbances, interpersonal relationships, and problems in living. Without this comprehensive approach, there seems to be no question that these treatment strategies would not enjoy the success that they do. Even clinicians or students not working directly with addictive behaviors will benefit from being familiar with this new generation of successful psychological approaches to drug abuse.—D. H. B.

OVERVIEW

Drug use disorders represent a highly prevalent and costly public health problem in the United States and virtually all other industrialized countries. To get a sense of the scope of the U.S. problem, an estimated 126 million persons 12 years and older (51.8%) report current alcohol use (past 30 days), 71.5 million (29.4%) report current tobacco use, and 19.7 million (8.1%) report current use of illicit drugs (Substance Abuse and Mental Health Services Administration [SAMHSA], 2006). Of course, not all current users experience adverse effects, but a sizable proportion incur substantial problems. An estimated 22.2 million (9.1%) Americans 12 years and older meet formal diagnostic criteria for drug abuse or dependence within the past year, and 3.9 million (1.6%) report being treated for a drug use problem within the past year (SAMHSA, 2006). The annual costs to the U.S economy associated with these problems are estimated to be approximately $500 billion (Office of National Drug Control Policy, 2004).

Clearly there is a tremendous need for effective treatments for drug use disorders. This chapter focuses on psychosocial treatments for illicit drug use disorders. Treatments for alcohol problems are covered in McCrady, Chapter

12, this volume, and there are several excellent reviews available on treatments for tobacco use disorders (e.g., Kenford & Fiore, 2004; Schnoll & Lerman, 2006). Because the focus is on empirically based interventions, we largely cover behavioral and cognitive-behavioral therapies. That said, effective contemporary treatments for drug use disorders often entail combining psychological treatments with medications, and this is reflected in this chapter as well. We use a multielement intervention to illustrate details of treatment implementation, namely, the community reinforcement approach (CRA) plus vouchers intervention that our group developed for outpatient treatment of cocaine dependence. Lastly, the National Institute on Drug Abuse (NIDA, 1999) has published 13 principles of effective treatment for illicit drug abuse based on 25 years of research, and when applicable we underscore those principles throughout the chapter (Table 13.1).

DEFINING THE CLINICAL DISORDER

Before proceeding to discussions about treatment, we outline current criteria for diagnosing drug abuse and dependence. Shown in Tables 13.2 and 13.3 are the diagnostic criteria outlined in the fourth edition, text revised *Diagnostic and Statistical Manual of Mental Disorders* (DSM-IV-TR) of the American Psychiatric Association (2000). These criteria represent a cluster of behavioral and physiological signs and symptoms resulting from a pattern of continued drug use despite significant drug-related problems. To receive a diagnosis of drug abuse, a person must satisfy one or more of the four criteria listed within a 12-month period, and cannot currently or previously have satisfied a diagnosis of drug dependence (Table 13.2). The criteria for abuse are designed to focus on harmful consequences of drug use and not the pattern of drug use per se, or tolerance or withdrawal, which are the focus of the dependence diagnosis.

To receive a diagnosis of drug dependence, the person must have exhibited three or more of the seven criteria listed within a 12-month period (Table 13.3). Note that while tolerance and withdrawal are listed first among the seven criteria, neither is necessary for a dependence diagnosis. One simply must meet any three of the criteria listed within a 12-month period to satisfy the diagnosis. The phrase "with physio-

TABLE 13.1. Principles of Effective Treatment

1. No single treatment is appropriate for all individuals.
2. Treatment needs to be readily available.
3. Effective treatment attends to multiple needs of the individual, not just his or her drug use.
4. An individual's treatment and services plan must be assessed continually and modified as necessary to ensure that the plan meets the person's changing needs.
5. Remaining in treatment for an adequate period of time is critical for treatment effectiveness (i.e., 3 months or longer).
6. Counseling (individual and/or group) and other behavioral therapies are critical components of effective treatment for addiction.
7. Medications are an important element of treatment for many patients, especially when combined with counseling and other behavioral therapies.
8. Addicted or drug-abusing individuals with coexisting mental disorders should have both disorders treated in an integrated way.
9. Medical detoxification is only the first stage of addiction treatment and by itself does little to change long-term drug use.
10. Treatment does not need to be voluntary to be effective.
11. Possible drug use during treatment must be monitored continuously.
12. Treatment programs should provide assessment for HIV/AIDS, hepatitis B and C, tuberculosis and other infectious diseases, and counseling to help patients modify or change behaviors that place themselves or others at risk of infection.
13. Recovery from drug addiction can be a long-term process and frequently requires multiple episodes of treatment.

logical dependence" can be used to specify diagnoses in which tolerance or withdrawal was present, and the phrase "without physiological dependence," to specify those in which they were not present. The rationale for use of these specifiers is that tolerance and withdrawal may be associated with a higher risk for medical problems and a higher relapse rate. Evidence does support a position that, on average, more severe drug dependence is associated with poorer treatment outcome. Severity is influenced by frequency of use, amount of drug used, and route of administration, among other factors. There seems little doubt that these factors will be positively correlated with tolerance, and the number of untoward signs and symptoms exhibited following a period of re-

TABLE 13.2. DSM-IV-TR Criteria
for Substance Abuse

A. A maladaptive pattern of drug use leading to
clinically significant impairment or distress, as
manifested by one (or more) of the following,
occurring within a 12-month period:

(1) recurrent substance use resulting in a failure
to fulfill major role obligations at work,
school, or home (e.g., repeated absences or
poor work performance related to substance
use; substance-related absences, suspensions,
or expulsions from school; neglect of
children or household)

(2) recurrent substance use in situations in
which it is physically hazardous (e.g.,
driving an automobile or operating a
machine when impaired by substance use)

(3) recurrent substance-related legal problems
(e.g., arrests for substance-related disorderly
conduct)

(4) continued substance use despite having
persistent or recurrent social or
interpersonal problems caused or
exacerbated by the effects of the substance
(e.g., arguments with spouse about
consequences or intoxication, physical
fights).

B. The symptoms have never met the criteria for
Substance Dependence for this class of
substance.

Note. From American Psychiatric Association (2000).
Copyright 2000 by the American Psychiatric Association.
Reprinted by permission.

peated drug use, and to that extent merit attention in a diagnostic assessment.

Regarding the course specifiers, "full remission" indicates that none of the criteria for
abuse or dependence have been met for at least
1 month; "partial remission" indicates that one
or more criteria have been met, but the full criteria for dependence have not been met for at
least 1 month. The terms "early" and "sustained" are used to indicate whether remission
has been for less than or greater than 12
months, respectively. The clinical utility of
these course specifiers rests on evidence that
the probability of relapse decreases as an orderly function of the duration time the individual has been abstinent (e.g., Higgins, Badger, &
Budney, 2000). The specifier regarding "ago-
nist therapy" applies mostly to opioid dependence, for which treatment with methadone or
a related opioid pharmacotherapy is recommended. The specifier "in a controlled environment" is applicable because the evidence noted

earlier about the probability of relapse being
inversely related to the duration of abstinence
is based on individuals residing in environments wherein the opportunity for drug use is
present. This relationship between duration of
abstinence and the probability of relapse is not
likely to apply, or it will be significantly
weaker, when the period of abstinence is
achieved in an environment in which the drug
is not available. Practically speaking, this specifier is commonly needed in clinical practice
with individuals whose treatment has been
mandated by the criminal justice system as a
condition of release from prison, and whose
last drug use may have been months or years
prior to entering treatment.

This section outlined commonly used criteria
for diagnosing drug abuse and dependence.
Now we turn to the more challenging practical
matter of clinical management.

ASSESSMENT

A comprehensive assessment is an essential first
step in effective clinical management of drug
abuse and dependence. This section outlines
the assessment practices we use in our clinic
with cocaine-dependent adults. The assessment
framework is relatively generic and can be
readily applied to other types of drug abuse
and dependence by substituting the cocaine-
specific information with pertinent information on whatever other type of drug use disorder is the presenting problem.

All initial clinic contacts are handled by a re-
ceptionist, who establishes that the caller reports
problems related to drug use, is age 18 years or
above, and resides within the county in which
the clinic is located. The CRA plus vouchers
treatment that we use is intensive, requiring several clinic visits per week. Persons living outside
the county are often unable to follow such a demanding schedule. A broader geographical
range may be possible with other, less intensive
interventions. The important matter is to have
established the geographical range that is practical for the treatment being offered. Those who
do not satisfy our basic inclusion criteria are referred to an appropriate alternative clinic. Those
who meet the criteria receive an appointment for
an intake assessment.

Every effort is made to schedule the intake
assessment interview as soon as possible (Principle 2, Table 13.1). Scheduling the interview

TABLE 13.3. DSM-IV-TR Criteria for Substance Dependence

A maladaptive pattern of substance use, leading to clinically significant impairment or distress, as manifested by three (or more) of the following, occurring at any time in the same 12-month period:

(1) tolerance, as defined by either of the following:
    (a) a need for markedly increased amounts of the substance to achieve intoxication or desired effect
    (b) markedly diminished effect with continued use of the same amount of the substance

(2) withdrawal, as manifested by either of the following:
    (a) the characteristic withdrawal syndrome for the substance (refer to Criteria A and B of the criteria sets for Withdrawal from the specific substances)
    (b) the same (or a closely related) substance is taken to relieve or avoid withdrawal symptoms

(3) the substance is often taken in larger amounts or over a longer period than was intended

(4) there is a persistent desire or unsuccessful efforts to cut down or control substance use

(5) a great deal of time is spent in activities necessary to obtain the substance (e.g., visiting multiple doctors or driving long distances), use the substance (e.g., chain-smoking), or recover from its effects

(6) important social, occupational, or recreational activities are given up or reduced because of substance use

(7) the substance use is continued despite knowledge of having a persistent or recurrent physical or psychological problem that is likely to have been caused or exacerbated by the substance (e.g., current cocaine use despite recognition of cocaine-induced depression, or continued drinking despite recognition that an ulcer was made worse by alcohol consumption)

Specify if:
    With Physiological Dependence: evidence of tolerance or withdrawal (i.e., either Item 1 or 2 is present)
    Without Physiological Dependence: no evidence of tolerance or withdrawal (i.e., neither Item 1 nor 2 is present)

Course specifiers (see text for definitions):
    Early Full Remission
    Early Partial Remission
    Sustained Full Remission
    Sustained Partial Remission
    On Agonist Therapy
    In a Controlled Environment

Note. From American Psychiatric Association (2000). Copyright 2000 by the American Psychiatric Association. Reprinted by permission.

within 24 hours of clinic contact significantly reduces attrition between the initial clinic contact and assessment interview, which is a substantial problem among those with drug use disorders (Festinger, Lamb, Kirby, & Marlowe, 1996). Some patients cannot come in within 24 hours, so our secondary goal is to get them in within 72 hours.

Clients are informed that the intake interview will take about 3 hours. This initial session is one of the most important. Clinic staff should be aware of the client's potential un-easiness and try to make the person feel at ease. Being courteous, complimenting clients on taking this important first step toward change, anticipating that some clients might be physically ill or uncomfortable related to recent drug use and being respectful of that, being flexible with tardiness, and so forth, can help. Accommodating the need for brief breaks, food or drink, or a brief phone call can help as well. Throughout all interactions we seek to be empathic and to convey a very upbeat, "You can do it" message.

During the intake assessment, we collect detailed information on drug use, evaluate treatment readiness, and assess psychiatric functioning, employment/vocational status, recreational interests, current social supports, family and social problems, and legal issues (see Principle 3, Table 13.1). The following instruments that we use to obtain such information are listed in the order in which they are typically administered. Modifications can be readily made to our list depending on the population being treated. We offer it only to provide an example of what we have found to be an effective assessment package, along with associated clinical rationales.

Self-Administered Questionnaires

We use several questionnaires that can be completed by the client upon arriving at the clinic for an initial intake assessment. The intake worker greets the client, introduces him- or herself, brings the client into a private office, and briefly but carefully informs him or her about what to expect during the intake process. It is essential to ask about clients' reading ability prior to having them complete self-administered questionnaires. If there is doubt about reading capability, we discreetly ask clients to read several questions aloud to get an indication of whether they can complete the forms without staff assistance. With poor readers, the questionnaires can be read aloud by a staff member in a private setting. This must be done with care and positive regard for the discomfort that poor readers may feel under such circumstances. Competent readers are given approximately 45 minutes to complete the forms.

We have clients complete a routine, brief demographics questionnaire. Obtaining a client's current address and phone number is important, as is obtaining the number of someone who always knows the client's whereabouts. This information is important for purposes of outreach efforts during treatment should the client stop coming to scheduled therapy sessions or need to be contacted for other clinical purposes, and contacting clients for routine posttreatment follow-up evaluations.

The Stages of Change Readiness and Treatment Eagerness Scale (SOCRATES; Miller & Tonigan, 1996) provides information on clients' perceptions of the severity of their drug use problems and their readiness to engage in behavior to reduce their use. This questionnaire provides a quantitative index of motivation to change, which may be an important indicator of clients' willingness to comply with certain treatment goals. We use three versions of the SOCRATES that refer to specific substances (i.e., cocaine, alcohol, and other drug use), because the clients' motivations to reduce substance use are often drug-specific. For example, almost all who seek treatment in our clinic are ready to act toward changing their cocaine use, but many are more ambivalent about changing their alcohol or marijuana use, which are the two other forms of drug use we deal with most frequently. Our approach is to reinforce the action the patient is ready to take with cocaine and to share empathically our empirical knowledge regarding the influence of other forms of drug use on the probability of successfully discontinuing cocaine use. Our recommendation is that at least short-term abstinence from all intoxicating substance use is the path with the greatest chance of success. Use of alcohol can directly increase the probability of cocaine use and predicts poor outcome. Use of marijuana, which does not predict poor outcome with regard to cocaine use per se, is associated with problems of its own.

We use an adaptation of the Cocaine Dependency Self-Test (Washton, Stone, & Hendrickson, 1988) as an efficient means to collect specific information regarding the type of adverse effects of cocaine that clients have experienced. Systematically collected information on the adverse effects of drug use is important. Such information is useful in helping clients to problem-solve regarding the pros and cons of cocaine use as part of efforts to promote and sustain motivation for change during the course of treatment.

A sizable proportion of clients with illicit drug use disorders are also problem drinkers, making assessment of that problem essential. As part of our alcohol assessment we use the Michigan Alcoholism Screening Test (MAST), a widely used, brief alcoholism screening instrument (Selzer, 1975). Considering that almost all clients entering treatment for cocaine abuse and dependence use alcohol and approximately 60% meet diagnostic criteria for alcohol dependence, the MAST is useful for flagging clients with alcohol problems.

Depressed mood is another common problem among those presenting for treatment for drug use disorders. We use the Beck Depression

Inventory (BDI) to screen for depressive symptomatology (Beck, Ward, Mendelson, Mock, & Erbaugh, 1961) and readminister it on a regular basis to monitor progress with those clients who score in the clinical range at intake. The average BDI scores of cocaine abusers entering treatment fall in the clinical range of that scale (average BDI intake score in our clinic is 19.8 $\pm$ 11.9). For most clients, those scores decrease precipitously after 1 or 2 weeks in treatment. However, that is not true for all clients. Therefore, it is important to assess carefully and monitor depressive symptomatology, and to refer or intervene when symptoms do not remit. Assessing and monitoring for suicide risk is important as well. We do so using a protocol we developed in collaboration with our local mental health crisis service.

The Symptom Checklist 90—Revised (SCL-90-R; Derogatis, 1983) is also used to screen for psychiatric symptomatology more broadly and is helpful in determining whether a more in-depth psychiatric evaluation is warranted. The SCL-90-R also can be easily readministered to monitor progress or change in psychiatric status.

After clients complete these self-administered questionnaires, they are reviewed by clinic staff to be sure that all questions have been completed and that the information appears consistent. Any obvious inconsistencies are resolved with the client.

Program Description

We find it useful to break up the data-gathering aspects of the initial assessment between completion of the self-administered questionnaires and initiation of the structured interviews. We provide a brief description of the treatment program and its philosophy at this time. Clients are given the opportunity to ask questions or to express any concerns they may have. The goal here is to orient clients regarding what will happen in treatment, to create an atmosphere of optimism, and to help clients feel hopeful that they can succeed in treatment. This description and interaction is typically brief (10–15 minutes). A therapist provides more detailed rationales and descriptions during this same intake session, but after the structured interviews are completed. When asked questions about the treatment process, the intake worker provides brief answers and reassures the client that a therapist will soon be meeting with him

or her to provide much more information about the program and how it works.

In providing the brief description, the intake worker explains that our program is confidential and specifically designed for persons who have problems with cocaine. For obvious reasons, users of illicit drugs are often quite concerned about confidentiality. Clients are informed about the overall duration of treatment, the recommended frequency and duration of clinic visits, and the general foci and orientation of our treatment approach (i.e., lifestyle changes). We explain that the primary goals of such changes are that clients discontinue cocaine use and make positive changes that result in greater life satisfaction. Examples of what might occur during treatment are provided:

"If you are interested in finding a job, the therapists will help you with the search, with a resume, and with transportation and phone support, if necessary. If you would like to go back to school, we can help you obtain the applications, access funding and assistance, and even take you to an interview if you don't have transportation. If you are having relationship problems, relationship counseling is available. If you don't regularly participate in any fun activities, we have lots of suggestions and may even take you to some of these, like basketball, tennis, fishing, boating, arts and crafts classes, etc.

"Also, we provide coping skills training. So if you have problems controlling anger, we can help with anger management. If you have money problems, we can assist you with financial management. If you have difficulty with behavior problems with your children, we can assist you in get some help with that problem. If you have trouble relaxing, we can work on relaxation skills and stress management, etc."

In addition, the intake worker provides a very brief description of our clinic's incentive program:

"You also will participate in our incentive program. How this works is that if you stay clean, that is, if you provide urine samples that are cocaine-free, you earn points that can be used to support your goals. What that means is, if you stay clean, you will accumulate points that can be used to pay for activities like going to the movies, joining a gym, taking a class, buying a fishing rod, etc. Your therapist will tell you more about these things when you meet him or her after our interview."

Semistructured Interviews

A semistructured drug history interview (developed in our clinic) is used to facilitate collection of information on current and past drug use. Such detailed information is essential for proper treatment planning.

The goal in completing a drug use history is to obtain detailed information regarding the duration, severity, and pattern of the client's drug use. The accuracy of the client's report of drug use (amount and frequency) is facilitated by the use of an effective technique for reviewing recent use (i.e., the Timeline Follow-Back: Sobell & Sobell, 1992). Using a calendar as a prompt, clients are asked to recall on a day-by-day basis the number of days they used in the past week, and the amount used per occasion. Grams are typically the best metric for determining amount of cocaine used. The same assessment is conducted for the past 3 weeks and as far back in time as needed for diagnostic reasons. This technique results in a good overview of the client's pattern of drug use during the past 30 days. The intake worker asks for as much clarification as possible to help obtain an accurate assessment of drug use history. Diagnoses of abuse and dependence are made later by master's- or doctorate-level psychologists.

The Addiction Severity Index (ASI; McLellan et al., 1985) is designed to provide reliable, valid assessments of multiple problems commonly associated with drug use, and a quantitative, time-based assessment of problem severity in the following areas: alcohol and drug use; employment; and medical, legal, family, social, and psychological functioning. The information obtained in the ASI is quite useful for developing treatment plans that include lifestyle change goals. It is also a useful instrument for assessing progress at follow-up, in that it is time-based and yields quantitative composite scores for multiple problem areas. Training on ASI administration is necessary to ensure that the intake worker conducts a reliable ASI interview (for information on training in the use of the ASI, see *www.tresearch.org/training/asi_train.htm*).

A Practical Needs Assessment Questionnaire (developed in our clinic) determines whether the client has any pressing needs or crises that may interfere with initial treatment engagement (e.g., housing, legal, transportation, or child care). The intake worker asks specific questions regarding current housing, child care, legal circumstances, medical issues, and other matters that might be of current and serious concern to the client. Detailed information is collected on any identified crisis. The rationale here is to identify matters that may need immediate clinical attention. The lives of many individuals entering treatment for drug dependence are in chaos. The probability of engaging and keeping such clients in treatment may be compromised if swift attention is not provided to assist with certain acute needs, typically in the form of referrals to community agencies for assistance.

After completing these interviews, the intake worker informs clients that they will be meeting with their therapist in a few minutes. A brief break (5–10 minutes) is given.

During this break, the intake worker completes an intake summary sheet for the therapist taking on this new case, along with all of the supporting intake information. The intake worker meets briefly with the therapist to review the case. Patients are then introduced to their therapists. We try never to allow a patient to leave the intake interview without a brief meeting with a therapist, so that he or she can depart feeling that treatment has begun, and with concrete plans for abstaining from cocaine use until the next clinic visit.

In many ways this initial meeting is an orientation session used to establish rapport with the client and to provide further rationales for our treatment approach. Doing so permits clients to develop clear expectations about treatment. We continue with the "can do" approach, acknowledging how hard the client and clinic staff will have to work to succeed but conveying a very confident message that success can be achieved by working together. The therapist and patient collaboratively begin formulating an initial treatment plan during this session. Clients are oriented to the rigorous urinalysis testing regimen that is a central component of this treatment. If it appears that a medication is indicated, initial steps are taken toward implementing the relevant medical protocols for making that happen. With the cocaine-dependent population, we routinely use a regimen of clinic-monitored disulfiram therapy to address problem drinking, which also reduces cocaine use (Carroll, Nich, Ball, McCance, & Rounsaville, 1998). Recently we have begun using a regimen of clinic-monitored naltrexone therapy as the prevalence of prescription opioid abuse has increased.

BEHAVIORAL AND COGNITIVE-BEHAVIORAL THERAPIES FOR ILLICIT DRUG ABUSE AND DEPENDENCE

Conceptual Framework

Behavioral and cognitive-behavioral therapies are based largely on the concepts and principles of operant and respondent conditioning, and social learning theory. Within this conceptual framework, drug use is considered learned behavior that is maintained, at least in part, by the reinforcing effects of the pharmacological actions of drugs in conjunction with social and other nonpharmacological reinforcement derived from the drug-abusing lifestyle (Higgins & Katz, 1998). The reliable empirical observation that abused drugs function as reinforcers in humans and laboratory animals provides sound scientific support for that position (Griffiths, Bigelow, & Henningfield, 1980). Cocaine, other psychomotor stimulants, ethanol, opioids, nicotine, and sedatives serve as reinforcers and are voluntarily self-administered by a variety of species. Moreover, through respondent and operant conditioning, environmental events that previously have been paired with drug use reliably lead to drug-seeking behavior. Physical dependence is not necessary for these drugs to support ongoing and stable patterns of voluntary drug seeking and use in otherwise healthy laboratory animals or humans. Commonalities do not end there. Effects of alterations in drug availability, drug dose, schedule of reinforcement, and other environmental manipulations of drug use are orderly and have generality across different species and types of drug abuse (Griffiths et al., 1980; Higgins, 1997). These commonalities support a theoretical position that reinforcement and other principles of learning are fundamental determinants of drug use, abuse, and dependence.

Within this conceptual model, then, drug use is considered a normal, learned behavior that falls along a frequency continuum ranging from patterns of little use and few problems to excessive use and many untoward effects, including death. The same processes and principles of learning are assumed to operate across the continuum. All physically intact humans are assumed to possess the necessary neurobiological systems to experience drug-produced reinforcement; hence, they develop patterns of drug use, abuse, and dependence. Said differently, individuals need not have any exceptional or pathological characteristics to develop drug abuse or dependence. Clearly genetic or acquired characteristics (e.g., family history of substance dependence, other psychiatric disorders) can affect the probability of developing drug abuse or dependence (i.e., they are risk factors), but this model assumes that such special characteristics are not necessary for these disorders to emerge.

Treatment is designed to assist in reorganizing the physical and social environments of the user. The goal is to weaken systematically the influence of reinforcement derived from drug use and the related drug-abusing lifestyle, and to increase the frequency of reinforcement derived from healthier alternative activities, especially those that are incompatible with continued drug use. Below we describe the basic categories of empirically tested and efficacious behavioral and cognitive-behavioral therapies for achieving these overarching goals (Carroll & Onken, 2005).

Prototypical Behavioral and Cognitive-Behavioral Interventions and Empirical Support for Efficacy

At least four empirically based, prototypical behavioral and cognitive-behavioral interventions are used in the treatment of illicit drug use disorders (Carroll & Onken, 2005). First is cognitive-behavioral/relapse prevention therapy, which has been shown to be effective with cocaine, methamphetamine, and other types of drug use disorders (e.g., Carroll et al., 1994; Rawson et al., 2004). Typically this approach entails functional analysis training through which clients learn to identify environmental antecedents and consequences that influence their drug use. Functional analysis is typically accompanied by skills training on how to rearrange one's environment to alter the probability of drug use by either avoiding high-risk settings or managing them effectively when contact cannot be avoided. Cognitive strategies are often used to identify and modify unrealistic expectations about drug use, to cope with craving for drug use, and to change thinking patterns that increase the likelihood of drug use. Social skills training is often incorporated when clients have used drugs to cope with social anxiety or when particular skills deficits limit clients' access to alternative, healthier sources of reinforcement (e.g., Monti, Rohsenow, Michalec, & Abrams, 1997). Systematic training is included to prevent relapse, with sufficient emphasis that the terms "cognitive-behavioral therapy" and "relapse prevention therapy" are often used interchangeably. There is good evidence that this approach is efficacious in treating illicit drug use disorders (for a meta-analysis, see Irvin, Bowers, Dunn, & Wong, 1999).

Second, contingency management is an efficacious behavioral treatment strategy commonly used to treat cocaine, opiate, and other types of illicit drug use disorders (e.g., Higgins, Wong, Badger, Ogden, & Dantona, 2000; Petry et al., 2005; Silverman, Robles, Mudric, & Stitzer, 2004). With contingency management, reinforcing and punishing consequences are systematically used to increase abstinence from drug use or to improve other therapeutic goals, such as treatment attendance or medication compliance (Higgins, Silverman, & Heil, 2008). A particular form of contingency management, wherein clients receive vouchers that are exchangeable for retail items contingent on objective evidence of recent abstinence from drug use, has become a common intervention for clients with illicit drug use disorders. We know of at least two meta-analyses supporting the efficacy of contingency management with methadone maintenance patients (Griffith, Rowan-Szal, Roark, & Simpson, 2000) and in the treatment of drug use disorders more generally (Lussier, Heil, Mongeon, Badger, & Higgins, 2006).

Third, motivational interviewing, an efficacious intervention with problem drinkers (Vasilaki, Hosier, & Cox, 2006), is being used more frequently to treat illicit drug use disorders as well. Motivational interviewing is a brief intervention designed to facilitate behavior change by helping clients to identify personal values and goals, to examine whether drug use may conflict with those values and goals, and to explore how to resolve any ambivalence or conflict between personal goals and values, and ongoing drug use (Miller &

Rollnick, 2002). Results on the use of motivational interviewing with illicit drug use disorders are still mixed (e.g., Martino, Carroll, & Rounsaville, 2006), but it appears to have promise as a method to enhance entry into and engagement in more intensive treatment (Dunn, Deroo, & Rivara, 2001).

Fourth, behavioral couple therapy has been effective in the treatment of illicit drug use disorders (e.g., Fals-Stewart & O'Farrell, 2003; Fals-Stewart, O'Farrell, & Birchler, 2001; for a review, see O'Farrell & Fals-Stewart, 2002), although it has not been extensively investigated (Carroll & Onken, 2005). Therapy typically emphasizes improved communication skills. Couples are taught how to negotiate for change in each other's behavior to make the relationship more reinforcing. A contract wherein the designated client agrees to abstain from drug use and or to comply with a recommended medication regimen is typically involved. There is also evidence that behavioral family counseling has efficacy with adolescents who have illicit drug use disorders (e.g., Azrin, Donohue, Besalel, Kogan, & Acierno, 1994) as do other family therapy interventions (e.g., Henggeler, Pickrel, Brondino, & Crouch, 1996; Liddle et al., 2001).

It is a common practice to provide multielement treatments for illicit drug use disorders that incorporate many of the specific interventions we have outlined (e.g., Bellack, Bennett, Gearson, Brown, & Yang, 2006). Indeed CRA plus vouchers, which we use to treat cocaine dependence, incorporates all of the interventions outlined earlier except for family therapies with adolescents. Below we describe the CRA plus vouchers intervention and its implementation in the treatment of cocaine dependence. With regard to efficacy, the meta-analysis supporting the efficacy of vouchers was noted earlier (Lussier et al., 2006). A meta-analysis supports the efficacy of CRA, with and without vouchers in the treatment of drug use disorders (Roozen et al., 2004), and a randomized trial has demonstrated that the CRA component is an active element of the CRA plus vouchers treatment (Higgins et al., 2003).

CRA plus Vouchers

The recommended duration of CRA plus vouchers therapy is 24 weeks of treatment and 24 weeks of aftercare (Budney & Higgins, 1998). The influence of treatment duration has not yet been examined experimentally with this or other efficacious psychosocial treatments for drug use disorders, but a duration of 3 or more months of care is generally recommended (Principle 5, Table 13.1).

CRA therapy in this model is delivered in individual sessions, although CRA has been delivered effectively in a group therapy format with alcohol-dependent clients (Azrin, 1976). As we noted earlier, the treatment involves two main components: CRA and vouchers.

The Community Reinforcement Approach

Before we get into the specific elements of CRA, more general characteristics of the therapy style are worth mentioning. Therapists try to be flexible in appointment scheduling and goal setting, which we believe facilitate treatment retention and progress toward target goals. Particularly in the early stages of treatment, therapists try to work around client's schedules and generally make participation in treatment convenient. We try to tolerate tardiness to sessions, early departure from sessions, flexibility in the time of day that sessions are scheduled, and we even meet with clients outside the office, if necessary. With especially difficult clients, improvements in these areas become part of the treatment plan.

Therapists must exhibit empathy and good listening skills. They need to convey a sincere understanding of the client's situation and its inherent difficulties. Throughout treatment, therapists avoid making value judgments, and instead exhibit genuine empathy and consideration for the difficult challenges that the client faces.

Last, CRA requires both therapists and patients to develop an active, make-it-happen attitude throughout treatment. Active problem solving is a routine part of the therapeutic relationship. Within ethical boundaries, therapists are committed to doing what it takes to facilitate lifestyle changes on the part of clients. Therapists take clients to appointments or job interviews. They initiate recreational activities with clients, and schedule sessions at different times of day to accomplish specific goals. They have clients make phone calls from their office, and search newspapers for job possibilities or ideas for healthy recreational activities in which clients might be able to participate. In summary, the CRA therapists' motto is "We

can make it happen," and they try their best to model that approach for patients.

CRA is delivered in twice-weekly 1–1.5 hour therapy sessions during the initial 12 weeks and once-weekly sessions of the same duration during the final 12 weeks of treatment. Sessions focus on the following seven general topics, depending on the needs of the individual client.

First, clients are instructed in how to recognize antecedents and consequences of their cocaine use, that is, how to functionally analyze their cocaine use. They are also instructed in how to use that information to reduce the probability of using cocaine. A twofold message is conveyed to the client: (1) His or her cocaine use is orderly behavior that is more likely to occur under certain circumstances than others, and (2) by learning to identify the circumstances that affect one's cocaine use, one can develop and implement plans to reduce the likelihood of future cocaine use. Our methods for teaching functional analysis are based on the work of Miller and Munoz (e.g., 2005) and McCrady (Chapter 12, this volume), whose methods are used widely in substance abuse treatment.

Using the form shown in Figure 13.1, we help clients analyze instances of their own cocaine use. We explain the following:

"A functional analysis allows you to identify the immediate causes of your cocaine use. You have probably noticed that in certain situations you use cocaine, whereas in others you do not. The situations around us can powerfully control cocaine use, particularly if we are unaware of their influence.

"Some of the situations that can influence cocaine use are people you are with, places you go, time of day, the amount of money you have with you, how much alcohol you have consumed, and how you are feeling. The first step in understanding your cocaine use is to identify the situations in which you are likely to use. We call that identifying your 'triggers.' You will also want to identify consequences of your use; that is, identify the immediate, usually positive consequences (getting high, having fun), and the delayed, often negative consequences (blowing your money, unwanted sexual encounters, fights with your spouse). As you identify triggers and consequences, you will

Trigger	Thoughts and feelings	Behavior	Consequences	
			Positive	Negative

FIGURE 13.1. Form for functional analysis of substance use.

discover certain patterns to your cocaine use that are important targets for intervention."

Clients are assigned the task of analyzing at least three recent episodes of cocaine use. Learning to analyze one's cocaine use is emphasized during initial treatment sessions, but the exercise is used throughout the treatment process to help clients understand and modify any lapses to cocaine use, as well as to address problems with cocaine craving.

In conjunction with functional analysis, clients are taught self-management plans for using the information revealed in the functional analyses to decrease the chances of future cocaine use. Using the self-management planning

sheet shown in Figure 13.2, clients are counseled to restructure their daily activities to minimize contact with known antecedents of cocaine use, to find alternatives to the positive consequences of cocaine use, and to make explicit the negative consequences of cocaine use.

A key part of self-management planning that is implemented with most clients is drug-refusal training. Most cocaine abusers who are trying to quit cocaine use continue to have contact, either planned or inadvertent, with individuals who are still using. Turning down cocaine or opportunities to go places where cocaine is available is more difficult than most clients anticipate. We approach this as a special case of assertiveness training (e.g., McCrady,

Trigger	Plans	± Consequences	Difficulty (1–10)
1.	a		
	b		
	c		
	d		
	e.		

FIGURE 13.2. Self-management planning sheet. From Budney and Higgins (1998).

Chapter 12, this volume; Meyers & Smith, 1995). The key components of effective refusal are shown in Table 13.4. Therapists should explain the rationale for drug-refusal skills training, engage the client in a detailed discussion of the key elements of effective refusal, assist the client in formulating his or her own refusal style (incorporating the key elements), and role-play some scenes in which the client is offered cocaine. The role-played situations should be very specific and realistic for the client in terms of people, times of day, location, and so forth. Client and therapist should alternate roles, so that the former has the opportunity to practice while receiving constructive feedback, and the latter has the opportunity to model effective refusal skills.

Second, developing a new social network that supports a healthier lifestyle and getting involved with enjoyable recreational activities that do not involve cocaine or other drug use are addressed with all clients. Systematically developing and maintaining contacts with "safe" social networks and participation in "safe" recreational activities remain a high priority throughout treatment for the vast majority of clients. Specific treatment goals are set, and weekly progress on specific goals is monitored (Principle 4, Table 13.1).

Clearly, plans for developing healthy social networks and recreational activities must be individualized depending on the circumstances, skills, and interests of clients. For clients who

TABLE 13.4. Components of Effective Refusal

1. *No* should be the first thing you say.
2. Tell the person offering you drugs or asking you to go out *not to ask you now or in the future* if you want to do cocaine. Saying things like "maybe later," "I have to get home," or "I'm on medication," and so forth, just make it likely that he or she will ask again.
3. Body language is important:
   a. Making good eye contact is important; look directly at the person when you answer.
   b. Your expression and tone should clearly indicate that you are serious.
4. Offer an alternative, if you want to do something else with that person. Make sure that it is something that is incompatible with cocaine use (taking your children for a walk or to the park, going to work out, etc.).
5. Change the subject to a new topic of conversation.

are willing to participate, self-help groups (Alcoholics or Narcotics Anonymous) can be an effective way to develop a new network of associates that supports a sober lifestyle. A clinic staff member often accompanies a client to his or her first self-help meeting or two. By no means do we focus exclusively on or mandate self-help involvement. We assist clients with getting involved in a wide variety of social groups that reinforce a healthy lifestyle (e.g., church groups). Clinic staff accompany clients who are trying new, healthy activities. Some clients wish to reinitiate activities in which they engaged prior to becoming involved with cocaine use, or have clear ideas about activities they would like to pursue. We assist those clients in renewing or initiating participation in those activities. Many others either never learned to recreate as adults without drug involvement or are simply unable to identify any activities they would currently like to pursue. We often have these clients complete a leisure–interest inventory to prompt ideas about activities they might have liked previously or otherwise want to explore. We encourage clients to sample new activities even if they are unsure whether they will find them enjoyable. As we describe below, vouchers may be used to support costs of initiating recreational and other activities that support a healthy lifestyle.

Third, various other forms of individualized skills training are provided, usually to address some specific skills deficit that may influence directly or indirectly a client's risk for cocaine use (e.g., time management, problem solving, assertiveness training, social skills training, and mood management). For example, essential to success with the self-management skills and social/recreational goals discussed earlier is some level of time-management skills. All clients are given daily planners to facilitate planning. Because clients may lose or forget their planners, providing photocopies to cover the next week of treatment is a good strategy. Therapists provide the following rationale:

"This part of your treatment involves learning to plan, schedule, and prioritize the events and activities in your life. Solving your cocaine problem requires making substantial lifestyle changes; it is important to develop efficient ways to do this. Some patients say they don't like to plan—they like to be spontaneous. But if they don't find a way to schedule and organize their lives, they often get overwhelmed and don't achieve their goals."

With most clients, time management in some form is worked on throughout treatment. The importance of writing down a schedule of activities that will help to promote cocaine abstinence between therapy sessions is emphasized in each session. Planning for "high-risk" times is particularly important. Use of "to do" lists, daily planning, and prioritizing activities is addressed.

As other examples of skills training, we implement protocols on controlling depression (Lewinsohn, Munoz, Youngren, & Zeiss, 1986; Munoz & Miranda, 2000) with those clients whose depression continues after they discontinue cocaine use (see Principle 8, Table 13.1). We sometimes implement social skills and relaxation training with individuals who report social anxiety about meeting new people, dating, and so forth (Rodebaugh, Holaway, & Heimberg, 2004). Many clients report persistent problems with insomnia following discontinuation of drug use. With them we often implement a protocol based on those developed by Morin (2004). We often work with clients regarding money management. With many clients that might simply involve helping them arrange direct deposit for their paycheck, so that they are not tempted to use because they have a large sum of cash on hand. For others, this might involve a plan to get out of debt, which can help to reduce stress. Because clients often have so many problems that could benefit from our assistance, we follow a rule of only treating those problems that we feel directly or indirectly affect the probability of initial and longer-term cocaine abstinence for individual clients. Here we rely heavily on functional analysis and other available information regarding the client's cocaine use. For problems that do not appear to be related to cocaine use but warrant professional attention, we generally make a referral. We work very hard to keep treatment focused on resolving the problem of cocaine use, and against being sidetracked by other pressing problems that may have no direct or indirect effect on the presenting problem of cocaine dependence.

Fourth, unemployed clients are offered Job Club, which is an efficacious method to help chronically unemployed individuals obtain employment (see the Job Club manual, Azrin & Besalel, 1980). The majority of clients who seek treatment for cocaine dependence are unemployed, so we offer this service to many of our clients. We assist others in pursuing educational goals or new career paths. A meaningful vocation is fundamental to a healthy lifestyle, and we recommend goals directed toward vocational enhancement for all clients. Rules that we follow for several common types of vocational problems are outlined in Table 13.5.

Fifth, clients with romantic partners who were not drug abusers are offered behavioral couple therapy, an intervention designed to teach couples positive communication skills and how to negotiate reciprocal contracts for desired changes in each other's behavior (see O'Farrell & Fals-Stewart, 2002). We attempt to deliver relationship counseling across eight sessions, with the first four sessions delivered across consecutive weeks and the next four delivered on alternating weeks. We introduce this aspect of therapy with the following rationale:

"As you well know, an important area of your life that is negatively affected by cocaine problems is your relationship with your

TABLE 13.5. Examples of Goals Set in Vocational Counseling

For the unemployed client:
- Eight job contacts per week.
- Develop a resume.
- Send out two resumes with a cover letter per day.
- Go to the job service twice per week.
- Enroll in a job training program.
- Enroll in a vocational exploration program.
- Take a job-skills-related class.
- Consider and collect information on educational possibilities.

For the client who works "too many" hours or has irregular schedule:
- Keep work hours between 35 and 50 hours per week.
- Establish a more regular schedule.
- Explore alternative work schedules.

For the person working in a "high risk" for drug use environment or the dissatisfied employee:
- Consider a job change.
- Submit applications for alternative employment while continuing to work.
- Modify the work environment to reduce risk of drug use or improve working conditions.
- Enroll in a career exploration class.
- Enroll in job-skills or alternative, career-related educational classes.

partner. Those close to the person with the problem are typically most adversely affected by the problem. Many partners of cocaine-dependent individuals have tried many times to help their mate to stop using. Strategies for trying to help vary. Anger and frustration usually build up, and feelings of hopelessness and helplessness arise. Sometimes attempts to help are met with resentment and anger from the partner with the problem.

"In this part of treatment, we focus on how cocaine use has affected your relationship and how we can work to increase the positive aspects of your relationship. We also discuss ways that your partner can assist you in achieving and maintaining abstinence. We hope to be able to help you both deal more effectively with this cocaine problem.

"We have found that where there are drug abuse problems, there are usually communication problems. Usually, we see communication that is filled with anger, silence, apathy, or resentment, and many times partners try to get their needs met outside the relationship. By the time patients come to see us, there is little, if any, enjoyment left in the relationship."

The intervention involves a related series of exercises. Partners independently rate their current level of happiness across household responsibilities, child rearing, social activities, money, communication, sex and affection, academic progress, personal independence, partner's independence, general happiness. Those ratings are shared and discussed, and then rerated weekly to monitor progress. Next, a system of "daily reminders to be nice" (i.e., express appreciation and affection toward one's spouse) is implemented. The obvious goal is to get the couple to take the time to be positive with each other. Each partner is expected to engage in a daily practice of "nice" gestures toward his or her spouse and to keep a daily compliance record of his or her own behavior—not the spouse's compliance. That information is reviewed and shared during sessions. After some level of positive interaction is established, partners independently identify what a "perfect relationship" would entail in terms of the key elements of their relationship that were mentioned earlier—what that perfect relationship would look like. Finally, the couple begins to work on using positive communication skills to

negotiate for reciprocal changes in each other's behavior to move toward that "perfect relationship." The terms "positive" and "reciprocal" are fundamentally important here. Requests are stated exclusively in positive terms and both members have to be willing to make changes.

Sixth, HIV/AIDS education is provided to all clients in the early stages of treatment, along with counseling that addresses any specific needs or risk behavior of the individual patient (Heil et al., 2005). We address with all clients the potential for acquiring HIV/AIDS from sharing injection equipment and through sexual activity. This involves at least two sessions. First, clients complete an HIV/AIDS knowledge test. They next watch and discuss with their therapist a video on HIV/AIDS. Points emphasized by therapists during the discussion are shown in Table 13.6. Clients are also provided HIV/AIDS prevention pamphlets and free condoms (if desired). The HIV/AIDS knowledge test is repeated and any remaining errors discussed and resolved. Finally, clients are given information about being tested for HIV antibodies and hepatitis B and C, and are encouraged to get tested (Principle 12, Table 13.1). Those interested in testing are assisted by clinic staff in scheduling an appointment.

Seventh, all who meet diagnostic criteria for alcohol dependence or report that alcohol use is involved in their use of cocaine are offered disulfiram therapy (see Principle 7, Table 13.1), which is an integral part of the CRA treatment for alcoholism (Meyers & Smith, 1995), and decreases alcohol and cocaine use in clients who are dependent on both substances (Carroll et al., 1998). Clients generally ingest a 250 mg daily dose, observed by clinic staff on urinalysis test days, and, when possible, by a significant other on the other days. We encourage clients to sign a disulfiram contract, shown in Figure 13.3. Disulfiram therapy is only effective when implemented with procedures to monitor compliance with the recommended dosage of medication. We find that having staff monitor compliance on days that clients report to the clinic works very well. Having a significant other monitor compliance on the other days works well if the appropriate person is available to do so at the frequency needed. When that is not possible, we sometimes adopt a practice of having the client ingest a larger dose (500 mg) on days when he or she reports to the clinic and skip dosing on the intervening days.

TABLE 13.6. Points Emphasized in Discussions of HIV/AIDS

1. The fastest-growing risk group for HIV/AIDS is made up of people who use intravenous (IV) drugs and their sexual partners. At the start of the epidemic, this group made up just a small proportion of those getting infected, but these numbers are increasing rapidly at the present time. Not just gay men get infected!
2. Review the three ways that HIV is transmitted: (a) through sexual contact with an infected person, (b) through blood (as in needle sharing), and (c) from infected mothers to their babies during pregnancy or at the time of birth. Explain that the most efficient way for HIV to be transmitted is through blood (blood contains the highest concentration of the virus) and that sharing needles ("works") is an "easy" way for the virus to get from the system of one person to that of another.
3. Emphasize the point that people who are infected with HIV do not necessarily look sick and might not even know they are infected. You cannot tell by looking at someone whether that person has the virus.
4. If clients are currently using IV drugs, point out that the only safe thing to do if they tend to share needles is to use new needles or to clean them, if they are still using. Review the steps necessary for appropriate syringe cleaning.
5. Unprotected sexual intercourse with the exchange of body fluids (blood, vaginal fluids, semen, preejaculatory fluid) is also an efficient means of giving or receiving the virus. Sex can be made safer by using latex condoms for each and every sexual encounter (this includes oral, vaginal, and anal sex).
6. Point out that alcohol and other drug use contribute to risk because of (a) possible suppression of the immune system, and (b) impaired judgment, which can lead to increased risk taking (e.g., drug use, unsafe sex).

Use of substances other than tobacco and caffeine is discouraged as well in CRA therapy. Anyone who meets criteria for physical dependence on opiates is referred to an adjoining service located within our clinic for methadone or other opioid replacement therapy (see Bickel, Amass, Higgins, Badger, & Esch, 1997). We recommend marijuana abstinence because of the problems associated with its abuse, but we have found no evidence that marijuana use or dependence adversely affects treatment for cocaine dependence (Budney, Higgins, & Wong, 1996). Importantly, we never dismiss or refuse to treat a client due to other drug use. We recommend cessation of tobacco use, but usually not during the course of treatment for

I, _____ , agree to take disulfiram at the regularly scheduled time outlined below. I agree to do this for _____ days. After this time, I agree to talk to my therapist and to discuss whether or not to continue taking disulfiram. I also agree to have the person designated below witness the administration of the disulfiram each time it is scheduled.

I, _____ , agree to be present and witness each take-home administration of disulfiram.

Time: _____

Days: _____

Where: _____

In response to _____ taking disulfiram as scheduled, I agree to _____ as a means of reinforcing the taking of disulfiram.

_____   _____
Patient's Signature   Partner's Signature

_____   _____
Therapist's Signature   Date

FIGURE 13.3. Disulfiram contract.

cocaine dependence. That practice may change as new research begins to demonstrate that smoking cessation can be successfully integrated into simultaneous treatment for other substance abuse or dependence disorders.

Upon completion of the 24 weeks of treatment, clients are encouraged to participate in 6 months of aftercare in our clinic, which involves at least a once-monthly brief therapy session and a urine toxicology screen. More frequent clinic contact is recommended if the therapist or the client deem it necessary. These clinic visits might be considered booster sessions that monitor progress and address problems with cocaine use or other aspects of the lifestyle changes initiated during treatment. They also allow for a gradual rather than abrupt ending of the client's involvement with the clinic.

Voucher Program

As was noted earlier, the voucher program is a contingency management intervention designed to increase retention and abstinence. Many cocaine- and other drug-dependent individuals arrive in treatment with their lives in disarray. A reasonable assumption is that some time will be needed to assist these individuals in stabilizing and restructuring their lives, so that naturalistic sources of reinforcement for abstinence can exert some influence over their behavior. A protected environment is an option, but the voucher program is deemed a less expensive alternative. The goal is to have this incentive program play a major role during the initial 12 weeks of treatment, during which time CRA therapy is ongoing as well. CRA is used to assist clients in restructuring their lifestyle, so that naturalistic reinforcers are in place to sustain cocaine abstinence once the vouchers are discontinued.

The voucher program is implemented in conjunction with a rigorous urinalysis monitoring program (see Principle 11, Table 13.1). We ask patients to sign an Abstinence Contract (Figure 13.4), which describes the voucher program and the urinalysis testing schedule. Urine specimens are collected from all participants according to a Monday, Wednesday, and Friday schedule during Weeks 1–12 and a Monday and Thursday schedule during Weeks 13–24 of treatment. Specimens are screened immediately via an onsite enzyme multiplied immunoassay technique (EMIT, Syva Company, San Jose, CA) to

minimize delays in delivering reinforcement for cocaine-negative specimens. To decrease the likelihood of submitting bogus specimens, all specimens are collected under the observation of a same-sex staff member, and staff members always reserve the right to request another specimen if they have any concerns regarding the integrity of a specimen. All specimens are screened for benzoylecgonine, a cocaine metabolite, and one randomly selected specimen each week also is screened for the presence of other abused drugs. Breath alcohol levels (BALs) are assessed at the time urine specimens are collected. Failure to submit a scheduled specimen is treated as a cocaine-positive result. Participants are informed of their urinalysis and BAL results within several minutes after submitting specimens.

Urine specimens collected during Weeks 1–12 that test negative for benzoylecgonine earn points that are recorded on vouchers and given to participants. Points are worth the equivalent of $0.25 each. Money is never provided directly to clients. Instead, points are used to purchase retail items in the community. A staff member makes all purchases. The first negative specimen is worth 10 points at $.25/point or $2.50. The value of vouchers for each subsequent consecutive negative specimen increases by 5 points (e.g., second = 15 points, third = 20 points, etc.). To further increase the likelihood of continuous cocaine abstinence, the equivalent of a $10 bonus is earned for each three consecutive negative specimens. Specimens that are cocaine positive or failure to submit a scheduled specimen reset the value of vouchers back to the initial $2.50 value from which they can escalate again according to the same schedule. Submission of five consecutive cocaine-negative specimens following submission of a positive specimen returns the value of points to where they were prior to the reset. Points cannot be lost once they are earned.

Patients and therapists jointly select retail items to be purchased with points. The items commonly obtained are quite diverse, including YMCA passes, continuing education materials, fishing licenses, gift certificates to local restaurants, hobby materials, and so forth. Therapists retain veto power over all purchases. Purchases are only approved if therapists deem them to be in concert with individual treatment goals of increasing drug-free, healthy activities.

The voucher program is discontinued at the end of Week 12. During Weeks 13–24, partici-

This is an agreement between _____ (the client) and
_____ (the therapist) to help the client maintain abstinence
from cocaine. By this agreement I direct my therapist to establish a schedule for collecting urine
specimens from me for 24 weeks. I will provide urine samples three times per week on a Monday,
Wednesday, and Friday schedule during the first 12 weeks of treatment. During the second 12 weeks of
treatment (Weeks 13–24), urine samples will be collected two times per week on a Monday and
Thursday schedule. A clinical staff member of my same sex will observe the urination. Half of each urine
sample will be submitted for immediate analysis and half will be saved at the clinic. Samples will be
assayed for a variety of drugs of abuse, among which are cocaine, amphetamines, opioids, marijuana,
and sedatives.

Each specimen collection requires 3.0 ounces of urine. If the quantity is insufficient for analysis, that will
be considered a failure to provide a scheduled sample.

If I travel out of town due to an emergency, I will inform my therapist in advance of leaving. My therapist
is authorized to verify such absences with _____ . If I require hospitalization,
my therapist will arrange to collect urine in the hospital. If I am sick and do not require hospitalization, I
will still arrange to produce scheduled urine specimens. If I have difficulty with transportation, or
inclement weather makes it difficult to travel, I will work out (with the assistance of the clinical staff) a
way to get to the clinic for urine collection. On certain major holidays the clinic will be closed. My
therapist and I will mutually agree to altered urine schedules on these occasions.

If for appropriate medical reasons a prescription for one of the drugs which sometimes is abused is
written, I will supply my therapist with copies of that prescription. The appearance of that drug in the
urine will not be counted as a relapse to drug use. I hereby direct my therapist to communicate by mail
or telephone with the prescribing physician or dentist when my therapist deems that action to be
appropriate.

Cocaine-Free Urines: For each cocaine-negative urine sample collected during Weeks 1–12 of
treatment, points will be earned. Each point is worth the monetary equivalent of $0.25, although they
may **not** be exchanged directly for cash. A voucher stating the earned point value will be presented to
me following the collection of a cocaine-negative sample. This voucher will specify the number of points
earned for that day, as well as the cumulative points earned to date and their monetary equivalent.

During the first 12 weeks of treatment, the first cocaine-free urine sample will earn 10 points, with each
consecutive cocaine-free sample collected thereafter earning an increment of 5 points above the
previously earned amount. For example, if 10 points are received on Wednesday for a cocaine-free
urine sample, Friday's cocaine-free sample will earn 15 points, Monday's will earn 20, and so on. As an
added incentive to remain abstinent from cocaine, a $10 bonus will be earned for each week of three
consecutive cocaine-negative urine samples collected at our clinic. Assuming there are no cocaine-
positive urine samples collected, the monetary equivalent of $997.50 can be earned during the first 12
weeks of treatment. Since a major emphasis in our program is on lifestyle changes, primarily increasing
activities that effectively compete with drug use, the money earned on this incentive system must be
used toward social or recreational goods and activities agreed upon by my therapist and myself. A list of
acceptable uses of vouchers has been developed for this purpose and will be shared with me. During
the second 12 weeks of treatment, the incentive program will be changed. Rather than earning vouchers
for cocaine-negative samples, I will be earning lottery tickets for clean samples.

For the entire 24 weeks of treatment, immediately after the urinalysis test results indicate that the urine
sample is cocaine-negative, the following will happen. The vouchers (Weeks 1–12) or lottery tickets
(Weeks 13–24) will be delivered. Following the presentation of each voucher, I will be asked if I would
like to "purchase" any goods or services. Vouchers may be used at any time during the 24-week
program. Earned vouchers cannot be taken away from me under any circumstances. The procedure for
dealing with cocaine-positive urine samples is discussed below.

(continued)

FIGURE 13.4. Sample abstinence contract.

Cocaine-Positive Urines: All urine samples will be screened for drug use. A record will be kept of all drugs screened positive, although this contract will be in effect for cocaine only. For each cocaine-positive urine sample collected I will not receive a voucher. In addition, the voucher earned for the next cocaine-free urine sample will be reset to 10. To reset the voucher value to where it was prior to the cocaine "slip," I must provide five *consecutive* cocaine-free samples. The fifth "clean" sample will then earn me the same monetary equivalent as that earned for the sample preceding the cocaine-positive one, and the system outlined earlier will continue to be in effect (i.e., each clean sample will earn 5 points more than the previous one).

Failure to Provide a Urine Sample: Failure to provide a urine sample on the designated date (without prior approval of my therapist) will be treated as a cocaine-positive sample and the procedures noted earlier will be in effect. Although clinic staff will make an attempt to obtain the sample by coming to my home (with my permission, of course), cocaine-negative urine samples collected in this manner will not earn voucher points, nor will they reset my voucher value to 10. In effect, cocaine-negative samples collected outside of our clinic (except in the case of hospitalization) are "neutral." On the other hand, if clinic staff obtain a sample from me outside of the clinic, and the sample is cocaine-positive, it will be treated in the manner outlined above for cocaine-positive urine samples.

My signature below acknowledges that I agree to the urinalysis monitoring system outlined above. This system has been carefully explained to me, and I understand the outcome of providing both cocaine-negative and cocaine-positive urine samples while I am a client at the clinic.

_____

Client

_____

Date

_____

Therapist

FIGURE 13.4. *(continued)*

pants receive a single $1.00 Vermont State Lottery ticket per cocaine-negative urinalysis test. Across the 24 weeks of treatment, patients can earn a maximum of $997.50 in vouchers during Weeks 1–12 and $24 in lottery tickets during Weeks 13–24. No material incentives are delivered during the recommended 6-month aftercare period. There is strong evidence that vouchers worth only several hundred dollars over the 12-week course of treatment are efficacious, although the magnitude of the treatment effect decreases significantly as the size of the incentive decreases (Lussier et al., 2006).

Getting Therapy Underway

The therapist has many tasks to accomplish during the first two sessions (Week 1) of treatment, in addition to simply getting to know the client and developing rapport. These sessions are critical to enhancing motivation and setting the tone for treatment. Hence, we provide detailed descriptions of the specific tasks to accomplish during initial therapy sessions.

As discussed earlier, urinalysis and cocaine use test results are the first areas addressed. By starting the session with a direct assessment of cocaine use, the therapist provides a clear message that the focus of this treatment is cocaine dependence.

After a discussion of cocaine use and voucher earnings, the therapist should make sure that the client has completed all the intake materials. Here the therapist can also answer any new questions the client may have.

If practical needs, such as housing, transportation, or child care, are issues for treatment attendance, these needs should be a primary focus of the first session. Therapists should do everything possible to assist clients in finding solutions to these problems.

The therapist should discuss alternative activities or strategies for coping with high-risk situations for cocaine use, especially situations that are likely to arise during the upcoming week. As discussed earlier, having the client use appointment books or photocopies provided by the clinic are very helpful for scheduling alternative plans or activities. The next session should also be scheduled, and the client should record the day and time in the appointment book.

The therapist should begin to formulate a comprehensive treatment plan with specific goals and methods. The therapist might introduce this task in the following way:

"A treatment plan will allow us to write down the things you and I think are important to accomplish and how we plan to go about trying to accomplish them. We will use the plan to keep us focused on the task at hand—that is, making lifestyle changes that will help you stop using cocaine and other drugs, and also increase your satisfaction with other important areas of your life. The treatment plan will be developed through a cooperative effort between you and me. It is important that you think the goals we set are important and will help you achieve what you want in life. My job in this process is to assist you in coming up with meaningful, effective goals, and to offer advice based on my knowledge and experience with treating persons with cocaine and other drug problems."

The therapist should then present ideas about which areas of the client's life need changes. For each suggested change, it is important that the therapist provide a rationale that draws from the information collected from the client, as well as from research findings and clinical experience. An open discussion and exchange of ideas should then follow.

If the client is reluctant to participate, the therapist should ask for his or her thoughts on each potential area for change. The therapist can facilitate client participation with questions, such as "What do you think?"; "Do you have any thoughts on this?"; "Does this make sense to you?"; "Do you think this is important?"; and "Is this type of change possible?" It is important for therapist and client to agree on which areas of life present problems and should be changed. If a client disagrees with the therapist's opinion, those areas should be dropped and discussed later in treatment if they continue to pose problems.

After the areas for change are agreed upon, therapist and client should discuss each one. Therapists should use active listening skills (reflection and empathy) and try to keep the focus on the specific areas. They should inform clients that they will focus on these problem areas in each session. Progress and problems are openly discussed, and additions or deletions to the plan are decided upon by the therapist and client together.

Next, the therapist and client together decide the order in which these problem areas should be addressed, always remembering that increasing cocaine abstinence is the primary goal. Mutual agreement is important, and a therapist may need to compromise to achieve such agreement.

Specific goals should then be set for each problem area. It is important that the therapist provide a rationale for setting specific goals:

"Setting specific goals is important. They will help us stay focused on the primary changes we agreed are important for stopping your drug use and achieving a more satisfying life without drugs. Specific goals also provide a way to measure progress. This can be very important, because many times progress can be slow. You may feel you are getting nowhere. In reality, you may be progressing in making changes, but you don't feel much different. Information about specific goals will help us both see more clearly whether we are heading in the right direction, even if the progress is slow.

"This information can also show when you are not progressing as we planned and can lead us to either reconsider the goal or find other ways to meet the goal. Keeping track of progress on specific goals also provides us with a reminder to reward or praise you for the hard work you are doing. Lifestyle changes are often difficult to make. We would also like you to learn to pat yourself on the back and take credit if you are doing well."

These goals should be quantifiable, so that progress can be graphed. Targets for change should be set in the priority areas listed in the treatment plan and categorized as primary or secondary behavior change goals. Examples of typical goals are as follows:

- Five job contacts per week or making an appointment for vocational rehabilitation.
- Engaging in three recreational activities each week during high-risk times.
- Spending 4 hours each week engaging in fun activities with a family member or friend.

- Attending class one night each week.
- Doing 2 hours of homework toward obtaining a general equivalency diploma (GED).
- Planning and doing activities with a person who does not use drugs on nights when one typically used cocaine.

A therapist and client should mutually decide on these goals. Basic principles of effective goal setting should be followed:

- Set relatively low goals at first, so that the client can experience success early.
- Thoroughly analyze all possible barriers to achieving selected goals, so that unrealistic goals are avoided.
- Make sure that the client understands how a goal relates to the overall treatment plan.

It is essential to maximize the probability that the client will carry through and achieve the desired behavior change. The therapist's responsibility is to use the appropriate counseling style and behavioral procedures to increase the probability of compliance with a targeted behavior.

The treatment plan should be updated regularly, because treatment planning is a process of constant reevaluation, assessment, and change based on objective indices of progress (Principle 4, Table 13.1). The client and therapist together should review, discuss, and assess the treatment plan frequently as goals are achieved or as interventions fail, or as new information becomes available. These changes should also be reviewed at the regular clinical supervision meeting.

Implementing the treatment plan, monitoring progress, and modifying and updating the treatment plan according to client needs, progress, and problems are the "meat" of the remainder of treatment.

Clinical Supervision

Doctorate-level psychologists who have expertise in behavioral psychology and substance abuse treatment provide supervision in our clinic. Supervisors provide significant input into treatment plans and selection of targets for behavior change. The supervisor provides guidance about how to monitor progress.

Supervision is provided weekly in sessions that usually last 2–3 hours, during which all cases are reviewed. Therapists update the supervisor and other clinic therapists on each patient's progress based on specific treatment goals and whether progress has been made since last supervision meeting. Progress is presented graphically for all goals.

A supervisor's style in this model should include a balance of support, feedback, problem solving, and instruction. Considering that CRA plus vouchers requires an active therapeutic approach that can be effortful, the supervisor must serve as a stable source of support, encouragement, and direction in implementing the treatment plan.

We follow a fixed protocol in reviewing cases. First, review begins with examination of a graph of the patient's cocaine urinalysis results from the start of treatment. Second, we review alcohol or any other drugs that are being targeted for change. Then we review attendance at therapy sessions, primary goals for lifestyle changes, and secondary goals for the same. Once those treatment targets have been reviewed and modified as necessary, any recent crises or relevant clinical issues, such as suicidal ideation or newly identified problem behaviors, are discussed.

At any point in treatment, treatment goals and targets may be changed. Changes in goals may be precipitated by achievement of prior goals, failure to make any progress toward a specific goal, and clear indication that the goal is not functionally related to cocaine use.

IMPLEMENTING THE CRA PLUS VOUCHERS TREATMENT: A CASE STUDY

In this section we review the case of a client treated in our clinic with the CRA plus vouchers treatment. We chose this case because it illustrates well a number of different aspects of using this treatment approach. Outcome was quite good but certainly not perfect, which is to be expected with this population. The case also illustrates the multifaceted problems with which cocaine-dependent clients present.

Bill, a 24-year-old, single (never married), European American male, was self-referred to the clinic for help with problems with cocaine use. He had been living with a friend, who also used cocaine, until several weeks prior to the intake interview, when Bill moved in with his parents. He had a 5-year-old daughter who lived with an estranged romantic partner. The client currently was without legal visitation rights with his daughter because of her mother's concerns over Bill's record of drug use.

Bill, a high school graduate, had been employed full time in a retail business for the past 3 years. He reported that most of the individuals with whom he associated were drug abusers. Bill reported a history of healthy social and recreational activities, including golf and skiing, but he had not engaged in those activities with regularity for a number of years.

He had a history of involvement with the criminal justice system, with one conviction for a weapons offense. Bill was incarcerated for 3 months related to that charge but was not under criminal justice supervision at the time he sought treatment.

Presenting Complaint

Bill reported being on a 3-day binge prior to intake and wanted help with stopping cocaine use. He reported numerous prior attempts to stop on his own, but with minimal success. Bill reported being "fed up" with how he felt following episodes of binge cocaine use and was concerned about the financial problems his cocaine use caused. He also expressed serious concerns that his drug use and related lifestyle had resulted in a strained relationship with his child and ex-girlfriend that interfered with his getting visitation privileges.

Assessment

Cocaine Use

Bill met DSM-IV-TR criteria for cocaine dependence. He reported a 6-year history of intranasal cocaine use. In his most recent use, 7 days prior to intake, Bill used 10.5 grams of cocaine at home with friends, reporting that this was his typical pattern of use. At intake, Bill reported three episodes of cocaine use during the prior 30 days, with each episode lasting approximately 48 hours, usually during weekends. He typically used cocaine with friends at bars or at friends' houses.

His cocaine use was often preceded by spending time in bars or working excessive hours, or by certain moods, including feeling bored, depressed, anxious, or upset. Bill reported a number of serious consequences as a result of his cocaine use, including physical and financial problems, a relationship breakup, and psychiatric symptoms such as depression, anxiety, suicidal ideation, and violent impulses.

Other Drug Use

Bill's first use of alcohol was at age 16. He reported a pattern of weekly binge drinking during which he would ingest 13–15 shots of hard liquor. He reported drinking 5 days out of the past 30 days. Bill's first use of cannabis was at age 14. He reported 10 years of daily use and having used cannabis on 30 of the prior 30 days. He reported limited prior use of amphetamines and hallucinogens but no regular or current use of those substances. A regular cigarette smoker, Bill smoked approximately 20 cigarettes per day. Bill reported no previous treatment episodes for substance abuse.

Bill also met DSM-IV-TR criteria for alcohol, cannabis, and nicotine dependence.

Other Psychiatric Problems

Bill reported a history of depression and suicidal ideation. He also noted problems with anger management, which he agreed had been a significant problem for him, and for which he previously received counseling. His BDI score was 23 at intake, but he reported no suicidal ideation.

Motivation to Change

Bill's score on the SOCRATES at intake indicated a strong commitment to cocaine abstinence. He expressed a moderate commitment to alcohol abstinence but agreed to disulfiram therapy for the duration of treatment. He noted plans to return to social drinking after completion of treatment. He was uninterested in discontinuing marijuana use, which he did not consider a problem, and was not currently interested in discontinuing cigarette smoking.

Conceptualization of the Case

Bill worked long hours, sometimes holding several jobs simultaneously. That practice left little time for other types of activities and, as might be expected, he reported minimal involvement in any form of ongoing recreational activities. Aside from work, then, there were few alternative sources of reinforcement to compete with the reinforcing effects of Bill's cocaine and other drug use. These situations typically snowball, so that cocaine and related drug abuse monopolize more and more the person's activities. In this case, Bill's practices of working long hours, frequenting bars, and using drugs, and his difficulties with anger management, were sufficient to destroy his relationship with his romantic partner, thereby greatly restricting his time with his daughter. Losing those relationships further eliminated any competing sources of reinforcement and also freed up additional time and resources to allocate to the bar and cocaine use scenes. While we deemed Bill's long work hours to have likely increased his vulnerability to the drug-abusing lifestyle, his full-time employment also likely provided some protection against cocaine gaining even greater control over his behavior. Full-time employment is a positive prognostic variable with this and other treatments for cocaine dependence, as is the use of an intranasal route of cocaine administration, which was Bill's preferred route.

Treatment Plan

Cocaine abstinence was the first priority in Bill's treatment plan and is always the main focus in this treatment approach. Next, we recommended alcohol abstinence due to the close relationship between Bill's cocaine and alcohol use. As mentioned earlier, Bill was unwilling to change his use of marijuana despite the rationales we provided regarding both the benefits of doing so and potential adverse consequences of continuing to smoke. Our clinical approach was to look for opportunities during the course of treatment to reinforce any movement toward reducing or discontinuing marijuana use, but not to make Bill's reluctance to change this problem behavior a point of contention. Reestablishing a regular pattern of involvement in healthy recreational activities, especially activities that might substitute for cocaine and alcohol use on weekends, was a high-priority goal. The therapist provided the following rationale to Bill as to why we deemed participation in these activities to be a high priority:

THERAPIST: Many times, when cocaine or other drugs become a regular part of someone's life, they stop doing many of the nondrug activities they used to enjoy. That seems to be true in your case. You used to do lots of healthy recreational activities, but after getting into cocaine use you got away from those other activities.

BILL: No doubt. It's funny too, because I'm not even sure how that happened. Just gradually got off into different things. Never really stopped liking the other stuff. Just seems like I sort of drifted away from them.

THERAPIST: That's a pretty common report. You have a lot going for you though, Bill. You have a history of doing these healthier activities and having liked them. That's a strength that you'll be able to build upon during treatment.

BILL: Good, haven't felt like I've had too many strengths lately. But how do we do this? What's the connection to my cocaine use?

THERAPIST: Healthy social and recreational activities are important in people's lives. They provide something positive to look forward to after work, a way to decrease boredom and to feel healthy, and a chance to be with people you like. Such activities can play an important part in becoming and staying cocaine free. When you give up using drugs, you have to do something else during the times you used to use. If the things you do are not satisfying or enjoyable, or you don't do anything but sit around and feel lonely or bored, you are more likely to use drugs. That is why we have a specific treatment component to assist you in developing a regular schedule of healthy social and recreational activities.

BILL: Yeah, that could be important for me. I don't find it easy to hang out around the house. I get bored, pretty antsy.

THERAPIST: OK, lets go right to work on these now. We gave you a daily planner. Lets plan some activities to do between today and your next clinic visit. We really have to think carefully about Friday night, because that's a high-risk night for you. We'll be doing a lot of this throughout therapy.

Another high priority was to assist Bill in finding an alternative source of employment that would permit him to have a more reasonable work schedule, and that paid well enough that he would not feel compelled to hold several jobs simultaneously. To further increase Bill's involvement in activities that were incompatible with the cocaine-abusing lifestyle, we assisted Bill in petitioning for visitation privileges with his daughter. Regarding other psychiatric problems, we decided to monitor Bill's BDI scores weekly to see whether they followed the precipitous decline that typically occurs with cocaine-dependent patients within a couple of weeks of entering treatment. Because anger management had been a problem for Bill previously in dealing with his estranged partner, and because he would have to interact with her if he was to obtain visitation privileges, we deemed anger-management treatment appropriate.

Below we outline the progress made in implementing this treatment plan.

Cocaine Abstinence

Contingent vouchers, as the primary intervention for promoting initial abstinence, were made available to Bill according to our standard 12-week protocol. Functional analysis was also implemented with Bill during Sessions 1 and 2. Circumstances that increased the likelihood that Bill would use were being at a bar or certain friends' houses, using alcohol, ending a particularly long work week, and experiencing depression or boredom. He identified going to the movies or a safe friend's house, hunting, fishing, and skiing as circumstances that decreased his likelihood of using. That information was updated and used throughout Bill's course of treatment in self-management planning and in planning for social and recreational activities.

Shown in Figure 13.5 is a cumulative record of Bill's cocaine use and urinalysis results during the 24-week treatment. His only instance of use occurred 7 weeks into treatment. Bill reported being surprised by the results and said that he had smoked marijuana with several friends, and that perhaps some cocaine had been in the pipe.

THERAPIST: Hi, Bill. How have things been going?

BILL: Pretty good.

THERAPIST: Look, the lab just called with your urinalysis results. You're positive for cocaine.

BILL: No way. That can't be right. Wow, I have-

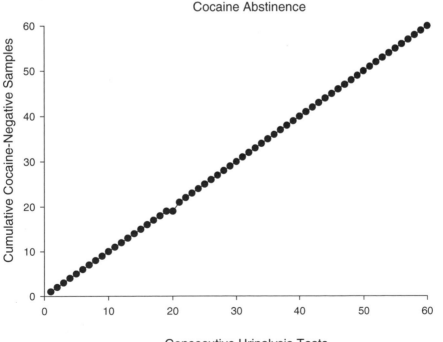

FIGURE 13.5. Shown is a cumulative record of Bill's urinalysis test results (*Y* axis) across 60 consecutive urinalysis tests (*X* axis) conducted during 24 weeks of treatment.

n't used cocaine. Didn't do much of anything over the weekend.

THERAPIST: That's how the machine read the sample. Let's talk more specifically about what you did over the weekend. Let's review what did you on each of the days, and perhaps that will give us some insights into what might be going on.

BILL: Just shut down the shop around midnight and went home and went to bed on Friday night. I worked Saturday morning. After I got off work, I hung out with some friends for a while.

THERAPIST: No gym like you planned?

BILL: Nah. Should have, but got sidetracked by running into some buddies I hadn't seen in a while.

THERAPIST: Any of those guys use cocaine?

BILL: Yeah, one does, but he knows I'm in treatment. I used to use cocaine with him. He doesn't do any cocaine around me now though.

THERAPIST: What exactly did you guys do?

BILL: Just hung out at this one buddies house, played video games, and watched some television. We smoked a couple of bowls of pot. You know I'm still smoking. Could be that the bowl we used had been used to smoke cocaine in recently. Bet that was it.

THERAPIST: Could be. What is pretty clear is that by getting off track of what you had planned, you increased your vulnerability for problems.

BILL: Yeah, I agree. I'm not sure I understand why I did that. I've been doing really well with sticking with my plans even when I run into the guys. Was supposed to get a ride to the gym from my mom, but it was a nice day, so I told her I'd walk. Saw these dudes, started talking, and just sort of bagged my plans for the gym.

THERAPIST: I have no doubt about that you've been doing a great job up to now with sticking with your plans. Bill, you've been doing terrific with abstaining from cocaine. That is not easy to do and you deserve a tremendous amount of credit for all of the work you've been doing.

BILL: Shoot, kind of blew it here.

THERAPIST: Important thing is to try to learn from what happened. As you know, my rec-

ommendation from the start of treatment has been to abstain from marijuana use. Marijuana has its own problems, plus it puts you into contact with other drug abusers, sometimes including cocaine users.

BILL: I agree with that to some extent, but I don't really think that marijuana was the problem here. I've been smoking regularly since starting treatment and have been able to stay away from cocaine. What is different here is that I hung out all day instead of sticking with my plan to go to the gym. That's where I screwed up. That's the big difference from what I had been doing on the other weekends.

THERAPIST: Good job with your analysis. Keep in mind though, if you weren't still smoking, you wouldn't have had any need to use a pipe—yours or theirs. Nevertheless, your point is well taken regarding what you did differently this weekend compared to the others since you've been in treatment. Sticking with the plans for alternative activities rather than just hanging out has really been working for you. I agree with you about that. The most important thing to do here is to learn from this situation and move on. What do you think you need to do to be sure you'll be cocaine-negative on Wednesday?

BILL: Well, I guess just keep doing what I've been doing—sticking to my plans: work, visit Mom, and I have a date tomorrow night. I'm scheduled to go to the gym tonight, and I'm definitely sticking with that. Being clean next time won't be a problem.

THERAPIST: How about minimizing your contact with any drug users, especially people you've used cocaine with in the past? We could even role-play how you might tell the guys how you have to be going, in case you run into them again.

BILL: I guess I could do that. I don't see most of those guys that often anyway. Yeah, sure.

THERAPIST: Good. As you know, we have to go by the urinalysis results. So you won't earn a voucher today and their value gets reset back to the original low value because of today's positive result. However, if you can get back on track with providing negative samples, five consecutive negatives mean that the value of the vouchers get reset back to where they were before today's positive.

BILL: That's fair enough.

Our experience is that there is little need to quibble over a client's denial of a single instance of cocaine use. If the client has resumed regular cocaine use, a pattern of positives will soon emerge. Instead, the therapist reviewed with Bill the risks of continuing to smoke marijuana while working on maintaining cocaine abstinence (continuing contact with drug-using friends, high-risk places, using marijuana rather than other possible activities or way to relax). They also reviewed the importance of sticking with planned activities and prepared to role-play some social skills that Bill could use to resist changing his plans should he run into drug-using friends again. Bill was very insightful about how he had deviated from what had been working for him up to this point—planning activities and sticking to the plans—and the therapist reinforced his analysis. The matter of denying cocaine use was not pursued further. Bill and the therapist carried on with implementing the treatment plan, with the few modifications mentioned. There were no further instances of cocaine use during Bill's 24 weeks of treatment. His record of documented cocaine abstinence was excellent.

Alcohol Abstinence

During the first session, the therapist discussed with Bill the rationale for disulfiram therapy:

THERAPIST: Bill, we want to go over at a few reasons for you to give disulfiram therapy and alcohol abstinence a try. First, your history indicates that if you drink, you are more likely to use cocaine. You're not alone in that regard. The scientific evidence is very clear that, for many individuals who seek treatment for cocaine dependence, alcohol and cocaine use are closely linked.

BILL: I don't want to get drunk any more. What about just a few drinks? Is that a problem too?

THERAPIST: Use of even modest doses of alcohol, even just a few drinks, can significantly decrease your chances of successfully abstaining from cocaine use. Our experience, and the experience in other clinics elsewhere around the country, is that you can make greater progress with cocaine abstinence by using disulfiram and abstaining from alcohol use than if you continue to drink.

BILL: How long are you suggesting I take the medicine? Are you saying I can never drink again?

THERAPIST: I'm not saying that you'll have to take this medicine forever or for years, or anything of that nature, or even that you can never go back to drinking. We can cross those bridges a ways down the road. But for now, if you want to give yourself the best chance to succeed with quitting cocaine, I recommend that you give disulfiram therapy a sincere try.

BILL: I'm not sure how much of a problem drinking is for me. I know it's caused some problems, but I'm just not so sure.

THERAPIST: Bill, the second thing I wanted to emphasize is that you also reported a history of depression and suicidal ideation. Substance use, particularly alcohol use, is a depressant and can worsen depressive symptoms and suicide risk. A period of abstinence may help a good deal with those problems. And still another point to consider is that agreeing to disulfiram therapy represents a concrete demonstration of your commitment to drug abstinence and substantial lifestyle changes. This would be helpful in general, but it could also be helpful in your pursuit of visitation privileges with your daughter.

BILL: Hey, I'm looking to make some progress here. When I've tried to quit cocaine on my own, it's not worked for beans. Maybe it's because I kept drinking, I'm not sure. I can't continue like this. How about I take the medicine during treatment? That's a pretty good commitment. What did you say, treatment is for 24 weeks? Lets say I'll go on the medicine for that amount of time.

Bill agreed to disulfiram therapy for the duration of treatment. A schedule was set up for Bill to ingest a 250 mg dose three times per week, under the observation of clinic staff, and to ingest the same dose under the observation of his father at home on alternating days.

In addition to disulfiram therapy, the therapist worked with Bill to functionally analyze his alcohol use, similar to the preceding process for cocaine. They reviewed specific circumstances under which Bill was more likely to drink or less likely to drink, and listed the negative consequences he had previously experienced from his alcohol use. The therapist and Bill then began to develop a plan for finding alternative ways to relax that did not involve the bar or drinking, as well as to rehearse how to refuse alcohol when it was offered, and how to identify times that Bill might be tempted to have a drink.

Bill was compliant with disulfiram therapy throughout treatment. He reported only one instance of alcohol use while on disulfiram therapy, when he did not take the medication on a Sunday morning and drank two beers at home that afternoon. On Monday, the therapist did a functional analysis with Bill to identify what set up the occasion for him to drink, and what had happened with his father serving as disulfiram assurance monitor. The therapist and Bill reviewed again his history of alcohol use and the negative consequences he had experienced in the past. Bill recommitted to alcohol abstinence and resumed disulfiram therapy.

When the end of the 24-week treatment approached (Week 23), Bill expressed a desire to "be able to have a drink if he wanted" and asked to discontinue disulfiram therapy, as planned. The therapist expressed his concerns about jeopardizing the substantial progress Bill had made.

THERAPIST: So you're due to end disulfiram therapy this week?

BILL: Yep, stuck to it like I promised, but now I'd like to be able to drink if I want to, like having a beer after work to relax. Nothing major.

THERAPIST: Bill, you've done really well so far with this current plan. Most folks are not as successful as you've been in stopping cocaine use.

BILL: Oh, I agree. I just feel like I've done really well in treatment and now that it's almost over, I'd like to be able to have that choice to drink if I want to.

THERAPIST: How risky do you think going off disulfiram is going to be for you in terms of continuing your success with abstaining from cocaine?

BILL: I really don't think it's going to be a problem. I'm feeling pretty confident about that.

THERAPIST: Bill, that's great. That sort of confidence is important to success. Let's talk about some specifics though. Remember, your alcohol history is still with you. In the past you've had periods of binge drinking combined with cocaine use. What's going to be different now from that past history?

BILL: Well, first of all, I don't plan on drinking like I used to. I'm not looking to get drunk. I'm not even sure I want to drink very often. Also, I'm not going to drink in bars. That's how I've gotten into trouble in the past. And I'm not going to drink with the same old crowd. I just want to know that if I go out to dinner on a date or something and want to have a drink, I can do that.

THERAPIST: You've given this careful consideration, which is good. Those kind of plans are important to continuing your success. Let's talk a bit more about how you can reduce your risk as much as possible if you're going to resume drinking. By that, I mean how often you drink, how much you drink per occasion, where and with whom you drink—more or less, anything you can do to protect yourself from excessive drinking and, subsequently, cocaine use. Does this sound reasonable to you?

BILL: Yeah, sure, that sounds really good.

At this time, the therapist began the clinic's controlled drinking protocol (see Miller & Munoz, 2005). Our primary clinical recommendation was abstinence, but Bill was not going to follow that recommendation. Hence, we felt that attempting systematically to provide him with some skills to decrease the likelihood of abusive or harmful drinking was indicated. The Miller and Munoz (2005) approach aims to teach skills that enable the client to drink in a controlled manner. Some of these skills are the same as those used with cocaine use, including functional analysis to identify the circumstances (location, people, times, feeling states) associated with heavy drinking. Others are specific to alcohol consumption (e.g., providing information about the alcohol content of common drinks, relationship between drinks consumed, body weight, and the blood alcohol curve). Bill and the therapist worked through some of the core elements of the controlled-drinking protocol during the final week of treatment, then covered the remaining parts during aftercare. Bill reported one instance of alcohol use during he final week of treatment. He had only two drinks and did not use cocaine. As we note below, Bill also has reported little drinking during posttreatment follow-up.

Other Drug Use

Bill continued the same pattern of marijuana use that he reported in the intake interview. He repeatedly asserted that marijuana use was not interfering with his other treatment goals. In turn, the therapist provided rationales for stopping or reducing marijuana use on numerous occasions but was not successful in initiating abstinence.

Recreational Activities

During the first several sessions, the therapist and Bill discussed the importance of developing new recreational activities. They decided on a goal of participating in four of these activities per week, as well as a plan to sample some new activities in the company of clinic staff. The therapist reminded Bill that the vouchers he would be earning during treatment for cocaine abstinence could be used to help pay for these activities.

During treatment, Bill consistently met his goal of four recreational activities per week. Those activities included movies, hunting, golf, and dinners at local restaurants. He used his vouchers to buy tickets to a performance at a local theater, greens fees to play golf, a gym membership, hunting and fishing licenses, and gift certificates to a local restaurant for dinner with a new girlfriend.

Family/Social Support

During the first few sessions, the therapist discussed with Bill the need for him to expand his social network to include family, friends, and other social contacts with non-drug-using people. Bill expressed a desire for increased contact with his daughter. Towards that end, Bill and his therapist completed a task analysis identifying the sequence of steps that would have to be taken to try to attain visitation privileges. These included requesting and completing legal forms from the court, helping Bill to discuss his wishes appropriately with his former partner, role plays in preparation for the court date, and accompanying him to court.

Bill succeeded in obtaining visitation privileges. His goal then became twice-weekly contact with his daughter, which he maintained consistently throughout the remainder of treatment.

Regarding other types of social support, Bill also increased contact with a couple of safe friends during the course of treatment. He also was able to meet several women through his new employment (discussed below), one of whom he began dating regularly.

Employment/Education

Bill came to treatment with a history of full-time employment, which is a good prognostic indicator in itself. However, his job upon entering treatment did not pay well and involved being around drinking. He expressed a desire to find a job that offered better pay, thereby allowing him to work fewer hours per week, to spend more time with his daughter, and to be at reduced risk for alcohol use. Therefore, Bill began participating in Job Club, coming to the clinic three times per week to go through local employment classifieds, complete a resume and cover letters with the help of staff, fill out job applications, and rehearse for job interviews. Bill successfully obtained a better paying job with fewer risks for alcohol use. Thereafter, his vocational goal was focused on avoiding excessive hours.

Bill also expressed concern regarding the extensive debt that he had accumulated during this prolonged cocaine use. The therapist began the clinic's money-management protocol, including developing a budget for repayment of outstanding loans and skills for managing personal finances. Bill opened a savings account at a nearby bank and arranged for direct deposit of his paychecks. Bill used the phone in his therapist's office to arrange payback plans with several debtors. He consistently made payments on his debt throughout treatment, which the therapist graphed weekly and, by the end of treatment, had eliminated all back debt and was now paying current bills.

Bill had a long-term vocational goal of eventually opening his own retail business. He and his therapist completed a preliminary task analysis (see Sulzer-Azaroff & Meyer, 1991) related to that goal. They agreed that taking accounting and computer courses would be a good start. The therapist helped Bill collect information from the local community college on the classes being offered. Bill requested financial aid applications from the community college for assistance with tuition, which his therapist helped him complete.

Psychiatric Monitoring

Recall that Bill's BDI score at intake was 23. His BDI score had dropped precipitously by the second week of treatment, and reached a score of 2 by the end of treatment.

Bill and his therapist worked through an anger management protocol for substance abusers (Monti, Kadden, Rohsenow, Cooney, & Abrams, 2002). This protocol helped Bill identify situations that would likely make him angry, develop coping skills to better deal with those triggers, and role-play those coping skills to gain proficiency. The therapist had Bill document when potential anger-provoking situations arose outside of the clinic and how he handled them. The therapist reviewed that information weekly, provided social reinforcement for those situations that were handled well, and problem-solved and role-played alternatives when Bill needed assistance.

Summary of Treatment Progress

Bill made substantial progress toward establishing a stable record of cocaine abstinence, eliminating problem drinking, increasing his involvement in social and recreational practices, improving his job situation, increasing his skill in managing anger, and in improving his relationship with his daughter. The one area in which we were unable to make progress was Bill's use of marijuana and associated involvement with the illicit drug abuse community. This progress is reflected in the pre- to posttreatment changes in ASI composite scores shown in Table 13.7. Composite scores range

from 0, representing no problems in the past 30 days to 1, representing severe problems. Bill's scores at the end-of-treatment assessment generally reflected substantial improvements.

Follow-Up

Following completion of the 24-week treatment protocol, Bill participated in a 6-month aftercare program and completed periodic follow-up assessments for 4 years after treatment entry (see Table 13.7). Thus, we have a relatively good picture of his progress.

Bill largely sustained the excellent progress he made during treatment toward resolving his cocaine-use problems. All urine toxicology tests conducted during follow-up were negative for cocaine use. He reported two instances of cocaine use during the 3.5-year follow-up period, but they were separated in time, and neither resulted in a full-blown relapse. He reported moderate use of alcohol throughout follow-up, with only one instance of drinking to intoxication. He continued to smoke marijuana regularly, as he had done during treatment.

Regarding other areas of functioning, Bill sustained full-time employment throughout the follow-up period. There was an episode of criminal justice involvement at the 12-month assessment that according to Bill was unrelated to substance abuse and was resolved before the later assessments. His depressive symptomatology remained well below intake levels throughout the follow-up period. Progress in other areas of functioning largely was sustained through follow-up, until the 48-month assess-

TABLE 13.7. ASI Subscale and BDI Scores at Intake, End of Treatment, and Posttreatment Follow-Up Assessments

Score	Intake	End of treatment	12 months	24 months	36 months	48 months
ASI subscales						
Medical	0.42	0.09	0.09	0.18	0.00	1.00
Employment	0.07	0.10	0.09	0.11	0.13	0.08
Alcohol	0.13	0.00	0.06	0.00	0.05	0.11
Drug (other than cocaine)	0.28	0.07	0.08	0.08	0.09	0.19
Cocaine	0.66	0.00	0.00	0.00	0.00	0.00
Legal	0.00	0.00	0.40	0.00	0.00	0.00
Family/Social	0.22	0.10	0.00	0.00	0.00	0.22
Psychological	0.36	0.00	0.09	0.09	0.18	0.53
BDI	23	1	3	5	10	6

ment, when a medical crisis arose. Bill developed a neuromuscular condition involving periodic episodes of full paralysis. He was also experiencing more routine but nevertheless painful dental problems. At the time of that assessment, Bill was still undergoing testing for the neuromuscular problem and did not have a diagnosis. This crisis had not precipitated a relapse back to cocaine or other drug abuse, which underscores the substantial progress he made with those problems. The increases in ASI drug scale scores at that 48-month assessment were related to taking pain medication for the dental problems. Clearly, though, the medical conditions were having a destabilizing effect on Bill physically and psychologically. Although he recognized that the situation put him at increased risk for relapse, he did not deem the situation at that time to warrant reentry into treatment. Treatment staff commended Bill on his sustained progress in abstaining from cocaine and alcohol abuse and reassured him that he could return to treatment if the need arose.

CONCLUDING COMMENTS

In this chapter we have presented the most up-to-date scientific information available on effective clinical management of illicit drug use disorders. In the process, we have tried to illustrate what have come to be considered principles of effective treatment for illicit drug use disorders in general, using cocaine dependence as a specific exemplar. We have emphasized one efficacious, multielement treatment approach but have underscored how it contains elements of all of the empirically based behavioral and cognitive-behavioral therapies except behavioral family therapy. We realize that limitations in resources and other practical constraints will prevent many clinicians from utilizing the treatment practices just as we have outlined them in this chapter. Costs for the treatment provided to Bill were covered exclusively through a research grant. However, we hope that this information offers insights into the important elements of effective treatment for illicit drug use disorders. We also hope that this information makes the job of clinicians who are out there in the trenches treating the drug-dependent population a little easier and, we hope, their practices more effective.

ACKNOWLEDGMENT

Preparation of this chapter was supported in part by National Institute on Drug Abuse Grant Nos. DA09378, DA07242, and DA08076.

REFERENCES

American Psychiatric Association. (2000). *Diagnostic and statistical manual of mental disorders* (4th ed., text rev.). Washington, DC: Author.

Azrin, N. H. (1976). Improvements in the community-reinforcement approach to alcoholism. *Behaviour Research and Therapy, 14*, 339–348.

Azrin, N. H., & Besalel, V. A. (1980). *Job club counselor's manual*. Baltimore: University Park Press.

Azrin, N. H., Donohue, B., Besalel, V. A., Kogan, E. S., & Acierno, R. (1994). Youth drug abuse treatment: A controlled outcome study. *Journal of Child and Adolescent Substance Abuse, 3*, 1–16.

Beck, A. T., Ward, C. H., Mendelson, M., Mock, J., & Erbaugh, J. (1961). An inventory for measuring depression. *Archives of General Psychiatry, 4*, 561–571.

Bellack, A. S., Bennett, M. E., Gearson, J. S., Brown, C. H., & Yang, Y. (2006). A randomized clinical trial of a new behavioral treatment for drug abuse in people with severe and persistent mental illness. *Archives of General Psychiatry, 63*, 426–432.

Bickel, W. K., Amass, L., Higgins, S. T., Badger, G. J., & Esch, R. A. (1997). Effects of adding behavioral treatment to opioid detoxification with buprenorphine. *Journal of Consulting and Clinical Psychology, 65*, 803–810.

Budney, A. J., & Higgins, S. T. (1998). *The community reinforcement plus vouchers approach: Manual 2: National Institute on Drug Abuse therapy manuals for drug addiction* (NIH Publication No. 98-4308). Rockville, MD: National Institute on Drug Abuse.

Budney, A. J., Higgins, S. T., & Wong, C. J. (1996). Marijuana use and treatment outcome in cocaine-dependent patients. *Journal of Experimental and Clinical Psychopharmacology, 4*, 1–8.

Carroll, K. M., Nich, C., Ball, S. A., McCance, E., & Rounsaville, B. J. (1998). Treatment of cocaine and alcohol dependence with psychotherapy and disulfiram. *Addiction, 93*, 713–727.

Carroll, K. M., & Onken, L. S. (2005). Behavioral therapies for drug abuse. *American Journal of Psychiatry, 162*, 1452–1460.

Carroll, K. M., Rounsaville, B. J., Nich, C., Gordon, L. T., Wirtz, P. W., & Gawin, F. (1994). One-year follow-up of psychotherapy and pharmacotherapy for cocaine dependence: Delayed emergence of psychotherapy effects. *Archives of General Psychiatry, 51*, 989–997.

Derogatis, L. R. (1983). *SCL-90-R: Administration,*

scoring and procedures manual—II. Towson, MD: Clinical Psychometric Research.

Dunn, C., Deroo, L., & Rivara, F. P. (2001). The use of brief interventions adapted from motivational interviewing across behavioral domains: A systematic review. *Addiction, 96,* 1725–1742.

Fals-Stewart, W., & O'Farrell, T. J. (2003). Behavioral family counseling and naltrexone for male opioid-dependent patients. *Journal of Consulting and Clinical Psychology, 71,* 432–442.

Fals-Stewart, W., O'Farrell, T. J., & Birchler, G. R. (2001). Behavioral couples therapy for male methadone patients: Effects on drug-using behavior and relationship adjustment. *Behavior Therapy, 32,* 391–411.

Festinger, D. S., Lamb, R. J., Kirby, K. C., & Marlowe, D. B. (1996). The accelerated intake: A method for increasing initial attendance to outpatient cocaine treatment. *Journal of Applied Behavior Analysis, 29,* 387–389.

Griffith, J. D., Rowan-Szal, Roark, R. R., & Simpson, D. D. (2000). Contingency management in outpatient methadone treatment: A meta-analysis. *Drug and Alcohol Dependence, 58,* 55–66.

Griffiths, R. R., Bigelow, G. E., & Henningfield, J. E. (1980). Similarities in animal and human drug taking behavior. In N. K. Mello (Ed.), *Advances in substance abuse: behavioral and biological research* (pp. 1–90). Greenwich, CT: JAI Press.

Heil, S. H., Sigmon, S. C., Mongeon, J. A., & Higgins, S. T. (2005). Characterizing and improving HIV/AIDS knowledge among cocaine-dependent outpatients. *Experimental and Clinical Psychopharmacology, 13,* 238–243.

Henggeler, S. W., Pickrel, S. G., Brondino, M. J., & Crouch, J. L. (1996). Eliminating (almost) treatment dropout of substance abusing or dependent delinquents through home-based multisystemic therapy. *American Journal of Psychiatry, 153,* 427–428.

Higgins, S. T. (1997). The influence of alternative reinforcers on cocaine use and abuse: A brief review. *Pharmacology Biochemistry and Behavior, 57,* 419–427.

Higgins, S. T., Badger, G. B., & Budney, A. J. (2000). Initial abstinence and success in achieving longer term cocaine abstinence. *Experimental and Clinical Psychopharmacology, 8,* 377–386.

Higgins, S. T., & Katz, J. L. (Eds.). (1998). *Cocaine abuse: Behavior, pharmacology, and clinical applications.* San Diego, CA: Academic Press.

Higgins, S. T., Sigmon, S. C., Wong, C. J., Heil, S. H., Badger, G. J., Donham, R., et al. (2003). Community reinforcement therapy for cocaine-dependent outpatients. *Archives of General Psychiatry, 60,* 1043–1052.

Higgins, S. T., Silverman, K., & Heil, S. H. (2008). *Contingency management in substance abuse use treatment.* New York: Guilford Press.

Higgins, S. T., Wong, C. J., Badger, G. J., Ogden, D. E., & Dantona, R. L. (2000). Contingent reinforcement increases cocaine abstinence during outpatient treatment and 1 year of follow-up. *Journal of Consulting and Clinical Psychology, 68,* 64–72.

Irvin, J. E., Bowers, C. A., Dunn, M. E., & Wong, M. C. (1999). Efficacy of relapse prevention: A meta-analytic review. *Journal of Consulting and Clinical Psychology, 67,* 563–570.

Kenford, S. L., & Fiore, M. C. (2004). Promoting tobacco cessation and relapse prevention. *Medical Clinics of North America, 88,* 1553–1574.

Lewinsohn, P. M., Munoz, R. F., Youngren, M. A., & Zeiss, A. M. (1986). *Control your depression.* New York: Simon & Schuster.

Liddle, H. A., & Dakof, G., Parker, K., Diamond, G. S., Barrett, K., & Tejeda, M. (2001). Multidimensional family therapy for adolescent drug abuse: Results of a randomized clinical trial. *American Journal of Drug and Alcohol Abuse, 27,* 651–688.

Lussier, J. P., Heil, S. H., Mongeon, J. A., Badger, G. J., & Higgins, S. T. (2006). A meta-analysis of voucher-based reinforcement therapy for substance use disorders. *Addiction, 101*(2), 192–203.

Martino, S., Carroll, K. M., & Rounsaville, B. J. (2006). A randomized controlled pilot study of motivational interviewing for patients with psychotic and drug use disorders. *Addiction, 101,* 1479–1492.

McLellan, A. T., Luborsky, L., Cacciola, J., Griffith, J., Evans, F., Barr, H., et al. (1985). New data from the Addiction Severity Index. *Journal of Nervous and Mental Disease, 173,* 412–423.

Meyers, R. J., & Smith, J. E. (1995). *Clinical guide to alcohol treatment: The community reinforcement approach.* New York: Guilford Press.

Miller, W. R., & Munoz, R. F. (2005). *Controlling your drinking: Tools to make moderation work for you.* New York: Guilford Press.

Miller, W. R., & Rollnick, S. (2002). *Motivational interviewing: Preparing people for change* (2nd ed.). New York: Guilford Press.

Miller, W. R., & Tonigan, J. S. (1996). Assessing drinkers' motivation for change: The Stages of Change Readiness and Treatment Eagerness Scale (SOCRATES). *Psychology of Addictive Behaviors, 10,* 81–89.

Monti, P. M., Kadden, R. M., Rohsenow, D. J., Cooney, N. L., & Abrams, D. B. (2002). *Treating alcohol dependence: A coping skills training guide* (2nd ed.). New York: Guilford Press.

Monti, P. M., Rohsenow, D. J., Michalec, E., Martin, R. A., & Abrams, D. B. (1997). Brief coping skills treatment for cocaine abuse: Substance use outcomes at three months. *Addiction, 92,* 1717–1728.

Morin, C. M. (2004). Cognitive-behavioral approaches to the treatment of insomnia. *Journal of Clinical Psychiatry, 65,* 33–40.

Munoz, R. F., & Miranda, J. (2000). *Individual therapy manual for cognitive behavioral treatment for depression.* Santa Monica, CA: RAND Corporation.

National Institute on Drug Abuse (NIDA). (1999). *Prin-*

ciples of addiction treatment: A research-based guide (NIH Publication No. 99-4180). Rockville, MD: National Institute on Drug Abuse.

O'Farrell, T. J., & Fals-Stewart, W. (2002). Behavioral couples and family therapy for substance abusers. Current Psychiatry Reports, 4, 371–376.

Office of National Drug Control Policy. (2004). The economic costs of drug abuse in the United States, 1992-2002 (Publication No. 207303). Washington, DC: Executive Office of the President.

Petry, N. M., Peirce, J. M., Stitzer, M. L., Blaine, J., Roll, J. M., Cohen, A., et al. (2005). Effect of prize-based incentives on outcomes in stimulant abusers in outpatient psychosocial treatment programs: A national drug abuse treatment clinical trials network study. Archives of General Psychiatry, 62, 1148–1156.

Rawson, R. A., Marinelli-Casey, P., Anglin, M. D., Dickow, A., Frazier, Y., Gallagher, C., et al. (2004). A multi-site comparison of psychosocial approaches for the treatment of methamphetamine dependence. Addiction, 99, 708–717.

Rodebaugh, T. L., Holaway, R. M., & Heimberg, R. G. (2004). The treatment of social anxiety disorder. Clinical Psychology Review, 24, 883–908.

Roozen, H. G., Boulogne, J. J., van Tulder, M. W., van den Brink, W., De Jong, C. A., & Kerkhof, A. J. (2004). A systematic review of the effectiveness of the community reinforcement approach in alcohol, cocaine and opioid addiction. Drug and Alcohol Dependence, 74, 1–13.

Schnoll, R. A., & Lerman, C. (2006). Current and emerging pharmacotherapies for treating tobacco dependence. Expert Opinion on Emerging Drugs, 11, 429–444.

Selzer, M. L. (1971). The Michigan Alcoholism Screening Test. American Journal of Psychiatry, 127, 89–94.

Silverman, K., Robles, E., Mudric, T., & Stitzer, M. L. (2004). A randomized trial of long-term reinforcement of cocaine abstinence in methadone-maintained patients who inject drugs. Journal of Consulting and Clinical Psychology, 72, 839–854.

Sobell, L. C., & Sobell, M. B. (1992). Timeline followback: A technique for assessing self-reported alcohol consumption. In R. Z. Litten & J. P. Allen (Eds.), Measuring alcohol consumption: Psychosocial and biochemical methods (pp. 41–72). Totowa, NJ: Humana Press.

Substance Abuse and Mental Health Services Administration (SAHMSA). (2006). Results from the 2005 National Survey on Drug Use and Health: National Findings (Office of Applied Studies, NSDUH Series H-30, DHHS Publication No. SMA 06-4194). Rockville, MD: Author.

Sulzer-Azaroff, B., & Meyer, G. R. (1991). Behavior analysis for lasting change. Fort Worth, TX: Holt, Rinehart & Winston.

Vasilaki, E. I., Hosier, S. G., & Cox, W. M. (2006). The efficacy of motivational interviewing as a brief intervention for excessive drinking: A meta-analytic review. Alcohol and Alcoholism, 41, 328–335.

Washton, A. M., Stone, N. S., & Hendrickson, E. C. (1988). Cocaine abuse. In D. M. Donovan & G. A. Marlatt (Eds.), Assessment of addictive behaviors (pp. 364–389). New York: Guilford Press.

CHAPTER 14

Eating Disorders
A TRANSDIAGNOSTIC PROTOCOL

CHRISTOPHER G. FAIRBURN
ZAFRA COOPER
ROZ SHAFRAN
G. TERENCE WILSON

The fourth edition of the *Diagnostic and Statistical Manual of Mental Disorders* (DSM-IV) clearly defined and separated anorexia nervosa and bulimia nervosa, and described for the first time a provisional new eating disorder termed "binge-eating disorder." But we now know that many people with serious eating disorders do not quite fit the current diagnostic criteria and are lumped into a "not otherwise specified" (NOS) category. It is also the case that individuals with eating disorders change from one category to another over time. This chapter is written by authors involved in the creation of the DSM-IV eating disorder categories, who are also among the originators of the most successful treatment yet devised for these disorders. Thus, it is significant that Fairburn and colleagues have moved ahead of the curve and created a "transdiagnostic" unified theory and treatment protocol applicable to all eating disorders. (For a similar approach to anxiety disorder, see Chapter 5) In this chapter they describe this state-of-the-art treatment for the first time. In what may be a surprising departure to some readers, the authors note that the central problem requiring intervention is not necessarily dieting, bingeing, or purging, but rather the culturally reinforced abnormal attitudes and beliefs regarding shape and weight. The recommendation for applying various treatment components in a "modular" fashion speaks to the art of administering this treatment. The detailed explication of cognitive-behavioral therapy as applied to eating disorders should be extraordinarily useful to clinicians working with these difficult problems.—D. H. B.

Clinical eating disorders such as anorexia nervosa and bulimia nervosa are a cause of substantial physical and psychosocial morbidity among adolescent girls and young adult women. They are much less common among men. They typically begin in adolescence and may run a chronic course. Their effect is pervasive because they interfere with psychological, physical, and social functioning. Once established, they are difficult to treat and impose a significant burden on health services. In this chapter we describe the psychopathology of the eating disorders and the mechanisms that cause them to persist. We then describe a transdiagnostic cognitive-behavioral treatment designed to disrupt these mechanisms.

CLASSIFICATION AND DIAGNOSIS

The DSM-IV scheme for classifying and diagnosing eating disorders recognizes two specific disorders: anorexia nervosa and bulimia nervosa. In addition, there is a residual category termed "eating disorder not otherwise specified" (eating disorder NOS; American Psychiatric Association, 1994).

In essence, three features need to be present to make a diagnosis of anorexia nervosa:

1. The overevaluation of shape and weight; that is, judging self-worth largely, or even exclusively, in terms of shape and weight. This is often expressed as a strong desire to be thin combined with an intense fear of gaining weight and becoming fat.
2. The active maintenance of an unduly low body weight (e.g., maintaining a body weight less than 85% of that expected or a body mass index (BMI) $\leq 17.5^1$).
3. Amenorrhea (in postpubertal females). The value of this criterion is questionable since the majority of female patients who meet the other two diagnostic criteria are also amenorrheic, and those who are not closely resemble those who are.

Three features also need to be present to make a diagnosis of bulimia nervosa:

1. The overevaluation of shape and weight, as in anorexia nervosa.
2. Recurrent binge eating. A "binge" is an epi-sode of eating during which an objectively large amount of food is eaten and there is a sense of loss of control at the time.
3. Extreme weight-control behavior, such as strict dietary restriction, recurrent self-induced vomiting, or marked laxative misuse.

In addition, there is an exclusionary criterion, namely, that the diagnostic criteria for anorexia nervosa should not be met. This criterion ensures that it is not possible for patients to receive both diagnoses at one time.

There are no diagnostic criteria for eating disorder NOS. Rather, it is a residual category for eating disorders of clinical severity that do not meet the diagnostic criteria for anorexia nervosa or bulimia nervosa. Eating disorder NOS is the most common eating disorder diagnosis. In outpatient settings it typically constitutes about half the cases, with bulimia nervosa constituting about a third, and the remainder being cases of anorexia nervosa (Fairburn & Bohn, 2005). In inpatient settings the great majority of cases are either underweight forms of eating disorder NOS or anorexia nervosa, with relatively few cases of bulimia nervosa (Dalle Grave & Calugi, 2007).

The relationship among the three diagnoses is represented diagrammatically in Figure 14.1. The two overlapping inner circles represent an-

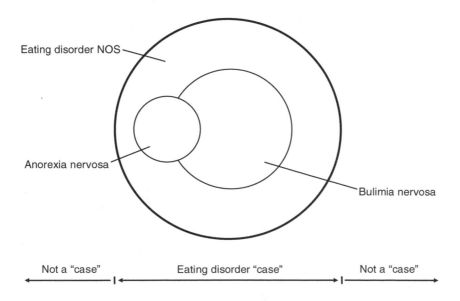

FIGURE 14.1. A schematic representation of the relationship between anorexia nervosa, bulimia nervosa, and eating disorder NOS. From Fairburn and Bohn (2005). Copyright 2005 by Elsevier. Reprinted by permission.

orexia nervosa (the smaller circle) and bulimia nervosa (the larger circle), respectively, with the area of potential overlap representing those people who would meet the diagnostic criteria for both disorders were it not for the DSM-IV "trumping" rule mentioned earlier. Surrounding these two circles is an outer circle that defines the boundary of eating disorder "caseness"; that is, the boundary between having an eating disorder, a state of clinical significance, and having a lesser, nonclinical eating problem. It is this boundary that demarcates what is, and is not, an eating disorder. Within the outer circle, but outside the two inner circles, lies eating disorder NOS.

In DSM-IV a new eating disorder diagnosis was proposed, termed "binge-eating disorder," to denote an eating problem characterized by recurrent binge eating in the absence of the extreme weight control behavior seen in bulimia nervosa. Because binge-eating disorder is a provisional diagnostic concept, it is currently an example of eating disorder NOS.

CLINICAL FEATURES

Anorexia nervosa and bulimia nervosa, and most cases of eating disorder NOS, share a distinctive "core psychopathology" that is essentially the same in females and males, adults and adolescents. This is the overevaluation of shape and weight. Whereas most people evaluate themselves on the basis of their perceived performance in a variety of domains of life (e.g., the quality of their relationships; their work performance; their sporting prowess), people with eating disorders judge their self-worth largely, or even exclusively, in terms of their shape and weight, and their ability to control them. This psychopathology is peculiar to the eating disorders (and to body dysmorphic disorder) and is rarely seen in the general population. It should be distinguished from body shape dissatisfaction, which refers to dislike of aspects of one's appearance. Body shape dissatisfaction is widespread, and its presence is sometimes referred to as "normative discontent."

The overevaluation of shape and weight results in the pursuit of weight loss—note that weight loss is sought, not a specific weight—and an intense fear of weight gain and fatness. Most other features of these disorders are secondary to this psychopathology and its conse-

quences (e.g., undereating; becoming severely underweight). Thus, in anorexia nervosa, a sustained and successful pursuit of weight loss results in patients becoming severely underweight. This pursuit is not seen as a problem: Rather, it is viewed as appropriate and, as a consequence, patients have little desire to change. Often it is other people who are responsible for these individuals' entry into treatment. In bulimia nervosa, equivalent attempts to restrict food intake are punctuated by repeated episodes of loss of control over eating (binges). Generally these binges are aversive and a source of distress, and they lead the patient to seek help. Consequently, patients with bulimia nervosa are easier to engage in treatment, although because of the accompanying shame and secrecy, there is typically a delay of many years before they divulge their eating problem and enter treatment.

The core psychopathology of anorexia nervosa and bulimia nervosa has other expressions too. Many patients mislabel adverse physical and emotional states as "feeling fat" and equate this with actually being fat. In addition, many repeatedly scrutinize their bodies, focusing on parts that they dislike. This may contribute to them overestimating their size. Others actively avoid seeing their bodies, assuming that they look fat and disgusting. Equivalent behavior is seen with respect to weighing (weight checking), with many patients weighing themselves frequently and as a result becoming preoccupied with trivial, day-to-day fluctuations, whereas others actively avoid knowing their weight but nevertheless remain highly concerned about it.

Anorexia Nervosa

In anorexia nervosa the pursuit of weight loss leads patients to engage in a severe and selective restriction of food intake, avoiding foods viewed as fattening. Generally there is no true "anorexia" (loss of appetite). The undereating may also be an expression of other motives, including asceticism, competitiveness, and a desire to attract attention from others. In the early stages of the disorder, undereating may be a goal in its own right, with the patient valuing the sense of self-control that it imparts. Some patients also engage in a driven type of exercising that contributes to their weight loss. This is characterized by a strong drive to exercise, a tendency to overexercise, and giving exercise precedence over other aspects of life. Self-induced vomiting and other extreme forms of weight control (e.g., the misuse of laxatives or diuretics) are practiced by a subgroup of these patients and an overlapping group have episodes of loss of control over eating, although the amount eaten may not be objectively large ("subjective binge eating"). Depressive and anxiety features, irritability, lability of mood, impaired concentration, loss of sexual appetite and obsessional symptoms are also frequently present. Typically these features get worse as weight is lost and improve with weight regain. Interest in the outside world also wanes as patients become underweight, with the result that most become socially withdrawn and isolated. This too tends to reverse with weight regain.

Bulimia Nervosa

The eating habits of individuals with bulimia nervosa resemble those seen in anorexia nervosa. The main distinguishing feature is that the attempts to restrict food intake are punctuated by repeated episodes of binge eating. The frequency of these episodes ranges from once or twice a week (the diagnostic threshold) to several times a day, and the amount eaten per episode varies but is typically between 1,000 and 2,000 kcal. In most cases, each binge is followed by compensatory self-induced vomiting or laxative misuse, but there is a subgroup of patients who do not "purge" (nonpurging bulimia nervosa). The weight of most patients with bulimia nervosa is in the healthy range (BMI between 20.0 and 25.0) due to the effects of undereating and overeating canceling each other out. As a result, these patients do not experience the secondary psychosocial and physical effects of maintaining a very low weight. Depressive and anxiety features are prominent in bulimia nervosa—indeed, more so than in anorexia nervosa—and there is a subgroup who engage in substance misuse or self-injury, or both. This subgroup, which is also present among some anorexia nervosa patients who binge eat, often attracts the diagnosis of borderline personality disorder.

Eating Disorder NOS

The psychopathology of eating disorder NOS closely resembles that seen in anorexia nervosa and bulimia nervosa. It is also of comparable duration and severity (Fairburn et al., 2007).

Conceptually, it is helpful to distinguish three subgroups within eating disorder NOS, although there is no sharp boundary between them. The first comprises cases that closely resemble anorexia nervosa or bulimia nervosa but just fail to meet their diagnostic criteria; for example, body weight may be marginally above the threshold for anorexia nervosa, or the frequency of binge eating may be too low for a diagnosis of bulimia nervosa. These cases may be viewed as "subthreshold" forms of anorexia nervosa or bulimia nervosa, respectively, and might be better included within these diagnoses. The second and largest subgroup comprises cases in which the clinical features of anorexia nervosa and bulimia nervosa are combined in a different way than that seen in the two prototypic disorders. Such states may be described as "mixed" in character. Patients with binge-eating disorder form the third subgroup. They report recurrent binge eating, much as in bulimia nervosa, but their eating habits outside the binges are quite different. As noted earlier, there is a high level of dietary restraint in bulimia nervosa, with most patients adhering to a highly restricted diet when not binge eating; in contrast, in binge-eating disorder there is a tendency to overeat outside the binges. Indeed, the eating habits of patients with binge-eating disorder resemble those of people with obesity, albeit with binges superimposed. Thus, self-induced vomiting and laxative misuse are not present, nor is there any tendency to overexercise. Most patients with binge-eating disorder are overweight or meet criteria for obesity (BMI ≥ 30.0).

DEVELOPMENT AND SUBSEQUENT COURSE

Anorexia nervosa typically starts in midteenage years with the onset of dietary restriction that becomes progressively more extreme and inflexible. In its early stages the disorder may be self-limiting and treatment-responsive, but if it persists, then it tends to become entrenched and requires more intensive treatment. In 10–20% of cases, it proves intractable and unremitting. Even in patients who recover, residual features are common, particularly some degree of overconcern about shape, weight, and eating. A frequent occurrence is the development of binge eating and, in about half the cases, progression to full bulimia nervosa. Most prominent among the favorable prognostic factors are an early age of onset and a short history, whereas unfavorable prognostic factors include a long history, severe weight loss, and binge eating and vomiting. In anorexia nervosa, the one eating disorder associated with a raised mortality rate, the standardized mortality ratio over the first 10 years from presentation is about 10. The majority of deaths are either a direct result of medical complications or suicide.

Bulimia nervosa has a slightly later age of onset, typically in late adolescence or early adulthood. It usually starts in much the same way as anorexia nervosa—indeed, in about one-fourth of cases the diagnostic criteria for anorexia nervosa are met for a time. Eventually, however, episodes of binge eating interrupt the dietary restriction and as a result body weight rises to normal or near normal levels. The disorder is highly self-perpetuating. Thus, patients often present with an unremitting history of 8 or more years of disturbed eating, and even 5 to 10 years after presentation between one-third and one-half still have an eating disorder of clinical severity, although in many cases it is a "mixed" form of eating disorder NOS. No consistent predictors of outcome have been identified, although there is evidence that childhood obesity, low self-esteem, and signs of personality disturbance are associated with a worse prognosis.

Almost nothing is known about the development and course of eating disorder NOS. Most patients present in their adolescence or 20s, as in bulimia nervosa, and with a comparable length of history. Between one-fourth and one-third have had anorexia nervosa or bulimia nervosa in the past; their present state is simply the latest expression of an evolving eating disorder.

Binge-eating disorder has a rather different age of presentation and course. Most of these patients are middle-aged, and one-third or more are male, quite unlike patients with anorexia nervosa, bulimia nervosa, and other forms of eating disorder NOS, who are generally adolescents or young adults and female (about 10% are male). Clinical experience suggests that binge-eating disorder also differs in its course, in that it tends to be phasic rather than persistent, with most patients describing sustained periods in which they are prone to binge eat and other times they are in control of their eating. Throughout, these patients have a general tendency to overeat and gain weight; few report a history of anorexia nervosa or bulimia nervosa.

THE "TRANSDIAGNOSTIC" PERSPECTIVE

The DSM-IV scheme for classifying eating disorders encourages the view that anorexia nervosa and bulimia nervosa are distinct clinical states, each requiring their own form of treatment. It should be clear from consideration of their clinical features and course over time that the evidence does not support this (Fairburn & Harrison, 2003). Binge eating disorder aside, patients with anorexia nervosa, bulimia nervosa and eating disorder NOS have many features in common, most of which are not seen in other psychiatric disorders, and studies of their course indicate that patients migrate between these diagnoses over time: indeed, temporal migration is the norm rather than the exception. This temporal movement, together with the fact that the disorders share the same distinctive psychopathology, suggests that common "transdiagnostic" mechanisms are involved in the persistence of eating disorder psychopathology (Fairburn, Cooper, & Shafran, 2003). If correct, this implies that treatments that are capable of successfully addressing these maintaining mechanisms should be effective with all forms of eating disorder rather than just one.

THE COGNITIVE-BEHAVIORAL THEORY OF THE MAINTENANCE OF EATING DISORDERS

Bulimia Nervosa

In common with most evidence-based cognitive-behavioral treatments, the theory that underpins cognitive-behavioral therapy for bulimia nervosa (CBT-BN) is primarily concerned with the processes that maintain bulimia nervosa rather than those responsible for its development. According to the theory, central to the maintenance of bulimia nervosa is these patients' dysfunctional scheme for self-evaluation. As noted earlier, whereas most people evaluate themselves on the basis of their perceived performance in a variety of domains of life, people with eating disorders judge themselves largely, or even exclusively, in terms of their shape and weight and their ability to control them. As a result, their lives become focused on their shape, weight, and eating, with dietary control, thinness, and weight loss being actively pursued while overeating, "fatness," and weight gain are assiduously avoided. Most of the other features of bulimia nervosa may be understood as stemming directly from this "core psychopathology," including the weight control behavior, the various forms of body checking and avoidance, and the preoccupation with thoughts about shape, weight, and eating. Figure 14.2 provides a schematic representation (or "formulation") of the main processes involved.

The only feature of bulimia nervosa that is not obviously a direct expression of the core psychopathology is these patients' binge eating. The cognitive-behavioral theory proposes that binge eating is largely a product of the particular way that these patients attempt to restrict their eating (i.e., their form of dietary restraint), irrespective of whether or not there is an actual energy deficit. Rather than adopting general guidelines about how they should eat, these patients try to adhere to multiple extreme and highly specific dietary rules. Accompanying these dietary rules is a tendency to react in a negative and extreme fashion to the (almost inevitable) breaking of them, such that even minor dietary slips are interpreted as evidence of lack of self-control. The result is that

patients respond by temporarily abandoning their efforts to restrict their eating and give in to the urge to eat. This produces a highly distinctive pattern of eating in which attempts to restrict eating are repeatedly interrupted by episodes of binge eating. The binge eating maintains the core psychopathology by intensifying patients' concerns about their ability to control their eating, shape, and weight. It also encourages yet greater dietary restraint, thereby increasing the risk of further binge eating.

It should be noted that these patients' dietary slips and binges do not come out of the blue; rather, they are particularly likely to occur in response to difficulties in patients' lives and associated changes in mood, in part because binge eating temporarily ameliorates negative mood states, and in part because it distracts patients from thinking about their difficulties.

A further process maintains binge eating among those patients who practice compensatory "purging" (i.e., those who induce vomiting or take laxatives in response to specific episodes of binge eating). Patients' faith in the ability of purging to minimize weight gain undermines a major deterrent against binge eating. They do not realize that vomiting only retrieves part of what has been eaten, and laxatives have little or no effect on energy absorption (see Fairburn, 1995).

This cognitive-behavioral account of the maintenance of bulimia nervosa has clear im-

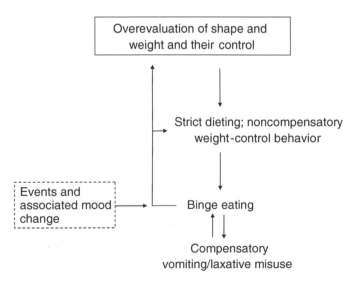

FIGURE 14.2. The cognitive-behavioral formulation of bulimia nervosa. From Fairburn (2008). Copyright by The Guilford Press. Adapted by permission.

plications for treatment. It suggests that if treatment is to have a lasting impact on the binge eating and purging, it also needs to address these patients' extreme dieting, their overevaluation of shape and weight, and their tendency to eat in response to adverse events and negative moods.

Anorexia Nervosa and Eating Disorder NOS

The cognitive-behavioral account of the maintenance of bulimia nervosa can be extended to all eating disorders. As noted earlier, the "transdiagnostic" theory of Fairburn and colleagues (2003) highlights the fact that anorexia nervosa and bulimia nervosa have much in common. They share essentially the same core psychopathology, with both groups of patients overevaluating shape and weight, and their control, and this psychopathology is expressed in similar attitudes and behavior.[2] Thus, patients with anorexia nervosa restrict their food intake in the same rigid and extreme way as do patients with bulimia nervosa, and they too may vomit, misuse laxatives or diuretics, and overexercise. Nor does binge eating distinguish between the two disorders for there is the subgroup of patients with anorexia nervosa who binge eat (with or without compensatory purging). As discussed earlier, the major difference between the two disorders lies in the relative balance of the under- and overeating, and its effect on body weight. In bulimia nervosa, body

weight is usually unremarkable, whereas undereating predominates in anorexia nervosa, with the result that body weight is extremely low and features of starvation contribute to the clinical picture and its maintenance. Particularly important in this regard is the pronounced social withdrawal seen in starvation that encourages self-absorption while isolating patients from external influences that might diminish their overconcern with eating, shape, and weight. Figure 14.3 shows the cognitive-behavioral formulation of the classic "restricting" form of anorexia nervosa.

The processes that maintain bulimia nervosa and anorexia nervosa also appear to maintain the clinical presentations seen in eating disorder NOS. Figure 14.4 shows a composite transdiagnostic formulation that is essentially a combination of the bulimia nervosa and restricting anorexia nervosa formulations. In our experience, this composite formulation represents well the core processes that maintain any eating disorder, whatever its exact form. The specific maintaining processes operating in any individual patient depend on the nature of the eating disorder psychopathology present. In some cases only a limited number of these processes are active (as in most cases of binge-eating disorder), whereas in others (e.g., cases of the binge-eating–purging type of anorexia nervosa) most of the maintaining processes are operating. As with the cognitive-behavioral account of the maintenance of bulimia nervosa, the transdiagnostic account highlights the pro-

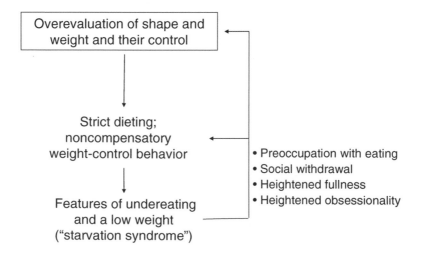

FIGURE 14.3. The cognitive-behavioral formulation of anorexia nervosa. From Fairburn (2008). Copyright by The Guilford Press. Adapted by permission.

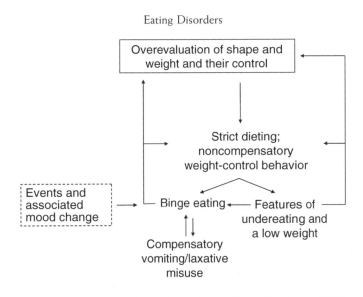

FIGURE 14.4. The transdiagnostic "template" formulation. From Fairburn (2008). Copyright by The Guilford Press. Adapted by permission.

cesses that need to be addressed in treatment, thereby helping the clinician design a bespoke treatment to fit the particular patient's psychopathology.

THE RESEARCH ON TREATMENT

Consistent with the current way of classifying eating disorders, research on their treatment has focused on the particular disorders in isolation. This research has been reviewed by Wilson, Grilo and Vitousek (2007) and an authoritative meta-analysis has been conducted by the U.K. National Institute for Health and Clinical Excellence, or NICE (National Collaborating Centre for Mental Health, 2004). The majority of the randomized controlled trials have focused on adults with bulimia nervosa, with the treatment of adolescents receiving little attention. The findings indicate that there is a clear leading treatment, a specific form of cognitive-behavioral therapy (CBT-BN). However, this treatment is far from being a panacea: At best, half the patients who complete treatment make a full and lasting response. Interpersonal psychotherapy (IPT) is a potential alternative to CBT-BN, but it takes 8–12 months longer to achieve a comparable effect. Antidepressant medication (especially fluoxetine at a dose of 60 mg in the morning) also has a beneficial effect, but not as great as that obtained with CBT-BN, and the limited available evidence suggests it is

often not sustained. Combining CBT BN with antidepressant medication conveys little, if any, advantage over CBT-BN alone.

There has been much less research on the treatment of anorexia nervosa, and no treatment is supported by robust research evidence. In this case, most of the work has focused on adolescents, and much of it has been concerned with a highly specific form of family-based treatment (Lock, le Grange, Agras, & Dare, 2001). Despite widespread enthusiasm for this treatment (often described as the "Maudsley method"), there is little evidence that it has a specific beneficial effect (Fairburn, 2005).

This is a growing body of research on the treatment of binge-eating disorder. Various approaches have shown promise, but the greatest support is for an adaptation of CBT-BN. This treatment has a marked effect on the binge eating of these patients but little effect on their body weight. Binge-eating disorder aside, there has been no research on the treatment of eating disorder NOS, a remarkable omission given the disorder's prevalence.

Enhanced Cognitive-Behavioral Therapy

A transdiagnostic form of cognitive-behavioral therapy has been developed for the full range of clinical eating disorders seen in adults, including eating disorders NOS (Fairburn et al., 2003). It is based on the transdiagnostic theory outlined earlier and was derived from CBT-BN

(Fairburn, Marcus, & Wilson, 1993). The treatment—enhanced cognitive-behavioral therapy (CBT-E)—is described as "enhanced" because it uses a variety of new strategies and procedures designed to improve treatment adherence and outcome, and because it has modules that address certain obstacles to change that are "external" to the core eating disorder, namely, mood intolerance, clinical perfectionism, low self-esteem, and interpersonal difficulties. There are two forms of CBT-E: a focused form (CBT-F) that focuses exclusively on eating disorder psychopathology, and a broad form (CBT-B) that also addresses the four external obstacles to change. The treatment also exists in two lengths, a 20-week version for patients who are not significantly underweight, defined as having a BMI over 17.5, and 40-week version for patients with a BMI of 17.5 or below, a commonly used threshold for anorexia nervosa.

CBT-E is an outpatient-based treatment designed to be delivered on an individual rather than group basis. Adaptations have been devised for adolescents (Cooper & Stewart, 2008) and for inpatients (Dalle Grave et al., 2008; Fairburn, 2008). The remainder of this chapter is devoted to individual CBT-E for adults. Limitations on space preclude the description of the 40-week variant for patients who are significantly underweight and the CBT-B version, which also addresses the four "external" maintaining mechanisms. Readers who want to learn more about the treatment and its implementation are referred to the complete treatment guide (Fairburn, 2008).

THE CONTEXT OF TREATMENT

The Patient

CBT-E is a treatment for patients with an eating disorder of clinical severity (i.e., the disturbance is persistent and significantly interferes with the patient's psychosocial functioning or physical health). The adult version of the treatment is designed for patients aged 18 years or older. It is equally suitable for men or women. Because it is an outpatient-based treatment, it is essential that it is safe for the patient to be managed this way, both in physical terms and from the psychiatric point of view. In practice this means that the patient's physical state must be stable and that he or she must not be at risk of suicide. The treatment has not been used

with patients at the extremes of the weight spectrum: rather, it is designed for patients with a BMI between 15.0 and 40.0. Although some patients with a BMI below 15.0 can be managed with CBT-E, this is probably best left to experienced therapists. Patients with a BMI over 40.0 have very specific treatment needs and may be candidates for obesity surgery.

The Therapist

There is no specific professional qualification required to practice CBT-E, but certain background knowledge and experience are desirable. Ideally, the therapist should be well informed about psychopathology in general and eating disorder psychopathology in particular; in practical terms, the therapist should have had training in CBT and prior experience working with patients with eating disorders.

In contrast to many other applications of CBT, the gender of the therapist is of some relevance to treatment. Most patients with eating disorders are female and as a result female therapists may have certain advantages. They may be viewed by patients as being more likely to understand their difficulties and, in addition, may serve as a role model in terms of acceptance of shape and weight. This said, however, the main point to stress is that therapist competence at delivering CBT-E is the critical issue and of far greater importance than therapist gender.

A subject rarely discussed is the appearance of the therapist. This is of little relevance if the therapist is middle-aged or of the opposite gender because the patient is unlikely to be interested in his or her appearance, but it is of relevance if patient and therapist are the same gender and similar in age. Patients with eating disorders are acutely aware of relevant other people's shapes, and this may include their therapists. Therapists who are very thin may find themselves at a disadvantage when trying to help underweight patients regain weight because patients may challenge them about their own eating habits and weight. Therapists who are overweight may find some patients hard to engage as a result of their prejudice against people who are large.

Although the overriding issue is the therapist's competence at delivering CBT-E, another matter that merits thought is whether the therapist has an eating disorder or a recent history of one. Two perspectives should be taken: the well-being of the patient and that of the therapist. With regard to the former, it makes little difference to the patient whether the therapist has, or has had, an eating disorder because it would not be appropriate for the therapist to disclose his or her psychiatric history. This said, such a history might well render the therapist more sensitive to the types of difficulty the patient is facing. The well-being of the therapist must not be neglected, however. One of the distinctive characteristics of people with eating disorders is the level of interest they have in issues related to food, eating, shape, and weight. The tendency of patients with anorexia nervosa to read recipe books and cook for others is well known, but similar behavior is seen across the eating disorders and is, of course, an expression of the core psychopathology. This psychopathology may also influence career choice: For example, it may lead people with eating disorders, or histories of them, to work as personal trainers, beauty therapists or dieticians, or indeed as therapists for patients who have an eating disorder. If this applies, the therapist in question might want to consider whether it is in his or her interests to engage in this type of work because doing so can maintain preoccupation with eating, shape, and weight, and serve as an obstacle to the broadening of his or her horizons.

ASSESSING PATIENTS AND PREPARING THEM FOR TREATMENT

The Initial Evaluation Interview(s)

The initial interview has two interrelated goals. The first is to put the patient at ease and begin to forge a positive therapeutic relationship. This is important for a number of reasons. First, many patients referred because of a possible eating disorder are highly ambivalent about treatment because of either the "ego-syntonic" nature of their psychopathology (especially true of underweight patients) or shame (especially true of those who are binge eating), or adverse treatment experiences in the past. The assessing clinician needs to be sensitive to and ask about the patient's attitude toward treatment. The goal is that the assessment interview be a collaborative enterprise that ends with the clinician giving the patient an expert opinion as to the nature of his or her problems and, if indicated, the treatment options. The patient

should also have ample opportunity to ask questions.

The other goal is to establish the diagnosis. An apparent eating disorder may, for example, turn out to be an anxiety disorder (e.g., difficulty eating with others due to a social phobia), a presentation of a mood disorder (e.g., severe weight loss resulting from a clinical depression), or simple overeating in cases of obesity. It is therefore critical to evaluate the problem thoroughly, both in terms of the diagnosis (or diagnoses, if there is current comorbidity) and the severity of the problem, to decide what is the most appropriate next step, if treatment is indeed indicated. It is not our practice to take an exhaustive personal history at this stage, nor do we attempt to provide patients with our understanding of the nature of their problem in psychodynamic or cognitive-behavioral (or other) terms. Rather, we focus on our two goals and do our utmost to achieve them.

Patients are invited to bring others to the appointment if they wish. Others may simply provide moral support (and stay in the waiting area), or they may also serve as informants, in which case we see them with the patient once we have conducted a one-to-one assessment with the patient alone, but only if the patient wishes us to do so. One of main priorities is to ensure that the patient feels that he or she is in control of the assessment process.

The perspective of informants is of interest in that it can provide a different perspective on the patient's difficulties. Problems may be described that were not disclosed by the patient (e.g., that the patient takes an inordinate time to eat meals or has extremely small portions), or difficulties between the patient and the informant may become evident. It is not appropriate to insist upon the presence of informants because some adult patients who have kept their eating problem hidden from others would not attend if disclosure were required. The situation is different with younger patients living at home, where involvement of the parents is essential.

Towards the end of the interview we weigh patients and measure their height. This is an extremely sensitive matter for most patients and some are resistant to it. Nevertheless, the patient must be weighed for the assessment to be complete. It is not appropriate to rely upon patients' self-reported weight or height because they can be inaccurate. We explain this to patients and say that we *must* check their weight to complete the assessment. In our experience patients know this and expect it, although they might prefer not to be weighed if they could get away with it! At this point we do not insist upon patients knowing their weight if they do not wish to, but we like to tell them their BMI when discussing the outcome of the assessment.

We are not in favor of lengthy assessment appointments because they are exhausting for the patient and, in our view, unnecessary. Ninety minutes is our maximum. On the other hand, we routinely see patients twice as part of the assessment process: We find that a second appointment 1 or 2 weeks later often adds new information of value. On this second occasion patients are more relaxed and sometimes disclose material they previously withheld, and we have an opportunity to pursue matters that require particularly careful exploration (e.g., the nature and extent of any comorbid depressive features). The second appointment is also a good time to discuss treatment options.

We routinely ask patients to complete certain questionnaires prior to the initial appointment. This is useful because it gives us standardized information on the nature and severity of patients' problems. The two questionnaires we favor are the Eating Disorder Examination Questionnaire (EDE-Q; Fairburn & Beglin, 1994) and the Clinical Impairment Assessment (CIA; Bohn & Fairburn, 2008). The EDE-Q provides a measure of current eating disorder features, and the CIA assesses the impact of this psychopathology on psychosocial functioning. Both questionnaires are short and easy to fill in, both focus on the previous 28 days, and both are sensitive to change. In addition, we include one of the well-established measures of general psychiatric features. For a thorough assessment of current eating disorder features, most experts recommend the Eating Disorder Examination (EDE; Fairburn & Cooper, 1993). This is a semistructured clinical interview, but it is probably too exhaustive to use on a routine clinical basis.[3]

Outcome of the Evaluation

By the end of the second appointment, it should be possible to decide on the best treatment options. Generally these are one or more of the following:

1. *Do "nothing."* This is appropriate with minor eating problems that are likely to be self-limiting.
2. *Observe.* This is appropriate if the nature or severity of the problem is not clear; for example, if the problem seems to be remitting.
3. *Recommend CBT-E.* This is appropriate for the vast majority of cases. We recommend CBT-E for virtually all patients with an eating disorder who have a BMI between 15.0 and 40.0; exceptions are patients whose medical or psychiatric state make management on an outpatient basis inappropriate. From the psychiatric point of view, it is primarily the risk of suicide that needs to be considered when deciding whether outpatient treatment is appropriate. This risk is largely, but not exclusively, restricted to patients who are clinically depressed, although heightened suicide risk is also present in patients who feel hopeless about the prospect of recovery. All eating disorder therapists should be competent at assessing suicide risk.
4. *Recommend more intensive treatment.* We recommend more intensive treatment (i.e., day patient or inpatient treatment) for patients whose BMI is below 14.0 and for those whose physical state is not stable. Such treatment can be followed by outpatient-based CBT-E. We may also recommend more intensive treatment when CBT-E fails to be of benefit to the patient.

Contraindications to CBT-E

There are certain contraindications to embarking upon CBT-E straightaway. Most of these apply to any psychological treatment for an eating disorder. They have in common the effect of substantially undermining the patient's concentration, motivation (which, in any case, may be a problem in some patients), or their ability to work on treatment between sessions. The main contraindications are as follows:

Comorbid Clinical Depression

Most patients with an eating disorder have secondary depressive features, but a subgroup has an independent but interacting clinical depression. Suggestive features include the following:

- Intensification of depressive features (in the absence of any change in the eating disorder or the patient's circumstances).
- Pervasive and extreme negative thinking (i.e., broader in content than concerns about eating, shape, and weight).
- Hopelessness in general (i.e., seeing the future as totally bleak; seeing no future; resignation).
- Recurrent thoughts about death and dying.
- Suicidal thoughts (e.g., thoughts that one would be better off dead).
- Guilt over events in the far past.
- Decrease in involvement with others over and above any impairment that already accompanied the eating disorder (e.g., stopping seeing friends).
- Loss of interest in activities that had been pursued despite the eating disorder (e.g., ceasing to listen to music or to read newspapers, or to follow the news).
- Decrease in drive and initiative.

The presence of a clinical depression interferes with psychological treatment in a number of ways. Depressive thinking results in patients being unduly negative about the possibility of change, which undermines their efforts to change. The reduction in drive that is seen in depression has a similar effect. Concentration impairment is also a problem because it results in the patient not retaining information.

Once the depression has been treated, then CBT-E can start. We favor treating the depression with antidepressant medication because doing so usually brings about a rapid and striking response. Guidelines for doing this are provided elsewhere (Fairburn, 2008). Rarely does the lifting of the clinical depression result in a significant change in the eating disorder. Patients who binge eat may experience a decrease in the frequency of their binge eating, but generally they continue to diet to an extreme degree and remain overly concerned about their shape and weight. Patients who are underweight may find that they become more successful at undereating. Whatever the change, when patients are no longer depressed, they are in a better state to address their eating disorder.

It is important to add that other, co-occurring forms of psychopathology (e.g., anxiety disorders, personality disorders) are not contraindications to CBT-E. Thus, the research on CBT-BN has typically included patients with coexisting Axis I and Axis II disorders, neither of which has been shown to be consistent predictors of outcome.

Persistent Substance Misuse

Intoxication in treatment sessions renders the sessions virtually worthless, and persistent intoxication outside sessions severely undermines the patient's ability to utilize the treatment. Once the substance misuse has been addressed, CBT-E can start.

Major Life Difficulties or Crises

These are distracting and interfere with treatment. For example, it is best not to start treatment with students who are about to take major examinations. Some life difficulties are more pressing than the eating disorder.

Inability to Attend Treatment

A central feature of CBT-E is establishing and maintaining "therapeutic momentum." This requires that appointments be frequent (especially in the early stages) and regular. We ask patients to guarantee that there will be no breaks in their attendance in the first 6 weeks and no breaks longer than 3 weeks throughout the whole of treatment. If this is impossible, say, because of a prebooked vacation, we prefer to defer starting treatment. Patients generally understand and respect the rationale behind this firm stance. They can see that we are taking their treatment seriously and do not want them to have a "false start."

Lack of Success of CBT-E in the Past

This is a relative contraindication rather than an absolute one. If patients have not benefited from a specific, well-delivered treatment in the past, then whether it is appropriate to offer them the same treatment a second time does merit thought. On the other hand, it is possible that the patient's circumstances may be more conducive to a good outcome than they were or that the patient may be more motivated than before.

It is important to point out that whereas it may appear that the patient had the same treatment before, it often turns out that the earlier treatment was quite different. Treatments referred to as "CBT" can differ remarkably because they were either different forms of CBT or mislabeled. It is always worth finding out exactly what the prior treatment involved.

OVERVIEW OF TREATMENT

Length of Treatment

CBT-E is a short-term, time-limited, psychological treatment for patients with eating disorders. Because it is highly individualized, CBT-E is best delivered on a one-to-one basis. For patients who are not significantly underweight (defined in this context as having a BMI above 17.5) an initial assessment appointment followed by 20 treatment sessions over 20 weeks is generally sufficient. For patients below this weight, treatment needs to be longer. (The treatment of underweight patients is described in the complete treatment guide; Fairburn, 2008.) The fact that CBT-E is time-limited might be thought to be inconsistent with the claim that it is individualized. To an extent this is true, but our experience is that 20 treatment sessions are sufficient, but not excessive, for the great majority of patients.

There are major advantages working within a fixed time frame and, in our view, these outweigh the potential disadvantage of standardizing the length of treatment. The main advantage is that a fixed time frame concentrates the mind of both the patient and the therapist. It encourages establishment of the therapeutic momentum needed early on and helps to ensure that the therapist and patient keep working hard at helping the patient change. It also makes it much more likely that treatment will have a formal ending rather than fizzling out, as sometimes happens in open-ended treatment. Having a definite endpoint ensures that important future-oriented topics are covered in the final sessions.

There are circumstances under which it is appropriate to adjust the length of treatment. It rarely needs to be shortened, although this does apply in those occasional cases in which change is so profound and rapid that there is little or no remaining psychopathology to address. Somewhat more often there is a case for extending treatment. The indications for doing this are described toward the end of the chapter.

Implementing CBT-E

CBT-E is designed to be a complete treatment in its own right. In our view it should not be combined with other forms of therapy, nor should it coexist with them. Both can detract from treatment (see Wilson, 2005). Whatever happens, CBT-E remains focused on the eating disorder more or less. If the patient experiences a crisis during treatment that cannot be ignored (e.g., the parents of one our younger patients disappeared unexpectedly, leaving the patient at a loss as to what to do), we arrange one or more "crisis sessions" to address the problem in question, in addition to the CBT-E sessions. This rarely happens, however. Very occasionally we suspend CBT-E for a few weeks, if continuing seems inappropriate. We have observed that some therapists are tempted to change therapeutic tack if progress is slow or difficult. We think that this is rarely appropriate. Whereas it might be tempting to switch over to another therapeutic modality (e.g., schema-based therapy), or to add or try to "integrate" other techniques, we recommend that the therapist continue to work within the framework of CBT-E, while trying to understand the basis for the relative lack of progress.

THE TREATMENT PROTOCOL

Stages of Treatment

The treatment has four stages:

- *Stage 1*—This is most important. The aims are to engage the patient in treatment and change, to create jointly a formulation of the processes maintaining the eating disorder, to provide education, and to introduce both weekly weighing and a pattern of regular eating. Appointments are twice weekly for 4 weeks.
- *Stage 2*—The aim of this stage is for therapist and patient to take stock, review progress, identify barriers to change, modify the formulation as needed, and plan Stage 3. This stage generally comprises two appointments, a week apart.
- *Stage 3*—This is the main body of treatment. The aim is to address the key mechanisms that are maintaining the patient's eating disorder. There are eight weekly appointments.
- *Stage 4*—This is the final stage in treatment,

and the focus is on the future. There are two aims: The first is to ensure that the changes made in treatment are maintained over the following months, and the second is to minimize the risk of relapse in the long term. There are three appointments, each 2 weeks apart.

In addition to these sessions, there is a single review appointment 20 weeks after treatment has finished.

Stage 1

This is the initial, intensive stage of treatment. A number of interrelated goals apply regardless of the exact nature of the patient's eating disorder psychopathology.

Engaging the Patient in Treatment and the Prospect of Change

A particular challenge in working with patients with eating disorders is to engage them in treatment. There may be aspects of their disorder that they would like to change (e.g., binge eating) but generally there are other elements that they value and may even identify with (e.g., maintaining strict control over eating, losing weight). Many come to treatment with misgivings and varying degrees of reluctance. It is essential that the therapist understand this and is sensitive at all times to patients' likely ambivalence.

The initial treatment session is especially important in this regard. The patient is evaluating the therapist just as much as the therapist is evaluating the patient. The therapist's manner, apparent attitudes, and choice of words are all being scrutinized and therefore merit the therapist's attention.

Much has been written about engaging these patients in treatment. We particularly recommend the article by Vitousek, Watson, and Wilson (1998). Some clinicians advocate an initial phase of "motivational enhancement." We agree that engagement in treatment, and especially in change, is crucial, but we contend that competently administered CBT-E enhances motivation for change and overlaps significantly with the strategies of motivational interviewing (Wilson & Schlam, 2004). We do not view special, non-CBT procedures as being required.

Therapists can enhance engagement early on by following these guidelines:

- Be "engaging" in interpersonal style, and empathetic.
- Be professional but not intimidating. Convey understanding of eating problems and expertise in their assessment and treatment.
- Actively involve the patient in the assessment process and in the creation of the formulation.
- Instill hope.
- Avoid being controlling or paternalistic.

Certain additional strategies and procedures that help to engage underweight patients are described in the complete treatment guide (Fairburn, 2008).

Integral to engaging patients is explaining what treatment involves. With this in mind, it is important that patients be fully informed about the treatment upon which they are embarking. Various topics need to be covered:

1. *Nature and style of the treatment.* Clearly, patients need to be told the name, nature, and style of the treatment.

2. *Practicalities.* Patients should also be told the number, duration, and frequency of the treatment sessions. It may be useful to arrive at an agreement about the time of day that sessions should take place. We do our best to accommodate patients' commitments, the difficulties they face in traveling, and, in some cases, their desire for secrecy.

3. *In-session weighing.* Patients need to be forewarned about the in-session weighing that becomes an element of treatment from Session 1 onward. The rationale for this needs to be explained (see "Establishing Weekly Weighing"). We are often asked whether patients ever refuse to be weighed. The answer is that the occasional patient is very reluctant, but in the context of an "engaging" initial session and the rationale being well explained we find that refusal is not a problem. However, we do occasionally have to be quite insistent. Our experience is that if one gives in to the patient's fear of weekly weighing at this stage, it is rarely, if ever, possible to introduce the procedure later on, which is unfortunate as in our view it is one of the most valuable new elements of the treatment. This view is shared by many patients, who report at the end of treatment that

regular in-session weighing in collaboration with the therapist was extremely helpful.

4. *Instillation of "ownership," enthusiasm, and hope.* The notion that it is the patient's treatment, not the therapist's, also needs to be mentioned. Throughout treatment, patients should feel clear about what is happening and why. They should be told that if they do not understand anything, they should ask. Similarly, the same applies in session should they disagree with anything.

Because many patients are keen to overcome their eating problem (including some underweight ones) and eager for treatment to start, it is important to maximize enthusiasm and hope. This in part involves conveying that one is knowledgeable about eating disorders in general and the patient's type of eating problem in particular. Not infrequently we come across patients who have been told that they will never overcome their eating disorder. Rarely have we felt that such a statement is warranted. Saying something like this is a self-fulfilling prophecy that undermines any hope of recovery that the patient might have. Research has not generated reliable predictors of treatment outcome, and our clinical experience over the years has taught us not to trust our clinical judgment in this regard. We are continually surprised (usually favorably) at our patients' response to treatment. Because it is unusual for us not to help patients, at least to some extent, we say to patients who are extremely pessimistic about the prospect of change, "I am sure we can help. It is good that you are here."

Assessing the Nature and Severity of the Psychopathology Present

Depending on the context within which one works, the person who conducts the initial evaluation interview(s) may or may not be the person who subsequently treats the patient. In our context, the therapist often is meeting the patient for the first time. This means that a second assessment of the eating disorder needs to take place so that the therapist is fully in the picture. Inevitably, this assessment overlaps to an extent with the initial one. This cannot be avoided.

Jointly Creating the Formulation

The next step is the creation of the "formulation"; that is, a personalized visual representation (i.e., a diagram) of the processes that appear to be maintaining the patient's eating problem. This is done in the initial session, unless the patient is significantly underweight or the eating disorder is unusual and difficult to understand. In such cases it is best to delay completing the formulation until the next session so that the therapist has ample time to think over its likely form.

The creation of the formulation has a number of purposes:

1. Done well, it can greatly help engage the patient in treatment.
2. The process of creating the formulation distances patients from their problems. Rather than simply having an eating problem, patients learn to step back and try to understand the problem and how it persists. The adoption of this "decentered" stance is central to helping patients change, but at this stage one simply wants to them to get interested in, and intrigued by, their eating problem.
3. The formulation conveys the notion that eating problems are understandable and are maintained by a variety of interacting, self-perpetuating maintaining mechanisms. When discussing this, therapists can point out (if applicable) that it is not surprising that patients have found it difficult to change.
4. By highlighting the main mechanisms that maintain patients' eating problem, the formulation provides a guide as to what needs to be targeted in treatment.

The composite transdiagnostic formulation shown in Figure 14.4 should be used as a template to derive a personalized formulation that matches the patient's particular clinical features. The more familiar the therapist becomes with the template formulation, the easier it is to create an individualized one. We have not encountered any patients who eating problems cannot be formulated in this way.

The following points should be kept in mind in creating the formulation:

- It should be simple.
- It should focus on the main mechanisms that appear likely to be maintaining the patient's eating problem. It need not be comprehensive (this runs the risk of being overdetailed and confusing), and it is not concerned with the origins of the problem.

The creation of the formulation—best referred to as the "diagram" or "picture"—is a skill worth practicing because it is important that it is done well. The formulation should be drawn out, step-by-step, in an unhurried manner, with the therapist taking the lead but the patient actively involved. It is best to start with something that the patient either wants to change (e.g., binge eating) or is clearly a problem (e.g., very low weight). Whenever possible and appropriate, the patient's own terms should be used. Because the formulation is based on information only just obtained, the therapist should clearly indicate that it is provisional and will be modified as needed during treatment. It is important that the patient accept the formulation as a credible explanation of the eating problem. Most resonate with it. In those rare instances when a patient remains unconvinced and holds a conflicting explanation (e.g., a psychodynamic or addiction-based one), the therapist should encourage the patient to reflect on the utility and validity of his or her current perspective (without making him or her defensive), while contrasting it with the well-supported cognitive-behavioral perspective.

Once the formulation has been created the therapist should discuss its implications for treatment. The points to be made are that to overcome the eating disorder the patient will need to address not only the things that he or she would like to change (e.g., loss of control over eating) but also the mechanisms responsible for maintaining them (the "vicious circles"). Thus, for example, with patients who binge eat, treatment commonly needs to focus on more than simply stopping binge eating; instead, it may also need to address the patient's various forms of dieting, his or her ability to deal with adverse events and moods without binge eating, and his or her concerns about shape and weight. Not addressing the range of maintaining processes markedly increases the likelihood of relapse.

Establishing Real-Time Self-Monitoring

Real-time self-monitoring is the ongoing "in-the-moment" recording of relevant behavior, thoughts, feelings, and events. It needs to be initiated from the outset of treatment and fine-tuned in Session 1. It continues throughout treatment and is central to it, and should be explained along the following lines:

"Self-monitoring is central to treatment. It has two main purposes.

1. First, it will help you identify precisely what is happening on a day-to-day basis. We need to know exactly what you are doing, thinking, and feeling at the very time that you are doing, thinking, and feeling things. We need to know the details; then we can work out how you can make changes and thereby break into your eating problem. So you need to start to notice and to record key things of importance. Self-monitoring is designed to help you do this.

2. Second, self-monitoring will help you change. By becoming acutely aware of what you are doing, thinking, and feeling *at the very time that things are happening*, you will learn that you have choices, and that some things you thought were automatic and outside your control (and perhaps awareness) can be changed with attention, effort, and practice. But you can only achieve this with accurate, real-time monitoring. Simply recalling how things were hours ago won't, of course, work."

The self-monitoring record that we employ is simple to complete and use. Exactly what is recorded evolves during treatment. At the beginning the emphasis is largely on the patient's eating habits. When describing how to monitor it is our practice to go over an example (created for this purpose) that roughly matches in form the eating habits of the patient in question. Figure 14.5 shows our instructions for self-monitoring and Figure 14.6 shows a completed self-monitoring record.

Fundamental to establishing accurate, real-time recording is going over the patient's records in detail, especially in Session 1, when the patient brings in the completed forms for the first time. Reviewing the records should be a joint process, with the patient taking the therapist through each day's record in turn. There are two aspects to the review in Session 1: assessing the quality of monitoring and the information gained about the patient's eating habits. In subsequent sessions, the focus is largely on what has been recorded, although the therapist should intermittently ask the patient about the recording process and the accuracy of the records. In these subsequent sessions the review of the records should generally take no longer than 10 minutes. Therapists need to remember not to address identified problems while doing

The purpose of self-monitoring is twofold: First, it provides a detailed picture of how you eat, thereby bringing to your attention and that of your therapist the exact nature of your eating problem; and second, by making you more aware of what you are doing at the very time that you are doing it, self-monitoring helps you change behavior that previously seemed automatic and beyond your control. Accurate "real-time" monitoring is central to treatment. It will help you change.

At first, writing down everything that you eat may be irritating and inconvenient, but soon it will become second nature and of obvious value. We have yet to encounter anyone whose lifestyle makes it truly impossible to monitor. Regard it as a challenge.

Your therapist will give you a sample monitoring sheet. A new sheet (or sheets) should be started each day.

- The first column is for noting the time when you eat or drink anything, and the second is for recording the nature of the food and drink consumed. Calories should not be recorded; instead, you should write down a simple (nontechnical) description of what you ate or drank. Each item should be written down as soon as possible after it is consumed. Recalling what you ate or drank some hours afterwards will not work because it will not help you change your behavior at the time. Obviously, if you are to record in the way that you are being asked, you will have to carry your monitoring sheets with you.
- Episodes of eating that you view as meals should be identified with brackets. Snacks and other episodes of eating should not be bracketed.
- The third column should specify where the food or drink was consumed. If this was in your home, the room should be specified.
- Asterisks should be placed in the fourth column, adjacent to any episodes of eating or drinking that you felt (at the time) were excessive. It is essential to record all the food that you eat during "binges."
- The fifth column is for recording when you vomit, take laxatives or diuretics (water tablets), or "overexercise."
- The last column is used in various ways during treatment. For the moment, it should be used as a diary to record events and feelings that have influenced your eating: For example, if an argument precipitated a binge or led you not to eat, you should write that down. You may wish to record other important events or circumstances in this column, even if they had no effect on your eating. The last column should also be used to record your weight each time you weigh yourself.

Every treatment session will include a review of your latest monitoring sheets. You must therefore remember to bring them with you.

FIGURE 14.5. Instructions for Self-Monitoring. From Fairburn (2008). Copyright by The Guilford Press. Adapted by permission.

Day ......Thursday...........   Date .....March 21...........

Time	Food and drink consumed	Place	*	p	Context and comments
7.30	Glass water	Kitchen			[118 pounds—really gross] Thirsty after yesterday
8:10	Whole cinnamon raisin bagel Light cream cheese Black coffee	Cafe	*		Should have only had half the bagel. Must not binge today.
10:35	Half banana Black coffee	Work—at desk			Better—on track
11:45	Smoked turkey on wheat bread Light mayo Diet coke	Cafe			Usual lunch
6:40 to 7:30	Piece of apple pie 1/2 gallon ice cream 4 slices of toast with peanut butter Diet coke Raisin bagel 2 slices of toast with peanut butter Diet coke Peanut butter from jar Raisin bagel Snickers bar Diet coke—large	Kitchen	* * * * * * * *	V V	Help—I can't stop eating. I'm completely out of control. I hate myself. I am disgusting. Why do I do this? I started as soon as I got in. I've ruined another day.
9:30	Rice cake with fat-free cheese Diet coke	Kitchen			Really lonely. Feel fat and unattractive. Feel like giving up.

FIGURE 14.6. A completed self-monitoring record.

this, but to acknowledge and to put them on the session agenda. Table 14.1 summarizes typical session structure and allocation of time.

TABLE 14.1. Typical Approximate Allocation of Time within Sessions

1. Collaborative weighing; updating and interpreting the weight graph (5 minutes)
2. Reviewing the latest monitoring records and any homework assignments (10 minutes)
3. Collaboratively setting the agenda for the session (3 minutes)
4. Working through the agenda and agreeing on any homework tasks (30 minutes)
5. Summarizing the session (2 minutes)

Note. From Fairburn (2008). Copyright by The Guilford Press. Adapted by permission.

Establishing Weekly Weighing

The "weekly weighing" intervention has a number of purposes. First, as patients' eating habits change in treatment, they are likely to be anxious about resulting changes in their weight. In-session weighing provides them with good, week-by-week data on their weight. Second, regular in-session weighing provides the therapist an opportunity to help patients interpret the number on the scale—a number that they otherwise are prone to misinterpret. Third, weekly weighing addresses one form of body checking, namely, weight checking. Because many patients with eating disorders weigh themselves at frequent intervals, sometimes many times a day, they become concerned with day-to-day weight fluctuations that would otherwise pass unnoticed. Others actively avoid knowing their weight but remain highly concerned about it. Generally these patients weighed themselves frequently in the past but switched to avoidance when they found frequent weight checking too aversive. Avoidance of weighing is as problematic as frequent weighing because it results in patients having no data to confirm or to disconfirm their fears about weight gain.

Patients need to learn how to assess and interpret their weight. They should be informed that body weight fluctuates through the day and from day to day according to their state of hydration, bowels and bladder, their point in the menstrual cycle, and other factors. Frequent weighing results in preoccupation with inconsequential fluctuations in weight that tend to be misinterpreted. This leads many patients to restrict their eating, whatever the reading on the scales. This important maintaining process is disrupted by the weekly weighing intervention.

Weekly weighing starts with what we term "collaborative weighing," in which therapist and patient together check the patient's weight at the beginning of the session.[4] This is done once a week (except with underweight patients with whom it is done every session). The therapist and patient plot the latest data point onto an individualized weight graph and jointly interpret the emerging pattern, placing particular emphasis on *trends over the past 4 weeks* rather than focusing on the latest reading. A crucial element of the intervention is that patients do not weigh themselves outside these times—but if they do, they should record this on their monitoring record. Patients who have a scale at home should be encouraged to make it inaccessible.

Patients are also educated about the BMI. They are told their BMI and its significance from a medical point of view. They are advised against having an exact desired weight that does not allow for natural day-to-day fluctuations. Instead they are advised to accept a weight range of approximately 6 pounds (or 3 kilograms).

Almost all patients are anxious about the effect treatment will have on their weight. Patients with bulimia nervosa or eating disorder NOS (other than those who are underweight) generally do not change much in weight. Nevertheless, some patients gain weight and others lose weight, and it is not possible to predict exactly what will happen to the individual patient. Patients should be told that the aim of treatment is to give them control over their eating; thus, they will have as much control over their weight as is possible. It is best that patients postpone deciding on a specific weight-range goal until near the end of treatment, when their eating habits have stabilized and they are less sensitive about their weight and shape. Later in treatment, patients are advised against having a goal weight (range) that necessitates anything more than slight dietary restraint because such restraint maintains preoccupation with food and eating and increases the risk of binge eating.

Educating the Patient about Eating Problems

Myths abound about eating and weight control. Patients with eating disorders are assiduous readers of articles and books about diets and dieting, and may acquire an idiosyncratic, ill-founded body of knowledge. They are also understandably ignorant about some topics; for example, the effects of vomiting and laxative misuse on calorie absorption.

To ensure that patients have a reliable source of information, we recommend that they read one of the authoritative books on eating disorders. We routinely use *Overcoming Binge Eating* (Fairburn, 1995) because it provides all the information needed and it is popular with patients.[5] In addition, its cognitive-behavioral orientation is highly compatible with CBT-E. Part I of the book is exclusively educational. With patients who are comfortable reading, the whole of Part I may be recommended. With patients who are less used to reading, certain sections should be highlighted (especially Chapters 1, 4, and 5). It should be noted that *Overcoming Binge Eating* is relevant to all patients with eating disorders, whether or not they binge eat, because it discusses eating disorder psychopathology in general, and not just binge eating.

It is our practice to provide the patient with a copy of the book; in this way, we can ensure that they have it at exactly the right point in treatment (generally Week 2). We ask patients to put check marks in the margins by sections that particularly apply to them, crosses by sections that do not, and question marks by sections that they do not understand or would like to discuss. We term this procedure "guided reading." It allows patients to be educated in an efficient, thorough, and personalized way.

Establishing "Regular Eating"

The "regular eating" intervention is fundamental to successful treatment, whatever the form of the eating disorder. For patients who binge eat, it reliably results in a rapid decrease in the frequency of binge eating. For patients who have a high level of dietary restraint, it addresses an important type of dieting, so-called "delayed eating"; that is, putting off eating during the day. And for patients who are underweight, it introduces regular meals and snacks that can be subsequently increased in size.

Regular eating is introduced around Session 3. It is the first time that patients are asked to change the way that they eat. There are two aspects to the intervention:

1. Patients should eat three planned meals each day, plus two (if underweight, three) planned snacks.
2. Patients' eating should be largely confined to these meals and snacks.

A number of points about the intervention need to be stressed:

• Patients should be allowed to choose what they eat in their planned meals and snacks. The only condition is that the meals and snacks must not be followed by vomiting, laxative misuse, or any other compensatory behavior. Patients should not be put under pressure to change what they eat at this point in treatment because doing so tends to result in them being unable to adopt the pattern of regular eating.

• The new eating pattern should take precedence over other activities and be adhered to, whatever patients' circumstances or appetite. On the other hand, it should be adjusted to suit patients' day-to-day commitments. Usually it will differ on weekdays and weekends.

• Patients should plan ahead. They should always know when they are going to have their next meal or snack, and there should rarely be more than a 4-hour interval between the meals and snacks. Each morning patients should write out (in outline) their plan for the day on the back of the day's monitoring record. If the day is going to be unpredictable, they should plan ahead as far as possible and identify a time when they can take stock and replan the rest of the day if need be.

• Patients whose eating habits are chaotic and those whose eating is highly restrictive may need to introduce this pattern in stages. At first they should be asked to focus on the part of the day when their eating is least problematic, usually the mornings, then gradually extend the regular eating pattern until it encompasses the entire day. This may take several weeks.

• Patients may seek advice about quantities they should eat and, in particular, whether they should eat until they feel full. They should be told that because their sensations of appetite, hunger, and fullness are all likely to be disturbed at present, they should not allow these sensations to determine what they eat. Instead, patients should adhere to the agreed pattern of eating and consume no more than average-size portions of food. The size of an average portion can be determined from the eating habits of friends or relatives, from recipes, and from the instructions on food packages.

• Patients who seek advice on what to eat should be told that the priority is their pattern of eating, not what they eat. If they nevertheless want guidance, they are told that the ideal is to adopt a varied diet, with the minimum number of avoided foods. Patients should be discouraged from counting calories, especially any tendency to keep a running total.

Three difficulties commonly arise when helping patients adopt this pattern of eating:

1. It is not uncommon for patients to say that they have never eaten in this way, and nor do their family or friends. Therapists should respond that although this may well be the case, adopting this pattern of eating will help them overcome their eating problem—and it will be the foundation upon which other important changes will be built. Once patients have overcome their eating problem, exactly how they eat will be up to them, but in the meantime it is in their best interests to follow this pattern of eating. Some patients are particularly reluctant to eat breakfast fearing that if they start the day by eating then they will not be able to stop. Implementing both aspects of the "regular eating" intervention properly provides an opportunity for them to test, and to disconfirm, this belief.

2. Some patients are reluctant to eat meals and snacks because they think that this will result in weight gain. Patients can be reassured

that this rarely occurs because they have not been asked to change the amount that they eat or what they eat. Also, with patients who binge eat, it should be pointed out that regular eating results in a decrease in the frequency of binge eating, thereby reducing significantly their overall energy intake (even if patients vomit, they absorb a significant amount of energy each time they binge). Despite such assurances, it is common for patients to select meals and snacks that are low in energy. There need be no objection to this: At this stage, the focus is on establishing a pattern of regular eating (i.e., the emphasis is on *when* patients eat rather than *what* they eat).

3. A common problem is that some patients are liable to feel full after eating relatively little, and that this feeling produces a desire to vomit or to take laxatives after eating. Feelings of fullness are especially prominent in underweight patients and may be attributed to the delayed gastric emptying that is a feature of starvation. With some patients, feelings of fullness are especially likely after they have eaten foods that they perceive as fattening. This reaction is likely to be largely cognitive in nature and the result of paying undue attention to abdominal sensations that normally pass unnoticed.

Patients who are troubled by feelings of fullness benefit from not wearing tight clothes at mealtimes and from engaging in distracting activities afterwards. They should be reassured that feelings of fullness generally subside within an hour and that their propensity to feel full will gradually decline with the adoption of this pattern of regular eating.

Two rather different strategies may be used to help patients resist eating in the time periods between the planned meals and snacks. The first is to help them identify activities that are incompatible with eating, or that make it less likely. These may include telephoning or visiting friends, going for a walk, exercising, e-mailing, searching the Internet, or having a bath or shower. As always, patients should be advised to plan ahead. They should try to predict when difficulties are likely to arise and intervene early by arranging activities that are likely to help them adhere to the regular eating pattern. The other strategy is very different. It involves asking patients to focus on the urge to eat and recognize that it is a temporary phenomenon—one to which they do not have

to give in. In this way patients learn to decenter from the urge, and simply observe it rather than try to eliminate it. As with feelings of fullness, they will find that the urge dissipates over time. This latter strategy is difficult for most patients, especially in the early stages of treatment. If it is to be used at all, it is best left until later on in treatment when urges to eat between meals and snacks are intermittent and less overwhelming.

Involving Significant Others

CBT-E was developed as an individual treatment for adults; hence, it does not actively involve others. Despite this, it is our practice to see "significant others" if this is likely to facilitate treatment and the patient is willing for this to happen. We do this with the aim of creating the optimum environment for the patient to change. There are two specific indications for involving others:

1. If others may be of help to the patient in making changes.
2. If others are making it difficult for the patient to change, for example, by commenting adversely on the patient's appearance or eating.

Typically the sessions with others last about 45 minutes and take place immediately after a routine session. Preparation in advance is important and involves discussing with the patient the aim and format of the meeting, and agreeing on who will do what. Generally the meeting involves the following:

- An introduction by the therapist and a statement about the aims of the meeting.
- The patient explaining something about treatment and its rationale, and what he or she is currently trying to do.
- Listening to the point of view of the significant other(s) and answering their questions.
- Discussing how they could be of practical help to the patient:
  - By responding to requests for help when the patient is having difficulty coping with urges to eat in the time periods between planned meals or snacks.
  - By helping underweight patients choose what and how much to eat and, later on, by stepping back and letting patients make these decisions themselves.

We hold up to three such sessions with about three-fourths of our patients (and sometimes more with underweight patients). Topics outside the eating disorder are not usually addressed. With adolescent patients there is far greater involvement of others (Cooper & Stewart, 2008).

Stage 2

Stage 2 is a transitional stage in treatment. It has three aims:

1. To conduct a joint review of progress
2. To revise the formulation, if need be
3. To design Stage 3

At the same time, the therapist continues to implement the procedures introduced in Stage 1. Session are now once weekly, except in the case of underweight patients whose appointments continue to be twice weekly.

The reason for conducting this formal review of progress is the strong evidence across a variety of psychiatric disorders (Wilson, 1999b), including bulimia nervosa (Agras et al., 2000; Fairburn, Agras, Walsh, Wilson, & Stice, 2004), that the amount that the patient changes during first few weeks of treatment is a potent predictor of outcome. This being so, it is crucial that the initial stages of treatment are implemented well. It also suggests that limited progress needs to be recognized early on and its explanation sought, so that treatment can be adjusted to overcome the identified obstacle(s) to change.

Conducting a Joint Review of Progress

The review of progress is best done systematically with the patient completing once again the EDE-Q, the CIA, and the measure of general psychiatric features. In this way patient and therapist can both review the extent of change. Reviewing the patient's monitoring records may also be helpful. In addition, patient and therapist should consider the degree to which the patient has been complying with the various elements of treatment.

Generally patients' views on their progress are unduly negative. An important task for the therapist, therefore, is to help the patient arrive at a balanced appraisal of what has changed and what has not. Typically there will have been a decrease in the frequency of any binge eating and compensatory purging, and an im-

provement in the pattern of eating, whereas concerns about shape will not have changed (to a large extent because they will not have been addressed).

One important and sometimes overlooked reason for progress not being as great as might be expected is the presence of a clinical depression. Ideally such depressions should be detected and treated before treatment is started, but inevitably some are missed and others develop afresh. If there appears to be a clinical depression, it is our practice to treat it with antidepressant medication and consider suspending CBT until the patient has responded.

Revising the Formulation (If Need Be)

It is important to review the formulation in light of what has been learned during Stage 1. Often no change is indicated, but sometimes problems and processes have been detected that were not obvious in Session 0, when the formulation was originally created. For example, it may have emerged that overexercising is a far greater problem than had been thought. If so, the formulation may need to be revised. Also, if the patient is receiving the "broad" form of CBT-E, it is at this point that the contribution of mood intolerance, clinical perfectionism, core low self-esteem, and interpersonal difficulties is considered (see Fairburn, 2008).

Designing Stage 3

Last, Stage 2 is the time when Stage 3 should be designed. It is at this stage that the treatment becomes highly individualized. The therapist has to decide which elements of Stage 3 will be most relevant to the patient and in what order they should be implemented (see below).

Stage 3

This is the main part of treatment, and its exact form differs from patient to patient. The focus is on the mechanisms that are maintaining the particular patient's eating disorder. These may be categorized under four broad headings:

1. The overevaluation of shape and weight and its various expressions
2. Dietary restraint
3. Residual binges
4. Undereating and being underweight

The first three are described below in turn; the fourth is beyond the scope of this chapter, and is described in the complete treatment guide (Fairburn, 2008). The order in which they are addressed depends on their relative importance in maintaining the patient's psychopathology. Generally it is best to start by addressing the concerns about shape and weight because this is the most complex and takes the longest. It is also the "core psychopathology." After a few weeks, the therapist also starts addressing one of the other mechanisms and, after a few more weeks, perhaps one of the others too. Meanwhile the therapist will be continuing to implement the procedures introduced in Stage 1. If the patient is receiving the broad form of CBT-E, one or more of the four additional treatment modules will also be used (see Fairburn, 2008).

Addressing the Overevaluation of Shape and Weight

At the heart of most eating disorders is the distinctive "core psychopathology," the overevaluation of shape and weight; that is, the judging of self-worth largely, or even exclusively, in terms of shape and weight, and the ability to control them. As described earlier, most of the other features of these disorders are secondary to this psychopathology and its consequences. For this reason, this psychopathology occupies a central place in most patients' formulation and is a major target of treatment. Clinical experience and research evidence suggest that unless this psychopathology is successfully addressed, patients are at substantial risk of relapse.

Five of the main elements of this aspect of treatment are now described in turn:

1. Identifying the overevaluation and its consequences
2. Developing marginalized self-evaluative domains
3. Addressing body checking and avoidance
4. Addressing "feeling fat"
5. Exploring the origins of the overevaluation

Other than the initial element, these are not necessarily introduced in this order.

IDENTIFYING THE OVEREVALUATION AND ITS CONSEQUENCES

The starting point is educating the patient about the notion of self-evaluation. The thera-pist then helps the patient identify his or her scheme for self-evaluation. Finally the implications of this scheme are discussed and a plan for addressing the expressions of the overevaluation is devised.

Because therapists are often unsure how to broach the subject of self-evaluation, an illustrative dialogue is provided below (adapted from Fairburn, 2008):

THERAPIST: We've decided that today we are going to focus primarily on the shape side of things. I'd like to go back to why we are doing this. If we look back at the diagram that shows the things that are driving your eating problem (*referring to the patient's formulation*), you can see that at the top are your concerns about your shape and weight. Clearly we need to focus on them since they seem important in keeping your eating problem going and they really worry you.

PATIENT: Yes, my shape is the main thing I worry about. It really bothers me—the fact that I can't get it off my mind—and it is so awful. I hate it.

THERAPIST: Well, to start with, we need to talk about the way we all evaluate or judge ourselves, something most of us don't even think about. All of us have a system, or way, of judging ourselves, and if we are meeting our personal standards in this respect, we feel reasonably good about ourselves, whereas if we are not, we feel bad. So if we take a typical person, there will be various things that he or she will judge him- or herself by. For example, relationships with others are often important—say, one's relationships with one's parents (and children, if one has some) and one's relationships with friends. Other things that are likely to be important may be how one is getting on at work, and at important pastimes—say, sports or singing, music, cooking, or whatever. And one's appearance, too, may be important. Now, if things are going well in these various areas of life, one feels fine, but if they are not, one feels bad—indeed, feeling bad is the best clue as to an area's importance. If one feels really bad when an aspect of life is not going well, this strongly suggests that this aspect is very important to one's self-evaluation. Does this make sense?

PATIENT: Yes, I think so. The way I look, for example, makes me feel really bad. I won't go out some days.

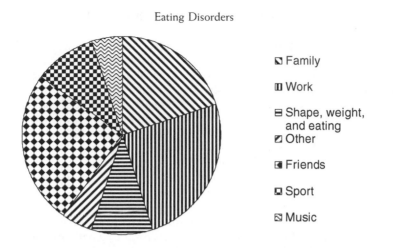

FIGURE 14.7. A "balanced" pie chart. From Fairburn (2008). Copyright by The Guilford Press. Adapted by permission.

THERAPIST: Exactly. So this indicates that your appearance is very important in how you see, or judge, yourself. Now a good way of representing all this is to draw a pie chart, with the various slices representing the various aspects of life that are important to you, and the bigger the slice, the more important that aspect is. Let me show you. (*Sketches out a "balanced" pie chart [see Figure 14.7].*) Now what I would like us to do together is to try to draw your pie chart. What we first need to do is list the things that are important in the way you judge, or evaluate, yourself. What might they be?

The therapist then helps the patient to generate a list of areas of life that are important to him or her. Almost invariably this includes appear-

ance and perhaps also control of eating. The therapist then goes on to explore the relative importance of these domains of self-evaluation; the clue to their relative importance is the magnitude (in terms of intensity and duration) of the patient's response to things going badly in the area. In this way the various areas of life that have been listed can be ranked. Finally, therapist and patient draw out a preliminary pie chart, with the size of each slice representing the relative importance of that area in the patient's scheme for self-evaluation. A typical pie chart is shown in Figure 14.8; the pie charts of patients with eating disorders are typically dominated by a large slice representing their overevaluation of shape and appearance.

A useful thing for patients to do is to review their pie chart each day and think whether it re-

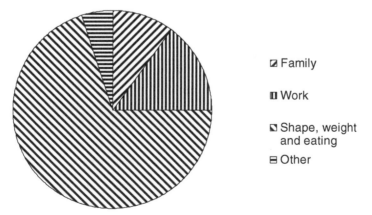

FIGURE 14.8. An "unbalanced" pie chart. From Fairburn (2008). Copyright by The Guilford Press. Adapted by permission.

ally represents the true state of affairs. At the next session, the pie chart is discussed further and adjusted as needed. Generally, any revision takes the form of expanding the size of the slice representing the importance of shape and weight.

The next step is to ask the patient to consider the implications of his or her scheme for self-evaluation (as represented by the pie chart) and to think whether any problems might be inherent to it. This discussion generally leads to the identification of two main problems:

1. Having a pie chart with a dominant slice is "risky." In this context the therapist might say:

   "It is like having all your eggs in one basket. It's fine so long as everything is going well in this regard, but if it isn't, you are in trouble. A parallel can be drawn with top athletes who also tend to have a dominant slice in their pie chart, one that is concerned with their athletic performance. If, unexpectedly, they can no longer compete—say, as a result of an car accident or an illness—they tend to have great trouble adjusting to this."

2. Judging oneself largely on the basis of appearance is also problematic. The therapist might go on to say:

   "In your case the problem lies not only in having most of your eggs in one basket but also in the nature of the basket itself. It is not a good one, because success in this area of life is elusive, and apparent failure is ever present for a number of reasons, some of which we will discuss later. Briefly, it is problematic to base your self-evaluation on appearance, since there is no objective index of success, and there will always be lots of people who seem more attractive (i.e., successful) than

you. Also, shape and weight are only controllable to a limited extent, and then only in the short term. Another problem is that judging yourself in this way may lead you to engage in forms of behavior that are unhelpful and may even do harm, making yourself sick being one example."

This discussion leads naturally to the final step in the examination of self-evaluation, namely, the creation of a formulation that includes the consequences of the overevaluation (the "extended" formulation). The therapist starts by asking patients what they do, or experience, as a result of the importance they place on shape and appearance, the goal being to derive a figure resembling that shown in Figure 14.9, with the therapist adding the upward feedback arrows saying something along the following lines:

"These things that you do, or that happen, as a result of your concerns about shape are themselves likely to maintain your concerns about shape—for example, repeatedly checking your body will intensify your unhappiness with your shape; similarly avoiding seeing your body will result in your fears and concerns persisting unchallenged; the experience of "feeling fat" often tends to be equated with being fat, yet it is something quite different. The point I am making is that it is vital that we tackle these consequences of your concerns because they are one of the main things that keep you so unhappy about your appearance. It's a vicious circle, and one that is hard to get out of."

In collaboration with the patient, the therapist needs to devise a plan for addressing the concerns about shape and weight, there being two overarching strategies: one being to de-

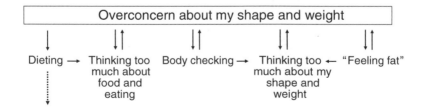

FIGURE 14.9. An "extended" formulation. From Fairburn (2008). Copyright by The Guilford Press. Adapted by permission.

velop other domains for self-evaluation and the other being to reduce the importance attached to shape and weight. Both are important and complement each another.

DEVELOPING MARGINALIZED DOMAINS FOR SELF-EVALUATION

Tackling the expressions of the overevaluation of shape and weight gradually reduces the extent of the overevaluation: The shape- and weight-related "slice" of the pie chart begins to shrivel. But at the same time, the corollary is important: to increase the number and importance of other domains for self-evaluation, which further diminishes the relative importance placed on shape and weight. The goal is that patients begin to get actively involved with other aspects of life.

There are six steps in encouraging patients to value other aspects of life:

1. The therapist explains the rationale for developing new domains for self-evaluation.

2. The therapist then helps the patient identify new activities that might be engaging. A clue may come from the patient's activities or interests in the past. The patient might have been a tennis player or might have painted, or might have liked hiking or pottery. It does not matter what the activity was or how good the patient was at it: It is simply valuable to know what types of things the patient used to like.

3. Next, the therapist and patient need to consider what activity or activities the patient might consider taking up now. A "brainstorming" approach is best, listing all possibilities, even if the patient views some of them as silly or intimidating. Good ideas may come from considering what others in the patient's peer group are doing.

4. Then, the therapist and patient need to agree on one, or possibly two, activities that the patient will try. These can be anything, so long as they are feasible and ongoing rather than on–off events. It is ideal if they involve others because they are then more likely to become self-perpetuating; furthermore, contact with others can help patients "catch up" interpersonally because some patients have missed out on age-appropriate experiences. (This is particularly true of underweight patients.)

5. Next, the therapist ensures that the patient actually does the activity identified. Barriers to starting should be reviewed and solutions sought. Here, a problem-solving approach is often of value (described later in the chapter).

6. Progress should be reviewed week-by-week with the therapist being encouraging and facilitative. Patients should be helped to use the problem-solving strategy to overcome any difficulties they may encounter. Over the course of treatment, as additional new activities are identified and adopted, others may be dropped.

Simultaneously, the therapist targets directly the patient's overevaluation of shape and weight, often starting with body checking, which often is of central importance in maintaining the patient's concerns.

ADDRESSING BODY CHECKING AND AVOIDANCE

The importance of body checking and avoidance has only recently been appreciated. The reason is quite simple: Few clinicians were aware of it because patients do not disclose the behavior unless asked, and many are not even aware of it.

The first step in addressing body checking is to provide information about body checking, body avoidance, and their consequences, stressing the following two points:

1. All people check their body to some extent, but many people with eating problems repeatedly check their bodies, and often in a way that is unusual. Such checking can become so "second nature" that they may not be aware of doing it. This checking needs to be addressed in people with eating problems because it can maintain dissatisfaction with body and appearance.

2. Some people with eating problems avoid seeing their bodies and dislike having other people seeing them too. Usually these people engaged in body checking in the past, but switched over to avoidance because the repeated checking became intolerable. Body avoidance is also problematic in that it allows one's concerns and fears about shape and appearance to persist in the absence of any information about how one actually looks. Therefore it needs to be tackled too.

Next, the therapist needs to find out the checking behaviors in which the patient engages. An adaptation of the usual monitoring record may be used for this purpose, with an extra "body checking" column inserted in the middle. Because recording body checking is highly distressing for some patients, it is best to ask patients to do it for only two 24-hour periods, one a working day and the other a day off work. The therapist may say something along these lines:

"To find out what you are doing, I would like you to record every time you check your body or compare someone else's body with your own. Please do this on one work day and on one day off work since they may differ. Here is an adaptation of our usual record for doing this. You may find that you have a lot to write down—don't worry about this—and you may feel like omitting some things. Try to write everything down because we need to know exactly what you are doing if we are going to tackle this."

It is common for patients to be taken aback at how often they check their shape.

The therapist and patient then categorize the various forms of body checking into two groups: forms of behavior that are best stopped, and behaviors that are better adjusted. The strategies used to achieve these goals differ. In addition the therapist will want to discuss in some detail mirror use and comparison-making.

Addressing Unusual Forms of Body Checking. Highly unusual forms of body checking are best stopped altogether. Patients can usually do this if the rationale is well explained and they are provided with support. The points to emphasize are as follows:

• Rarely do people feel better after body checking, because they are focusing on aspects of their appearance that they dislike.
• Stopping unusual forms of checking is generally experienced (after a week or so) as a relief.

Addressing More Normative Forms of Body Checking. A different strategy needs to be adopted with more normative forms of body checking. Here the problem is the frequency of the checking, the way that it is done, and patients' interpretation of what they find. The therapist needs to help patients consider the following questions each time that they are about to check themselves:

• What am I trying to find out?
• Do I need to find this out just now?
• Can I find this out in this way?
• Might there be adverse effects from checking myself in this way?
• Is there a better alternative?

Mirror use deserves particular attention given that mirrors have the potential to provide misleading, but highly credible, information and it is likely that they play an important role in the maintenance of many patients' body dissatisfaction. Education about mirrors and mirror use is therefore of importance. The main point to stress is that, as with other forms of body checking, what patients find out depends to an extent upon how they look. If patients study aspects of their appearance that they dislike, apparent flaws that normally go unnoticed are drawn to one's attention, and once noticed, they are hard to forget and ignore. Thus, scrutiny is prone to magnify apparent defects. Patients therefore need to question their use of mirrors as they are the main way that we determine how we look. Women need mirrors to put on makeup and to adjust their hair, and men need them for shaving. Full-length mirrors are also useful to see whether clothes go well together. But therapists should ask patients whether there is ever a case for looking at oneself naked in a full-length mirror. If one is already dissatisfied with one's appearance, doing so is likely to risk increasing one's dislike of one's shape through the magnification process mentioned earlier. This is not to say that total avoidance is to be recommended; rather, the advice is (for a time) to restrict the use of mirrors to the purposes listed above.

Another form of body checking that actively maintains dissatisfaction with shape involves comparing oneself with other people. The nature of these comparisons generally results in patients concluding that their bodies are unattractive relative to those of others. As noted earlier, patients' appraisals of their shape often involve scrutiny and selective attention to disliked body parts. The scrutiny is liable to result in the magnification of perceived defects, and the selective attention increases overall dissatisfaction with shape. In contrast, patients' assessment of others is very different. They tend to make superficial and often uncritical judgments about others. Furthermore, when making these comparisons, they tend to choose biased reference groups: One is selected people they encounter in their day-to-day life, generally those of the same age and gender who are thin-looking; and the other is people in the media. They fail to notice people who are not good-looking. Thus, the playing field is uneven, with an inherent unfavorable bias in the nature of the comparisons being made.

The steps involved in addressing patients' comparison-making are as follows:

1. The therapist helps patients identify when and how they make comparisons. Information of the following type is needed:

- The subject of the comparison. Who were they? How were they selected? Were they representative of people the patient's age and gender, or were they a select and atypical subgroup?
- How the person was assessed. What body parts were the focus of the comparison, and how were they evaluated?

2. Once this information has been collected, the therapist helps the patients to consider whether the comparison was inherently biased in terms of the person chosen and how his or her shape was evaluated. Two points are worth highlighting:

- Comparing oneself with people portrayed in the media (models, film stars, and other celebrities) is problematic because they are an unusual subgroup and images of them may well have been manipulated.
- Most ways of assessing one's body are idiosyncratic: it is difficult, if not impossible, to get the same perspective on someone else's body. For example, looking down at how much one's thighs splay out when sitting is a view one can only have of oneself: One never sees another person's thighs from this vantage point. The same applies to looking in the mirror, feeling one's stomach, touching one's bones, and pinching one's flesh.

3. Certain homework tasks usefully complement these discussions; for example, patients may be asked:

- To be more scientific when choosing someone to compare themselves with. Instead of selecting thin people, the therapist may ask them to select every third person (of their age and gender) that they encounter. What they

will discover is that people's bodies vary a great deal and that attractiveness is not directly related to thinness.

- To scrutinize other people's bodies. The goal is to demonstrate the point that "What you see depends (to an extent) upon how one looks." One way a patient may do this is to go to a changing room (e.g., of a swimming pool or gym), select someone nearby of about the same age and level of attractiveness, then unobtrusively scrutinize that person's body, focusing exclusively on the parts that the patient is most sensitive about. The longer the scrutiny, the better. Patients discover that even attractive people have apparent flaws—dimpled thighs or buttocks ("cellulite"), a protruding stomach, or wobbling flesh.

4. Assuming that the patient's comparison-making is biased (as it almost invariably is), the therapist should explore the implications of this bias in terms of the validity of the patient's views on his or her appearance. The goal is that patients become aware that their comparison-making has yielded misleading information about other people's bodies in relation to their own.

Addressing Body Avoidance. "Exposure" in its technical and literal sense is the strategy here. Therapists need to help patients get used to the sight and feel of their bodies, and to learn to make even-handed comparisons with those of others. They may need to get used to seeing their own bodies and letting others see them too. Patients need to stop dressing and undressing in the dark, and should abandon wearing baggy, shape-disguising clothes. Participation in activities that involve a degree of body exposure can be helpful, for example, swimming. Depending on the extent of the problem, tackling body avoidance may take many successive sessions. Because of the risk that the patient may return to repeated body checking, the therapist needs to help the patient adopt normative and risk-free forms of checking.

ADDRESSING "FEELING FAT"

"Feeling fat" is an experience reported by many women but the intensity and frequency of this feeling appears to be far greater among people with eating disorders. Feeling fat is an important target for treatment because it tends to be equated with being fat, whatever the patient's actual weight and shape. Hence, feeling fat maintains body dissatisfaction.

There has been almost no research on feeling fat, and little has been written about it. What is striking is that it tends to fluctuate markedly from day to day and even within a single day. This is quite unlike many other aspects of these patients' core psychopathology, which is relatively stable. Our impression is that in people with eating disorders, feeling fat is either an expression of body dissatisfaction or a result of mislabeling certain emotions and bodily experiences. It is important to stress that "feeling fat" and "being fat" are quite different, but they can co-occur. Many people with obesity are not troubled by feeling fat, but some are, and in the same way as people with an eating disorder. For them, feeling fat contributes to the maintenance of body dissatisfaction. It is therefore essential that feeling fat be addressed in these patients, too.

Addressing feeling fat is an important element in tackling patients' concerns about shape. In general it is best to focus on feeling fat once the patient has begun to make inroads into body checking and avoidance, but this is not invariably the case. In patients in whom feeling fat is a particularly prominent feature it is best to address it before tackling body checking and avoidance.

The steps in addressing feeling fat are as follows:

1. First, the therapist determines whether the patient feels fat at times and whether this is a problem. It is almost invariably seen as such. The therapist then explains that it is useful to learn more about this phenomenon because it may mask other feelings or sensations that occur at the same time. It should also be stressed how important it is not to equate feeling fat with being fat (i.e., the shape of one's body) because the two are quite different. Even very thin people can feel fat. The therapist should point out that whereas feelings of fatness fluctuate from day to day and within each day, body shape barely changes within such a short time frame. Therefore, something else must be responsible for the fluctuations in the feelings of fatness.

2. Next, patients should be asked to record when they have particularly intense feelings of fatness. Asking them to monitor whenever they

feel fat does not work because the feeling tends to be ever-present. This monitoring can be part of patients' normal recording process, using the right-hand column of the recording sheet for this purpose. When patients record feeling fat, they should also think about (and record) what else they are feeling at the time.

3. In the next session, each recorded occurrence of feeling fat should be reviewed in terms of the context in which it occurred and the presence of any potentially masked feelings or sensations.

4. Over the following week the patient should be asked to record in even greater detail the context in which subsequent feelings of fatness occur, the goal being to improve their identification of disguised feelings and experiences, and their triggers.

5. By the next session it should be clear that the patient's experience of feeling fat tends to be triggered either by the occurrence of certain negative mood states or by physical sensations that heighten body awareness. Examples of these two types of stimulus include the following:

- Feeling bored, depressed, lonely, or tired
- Feeling full, bloated, sweaty; feeling one's body wobble or one's thighs rub together; the sensation that one's clothing is tight

The therapist should help patients see these possible associations.

6. Over the subsequent week patients should attempt to identify these triggers in real time. Thus, the patients' task changes to asking "What am I really feeling just now?" every time they have strong feelings of fatness. In addition, patients should be asked to address the masked problem (e.g., feeling bored) using the problem-solving approach. [Problem solving is described later in the chapter. Some patients will have already been taught problem solving in the context of addressing event-triggered changes in eating. For others, the approach needs to be introduced at this point.]

7. Thereafter patients should repeatedly practice:

- Identifying when they have intense feelings of fatness
- Asking themselves the question "What am I really feeling just now?"
- Addressing the trigger using the problem-solving approach

With regard to tackling patients' responses to heightened body awareness, therapists should help them appreciate that the problem is their negative interpretations of these sensations rather than the sensations themselves.

To address feeling fat typically takes many weeks and will be a recurring item on the agenda of each session. What generally happens is that the frequency and intensity of feeling fat progressively decline and patients' "relationship" to the experience changes, such that it is no longer equated with being fat. This metacognitive change is important because, once it has happened, feeling fat ceases to maintain body dissatisfaction.

EXPLORING THE ORIGINS
OF THE OVEREVALUATION

Toward the end of Stage 3 it is often helpful to explore the origins of the patient's sensitivity to shape, weight, and eating. This helps the patient make sense of how the problem developed and evolved, and highlights how it might have served a useful function in its early stages—for example, exerting strict dietary control gives some people a sense of self-control when other aspects of their life feel beyond their influence. Occasionally specific events are identified that appear to have played a critical role in the development of the eating problem. These commonly involve the patient having been humiliated about his or her appearance. In such instances, the therapist needs to help the patient reappraise the critical event from the vantage point of the present.

Addressing Dietary Restraint

A major goal of treatment is to reduce, if not eliminate altogether, these patients' strong tendency to diet. This dieting has two aspects: attempting to curtail one's eating, which is termed "dietary restraint," and actual undereating in physiological terms, which may be termed "dietary restriction." The latter always coexists with the former, whereas the opposite is not the case. Dietary restriction may occur only during parts of the day—typically, the first half, as a result of delaying eating until late in the day—or there may be sustained undereating that results in the patient either losing weight or maintaining an unhealthily low weight. The "regular eating" intervention of

Stage 1 addresses the former ("delayed eating"). Addressing dietary restriction is beyond the scope of this chapter (for details, see Fairburn, 2008).

The dietary restraint of patients with eating disorders is both extreme in intensity and rigid in form. These patients set themselves multiple, demanding dietary rules concerning when they eat (e.g., not after 6:00 P.M.), how much they should eat (e.g., less than 600 kcal per day) and, most especially, what they should eat; most patients have a large number of foods that they attempt not to eat at all ("food avoidance"). Many attempt to follow all three types of dietary rules and as a result their eating is inflexible and restricted in nature. Despite this, dietary restraint is valued: Patients view it as desirable and tend to be oblivious to its adverse effects.

An important first step when addressing dietary restraint is for the therapist to bring the adverse effects of dieting to the patient's attention. This is best done with reference to the formulation and perhaps by asking the patient to complete a further CIA. The main adverse effects are as follows:

• *Dietary restraint is a major cause of the intense preoccupation with thoughts about food and eating experienced by many patients.* This preoccupation interferes with concentration and many aspects of day-to-day life (e.g., patients may find it difficult to read, to follow conversations, or to keep their mind on the plot of films). It is generally experienced as aversive.
• *Dietary restraint restricts the ways in which patients can eat.* For example, many patients find it difficult to eat unless they know the exact composition of what they are eating, and some cannot tolerate eating in front of others because they fear it will be interpreted as a sign of weakness or indulgence. As a result social eating is difficult, if not impossible. This is severely impairing given that eating is a highly social activity.
• *Dietary restraint is one major contributory factor to binge eating.* It is essential that patients understand this because many view restraint as simply their response to binge eating rather than as a cause of it. Generally dietary restraint leads to binge eating through cognitive mechanisms rather than physiological ones stemming from undereating, although both may contribute in patients in whom there is both dietary restraint and dietary restriction.

The basis for the cognitive mechanism is the dichotomous thinking (black-and-white thinking) present in most of these patients. Thus, they view any dietary slip, however minor, as a complete failure of dietary control ("I've broken my diet") and their response is to abandon temporarily attempts at dietary control and to binge eat instead, only to resume dietary restraint later in the day or on the next day. This response to dietary slips accounts for their distinctive pattern of eating, whereby dietary restraint is repeatedly punctuated by episodes of binge eating. Many patients who binge eat recognize this phenomenon and may even have terms for aspects of it; thus, some foods may be described as "trigger foods" as the patient knows that eating them is likely to trigger binge-eating, and one patient described her response as her "Sod it" reaction.

Patients who do not binge (especially those who are underweight) may dismiss this potential adverse effect of dieting as being of no relevance to them. In this case, the therapist needs to explain that this attitude is unwise because many patients who are underweight will end up binge eating, a development that is tantamount to their worst fears coming true.

- *Dietary restraint may result in dietary restriction, which in turn may lead to weight loss or the maintenance of an unduly low weight.* Although this is exactly what many patients want, they need to understand the immense price they would pay for this (see Fairburn, 2008).

Once it has been agreed that dietary restraint is a problem that needs to be tackled in treatment, the therapist and patient need to identify the patient's various dietary rules. Many rules will be evident by this stage in treatment, although some may not have come to light and others may have developed. In each case the therapist needs to identify the exact nature of the rule present and the patient's concerns that are driving it. The patient should then be helped to break the rule, possibly in the form of a behavioral experiment designed to test the concern in question. For example, the patient may believe that eating a certain food (e.g., chocolate) will inevitably lead them to binge eat. This belief can be disconfirmed by asking patients to introduce the avoided food into one of their planned meals or snacks on days when they are feeling in control over their eating and are able to resist binge eating. (They do not

need to each much of the avoided food; eating even a small quantity of it breaks the dietary rule.) By doing this repeatedly patients learn that the feared consequence that has been driving the dietary rule is not an inevitable result of breaking the rule. This has the effect of undermining and eroding the rule, thereby allowing the patient's eating to become more flexible.

With patients who binge eat it is important to pay particular attention to food avoidance and dichotomous thinking. The first step is to identify the avoided foods. A good way of doing this is to ask patients to visit a local supermarket and note all foods that they would be reluctant to eat because of their possible effect on their shape or weight, or because they fear that eating them might trigger a binge. Then patients should be asked to rank these foods (often 40 or more items) by dividing them into groups of foods they would find increasingly difficult to eat. Usually four or five groups are sufficient. Over the following weeks patients should progressively introduce these foods into their diet, starting with the easiest group and moving on to the most difficult. As noted earlier, the amount eaten is not important, although the eventual goal is that patients should be capable of eating normal quantities with impunity. The systematic introduction of avoided foods should continue until patients are no longer anxious about eating them. Patients may thereafter elect to eat a narrower diet. The tendency to think dichotomously should be tackled along conventional cognitive-behavioral lines.

Other dietary rules should be tackled in a similar fashion, with a focus both on the belief that is maintaining the rule and on breaking the rule itself. It is especially important to address rules that interfere with social eating. A small number of patients find it impossible to break their dietary rules; for example, they may be unable to introduce "banned foods" into their diet, or they may go on to binge and perhaps purge afterwards. With such patients some form of therapist-assisted eating may be helpful (see Dalle Grave et al., 2008).

Analyzing Changes in Eating

Among patients with eating disorders, eating habits may change in response to outside events. The change may involve eating less, stopping eating altogether, or overeating or frank binge eating (subjective or objective).

The variety of different mechanisms that may be involved include the following:

- Patients may eat less or stop eating to gain a sense of personal control when external events feel outside their control. This is seen most often in underweight patients.
- Another cause of eating less is to influence others; for example, it may be a way to exhibit feelings of distress or anger, or it may be an act of defiance.
- Overeating may be used by patients as a way to give themselves a "treat." This tends to be most characteristic of overweight patients.
- Binge eating may occur in response to adverse events and associated changes in mood. Binge eating has two properties that help people cope with negative events. First, the act of binge eating is distracting, so it takes the person's mind off the stimulus. Second, it has a direct mood-modulatory effect in that it dampens down strong mood states, possibly because it is somewhat sedating. Often both mechanisms operate in tandem.

Event-triggered changes in eating are common, but they decrease in response to the introduction of "regular eating." If they persist into Stage 3, they should be directly addressed. The first step with most patients is to identify such changes through the use of a real-time recording, and in the following session go over in detail one or more examples highlighting the processes involved. Then, depending on what appear to be the main mechanisms operating, the therapist will generally focus on one or more of the following:

- Enhancing patients' ability to deal with, and ideally to forestall, day-to-day problems by training them in proactive problem solving (see below).
- Helping patients accept the triggering moods states, and introducing the notion that they do not necessarily have to be neutralized.
- Identifying nonharmful ways patients can modulate their mood (unlike binge eating, substance misuse, or self-harm).

With most patients this is sufficient to address the phenomenon. However, a subgroup of patients either experiences particularly intense mood states or is unusually sensitive to them. These patients need more intensive focus on their moods and how to cope effectively with

them. The "mood intolerance" module of the broad form of CBT-E is designed for them (see Fairburn, 2008; Fairburn et al., 2003).

Thus, with the majority of patients, the core procedure is as follows:

1. The therapist should identify a recent example of an event-related change in eating. If one is not available, identify a specific example from the recent past (e.g., pressure at work, an argument, having nothing to do all day, coming home to an empty house).
2. The sequence of events that led to the change should be examined. This requires a detailed reconstruction of the sequence of events in terms of feelings, thoughts, and behavior.
3. Therapist and patient should identify possible alternatives to what happened, thereby introducing the notion that such changes in eating are not inevitable (e.g., someone might have called the patient and invited him or her out to see a film).
4. The patient should be taught how to use proactive "problem solving" to avoid event-triggered changes in eating. We do this with reference to the relevant section from *Overcoming Binge Eating* (Fairburn, 1995). The therapist explains that whereas many problems may seem overwhelming at first, they usually turn out to be manageable or even preventable if they are approached systematically. By becoming effective problem solvers, most patients can successfully tackle events of the type that have in the past disrupted their eating. Effective problem solving involves the following commonsense steps:

- *Step 1. Identifying the problem as early as possible.* Spotting problems early is of great importance. Almost invariably problems are easier to address if they are caught early on.
- *Step 2. Specifying the problem accurately.* Working out the true nature of the problem is essential if the best solution is to be found. Doing so may lead to the realization that two or more separate problems coexist, in which case each should be addressed individually. Rephrasing the problem is often helpful.
- *Step 3. Considering as many solutions as possible.* All ways of dealing with the problem should be considered. The patient should generate as many potential solutions as possible. Some solutions may seem nonsensical or impractical. Nevertheless, they should be included in the list of possible al-

ternatives. The more solutions that are generated, the more likely a good one will emerge.

- Step 4. *Thinking through the implications of each solution*. The likely effectiveness and feasibility of each solution should be considered.
- Step 5. *Choosing the best solution or combination of solutions*. Interestingly, if Step 4 has been thorough, choosing the best solution (or combination of solutions) is usually straightforward.
- Step 6. *Acting on the solution*. The final step is to act on the solution.

5. The therapist and patient should go through the identified problem using the six problem-solving steps. This is crucial and it should be collaborative, with the patient being encouraged to take the lead whenever possible. If time allows, another recent example should be identified and approached in the same way.

6. The therapist should help the patient consider potential alternative ways of responding to events. The therapist should introduce the notion that urges to eat are a temporary phenomenon and patients do not have to accede to them. Patients can learn to decenter from the urge, simply observing it rather than trying to eliminate it. (With some patients this notion will have been raised in the context of establishing a pattern of regular eating.) Alternatively, patients can experiment with response delay (or "urge surfing"); that is, dealing with urges to eat by waiting for the urge to subside. Response delay is of most relevance to event-triggered overeating or binge eating. Potential delaying activities should be identified with the patient. To be effective, the chosen activity needs to be engaging and of a type that tends to put the patient in a different frame of mind.

7. As homework, patients should be asked to practice their problem-solving skills. Over the following 7 days patients should identify events of the type that are liable to trigger changes in eating and address them by using the problem-solving procedure they have been taught. The following day, patients should review their attempts at problem solving. The aim is that they focus not on whether the problem was successfully solved but on their use of the problem-solving procedure. In other words, they should focus on enhancing their problem-solving skills.

8. *This homework should be reviewed at the next session, and further practice encouraged*. Throughout, the emphasis should be on acquiring the ability to address, or prevent, events that would previously have triggered changes in eating.

A variant of this procedure is used to tackle any residual binges. Termed "binge analysis," it is described in the complete treatment guide (Fairburn, 2008).

Stage 4

This is the final stage in treatment. With patients who are receiving 20 sessions of treatment, it comprises three sessions over 5 weeks (i.e., the sessions are 2 weeks apart). It has two broad aims:

1. To ensure that the changes made in treatment are maintained and built upon.
2. To minimize the risk of relapse in the future.

At the same time, patients discontinue self-monitoring and transfer from in-session weighing to weighing themselves at home.

Ensuring That the Changes Made in Treatment Are Maintained and Consolidated

The first step in doing this is to review in detail the patient's progress and what problems remain. This is done in much the same way as in Stage 2, with the EDE-Q and CIA as a guide. Then, depending on what problems remain, the therapist and patient jointly devise a specific plan for the patient to follow over the following 5 months (i.e., until the posttreatment review appointment). Typically this includes further work on body checking, food avoidance, and perhaps further practice at problem solving. In addition, the therapist encourages patients to maintain their efforts to develop new interests and activities.

Minimizing the Risk of Relapse in the Future

Eating disorders are conditions in which there is a risk of relapse. Our emerging experience with CBT-E (with over 300 patients) suggests that although full-scale relapse is uncommon, setbacks do occur and it is important that they are dealt with effectively.

Relapse is not an all-or-nothing phenomenon. It occurs in degrees and may start as a "slip," which then escalates. Commonly the slip comprises the resumption of dietary restraint, often triggered by an adverse shape-related event (e.g., a critical comment, clothes feeling tighter than usual). In patients who were previously prone to binge eat, this return of dietary restraint may lead to an episode of binge eating through the mechanisms described earlier, which in turn encourages yet greater dietary restraint, thereby increasing the risk of further episodes of binge eating. Within days, most aspects of the eating disorder may have returned, including delayed eating, food avoidance, and body checking. The patient's reaction to this sequence of events is crucial in determining what happens. The return of dietary restraint is not generally detected by the patient, but the resumption of binge eating is both noticeable and highly aversive, and may be experienced by the patient as "having gone back to square one." If the patient adopts a passive stance to the unfolding problem, what started as a lapse can develop rapidly into a full-scale relapse.

With patients whose eating disorder was characterized primarily by dietary restriction, and perhaps by being underweight, the sequence of events tends to be somewhat different. Again, the initial event is generally a return of dietary restraint, but this rapidly leads to dietary restriction and weight loss. Because none of this may be detected by the patient, the result is that the deterioration in eating habits may be well established before it comes to the patient's attention. Indeed, others often notice the problem first.

Clinical experience suggests that the following features are associated with an increased risk of relapse:

- Residual eating disorder features (especially overconcern with shape, continuing dietary restraint or restriction, being underweight)
- Having had an eating disorder characterized primarily by dietary restriction
- The occurrence of adverse shape-related events
- The development of a clinical depression
- Negative life events (e.g., interpersonal problems)

The therapist needs to do the following to minimize the risk of relapse:

1. *Educate the patient about the risk of relapse*, highlighting common triggers and the likely sequence of events in the patient's case. There is a tendency among some patients to hope that they will never have an eating problem again. This is especially common among those who have ceased to binge eat, but it is seen in other patients too. Without casting a negative light on patients' hopes for the future, therapists need to ensure that patients' expectations are realistic; otherwise, there is a risk that they will not take seriously the need to devise a "maintenance plan." Also, they will be vulnerable to reacting negatively to any emerging setback. Patients should be taught to view their eating disorder as their Achilles' heel; that is, their response to stress in general, and their response to certain triggers in particular.

2. *Stress the importance of detecting problems early*, before they become entrenched. With this in mind, therapist and patient should identify likely early warning signs of an impending relapse. Patients who are prone to binge or purge are fortunate in that these forms of behavior occur early on in the course of any setback and are noticeable. Patients whose eating disorder is primarily characterized by dietary restriction need help to spot ominous signs. It is best to bring to the patient's attention easily detected changes. Examples include the following:

- Cutting back on eating (e.g., skipping meals or snacks; the resumption of food avoidance)
- The avoidance of social events that involve eating
- An increase in exercising
- Changes in body checking or avoidance (e.g., a change in mirror use or weighing)
- Weight falling below an agreed threshold (e.g., a weight equivalent to a BMI of 19.0)

3. *Construct with the patient a plan of action (a written personalized "maintenance plan") for use in the future should a problem arise*. This comprises two elements. First is a focus on the emerging eating problem and how to correct it. In general this involves "doing the right thing"; that is, the patient forces him- or herself to do what was learned in treatment (e.g., regular eating, eating enough, weighing weekly, etc.). The cognitive-behavioral self-help program described in the second half of *Overcoming Binge Eating* (Fairburn, 1995) may be used for guidance in this regard. The

second aspect of the intervention is to address what triggered the setback. This is best done with the problem-solving procedure the patient learned in treatment. Again patients can refer to *Overcoming Binge Eating* to refresh their memory of what this involves.

4. *Discuss when the patient should seek further help.* It is important that patients seek further help if it is needed. The strategy described earlier should get patients back on track within a few weeks. If, after 3 weeks of trying to correct matters, the problem has not substantially resolved, the patient should seek outside help.

Ending Treatment

It is unusual not to end CBT-E as planned. As noted earlier, so long as patients have reached the point where the main maintaining mechanisms have been disrupted, then treatment can and should finish. Otherwise, patients (and therapists) are at risk of ascribing continuing improvement to the ongoing therapy rather than to the natural resolution of the eating disorder. In practice this means that it is acceptable to end treatment with patients still dieting to an extent, perhaps binge eating and vomiting on occasions, and having residual concerns about shape and weight.

At times, there are grounds for extending treatment. In our view, the main indication for doing this is the presence of eating disorder features that continue to interfere significantly with the patient's functioning and are unlikely to resolve of their own accord. Another reason to extend treatment is to compensate for the deleterious impact of disruptions to treatment, generally due to the emergence of a clinical depression or the occurrence of a life crisis.

The occasional patient benefits little from CBT-E. It is our practice to refer such patients for day patient or inpatient treatment.

The Posttreatment Review Appointment

We routinely hold a posttreatment review appointment about 20 weeks after the completion of treatment. During the intervening period patients do not receive any further therapeutic input. Instead, our intention is that they implement the agreed-upon short-term plan, so that they can maintain and consolidate the changes made in treatment. Patients who have experienced any setbacks are expected to have implement their maintenance plan.

In most cases we find that patients are managing well and have maintained the changes made in treatment. Patients may report having had minor setbacks that may or may not have required them to take action. Of course, the occasional patient will have experienced more major difficulties and may have sought help, but this is unusual.

CONCLUDING REMARKS

A common misconception is that manual-based treatments are "rigidly structured" protocols that are inconsistent with the provision of individualized treatment, undermine clinical judgment, and preclude dealing with co-occurring problems (e.g., Westen, Novotny, & Thompson-Brenner, 2004). In reality, even the early manual-based treatments allowed therapists to individualize treatment in several different ways, including developing a treatment plan for the individual patient within the overall treatment model, and providing session-to-session assessment (based on self-monitoring) to determine the timing and targets of interventions. Nevertheless, the challenge is to do still more in formulating manual-based treatments that are capable of addressing in a flexible manner the often multiple needs of individual patients. It is our hope that CBT-E represents a step forward in this regard.

A major limitation of some manual-based treatments is that the form that treatment takes is determined almost exclusively by the patient's DSM-IV diagnosis. This ignores the heterogeneity that exists within most DSM categories. By contrast, CBT-E is derived from a transdiagnostic theory, and its exact form depends on a highly personalized formulation rather than a DSM-IV-based one. Thus, whereas the treatment has much in common with functional analysis, a defining feature of behavior therapy, it is also derived from an empirically supported treatment for bulimia nervosa.

A major challenge in emphasizing greater individualization of treatment is to balance clinically appealing flexibility with the more structured and specified style of manual-based treatments. CBT-E attempts to achieve this synthesis by identifying the mechanisms that maintain the specific patient's eating disorder, then targeting them with evidence-based treatment procedures. In this way CBT-E attempts to integrate clinical research findings with therapist judgment (Wilson, 1999a).

It is often argued that clinical practice in the "real world" is self-correcting - if one method is unsuccessful, another is adopted (Seligman, 1995). In contrast, it is alleged that manual-based treatment proceeds in an unchanging, lock-step fashion. In fact, there is little evidence to indicate that routine clinical practice is self-correcting. A potential strength of CBT-E is that it contains a built-in self-correcting process in Stage 2, as described above. This formal evaluation of initial progress, or lack thereof, allows treatment to be adjusted as needed. It also fits well with the evidence that early response to treatment is a robust predictor of outcome, and that therefore this is the ideal time to conduct a thorough reassessment.

CBT-E has implications for psychological treatment beyond the field of eating disorders. In more general terms, it is consistent with emerging evidence on the role of common psychopathological processes across different diagnostic categories (Harvey et al., 2004). The transdiagnostic approach could be applied to other groups of related clinical disorders: consider, for example, Barlow, Allen, and Choate (2004) proposal for a unified treatment protocol for anxiety and mood disorders (see Chapter 5, this volume). The specific way that the transdiagnostic treatment for eating disorders has been operationalized might provide a model for designing treatments for other groups of functionally related conditions.

ACKNOWLEDGMENTS

A substantial proportion of this chapter has been reproduced (with permission) from the complete description of CBT-E (Fairburn, 2008). We are grateful to the Wellcome Trust for its support: C. G. F. is supported by a Principal Research Fellowship (No. 046386); Z. C. is supported by a program grant (No. 046386); and R. S. is supported by a Research Career Development Fellowship (No. 63209). We are also grateful to Suzanne Straebler for her help preparing the manuscript.

NOTES

1. BMI is a widely used way of representing weight adjusted for height. It is weight (in kilograms) divided by height squared (in meters) (i.e., weight/height^2). The healthy range for adults (of either sex) is 20.0 to 25.0.
2. If there is a difference in their core psychopathology,

it is that some patients with anorexia nervosa are primarily concerned with controlling their eating per se, rather than their shape and weight. This is especially true of younger patients whose disorder is of short duration. (See Fairburn, Shafran, and Cooper, 1999, for discussion of the issue of control in anorexia nervosa.)
3. Readers may find the EDE schedule of interest because it provides widely accepted definitions of many eating disorder concepts (e.g., binge eating, or in EDE terms, "objective bulimic episodes,"; driven exercising, overevaluation of shape and weight).
4. We favor medical beam balance scales, which are robust, accurate, and give sufficient precision. We recommend not using scales that provide a digital readout because their apparent accuracy reinforces concern with trivial changes in weight.
5. C. G. F. acknowledges the obvious conflict of interest.

REFERENCES

Agras, W. S., Crow, S. J., Halmi, K. A., Mitchell, J. E., Wilson, G. T., & Kraemer, H. C. (2000). Outcome predictors for the cognitive behavior treatment of bulimia nervosa: data from a multisite study. *American Journal of Psychiatry, 157*, 1302–1308.

American Psychiatric Association. (1994). *Diagnostic and statistical manual of mental disorders* (4th ed.). Washington, DC: Author.

Barlow, D. H., Allen, L. B., & Choate, M. L. (2004). Towards a unified treatment for emotional disorders. *Behavior Therapy, 35*, 205–230.

Bohn, K., & Fairburn, C. G. (2008). The Clinical Impairment Assessment Questionnaire. In C. G. Fairburn (Ed.), *Cognitive-behavior therapy and eating disorders*. New York: Guilford Press.

Cooper, Z., & Stewart, A. (2008). CBT-E for adolescents. In C. G. Fairburn (Ed.), *Cognitive-behavior therapy and eating disorders*. New York: Guilford Press.

Dalle Grave, R. (2008). Inpatient CBT-E. In C. G. Fairburn (Ed.), *Cognitive-behavior therapy and eating disorders*. New York: Guilford Press.

Dalle Grave, R., & Calugi, S. (2007). Eating disorder not otherwise specified on an inpatient unit. *European Eating Disorders Review, 15*, 340–349.

Fairburn, C. G. (1995). *Overcoming binge eating*. New York: Guilford Press.

Fairburn, C. G. (2005). Evidence-based treatment of anorexia nervosa. *International Journal of Eating Disorders, 37*, S26–S30.

Fairburn, C. G. (Ed.). (2008). *Cognitive-behavior therapy and eating disorders*. New York: Guilford Press.

Fairburn, C. G., Agras, W. S., Walsh, B. T., Wilson, G. T., & Stice, E. (2004). Prediction of outcome in bulimia nervosa by early change in treatment. *American Journal of Psychiatry, 161*, 2322–2324.

Fairburn, C. G., & Beglin, S. J. (1994). Assessment of

eating disorder psychopathology: interview or self-report questionnaire? *International Journal of Eating Disorders, 16,* 363–370.

Fairburn, C. G., & Bohn, K. (2005). Eating disorder NOS (EDNOS): An example of the troublesome "not otherwise specified" (NOS) category in DSM-IV. *Behaviour Research and Therapy, 43,* 691–701.

Fairburn, C. G., & Cooper, Z. (1993). The Eating Disorder Examination (12th ed.). In C. G. Fairburn & G. T. Wilson (Eds.), *Binge eating: Nature, assessment, and treatment* (pp. 317–360). New York: Guilford Press.

Fairburn, C. G., Cooper, Z., Bohn, K., O'Connor, M. E., Doll, H. A., & Palmer, R. L. (2007). The severity and status of eating disorder NOS: Implications for DSM-V. *Behaviour Research and Therapy, 45,* 1705–1715.

Fairburn, C. G., Cooper, Z., & Shafran, R. (2003). Cognitive behaviour therapy for eating disorders: A "transdiagnostic" theory and treatment. *Behaviour Research and Therapy, 41,* 509–528.

Fairburn, C. G., & Harrison, P. J. (2003). Eating disorders. *Lancet, 361,* 407–416.

Fairburn, C. G., Marcus, M. D., & Wilson, G. T. (1993). Cognitive-behavioral therapy for binge eating and bulimia nervosa: A comprehensive treatment manual. In C. G. Fairburn & G. T. Wilson (Eds.), *Binge eating: Nature, assessment, and treatment* (pp. 361–404). New York: Guilford Press.

Fairburn, C. G., Shafran, R., & Cooper, Z. (1999). A cognitive behavioural theory of anorexia nervosa. *Behaviour Research and Therapy, 37,* 1–13.

Harvey, A., Watkins, E., Mansell, W., & Shafran, R. (2004). *Cognitive behavioural processes across psychological disorders: A transdiagnostic approach to research and treatment.* Oxford, UK: Oxford University Press.

Lock, J., le Grange, D., Agras, W. S., & Dare, C. (2001). *Treatment manual for anorexia nervosa: A family-based approach.* New York: Guilford Press.

National Collaborating Centre for Mental Health. (2004). *Eating disorders: Core interventions in the treatment and management of anorexia nervosa, bulimia nervosa and related eating disorders.* London: British Psychological Society and Royal College of Psychiatrists.

Seligman, M. E. P. (1995). The effectiveness of psychotherapy. *American Psychologist, 50,* 965–974.

Vitousek, K. M., Watson, S., & Wilson, G. T. (1998). Enhancing motivation for change in treatment-resistant eating disorders. *Clinical Psychology Review, 18,* 391–420.

Westen, D., Novotny, C. M., & Thompson-Brenner, H. (2004). The empirical status of empirically supported psychotherapies: Assumptions, findings, and reporting in controlled trials. *Psychological Bulletin, 130,* 631–663.

Wilson, G. T. (1999a). Cognitive behavior therapy for eating disorders: Progress and problems. *Behaviour Research and Therapy, 37,* S79–S95.

Wilson, G. T. (1999b). Rapid response to cognitive behavior therapy. *Clinical Psychology: Science and Practice, 6,* 289–292.

Wilson, G. T. (2005). Psychological treatment of eating disorders. In S. Nolen-Hoeksema (Ed.), *Annual review of clinical psychology* (Vol. 1, pp. 439–466). Palo Alto, CA: Annual Reviews, Inc.

Wilson, G. T., Grilo, C. M., & Vitousek, K. M. (2007). Psychological treatment of eating disorders. *American Psychologist, 62.*

Wilson, G. T. & Schlam, T. R. (2004). The transtheoretical model and motivational interviewing in the treatment of eating and weight disorders. *Clinical Psychology Review, 24,* 361–378.

CHAPTER 15

Sexual Dysfunction

JOHN P. WINCZE
AMY K. BACH
DAVID H. BARLOW

Psychological treatments that have emerged during the past several decades for the various sexual dysfunctions have a particularly strong empirical base. We now have psychological procedures, with or without new medications, that are highly effective for the overwhelming majority of individuals whose sexual dysfunctions have a psychogenic component. But, as the authors point out, the organic–psychogenic distinction is no longer particularly useful in the assessment of these problems. For this reason, the development of new and effective medications for one sexual dysfunction, male erectile disorder, has overshadowed the fact that psychological interventions are often necessary even in cases in which medication is effective. This aspect of treatment has been neglected to some extent by primary care physicians with less experience in these matters. In this chapter, after an up-to-date review of important advances in sexuality research, a biopsychosocial model is presented that integrates consideration of medical and psychological factors in diagnosis and treatment. This section is followed by two cases, new to this edition, that illustrate nicely the integration of many of these procedures. Frank and Anna are an older couple, and Frank suffers from low sexual desire. Kara, a 31-year-old law student with sexual aversion disorder, has never dated. The reader may be struck by the twists and turns that the therapist took with these cases and the particular therapeutic strategies required. In covering specific approaches to all sexual dysfunctions, the authors not only highlight individual behavioral approaches required by each condition but also note common therapeutic factors that cut across conditions (e.g., providing sexual education, facilitating communication, and identifying important emotional and cultural factors that may contribute to sexual dysfunction). In sex therapy, we see some of the best illustrations of the integration of cognitive-behavioral, medical, and interpersonal systems approaches, and these case studies illustrate some of the ways in which this happens.—D. H. B.

Our purpose in this chapter is to outline a cognitive-behavioral approach to the assessment and treatment of sexual dysfunction. Cognitive-behavioral therapy (CBT) for sexual dysfunction can serve as a sole treatment or as an adjunct to a medical or surgical intervention. In either case, the techniques and information we present should be adapted to the particular needs of the individual or couple and the nature of the sexual difficulty. Before describing our approach to clinical work, we begin by addressing two key developments in sexuality research.

IMPORTANT ADVANCES IN SEXUALITY RESEARCH

The Prevalence of Sexual Dysfunction

Over the last 15 years, a number of important studies have examined the prevalence of sexual dysfunction (DeLamater & Sill, 2005; Feldman, Goldstein, Hatzichristou, Krane, & McKinlay, 1994; Rosen, Wing, Schneider, & Gendrano, 2005). Feldman and colleagues (1994) looked at minimal, moderate, and severe impotence in a sample of 1,290 men and found a combined prevalence of 52% in men ages 40–70. This study identified a higher prevalence of impotence with increasing age. Laumann, Paik, and Rosen (1999) published a landmark study in which they surveyed 1,410 men and 1,749 women between ages 18 and 59 years regarding the presence of various sexual difficulties. Demographics of the sample was representative of the U.S. population. Respondents were surveyed in person by experienced interviewers, who found that 43% of women and 31% of men endorsed some form of sexual dysfunction, making sexual dysfunction more prevalent than anxiety disorders, mood disorders, or substance use disorders (Kessler et al., 1994). These data received nationwide attention and validated clinicians' claims that sexual dysfunction is a widespread problem affecting a significant proportion of the population.

Rosen and colleagues (2005) reviewed evidence from worldwide epidemiological studies and concluded that erectile dysfunction (ED) is highly prevalent and affects approximately 60% of men older than age 60. Furthermore, the prevalence of ED is highly correlated with medical conditions such as diabetes, cardiovascular disease, and lower urinary tract symptoms, as well as lifestyle factors such as obesity, smoking, and lack of exercise. In another recent study, DeLamater and Sill (2005) looked at sexual desire in 639 men and 745 women ages 45–94, and found a decrease in desire as men and women aged, but sexual desire was maintained at relatively high levels until about age 75.

The publication of methodologically sound prevalence studies is one of at least two major developments in sexuality research to have emerged over the past decade. The second major development is, of course, the introduction of oral medications for enhancing erectile response: sildenafil (Viagra), tadalafil (Cialis), and vardenafil (Levitra). Sildenafil was introduced in 1998, and since then, tadalafil and vardenafil have entered the market. All three have proven to be effective treatments for ED (Carson & Lue, 2005; Segraves, 2003). These oral medications have successfully restored erectile functioning in millions of men with either psychogenic or organic etiologies. Research to date, has not shown any of these medications to be helpful to women (Segraves, 2003).

Pharmacology: Integration with Sex Therapy

The introduction of sex-enhancing medications has in some respects sparked a revolution in the treatment of sexual dysfunction. Once discussed only reluctantly with health professionals, sexual problems and their pharmacological treatments are now more widely addressed and advertised in the media. Mass media attention surrounding these medications has resulted in a dramatic increase in public awareness and acceptance of sexual dysfunction. Moreover, the treatment success has fueled patients' hopes and expectations that their sexual difficulties can be easily remedied. The result has been a sharp rise in the number of patients seeking treatment for sexual problems.

Some wondered whether the advent of drugs would mark the beginning of the end for sex therapy. On the contrary, sex therapists are treating more patients than ever. Although these drugs have benefited countless couples, they, like all "wonder drugs," have limitations. The most obvious drawbacks include serious risk to patients taking nitrates; side effects such as headaches, flushing, and dyspepsia; high cost; and the fact that these drugs do not significantly improve sexual functioning for 16–44% of men and as many as 82% of postmenopausal women (Conti, Pepine, & Sweeney, 1999; Goldstein et al., 1998; Kaplan et al., 1999). A more subtle issue is the fact that studies on the efficacy of ED medications focus primarily on the drug's ability to restore physiological sexual responding. Firm erections and adequate lubrication do not always lead to a satisfying sexual relationship. Thus, couples with poor communication, negative attitudes, and faulty beliefs regarding sexual function may find that a pill cannot do all that they hoped it would. These couples may find that CBT is an appealing alternative or a necessary adjunct to medical treatment. The challenge, then, is to identify the best treatment option for each patient and couple: medication alone, psychosocial treatment alone, psychosocial treatment in conjunction with medication, or no treatment for sexual dysfunction.

Before one can identify the appropriate treatment options, it is necessary, of course, to determine the nature of the sexual problem. Following is a brief description of each sexual dysfunction as defined in the fourth edition, text revision, of the *Diagnostic and Statistical Manual of Mental Disorders* (DSM-IV-TR; American Psychiatric Association, 2000).

THE SEXUAL DYSFUNCTIONS DEFINED

The four phases of the sexual response cycle are desire, excitement, orgasm, and resolution. DSM-IV-TR defines "sexual dysfunction" as a disturbance in one of these phases or as pain associated with intercourse. Most people occasionally experience a lack of interest in sexual activity, difficulty becoming aroused, or problems related to orgasm. A diagnosis of sexual dysfunction is reserved for cases in which difficulties with sexual functioning occur persistently and cause significant distress or problems for the individual or couple. In determining whether sexual difficulties warrant a clinical diagnosis, one must consider the patient's age and culture, as well as the course of the problem. Once a diagnosis of sexual dysfunction is assigned, the clinician should consider whether the problem occurs across all situations (generalized) or only in certain circumstances (situational). The clinician should also note whether the problem has always been present (lifelong) or whether it developed after a period of healthy functioning (acquired). Finally, the clinician should specify whether the problem is due to psychological factors or to combined (psychogenic and organic) factors. DSM-IV-TR recommends that clinicians use these specifiers, because they provide the treating therapist with useful information regarding the nature and course of the dysfunction and may have implications for treatment.

A useful assessment model for all sexual dysfunctions is the biopsychosocial model (DeLamater & Sill, 2005; Wincze & Carey, 2001). When diagnosing a sexual dysfunction, there must be consideration of the following influences: *biological* (e.g., hormonal system, vascular system, illness, medication, age); *psychological* (e.g., sexual knowledge, sexual attitude [positive or negative], sexual experience, mental health); *social* (e.g., availability of a partner, partner's health, partner's sexual en-

thusiasm/comfort, quality and length of relationship, privacy and conditions under which sex occurs). By considering these influences during the assessment, a comprehensive understanding of any sexual dysfunction is elucidated. More detailed implications of this model for etiology, assessment, and treatment are presented below.

Desire Disorders

Hypoactive Sexual Desire Disorder

DSM-IV-TR defines "hypoactive sexual desire disorder" as a lack or absence of sexual fantasies and desire for sexual activity (although there is no universally accepted definition of sexual desire; DeLamater & Sill, 2005). Beck (1995) argued that because the definition of low desire is ambiguous in DSM-IV-TR, some researchers operationalize it based on the frequency of sexual activity. Beck suggested that this is problematic, because people may engage in sexual activity when they do not have a desire to do so (e.g., to please a partner). More reliable measures of sexual desire may be the frequency of sexual thoughts, urges, and fantasies, and the extent to which the person takes advantage of opportunities for sexual activity (Wincze & Carey, 2001). It is, of course, important to consider these variables in the context of the person's age, culture, and gender. Undergraduate males, for example, report significantly more urges and masturbatory fantasies than their female counterparts (Jones & Barlow, 1990).

Low desire may be a primary problem, or it may be secondary to another sexual dysfunction (e.g., a man may lose interest in sex because he is frustrated by ED). Laumann and colleagues (1999) report that 5% of men and 22% of women have difficulties with low sexual desire. Surveys of women in gynecological clinics have yielded similar estimates of 17% (Osborn, Hawton, & Gath, 1988) and 21% (Bachmann, Leiblum, & Grill, 1989). Low desire appears to be one of the most common problems in patients seeking treatment for sexual difficulties. Segraves and Segraves (1991) examined the diagnoses of 906 participants recruited for a multisite pharmaceutical study of sexual dysfunctions. They found that 65% had a primary diagnosis of hypoactive sexual desire disorder; of these, 81% were female. A decline in sexual desire is significantly associated with age (DeLamater & Sill, 2005). This age-related decline in desire is strongly influenced by medical factors such as diabetes, prostate disease, cardiovascular disease, and arthritis that concomitantly increase with age. Older individuals are also less likely to have an available sexual partner and, for those who do, sexual monotony and overfamiliarity may contribute to loss of desire. Delamater and Sill point out, however, that sexual desire remains intact in healthy, educated older men and women with an available partner who is interested in sex.

Sexual Aversion Disorder

Whereas patients with hypoactive sexual desire disorder express a feeling of indifference, patients with sexual aversion disorder describe a very negative response to sexual activity. Fear or disgust usually characterizes their response to sexual activity. As a result, a person with sexual aversion disorder often avoids sexual activity (American Psychiatric Association, 2000). Unfortunately, there are limited data on the prevalence of this dysfunction. Clinical experience suggests that the majority of patients seeking treatment for sexual aversion disorder are women. People with sexual aversion disorder most often fear or feel repulsed by sexual intercourse. Women may report thoughts that they will feel significant pain or bleed a great deal upon penetration. Sexual aversion can be associated with any form of vaginal penetration (e.g., use of tampons, gynecological exam) and any aspect of sexual activity. One of us (A. K. B) recently treated a woman who was comfortable with kissing and fondling, but very uncomfortable when hugging or holding hands with a partner. Finally, in some cases, sexual aversion may be secondary to panic disorder. In such cases, the patient avoids sexual activity because of a conditioned fear response to physical sensations such as increased heart rate and rapid breathing (Sbrocco, Weisberg, Barlow, & Carter, 1997).

Arousal Disorders

Male Erectile Disorder

The introduction of ED medication has rendered male erectile disorder the most widely recognized sexual dysfunction. Male erectile disorder, which is also referred to as ED or "impotence," is defined as a persistent or recurrent inability to get or keep an adequate erection until the completion of sexual activity (American Psychiatric Association, 2000). Laumann and colleagues (1999) report a prevalence rate of 5% for ED. This rate is most likely an underestimation, because their sample did not include men age 60 years and older, the group in which male erectile disorder is most common. Feldman et al. (1994) surveyed 1,290 men between the ages of 40 and 70 years, living in Massachusetts. They found that whereas the prevalence of complete erectile failure was 5% at age 40, it rose to 15% at age 70. The probability of moderate erectile difficulties was 17% at age 40 and 34% by age 70. The National Institutes of Health (NIH) Consensus Conference (1993) on impotence also found ED to be very widespread, indicating that it affects 10–20 million men in the United States.

Men with ED often report that they cannot perform, or that "nothing happens." Research suggests that these men may actually underestimate their erectile response during sexual activity (Abrahamson, Barlow, Sakheim, Beck, & Athanasiou, 1985). A psychophysiological assessment of male sexual arousal is very useful, because it provides an objective measure of the patient's erectile function.

Men without any organically based ED normally experience full erections during sleep. Such erections, referred to as nocturnal penile tumescence, or NPT, can be detected with a RigiScan, a medical device that is attached to the penis and worn during sleep. The RigiScan, available in urology clinics that evaluate sexual dysfunction, is used to differentiate between organically and psychogenically based ED. If full erections are present during sleep, then the etiology of ED is most likely psychogenic.

Female Sexual Arousal Disorder

DSM-IV-TR defines "female sexual arousal disorder" as a persistent or recurrent inability to attain or maintain adequate lubrication and swelling until the completion of sexual activity. Women with this disorder may experience little or no subjective sense of arousal. Laumann and colleagues (1999) report that 20% of women ages 18–59 years have difficulty becoming physiologically aroused during sexual activity.

Female sexual arousal disorder is most commonly associated with menopause (Dennerstein & Hayes, 2005; Phillips, 2000) and with diabetes (Muniyappa, Norton, Dunn, & Banerj, 2005; Rutherford & Collier, 2005). Diabetes also contributes to decreased genital sensations in women and an increase in vaginal infections (Muniyappa et al., 2005). Women may be unlikely to seek professional help for difficulty becoming aroused because they can remedy the problem with a lubricant. Without any form of intervention, female sexual arousal disorder may result in painful intercourse, avoidance of sexual activity, and relationship problems.

Orgasmic Disorders

Premature Ejaculation

"Premature ejaculation" is somewhat loosely defined in DSM-IV-TR as ejaculation with limited stimulation that occurs before, on, or shortly after penetration and sooner than the person would like (American Psychiatric Association, 2000). Strassberg, Kelly, Carroll, and Kircher (1987) operationally defined the problem as ejaculation that occurs within 2 minutes of penetration on 50% or more of occasions, a feeling of being unable to control the latency to ejaculation, and a belief that this is a problem. Rowland, Cooper, and Schneider (2001) pointed out the wide discrepancies that exist in published research studies in defining premature ejaculation. In fact, over 50% of all published studies report no criteria at all for defining this disorder. The absence of a consistent definition has made treatment outcome studies almost impossible to compare and has resulted in widely disparate prevalence estimates. Ultimately, the most important criterion may be a man's subjective sense that he cannot control the timing of his orgasm. Men with premature ejaculation may report that they ejaculate just as they are beginning to feel aroused. Although the latency to ejaculation alone cannot be used as a deciding criterion, it is important to ask men presenting with this problem how soon is "too soon." Some men mistakenly endorse premature ejaculation because they cannot engage in sexual intercourse for 20–30 minutes before ejaculating. A focus on premature ejaculation may also be a "smoke screen" for other problems within the relationship. In such cases, a diagnosis of premature ejaculation is not warranted, and the person or couple can benefit

from education regarding normative latencies to ejaculation. Laumann and colleagues (1999) suggest that premature ejaculation affects 21% of men. Spector and Carey (1990) report a higher estimate of 36–38%.

Male Orgasmic Disorder

"Male orgasmic disorder" refers to a delay in or absence of orgasm following a normal phase of excitement and an adequate degree of stimulation (American Psychiatric Association, 2000). Laumann and colleagues (1999) report that this problem affects 8% of men. Spector and Carey (1990) provide a similar estimate of 4–10%. Male orgasmic disorder is most often situational; the person often has difficulty reaching orgasm with a partner, but not during masturbation (Wincze & Carey, 2001). Delayed or absent orgasm may also be related to masturbatory habits. A common example is a man who has masturbated all of his life by rubbing his penis against an object (i.e., sheets, pillow) and has become dependent on the sensations and mechanics associated with this object.

Female Orgasmic Disorder

Similar to the definition of male orgasmic disorder, "female orgasmic disorder" is the delay or absence of orgasm following a normal sexual excitement phase and adequate stimulation (American Psychiatric Association, 2000). Laumann and colleagues (1999) indicate that 26% of women have significant difficulty reaching orgasm. Osborn and colleagues (1988) surveyed a community sample of 436 women between the ages of 35 and 59 years regarding their sexual functioning. They defined "infrequency of orgasm" as the complete absence of orgasm during sexual activity over the previous 3 months. According to this conservative definition, 16% of the women in their sample reported difficulty related to orgasm. The frequency with which women achieve orgasm may vary considerably across individuals. LoPiccolo and Stock (1987) suggest that only 50% of women experience reasonably regular orgasms during sexual intercourse. Thus, in evaluating a woman for the presence of female orgasmic disorder, the actual frequency of orgasm may be less important than the extent to which she considers it a problem.

Pain Disorders

Dyspareunia

A person with dyspareunia experiences pain in the genital area before, during, or after sexual intercourse (American Psychiatric Association, 2000). The nature, duration, and intensity of the pain vary across individuals, but it is most often experienced during sexual intercourse (Wincze & Carey, 2001). In a survey of 329 women at a gynecological clinic, Rosen, Taylor, Leiblum, and Bachmann (1993) found that 7.7% of women experienced painful intercourse on most or all occasions. Osborn and colleagues (1988) provided a very similar estimate of 8%. Unfortunately, we have very few data on the prevalence of this problem in men. Our clinical experience suggests that when this problem occurs in men, it is most often the result of a medical problem (e.g., a urinary tract infection). Dyspareunia in women is more apt to result from a medical problem, psychological factors, or a combination of the two. Laumann and colleagues (1999) reported that overall, 14.4% of women and 3.0% of men report pain during intercourse. Health status and happiness appear to be negatively correlated with the experience of pain during intercourse; more pain in sex is associated with individuals who report a "poor health status" and who are "unhappy most of the time" at a rate approximately three times that of individuals who report themselves as having "excellent health" and/or "extremely happy" (Laumann et. al., 1999). It should be noted that Binik (2005) presents a compelling argument that dyspareunia should not be classified as a sexual dysfunction; rather, it should be classified as a "urogenital pain disorder." Binik supports his argument with theoretical and empirical evidence, and feels that such a reclassification would focus therapy on pain control and illness reduction, as well as sex promotion.

Vaginismus

DSM-IV-TR defines "vaginismus" as an involuntary spasm of muscles surrounding the outer one-third of the vagina in response to attempted penetration. This problem most often occurs in response to attempted intercourse. A woman may report that her partner "hits a wall" when attempting penetration. The problem may also occur, however, in response to penetration by a finger, tampon, or speculum.

Reissing, Binik, and Khalife (1999) raise a number of interesting issues regarding the definition of vaginismus. They point out that although vaginismus is listed as a pain disorder in DSM-IV-TR, pain is neither a central nor a necessary criterion for the diagnosis. Instead, the diagnosis of vaginismus focuses on the involuntary muscle spasm. Reissing and colleagues disagree with this approach and suggest that vaginismus may be best defined either as a phobic/aversive response to vaginal penetration (often not specific to intercourse) or as a pain disorder. They suggest that this definition more accurately reflects the nature of the problem.

Rosen and colleagues (1993) found that vaginismus was a common problem for 6.8% and an intermittent problem for 21.6% of the women in a gynecological clinic. Consistent with these estimates, Reissing and colleagues (1999) reported that rates of vaginismus range from 5 to 17%. Most recently, Crowley, Richardson, and Goldmeir (2006) found that about 25% of women who report some sexual dysfunction experience vaginismus.

BIOPSYCHOSOCIAL MODEL OF CAUSAL FACTORS

Over the last three decades, there have been dramatic shifts in beliefs about what causes sexual dysfunction. In the 1970s, the work of William Masters and Virginia Johnson led to a widespread belief that, in the majority of cases, sexual dysfunction resulted from psychological factors. The 1980s marked the introduction of several medical treatments for sexual dysfunction. This caused a shift to the idea that sexual dysfunction was largely a biological problem. In the 1990s, there continued to be some debate regarding the respective roles of psychogenic and organic factors. Nevertheless, the majority of professionals now acknowledge that both psychological and biological factors play a significant role in the etiology of sexual dysfunction. The assessment of sexual dysfunction often requires a multidisciplinary approach. Ideally, the clinician and physician collaborate to evaluate and identify social, psychological, and biological factors that may be causing sexual difficulties. These factors often interact, affecting one another. Thus, it is necessary to evaluate each case as a whole rather than focusing on only one component of the etiological picture. A failure to consider the respective roles of both biological and psychosocial factors may significantly compromise the potential benefits of treatment.

Biological Risk Factors

A number of biological factors may contribute to sexual difficulties. These factors may directly affect sexual functioning, as in the case of vascular disease that causes insufficient blood flow to the penis. Alternatively, they may indirectly affect sexual functioning, as in the case of pain that does not interfere physiologically but limits the person's enjoyment of sexual activity.

Direct Biological Risk Factors

Some of the most common direct biological risk factors for sexual dysfunction are diabetes, vascular disease, alcohol, and medications. Before discussing these factors in greater detail, it is important to note that mild to moderate medical problems may simply predispose someone to sexual dysfunction. The presence of positive psychosexual factors may override the effects of such conditions and allow a person to retain healthy sexual functioning. Alternatively, if more severe, or if combined with negative psychosexual conditions, then the following factors may lead to sexual difficulties.

VASCULAR DISEASES

Vascular diseases may negatively affect sexual functioning in one of two ways. They may limit arterial inflow, preventing sufficient blood supply from entering the genitalia. Alternatively, they may disturb the venous system, allowing blood that has entered the genitalia to leak out slowly (Wincze & Carey, 2001). Erections in men and vaginal engorgement in women are dependent upon increased blood flow to the genital area. Thus, vascular problems may disrupt the arousal phase of sexual functioning. Atherosclerosis, a common risk factor, may be present in as many as 70% of cases of male erectile disorder in men age 60 years and older in the United States (Kellett, 1996; Korenman, 1998). Other vascular disorders that may negatively affect sexual functioning are peripheral vascular disease, cardiovascular disease, and hypertension (Feldman et al., 1994; Korenman, 1998; NIH Consensus Conference, 1993).

There is increasing evidence that coronary artery disease and ED frequently coexist (Rodriquez, Dashti, & Schwartz, 2005). In fact, the comorbidity is so high that it is now recommended that men presenting with ED should undergo a screening test for cardiovascular disease, because ED may be an early sign of vascular risk (Jackson, Rosen, Kloner, & Kostis, 2006; Sadovsky & Miner, 2005).

DIABETES AND OTHER DISEASES AFFECTING THE CENTRAL AND PERIPHERAL NERVOUS SYSTEMS

Feldman and colleagues (1994) reported that the rate of complete erectile failure is 28% in men who are treated for diabetes. Those with poorly regulated diabetes may be at particularly high risk for sexual dysfunction (Bemelmans, Meuleman, Doesburg, Notermans, & Debruyne, 1994). Thomas and LoPiccolo (1994) suggested that the physiological effects of diabetes on sexual functioning are not as severe for women as they are for men. Schreiner-Engel, Schiavi, Vietorisz, and Smith (1987) found that the effects of diabetes on female sexual functioning may vary, depending on the type of diabetes. They observed no differences in the rate of sexual dysfunction for women with type I diabetes and a group of healthy controls. By contrast, women with type II diabetes were significantly more likely to experience difficulties related to sexual desire, arousal, orgasm, and sexual satisfaction. Results of at least one study conflict with this finding. Wincze, Albert, and Bansal (1993) examined physiological and subjective sexual arousal in response to erotic films among women with type I diabetes and a group of women without diabetes. They found that although there were no differences in levels of subjective arousal, women with type I diabetes evidenced significantly lower levels of physiological arousal in response to the films. Results of this study suggest that women with type I diabetes may in fact be at increased risk for sexual difficulties. Although the link between diabetes and sexual dysfunction is not as clear cut in women as it is in men, there is certainly an association of increased female sexual dysfunction with diabetes, and this association should not be ignored (Muniyappa et al., 2005).

It is believed that neuropathy and vascular problems often account for sexual dysfunction in patients with diabetes (Bemelmans et al.,

1994; Korenman, 1998). Takanami, Nagao, Ishii, Miura, and Shirai (1997), however, found that ED is not organically based in all patients. The authors measured physiological arousal to an erotic film in 24 men with diabetes and erectile disorder, and found that 25% of the men evidenced a significant increase in penile circumference (i.e., 20% or greater increase) without the aid of a medical intervention. Takanami and colleagues hypothesize that there is a psychogenic basis to erectile disorder in these cases. They suggest that diabetes serves as a source of considerable stress, and that the stress may in turn negatively affect sexual functioning in this subgroup of patients. Other diseases that affect the central and peripheral nervous systems and may lead to sexual dysfunction include epilepsy, multiple sclerosis, and renal disease (Hakim & Goldstein, 1996; Wincze & Carey, 2001). Along with neurological diseases, trauma such as pelvic surgery, injury or surgery to the perineum, and spinal cord injury may interfere with normal sexual responding (Korenman, 1998).

HORMONE LEVELS

Low levels of testosterone are associated with low levels of sexual desire in men (Meston, 1997). Research suggests, however, that low testosterone alone does not lead to ED. Korenman (1995) argued that a testosterone deficiency does not preclude normal erectile functioning in response to an erotic stimulus. Consistent with this finding, results of several studies (e.g., Schiavi, White, Mandeli, & Levine, 1997) suggest that although testosterone supplements may enhance sexual desire, they do not lead to significant improvements in erectile functioning. Findings on the relationship between hormones and sexual functioning in women are less consistent (Sherwin, 1988). In summarizing the results of several studies, Beck (1995) concluded that testosterone may increase sexual desire and subjective pleasure in women; low estrogen may be linked to vaginal tissue atrophy, which can result in dryness and discomfort during sexual activity.

ALCOHOL

Several researchers have identified heavy alcohol use as a risk factor for sexual dysfunction (e.g., Benet, Sharaby, & Melman, 1994; Hirschfield, 1998). In a review of studies on the relationship between sexual dysfunction and alcohol abuse, Schiavi (1990) reported that 8–54% of men with alcoholism have ED, and 31–58% suffer from low desire. Schiavi points out that although there is much evidence for a relationship between sexual functioning and alcohol use, many studies fail to control for the stage of the disorder (e.g., still abusing, in the midst of detoxification) and the effects of medication, age, and physical illness. Studies focusing on women also suggest a relationship between alcohol misuse and sexual dysfunction. Klassen and Wilsnack (1986) surveyed 917 women in the United States and found a positive correlation between heavy drinking and sexual problems. Malatesta, Pollack, Crotty, and Peacock (1982) examined the immediate effects of heavy alcohol consumption on female orgasm. They found that women with higher blood alcohol levels tended to have a longer latency to orgasm and a decrease in the subjective intensity of orgasm.

It is believed that chronic, excessive alcohol use may contribute to sexual difficulties through its effects on hypothalamic–pituitary function (e.g., decline in testosterone levels), the liver, and both central and peripheral neurological processes (e.g., neuropathy) (Schiavi, 1990). It has also been suggested that alcohol abuse contributes to sexual dysfunction by disrupting interpersonal relationships. O'Farrell, Choquette, Cutter, and Birchler (1997) found that men with alcoholism had a significantly higher rate of ED than maritally conflicted and maritally nonconflicted men without alcoholism. Interestingly, however, the men with alcoholism did not differ from the maritally conflicted men without alcoholism in their level of sexual desire, rate of premature ejaculation, and prevalence of sexual pain in their wives. Both groups reported significantly more problems in these areas than did the maritally nonconflicted men without alcoholism. Results of this study suggest that aside from erectile difficulties, the higher rate of sexual problems in men with alcoholism may be due in great part to the relationship problems associated with alcoholism.

MEDICATIONS

A number of medications may contribute to disorders of desire, arousal, or orgasm in men and women. The medications that are most often implicated in the etiology of sexual dysfunction are antihypertensives, antidepressants, and antipsychotic drugs (Finger, Lund, & Slagle, 1997; Gitlin, 2003). Hogan, Wallin, and Baer (1980) reported that 9–23% of men taking antihypertensive medication experienced sexual dysfunction, relative to 4% of men in a healthy control group. Chang and colleagues (1991) found that the rate of sexual dysfunction was particularly high in men who were taking diuretics. Hodge, Harward, West, Krongaard-DeMong, and Kowal-Neely (1991) conducted one of the few studies focusing specifically on the effects of antihypertensive medication on female sexual functioning. They failed to find any significant differences between women taking antihypertensive medications and a group of healthy controls. Unfortunately, the findings of this study were limited by a small sample size.

The antidepressant class known as selective serotonin reuptake inhibitors (SSRIs) includes drugs such as Prozac, Zoloft, and Paxil. In a prospective study of 192 women and 152 men taking SSRIs, Montejo-Gonzalez and colleagues (1997) found that 14% of the patients spontaneously reported sexual dysfunction to their physicians, and 58% endorsed sexual problems when directly asked. Results of this study indicate that sexual side effects occur in a significant proportion of patients taking SSRIs. The data also suggest that studies based on spontaneously reported side effects may significantly underestimate the rate of sexual side effects associated with a particular medication. Segraves (1998) reviewed the effects of antidepressant medication on sexual functioning. He found that the rate of orgasmic disturbance alone is 20–75% in people taking antidepressant medication. Segraves reported that delayed orgasm and premature ejaculation are the two most common side effects. Other drugs associated with sexual difficulties include minor tranquilizers, anticonvulsants, and anticholinergics. (For a complete list of medications with sexual side effects, see Finger et al., 1997.)

OTHER DIRECT RISK FACTORS

In their review of the literature on vaginismus, Reissing and colleagues (1999) suggest that the following factors or conditions may lead to painful attempts at penile–vaginal intercourse: hymeneal abnormalities; congenital abnormalities; vaginal atrophy and adhesions due to atrophy, vaginal surgery, or intravaginal radiation;

prolapsed uterus; vulvar vestibulitis syndrome; endometriosis, infections; vaginal lesions and tumors; sexually transmitted diseases; and pelvic congestion.

Indirect Biological Risk Factors

AGE

One of the most common indirect risk factors for sexual dysfunction is aging. Many people believe that sexual dysfunction is a natural consequence of aging. In fact, sexual functioning may be qualitatively different for older men and women. Aging men may find that it takes more time and more stimulation to attain an erection, that the erection may not be as firm as it was in the past, that the duration of orgasm and the intensity of ejaculation may diminish, and that sexual desire may decline (Leiblum & Segraves, 1995; Meston, 1997). During and after menopause, women may experience increased latency to lubrication, less and thinner vaginal lubrication, and reduction in the fullness of the labia majora (Bachmann, 1995; Leiblum & Segraves, 1995). Although some of these changes may contribute to sexual difficulties, age alone is not a direct cause of sexual dysfunction in the majority of cases. In support of this, in a large sample study on aging in men and women, DeLamater and Sill (2005) found that the most significant factors influencing sexual functioning were psychological (positive attitude) and relational (availability of a sexual partner). As people age, they are also more apt to develop medical conditions that serve as risk factors for sexual dysfunction (Korenman, 1998; NIH Consensus Conference, 1993). Thus, age is an indirect, rather than a direct, risk factor for sexual dysfunction.

CIGARETTE SMOKING

Cigarette smoking may indirectly affect sexual functioning by amplifying the effects of risk factors such as treated heart disease; treated hypertension; untreated arthritis; and use of cardiac and antihypertensive drugs, and vasodilators (Feldman et al., 1994; NIH Consensus Conference, 1993). There is also evidence that cigarette smoking serves as an independent risk factor for sexual dysfunction. Mannino, Klevens, and Flanders (1994) controlled for the effects of risk factors such as vascular disease, hormonal factors, and substance misuse in a group of 4,462 male Army veterans. They found that cigarette smoking alone was associated with a significantly higher rate of ED.

OTHER INDIRECT RISK FACTORS

A number of additional medical factors or conditions can lead indirectly to sexual dysfunction. Pain, particularly chronic pain, may cause a person significant discomfort or anxiety during sexual activity; this may result in difficulty becoming aroused or a loss of interest in sexual activity. Chronic or serious medical conditions, such as heart disease or cancer, may also lead to changes in sexual arousal or desire. Patients who have had a heart attack may fear that the physical exertion of sexual activity will cause another heart attack. Unpleasant symptoms associated with an illness or its treatment (e.g., nausea resulting from chemotherapy) may interfere with positive sexual functioning. Finally, medical conditions or procedures that involve changes in one's physical appearance (e.g., mastectomy) can lead to body image issues that interfere with healthy sexual functioning.

Psychosocial Risk Factors

In the context of the popularity of Viagra, Levitra, and Cialis, the mass media have promoted the notion that sexual dysfunction is almost always caused by organic factors such as those we presented earlier. Indeed, biological risk factors are present in many cases. Nevertheless, psychosocial factors, whether alone or in combination with biological factors, play some role in the majority of cases. Psychosocial risk factors may be classified into two broad categories: individual factors and relationship factors. Individual risk factors involve the individual and are independent of the relationship (e.g., faulty beliefs regarding sexual functioning). Relationship factors involve both the individual and the partner (i.e., problems or limitations within the relationship). In general, relationship factors are best addressed by working with the couple rather than with each person individually.

Individual Risk Factors

PSYCHOLOGICAL DISORDERS

One of the most common individual risk factors for sexual dysfunction is the presence of psychological disorders, including mood disorders, anxiety disorders, alcohol or other substance use disorders, and eating disorders. Depression often involves "anhedonia," a lack of pleasure or interest in activities the person normally enjoys. Thus, it is not surprising that depression may be associated with a loss of sexual desire and difficulty in becoming aroused (Cyranowski et al., 2004; Hirschfield, 1998). Angst (1998) prospectively compared the rate of sexual dysfunction in 591 men and women categorized as nondepressed, nontreated depressed, or treated depressed. Angst found that the rates of sexual dysfunction in these groups were 26, 45, and 62%, respectively. Results of this study support the hypothesis that rates of sexual dysfunction are higher among depressed men and women. It is possible that the rate of sexual dysfunction was highest in the third group studied by Angst, because patients who sought treatment were those whose depression was more severe and, consequently, more likely to affect their sexual functioning. A person with panic disorder fears physiological sensations such as rapid heartbeat, shortness of breath, sweating, and hot flushes. Many of these symptoms occur during sexual activity. Thus, a person with panic disorder may respond to sexual activity with anxiety, discomfort, difficulty in becoming aroused, or aversion (Kaplan, 1988; Sbrocco et al., 1997).

EMOTIONS

Given the potential impact of mood and anxiety disorders on sexual functioning, it follows that emotions affect sexual arousal. Kaplan (1979) asserted that "the sexual dysfunctions . . . are caused by a single factor: anxiety" (p. 24). Empirical examinations of the effects of anxiety on sexual arousal indicate that the relationship is not as simple as Kaplan suggested. Through a series of studies, researchers have demonstrated that anxiety negatively affects sexual arousal in people with sexual dysfunction but may enhance arousal in people who do not have sexual difficulties (e.g., Barlow, Sakheim, & Beck, 1983; Hoon, Wincze, & Hoon, 1977). Barlow (1986; Cranston-Cuebas & Barlow, 1990) hypothesizes that when sexually functional men and women become anxious during sexual activity, their level of autonomic arousal increases, they focus more efficiently on erotic cues, and they become increasingly aroused. By contrast, when people with sexual dysfunction become anxious, their level of autonomic arousal increases, and they focus more intently on the consequences of not performing. Not surprisingly, they then fail to become aroused. Mitchell, DiBartolo, Brown, and Barlow (1998) used a musical mood induction to examine the effects of positive and negative mood states on sexual arousal in sexually functional males. They found that negative mood states were associated with significantly lower levels of physiological arousal. Anger is another emotion that may negatively affect sexual functioning. Feldman and colleagues (1994) found that suppression and expression of anger were correlated with significantly higher rates of ED.

MALADAPTIVE COGNITIONS

Maladaptive cognitions (e.g., negative expectations) may negatively affect sexual functioning. Barlow (1986; Cranston-Cuebas & Barlow, 1990) hypothesized that men and women with sexual dysfunction respond to sexual stimuli by focusing on negative, self-focused cognitions that distract them from erotic cues and interfere with their ability to become aroused. Results of several studies suggest that distraction from erotic cues is associated with lower levels of physiological arousal (e.g., Abrahamson et al., 1985; Geer & Fuhr, 1976). Moreover, more recent studies suggest that negative expectations and internal attributions for past erectile failure may lead to lower levels of physiological arousal (Bach, Brown, & Barlow, 1999; Weisberg, Brown, Wincze, & Barlow, 2001).

Maladaptive thoughts may also come in the form of negative attitudes or misconceptions regarding sexual functioning. Patients are not born with ideas and beliefs regarding sexuality; they develop them as they grow up. Thus, the messages and information that patients receive as children or adolescents may have a significant impact on their attitudes as adults. These attitudes in turn affect sexual functioning. Individuals who are raised in very conservative cultures may learn that premarital sex is wrong, that masturbation is dirty, and that sex within a marriage is solely for the purpose of procreation. Men may learn that they should be able to get an erection under any circumstances. Women may be taught that intercourse is very painful. Such ideas can interfere with healthy sexual functioning. McCabe and Cobain

(1998) found that women with sexual dysfunction were more likely than women without sexual difficulties to report having had negative attitudes toward intercourse as adolescents. Moreover, men and women with sexual dysfunction were more likely than those without sexual problems to have negative attitudes toward sex as adults. Nobre and Pinto-Gauveia (2003) developed a questionnaire to measure maladaptive cognitions in men and women experiencing sexual dysfunction. Their Sexual Modes Questionnaire was found to be valid and reliable in discriminating between sexually dysfunctional and sexually functional individuals. This research strongly supports the association of maladaptive cognitions and sexual dysfunction. Further identification of this association is elaborated in Nobre's (2006) book.

CULTURAL FACTORS

Racial, ethnic, and religious background often affect a person's beliefs, expectations, and behaviors in sexual relationships. Moreover, definitions of and reactions to sexual problems are often culturally determined. For example, Verma, Khaitan, and Singh (1998) reported the frequency of various sexual dysfunctions in 1,000 consecutive patients presenting to a psychosexual clinic in India. They found that 77% of male patients reported difficulties with premature ejaculation—a rate significantly higher than that reported in the United States. Moreover, 71% of male patients presented with concern about nocturnal emission associated with erotic dreams. The authors suggest that the high rate of problems associated with ejaculation is due in part to a widely held belief in India that loss of semen causes depletion of physical and mental energy. It is interesting to note that only 36 of these 1,000 patients were female. The authors suggest that this may be due to the religious, social, and cultural background of India, in which it is considered immoral for women to seek treatment for sexual problems.

LACK OF EDUCATION
REGARDING SEXUAL FUNCTIONING

Finally, limited information regarding sexual functioning is a risk factor for sexual dysfunction. In our clinical experience, a person's level of education does not necessarily correlate with his or her degree of knowledge regarding sexual functioning; that is, an attorney is as likely as a person who dropped out of high school to have faulty ideas and information regarding sexual functioning. Thus, it is important for the clinician not to presume that a given patient has an adequate base of knowledge from which to work. One of us (A. K. B.) once assessed a college-educated professional who reported that he was having erectile difficulties. The interview revealed that he was engaging in oral sex to the point of ejaculation; when, after ejaculating, he was unable to maintain an erection sufficient for intercourse, he believed that he had ED. Unfortunately, he was so distressed by this belief that he eventually developed erectile difficulties.

Relationship Factors

COUPLE DISTRESS

Sexual problems are sometimes secondary to couple distress. When couple distress is severe, treatment of sexual dysfunction should be postponed. When and if the relationship problems are resolved, the remaining sexual difficulties may be directly addressed. Sexual problems may cause frustration, distress, and tension within a relationship. Thus, many couples who present for treatment of sexual dysfunction have mild relationship problems. If these problems are primarily a consequence rather than a cause of the sexual dysfunction, they may be addressed within the context of sex therapy.

POOR COMMUNICATION

Poor communication may negatively affect a sexual relationship. Patients who cannot communicate effectively with their partners may harbor anger, resentment, or other negative feelings that interfere with sexual functioning. The ability to address disagreements in a constructive manner may be particularly important. McCabe and Cobain (1998) found that men with sexual dysfunction argued with their partners significantly more than did men without sexual difficulties. Hawton and Catalan (1986) found that ease of communication of anger was associated with a better outcome for couples participating in sex therapy. Along with general communication problems, an inability to communicate about sex may contribute to sexual difficulties. Some couples communicate effectively about other aspects of their relationship but have difficulty talking comfortably about sex. Partners who fail to communicate about their sexual relationship allow false assumptions to go unchallenged (e.g., "My partner is not aroused because he is not attracted to me"). Moreover, they lack a forum in which they can express their preferences regarding different types of stimulation. It is not uncommon to work with a couple in which partners who have been married for years have never discussed what sexual activities they like and dislike. Such a couple may believe that a good lover simply knows what his or her partner wants. Alternatively, they may feel uncomfortable initiating such a conversation.

LACK OF PHYSICAL ATTRACTION

All men and women, whether they are in their first month of dating or their 30th year of marriage, need to feel attracted to their sexual partners. Couples sometimes underestimate the importance of this factor. They may believe that mutual love and respect are sufficient for a satisfying sexual relationship (Wincze & Barlow, 1997b). This is not the case. Physical attraction is an important part of a relationship. The absence of such feelings is an obstacle to healthy sexual functioning. If sexual feelings were never present in a relationship, then it is difficult to manufacture such feelings no matter how desireable a person's partner may be on nonsexual dimensions. Partners who once had very strong sexual feelings but who have lost those feelings can make efforts to restore them. Recognizing the importance of being attracted to one another, rather than thinking it no longer matters, marks the first step toward addressing this issue.

Feeling attractive is also of great importance to one's sexual experience. Koch, Mansfield, Thurau, and Carey (2005) found that the more a woman perceives herself as less attractive than before, the more likely she is to report a decline in sexual desire and in the frequency of sexual activity. Clearly, the physical attractiveness of one's partner and one's self-perception are important variables affecting sexual activity.

RESTRICTED SEXUAL REPERTOIRE

Occasional sexual difficulties are normative experiences. Partners who engage in various forms of stimulation are not unduly affected by occasional problems related to intercourse; they have more than one means of satisfying each other sexually. Many couples, however, equate sex with intercourse. For these couples, inability to have intercourse means that physical intimacy is not possible. Performance demands and fear of failure are higher for these couples (Rosen, 1996). Thus, they are at greater risk of developing persistent sexual difficulties. Consistent with this hypothesis, McCabe and Cobain (1998) found that women with sexual dysfunction were more likely than women without sexual difficulties to report a restricted sexual repertoire. Similarly, Wiegel, Bach, Brown, Rhein, and Barlow (1997) found that men with ED reported a more restricted range of sexual behaviors than men without erectile difficulties.

CONTEXT OF ASSESSMENT AND TREATMENT

Having defined sexual dysfunction and identified risk factors for it, we now consider the context in which the assessment and treatment of these problems occur.

Setting

Over the past decade, the media have widely promoted the notion that people with sexual problems should seek help from their physicians (Tiefer, 1996). Thus, a medical center is often the ideal base for a sex therapist. In this setting, a therapist is available to a significant proportion of patients. Moreover, working closely with urologists, gynecologists, and primary care physicians helps to ensure a multidisciplinary approach to the assessment and treatment of sexual problems. Other clinicians may see patients in university-based outpatient clinics, community mental health centers, or private practices. In these instances, it is helpful for clinicians to develop working relationships with local physicians. This facilitates the use of a multidisciplinary approach and enables the exchange of referrals. Patients seeking treatment for sexual difficulties may initially feel very nervous and uncomfortable discussing such a personal subject. An office that is professional and a therapist who is neatly and professionally dressed may help to put a patient or couple at ease. The office should be large enough to seat comfortably a couple and one or two therapists. In settings where psychophysiological assessments are an option, two adjoined rooms are needed: a private room for the patient and another for the therapist.

Spacing of Sessions and Length of Therapy

Masters and Johnson's treatment program for sexual dysfunction served as the model for sex therapy for two decades. Their approach involved daily therapy sessions conducted over a 2- or 3-week period. Thus, a schedule of daily sessions was once considered ideal. Heiman and LoPiccolo (1983) compared the relative efficacy of 15 daily versus 15 weekly therapy sessions. They found that on the majority of measures the differences between the two formats were nonsignificant. To the extent that either approach had an advantage, it was a schedule of weekly sessions. We typically conduct therapy on a weekly basis, at least until the patient or couple is working on behavioral assignments (e.g., sensate focus exercises) between sessions (Wincze & Barlow, 1997b; Wincze & Carey, 2001). At that time, the frequency of sessions may be decreased to once every 2 or 3 weeks to allow a couple more time to practice assigned exercises. We have found that it is often not helpful to conduct treatment less than once every 3 or 4 weeks. Conducting sessions too infrequently may break the continuity of treatment and seems to reduce the patient's or couple's motivation to practice skills routinely between sessions. The length of treatment varies from one case to the next. Some patients benefit from three or four sessions that comprise mainly psychoeducation. Others require a full course of treatment (i.e., 10–12 or more sessions). In the majority of cases, we tell patients that we will review treatment goals after 10–12 sessions and determine whether additional sessions would be useful. We find it helpful to frame the treatment plan in this manner, so that patients who have not attained their goals after 12 sessions do not consider themselves treatment failures. The majority of patients can achieve their treatment goals within 15 sessions. Although Masters and Johnson (1970) recommended the use of male and female cotherapists, we have found that this approach is neither necessary nor practical. In the era of managed care, such an approach is rarely an option. Thus, unless we are training interns or graduate students, we generally work individually.

Working with Couples or with Individuals

Although we do not require it, we strongly encourage every patient with a partner to undergo an assessment and treatment as a couple. This is helpful for several reasons. An interview with the partner may provide additional insight into psychosocial factors that are contributing to the sexual difficulty. Moreover, the partner's participation in the assessment gives the clinician an opportunity to observe the couple's interactions. Inclusion of the partner in treatment ensures that both partners understand the treatment plan and helps to promote compliance. Finally, working with the couple rather than the individual helps us to restructure the notion that sexual dysfunction is the patient's problem and that he or she needs to be "fixed." The value of working with a couple versus the patient alone is supported by recent empirical findings. Hirst and Watson (1997) examined the relative efficacy of individual versus couple treatment of sexual dysfunction. They found that attendance was the best predictor of outcome; patients who had partners but underwent individual treatment attended fewer sessions and canceled more appointments. Ultimately, 84% of patients who received couple treatment had a good outcome, relative to 51% of patients whose partners did not attend. Consistent with results of this study, Wylie (1997) examined outcome in 37 couples undergoing psychosocial couple treatment for male erectile disorder. He reported a trend toward remaining in therapy for patients whose partners attended the assessment interview. When assessing a couple, we find it helpful to meet with each person individually, along with meeting with them as a pair. Sometimes information that is essential to an understanding of the case is not revealed when a therapist meets with the patient and partner as a couple. We also find it useful to meet periodically with each person individually over the course of treatment. This gives the therapist an opportunity to devote more time to each partner and his or her individual issues. At the same time, it allows each person to speak privately with the therapist and share issues or concerns that he or she does not feel comfortable addressing when the three meet together. When speaking with each person individually, the therapist should explicitly ask which, if any, issues should not be shared with the partner. It is important for both the patient and partner to understand that information they share with the clinician will be kept confidential and will not be shared with the other person if he or she wishes to keep it private. If a person thinks that sensitive information will be shared with the partner, he or she may not disclose details that are central to the case.

Cognitive-behavioral treatment can certainly be beneficial for a patient who does not have a partner. In such cases, treatment focuses on providing psychoeducation, challenging thoughts that may interfere with sexual functioning, and assigning behavioral exercises that may be completed independently. This treatment may involve fewer sessions than that for a couple, because there are certain exercises that cannot be practiced and issues that cannot be addressed in the absence of a partner. Thus, in such a case, we cover as much as possible with the individual, develop a plan for how he or she might further address problems or concerns in the context of a future relationship, and give the patient the option of resuming treatment once he or she has a steady partner. A single patient may sometimes suggest involving a casual partner in the assessment and treatment process. Alternatively, a younger patient (e.g., a college student) may wish to include a steady partner in therapy. In both cases, we explain to the patient that because very sensitive information will be revealed over the course of the assessment and treatment, it may be prudent to work individually with a therapist. This protects the confidentiality of the patient and ensures that he or she will not ultimately regret having shared such private information with someone other than the therapist. Periodically including the partner in relevant treatment sessions can serve as a compromise in such cases.

Patient Variables

Hawton and Catalan (1986) conducted one of the earliest studies that examined prognostic variables in sex therapy. They found that the quality of the couple's sexual relationship, the quality of the overall relationship, the patient's motivation, and homework compliance by the third treatment session were significant predictors of treatment outcome. Hawton, Catalan, and Fagg (1992) found that the quality of pretreatment communication, general sexual adjustment, the presence of mental illness in the female partner, socioeconomic status, and the couple's early engagement in treatment were significant predictors of treatment outcome. Sarwer and Durlak (1997) found that the number of sensate focus exercises completed in the last week of treatment was a significant predictor of treatment outcome. Finally, as noted earlier, Wylie (1997) examined outcome in 37 couples undergoing psychosocial treatment for male erectile disorder. He found that patient dropout was associated with lower scores on a measure of relationship satisfaction at pretreatment. Moreover, he found that a history of mental illness in the male partner was associated with a poor outcome. These studies are consistent in suggesting that the quality of the relationship at pretreatment is positively correlated with treatment outcome. Moreover, these studies indicate that patients who are more compliant with treatment (i.e., engage in assigned exercises between sessions) tend to have a better outcome.

Religious, ethnic, and cultural variables often play a central role in sex therapy. These factors may strongly influence a patient's values and beliefs regarding sexual activity. If the patient's ideas are consistent with those of his or her subculture, the therapist needs to respect them and not impose his or her own value system. In some instances, however, a patient misinterprets the teachings of his or her religion or subgroup. In such cases, it can be helpful to refer the patient to a member of the clergy or religious group. This person will help the patient develop a more accurate understanding of the religion's teachings. A therapist may not always be aware of the unique issues that are relevant for patients from a particular subgroup. Thus, the therapist must be prepared to educate himor herself and seek consultation when necessary.

Therapist Variables

There are limited data on the effects of therapist variables on the treatment of sexual dysfunction (Mohr & Beutler, 1990). In one of the few studies in this area, LoPiccolo, Heiman, Hogan, and Roberts (1985) found that the number of therapists (i.e., one vs. two) did not significantly affect treatment outcome. Moreover, they found no effect for the gender of the therapist. Although research suggests that the gender of the therapist does not significantly

affect treatment outcome, some patients may express a strong preference for either a male or a female therapist. In such cases, we try to accommodate patients' wishes. Although additional research on the effects of therapist variables is limited, our clinical experience suggests that a supportive yet direct style is effective. It is also important for the therapist to be sensitive and nonjudgmental when discussing such a personal aspect of patients' lives.

ASSESSMENT AND TREATMENT

The remainder of the chapter outlines our approach to the assessment and treatment of patients with sexual dysfunction. The information and techniques presented are discussed in greater detail by Wincze and Barlow (1997a, 1997b) and Wincze and Carey (2001).

Goals of Assessment

Although patients are often eager to begin treatment, we feel it is important to allot an adequate number of sessions to the assessment process. Sufficient background information, details regarding the nature and extent of the sexual difficulties, and working knowledge of etiological and maintaining factors are necessary before the therapist can develop an effective treatment plan. We typically use the first three sessions for assessment before beginning the intervention. The first goal of the assessment is to understand and to characterize accurately the nature of the presenting problem. As indicated earlier, patients presenting with sexual problems may ultimately be diagnosed with a sexual dysfunction, a mood or anxiety disorder, a substance use disorder, another mental disorder, or couple distress. Alternatively, patients presenting with sexual concerns may simply lack information regarding normative sexual functioning. For example, a woman may believe that she has low sexual desire because her interest in sex does not match that of her husband. In such cases, patients benefit from psychoeducation regarding normative sexual functioning and individual variability.

If sexual dysfunction is present, the therapist must determine the history, frequency, antecedents, and consequences of the sexual difficulty. The second goal of an assessment is to identify (1) predisposing biological and psychosocial factors (e.g., diabetes, negative messages about sex in childhood); (2) immediate precipitants (e.g., use of alcohol, arguments); and (3) maintaining factors (e.g., neuropathy, performance-related concerns). Identification of these factors often requires an integration of information obtained through a comprehensive psychosocial evaluation and a recent medical examination. The third goal of the assessment process is to determine a pretreatment baseline for the patient's sexual functioning. Baseline data allow the therapist to measure progress over the course of treatment.

Throughout the assessment, the therapist will have opportunities to provide psychoeducation and address patients' faulty beliefs or misconceptions regarding sexual functioning. In this respect, the intervention begins in the context of the assessment. The provision of basic information can often have immediate positive effects on the couple's sexual relationship. This helps the couple to feel that although the intervention has not yet begun, both partners already have benefited from addressing their difficulties with a professional. Over the course of the assessment, the therapist helps the couple to identify conditions under which sexual problems are most likely to occur. This process benefits the partners in at least two ways. It allows them to view the sexual problem as a condition that is subject to change depending on various factors; thus, it helps them to be optimistic regarding the potential benefits of treatment. In addition, it helps to separate the patient from the problem, and diminishes the sense of blame and guilt that may be present at the outset of therapy. Finally, the assessment provides an opportunity for the patient and partner to learn how to discuss their sexual relationship with the therapist. By openly and comfortably discussing sexual functioning, the therapist normalizes the process, provides a useful model, and implicitly gives both partners permission to talk about a very intimate and private aspect of their lives.

Process Issues in Assessment

Wincze and Carey (2001) define "process" as the interaction between the therapist and the patient. Certain process issues are significant in any form of psychotherapy; these include the gender, age, race or ethnicity, and religion of the therapist and the patient. Differences between the therapist and patient on any of these factors may have a significant impact on the

therapy process. The therapist should be sensitive to ways in which his or her background differs from that of the patient. The therapist might consider acknowledging these differences and asking the patient how he or she feels about them. At the very least, the therapist should consider ways in which these factors might facilitate or interfere with the therapy process.

Other process issues are particularly significant in the treatment of sexual dysfunction. Therapists who do not specialize in the assessment and treatment of sexual functioning may be uncomfortable discussing it with patients. Discomfort on the part of the therapist is evident to a patient and may impede the therapy process. Alternatively, therapists who routinely treat patients with sexual dysfunction may forget that their patients are not in the habit of discussing sexual activity in this context; consequently, they may be insensitive to patients' embarrassment or discomfort. Ideally, of course, the therapist feels comfortable discussing sexual matters and is sensitive to discomfort on the part of the patient. When working in the area of sexual dysfunction, it is particularly important for therapists to draw and retain appropriate professional boundaries. A therapist who finds him- or herself attracted to a patient should seek consultation from a colleague. Consulting with peers can help a therapist to be mindful of blurred boundaries. If a therapist is unable to retain a strictly professional role or suspects that the patient reciprocates feelings of attraction, the patient should be referred to another therapist.

Along with these process issues, Wincze and Carey (2001) outline a series of assumptions that are useful in assessing sexual functioning:

• Patients are usually embarrassed and have difficulty discussing sexual matters. This embarrassment may cause them to withhold information, to miss sessions, and generally to avoid discussing their concerns. The clinician may help by normalizing (and even "predicting") patients' discomfort and modeling comfortable discussion of sexual functioning.

• Many patients do not understand medically correct terminology such as "intercourse," "ejaculation," and "vagina." Moreover, even patients who use these terms may not use them correctly. It is sometimes helpful for the clinician to follow medically correct terms with more commonly used lay terms such as "cum" or "wet." This ensures that the patient knows the meaning of the clinician's questions; it teaches the patient the meaning of medically correct terms; and it may increase the patient's comfort level by suggesting that it is acceptable to use lay terms.

• Even the most well-educated patients may be misinformed about sexual functioning. Some women believe that they will bleed very heavily on their first attempt at intercourse. Men may believe that they should be able to engage in intercourse for 30 minutes before ejaculating. Identifying and correcting these misunderstandings can often lead to rapid and significant clinical improvement.

• Some patients may be in crisis and may be suicidal. A clinician should not assume that sexual dysfunction is the primary problem for a patient presenting with sexual difficulties. An assessment of general psychological functioning may reveal that the patient is very depressed, perhaps suicidal. In such cases, the clinician must attend to issues other than sexual functioning and ensure that proper treatment is provided.

• Partners often have not been open with each other and do not freely discuss sexual matters. It is safest to assume that partners have withheld significant information, thoughts, or feelings from each other. Therapy can serve to promote more open communication. As indicated earlier, many couples do not comfortably discuss their sexual relationship. This area of communication must also be addressed.

• When patients discuss sexual problems with a therapist, it may be for the first time. Sexual functioning is an extremely private aspect of people's lives. At the same time, our culture places a great deal of emphasis on the importance of sexual activity and a person's "performance" in this domain. For both of these reasons, patients are often reluctant to discuss or to acknowledge sexual difficulties. Some patients are not even comfortable addressing the difficulty with their sexual partners. Thus, for many patients, the first appointment with a therapist is the first time they have talked about their sexual difficulty.

• A couple often may have avoided sex because of the partners' fear and discomfort. Many couples who experience sexual difficulties begin to avoid sexual activity, because it becomes a source of frustration, disappointment, anxiety, or physical discomfort. Partners who are unable to engage in intercourse may report that they have ceased sexual relations because their attitude is "Why bother?" In some couples with sexual dysfunction, partners stop being affectionate with one another because of reluctance to "start something they cannot finish."

Assessment Methods

Psychosocial assessment of sexual dysfunction typically involves a clinical interview. It may also involve the use of self-report measures or a psychophysiological assessment.

Clinical Interview

Talking to patients about their psychological functioning can be difficult; it requires a sensitive, empathic, and skilled therapist. This is particularly true when patients are presenting with sexual difficulties. Patients who undergo an assessment of their sexual functioning must discuss the most intimate, private aspects of their lives with the therapist. They are typically uncomfortable talking about sex and may be embarrassed to divulge information regarding their own sexual functioning. The therapist must combine a gradual approach to asking highly personal questions and a time-efficient strategy for obtaining necessary information. The use of an outline structures the clinical interview and helps the clinician to obtain necessary information in an organized, time-efficient manner. The outline we follow is described below. Alternatively, clinicians may choose to use a semistructured interview (e.g., Sbrocco, Weisberg, & Barlow, 1992). Commonly used in research settings, semistructured interviews provide a clear framework for clinical interviews and guide the clinician through the assessment of sexual functioning. As indicated earlier, we typically reserve three sessions for the assessment process. We interview the patient alone for the first session, interview the partner alone for the second session, and then meet with the couple together for the third session.

FIRST SESSION:
INTRODUCTION AND PATIENT INTERVIEW

We begin the first session with an explanation of the assessment process. A proper orientation to the purpose of the assessment is particularly important for patients who have been referred by physicians. These patients sometimes schedule an appointment with a therapist simply because a doctor recommended it. They may not know why they are meeting with a therapist or what they can expect. At the start of the first session, we talk briefly with the patient and partner together. This gives us an opportunity to explain the assessment process and to address the couple's questions and concerns. Providing this information to the couple rather than to each person individually reinforces the notion that although one person is the identified "patient," the partners undergo the assessment and treatment as a couple. This brief meeting also provides an opportunity for the therapist to observe directly the way the partners interact and communicate.

Once the assessment process is explained and the couple's questions and issues have been addressed, the remainder of the first session should be devoted to interviewing either the patient or the partner (often the patient) individually. The therapist should explain to the couple that individual interviews help to develop the clearest understanding of the sexual difficulty by providing as much information as possible from each individual. The couple may be informed that periodical meetings with each person individually may also be useful during treatment, allowing the therapist to spend more time focused on each person and to work through individual issues. The couple may need to be reminded of the rationale for meeting with each person individually once treatment begins. Nevertheless, by explaining this at the outset, the therapist instills the notion that individual meetings are routine when working with couples.

Objectives of the patient interview include establishing rapport, collecting demographic information, obtaining a description of the presenting problem, conducting an assessment of general psychological functioning, and assessing the patient's psychosexual history. Although it is helpful to use an outline when conducting the interview, the therapist must be willing to deviate from a standard set of questions to focus on more primary problems or important background information. Given this caveat, we find the following general approach to clinical interviews useful.

Because patients may initially feel nervous and uncomfortable, it is often helpful to begin by gathering nonthreatening information, such as demographics. The therapist may then continue with open-ended questions or statements, such as "Tell me a little bit about the difficulties you have been having recently." The therapist can observe how freely and comfortably a patient discusses his or her sexual problems. For those who seem embarrassed or defensive, it may be helpful to gather other, necessary information before further discussing the sexual difficulty. This gives such patients more time to relax and feel comfortable with the therapist.

It is often helpful to obtain a psychosexual and psychosocial history. The therapist may want to gather information regarding the patient's childhood. Important data include details regarding the patient's family structure, the parents' relationship with each other and with the patient (including demonstrations of affection), childhood sexual or physical abuse, early messages about sex, and early sexual experiences (pleasant or unpleasant). Adolescence marks a very significant period in psychosexual development; thus, information on the patient's experiences as an adolescent may be very useful. Relevant details include treatment of the patient by his or her peers (e.g., ridicule for physical attributes such as acne, weight, and facial features), dating experiences, body image, and history of alcohol or other substance misuse. The therapist will then want to gather information regarding the person's history and experiences as an adult. The most important areas to address are the following:

• *A relationship history after the age of 20.* This includes a history of sexual relationships, long-term relationships, and prior marriages.
• *History of any unusual experiences.* This includes a brief assessment for the presence of paraphiliac fantasies or behaviors such as sexual arousal associated with children or inanimate objects. For patients who endorse atypical sexual fantasies, it is important to determine whether they have acted on these fantasies, whether they intend to do so, and whether they can become sexually aroused in the absence of these stimuli/situations.
• *Medical history.* Regardless of whether the patient has had a recent medical evaluation, the therapist should inquire about a childhood/teenage history of diseases, surgery, medical care, congenital disorders, and other significant medical problems. Information regarding the patient's medical history since the age of 20 is

particularly important. Again, relevant information includes a history of diseases, surgery, medical care, and significant health problems. Finally, the therapist should determine whether the patient has had regular medical care (if not, he or she should be referred for a medical evaluation), is currently taking prescribed medication, or is currently being treated for any medical problem. It is also not at all unusual for male patients already to have tried using one or more of the erection-enhancing medications now available. Very careful exploration of which medications, dosage levels, number of times the medication was tried, and circumstances under which it was used must occur to determine whether the medication was properly used. Careful inquiry often reveals that many individuals have been misinformed about the medication or have misused the medication.

• *Current psychological functioning and mental health history.* An assessment of general psychological functioning is necessary to deter-

mine whether it is appropriate to focus specifically on sexual dysfunction. If sexual difficulties are secondary to problems such as depression, anxiety, severe couple distress, or a substance use disorder, the person is unlikely to benefit from starting with treatment for sexual dysfunction. Instead, the patient should begin by addressing the primary problem. When this problem is successfully treated or stabilized, the person may effectively focus on treatment for residual sexual difficulties. Figure 15.1 is a decision tree that aids the therapist in deciding when treatment focused specifically on sexual dysfunction is appropriate for various patients (Wincze & Barlow, 1997b). The therapist should also obtain a history of past mental health treatment.

• *Information regarding the patient's current sexual and overall relationship.* Relevant information includes satisfaction with the current sexual and overall relationship, commitment to the relationship, activities the partners enjoy engaging in together, and strengths and

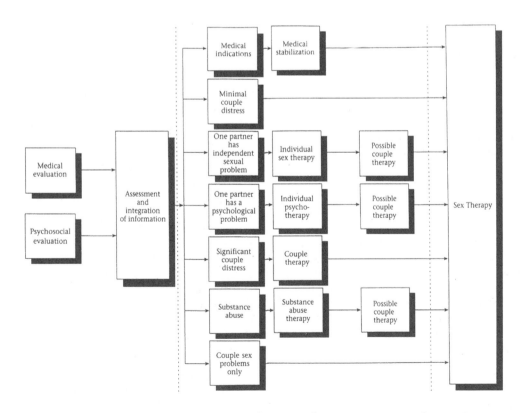

FIGURE 15.1. Clinical assessment, diagnostic conclusion, and prerequisites to sex therapy: Seven critical pathways. From Wincze and Barlow (1997b). Copyright 1997 by Oxford University Press. Reprinted by permission.

weaknesses of the relationship. The therapist also assesses the impact of the sexual difficulty on the relationship, each partner's reactions to the sexual difficulties, the extent and nature of sexual activity since the sexual difficulty developed, and thoughts and beliefs related to sexual activity. Last, the therapist ensures that adequate information regarding the nature, onset, severity, and course of the sexual difficulty has been obtained. The therapist should be clear on the circumstances in which the difficulty occurs, and can inquire about the patient's attributions for the problem. Throughout the assessment, the therapist needs to be sensitive to information the patient is concerned about keeping private. As indicated earlier, the therapist should clarify with the patient which, if any, issues should not be shared with the partner. The first session may end with an open-ended question that allows the patient to add information about which the therapist has not asked. The therapist may directly ask, "Is there anything we have not talked about that might be helpful for me to know?"

SECOND SESSION: PARTNER INTERVIEW

The second session is devoted to interviewing the partner, unless for some reason the partner has been interviewed in the first session. The therapist may start by asking whether anything has changed since the last appointment. It is always helpful to ask this in the event that significant events (e.g., death in family, loss of job, argument) have positively or negatively affected the couple. It is important to know whether the couple is preoccupied with such events and distracted from the focus of therapy. The therapist may also ask whether the partners discussed the first session. Answers to this question may provide information regarding the couple's interaction pattern and openness in communication. In some couples, partners may willingly discuss sensitive subjects with one another in the therapist's office but completely avoid doing so at home. Thus, it is helpful to determine how partners communicate not only in the company of the therapist but also when they are alone. Before initiating further questions, the therapist may ask the patient's partner whether there is anything he or she would like to ask or discuss. This open-ended question gives the partner an opportunity to introduce process issues or personal factors that may have an impact on therapy. Once the therapist

and partner have discussed these issues, the partner interview then follows a format similar to that of the patient interview.

In some cases, after finishing the patient and partner interviews, the therapist decides that additional portions of the assessment are needed before he or she makes treatment recommendations. This information may include a physiological assessment or a medical evaluation. In such cases, the therapist should explain to the couple why additional information is needed and what value the added information may have. If both partners understand the potential importance of additional information, they are less likely to feel frustrated by the delay of disposition. The therapist should also explain what effect the additional portions of the assessment may have on the ultimate plan for treatment.

THIRD SESSION: FEEDBACK

The third session typically includes both partners. In some instances, however, the therapist may decide that individual therapy is needed before the partners can jointly address their sexual difficulties. He or she may meet with the couple briefly and indicate that this is the recommendation, then meet with the patient individually for the remainder of the session to explain in greater detail why individual therapy is indicated. We assume here that the therapist meets with the couple together for the entire third session.

The therapist may start by asking both partners whether anything new has happened since they last met, or whether they wish to discuss any issues related to the previous sessions. The partners' responses to an open-ended question allows the therapist to observe how they communicate, who raises questions or issues, how the other person responds, and how well each person communicates his or her needs. As indicated earlier, beginning this way also prompts discussion of personal issues other than sexual difficulties that are consuming time or emotional energy (e.g., problems with the couple's children). It is important for the therapist to be aware of such issues, because they may interfere with sex therapy.

Once the issues raised by the couple have been addressed, the therapist should present his or her case conceptualization. After outlining the factors that seem to be contributing to the sexual dysfunction, the therapist may work with the couple to identify appropriate treatment goals. Once treatment goals have been identified and agreed upon, the therapist can present a rough treatment outline to the couple and discuss the initial stages of therapy. (Please see later sections titled "Integration of Data across Methods" and "Goals of Treatment" for further discussion.)

Self-Report Questionnaires

A self-report questionnaire is a standardized, paper-and-pencil measure that is generally inexpensive, brief, and easy to administer and to score. There are several advantages to using self-report questionnaires. They may supplement information obtained in the interview and may provide information a patient is unwilling to reveal in person. With the use of norms, a standardized questionnaire may provide a comparison of the patient's symptoms or thoughts and those of others in the same age group. Finally, because they are brief, most self-report measures can be administered on multiple occasions. Repeated administrations may help the clinician to evaluate a patient's progress more objectively over the course of treatment. There are a number of self-report questionnaires; some focus specifically on sexual functioning, whereas others focus more generally on overall psychological functioning. Following are some of the self-report questionnaires we often use in our clinical work.

The Derogatis Sexual Functioning Inventory (DSFI) is intended to provide an "omnibus" measure of sexual functioning (Derogatis & Melisaratos, 1979). The instrument comprises 10 subscales: Information, Experience, Drive, Attitudes, Psychological Symptoms, Affect, Gender Role Definition, Fantasy, Body Image, and Sexual Satisfaction. The subscales demonstrate good to very good internal consistency and test–retest reliability (Derogatis & Melisaratos, 1979). The DSFI evidences good discriminant validity. Nine of 10 subscales differentiate between men with and without sexual dysfunction; 5 of 10 subscales differentiate between women with and without sexual dysfunction. The DSFI serves as a useful means of measuring a range of factors involved in sexual functioning. Disadvantages of the scale include its length (245 items) and somewhat complicated scoring.

The Dyadic Adjustment Scale (DAS), a widely used, 32-item self-report instrument, provides an overall measure of dyadic adjustment, as well as scores on four subscales: Dyadic Satisfaction, Dyadic Cohesion, Dyadic Consensus, and Affectional Expression. The DAS has demonstrated good discriminant validity, very good construct validity, and very high internal consistency (Spanier, 1976; Spanier & Thompson, 1982).

The Sexual Opinion Survey (SOS; Fisher, 1988; Fisher, Byrne, White, & Kelley, 1988) comprises 21 items designed to assess affective and evaluative responses to a variety of sexual stimuli. Each item describes a sexual situation and an associated negative or positive response. Patients rate the extent to which they agree with each response. We use the SOS to aid in our understanding of individuals and their comfort with a range of sexual situations. Research suggests that the SOS is valid and reliable, and norms are available (Fisher et al., 1988). The SOS can typically be completed and scored in less than 20 minutes.

Most recently, brief questionnaires have been developed that are easy to administer, valid, and reliable measures of male sexual difficulties: The International Index of Erectile Function (IIEF; Rosen et al., 1997) is a widely used self-administered measure of erectile function, and the Erection Quality Scale (EQS; Wincze et al., 2004) is a measure that focuses specifically on the quality of the male erectile response. Such tools can be used as effective pre- and posttreatment measures of either research outcome studies or treatment effectiveness.

A portion of the clinical interview focuses on the assessment of psychological functioning. Self-report measures may provide valuable additional information in areas such as mood, anxiety, and substance use. The Brief Symptom Inventory (Derogatis & Melisaratos, 1983) is a useful measure of general psychopathology. The Depression Anxiety Stress Scales (DASS; Lovibond & Lovibond, 1993) provide separate measures of depression, anxiety, and stress symptoms. The brief version of the Michigan Alcohol Screening Test (Pokorny, Miller, & Kaplan, 1972) and the Drug Abuse Screening Test (Skinner, 1982) are useful screens of alcohol and other substance use, respectively.

Psychophysiological Assessment

A psychophysiological assessment can contribute unique and valuable information to the assessment of sexual functioning. A clinical interview may be biased by both the patient's report and the clinician's interpretation. Self-report measures may be biased by the patient's response style. The strength of a physiological assessment is that it can provide an objective measure of sexual arousal. These data can help to determine the nature and severity of a patient's functional impairment and also to delineate the etiology of the dysfunction (i.e., organic, psychogenic, or mixed type). The most widely used approach to the psychophysiological assessment of sexual arousal in men is to measure nocturnal penile tumescence (NPT)—that is, a man's erectile activity during sleep. In the past, it was often necessary for men to spend at least one night in a sleep laboratory to obtain measures of NPT. Technological advances, however, have now made it possible to measure NPT in the privacy of a patient's home. The RigiScan monitor (Timm Medical Technologies, Inc.; Eden Prairie, MN) is a small, portable measuring device worn during sleep that provides measures of both NPT and penile rigidity. A patient is sent home to wear the device during sleep and returns with data for the physician to interpret.

An additional approach is to measure a patient's physiological response to erotic stimuli in the laboratory. This method is used to measure sexual arousal in both men and women. The patient sits in a private room. A male patient may place either an electromechanical gauge, which is a soft metal clip (see, e.g., Barlow, Becker, Leitenberg, & Agras, 1970), or a mercury strain gauge, which is a flexible band, around his penis. These gauges measure changes in penile circumference. A female patient inserts a plastic cylinder approximately the size of a tampon in her vagina (Geer, Morokoff, & Greenwood, 1974). The small device emits light and measures the amount of light that is reflected back. As a woman becomes aroused, blood flow to the vaginal wall increases, and less light passes through it. The rationale for the laboratory assessment is that patients who have difficulties becoming aroused during sexual activity with a partner may become aroused to erotic stimuli when there is no demand to engage in sexual activity. If so, there is evidence that such patients are physically capable of becoming aroused; there are simply factors that make it difficult for them to become aroused in a natural situation (e.g., performance-related concerns). A failure

to become aroused during a psychophysiological assessment does not, however, necessarily indicate an organic basis to the sexual dysfunction. On occasion, patients experience anxiety in the laboratory, because it is a novel situation and they know their response is being monitored; this performance anxiety may interfere with their ability to become aroused. In such instances, a second assessment may be helpful, because patients will often feel more relaxed. Aside from considerable money, technical knowledge and skills are required to operate the equipment. Thus, although a psychophysiological assessment may provide important and valuable information, it is not a practical option in many clinical settings.

Medical Examination

In most instances, the patient should undergo a medical exam as part of an assessment to determine what, if any, biological factors are contributing to the sexual difficulty. If a medical evaluation has not been completed at the start of the psychosocial evaluation, the patient should be referred for one. In either case, the therapist should ensure that the patient has told the physician about his or her sexual difficulties. It is not uncommon for a patient undergoing such an evaluation never to tell the physician his or her reason for seeking medical care. Once it has been completed, results of the medical exam can be integrated with those of the interview and the psychophysiological assessment.

Integration of Data across Methods

One of the goals of the assessment is to develop a coherent case formulation (i.e., a working hypothesis of the etiology of the problem). This formulation should relate all aspects of the patient's complaints to one another and explain why the individual has developed these difficulties (Carey, Flasher, Maisto, & Turkat, 1984). The first purpose of this formulation is to aid the therapist in the development of a treatment plan. A second purpose is to communicate to patients that (1) their problem is an understandable one given their physiology, medical history, life experiences and so on; (2) there is reason for hope and optimism; and (3) there is a conceptual "road map" and rationale on which to build a therapeutic plan. Finally, developing a case formulation allows the therapist to check with the patient to see whether he or she has obtained all the necessary information and that the information is correct. One of the more challenging aspects of sex therapy is integrating multiple levels of influence (i.e., biological, psychological, dyadic, and cultural) into a coherent case formulation.

Despite its difficulty, a biopsychosocial case formulation captures the richness of sexual function and dysfunction. A patient is more likely to agree to try a psychosocial approach if the therapist recognizes that biological causes are not irrelevant, but inquires about and recognizes specific dyadic and sociocultural influences that might override or compensate for these. It is important to be sensitive to specific rituals and traditions that a couple has established, as well as ethnic, cultural, or religious issues. The case formulation should include biological, psychological, and social areas even if the therapist believes that one of the areas is not contributing to the problem at the moment. It is always hard to predict the future, and the groundwork should be laid in case additional information becomes available and/or future developments occur. Moreover, this comprehensive approach to case formulation gives the patient confidence that the therapist has considered all possibilities. Indirectly, the therapist communicates that the patient should also think about the problem in a multifaceted biopsychosocial framework.

Goals of Treatment

Many patients enter sex therapy with a performance-oriented treatment goal. For example, men with erectile disorder want to attain firm erections, and women with female orgasmic disorder want to reach orgasm. We feel that performance-oriented goals are problematic for a few reasons. They place pressure on patients and may increase performance anxiety; thus, they are usually self-defeating. In addition, performance-oriented goals are based on the belief that a sexual interaction is a "failure" if certain events (e.g., intercourse, orgasm) do not occur. These goals conflict with the notion that a couple may be physically intimate and sexually satisfied in multiple ways. We suggest that the primary goal of sex therapy should be to help a couple develop a more satisfying sexual relationship. We explain to both partners that there is nothing wrong with a desire to engage in intercourse or reach orgasm

(failure to acknowledge this may alienate the patient or partner and diminish the therapist's credibility). These goals, however, are secondary. If intercourse or orgasm occurs, that is fine; these events, however, are not necessary for sexual activity to be satisfying. The therapist can talk to the couple about the drawbacks of performance-oriented goals. Ultimately, it is important that the therapist and the couple come to some agreement regarding treatment goals. If the patient or couple is working toward a performance-oriented goal and the therapist is not, frustration with the therapy and with the clinician may result. We suggest that the therapist and the couple periodically review treatment goals over the course of therapy. This helps to ensure that the therapist and the couple remain in agreement regarding the objectives of therapy. It also provides an opportunity to assess progress and to modify goals as needed.

Process Issues in Treatment

Default Assumptions

As in the case of assessment, it is helpful to begin treatment with a set of default assumptions. Wincze and Carey (2001) suggest that the following assumptions may help to facilitate efficient and effective treatment:

1. A patient usually has a narrow definition of sex and will focus on performance as a marker of success.
2. A patient sometimes has stereotyped views of masculine and feminine roles that will interfere with the assimilation of new information.
3. A patient often does not understand the ingredients conducive to sexual arousal (e.g., favorable times to have sex and factors that may interfere).
4. A patient may have a pattern of avoidance of sexual interactions and, as a result, may unintentionally sabotage therapy.
5. A patient may be uninformed about sexually transmitted diseases and may not be using safe sex practices.

These assumptions help the therapist to anticipate potential obstacles to successful treatment. If certain assumptions prove not to be true, those issues may not need to be addressed. This indicates that the patient has one less barrier to achieving his or her treatment goals.

Challenges to Therapy

PREFERENCE FOR A SIMPLE PILL

Having heard of medication for treating ED, many patients expect that their sexual difficulties can be cured with a simple pill. They may see little point in investing the time and effort required for effective CBT. In such cases, it is helpful to remind couples that CBT is a long-term investment. It provides them with strategies they can use well after treatment ends to maintain a satisfying sexual relationship. It may also be useful to remind couples that all treatments (including both medication and sex therapy) have advantages and disadvantages. A patient and partner need to weigh the costs and benefits associated with each treatment option and decide which approach is best for them.

RIGID, FAULTY ATTRIBUTION FOR THE SEXUAL DIFFICULTIES

Patients sometimes cling to a single explanation of their sexual difficulty. For example, a male patient may insist that there is a medical basis to his ED. The therapist may need to reframe alternative explanations, so that they are more acceptable and less threatening to the patient. In the case of the man who firmly believes his ED is medically based, the therapist may emphasize that it is good that medical factors are not involved.

NONCOMPLIANCE WITH HOMEWORK ASSIGNMENTS

Cognitive-behavioral treatments typically involve homework assignments that allow patients to practice the skills they are learning between sessions. Homework plays a uniquely central role in sex therapy, because a number of treatment methods (e.g., sensate focus) can only be practiced or applied outside of sessions. For this reason, failure to comply with homework assignments presents a very significant challenge to treatment. Noncompliance may result from a number of factors, including fear and avoidance, an uncooperative partner, and busy schedules. We have found that it is important to anticipate potential obstacles to completing homework (e.g., a patient may feel un-comfortable or embarrassed completing certain exercises) and to address these issues proactively with the couple. If partners have difficulty making time for assigned exercises, it is sometimes helpful to schedule the exercises in advance. Of course, the partners should choose times when they can relax and will not be bothered. The therapist can remind the partners that they should respect scheduled time with each other just as they would respect time scheduled with someone else (e.g., a doctor or supervisor).

EXTRAMARITAL AFFAIRS

When working with a couple, a therapist may occasionally learn that one person is having an affair. In these cases, the therapist must try to remain objective and evaluate the impact of the affair on the couple's relationship and on treatment. If the affair is counterproductive to therapy (as is usually the case), the therapist may help the person evaluate his or her priorities and decide whether to end the affair. If the person does not end the affair and the therapist does not feel that treatment can be beneficial as long as the affair goes on, the therapy may be discontinued. The therapist may approach this in different ways, depending on the particular case. In all instances, however, the therapist should respect the confidentiality of both the patient and the partner.

CULTURAL OR RELIGIOUS OPPOSITION TO TREATMENT METHODS

Cultural or religious opposition to treatment methods can present a challenge to the therapy process. One of the most common examples of this is some patients' negative response to the idea of masturbation. Masturbation exercises are often used to help patients become more comfortable with their bodies and to help women with aversion or pain disorders become more comfortable with penetration. Some patients believe that masturbation is dirty or sinful, or that it is not something a married person should do. One way to help patients feel comfortable with the idea of masturbatory exercises is to explain that they serve a clinical purpose. The therapist may indicate that masturbation is not an activity a person must adopt on a permanent basis. Rather, it is a technique that may be used over the short term to help the patient achieve his or her treatment goals.

Treatment Methods

Education

Education can be one of the most important components of sex therapy. Faulty beliefs, unrealistic expectations, and lack of information regarding physiology, anatomy, and sexual functioning can play central roles in the etiology and maintenance of sexual dysfunction. As a result, psychoeducation sometimes leads to rapid improvement in the first few sessions. For example, men who do not know there is a refractory period following ejaculation are very relieved to learn that their "erectile failure" after orgasm is normal. Similarly, women are relieved to find that lack of lubrication is a natural consequence of menopause and can easily be remedied with a lubricant. Excerpts from textbooks on human sexuality can provide a helpful overview of sexual functioning. We also use pictures or diagrams of male and female genitalia to help patients develop a better understanding of the human anatomy. Information on the risks of unprotected sex and sexually transmitted diseases (including human immunodeficiency virus and hepatitis) is important in all cases and should be presented to couples routinely. Unfortunately, the task of re-educating patients in regard to normative sexual functioning is not always easy. We live in a culture that promotes a number of myths regarding sexual functioning. Thus, patients' faulty beliefs and unrealistic expectations are sometimes firmly entrenched and resistant to change. The following compilation of common myths of male and female sexuality is adapted from Heiman and LoPiccolo (1988), Wincze and Barlow (1997a), and Zilbergeld (1998).

Myths of male sexuality

1. A real man is not into sissy stuff like feelings and communicating.
2. A man is always interested in and always ready for sex.
3. A real man performs in sex.
4. Sex is centered on a hard penis and what is done with it.
5. A man should be able to make the earth move for his partner, or at the very least knock her socks off.
6. Men do not have to listen to women about sexual matters.
7. Real men do not have sex problems.
8. Bigger is better.
9. Men should be able to last all night.
10. Women will not like a man who cannot get it up.
11. If a man cannot get it up, he must not really love his partner.
12. If a man knows that he might not be able to get an erection, it is unfair for him to start sexual activity with a partner.
13. Focusing more intensely on one's erection—trying harder—is the best way to get an erection.

Myths of female sexuality

1. Sex is only for women under 30.
2. Normal women have an orgasm every time they have sex.
3. All women can have multiple orgasms.
4. Pregnancy and delivery reduce women's sexual responsiveness.
5. A woman's sex life ends with menopause.
6. There are different kinds of orgasms related to a woman's personality; vaginal orgasms are more feminine and mature than clitoral orgasms.
7. A sexually responsive woman can always be turned on by her partner.
8. Nice women are not aroused by erotic books or films.
9. A woman who does not like the more exotic forms of sex is frigid.
10. If a woman cannot have an orgasm quickly and easily, then there is something wrong with her.
11. Feminine women do not initiate sex or become wild and unrestrained during sex.
12. Double jeopardy: A woman is frigid if she does not want sex and wanton if she does.
13. Contraception is a woman's responsibility, and she's just making up excuses if she says contraception issues are inhibiting her sexually.
14. If a woman does not initiate sex, she is just not interested in sex.

Myths of Male and Female Sexuality

1. We are liberated folks who are very comfortable with sex.
2. All touching is sexual or should lead to sex.
3. Sex equals intercourse.
4. Good sex requires orgasm.
5. People in love should automatically know what their partners desire. Sex should be spontaneous, with no planning and no talking. It is not romantic if you ask your partner what he or she enjoys.
6. Too much masturbation is bad.

7. Someone with a sexual partner does not masturbate.
8. Fantasizing about something else means a person is not happy with what he or she has.

We typically review these myths with couples and ask them to indicate which statements they believe are true. This exercise helps couples to explore their attitudes about sexual functioning. Moreover, it helps the therapist to identify beliefs that need to be challenged in treatment. In some cases, patients' faulty beliefs regarding sexual functioning (e.g., sex equals intercourse) need to be challenged repeatedly over the course of therapy. Along with obtaining information from the therapist, patients often benefit from reading selected books. A number of books are helpful to patients; examples include those by Wincze and Barlow (1997a), McCarthy and McCarthy (1998), and Zilbergeld (1998). We do not recommend that therapists suggest any book to patients before reading it themselves. In addition, if a therapist assigns readings to a couple, we recommend that time be reserved in the subsequent session to discuss the reading. This provides an opportunity for the couple to address any questions or concerns. It also reinforces the couple for completing the assignment and promotes continued compliance in the future.

Stimulus Control

Many couples mistakenly believe that sexual functioning is an automatic process that requires nothing more than a willing partner. They may engage in sexual activity in very unfavorable conditions and have little insight into why they experience sexual problems. One of us (A. K. B.) recently interviewed a patient who indicated that he was not happy in his current relationship. When asked what he and his partner enjoyed doing together, he laughed and responded, "Spending time apart." Despite the obvious problems within the relationship, the patient was surprised and concerned that he was not able to maintain an erection during sexual activity with his partner. Positive interpersonal and environmental factors are necessary for healthy sexual functioning. "Stimulus control" is a treatment method that involves manipulating environmental factors to facilitate a particular behavior or outcome. In the context of sex therapy, stimulus control refers to an effort to create conditions that are condu-

cive to healthy sexual functioning. Biological, psychological, and interpersonal factors all affect sexual functioning. Positive and negative factors in each of these areas interact to affect sexual arousal (see Figure 15.2). Some examples of biological factors are disease, drugs, alcohol, cigarettes, or even fatigue. Psychological factors include self-esteem, mood, anxiety, thoughts, and attitudes. Interpersonal factors (included with the psychological factors in Figure 15.2) include physical attraction to and positive attitude toward the partner. The first objective with respect to stimulus control is to help the couple appreciate that certain conditions are necessary for healthy sexual functioning to occur (e.g., a partner with whom a person feels comfortable). It may be important to explain to patients that even a medical treatment may not lead to sexual arousal if favorable psychological and interpersonal conditions are not present. Additionally, as indicated earlier, a medical problem (e.g., hypertension) may place someone at risk for sexual difficulties, but with positive interpersonal and psychological conditions, the person may function

Psychological Factors	Good emotional health	Depression or PTSD
	Attraction toward partner	Lack of partner attraction
	Positive attitude toward partner	Negative attitude toward partner
	Positive sex attitude	Negative attitude toward sex
	Focus on pleasure	Focus on performance
	Newness	Routine, habit
	Good self-esteem	Poor self-esteem
	Comfortable environment for sex	Uncomfortable environment for sex
	Flexible attitude toward sex	Rigid, narrow attitude toward sex
Physical Factors	No smoking	Smoking
	No excess alcohol	Too much alcohol
	No medications that affect sex	Antihypertensive medication (heart)/Drugs
	Good physical health	Poor physical health
	Regular, appropriate exercise	Heart and blood-flow problems
	Good nutrition	Diabetes
	Successful Sexual Functioning	**Dysfunctional Sexual Functioning**

FIGURE 15.2. Positive and negative factors that affect sexual functioning. From Wincze and Barlow (1997b). Copyright 1997 by Oxford University Press. Reprinted by permission.

without a problem. Each member of a couple can generate a list of conditions or factors that positively affect his or her sexual arousal. The person may list factors such as the setting, time of day, his or her mood, the partner's mood, or the atmosphere (music, candles, lingerie). The couple can then work to maximize the number of positive factors in each sexual encounter. Partners should also determine what factors negatively influence their sexual functioning. Negative factors such as faulty beliefs, poor environmental conditions, and performance-related concerns may be addressed in the context of sex therapy. Alternatively, a referral to a marriage counselor, individual therapist, or physician can be made, if necessary.

Cognitive Restructuring

At the start of treatment, we typically ask patients what thoughts they have when they engage in sexual activity. If a couple is completely avoiding sexual activity, we ask what thoughts the partners have if they imagine engaging in sexual activity. Most readily identify negative thoughts such as "I wish it would work this time," "I am going to disappoint him or her again," "I don't feel like doing this," and "This is going to be painful." We point out to the couple that these thoughts are neither relaxing nor arousing; it is only natural that when these thoughts are running through partners' minds, they do not feel sexually aroused. Pointing this out serves to normalize the occurrence of sexual difficulties and helps both partners appreciate the impact of thoughts on sexual arousal. If a patient's sexual dysfunction is acquired, we ask the patient to describe the types of thoughts he or she had during sexual activity before the problem developed. The therapist can help the patient conclude that during pleasurable sexual activity, people focus on body parts, physical sensations, and other arousing aspects of sexual activity. The therapist can explain to the patient that one component of treatment is to challenge the negative thoughts that distract him or her during sexual functioning. This allows the patient to return his or her focus to the thoughts associated with pleasurable sexual activity.

As we indicated earlier, many patients readily identify the interfering thoughts they have during sexual activity. Others may have more difficulty identifying negative cognitions. In either case, we often ask patients to complete a simple self-monitoring form after engaging in sexual activity. They record the nature of the sexual activity (e.g., massage), the level of anxiety (on a 0- to 8-point Likert-type scale), and the thoughts they had. Self-monitoring helps patients to identify negative thoughts, facilitates discussion during sessions, and helps the therapist to track progress over the course of treatment.

Once negative thoughts are identified, the therapist can teach the patient to challenge them. One strategy for challenging negative thoughts is to provide education. As we noted earlier, education is a powerful tool in sex therapy. One of us (A. K. B.) worked with a woman who had an aversive response to semen. A discussion of this revealed that her husband had a family history of testicular cancer. During sexual activity, she worried that she might contract cancer through her husband's semen. Basic education helped to relieve this woman's fear and allowed her to feel more comfortable during sexual activity.

A second strategy for challenging patients' thoughts is to help them determine whether a negative thought has any factual basis. Patients often cling to negative assumptions or negative predictions despite the absence of supporting evidence. The therapist can teach patients to base their thoughts on facts rather than on fear. For example, a man with erectile disorder may believe that his partner will leave him if the problem does not improve. Couple therapy provides an excellent opportunity to address the patient's assumptions regarding his partner's thoughts or feelings. The session can be used to help the patient address his concerns with the partner. The partner's response often resolves misunderstandings and challenges false assumptions. The discussion also helps to promote better communication outside of the session. A woman with sexual aversion disorder may believe that intercourse will be extremely painful and unpleasant. The therapist can help her to challenge such negative thoughts by examining the evidence for and against them. The therapist can ask her to explain what evidence she has that a belief or negative prediction is valid. As the patient presents this evidence, the therapist can help to identify errors in her thinking. For example, the patient may state that when she was an adolescent, her mother told her sex was extremely painful and unpleasant. The therapist can point out that this does not necessarily mean it is true, or that it would apply to her; perhaps there are examples of other things about which she and her mother disagree. The therapist can then ask what further evidence might suggest that this belief is not true. The therapist can work with the patient to generate as much evidence as possible to counter the negative thought.

One final method of challenging patients' negative thoughts is to help them decatastrophize negative outcomes (i.e., understand that even if the outcome is negative, it will not be the end of the world). For example, a male patient may report that he would die of embarrassment if he lost his erection on his first attempt at intercourse with a partner. The therapist may help the patient see that if he lost his erection, it might be embarrassing or awkward, but he could cope with it. The therapist might elicit an example of a negative experience with which the patient has successfully coped in the past and help him to develop more realistic outcome expectations.

Along with challenging patients' negative thoughts, it is often necessary to address their partners' thoughts. Many people begin to have negative, interfering thoughts during sexual activity if their partners are experiencing sexual problems. Thus, we typically ask partners what thoughts they have during sexual activity. The same techniques can then be used to help the partners challenge the negative thoughts they endorse. Cognitive restructuring techniques are sometimes complex and may be difficult for some patients to grasp. Thus, the process of challenging a patient's thoughts should be simplified to suit the particular patient. For more information regarding the use of cognitive restructuring techniques, the therapist may wish to consult Beck (1976).

Once the patient has begun to challenge interfering thoughts, the next objective is to return his or her attention to erotic cues. The therapist may suggest that the patient focus on sensations or particular body parts during sexual activity. The therapist may also encourage the patient to employ fantasy. Some patients may be reluctant to use fantasy, fearing that this suggests their sexual relationship is unsatisfying. The therapist must approach this topic with care, but he or she may ultimately help to normalize the use of sexual fantasies. A couple may benefit from reading McCarthy's (1988) chapter on sexual fantasies.

Behavioral Techniques for Specific Disorders

AROUSAL DISORDERS

Sensate focus is a treatment method that was developed by Masters and Johnson (1966). It may be applied to patients with any sexual dysfunction, but it is most often used in the treatment of arousal disorders. Sensate focus involves placing a ban on intercourse and engaging in a series of increasingly sensual/sexual activities. The primary objectives of sensate focus are to remove the pressure to perform, to return a couple's focus to pleasurable sensations, to reintroduce the couple to the "basics" of sexual activity, and to encourage the couple to derive pleasure from various forms of stimulation. Many couples may be surprised and somewhat concerned by the notion that they are not supposed to engage in sexual intercourse. If they do not understand the rationale for these instructions, they may discontinue treatment prematurely. Thus, it is very important that the therapist clearly explain the purpose of sensate focus. The therapist may explain that sexual activity is most satisfying when each person focuses on sensations. Couples experiencing sexual problems often focus too much on performance and fail to focus on sensations. Sensate focus is intended to remove the pressure to perform and allow couples to enjoy pleasurable sensations again. Each week, the therapist and the couple agree to a specific sensate focus exercise. In assigning a sensate focus exercise, the therapist should be clear about the following:

- What the exercise will be
- How often it should be practiced (generally one to three times each week)
- How long it should last (generally 15–30 minutes)
- What the goals of the exercise are (e.g., to focus on physical sensations, to practice communicating about sexual activity)
- What the goals of the exercise are *not* (e.g., to become aroused, to reach orgasm, to engage in intercourse; it is OK if one or both partners become aroused, but the goal is pleasure, not specifically arousal)
- Who should initiate the exercise

The specific exercises employed vary depending on the particular needs and comfort level of each couple. In many cases, sensate focus begins with a nongenital massage. Couples may start by being clothed or unclothed, depending on their comfort level. The therapist may suggest that the partners express their preferences for different forms of touch and give each other positive feedback (not criticism) during the massage. This allows both partners to practice communicating about sexual activity. As the partners become comfortable with the nongenital massage, they may advance to a massage that involves genital contact. Once genital contact is introduced, the therapist should emphasize that the purpose is not to stimulate one another to the point of orgasm or even to become aroused. Again, the goals are to promote pleasure and intimacy. The couple should be clear on this point before beginning the exercise. The next step is often penetration without thrusting. At this stage, it may be helpful to remind the partners that if they are unable to complete penetration (e.g., the man cannot maintain a firm erection), they may continue sexual activity with other forms of stimulation. This helps to minimize performance demand and reinforces the notion that sexual satisfaction is not dependent on intercourse. The final stage of sensate focus is typically sexual activity that may include intercourse. By stating that sexual activity "may" include intercourse, the therapist continues to limit performance demands and reinforces the notion that the couple may not always *wish* to include intercourse. The therapist may remind the partners that they have learned to derive pleasure from various forms of stimulation. Thus, whereas intercourse may now be a part of sexual activity, it does not invariably play the central role.

The steps we just described can be broken down into a series of smaller exercises depending on a couple's particular needs. For example, nongenital massage may begin with holding hands while clothed and advance to back massage while unclothed. Each couple begins at a different point along the continuum. Some couples advance very slowly, working on one step for weeks or months before advancing to the next. In such cases, it is important periodically to remind both partners that they are working toward the long-term goal of having a satisfying sexual relationship. See Table 15.1 for an example of typical progression through sensate focus assignments.

TABLE 15.1. Sensate Focus: Sample Series of Assignments

Each assignment should be practiced one to three times between sessions for 15–30 minutes each time.

Assignment 1: Each partner gives the other a massage while dressed. The person receiving the massage can give feedback about what he or she likes or dislikes. The goal of the exercise is not to become aroused; it is simply to enjoy the time together. The couple agrees not to engage in intercourse.

Assignment 2: Each partner gives the other a massage while nude—with no genital contact and no intercourse. The person receiving the massage can give feedback about what he or she likes and dislikes. The goal of the exercise is not to become aroused; it is simply to enjoy the time together.

Assignment 3: Repeat Assignment 2.

Assignment 4: Each partner gives the other a massage while nude, with genital contact. Again, becoming aroused is not the goal; the goal is simply to enjoy the time together and focus on the sensations. No intercourse. No effort is focused specifically on reaching orgasm. Continue the practice of giving feedback. The therapist will not ask in the next session whether either partner became physically aroused (e.g., attained an erection). *This is stated ahead of time, to reinforce the notion that erections and lubrication are not the goal of the exercise.*

Assignment 5: Repeat Assignment 4.

Assignment 6: Repeat Assignment 4.

Assignment 7: The couple engages in sexual activity that includes penetration without thrusting. The goal of penetration is to enjoy the sensations.

Assignment 8: The couple engages in sexual activity that includes penetration with minimal thrusting. The goal of penetration is not to achieve orgasm; it is simply to enjoy the sensations. The couple should cease penetration and resume other forms of sexual activity after a brief time.

Assignment 9: The couple engages in sexual activity that may include intercourse—complete lift of the ban on intercourse.

Along with helping the couple to plan the exercises, it is the therapist's role to review the exercises in the following session. It maybe helpful to have each partner record the thoughts he or she experiences during assigned exercises, to facilitate discussion in the session. The therapist can help the couple restructure distorted thoughts, address problems that occurred, and identify and target avoidance behaviors.

INTEGRATING ED MEDICATIONS INTO COGNITIVE-BEHAVIORAL TREATMENT

As previously noted in this chapter, it is certainly common for men experiencing ED to have knowledge of or experience with Viagra, Levitra, or Cialis. Whereas these medications are often sufficient by themselves to treat ED effectively, it is not at all unusual for high levels of performance anxiety to persist and interfere with patients' erectile responding in spite of their use of the medication. Consequently, it is advisable to consider treatment for performance anxiety when medication is used. For some men, just knowing that the medication works and is available, if needed, is sufficient to overcome any performance anxiety. For many other men, however, the performance anxiety must be dealt with directly.

When medication to treat ED is used, it is advisable to direct men first to use the medication during masturbation, without the pressure of a partner. This strategy effectively removes performance anxiety in most cases and allows a man to gain confidence in the medication's effectiveness. In addition, dosage level can be established and side effects (if any) can be addressed. Following several masturbation experiences with the medication, sensate focus can then be utilized with the partner and the medication. Once erections are reliably occurring with the medication in partnered sexual activity, the medication can then be weaned. During weaning, couples are encouraged to begin sexual activity without the medication on *some* occasions. Therapists should work with couples to establish the most comfortable approach to using sensate focus in conjunction with medication.

PREMATURE EJACULATION

The first step in the treatment of premature ejaculation is often providing psychoeducation about normative latencies to ejaculation. The therapist may inform the patient that most men typically ejaculate within 2 to 8 minutes of penetration (Wincze & Barlow, 1997b). The patient's age and the length of time since the last ejaculation also affect latency to ejaculation. One option for men who ejaculate quickly is to modify their sexual routine. The couple may continue to engage in intercourse as long as possible after ejaculation. When ejaculation no longer signifies the end of intercourse, there is less emphasis on the man's ability to control his ejaculation. This reduces the man's performance-related concerns and may even increase the latency to ejaculation. A similar approach is to continue engaging in sexual activity once intercourse is no longer possible. Again, this reduces the pressure on the man, because it means that ejaculation does not signal the end of sexual activity. If premature ejaculation is severe (e.g., ejaculation occurs before penetration), or if the man must wear a condom during sexual activity, then continuing intercourse after ejaculation is not a viable option.

In severe cases of premature ejaculation, medication may be considered. Delays in ejaculation have been associated with many of the medications used for treatment of depression (Segraves, 2003). Consequently, antidepressant medication is commonly prescribed for treating premature ejaculation. In this strategy, the patient may be given antidepressant medication on an as-needed basis (about 6 hours before anticipated sexual relations) or daily (Segraves, 2003). The optimal pharmacological approach (type of medication, dosage level, and dosage regimen) can be experimented with and worked out with each patient. In some cases, antidepressant medication may be supplemented with Cialis, Levitra, or Viagra to ensure maintenance of the erection and delay of the ejaculation. Studies have shown the combination to be effective in increasing sexual satisfaction (Chen, Mabjeesh, Matzkin, & Greenstein, 2003; Salonia et al., 2002).

MALE AND FEMALE ORGASMIC DISORDERS

Therapists should ensure that couples have realistic expectations regarding orgasm (e.g., the degree of stimulation required, normative frequency and intensity) and an understanding of individual variations. Once a couple has realistic expectations, a therapist should discuss whether the patient with orgasmic disorder is receiving adequate stimulation during sexual activity. If not, the therapist can provide guidelines for increasing stimulation. Patients who achieve orgasm during masturbation, but not during sexual activity with a partner, may demonstrate for their partners the type of stimulation they find arousing. Patients who do not achieve orgasm during either masturbation or sexual activity with a partner may proceed through exercises, such as those in Table 15.2, to learn more about what they find arousing. In both cases, the therapist can help the person to

TABLE 15.2. Homework Assignments for Treatment of Orgasmic Disorders

- Instruct the patient and partner to construct a list of good and bad conditions for sexual activity. This helps both partners begin to consider the circumstances in which they become most aroused.

- Encourage the patient to read literature, peruse magazines, watch videos, or look at art that he or she finds arousing. This material may be used to aid the patient in formulating sexual fantasies. Normalize and encourage the use of sexual fantasy inside and outside of sexual activity.

- Assign a series of self-stimulation exercises. The person should engage in these exercises daily for approximately 10–20 minutes, depending on the exercise. The purpose of the exercises is to increase the patient's comfort with his or her body and learn more about what is most arousing to him or her. The goal is not specifically to reach orgasm, but more generally to increase enjoyment of sexual activity. The specific exercises vary depending on a patient's comfort level. A typical progression of exercises is as follows:
  - Patient views his or her body nude in the mirror.
  - Patient views his or her genitals nude in the mirror.
  - Patient rubs/stimulates areas of his or her body other than the genitals.
  - Patient stimulates his or her genitals. (Therapist should ensure that patient understands what types of genital stimulation are generally arousing for people; it should not be assumed that a person knows what is meant by "masturbation.")
  - Mirror exercises are repeated until the person feels comfortable doing them. Stimulation exercises are repeated until the person feels comfortable and has learned how that type of stimulation can be pleasurable for him or her ("pleasurable" may mean relaxing, arousing, or in any way positive).

- Patient demonstrates for partner the type of stimulation that he or she finds pleasurable.

challenge any distracting or negative thoughts that may be occurring during sexual activity with a partner. Finally, a couple may enhance arousal with the use of fantasies; sexy lingerie or underwear; sex toys and vibrators; and novel behaviors, positions, or settings.

Although the couple is working to enhance the patient's arousal, the therapist should be careful not to reinforce a performance-oriented approach to sexual activity. The therapist may explain to the couple that orgasm is not essential for satisfying sexual activity, and remind the couple that there are times when the most satisfying sexual encounters do not involve orgasm and the most disappointing sexual encounters do.

PAIN DISORDERS AND SEXUAL AVERSION DISORDER

When assessing a patient with a pain disorder or a sexual aversion disorder, the therapist should determine what activities are difficult or anxiety-provoking for the patient. Most patients with these disorders have problems with intercourse. Female patients may also have difficulty using tampons, undergoing a gynecological examination, or even looking at themselves nude in the mirror. At the start of treatment, the therapist may work with the patient to construct a hierarchy of 10–15 anxiety-provoking activities. The activities should range from moderately to very challenging. Treatment involves gradually working through this hierarchy using repeated exposure and cognitive restructuring. (Please see Figure 15.3 for an example of a typical fear and avoidance hierarchy.) The patient may begin by practicing moderately anxiety-provoking activities that do not involve a partner (e.g., a female patient looks at her nude breasts in the mirror for 5 minutes). The activity should be practiced several times before the next session. The patient may record the thoughts and anxiety level experienced during each exposure. In the next session, the therapist helps the patient challenge maladaptive thoughts and reviews her anxiety levels. Each step on the hierarchy should be repeated until the patient can perform it comfortably. Eventually, the patient can practice activities that involve the partner (e.g., a partner touches the exterior portions of the woman's genitalia). Again, each step should be repeated until the patient is comfortable with it. The patient should be in control of the expo-

Activity	Fear	Avoidance
Intercourse	8	8
Partner inserts penis into vagina—no thrusting	8	8
Partner inserts finger into vagina	8	7
Partner inserts tip of finger into vagina	7	7
Patient inserts her finger into her own vagina	6	6
Patient inserts tip of her finger into her own vagina	6	5
Partner touches exterior portions of patient's genitalia	6	5
Patient looks at her genitals in the mirror	5	5
Partner touches nude breasts	4	4
Patient touches exterior portion of her own genitalia	4	4
Patient looks at a photo of male genitalia	4	4
Patient looks at a photo of female genitalia	3	4
Patient watches video of sexual activity—actors nude	3	4
Patient watches video of sexual activity—actors clothed	3	3

FIGURE 15.3. Sample fear and avoidance hierarchy for treatment of sexual pain and aversion disorders. (This hierarchy is written for a female patient. Ratings are based on a 0–8 Likert-type scale, where 0 = *No fear or avoidance* and 8 = *Extreme fear or avoidance.*)

sure exercises at all times; thus, the patient may terminate an exposure if she feels too uncomfortable. The partner must agree to comply fully with this condition before exercises are begun.

HYPOACTIVE SEXUAL DESIRE DISORDER

The first step in treating hypoactive sexual desire disorder is to identify personal and interpersonal factors that may be inhibiting sexual desire. Examples of such factors include a history of sexual abuse, lack of physical attraction to the partner, and negative attitudes regarding sexual activity. Once identified, these factors can be addressed over the course of treatment. Table 15.3 lists strategies for targeting psychosocial factors that often contribute to low desire. Along with addressing personal or interpersonal issues, a patient may read or view erotic literature or art to enhance sexual desire. Different patients find different books, videos, and forms of art arousing. Thus, although suggestions can be offered, we find it is helpful to leave this assignment open-ended. This permits each patient to explore options that are most acceptable and arousing to him or her. When working with patients who are very religious or

conservative, the therapist may need to be creative in finding images that are arousing but not offensive to the patients. A patient may also jump-start his or her sexual desire with a vacation, a change in routine (different setting or different time of day for sexual activity), lingerie, or sexual props (e.g., vibrator, sex toys).

Communication Training

Some degree of communication training is necessary in nearly all sex therapy cases. Couples may need to work on general communication skills. Wincze and Barlow (1997a) present a checklist of positive communication skills (please see Figure 15.4). This checklist may be provided to a couple as a handout relatively early in treatment. The couple may practice using these skills in daily interactions. Improvement in overall communication may increase relationship satisfaction. Moreover, the use of these skills helps partners to discuss their sexual problems in a constructive manner.

The majority of couples have difficulty communicating about their sexual matters and should be encouraged to discuss their sexual relationship (Wincze & Barlow, 1997b). It is important to initiate such discussions at an op-

TABLE 15.3. Strategies for Addressing Factors That May Contribute to Low Desire

Boredom

Encourage both partners to add novelty and variety to their sexual relationship: new places, new sexual activities, new positions, addition of different "props" (e.g., sex toys, new lingerie). Normalize and encourage the use of sexual fantasy during and outside of sexual activity. Ask each partner to develop a "wish list" of activities, conditions, or scenarios that he or she would like to add to the sexual repertoire. The partners should share their lists and decide which items would be pleasing or agreeable to both of them. Instruct each person to write a list of good and bad conditions for sexual activity. The couple can use these lists to create situations that are most conducive to pleasurable sexual activity.

Lack of physical attraction to partner

Address the importance of physical attraction in a relationship. Encourage the partners to discuss factors that help them feel attracted to one another. Examples include using perfume or cologne, wearing one's hair a certain way, shaving, keeping the door closed when using the bathroom, wearing particular things during the day or to bed at night. Encourage the couple to attend to these factors and make efforts to be attractive to one another. Stress the relationship between physical health and fitness, and sexual functioning. Encourage the couple to adhere to a healthy diet and to exercise regularly. These lifestyle changes can be particularly helpful to patients who are dissatisfied with their own weight or that of their partners. Nevertheless, they can be beneficial for all couples.

Negative or faulty attitudes

Target maladaptive thoughts with psychoeducation and cognitive restructuring, as described in the chapter text.

Dissatisfaction with what a partner does or does not do during sexual activity

Normalize and encourage communication regarding what each person prefers during sexual activity. Explain that preferences for particular sexual activities vary not only between partners but also vary within each individual from one occasion to the next. Thus, without communication, it is very hard for one partner to know what the other wants or likes. Help the partners to discuss constructively what they do not like during sexual activity. This discussion should take place outside of sexual activity and be addressed in a sensitive, nonpunitive manner.

History of sexual abuse

If the person suffers from depression, posttraumatic stress disorder (PTSD), or another psychological problem as a result of the abuse, this problem should be addressed before focusing specifically on sexual dysfunction. Before enhancing positive feelings related to sex, it is necessary to address the person's negative feelings (e.g., fear, disgust, indifference related to sexual activity). Construct and work through a fear and avoidance hierarchy as described for treatment of sexual pain and aversion disorders. Address thoughts/fears that interfere with sexual activity through use of psychoeducation and cognitive restructuring. Once this is done, use the strategies listed above to enhance positive feelings regarding sexual activity.

portune time (e.g., not immediately after a negative sexual experience). The partners may specifically schedule times when they will not be bothered by distractions. Although it may be difficult to find such time, eliminating distractions and sitting down together help to promote constructive discussions. Scheduling and protecting such times also convey to each partner that the other considers the relationship a priority. Partners should be encouraged to discuss their sexual problems. If they do not, misunderstandings are likely to develop and remain unchallenged. Although discussing sexual problems is important, partners must be care-

ful not to blame each other, either subtly or overtly. This is destructive, can deter future discussion, and may serve to maintain the problem. The therapist can also encourage partners to express their preferences for different forms of stimulation or certain sexual activities. The partners may tell each other what they enjoyed following a particular encounter. They should not, however, provide criticism or negative feedback immediately following sexual activity. Some couples may resist the idea of providing feedback regarding sexual activity. They may feel that a "good lover" knows what his or her partner wants without having to ask. The ther-

If the statement describes what you do, place a check mark in the box.

Sender Skills (The *sender* is the person who wants to talk about an issue or problem.)

□ 1. Stay with the topic you wish to discuss. Do not bring into the discussion old topics or topics that are not related, which sidetrack the issue.

□ 2. Point out behaviors you would like changed and avoid general statements. For example, do not say, "You need a better attitude." Instead, say, "I wish you would focus more on the good things I do and less on what you feel I do wrong."

□ 3. Be honest and direct. Don't leave your partner guessing about what you mean.

□ 4. Talk about your feelings or thoughts without accusing or name calling.

□ 5. Talk in an adult way and do not "talk down" to your partner, as if he or she were a child. Be polite and talk to your partner as you would to anyone you respect.

□ 6. Do not use words like "never" or "always." Always try to use words that reflect a real situation or behavior. Doing this will give more meaning to your statements, and your partner will be more likely to listen to what you have to say.

□ 7. If you must say something negative to your partner, try to be helpful and not hurtful. Point out some good behaviors about your partner when you are also pointing out bad ones. In this way, you address your partner's behavior rather than his or her whole personality.

Receiver Skills (The *receiver* is the person with whom the sender wants to have the discussion.)

□ 1. Use behaviors that show you are interested. These include eye contact, nods of agreement, and body posture.

□ 2. Control your own behavior until it is your turn to talk. You do not interrupt or make faces.

□ 3. You make sure you understand what the sender is saying. To do this, say back in your own words statements that were unclear to you.

□ 4. Read the sender's nonverbal cues and respond to them. These are facial expressions, gestures, and other body language. For instance, you say, "You are frowning and seem upset." This shows you are paying attention and are sensitive to the sender's feelings.

FIGURE 15.4. Checklist of positive communication skills. From Wincze and Barlow (1997a). Copyright 1997 by Oxford University Press. Reprinted by permission.

apist can help such couples to challenge this notion and may incorporate practice in providing feedback into sensate focus exercises.

CASE STUDIES

Following are case studies of two patients that one of us (A. K. B) recently saw in our clinical practice. They demonstrate application of the principles and techniques we described earlier.

Case 1

Background

Frank, a 57-year-old, never married, engaged state employee, presented with his partner of 8 years, Anna, for treatment of his low desire. Anna, a 58-year-old divorced, white female,

worked at a public library. They had been living together for 3 years and were engaged to be married.

Frank had been taking antihypertensive medication for 8 years. During that time he had noticed a decrease in the firmness of his erections. This change did not preclude penetration, but Frank was upset by it. Frank indicated that his sexual desire had always been relatively low. Over the last 5–6 years his desire had further decreased, so that he had very little interest in sex.

Clinical Interview

The interview began with the therapist's explanation of her training, background, and therapeutic orientation. She explained the format of the assessment, then spent a few minutes talking to the couple about why they were coming in for treatment. This brief conversation gave the therapist a glimpse of the couple's dynamic and ensured that both partners were aware of/in agreement about the objective of seeking treatment.

The partners indicated that they were seeking treatment because of Frank's low desire. Frank said that he was not particularly bothered by his low desire, but he knew it was a problem for Anna; therefore, he wanted to address it. Both Frank and Anna seemed open to meeting with the therapist and motivated for treatment.

The therapist obtained demographic information, then met with Frank individually. She began by conducting an assessment of Frank's general psychological functioning. Frank did not endorse any Axis I disorders aside from sexual dysfunction, nor did he evidence significant character pathology. The therapist continued:

THERAPIST: Now I will ask questions focusing specifically on your sexual functioning. I understand that this is a very personal aspect of your life and that it can be difficult to discuss. If you feel uncomfortable at any point, please let me know.

FRANK: Sure.

THERAPIST: I know that you feel your desire for sex is too low. Can you tell me more about that?

FRANK: Yeah. I really don't care about having sex. It just isn't important to me. I don't feel a need for it.

THERAPIST: Do you ever have pleasant thoughts about sex when you are in a nonsexual situation?

FRANK: No, never.

THERAPIST: Do you ever have dreams about sex?

FRANK: No.

THERAPIST: And who typically initiates sexual activity in your relationship?

FRANK: For a while Anna initiated, but I think she got tired of me making excuses.

THERAPIST: How long would you say it has been that your interest has been low?

FRANK: It has never been high, but it has been really low for the last 5–6 years.

THERAPIST: Are there any situations in which your interest is higher? Under certain conditions or in relation to other women?

FRANK: No, no. I think Anna wonders whether I am more interested in other women. But my interest is just always low.

The therapist then assessed other areas of Frank's sexual functioning. Frank somewhat reluctantly acknowledged that he had noticed a change in the firmness of his erections over the last 8 years. He indicated that this did not interfere with his ability to engage in penetration, but he saw it as an indication that "the plumbing doesn't work as well as it used to." The therapist asked Frank whether this bothered him. He responded that this was "just part of getting older, nothing you can do about it." Frank continued to have what he described as "pretty firm" nocturnal (or morning) erections. He did not engage in self-stimulation, as is typical for someone with low desire.

The interview with Frank ended with questions regarding his satisfaction with the overall relationship and a discussion of his personal history. Frank indicated that he and Anna had a very happy relationship; they got along well, spent most of their free time together, and laughed a lot. He stated that they were both happier since moving in together.

Frank grew up as one of five children. He reported that his family rarely expressed affection—verbally or physically—when he was growing up. He had one serious relationship as a young adult. He reported enjoying his sexual relationship with this woman. He was disappointed when she ended the relationship. Following that, Frank devoted much of his personal time to caring for his aging parents. He did not have another romantic relationship until he met Anna. Frank indicated that he had not been an affectionate person until he and Anna had dated for some time. Even then, he described himself as a reserved person who was affectionate with Anna but not others. Moreover, he defined sex fairly strictly in terms of intercourse.

Partner Interview

The partner interview also began with an assessment of general psychological functioning. Anna had a history of depression and anxiety, but her mood had been stable for several years.

She had a prescription for a benzodiazepine, which she used on rare occasions.

The therapist then asked questions regarding Anna's sexual functioning and her sexual relationship with Frank. Anna denied any problems with sexual desire, arousal, pain, or orgasm. She reported that she was very frustrated with Frank's low desire. She explained that she was very happy in their relationship, but she could not remain in a long-term relationship devoid of sexual intimacy. The therapist validated her feelings but explained that treatment would require some additional patience on her part. (When a person seeks treatment for low desire, his or her partner is often fed up with the lack of sexual activity. Their willingness to invest the additional time and effort necessary for treatment should be addressed. This issue is further discussed below.)

Case Conceptualization

The therapist met with Frank and Anna together and gave feedback based on the following breakdown of factors that might be contributing to their sexual difficulties.

BIOLOGICAL/MEDICAL FACTORS

Results of a recent medical workup indicated that Frank's testosterone levels were within the normal range. Antihypertensive medication was identified as a factor that might be contributing to the change in the quality of Frank's erections. The therapist suggested that if this bothered Frank, then it may have further decreased his sexual desire. Thus, the antihypertensive medication might be an indirect causal factor in Frank's low desire.

PSYCHOLOGICAL FACTORS

Frank was personally reserved and was unaccustomed to physical expressions of love and affection. As an adult, he had limited exposure to situations or stimuli that might fuel sexual desire. The change in the quality of Frank's erections did not constitute erectile dysfunction, because he continued to have firm erections, sufficient for penetration. Nevertheless, Frank experienced the change in the quality of his erections as discouraging and a sign of aging.

SOCIAL FACTORS

Frank and Anna both felt they had a happy, trusting relationship. They enjoyed living together but set aside little couple time for fun activities. Although they communicated well about other aspects of their relationship, they had some difficulty communicating about intimacy.

The therapist recommended couple cognitive-behavioral sex therapy. She gave them an opportunity to ask questions about the treatment recommendations. Frank and Anna had few questions at this point and were eager to begin treatment. Their work schedules made it difficult for them to schedule therapy appointments. Therefore, it was agreed that they would meet with the therapist every other week.

Session 1

Psychoeducation was a primary component of the first session. The therapist encouraged the couple to hold realistic expectations regarding sexual functioning. She explained that no one is interested in sex all of the time (even those who profess to be find that upon consideration, that there are conditions under which they are more or less interested).

The therapist also discussed the normative effects of age on sexual functioning. She explained that medication rather than age might be the cause of the change in Frank's erections. She emphasized that even when there are changes in physiological response with age, couples can continue to enjoy healthy sexual functioning throughout their lives.

The therapist encouraged Frank and Anna to discuss their beliefs regarding sexual activity, so that she could challenge any maladaptive thoughts. Frank expressed the idea that sex was really for younger people, not for people "their age." The therapist challenged this, suggesting that they were not too old for other aspects of their relationship, such as laughing together, listening and supporting each other. She explained that sexual intimacy is simply one more component of a romantic relationship, one more way to enjoy being together.

Like many couples, Frank and Anna defined "sex" as intercourse. The therapist explained that this was typical, but that treatment would stress a broader definition of sex:

"Sex can consist of various forms of physical intimacy—a sensual massage, a shower, or intercourse. A broader definition of sex means that if one or both partners is not interested in intercourse on a given day, the couple has other ways of connecting physically. The end result is a greater frequency of sexual intimacy and higher sexual satisfaction."

The therapist also encouraged the couple to move away from a performance-oriented approach to sex—one that focused on erections and orgasm. Instead, she stressed the importance of a pleasure-oriented approach to sexual activity.

The session ended with a discussion of how sexual dysfunction had affected the overall relationship. Anna indicated that although she was very happy with Frank, the lack of sexual intimacy was very hurtful to her.

AANNA: The fact that Frank is not interested in being sexual with me makes me feel unattractive; I feel rejected. We get along really well, but it is so hurtful. I just can't stay in the relationship if that is how it will be.

THERAPIST: Frank, Anna feels as though your low desire means that you do not find her attractive. Is that true? [Pointed questions such as this allow the therapist to challenge assumptions that a person makes about his or her partner's thoughts or feelings. On sensitive issues such as this one, the therapist has generally asked the question in advance, during an individual meeting, so she knows how the person will answer. She asks it again with the couple, so that Frank can directly refute Anna's assumption.]

FRANK: I find Anna very attractive. I think that she is beautiful. I know that this whole thing upsets her. But I have tried to explain that it is not about my feelings for her. I don't feel interested in sex with other women either. It's just not something I care that much about.

THERAPIST: (addressing Anna) So it's true that Frank's desire is low, and that is frustrating for both of you. But it is important to realize that it is not because he finds you unattractive. On the contrary, he finds you very attractive, and I think that is part of why this problem is confusing and frustrating for him as well.

The couple indicated that Frank's low desire had not significantly impacted their level of affection. Anna explained that Frank was not very affectionate early in their relationship. Over time, he had grown more accustomed to holding hands, hugging, and snuggling. This physical affection continued despite the decrease in his desire. It was encouraging that Frank and Anna continued to be affectionate despite an issue with low desire. Couples in which one person has low desire often take an all-or-nothing approach—as intercourse decreases, so does the level of affection. The person with low desire is often reluctant to "start something he or she doesn't want to finish" and the person with healthy desire fears further rejection.

Other aspects of their relationship were not strongly affected. Again, they got along well and shared a number of mutually enjoyable activities.

Session 2

The therapist began by asking whether anything significant had happened since the last session. (Each session starts with this question in the event that an important event or issue has developed since the last session, consuming the couple's attention). The couple reported no such issues.

The therapist reviewed the importance of broadly defining sex and adopting a pleasure-oriented approach to sexual activity. She discussed with the couple the importance of creating positive conditions for sexual activity, emphasizing the importance of a trusting relationship in which there was mutual emotional and physical attraction. The therapist talked with the couple about planning dates on a regular basis to maintain emotional attraction. The couple responded:

FRANK: We don't plan dates, so to speak, but we spend almost all of our free time together.

THERAPIST: What do you do together during your free time?

FRANK: We get errands done and get the house picked up on Saturdays. A lot of times on Sundays we get together with family.

THERAPIST: What about during the week?

ANNA: We like watching TV together after dinner, then I usually fall asleep pretty early.

THERAPIST: So how often do you do fun things together just as a couple?

ANNA: Not that much. We did that more before we lived together.

THERAPIST: It is important to create couple time. I am going to ask that you schedule one date each week. A date could be taking a day trip or going out for ice cream, or a long walk. Whatever you'd both enjoy.

Frank and Anna agreed that this was a reasonable goal. The therapist then continued with a discussion of positive and negative conditions for sexual intimacy. She helped the couple to start a list of these (e.g., positive = morning, well rested; negative = dog in the room).

The therapist asked Frank and Anna each to complete a list of positive and negative conditions before the next session.

Session 3

The session began with a review of homework: scheduling dates and completing the list of positive and negative conditions. Frank and Anna reported that they had done well with scheduling dates. They took turns scheduling one fun activity for each week. They found this enjoyable and said they had not realized the extent to which they had fallen away from doing it. The therapist praised them for having scheduled and followed through on these dates.

The couple had spent some time working on the list of positive and negative conditions for sexual activity. The therapist pointed out that some of the conditions they listed were idealized (e.g., vacation), but others were easy to create (e.g., evening, relaxing music). She emphasized the importance of maximizing the positive conditions and minimizing the negative ones.

The therapist then talked to the couple about the use of sensate focus. She explained that the rationale for sensate focus was to reintroduce sexual intimacy into the relationship without tension and pressure, and indicated that she would assign a series of exercises designed to help the couple focus on the pleasure of touch without the pressure to perform. She asked whether the couple would agree to abstain from intercourse until asked to do otherwise. Frank and Anna were receptive to this. They indicated that this would not be a change, because they had not engaged in intercourse for quite a while. (This couple was amenable to a ban on intercourse. In other cases, this suggestion may be met with great frustration on the part of the partner with healthy sexual functioning. In these instances, it is very important to emphasize that the goal of treatment is to increase sexual satisfaction and the frequency of sexual activity. Continuing to engage in intercourse when one person is disinterested can worsen the problem. Intercourse may become aversive for the person with low desire, and stressful and frustrating for the couple. Although a ban on intercourse requires additional patience and sacrifice in the short term, the purpose is to move the couple toward the long-term goal. This discussion is a critical juncture in treatment. If the partners' reservations are not adequately addressed, the couple may terminate treatment prematurely.)

The therapist talked with Anna and Frank about the first sensate focus exercise.

THERAPIST: Usually the exercises begin with a massage. The purpose is for the massage to be pleasurable. If the massage is arousing, that is fine, but that is not necessarily the goal. The goal is simply for both of you to enjoy the experience. You can do the first massage fully clothed, partially clothed, or nude, depending on what feels comfortable to you.

FRANK: I know she wants me to stay nude, (*looking to Anna*) right?

ANNA: I didn't say that.

FRANK: That's fine with me. I just don't like to be cold. So I can put a blanket over me if I want. [It is possible that Frank's desire to use a blanket was less about being cold than it was about discomfort with being nude. Nevertheless, he is indicating that this is the place at which he feels comfortable starting the massage. In future sessions, the therapist will need to determine whether Frank's comfort level with nudity increases.]

THERAPIST: OK, so nude with the option of a blanket. Anna, does that sound OK to you?

ANNA: That's fine with me.

THERAPIST: OK, so I want you to limit the massage to back, arms, legs, and head. Genitals, breasts, and buttocks will be off limits for now. Are there any questions about that?

FRANK AND ANNA: No.

THERAPIST: Just to reiterate, the goal of the massage is not a particular physical response, such as arousal or orgasm. The goal is simply to enjoy what you are doing. In keeping with this, I would encourage you to give each other constructive feedback about what kind of touch you would like, what feels good, and what does not. [This gives the couple experience with communication during sexual activity.] So, between now and the next session, try to do two massages each week, devoting 30 minutes total each time. Most couples find that it works best to schedule the 30-minute blocks in advance. You can either take turns—giving each person one 30-minute massage per week. Or you can split each 30-minute block in half, giving each person a 15-minute massage each time. Do whatever works best for you. Any questions? If something is unclear, it is important to ask me now, so that there are no misunderstandings between you when you do the exercises.

Frank and Anna did not have any questions. They indicated that they felt ready to begin the exercises.

Session 4

Again, the therapist began with a general question regarding any new issues that might have arisen since the last session. The session then focused on a review of the homework. (From this point forward in treatment, a review of homework provides much of the structure for the session. If the individual or couple is noncompliant, much of the session is devoted to problem solving and addressing barriers to compliance.)

Frank and Anna had gone on one date since the last session. They found it difficult to do a date the second week, because their weeknights were busy, they did errands on Saturday, and they had a family obligation on Sunday. The therapist spoke with them about the importance of planning couple time in advance, making it a priority, and setting limits on other responsibilities to create free time. Frank and Anna enjoyed having Sunday mornings to themselves. They would go out for breakfast or take a walk along the beach. They agreed that they would begin to reserve this time for dates each week. If there was a conflict (e.g., a family function), they would

anticipate this and reserve a different block of time.

The couple completed one massage. Anna massaged Frank for 30 minutes. The therapist first focused on how this massage had gone. Both Frank and Anna felt it had gone well. They scheduled it in advance. Frank said that he enjoyed it, and Anna enjoyed giving it to him. Both denied feeling any anxiety during the massage. They incorporated some of the positive conditions, such as putting on relaxing music, and scheduling it for the evening, after their tasks for the day were done. They avoided some of the negative conditions (e.g., kept the a dog out of the room, turned off the ringer on the telephone).

The therapist told Frank and Anna that they had done a great job of scheduling and executing the massage. She noted the fact that they had enjoyed it. She asked what had made it difficult for them to do more than one. Frank and Anna listed a number of factors that had served as barriers (e.g., family visiting from out of town, other commitments, Anna falling asleep before the massage, Frank not wanting to give 30-minute massage). The therapist worked with the couple on problem solving. They agreed that they would schedule massages for earlier in the evening in the future, and they would split them in half, so each person would get/give a 15-minute massage. The couple also felt that two massages each week might not be realistic for them. They agreed to work toward a goal of one massage each week. (Although this was not ideal, it is important to set realistic goals, so that the couple does not repeatedly experience a sense of failure. It is a starting point for creating intimate time.)

Session 5

Frank and Anna continued to do well with scheduling dates. They took turns planning them and found that this worked well, indicating that they were more successful in planning the massages this time. They scheduled them for earlier in the evening—after daily tasks were done but before Anna was too tired. They split each massage into two 15-minute blocks. Both felt that this worked better, in that each massage was pleasurable for them both.

Both Frank and Anna reported that the massages were enjoyable. Frank denied any anxiety or tension and said he looked forward to the massages. (Relative to patients with sexual aversion disorder, those with low desire more often report that they enjoy touching if they know it will not lead to intercourse.) The therapist inquired as to whether Frank and Anna had attended to other positive–negative conditions. They indicated that they had. The therapist also asked whether they had given each other feedback during the massage. Anna said that she had told Frank what type of touch she was enjoying and what she wanted. She said that Frank had not given her any feedback, so she was happy to learn today that he had enjoyed it. The therapist asked Frank why he had not given Anna any feedback. He responded that he was enjoying the massage and saw no reason to say anything. The therapist suggested that telling Anna that he enjoyed what she was doing made it more likely that she would continue. It also would give her the satisfaction of knowing that what she did was pleasurable. The therapist encouraged Frank to work on giving more feedback in the future.

In the remainder of the session, the therapist discussed the use of fantasy. She normalized and encouraged its use and addressed reservations that people often have (e.g., "If I am fantasizing during sex with my partner, doesn't that mean that I am not happy where I am?"). She encouraged Frank and Anna to consider ways of fueling their sexual imagination. Options included erotic films, adult magazines, romantic novels, or certain forms of art. She emphasized that they could select a medium with which they were comfortable. They indicated that they had enjoyed watching adult films in the past.

The couple's homework after this session was to have one date each week, do one massage each week, and watch one adult film. The therapist kept the same guidelines in place for the massage, so that the couple could feel very comfortable before moving to the next step.

Sessions 6–10

Anna and Frank developed a routine of scheduling their massages in advance. They began achieving their goal of one massage per week. The couple grew very comfortable with the initial guidelines for the massage. The therapist encouraged them to start incorporating other areas of the body (i.e., breasts, buttocks), without genital contact. Both Anna and Frank initially avoided this, with both saying that they

feared it would go badly as it had in the past. The therapist challenged these concerns, citing the recent success of intimate time, and reinforced use of a pleasure-oriented approach. Frank and Anna eventually broadened the massage, and said they found this enjoyable. The therapist encouraged them to continue practicing this. Frank and Anna did a good job of scheduling dates. They also did well with devoting one night a week to watching an adult film. They initially had trouble finding a film they liked, but with some effort found a set that they enjoyed. They liked watching the film, and Frank thought that this sparked his desire for the next day or so.

Sessions 11–14

Once they were comfortable with the broader approach to massages, the therapist suggested that Frank and Anna lift the ban on intercourse. Coincidentally, the couple went on vacation the following week. They engaged in intercourse. Frank was not focused on the firmness of his erections, and both were very happy with the experience. The couple avoided engaging in intercourse again after returning from vacation. The therapist worked with Frank and Anna on how they could approximate the conditions that were so conducive to sexual activity on vacation. They recognized the importance of taking time to do fun, relaxing things on the weekend rather than getting caught up in commitments and responsibilities. The couple continued to schedule dates and to watch adult films each week. The therapist emphasized the need to continue doing these things to maintain an emotional connection and promote positive thoughts of sex. Frank indicated that his interest in sexual activity was higher when he and Anna adhered to their new routine. Anna was pleased that she and Frank were intimate more frequently. Frank sometimes initiated sexual activity, and both reported that intimate time was now pleasurable rather than tense and frustrating.

The therapist continued follow-up with the couple on a monthly basis for some time. Medical issues and a problem with Frank's job created stress that sometimes distracted them from the routine they had achieved. The therapist encouraged them to use intimacy as a means of connecting and comforting each other during times of stress. She suggested that they use Wednesday evenings (the time they typically met for therapy) as an opportunity to check in and schedule time together. This worked well. They got back into a good routine, and both reported that they were happier with their sexual relationship. The therapist suggested that they continue to communicate openly and work at any additional changes they felt were necessary.

Case 1 represents a typical application of cognitive-behavioral sex therapy for a couple seeking treatment. Following is a brief overview of treatment for a different sexual dysfunction, with an individual rather than a couple.

Case 2

Kara, a 31-year-old, single, white female law student, was self-referred for treatment of anxiety. Kara's primary diagnosis was generalized anxiety disorder. She received cognitive-behavioral treatment for this. As she learned to manage worry about her grades, finances, and her future, the focus of treatment shifted to her anxiety about dating. Kara expressed interest in men but avoided dating. Initially, it seemed that this was another sphere of worry, or a nongeneralized form of social anxiety. Further discussion revealed, however, that Kara avoided dating because she was very anxious about sexual intimacy.

Kara feared that penetration would be painful. She avoided other forms of sexual activity because they might lead to intercourse, and the idea of someone touching her body made her uncomfortable. As a teenager she had kissed two boys, but she had no other sexual experience. Kara had attempted to use a tampon once as an adolescent and found this awkward and uncomfortable. She had not used tampons since, and she had never met with a gynecologist. Kara wanted to be comfortable going to see a gynecologist, and wanted to address the negative feelings she had about sex and dating. She began CBT for sexual aversion disorder.

Case Conceptualization

BIOLOGICAL FACTORS

Kara was not taking any medications. A medical examination was necessary to rule out an anatomical abnormality or medical issue that

might cause pain with penetration. (There was no clear evidence that Kara did, in fact, experience pain with penetration. Information from the medical exam would be necessary, however, to address Kara's fear.)

PSYCHOLOGICAL FACTORS

Kara was one of four daughters. She indicated that her three sisters and her mother were all comfortable with nudity and talked fairly openly about sex. Kara described herself as more modest and reserved. When they were teens, her sisters teased her for not wanting to change clothes in front of them, and she typically left the room when they talked about sex. The contrast between their comfort level and hers made her feel like a "prude," and she worried that she would not be "good at sex."

Kara had a poor body image. She felt that she was somewhat overweight, and she was critical of other aspects of her appearance. She dressed in loose-fitting clothes that would not draw attention to her or her body. Kara was socially skilled and very intelligent, attending a highly competitive law school. She said, "I don't like doing things that I am not really good at." She had few male friends and had distanced herself from her closest male friend in college when he expressed romantic interest in her.

SOCIAL FACTORS

Kara devoted much of her time to studying and other work-related activities. She had several close female friends with whom she enjoyed spending time. She spent limited time with men socially.

Sessions 1–3

The therapist constructed a fear and avoidance hierarchy (FAH), with items ranging from Kara looking at her body nude in the mirror to intercourse or having a Papanicolaou (PAP) smear. The therapist helped Kara to identify her thoughts regarding penetration and intimacy. Four key thoughts were challenged early in the sessions:

- Kara believed she was overweight and that men found her unattractive.
- Kara believed that she was a "prude" and

would not be "good at sex," because she was not as open and comfortable as her family.

- Kara was embarrassed that she had never seen a gynecologist, and feared that the gynecologist would criticize or scold her for this.
- Kara was also concerned that the doctor would ask about her sexual history and might think she was a lesbian, because she had never had a boyfriend.

The therapist worked with Kara on challenging these thoughts.

- She encouraged Kara to move away from an "all-or-nothing" evaluation of her appearance, worked with her on identifying positive and negative aspects of her appearance, and suggested that Kara assumed men found her unattractive but did not have facts to support this.
- The therapist suggested that different people have different boundaries with respect to nudity and discussing sex. The fact that Kara's boundaries were different from those of her family did not mean that she could not enjoy healthy sexual functioning.
- The therapist helped Kara identify alternative reactions that a doctor might have when she went in for her first appointment (e.g., the doctor might be glad Kara had come). Last, the therapist helped Kara to decatastrophize the idea that the doctor would wonder why Kara had no sexual experience (i.e., even if the doctor wondered about this, it would not be the end of the world).

The therapist began working with Kara on practicing the items on her FAH. Kara started looking at her nude body in the mirror and progressed to touching the exterior portions of her genitals for 5–10 minutes each day. The therapist discussed with Kara the fact that these assignments might feel "weird" or embarrassing. She normalized these feelings and carefully explained the clinical benefit of Kara becoming more comfortable with her body.

The therapist talked to Kara about going to a gynecologist for an initial meeting and an external exam, until she felt comfortable undergoing the full examination. Kara was very reluctant to do this but agreed that it would be a good intermediate step to a full exam. Kara and the therapist did role plays to help Kara get comfortable answering the doctor's questions.

Sessions 4–6

The therapist continued to work with Kara on challenging negative beliefs. Kara feared that penetration would be painful. The therapist suggested that a medical exam could confirm whether there was any medical reason to expect discomfort. She also assured Kara that self-stimulation exercises would allow her to progress at her own pace in a relaxed way to minimize the possibility of discomfort.

Kara began to practice inserting the tip of her finger into her vagina. She returned saying that it was uncomfortable, so she had stopped after the first try. The therapist encouraged Kara to try again, and if she experienced discomfort, to hold her finger where it was, do deep breathing, and change positions or angles to see if that helped. Kara reported that this worked well. After repeated practice, she was able to insert the tip of her finger comfortably.

The therapist talked to Kara about scheduling an appointment to see a gynecologist. After several role plays in which Kara practiced her conversation with the gynecologist, she made an appointment. The therapist recommended a physician who had experience working with women who had sexual aversion disorder. The appointment went well, and the gynecologist encouraged Kara to continue with therapy and come back when she was ready to have a PAP smear.

Sessions 6–9

The gynecologist's external exam indicated no obvious reason that penetration would be painful for Kara. The therapist encouraged Kara to practice inserting one-fourth of her finger into her vagina for 5–10 minutes each day. She initially avoided this, using different excuses. The therapist addressed this avoidance and explained that only repeated practice would lead to a reduction in Kara's anxiety and an increase in physical comfort. The therapist and Kara identified a period in the day that would work well for practices. They set specific short-term goals between each session. Kara began to practice more regularly and slowly observed improvement, inserting one-half of her finger. She attempted to insert a tampon twice with some success, but she was too anxious to try again. The therapist reinforced Kara's efforts and encouraged her to continue with regular practice. The therapist also encouraged Kara to practice talking with men more often (e.g., at school, when out with a group of friends) and to wear some fitted clothes (in order to become more comfortable with her body).

Sessions 10–12

Kara progressed to inserting one finger comfortably into her vagina, and she continued to practice using tampons. The therapist indicated that it might take some time for Kara to feel completely comfortable with tampons, but she urged her to continue practicing. (Kara could ultimately decide whether she wanted to use tampons or not. She was urged to continue doing so at this point simply to increase her comfort with penetration.) The therapist encouraged Kara to consider returning to the gynecologist for a full examination. She challenged Kara's fears and suggested that she request that the doctor use a small speculum designed for children. Kara ultimately went for the evaluation. She reported that is was uncomfortable but not painful. Kara was glad she had finally gone, and said she was confident that it would be easier in another year, when she went again.

Kara and the therapist began to discuss strategies for helping Kara become more comfortable with dating. She had a good network of female friends at school. Kara said that she would inform them that she was open to dating, if they wanted to introduce her to potential partners.

Following Treatment

The therapist encouraged Kara to continue self-stimulation exercises and using tampons each month, so she would remain comfortable with penetration. She suggested that Kara begin moving her finger when she practiced self-stimulation, to determine what type of stimulation felt pleasurable.

Kara was still reluctant to go on a date, but she went out with potential partners in a group to get to know them better. She sometimes wore more fitted clothes and was less critical of her physical appearance. The therapist advised Kara that if she began dating someone, she could resume treatment to address issues that might result from being in a relationship and approaching intimacy. Kara still had goals she had not yet reached (e.g., feeling comfortable with sexual activity with a partner), but she

now had tools that would help her work toward these goals.

This cases above illustrate two of the many types of disorders one might see in the treatment of sexual dysfunction. Whereas these cases involve the use of cognitive-behavioral treatment alone, others involve the integration of medications such as Viagra, Cialis, and Levitra.

CONCLUDING COMMENTS

The case of Frank and Anna and that of Kara are intended to demonstrate the application of several key concepts and principles that are fundamental to effective cognitive-behavioral treatment of sexual dysfunction. The most central of these are as follows:

- Sexual dysfunctions may include disturbances in desire, arousal, and orgasm, or pain associated with sexual activity.
- A comprehensive assessment allows the therapist to identify etiological and maintaining factors for the sexual difficulty. Biological, psychological, cultural, and interpersonal factors should be considered; thus, to the extent possible, a multidisciplinary approach to treatment is recommended. Once the contributing factors have been identified, the therapist can formulate a case conceptualization and outline an effective treatment plan.
- The presence of organic factors does not dictate that a medical treatment alone is the most appropriate treatment option. Some attention to psychosocial factors is often essential to effective treatment.
- CBT for sexual dysfunction is a multicomponent treatment that involves psychoeducation, communication training, cognitive restructuring, and behavioral exercises.
- The primary goal of CBT for sexual dysfunction is not a functional one. Rather, the goal of treatment is to enhance partners' ability to derive satisfaction from their sexual relationship.

Some of these points were not central tenets of sex therapy 20 years or even a decade ago. Sex therapy as a field continues to evolve. Awareness and acceptance of sexual dysfunction may be higher than ever, thanks to the advent of Viagra and other medications. Likewise, the number of treatment options for sexual dysfunction is larger and still growing. As we indicated at the start of the chapter, with new medical treatment options and more refined cognitive-behavioral techniques, the challenge now facing clinicians and physicians is to determine which treatment option is best for each patient: medical treatment alone, psychosocial treatment alone, psychosocial treatment in conjunction with a medical treatment, or no treatment for sexual dysfunction. This decision will depend on many factors, including the etiology of the problem, the nature of maintaining factors, the patient's attitude toward treatment, and the resources available. In cases in which the clinician or physician decides that psychosocial treatment is appropriate, we hope that this chapter serves as a useful guide.

REFERENCES

Abrahamson, D. J., Barlow, D. H., Sakheim, D. K., Beck, J. G., & Athanasiou, R. (1985). Effect of distraction on sexual responding in functional and dysfunctional men. *Behavior Therapy, 16,* 503–515.

American Psychiatric Association. (2000). *Diagnostic and statistical manual of mental disorders* (4th ed., text rev.). Washington, DC: Author.

Angst, J. (1998). Sexual problems in healthy and depressed persons. *International Clinical Psychopharmacology, 13*(Suppl. 6), S1–S4.

Bach, A. K., Brown, T. A., & Barlow, D. H. (1999). The effects of false negative feedback on efficacy expectancies and sexual arousal in sexually functional males. *Behavior Therapy, 30,* 79–95.

Bachmann, G. A. (1995). Influence of menopause on sexuality. *International Journal of Infertility, 40*(Suppl. 1), 16–22.

Bachmann, G. A., Leiblum, S. R., & Grill, J. (1989). Brief sexual inquiry in gynecologic practice. *Obstetrics and Gynecology, 73,* 425–427.

Barlow, D. H. (1986). Causes of sexual dysfunction: The role of anxiety and cognitive interference. *Journal of Consulting and Clinical Psychology, 54,* 140–148.

Barlow, D. H., Becker, R., Leitenberg, H., & Agras, W. S. (1970). A mechanical strain gauge for recording penile circumference change. *Journal of Applied and Behavior Analysis, 3,* 73–76.

Barlow, D. H., Sakheim, D. K., & Beck, J. G. (1983). Anxiety increases sexual arousal. *Journal of Abnormal Psychology, 92,* 49–54.

Beck, A. T. (1976). *Cognitive therapy and the emotional disorders.* New York: International Universities Press.

Beck, J. G. (1995). Hypoactive sexual desire disorder: An overview. *Journal of Consulting and Clinical Psychology, 63,* 919–927.

Bemelmans, B. L. H., Meuleman, E. J. H., Doesburg, W. H., Notermans, S. L. H., & Debruyne, F. M. J. (1994). Erectile dysfunction in diabetic men: The neurological factor revisited. *Journal of Urology, 151,* 884–889.

Benet, A. E., Sharaby, J. S., & Melman, A. (1994). Male erectile dysfunction: Assessment and treatment options. *Comprehensive Therapy, 20,* 669–673.

Binik, Y. (2005). Should dyspareunia be retained as a sexual dysfunction in DSM-V?: A painful classification decision. *Archives of Sexual Behavior, 34*(1), 11–21.

Carey, M. P., Flasher, L. V., Maisto, S. A., & Turkat, I. D. (1984). The a priori approach to psychophysiological assessment. *Professional Psychology: Research and Practice, 15,* 515–527.

Carson, C., & Lue, T. (2005). Phosphodiesterase type 5 inhibitor for erectile dysfunction. *BJU International, 96,* 257–280.

Chang, S. W., Fine, R., Siegel, D., Chesney, M., Black, D., & Hulley, S. B. (1991). The impact of diuretic therapy on reported sexual function. *Archives of Internal Medicine, 151,* 2402–2408.

Chen, J., Mabjeesh, N., Matzkin, H., & Greenstein, A. (2003). Efficacy of Sildenafil as adjuvant therapy to selective serotonin reuptake inhibitors in alleviating premature ejaculation. *Adult Urology, 61*(1), 197–200.

Conti, C. R., Pepine, C. J., & Sweeney, M. (1999). Efficacy and safety of sildenafil citrate in the treatment of erectile dysfunction in patients with ischemic heart disease. *American Journal of Cardiology, 83,* 29C–34C.

Cranston-Cuebas, M. A., & Barlow, D. H. (1990). Cognitive and affective contributions to sexual functioning. *Annual Review of Sex Research, 1,* 119–161.

Crowley, T., Richardson, D., & Goldmeier, D. (2006). Recommendations for the management of vaginismus: BASHH special interest group for sexual dysfunction. *International Journal of STD and AIDS, 17,* 14–18.

Cyranowski, J. M., Bromberger, J., Youk, A., Matthews, K., Kravitz, H. M., & Powell, L. H. (2004). Lifetime depression history and sexual function in women at midlife. *Archives of Sexual Behavior, 33*(6), 539–548.

DeLamater, J., & Sill, M. (2005). Sexual desire in later life. *Journal of Sex Research, 42*(4), 138–149.

Dennerstein, L., & Hayes, R. D. (2005). Confronting the challenges: Epidemiological study of female sexual dysfunction and the menopause. *Journal of Sexual Medicine, 2*(Suppl. 3), 118–132.

Derogatis, L. R., & Melisaratos, N. (1979). The DSFI: A multidimensional measure of sexual functioning. *Journal of Sex and Marital Therapy, 5,* 244–281.

Derogatis, L. R., & Melisaratos, N. (1983). The Brief Symptom Inventory: An introductory report. *Psychological Medicine, 13,* 595–605.

Feldman, H. A., Goldstein, I., Hatzichristou, D. G., Krane, R. J., & McKinlay, J. B. (1994). Impotence and its medical and psychosocial correlates: Results of the Massachusetts Male Aging Study. *Journal of Urology, 151*, 54–61.

Finger, W. W., Lund, M., & Slagle, M. A. (1997). Medications that may contribute to sexual disorders: A guide to assessment and treatment in family practice. *Journal of Family Practice, 44*, 33–43.

Fisher, W. A. (1988). The Sexual Opinion Survey. In C. M. Davis, W. L. Yarber, & S. L. Davis (Eds.), *Sexuality-related measures: A compendium* (pp. 34–37). Lake Mills, IA: Graphic.

Fisher, W. A., Byrne, D., White, L. A., & Kelley, K. (1988). Erotophobia–erotophilia as a dimension of personality. *Journal of Sex Research, 25*, 123–151.

Geer, J. H., & Fuhr, R. (1976). Cognitive factors in sexual arousal: The role of distraction. *Journal of Consulting and Clinical Psychology, 44*, 238–243.

Geer, J. H., Morokoff, P., & Greenwood, P. (1974). Sexual arousal in women: The development of a measurement device for vaginal blood volume. *Archives of Sexual Behavior, 3*, 559–564.

Gitlin, M. (2003). Sexual dysfunction with psychotropic drugs. *Expert Opinion in Pharmacology, 4*(12), 2259–2269.

Goldstein, I., Lue, T. F., Padma-Nathan, H., Rosen, R. C., Steers, W. D., & Wicker, P. A. (1998). Oral sildenafil in the treatment of erectile dysfunction. *New England Journal of Medicine, 338*, 1397–1404.

Hakim, L. S., & Goldstein, I. (1996). Diabetic sexual dysfunction: Endocrinology and metabolism. *Endocrinology and Metabolism Clinics of North America, 25*, 379–400.

Hawton, K., & Catalan, J. (1986). Prognostic factors in sex therapy. *Behaviour Research and Therapy, 24*, 377–385.

Hawton, K., Catalan, J., & Fagg, J. (1992). Sex therapy for erectile dysfunction: Characteristics of couples, treatment outcome, and prognostic factors. *Archives of Sexual Behavior, 21*, 161–175.

Heiman, J. R., & LoPiccolo, J. (1983). Clinical outcome of sex therapy: Effects of daily versus weekly treatment. *Archives of General Psychiatry, 40*, 443–449.

Heiman, J. R., & LoPiccolo, J. (1988). *Becoming orgasmic: A sexual and personal growth program for women* (rev. ed.). Englewood Cliffs, NJ: Prentice-Hall.

Hirschfield, R. M. A. (1998). Sexual dysfunction in depression: Disease- or drug-related? *Depression and Anxiety, 7*(Suppl. 1), 21–23.

Hirst, J. F., & Watson, J. P. (1997). Therapy for sexual and relationship problems: The effects on outcome of attending as an individual or as a couple. *Sexual and Marital Therapy, 12*, 321–337.

Hodge, R. H., Harward, M. P., West, M. S., Krongaard-DeMong, L., & Kowal-Neeley, M. B. (1991). Sexual function of women taking antihypertensive agents: A comparative study. *Journal of General Internal Medicine, 6*, 290–294.

Hogan, M. J., Wallin, J. D., & Baer, R. M. (1980). Antihypertensive therapy and male sexual dysfunction. *Psychosomatics, 21*, 234–237.

Hoon, P., Wincze, J., & Hoon, E. (1977). A test of reciprocal inhibition: Are anxiety and sexual arousal in women mutually inhibitory? *Journal of Abnormal Psychology, 86*, 65–74.

Jackson, G., Rosen, R., Kloner, R., & Kostis, J. (2006). The second Princeton consensus on sexual dysfunction and cardiac risk: New guidelines for sexual medicine. *Journal of Sexual Medicine, 3*(1), 28–36.

Jones, J. C., & Barlow, D. H. (1990). Self-reported frequency of sexual urges, fantasies, and masturbatory fantasies in heterosexual males and females. *Archives of Sexual Behavior, 19*, 269–279.

Kaplan, H. S. (1979). *Disorder of sexual desire and other new concepts and techniques in sex therapy.* New York: Brunner/Mazel.

Kaplan, H. S. (1988). Anxiety and sexual dysfunction. *Journal of Clinical Psychiatry, 49*, 21–25.

Kaplan, S. A., Reis, R. B., Kohn, I. J., Ikeguchi, E. F., Laor, E., Te, A. E., et al. (1999). Safety and efficacy of sildenafil in postmenopausal women with sexual dysfunction. *Urology, 53*, 481–486.

Kellett, J. M. (1996). Sex and the elderly male. *Sexual and Marital Therapy, 11*, 281–288.

Kessler, R. C., McGonagle, K. A., Zhao, S., Nelson, C. B., Hughes, M., Eshleman, S., et al. (1994). Lifetime and 12-month prevalence of DSM-III-R psychiatric disorders in the United States. *Archives of General Psychiatry, 51*, 8–19.

Klassen, A. D., & Wilsnack, S. C. (1986). Sexual experience and drinking among women in a U.S. national survey. *Archives of Sexual Behavior, 15*, 363–392.

Koch, P., Mansfield, P., Thurau, D., & Carey, M. (2005). "Feeling frumpy": The relationship between body image and sexual response changes in midlife women. *Journal of Sex Research, 42*(3), 215–223.

Korenman, S. G. (1995). Advances in the understanding and management of erectile dysfunction. *Journal of Clinical Endocrinology and Metabolism, 80*, 1985–1988.

Korenman, S. G. (1998). New insights into erectile dysfunction: A practical approach. *American Journal of Medicine, 105*, 135–144.

Laumann, E. O., Paik, A., & Rosen, R. C. (1999). Sexual dysfunction in the United States. *Journal of the American Medical Association, 281*, 537–544.

Leiblum, S. R., & Segraves, R. T. (1995). Sex and aging. In *American Psychiatric Press review of psychiatry* (Vol. 14, pp. 677–695). Washington, DC: American Psychiatric Press.

LoPiccolo, J., Heiman, J. R., Hogan, D. R., & Roberts, C. W. (1985). Effectiveness of single therapists versus cotherapy teams in sex therapy. *Journal of Consulting and Clinical Psychology, 53*, 287–294.

LoPiccolo, J., & Stock, W. E. (1987). Sexual function, dysfunction, and counseling in gynecological practice. In Z. Rosenwaks, F. Benjamin, & M. L. Stone (Eds.), *Gynecology* (pp. 339–371). New York: Macmillan.

Lovibond, S. H., & Lovibond, P. F. (1993). *Manual for the Depression Anxiety Stress Scales (DASS)* (Psychology Foundation Monograph). (Available from the Psychology Foundation, Room 1005 Mathews Building, University of New South Wales, NSW2052, Australia)

Malatesta, V. J., Pollack, R. H., Crotty, T. D., & Peacock, L. J. (1982). Acute alcohol intoxication and female orgasmic response. *Journal of Sex Research, 18,* 1–17.

Mannino, D. M., Klevens, R. M., & Flanders, W. D. (1994). Cigarette smoking: An independent risk factor for impotence? *American Journal of Epidemiology, 140,* 1003–1008.

Masters, W. H., & Johnson, V. E. (1966). *Human sexual response.* Boston: Little, Brown.

Masters, W. H., & Johnson, V. E. (1970). *Human sexual inadequacy.* Boston: Little, Brown.

McCabe, M. P., & Cobain, M. J. (1998). The impact of individual and relationship factors on sexual dysfunction among males and females. *Sexual and Marital Therapy, 13,* 131–143.

McCarthy, B. W. (1988). *Male sexual awareness.* New York: Carroll & Graf.

McCarthy, B. W., & McCarthy, E. (1998). *Couple sexual awareness.* New York: Carroll & Graf.

Meston, C. M. (1997). Aging and sexuality. *Western Journal of Medicine, 167,* 285–290.

Mitchell, W. B., DiBartolo, P. M., Brown, T. A., & Barlow, D. H. (1998). Effects of positive and negative mood on sexual arousal in sexually functional males. *Archives of Sexual Behavior, 27,* 197–207.

Mohr, D. C., & Beutler, L. E. (1990). Erectile dysfunction: A review of diagnostic and treatment procedures. *Clinical Psychology Review, 10,* 123–150.

Montejo-Gonzalez, A. L., Liorca, G., Izquierdo, J. A., Ledesma, A., Bousono, M., Calcedo, A., et al. (1997). SSRI-induced sexual dysfunction: Fluoxetine, paroxetine, sertraline, and fluvoxamine in a prospective, multicenter, and descriptive clinical study of 344 patients. *Journal of Sex and Marital Therapy, 23,* 176–194.

Muniyappa, R., Norton, M., Dunn, M. & Banerj, M. (2005). Diabetes and female sexual dysfunction: Moving beyond "benign neglect." *Current Diabetes Report, 5*(3), 230–234.

National Institutes of Health (NIH) Consensus Conference. (1993). Impotence: NIH Consensus Development Panel on Impotence. *Journal of the American Medical Association, 270,* 83–90.

Nobre, P. (2006). *Disfuncoes sexuais: Teoria, investigacao, e tratamento* [Sexual dysfunction: Theory, investigation and treatment]. Lisboa: Climepsi Editores.

Nobre, P., & Pinto-Gouveia, J. (2003). Sexual modes questionnaire: Measure to assess the interaction among cognitions, emotions, and sexual response. *Journal of Sex Research, 40*(4), 368–382.

O'Farrell, T. J., Choquette, K. A., Cutter, H. S. G., & Birchler, G. R. (1997). Sexual satisfaction and dysfunction in marriages of male alcoholics: Comparison of nonalcoholic maritally conflicted and nonconflicted couples. *Journal of Studies on Alcohol, 58,* 91–99.

Osborn, M., Hawton, K., & Gath, D. (1988). Sexual dysfunction among middle aged women in the community. *British Medical Journal, 296,* 959–962.

Phillips, N. (2000). Female sexual dysfunction: Evaluation and treatment. *American Family Physician, 62,* 127–136.

Pokorny, A. D., Miller, B. A., & Kaplan, H. B. (1972). The brief MAST: A shortened version of the Michigan Alcohol Screening Test. *American Journal of Psychiatry, 129,* 342–345.

Reissing, E. D., Binik, Y. M., & Khalife, S. (1999). Does vaginismus exist? *Journal of Nervous and Mental Disease, 187,* 261–274.

Rodriquez, J., Dashti, R., & Schwartz, E. (2005). Linking erectile dysfunction to coronary artery disease. *International Journal of Impotence Research, 17,* 12–18.

Rosen, R., Riley, A., Wagner, G., Osterloh, I., Kilpatrick, J., & Mishra, A. (1997). The International Index of Erectile Function (IIEF): A multidimensional scale for assessment of erectile dysfunction. *Urology, 49,* 822–830.

Rosen, R., Wing, R., Schneider, S., & Gendrano, N. (2005). Epidemiology of erectile dysfunction: The role of medical comorbidities and lifestyle factors. *Urological Clinics of North America, 32,* 403–417.

Rosen, R. C. (1996). Erectile dysfunction: The medicalization of male sexuality. *Clinical Psychology Review, 16,* 497–519.

Rosen, R. C., Taylor, J. F., Leiblum, S. R., & Bachmann, G. A. (1993). Prevalence of sexual dysfunction in women: Results of a survey study of 329 women in an outpatient gynecological clinic. *Journal of Sex and Marital Therapy, 19,* 171–188.

Rowland, D. L., Cooper, S. E., & Schneider, M. (2001). Defining premature ejaculation for experimental and clinical investigations. *Archives of Sexual Behavior, 30*(3), 235–253.

Rutherford, D., & Collier, A. (2005). Sexual dysfunction in women with diabetes mellitus. *Gynecological Endocrinology, 21*(4), 189–192.

Sadovsky, R., & Miner, M. (2005). Erectile dysfunction is a sign of risk for cardiovascular disease: A primary care view. *Primary Care, 32*(4), 977–993.

Salonia, A., Maga, T., Colombo, R., Scattoni, V., Briganti, A., Cestari, A., et al. (2002). A prospective study comparing paroxetine alone versus paroxatine plus sildenafil in patients with premature ejaculation. *Journal of Urology, 168,* 2486–2489.

Sarwer, D. B., & Durlak, J. A. (1997). A field trial of the effectiveness of behavioral treatment for sexual dysfunctions. *Journal of Sex and Marital Therapy, 23,* 87–97.

Sbrocco, T., Weisberg, R. B., & Barlow, D. H. (1992). *Sexual Dysfunction Inventory (SDI).* Unpublished semistructured interview, Center for Anxiety and Related Disorders at Boston University.

Sbrocco, T., Weisberg, R. B., Barlow, D. H., & Carter, M. M. (1997). The conceptual relationship between panic disorder and male erectile dysfunction. *Journal of Sex and Marital Therapy, 23,* 212–220.

Schiavi, R. C. (1990). Chronic alcoholism and male sexual dysfunction. *Journal of Sex and Marital Therapy, 16,* 23–33.

Schiavi, R. C., White, D., Mandeli, J., & Levine, A. C. (1997). Effect of testosterone administration on sexual behavior and mood in men with erectile dysfunction. *Archives of Sexual Behavior, 26,* 231–241.

Schreiner-Engel, P., Schiavi, R. C., Vietorisz, D., & Smith, H. (1987). The differential impact of diabetes type on female sexuality. *Journal of Psychosomatic Research, 31,* 23–33.

Segraves, K. B., & Segraves, R. T. (1991). Hypoactive sexual desire disorder: Prevalence and comorbidity in 906 subjects. *Journal of Sex and Marital Therapy, 17,* 55–58.

Segraves, R. T. (1998). Antidepressant-induced sexual dysfunction. *Journal of Clinical Psychiatry, 59*(Suppl. 4), 48–54.

Segraves, T. (2003). Pharmacological management of sexual dysfunction: Benefits and limitations. *CNS Spectrums, 8*(3), 225–229.

Sherwin, B. (1988). A comparative analysis of the role of androgen in human male and female sexual behavior: Behavioral specificity, critical thresholds, and sensitivity. *Psychobiology, 16,* 416–425.

Skinner, H. A. (1982). The Drug Abuse Screening Test. *Addictive Behaviors, 7,* 363–371.

Spanier, G. B. (1976). Measuring dyadic adjustment: New scales for assessing the quality of marriage and similar dyads. *Journal of Marriage and the Family, 38,* 15–28.

Spanier, G. B., & Thompson, L. (1982). A confirmatory analysis of the dyadic adjustment scale. *Journal of Marriage and the Family, 44,* 731–738.

Spector, I. P., & Carey, M. P. (1990). Incidence and prevalence of the sexual dysfunctions: A critical review of the empirical literature. *Archives of Sexual Behavior, 19,* 389–408.

Strassberg, D. S., Kelly, M. P., Carroll, C., & Kircher, J. C. (1987). The psychophysiological nature of premature ejaculation. *Archives of Sexual Behavior, 16,* 327–336.

Takanami, M., Nagao, K., Ishii, N., Miura, K., &

Shirai, M. (1997). Is diabetic neuropathy responsible for diabetic impotence? *Urologia Internationalis, 58,*181–185.

Thomas, A. M., & LoPiccolo, J. (1994). Sexual functioning in persons with diabetes: Issues in research, treatment, and education. *Clinical Psychology Review, 14,* 61–86.

Tiefer, L. (1996). The medicalization of sexuality: Conceptual, normative, and professional issues. *Annual Review of Sex Research, 7,* 252–282.

Verma, K. K., Khaitan, B. K., & Singh, O. P. (1998). The frequency of sexual dysfunctions in patients attending a sex therapy clinic in North India. *Archives of Sexual Behavior, 27,* 309–314.

Weisberg, R. B., Brown, T. A., Wincze, J. P., & Barlow, D. H. (2001). Causal attributions and male sexual arousal: The impact of attributions for a bogus erectile difficulty on sexual arousal, cognitions, and affect. *Journal of Abnormal Psychology, 110*(2), 324–334.

Wiegel, M., Bach, A. K., Brown, T. A., Rhein, A. N., & Barlow, D. H. (1997, November). *Arousability and emotional response to sexual stimuli and behaviors: A comparison of sexually functional and dysfunctional males.* Poster presented at the annual meeting of the Association for Advancement of Behavior Therapy, Miami Beach, FL.

Wincze, J. P., Albert, A., & Bansal, S. (1993). Sexual arousal in diabetic females: Physiological and self report measures. *Archives of Sexual Behavior, 22,* 587–601.

Wincze, J. P., & Barlow, D. H. (1997a). *Enhancing sexuality: A problem solving approach (client workbook).* New York: Oxford University Press.

Wincze, J. P., & Barlow, D. H. (1997b). *Enhancing sexuality: A problem solving approach (therapist guide).* New York: Oxford University Press.

Wincze, J. P., & Carey, M. P. (2001). *Sexual dysfunction: A guide for assessment and treatment* (2nd ed.). New York: Guilford Press.

Wincze, J., Rosen, R., Carsons, C., Korenman, S., Niederberger, C., Sadovsky, R., et al. (2004). Erection Quality Scale: Initial scale development and validation. *Urology, 64,* 531–356.

Wylie, K. R. (1997). Treatment outcome of brief couple therapy in psychogenic male erectile disorder. *Archives of Sexual Behavior, 26,* 527–545.

Zilbergeld, B. (1998). *The new male sexuality* (rev. ed.). New York: Bantam.

CHAPTER 16

Couple Distress

ANDREW CHRISTENSEN
JENNIFER G. WHEELER
NEIL S. JACOBSON

The second edition of this book presented, for the first time, a substantially different approach to couple therapy—different both in conceptualization and in treatment strategies. It was noted that these changes in technique and conceptualization were profound enough to warrant a new name for the approach: "integrative behavioral couple therapy" (IBCT). As described in this fourth edition, IBCT has matured into a sophisticated and intuitively appealing set of strategies. These strategies are very nicely illustrated in this chapter in the context of the comprehensive treatment of one couple in substantial distress. Because these strategies require considerable clinical skill and talent, beginning therapists in particular should learn much from the case descriptions presented in this very readable and engaging chapter. As most readers will know, this new approach was initially conceptualized and developed by Andrew Christensen and the late Neil Jacobson, working in close concert with other colleagues and students such as Jennifer Wheeler. Tragically, Neil passed away in 1999, but the force survives him and continues to grow in influence.
—D. H. B.

Unlike other chapters in this *Handbook*, the term "couple distress" does not refer to a specific clinical or personality disorder. In DSM-IV-TR, couple distress is not a "mental disorder" but is relegated to the category of "other conditions that may be a focus of clinical attention" and assigned a presumably lesser "V code" of "partner relational problem." Yet it is certainly arguable that couple distress creates as much psychological and physical pain as many, if not most, of the DSM-IV-TR disorders (Burman & Margolin, 1992). Furthermore, couple distress can initiate, exacerbate, and complicate DSM-IV-TR disorders such as de-

pression, or trigger their relapse (Whisman, 1999; Whisman & Bruce, 1999). Furthermore, couple distress can have a major impact on children of the pair, triggering or exacerbating externalizing and internalizing disorders (Buehler et al., 1997). Indeed, there is a push to give relationship processes such as couple distress greater attention in the next edition of the DSM and even to include some relationship problems as disorders (Beach et al., 2006). Whatever the merits and outcome of these efforts, there is no doubt that couple distress has serious psychological consequences and is deserving of therapeutic attention.

In this chapter we describe one promising new approach to the treatment of couple distress called integrative behavioral couple therapy (IBCT; Christensen & Jacobson, 2000; Christensen, Jacobson, & Babcock, 1995; Jacobson & Christensen, 1998). We briefly review the development of this approach from its origins in traditional behavioral couple therapy, followed by a description of IBCT theories and techniques. Then we describe the application of IBCT, including the stages of therapy and the use of specific interventions. Finally, we discuss the empirical evidence in support of IBCT and provide a case example to demonstrate the application of IBCT to the treatment of couple distress.

TRADITIONAL BEHAVIORAL COUPLE THERAPY

The term "couple therapy" (as opposed to "individual" or "group" therapy) refers to clinical approaches for improving the functioning of two individuals within the context of their relationship to one another.[1] Although couple therapy is unique in its emphasis on a specific dyad, by its very definition, it is a contextual approach to the treatment of two *individuals*. Accordingly, successful treatments for couple distress have emphasized the assessment and modification of each individual's contribution and response to specific interactions in their relationship (e.g., Baucom & Hoffman, 1986; Gurman, Knickerson, & Pinsoff, 1986; Holtzworth-Munroe & Jacobson, 1991; Jacobson, 1978a, 1984; Jacobson & Holtzworth-Munroe, 1986; Jacobson & Margolin, 1979; Stuart, 1980; Weiss, Hops, & Patterson, 1973).

For over two decades, the "gold standard" for the treatment of couple distress has been behavioral couple therapy (for reviews of couple therapies, see Baucom, Shoham, Kim, Daiuto, & Stickle, 1998; Christensen & Heavey, 1999; Jacobson & Addis, 1993; Snyder, Castellani, & Whisman, 2006). First applied to couple distress by Stuart (1969) and Weiss and colleagues (1973), traditional behavioral couple therapy (TBCT) uses basic behavioral principles of reinforcement, modeling, and behavioral rehearsal to facilitate collaboration and compromise between partners. With an eye toward facilitating changes in the couple's behavior, TBCT teaches a couple how to increase or decrease target behaviors (behavior exchange), to communicate more effectively (communication training), and to assess and solve problems (problem solving) to improve overall relationship satisfaction. The monograph by Jacobson and Margolin (1979) is a commonly used treatment manual for TBCT.

In early studies, TBCT demonstrated significant empirical success (Jacobson 1977, 1978b) and soon became the focus of numerous treatment manuals, programs, and publications supporting the application of behavioral techniques to the treatment of couple distress (e.g., Floyd & Markman, 1983; Gottman, Notarius, Gonso, & Markman, 1976; Jacobson & Margolin, 1979; Knox, 1971; Liberman, 1970; Liberman, Wheeler, deVisser, Kuehnel, & Kuehnel, 1981; Stuart, 1980). Subsequent outcome research has consistently supported the efficacy of behavioral approaches for the treatment of couple distress (Baucom & Hoffman, 1986; Gurman et al., 1986; Jacobson, 1984; Jacobson, Schmaling, & Holtzworth-Munroe, 1987).

However, outcome research also revealed some limitations in the efficacy and generalizability of TBCT. For example, approximately one-third of couples failed to show measurable improvement in relationship quality following treatment with TBCT (Jacobson et al., 1987). Furthermore, many couples who initially responded to treatment relapsed within 1 or 2 years after therapy (Jacobson et al., 1984, 1987). Four years after therapy, Snyder, Wills, and Grady-Fletcher (1991) found a divorce rate of 37% in couples treated with TBCT.

Findings about the limited effectiveness of TBCT encouraged the development of additional therapeutic approaches. Various modifications and enhancements have been made to TBCT in an effort to improve its effectiveness (e.g., Baucom & Epstein, 1990; Baucom, Epstein, & Rankin, 1995; Epstein & Baucom, 2002; Floyd, Markman, Kelly, Blumberg, & Stanley, 1995, Halford, 2001), yet the existing comparative treatment studies have failed to demonstrate any incremental efficacy in various enhancements to TBCT, such as the addition of cognitive strategies. The addition of cognitive strategies created a treatment that was as good as but not better than TBCT (e.g., Baucom et al., 1998).

In addition to examining treatment outcome, couple therapy research aimed at understanding how "treatment successes" differed from "treatment failures." Early research on treatment response identified several factors that appeared to affect the success of TBCT. Compared to couples who responded positively to TBCT, couples who were regarded as "treatment failures" or "difficult to treat" were generally older, more emotionally disengaged, more polarized on basic issues, and more severely distressed (Baucom & Hoffman, 1986; Hahlweg, Schindler, Revenstorf, & Brengelmann, 1984; Jacobson, Follette, & Pagel, 1986; see Jacobson & Christensen, 1998, for a review). Despite the fact that these couples arguably had the greatest need for effective treatment, each of these factors has an obvious deleterious effect on their ability to collaborate, compromise, and facilitate behavioral change. Older couples, for example, have had more time than younger couples to become "stuck" in their destructive behavioral patterns. Couples who are more polarized on fundamental issues (e.g., how "traditional" they are with respect to their gender roles) may never be able to reach a mutually satisfying compromise. And extremely disengaged couples may be unable to collaborate. Each of these factors is likely to be associated with long-standing, deeply entrenched, and even "unchangeable" behavioral patterns. Thus, it should come as no surprise that the change-oriented techniques of TBCT are ineffective for these couples.

AN "INTEGRATIVE" THERAPY

These findings served as the impetus for the development of IBCT. Evidence on the limited success of TBCT, particularly during follow-up, spurred an effort to find a treatment with more enduring effects. Evidence on TBCT's failures spurred efforts to find treatments that would be applicable even to these difficult cases. Three developments in IBCT are directed toward making treatment more enduring and more broadly applicable: (1) a focus on the couple's relational "themes" rather than on specific target behaviors; (2) an emphasis on "contingency-shaped" versus "rule-governed" behavior; and (3) a focus on emotional acceptance.

The first aspect of IBCT that is intended to make its effectiveness more broadly applicable and more enduring is IBCT's focus on a cou-

ple's relational "themes," that is, their long-standing patterns of disparate yet functionally similar behaviors. Although this focus is similar to TBCT in that it requires a comprehensive assessment of the couple's behavioral patterns, it differs from TBCT in that multiple and complex behavioral interactions—and not just specific behavioral targets—are considered for therapeutic intervention.

A highlight of all behavioral approaches, and certainly of TBCT, is an assessment process that transforms broad, global complaints into specific, "pinpointed" behaviors. For example, a wife may come into therapy complaining that her husband does not love her, while her husband complains that his wife does not believe in him. The TBCT therapist would assist the wife in defining her general complaint into specific behavioral targets for her husband, such as kissing her and hugging her more often. The therapist would also assist the husband in defining his general complaint into specific behavioral targets for his wife, such as complimenting his achievements more often. However, IBCT suggests that valuable information may be lost in the transformation of a global complaint into a specific behavioral target. By quickly narrowing down global complaints into specific behavioral targets, TBCT inadvertently limits the means by which partners may satisfy each other. For example, if "feeling loved" is defined solely in terms of physical affection and the husband has difficulty in increasing and/or sustaining a higher level of physical affection, then his wife's needs will not be satisfied. Indeed, the husband could perform a variety of other behaviors in addition to physical affection that function to make his wife feel loved, such as calling her during work to see how she is doing, listening to her troubles with her family, or noticing that the air in her car tires is dangerously low. She may not be able to articulate many behaviors that might function in ways to make her feel loved, either because she is not aware of the desired behaviors or perhaps she feels too vulnerable to express this need. Without more elaborate exploration of and functional analysis of the wife's and husband's thoughts, feelings, and behaviors, such important opportunities for facilitating therapeutic change may be lost. Furthermore, these very specific behavioral definitions may have iatrogenic effects. In the previous example, the wife may begin to define her husband's love more and more in terms of his limited ability to be affectionate, because this is how "love" was operationalized in the context of the TBCT intervention. If the husband is unable to make her feel "loved" via physical affection alone, then her anger and sense of loss could be heightened rather than ameliorated by the treatment.

In contrast to TBCT's emphasis on specific behavioral targets, IBCT places its focus on broader "themes" in the couple's history; that is, developing a shared understanding of the many circumstances in which the wife has felt loved and unloved, and in which the husband has felt that his wife believed or did not believe in him. Certainly this shared understanding includes some specific behavioral examples illustrating what makes the wife feel unloved and what would make her feel loved, and what makes the husband feel that his wife does not believe in him and what would make him feel that she does. However, IBCT tries to keep open all possibilities of behaviors that function to provide each spouse with his or her desired emotional state. Thus, if one partner has difficulty performing a particular behavior (e.g., physical affection), he or she may still be able to perform other, perhaps less obvious behaviors that serve the same function (e.g., calling one's wife from work). By focusing on the broader behavioral "theme" (her history of feeling unloved, his history of feeling not believed in), rather than attempting to operationalize that theme completely into one specific behavior, IBCT maintains its functional roots, while increasing the chances that each partner is able to meet the other's needs.

A second development that is designed to make IBCT applicable to more couples and to create more enduring change is based on the distinction between "rule-governed" versus "contingency-shaped" behavior (Skinner, 1966). In the former, an individual is provided with a rule to guide his or her behavior and is then reinforced when he or she follows the rule. Using the previous example, a therapist could develop a list of possible affectionate behaviors for the husband, such as giving his wife a kiss when he leaves for work and when he returns, then encourage the husband to implement these behaviors. Upon implementing them, the husband would be reinforced by both his wife and the therapist. TBCT is largely based on employing "rule-governed" strategies to create positive change. Not only is behavioral exchange a "rule-governed" strategy, but even more important, the TBCT strategies of communication training and problem solving training are also dominated by "rule-governed" strategies. In both, the TBCT therapist teaches the couple certain rules of good communication or good problem solving to use during their discussions of problems. The guideline to use "I statements" or to "define the problem clearly before proposing solutions" are examples.

With "contingency-shaped" behavior, naturally occurring events in the situation serve to elicit and reinforce the desired behavior. For example, the husband would be affectionate with his wife when something in their interaction triggered a desire for him to hug or kiss her; the experience of closeness or physical contact in the affectionate gesture itself, or his wife's response to his gesture, would serve to reinforce his affectionate behavior. In contrast to TBCT, IBCT engages in "contingency-shaped" behavior change. IBCT therapists try to discover the events that function to trigger desired experiences in each partner, then attempt to orchestrate these events. For example, IBCT therapists might hypothesize that a wife's criticisms push her husband away, but that her expressions of loneliness could bring him toward her. The IBCT therapist listens to her criticisms (e.g., that her husband ignores her), suggests that she may be lonely (as a result of feeling "ignored"), and, if she acknowledges such a feeling, encourages her to talk about it. The therapeutic goal is that this "shift" in her conversation (from criticism to self-disclosure) might also "shift" her husband's typically defensive posture in listening to (or ignoring) his wife. Although such a strategy of emphasizing "contingency-shaped" behavior makes intervention more complicated and less straightforward than a purely "rule-governed" approach, IBCT suggests that a "contingency-shaped" approach leads to more profound and enduring changes in the couple's relational patterns.

A third development in IBCT that is designed to make it applicable to more couples and to create more enduring change is its focus on emotional acceptance. In TBCT, the approach to solving couple problems is to create positive change. If the husband in the couple we discussed could be more physically affectionate, and the wife more verbally complimentary, then the couple's problems would presumably be solved. However, if the husband is unable or unwilling to be more physically affectionate, and if the wife is unable or unwilling to be more complimentary, then the case will be a treatment failure. If the husband and wife are able to make these changes initially but are unable to maintain them over the long run, then the case becomes a temporary success followed by relapse.

In contrast to TBCT, the focus of IBCT is on emotional acceptance. Unlike the change-oriented goal of TBCT, the primary goal of IBCT is to promote each partner's *acceptance* of the other and their differences. Rather than trying to *eliminate* a couple's long-standing conflicts, a goal of IBCT is to help couples develop a new understanding of their apparently irreconcilable differences, and to use these differences to promote intimacy, empathy, and compassion for one another. With its focus on *acceptance* rather than *change*, IBCT creates an environment for couples to understand each other's behavior before deciding whether and how they might modify it. In the earlier example, IBCT would explore the husband's difficulties in expressing affection and the wife's difficulties in giving him compliments—difficulties that may have little to do with how much love they feel for one another. Through this exploration of the individuals, the partners may come to a greater understanding of one another and experience more emotional closeness, thus achieving the feelings of love they previously pursued by requesting changes in each other's behavior (i.e., increased physical affection and verbal compliments).

While there *is* an expectation of "change" in IBCT, this expectation differs significantly from that of TBCT in regard to *which* partner and *what* behavior is expected to change. In TBCT, the "change" only involves Partner A increasing–decreasing the frequency or intensity of a specified behavior in response to a complaint from Partner B. But in IBCT, it is hoped that the therapeutic "change" also involves Partner B modifying his or her *emotional reaction* to Partner A's "problem" behavior. When a difference is "irreconcilable," the therapeutic strategy of IBCT is to change the "complaining" partner's response to the "offending" partner's behavior, rather than directing all therapeutic efforts at attempting to change what has historically been an essentially "unchangeable" behavior. Ideally, through exploration of the thoughts and feelings underlying Partner A's behaviors, Partner B develops a new understanding of his or her partner's behavior, and the "complaint" is

transformed into a less destructive response. In turn, this change in Partner B's reaction often then has a salutary impact on the frequency or intensity of Partner A's behavior. Using this approach, as opposed to an exclusively change-focused approach, even the most polarized, disengaged, and "unchangeable" couples have an opportunity to increase their overall marital satisfaction.

It is important to note that in this context acceptance is not confused with resignation. Whereas "resignation" involves one partner grudgingly giving in to the other, perhaps unwillingly "tolerating" what is seen as an unyielding status quo, "acceptance" involves one partner "letting go" of the *struggle to change* the other. Instead of encouraging one partner to "give in" to the other, acceptance work focuses on transforming a couple's "irreconcilable" differences into a vehicle for promoting closeness and intimacy. Ideally, partners "let go" of the struggle not grudgingly but as a result of a new appreciation for their partner's experience. By understanding their couple distress in terms of their individual differences, and by learning to accept each other's differences, it is hoped that the distress that has historically been generated by their struggle to change one another will be reduced. Thus, for IBCT to be effective in treating couple distress, it is important for partners to understand the factors that have contributed to the development and maintenance of their distress.

THE ETIOLOGY OF COUPLE DISTRESS

IBCT interventions promote couples' understanding of the etiology and maintenance of their distress. According to IBCT, relationship distress develops as a result of two basic influences—reinforcement erosion and the emergence of incompatibilities. "Reinforcement erosion" refers to the phenomenon whereby behaviors that were once reinforcing become less reinforcing with repeated exposure. For example, demonstrations of physical affection may generate powerful feelings of warmth and pleasure for each partner during the early stages of their relationship. But after partners have spent many years together, the reinforcing properties of these affectionate behaviors may disappear. For some couples, once-reinforcing behaviors may become "taken for granted," whereas for others, once-reinforcing behaviors may actually become aversive. In some cases, behaviors that were once considered attractive, endearing, or pleasing become the very same behaviors that generate or exacerbate the couple's distress.

As with the erosion of reinforcing behaviors, "incompatibilities" may emerge as couples spend more and more time together. In the early stages of a relationship, differences in partners' backgrounds, goals, and interests may initially be downplayed or ignored. For example, if Partner A prefers to save money and Partner B prefers to spend money, this difference may not be apparent during courtship, when spending money is a tacit expectation of both partners. If this difference *is* detected early on, perhaps it is be regarded as a "positive" difference, in that each partner is encouraged to be a little more like the other in his or her spending habits. Or perhaps each partner expects the other to eventually compromise or change to his or her way of doing things. But over time, these incompatibilities and their relevance to the relationship are inevitably exposed. Differences that were once regarded as novel, interesting, or challenging may ultimately be perceived as impediments to one's own goals and interests. And in addition to any extant incompatibilities, further unanticipated incompatibilities may emerge with new life experiences (e.g., having children, changing careers). Thus, even those couples who had initially made a realistic appraisal of their differences may discover unexpected incompatibilities over time. One goal of IBCT is to identify and reframe a couple's incompatibilities in a way that minimizes their destructive nature, while maximizing the couple's level of intimacy and relationship satisfaction.

APPLICATION OF IBCT

The Formulation

The most important organizing principle of IBCT is the "formulation," which is the way the therapist conceives of and describes the couple's problem in terms of the partners' differences, incompatibilities, and associated discord. The formulation is based on a functional analysis of the couple's problems and comprises three basic components: a *theme*, a *polarization process*, and a *mutual trap*. The therapist refers back to the formulation and its components throughout the treatment process, whenever couples have conflicts during or between therapy sessions.

Simply put, one of the most basic goals of IBCT is for the partners to adopt the formulation as part of their relationship history. They can use the formulation as a context for understanding their relationship and their conflicts. It gives couples a language to discuss their problems, and allows partners to distance themselves from their problems. It is important to remember, however, that the formulation is a dynamic concept that may require alteration and modification (or "reformulation") throughout treatment.

The Theme

The "theme," the description of the couple's primary conflict, is usually described by a phrase that captures the nature of the couple's differences. The theme is a "shorthand" way of describing the function of each partner's behavior during typical conflicts. A couple's theme underlies both the partners' polarization process and their mutual trap. For example, a common theme of many distressed couples is that of "closeness–independence," in which one partner seeks greater closeness, whereas the other seeks greater independence.

IBCT suggests that partners have their primary conflict, or theme, because of differences between them and each partner's individual vulnerabilities. For example, in the theme of closeness–independence, Partner A may want more closeness and connection, and Partner B may want more independence simply because they are different people with different genes and different social learning histories. Perhaps this difference was not readily apparent early on, because both partners were enchanted by their developing relationship. Or perhaps there really was little difference in their desires for closeness and independence, until they had children or until one partner's career took off. Whatever the basis for the difference, it creates problems for the couple. Partners find that they cannot both get their needs fully satisfied. Compromise may be relatively easy unless vulnerabilities are also present, which provide emotional fuel for the differences. If Partner A wants greater closeness than Partner B and is emotionally vulnerable to easily feeling abandoned, then negotiations about closeness may be threatening to Partner A. Similarly, if Partner B wants greater independence and is emotionally vulnerable to easily feeling controlled and restrained, then negotiations about closeness may be threatening for Partner B as well. If both Partner A and Partner B are emotionally vulnerable to their differences, they are likely to engage in destructive communication that IBCT calls the "polarization process."

The Polarization Process

The "polarization process" refers to the destructive interaction that ensues when a distressed couple enters into a theme-related conflict. A natural response for partners confronted with their differences is for each partner to try to change the other. In many cases these efforts at changing each other may be successful. However, many times the result may be that their differences are exacerbated and the two partners become polarized in their conflicting positions. When a couple has become polarized on an issue, partners' further attempts to change each other only increase the conflict and perpetuate their polarized stance. For example, in a couple whose theme is closeness–independence, the polarization process is likely to occur when the independence seeker "retreats" from attempts by the closeness seeker to gain more intimacy, which then creates more "intrusive" efforts by the closeness seeker. The more the one partner "advances," the more the other partner "retreats"; the more that partner "retreats," the more the other partner "advances." As part of this pattern, partners may come to see their differences as deficiencies in the other. For example, the closeness seeker may see the other as being "afraid of intimacy"; the independence seeker may see the other as being "neurotically dependent." Furthermore, being deprived of a desired goal can make that goal seem even more important: Partners can become desperate, escalating their futile efforts, and their differences become magnified. It can begin to look like the closeness seeker has no needs for independence and the independence seeker has no needs for closeness. Though their interaction, they have become more different than they were originally.

The Mutual Trap

The mutual trap, which describes the outcome of the polarization process, is called a "trap" because it typically leaves the partners feeling "stuck" or "trapped" in their conflict. Partners in a mutual trap feel that they have done everything they can to change the other, and nothing seems to work. But they are reluctant to give up their efforts to change each other, because this would mean resigning themselves to a dissatisfying relationship. As a result, they become more entrenched in their respective positions.

The experience of partners who are so polarized is one of helplessness and futility, and this experience is rarely discussed openly between them. As a result, each partner may be unaware that the other also feels trapped. Making each partner aware of the other's sense of entrapment is an important part of acceptance work, and encouraging each partner to experience the other's sense of "stuckness" can sometimes be the first step toward promoting empathy and intimacy between partners.

Stages of Therapy

In IBCT there is a clear distinction between the assessment phase and the treatment itself. The *assessment* phase comprises at least one conjoint session with the couple, followed by individual sessions with each partner. The assessment phase is followed by a feedback session, during which the therapist describes his or her *formulation* of the couple and their problems. The feedback session is followed by the treatment sessions, the exact number of which should be determined on a case-by-case basis depending on each couple's treatment needs. However, the protocol used in a recent clinical trial of IBCT (to be discussed below) was a maximum of 26 sessions, including both the assessment and treatment phases.

The Use of Objective Measures

Objective assessment instruments (see Table 16.1) may be useful for both initial assessment and for monitoring a couple's progress at various points throughout treatment. Although such objectives measures are not necessary to conduct IBCT, they may provide additional information about areas of disagreement that have not been covered in the session, or they may provide objective data about a couple's levels of distress and satisfaction. For example, a couple's relationship satisfaction can be assessed using the

TABLE 16.1. Useful Assessment and Screening Instruments

- Dyadic Adjustment Scale (Spainer, 1976): Measures relationship distress and commitment. (To obtain this measure, contact Western Psychological Services, 12031 Wilshire Blvd., Los Angeles, CA 90025; *www.wpspublish.com*.)

- Marital Status Inventory (Crane & Mead, 1980; Weiss & Cerreto, 1980): Assesses commitment to the relationship and steps taken toward separation or divorce. (To obtain this measure, contact Robert L. Weiss, PhD, Oregon Marital Studies Program, Department of Psychology, University of Oregon, Eugene, OR 97403-1227; *darkwing.uoregon.edu/~rlweiss/msi.htm*.)

- Revised Conflict Tactics Scale (Straus, Hamby, Boney-McCoy, & Sugarman, 1996): Assesses domestic violence. (To obtain this measure, contact Multi-Health Systems, P.O. Box 950, North Tonawanda, NY 14120; *www.mhs.com*.)

- Frequency and Acceptability of Partner Behavior Inventory (Christensen & Jacobson, 1997; Doss & Christensen, 2006): Assesses acceptability of behavior at their current frequency for 24 categories of spouse behavior. (To obtain this measure, contact Andrew Christensen, PhD, UCLA Department of Psychology, Los Angeles, CA 90095; *christensen@psych.ucla.edu*.)

Dyadic Adjustment Scale (Spanier, 1976); partners' commitment to the relationship and steps taken toward separation or divorce can be assessed using the Marital Status Inventory (Crane & Mead, 1980; Weiss & Cerreto, 1980); partner's troubling behaviors can be assessed with the Frequency and Acceptability of Partner Behavior Inventory (Christensen & Jacobson, 1997; Doss & Christensen, 2006), and the couple's level of physical violence, with the Conflict Tactics Scale—Revised (Straus, Hamby, Boney-McCoy, & Sugarman, 1996). Ideally the couple completes any such questionnaires before coming in for the first session, so that the therapist has a preliminary idea of the couple's presenting problems and overall levels of distress. However, partners can also complete the questionnaires after their first joint session and before their individual sessions. In addition to being part of the assessment phase, the questionnaires can be administered later in treatment, at the end of treatment, and at follow-up to assess changes from partners' presenting baseline levels of distress and satisfaction.

Assessment of Domestic Violence

Objective measures are particularly useful in assessing a couple's history of physical violence. Assessing for domestic violence is a critical part of every couple's intake—not only to determine whether the personal safety of either partner is in imminent danger but also because couple therapy may actually be *contraindicated* for some violent couples (Jacobson & Gottman, 1998; Simpson, Doss, Wheeler, & Christensen, 2007). Couple therapy requires that both partners take some degree of responsibility for their problems, but such a perspective is inappropriate when a couple's problems include domestic violence, because perpetrators of violence must assume sole responsibility for their behavior. Furthermore, because therapy sessions can elicit strong emotions, the couple therapy itself may trigger postsession violence in some couples. In such cases, treatment that focuses on the violent behavior of the perpetrator—and not the interactive distress of the couple—is indicated. The Conflict Tactics Scale—Revised (Straus et al., 1996) is a useful screening tool for evaluating the frequency and severity of a couple's physical aggression, and to determine whether couple therapy is contraindicated. Finally, a couple's history of violence should be directly addressed during the assessment phase, primarily during the individual sessions, when each partner can talk freely without fearing consequences from the other.

Assessment

The *assessment* phase typically comprises one joint session with the partners (Session 1), followed by individual sessions with each partner (Sessions 2 and 3). The primary goal of the assessment phase is for the therapist to evaluate whether the couple is appropriate for therapy and, if so, to develop the *formulation*. However, the therapist should also use the assessment period to orient the couple to the therapy process. In addition, although the IBCT therapist is not actively intervening during the assessment phase, it is possible for the therapist to have a therapeutic impact in these first few sessions.

Orientation (Session 1)

After greetings and introductions, the couple is oriented to the upcoming therapy process. This orientation likely includes reviewing and signing an informed consent form, which explains billing procedures, defines confidentiality and its exclusions, and outlines the possible risks and benefits of participating in IBCT.

In addition to the general information provided during informed consent, the couple is also oriented to the specific process of IBCT. Therapists should explain the difference between the assessment and treatment phases of therapy, and ask the couple whether this is different from the couple's expectations in coming to therapy. Therapists should be prepared for couples' disappointment when they learn that therapy is not going to begin immediately. Therapists may need to explain to couples why an assessment period is needed before therapists can provide any useful help to them.

Also during the first session, couples are introduced to their manual *Reconcilable Differences* (Christensen & Jacobson, 2000). Couples are asked to complete Part I of this book prior to the feedback session. Ideally, this reading helps couples begin to conceptualize their problems in a way that is similar to how their therapist will portray them during the feedback session.

Therapists should be aware that at least one partner, if not both, is likely to be ambivalent about participating in therapy. Such ambivalence should be normalized and validated, and the therapist should explain to partners that the assessment period is also *their* opportunity to get to know the therapist and to determine whether this treatment is going to be a "good match" for them.

Problem Areas (Sessions 1, 2, and 3)

After the couple has been oriented to the therapy process, the therapist begins the evaluation by reviewing the couple's presenting problem(s). Much of this information can be gathered from objective measures and also during each partner's individual session, so this discussion during Session 1 should not consume the entire session. However, it is important during the first session that the partners feel heard and validated, and that their problems and distress are clearly understood by the therapist.

From the information gathered from objective measures and during the evaluation sessions, therapists should be able to describe the partners' problem areas and develop their formulation. The following six questions provide

a guideline for this assessment, and each should be answered by the end of the assessment period.

1. How distressed is the couple?
2. How committed is this couple to the relationship?
3. What issues divide this couple?
4. Why are these issues a problem for them?
5. What strengths keep this couple together?
6. What can treatment do to help them?

The first three questions can be addressed with objective questionnaires. However, even questions that can be addressed with questionnaires should usually be explored in further detail in interviews. For example, the individual sessions may be particularly useful for assessing whether distress is so great that separation is imminent, for assessing each partner's level of commitment to the relationship and the possible presence of affairs, and for assessing the couple's history of physical violence.

The assessment of a couple's problem areas should also include a determination of the couple's "collaborative set" (Jacobson & Margolin, 1979). This term refers to the couple's joint perspective that they *share* responsibility for the problems in their relationship, and that *both* will have to change if the relationship is to change. The strength of this set determines whether change- or acceptance-oriented interventions are indicated. The stronger the couple's collaborative set, the more successful change-oriented interventions are likely to be. But partners who lack this collaborative set—who enter therapy believing they are the innocent victim of the other's behavior—first need to focus on acceptance work.

The fourth question—why the partners' issues are a problem for them—requires a functional analysis that normally is based on information obtained in the individual and joint interviews. Because adults are often unaware of the contingencies controlling their behavior, or may be embarrassed to admit those contingencies even if they know them, a functional analysis involves much more than a simple, straightforward inquiry. The therapist must be particularly sensitive to the emotional reactions of partners, which may indicate important reinforcers and punishers. For example, let us assume that our partners with the closeness–iIndependence theme argue frequently about the amount of time they spend together. However, that specific issue may not be where the most powerful contingencies are found. Perhaps the wife's history includes having been abandoned by her family members at a time when she was in particular need of their support and comfort. Her fear in her marital relationship is that her husband may do likewise. For her, time they spend together is simply a poor proxy for her concerns that he may not always be there when she needs him. If she felt confident of that, then she could tolerate much less time together. For her husband's part, let us assume that his social learning history has led him to be especially sensitive to being controlled or restricted by another person. Therefore, he battles his wife over their time together not so much because he does not want the time together, but because he feels controlled by her and naturally resists. In such a situation, the IBCT therapist needs to move the discussion away from the repetitive arguments about time spent together toward the more important contingencies that affect each spouse's behaviors.

Answers to the fifth question, about the couple's strengths, also come from the joint and individual interviews. It is helpful for couples to keep their strengths in mind even as they focus on their difficulties. Sometimes there is an interesting relationship between a couple's strengths and problems, in that the latter may involve some variation of the former. For example, let us assume that two partners got together in part because of their different approaches to life. He is much more spontaneous; she is more deliberate and planful. Those differences may be attractive and helpful at times, but they can also be a source of irritation and conflict.

In answering the final question, what treatment can do to help, the therapist must first be sure the couple is appropriate for couple therapy. If the couple has serious violence or a substance dependence problem, for example, then couple therapy as usual will not be the recommendation. Treatment directed at those particular problems will be necessary. If the couple is appropriate for couple therapy, the therapist will need to outline the focus of the therapy and what it comprises.

The Couple's History (Session 1)

After the partners have been oriented to therapy and their problem areas have been assessed, the therapist then takes the history of the couple's relationship. The therapist's obvious objective for taking this history is to gain a good understanding of the partners' attachment to one another. Often the couple's distress has escalated to the degree that it has overshadowed the reasons the two became a couple in the first place. In addition, this history can provide some immediate therapeutic benefit to the couple. Generally, when partners discuss the earlier (and usually happier) stages of their relationship, their affect is likely to become more positive. They have been focused for so long on the negative aspects of their relationship that they probably have not thought about their early romance, courtship, and attraction to each other for a very long time. In this way, having couples describe the evolution of their relationship can be therapeutic in and of itself. Although some couples may be in too much pain to discuss their history without blaming and accusatory remarks (in which case the therapist should abandon the following guidelines and instead use the session to validate their pain), most couples enjoy reminiscing about their happier times.

The following series of questions provide the therapist with useful information about the couple's history and allow the partners an opportunity to reflect upon the reasons they fell in love in the first place:

- How did they get together?
- What was their courtship like?
- What attracted each of them to the other?
- What was their relationship like before their problems began?
- How is their relationship different *now* on days when they are getting along?
- How would the relationship be different if their current problems no longer existed?

These and other, related questions may also reveal useful information about each partner, such as his or her hopes and dreams for the future. Information about the couple's history is useful for the therapist in developing the couple's formulation, which is presented to them during their feedback session.

Individual History (Sessions 2 and 3)

Each partner's individual history can often provide useful information for the formulation, in that it provides a context for each partner's behavior and illuminates possible vulnerabilities in each. For example, perhaps the husband experienced his mother as very demanding of him and learned to cope with this through withdrawal, so the withdrawal continues in response to his wife's demands. Or perhaps the wife had two previous boyfriends who cheated on her, so she is sensitive to any indication of betrayal by her husband.

The following questions may be useful in guiding a discussion of each partner's individual history:

• What was your parents' marriage like?
• What was your relationship with your father like?
• What was your relationship with your mother like?
• What were your relationships with your siblings like?
• What were your relationships with previous important romantic partners like?

Each of these questions could potentially take an inordinate amount of time. The IBCT therapist tries to elicit features of these early relationships that are similar to or may inform the current relationship. For example, if the therapist were aware of a difference between husband and wife in how open to be about their disagreements, he or she would guide the husband away from details about where his family lived and focus on the suppression of conflict that occurred in his family.

Feedback

From the information gathered during the assessment sessions and the questionnaires, the therapist develops the couple's formulation. The formulation is discussed with the couple in the feedback session (usually the fourth session). The feedback session can follow the outline of the six questions used to assess the couple's problem areas. It is important that the feedback session be a dialogue and not a lecture from the therapist—with the therapist continually getting feedback from the couple about the formulation being presented. The partners are the experts on their relationship and should be treated as such.

The feedback session is also used to describe the proposed treatment plan for couples, based on their formulation. The therapist describes for the couple the goals for treatment and the procedures for accomplishing these goals. The goals for therapy are to create an in-session environment in which the couple's problems can be resolved through some combination of acceptance and change techniques. The procedures for meeting these goals are usually (1) in-session discussions of incidents and issues related to the formulation, and (2) homework to be conducted outside the session to further the in-session work.

The purpose of the feedback session is to orient partners to the goals of change and acceptance through open communication and finding new ways of looking at their problems. In addition, the feedback session is used to give partners some idea of what they can expect from therapy, and to elicit their willingness to participate. Finally, the feedback session may be used to implement some interventions. The first intervention is the therapist's description of the couple's strengths. From this discussion, partners may be able to see some solutions to their problems. The therapist can begin assigning relevant chapters from Part II of *Reconcilable Differences* (Christensen & Jacobson, 2000), which specifically address the topic of acceptance. After the formulation and treatment plan have been described to the couple, and the partners have agreed to proceed with therapy, the remaining sessions are devoted to building acceptance between partners and promoting change in each partner.

Treatment

IBCT Techniques for Building Emotional Acceptance

Typically, treatment begins with a focus on promoting acceptance. The exception is when partners are able to collaborate with one another ("the collaborative set") and both want to make specific changes in their relationship. In that case, the therapist begins with change strategies.

In the context of acceptance work, the actual content of each session is determined by the partners and what they "bring in" every week. The therapist looks for emotionally salient material that is relevant to the formulation. Recent negative or positive events related to the formulation are often the topics of discussion. For example, a couple with a closeness–independence theme might discuss a difficult incident in which the independence seeker wanted to spend the night out with friends and the closeness seeker protested that. Discussions also may be centered around upcoming events, such as a weekend trip for the couple in which the independence seeker fears that there will not be space for him or her to be alone. Broad issues related to the formulation are also appropriate for discussion, such as whether separate weekend trips apart with friends are acceptable for the couple.

Sometimes salient events relevant to the formulation occur between partners within the session, and the therapist should definitely focus on these. For example, when the independence seeker turns away as the closeness seeker gets emotionally agitated during a discussion, the IBCT therapist focuses on this "in the moment" example of their closeness–independence theme. The therapist might also structure interactions during the session that mimic their difficulties or create possibilities for a different kind of interaction. For example, the therapist may have the couple replay a recent, difficult interaction to learn from it, or encourage the couple to attempt a different and more positive interaction around the topic. All of these topics are useful means for implementing the three acceptance-building strategies of *Empathic Joining, Unified Detachment from the Problem*, and *Tolerance Building*. Because they can create greater closeness, as well as greater acceptance, the first two strategies are more commonly employed than the last one.

EMPATHIC JOINING

"Empathic joining" refers to the process by which partners cease to blame one another for their emotional suffering and instead develop empathy for each other's experience. To foster empathic joining, the IBCT therapist reformulates the couple's problem as a result of common differences rather than deficiencies in either partner. Partners' behaviors are described in terms of their differences from one another, and their responses to these differences are validated as normal and understandable, especially given the vulnerabilities that each may have.

In making this reformulation of each partner's behavior, it is important that the IBCT therapist emphasize the pain that each partner is experiencing rather than the pain each has delivered. One strategy for building empathy between partners is though the use of "soft disclosures." Often partners express their emotional pain by using "hard" disclosures of feelings such as anger or disgust. Although hard disclosures are easier to make, because they do not reveal vulnerability, they are more difficult for the other partner to hear, because they imply blame. It is the combination of "pain and blame" that results in discord. But if the therapist can encourage partners to express their pain *without* expressing blame, the result may be increased acceptance from the other partner. IBCT therapists often encourage soft disclosures by suggesting "soft" feelings, such as the fear, hurt, and shame that may underlie each partner's behavior. Although soft disclosures are more difficult to make, because they reveal vulnerability, they are easier for the other partner to hear and arouse more empathy. Thus, empathic joining is promoted by (1) *reformulation* of a couple's discord as a result of partners' common *differences* and their understandable reactions to those differences, and (2) the use of *soft disclosures* to express painful emotions.

UNIFIED DETACHMENT FROM THE PROBLEM

This IBCT technique allows partners to "step back" from their problems and describe them without placing blame—or responsibility for change—on either partner. In this way, partners engage in *unified detachment* from their problematic interactions. The therapist engages partners in a dialogue in which they use nonjudgemental terms to describe the sequence of a particular conflict, including what factors typically trigger their reactions, how specific events are connected to one another, and how they can defuse or override the conflict in the future. The approach is an intellectual analysis of the problem that is described in an emotionally detached manner as a third-party "it" rather than in terms of "you" or "me." When possible, the therapist should give the couple's theme, polarization process, and mutual traps a name, and use this name to define the problem further as an "it." By detaching themselves from the problem, partners have an opportunity to discuss their conflict without becoming emotionally "charged" by it. In this way, they can try to understand the conflict from a more neutral, objective stance. They engage in a kind of joint mindfulness about their problem. The therapist can also use metaphor and humor to distance the couple emotionally from the problem, as long as the humor does not in any way belittle either partner.

TOLERANCE BUILDING

Building acceptance may be most challenging when one partner experiences intense emotional pain as a result of the other partner's behavior. In these circumstances, the IBCT therapist must help one partner build tolerance for the other partner's "offending" behavior. By building tolerance, partners ideally experience a reduction in the pain caused by the behavior. To build tolerance, however, partners must cease efforts to prevent, avoid, or escape the "offending" partner's behavior. Instead, by exposing themselves to the behavior without the associated struggle, partners reduce their sensitivity to the behavior and, ideally, experience the "offending" behavior as less painful.

One strategy for building tolerance is through positive reemphasis, or focusing on the *positive aspects of a partner's negative behavior*. This strategy may be relatively easy when a negative behavior is in some way related to a quality the partner once found attractive about the other. For example, what she sees as her partner's "uptightness" might be the "stability" that first attracted her. Alternatively, what he sees as her "flakiness" or "irresponsibility" might be the "free-spiritedness" or "rebelliousness" that so attracted him in the beginning of their relationship. The positive reemphasis does not deny the negative qualities of the behavior in question but helps partners gain the perspective that any quality often has both good and bad features.

Another strategy for building tolerance for differences is to focus on the *ways these differences complement each other*, and to present these differences as part of what makes the relationship "work." One partner's stability might balance the other's free-spiritedness. The therapist might describe for the partners the ways they would be "worse off" if those differences did not exist. The differences can become a positive aspect of the couple's relationship, something in which the partners take pride rather than something they see as a destructive threat.

A third technique for building tolerance to a partner's behavior is to *prepare couples for inevitable slipups and lapses* in behavior. This is especially important when couples first begin to detect changes in their behavior and begin to feel positive about the progress they are making in therapy. It is during this time that the therapist should congratulate couples for their hard work and progress, then warn them that "backsliding" is still a likely occurrence. The couples should be asked to imagine some of the circumstances in which a slipup is likely to occur, and to consider possible responses to the slipup in advance. Working out how they will face such lapses helps partners build their tolerance for them.

A related strategy for building tolerance is to instruct couples *to fake negative behavior* while they are in session or at home. Each partner is instructed to engage in a designated "bad behavior"—with the stipulation that the couple is to engage in this behavior only when partners do not feel like doing so. The instructions are given to the couple, so that each partner knows that a bad behavior he or she is about to witness in session or may see in the future might actually be faked. Ideally this introduces an ambiguity about future negative behaviors that may mitigate the partner's emotional response to them. More importantly, however, is that faking behavior gives both partners an opportunity to observe the effects of their negative behavior on the other. Specifically, because they are performing the "bad behavior" during a time when they do not feel like it, they make these observations when they are in a calm emotional state that allows them to be more sympathetic. When done in session, the therapist can help debrief the reactions to the "bad" behavior. When done at home, the faker is instructed to let the other partner know about the faked behavior soon after is it performed, so the situation does not escalate and the couple has an opportunity to "debrief" following their "experiment."

One unavoidable source of pain for many partners is the feeling that the other fails to meet their needs in some important way. However, rarely is a partner able to fulfill all of the needs of the other. An important aspect of acceptance building is for partners to increase their own self-reliance, or *self-care*, in getting their needs met. They should be encouraged to find alternative ways to care for themselves when their partners are not able to do so. Partners may need to learn to seek support from friends and family in times of stress, or to find new ways to define and solve a problem on their own. As their self-reliance increases, reliance on partners to meet all of their emotional needs decreases. Ideally, this results in decreased sensitivity to their partners' failure to meet their needs, thereby reducing conflict.

Traditional Strategies for Promoting Change

For some couples, change interventions may be indicated. Whether an IBCT therapist begins by implementing "acceptance" rather than "change" techniques depends primarily on the couple's collaborative set and on their specific treatment needs. In general, however, change techniques are most effective if implemented later in therapy, after acceptance work has been done. Often acceptance work is sufficient for bringing about acceptance and change, and no deliberate change strategies need to be employed.

BEHAVIOR EXCHANGE

The primary goal of behavior exchange (BE) is to increase the proportion of a couple's daily positive behaviors and interactions. These techniques are instigative, in that they are intended to increase each partner's performance of positive behaviors. Because BE requires a great deal of collaboration between partners, it is best implemented later in therapy after acceptance work has been done. In addition to using BE to increase a couple's positive interactions, the IBCT therapist should also consider BE a diagnostic tool for assessing possible areas in need of more acceptance work.

The three basic steps in BE are (1) to identify behaviors that each partner can do for the other that would increase relationship satisfaction, (2) to increase the frequency of those behaviors in the couple's daily behavioral repertoire, and (3) to debrief the experience of providing and receiving positive behaviors. Partners are often given a homework assignment to generate a list of actions they can do for the other to increase his or her partners' satisfaction. Partners are instructed not to discuss these lists with each other to reduce the threat of criticism from the other and to keep each partner focused on his or her own assignment. In the next session, partners' lists are reviewed and discussed. Their next assignment might be to perform one or more of the actions on the list during the next week, but they are not to tell the partner which action they are performing. In the subsequent therapy session, partners review the success of their assignment and whether it had the desired effect on the other. The list can be modified to eliminate items that do not seem to have an effect, and in later sessions each partner can elicit feedback from the other to optimize the benefit of the actions on the list.

COMMUNICATION AND PROBLEM-SOLVING TRAINING

Although many couples are effective communicators without having had any formal "training," poor communication may exacerbate or even cause many problems for distressed couples. In their attempts to get the other to change, partners may resort to maladaptive communication tactics such as coercion (crying, threatening, withholding affection). Although coercion may be effective in the short term, in that the other may eventually comply with the demand, the use of coercion is likely to escalate such that increasingly coercive tactics are required to achieve the desired effect. Also, coercion tends to beget coercion, so that coercion by one partner leads to coercion by the other. The inevitable result of such interactions is that couples become extremely polarized. The goal of communication and problem solving training is to teach couples how to discuss their problems and to negotiate change without resorting to such destructive tactics. Ideally, these skills will be useful to couples even after therapy has ended.

As part of communication training, couples are taught both "speaker" and "listener" skills. To become more effective "speakers," couples are instructed to (1) focus on the self by expressing "I statements"; (2) focus on expressing emotional reactions, such as "I feel disappointed . . . "; and (3) focus on the partner's specific behaviors that lead to emotional reactions, such as "I feel disappointed when you don't call me when you are away." To become more effective listeners, partners are instructed to paraphrase and reflect what the other has just said. Paraphrasing ensures that neither partner is being misread during the conversation, and it decreases a couple's tendency to jump to conclusions about what is being said, in addition to generally slowing down the interaction.

Once couples have been given some instruction in these communication skills, they are directed to use these skills in practice conversations in the therapy session. Communicating with these guidelines may feel awkward during practice conversations, so therapists should try to adapt the guidelines to the couple's style of conversation and explain that following the guidelines will feel more natural with increased use. The therapist should be prepared to interrupt and make corrections if the couple deviates from the guidelines and engages in destructive communication. The therapist should provide the couple with feedback after each practice session, and the exercise should be adequately debriefed. When the therapist is confident that the partners have improved their in-session communication skills, he or she then encourages them to practice these skills as homework.

These basic communication skills often enable partners' to share their feelings with one another and to discuss difficult issues that arise, such as when one partner gets upset with the other's action. However, sometimes partners need to do more than share feelings or debrief an event. They need to solve an upcoming or recurrent problem. Often what is more damaging in their struggles around daily problems than the problems themselves is their destructive attempts to solve them. These attempts may begin with an accusation by one partner, which is met by defensiveness and anger from the other. Soon the argument may escalate to counterblaming and character assassination—and the problem itself gets lost in the conflict around it. In problem-solving training, couples are taught to have constructive problem-solving discussions while employing three sets of skills: problem definition skills, problem solution skills, and structuring skills.

First, partners are taught to *define* the problem as specifically as possible by specifying the behavior of concern and the circumstances surrounding it. Partners are encouraged to describe some of the emotions they experience as a result of the problem, in an effort toward increased emotional acceptance. Finally, both partners are asked to define their respective roles in perpetuating the problem.

Once the problem has been defined, the couple can begin working toward problem *solution*. The first step in problem solution is brainstorming, in which couples try to come up with as many solutions to the problem as possible. Couples are told that any and all solutions may be considered, even impossible or silly ones. Immediate evaluative comments about the brainstormed solutions are discouraged, and discussions of which options are actually viable are held off for later. Suggestions are written down so that they can be reviewed later. This exercise can be lighthearted and playful, often generating positive affect during the session. After the list has been generated, couples go through the list, eliminating those suggestions that are obviously impossible, silly, or unlikely to be effective. After the list is pruned, each item is considered for its potential to solve the problem. For each item the couple considers the pros and cons, and the list is further modified, until a final list of options has been generated. The remaining items are used to formulate a possible solution to the problem. The agreement that is made about this solution is written down and sometimes signed by each partner. Finally, couples are asked to consider any obstacles to executing the agreement, and to work out strategies for combating these. The partners are told to post the agreement in a place where they both can see it often, and a date is set to review their progress in solving the problem. During the next few sessions, the therapist checks in with them on their progress, and the agreement may be renegotiated, if necessary.

Finally, couples learn *structuring skills* for their problem-solving discussions. Couples structure these discussions by setting aside a specific time and place to have them. They are also instructed not to discuss the problem at the "scene of the crime," that is, to hold off discussing a problem until the designated time. Finally, couples are instructed to focus on only one problem at a time. Throughout their problem-solving discussions, partners are asked to follow the basic guidelines of paraphrasing each other's statements, avoiding negative inferences about each other's intent, and avoiding negative verbal and nonverbal communication.

The couple's first attempts at using these problem-solving skills should occur in session, under the supervision of the therapist. But after the partners have practiced and received feedback about their problem-solving skills, they are encouraged to apply these techniques at home to help discuss and negotiate their problems.

In implementing these behavior change skills, the IBCT therapist tries to adapt the strategies discussed earlier to the particular needs of the couple. For example, if a couple finds it helpful to go back and forth between definition and solution while discussing a problem, the therapist would eliminate the guideline specifying that the problem be carefully defined before solutions are considered. Or if a couple finds it distracting to generate silly or impossible solutions, the therapist would not encourage that. The therapist also tries to adapt these strategies to the formulation for the couple. For example, if the closeness seeker tends to dominate discussions and make proposals for solving a problem about time together, while the independence seeker tends to withdraw from the discussion, the therapist might shift the focus on problem solving to the independence seeker.

Therapist and Client Variables Relevant to IBCT

As in any therapy, it is important that IBCT therapists maintain a nonjudgmental stance toward their clients. But in the context of IBCT, it is particularly important that the therapist practice acceptance with both partners in the same way that they are asked to practice acceptance with one another. The IBCT therapist must validate the experiences and responses of both partners, and find ways to develop empathy and compassion for them no matter how challenging this may be.

In addition to practicing acceptance, it is important that IBCT therapists listen carefully to couples' in-session interactions and look for the functions of their various problematic behaviors. IBCT therapists must be particularly attentive to subtle verbal and nonverbal cues that may be relevant to the formulation of couples' problems. IBCT therapists must also be prepared to abandon any prescribed agenda to address the immediate needs of the couple at any given time. When destructive interactions occur in-session, the IBCT therapist must not only be able to maintain a nonconfrontational demeanor but also to stop the interaction effectively. Other important IBCT skills include using the couple's language and jargon when making interventions. Finally, it is not a goal of IBCT therapists to "cheerlead" for the success of the relationship; rather, they create an environment in which couples can safely discuss and evaluate their own relationships.

The Efficacy of IBCT

Three studies have been conducted that attest to the efficacy of IBCT—two small pilot investigations and one major outcome study. Wimberly (1998) randomly assigned eight couples to a group format of IBCT and nine couples to a waiting-list control group, and found superior results for the IBCT couples. Jacobson, Christensen, Prince, Cordova, and Eldridge (2000) randomly assigned 21 couples to either IBCT or TBCT. At the end of treatment, 80% of couples who had received IBCT showed clinically significant improvements in relationship satisfaction compared to 64% of couples who had received TBCT.

The largest study to date of couple therapy in general and of IBCT in particular was reported by Christensen and colleagues (2004). In a two-site clinical trial conducted at UCLA and the University of Washington, Christensen and colleagues randomly assigned 134 seriously and chronically distressed couples to either IBCT or TBCT. Couples received a maximum of 26 sessions of couple therapy delivered by professional PhD-level therapists, who provided both IBCT and TBCT treatments and were carefully supervised in both. Adherence and competence data provided evidence that treatments were delivered as expected. At termination, 70% of IBCT couples and 61% of TBCT couples had clinically significant improvements in relationship satisfaction. Although the termination results were not significantly different, the trajectory of change for both IBCT and TBCT couples was. IBCT couples improved steadily in satisfaction throughout treatment, but TBCT couples improved more rapidly early on in treatment, with their gains flattening out more than those of IBCT couples later in treatment.

Atkins and colleagues (2005) examined the predictors of response to treatment in the previous study. A variety of interpersonal variables, such as quality of communication, predicted the initial status of couples, but precious few variables predicted change from intake to termination. Couples who were married longer showed greater improvements in satisfaction, and exploratory analyses indicated that sexually dissatisfied couples showed slower initial gains but overall more consistent gains in IBCT than in TBCT.

Over a 2-year follow-up, couples showed a "hockey stick" pattern of change. Immediately after the end of treatment, couples in both conditions showed some deterioration, then reversed course and began improving throughout the follow-up period. IBCT couples improved at a significantly earlier point than did TBCT couples. Also, IBCT couples who stayed together were significantly happier than TBCT couples who stayed together. At 2-year posttreatment, 69% of IBCT couples and 60% of TBCT couples obtained clinically significant improvements over their pretreatment levels of satisfaction, a difference that was not significantly different (Christensen, Atkins, Yi, Baucom, & George, 2006). Thus, over two-thirds of seriously and chronically distressed couples who received IBCT showed significant improvement by 2-year posttreatment. The results compare favorably with previous long-term studies of couple therapy (Christensen et al., 2006).

It is important to note that this sample excluded couples in which one or both partners were experiencing bipolar disorder, schizophrenia, or serious suicidality; met criteria for current drug or alcohol abuse or dependence; met criteria for borderline, antisocial, or schizotypal personality disorders; or had a history of severe physical violence. The rationale for these exclusionary criteria is that for such individuals, a primary treatment other than couple therapy is likely to be indicated. However, the sample did *not* exclude couples in which one or both partners suffered from other psychological disorders, such as anxiety or depression. The rationale for including these couples is that their relationship can still be treated despite partners having such individual problems. Furthermore, some of the couples' relationship problems may even be *contributing* to these individual problems. Thus, preliminary data suggest that integrative couple therapy can be successfully applied to many couples, including those in which a partner has certain other psychological disorders. For example, the preceding predictor study found that indices of mental illness, including Structured Clinical Interview for DSM-IV diagnoses, were *not* related to improvements during couple therapy.

Doss, Thum, Sevier, Atkins, and Christensen (2005) recently analyzed the mechanisms of change in this study of couple therapy. Early in therapy, changes in the frequency of targeted behaviors were associated with increases in satisfaction for both treatment conditions. However, later in therapy, changes in the acceptance of targeted behaviors were associated with increases in satisfaction for both treatment conditions. TBCT generated significantly greater increases than IBCT in targeted behaviors early in treatment. However, IBCT generated significantly greater increases in the acceptance of targeted behaviors throughout treatment. Thus, the study validated some of the putative mechanisms of change and differences between the treatments in their impact on these mechanisms.

Ongoing research is collecting data on couples' outcome 5 years after the end of treatment and will examine the factors that predict this long-term outcome. Current studies are also examining observational data on change in the communication of couples over time and processes of change during couple therapy sessions through observational ratings, as well as linguistic analyses, of these sessions.

CASE STUDY

We use the case example of Anne and Mark[2] to demonstrate the application of IBCT. We have included excerpts from the assessment and feedback sessions, in addition to treatment sessions selected for their effective use of IBCT acceptance-building interventions.[3]

Anne and Mark were a middle-aged couple married for 10 years at treatment onset. Anne had three children from her previous marriage.

Assessment

Session 1

After greetings and introductions, Anne and Mark's therapist (Dr. S) began Session 1 by orienting them to the assessment process as follows:

"We'll be working together for the next 25 sessions. You have already done the first step of the assessment process by completing all of those questionnaires. Your next three visits, including today, will be the second step of the assessment phase. Today I'm meeting with the two of you to get to know your relationship, to hear about your relationship . . . as you share some of the history about meeting and dating, and bring us up until today. Then over the next two visits, I'd like to meet with the two of you individually. After that, at the fourth visit, I'll give you feedback. That's where I'll put together all of the information from the questionnaires and our time together today, as well as our time individually, to paint a picture to present some understanding of what could be going on."

Particularly if the couple expresses hesitation or ambivalence about being in therapy, the therapist should include the following:

"This assessment period is also your opportunity to get to know me and the kind of therapy we'll be doing, so that you can get a feeling for whether this is going to be a good match for your needs right now."

After checking in with Anne and Mark to see whether they understood this explanation, Dr. S elicited from them a brief description of their presenting problems:

"Before we get into your history, maybe you could give me a sense of some of the problems that have been going on that led you to decide, "Let's get some help."

After Mark and Anne took turns describing their side of the problems in the relationship, Dr. S gathered the couple's developmental history, using probing phrases such as the following:

"Let's start at the beginning. Why don't you tell me where and how the two of you met."
"Mark, what was it about Anne that attracted you initially? What about you, Anne?"
"Anne, how could you tell that Mark was interested in you? . . . What kinds of things did he say? . . . How did you flirt with him? Which one of you made the first move?"
"When you decided to go from living together to getting married, how did that happen?"

In the course of their description, Anne and Mark had many opportunities to say complimentary things about the other. Mark described Anne as sensual, a quality that he found very attractive, and Anne described Mark as very nice and easygoing. Dr. S was very thorough and behaviorally specific when eliciting

details of Mark and Anne's courtship, such as the fact that both partners agreed that their first kiss was very good.

Even during this part of the assessment phase, opportunities for building acceptance may present themselves. At one point during Session 1, Anne made a soft disclosure when she discussed a time when she had initially rejected Mark (who had asked her to dance). Anne said that when Mark did not get angry with her after she rejected him, she felt safe with him, because she could be herself and he would not get mad at her. She reported that this quality about Mark attracted her to him. Mark, who had initially reported feeling humiliated by Anne's rejection, responded to Anne's soft disclosure by saying, "I'm kind of surprised by that. I know that is an important feeling for her, but I didn't realize she was feeling that back then." Anne said that she had not realized she felt that way either, until describing the incident in the therapy session.

By the end of Session 1, Dr. S had a good understanding of Anne and Mark's history together, the qualities that first attracted each to the other, and some idea of their problem areas. The next two individual sessions helped Dr. S "fill-in" any missing information that he needed for their formulation.

Sessions 2 and 3

Dr. S introduced these individual sessions with a brief orientation, followed by an introduction to the ongoing assessment of the couple's problem areas:

"There are a lot of different topics that we'll be covering today as we go along. I'd like to spend some time clarifying some of the problems both you and [Anne/Mark] have had. In our first meeting, you described some problems that you've perceived about [problem area]. Can you tell me what you meant by that?"

In addition to the problems that Anne and Mark raised in their conjoint session, Dr. S used the individual sessions to address problem areas that Anne and Mark had indicated on the Frequency and Acceptability of Partner Behavior Questionnaire:

"When I looked over your list of problem areas, the item of most concern to you was [problem area]. Can you describe that to me?"

Dr. S was very specific in his efforts to get Anne and Mark to describe their disagreements and arguments. To encourage Mark and Anne to be behaviorally specific in these descriptions, Dr. S used probing questions:

"Do the two of you have fights about [problem area]? What do those fights look like?"

"When you are both angry, what do *you* tend to do?"

"Describe for me your most recent argument. Describe for me the worst argument you've ever had. If I had a video camera there with you, what would I have seen?"

In addition to understanding their conflict patterns, Dr. S also asked how problems were addressed in Anne's and Mark's families growing up ("How did your own parents deal with conflict?"). This information may be useful in understanding the developmental history and emotional vulnerabilities that each partner brings with him or her into a conflict, and the patterns each may risk repeating or trying to avoid (e.g., physical violence).

When eliciting descriptions of Anne and Mark's arguments, Dr. S also assessed whether the couple had ever engaged in physical violence. This assessment is a critical part of every couple therapy evaluation, and is a major rationale for conducting these individual interviews. A simple direct question is useful here:

"Have your arguments ever led to pushing, shoving, or any type of physical violence?"

If either partner endorses this question, or has indicated violence on a questionnaire such as the Revised Conflict Tactics Scale (CTS), a more thorough assessment of violence should be conducted and appropriate referrals should be made as indicated (Jacobson & Gottman, 1998). In this case example, violence was not an issue for Anne and Mark.[4]

Finally, the individual sessions provide a good opportunity for the therapist to assess each partner's level of commitment to the relationship. This assessment also includes inquiry as to whether one or both partners are en-

gaging in extramarital affairs. Affairs require special treatment in IBCT (Jacobson & Christensen, 1998), which is beyond the scope of this chapter. Fortunately, Anne and Mark's relationship was not troubled by affairs. With Anne and Mark, Dr. S asked:

"On a scale of 1 to 10, how would you rate your level of commitment to [Mark/Anne]?"

By the end of Anne's and Mark's assessment sessions, Dr. S had sufficient information about their problem areas, patterns of conflict (including their history of violence), relevant family history, and level of commitment to come up with their formulation and proceed with their feedback session.

FEEDBACK AND FORMULATION

Session 4

Dr. S began the feedback session by orienting Anne and Mark to what to expect, and also eliciting their participation in giving him feedback about his formulation and description of their problem areas:

"During this session, I'd like to share with you some feedback, as I mentioned in our first session together. I've spent some time looking over your questionnaires, and we've spent some time talking, which has been very helpful in helping me get a better sense of the two of you. As I go along, I'd really like your input, your reactions, because that's an important part of our work together—with you both responding, as opposed to me directing, interjecting any thoughts you have, as well as adding any information that fits or telling me when information doesn't fit."

Dr. S began giving Anne and Mark feedback by explaining the information gathered from questionnaires they completed:

"The measures we gave you were designed to give us a sense of where you are as a couple, in terms of the range of couples from the very happily married to those with "everyday," normal distress, to the other end of the spectrum—couples who are very similar to ones who have divorced. Both of you are in the area of couples who are experiencing distress, couples who would like things to be better. You are both distressed, although Anne reported higher levels of distress."

Dr. S moved on to summarize Anne's and Mark's levels of commitment, which he characterizes as a strength for their work on therapy:

"With regard to commitment, both of you are committed to the relationship, which is very important to both of you. And that is very important in couple work—that in spite of everything that has gone on, there is still the commitment. That is very telling—you've both shown and expressed that."

Dr. S then moved on to summarize the content of Anne and Mark's problem areas. Dr. S had distilled their questionnaire data and their in-session descriptions to the following three basic problem areas:

"So let's talk about the areas of your relationship that are troubling. One area is finances; that tends to be an area of dispute. For you, Anne, feeling resentful sometimes, feeling the burden of the responsibility, and for you Mark, feeling guilty about how things are financially. This area really brings out lots of different feelings—feelings of resentment, feelings of guilt, feelings of burden—and rather than feelings of closeness and togetherness, feelings of control. Does that sound accurate? Are their any other aspects of finances that the two of you can think of?

"The other area I saw was with regard to children—both the topic of Anne's children and the children that you won't have. You both feel very differently about the subject of Anne's children: Anne, you feel like Mark is not involved with your children, and Mark, you feel as though you have not been invited. For you, Mark, the experience of being rejected [by the children] is Anne's fault. This is an area that brings out very strong feelings for both of you, whether it gets expressed directly or not. You may not talk about it, but I definitely got the sense that this is a real pressure cooker for both of you. This is an area that I imagine will come up in different ways, especially with the holidays coming up.

"The third area I saw concerns responsiveness. 'How responsive are you to me?' Whether you are being physical ('You're not responsive enough' or 'You're too responsive'), listening ('Are you listening to me?'), touching, or asking a question, your actions can carry a message of what you want to express, or a feeling that you are having. So part of what we will work on is expressing those feelings you are having. Those may be a surprise for each of you."

Throughout each of his descriptions, Dr. S checked in with Anne and Mark for their feedback about each problem area, and the ways that they might add to his description.

Even during this part of the feedback session, an opportunity for acceptance work presented itself. When Mark discussed his relationship with Anne's children, he was initially making only "hard" disclosures, by describing her children as rude, and only able to talk about themselves. As Mark made such critical statements about Anne's children, Dr. S elicited from Mark some softer disclosures about his emotions with regard to Anne's children:

DR. S: Besides them being rude, what is the feeling you are left with when [Anne's children] don't talk to you?

MARK: The feeling I'm left with is being ignored.

DR. S: Besides being ignored, how did it feel?

MARK: Like I don't matter, like I am only there to serve them.

DR. S: Like you are not a part of the family.

MARK: Yeah. I think I've just resigned myself to hoping that they'll show their love for their mother.

DR. S: So it upsets you that they don't take an interest in their mother? So it isn't just about *you*, you have some feelings about how Anne's sons interact with *her*?

MARK: Yeah, yeah, I do.

DR. S: And that upsets you?

MARK: Yeah, it does. I feel protective. I'd like them to show more appreciation to her. But then, I'd like myself to show more appreciation to her. I don't think I show enough appreciation to her. Maybe they're related . . . it's a reminder of the things *I'm* not doing well.

By moving Mark from criticizing Anne's children and to making softer statements about his feelings, Dr. S gave Mark an unexpected opportunity to make important realizations about his own behavior.

After reviewing their problem areas, Dr. S proceeded to describe the two themes he had observed from his assessment of Anne and Mark:

"It seems to me from what you've both described in your individual sessions, your questionnaires, and even today, there are two themes that come up for you. When I say 'theme,' it's like in our sessions; whatever the topic is for the day, there's usually a theme. The theme is something I'll bring up from time to time. Again, it's clearly something that we'll work on together. It may take a different form, so I want to share it with you to make sure that it's on the mark, OK?

"I think the first theme is that you both have feelings of being unloved and unappreciated. You have an idea of what it means to be loved. You have an idea of what it means to be appreciated. But your definitions are different. And because of those different definitions, because of your different experiences, if something does happen, it leaves you feeling unappreciated and unloved. Within the arguments about finances or children, there is something about that—about feeling unappreciated. How does that sound to you?

"The second theme is that you both have your insecurities. You both have feelings of insecurity, for whatever reason. Some of the arguments, the differences, the conflicts, the big fights, come from that also. That feeling comes up and can create the whole battle. A concrete example is that you, Anne, described feeling insecure about yourself in relation to some of your family members. That affects how you feel about yourself in comparison to other women. Mark, you described feeling insecure about the fact that Anne has not annulled her previous marriage. That may affect how confident you feel in comparison to other men. Again, these feelings of insecurity, feeling not loved, unappreciated—these are the themes."

After Dr. S described each theme and received feedback from Anne and Mark about these themes, he moved on to discuss their polarization process and mutual trap:

"Now, what is what we call the 'trap' that you both get into? You each have different ways of responding to feeling unloved and insecure. The sense that I get is that, Mark, when you start to feel those things, you use distance. The sense I get from you, Anne, is that you become critical. Put the two of you together, and you have a cycle: The feelings come up, Mark gets distant, and Anne gets critical. Mark feels criticism, he gets distant. Anne experiences the distance, she gets critical. Distance, criticism, criticism, distance. That's what we call the trap. It may be that you take turns being critical and distant, and that each response makes the other person feel even more insecure."

After reviewing the polarization process and mutual trap, Dr. S proceeded to explain to Anne and Mark what they can expect from the upcoming therapy sessions:

"So this is what we're going to do in the upcoming weeks, the kinds of things we've talked about today. We'll talk about whatever is going on for the two of you on a given day. It isn't going to be structured in terms of things we *have* to do each day—it's up to you, whatever you bring in.

"What I hope to do is create in here a place of comfort, enough that you can both take risks in opening up, in sharing—sharing some of your reactions, your questions, your experiences. There is a desire for closeness here that is going to take some sharing and some risk taking. Now, there's no guarantee about how the other person is going to react. It may not always be pleasant. But on the other hand, that's the price we have to pay to get there, to open up. You can do some more thinking about this and from week to week we can reformulate, and we'll keep getting a clearer, better picture."

Having set the stage with the formulation, including the themes, polarization process, and mutual trap, Dr. S is prepared to begin work on building acceptance.

Treatment: Building Acceptance

Most of Anne and Mark's subsequent sessions were focused on building acceptance. Below are excerpts from a few sessions in which Dr. S helped Anne and Mark increase acceptance by using techniques such as empathic joining, unified detachment, and tolerance building.

Session 12

The content of this session was about Anne and Mark's search for a condominium, and some of the difficulties they were experiencing. The discussion included Mark's admission that he felt inadequate and insecure, because he did not make enough money for them to afford Anne's dream condo. This led to an opportunity to explore Anne and Mark's theme of insecurity:

MARK: If we settle for a condominium that we don't really want, it will forever be a monument to my inability to get the condo she wants.

DR. S: I'm wondering if there's another part that wonders, "Will I ever really be able to give her what she wants?"

MARK: Yeah. If she married somebody who had a lot of money, she could get whatever condo she wanted.

ANNE: But if you married someone who was gorgeous, who was 20 years younger, you could have a trophy wife, but that's not what happened. (*Both laugh.*)

DR. S: So that may be part of your insecurity, if you looked the way that you experience as "the way he wants things," then maybe he'd be happier.

MARK: (*to Dr. S*) I think that's how she feels about herself at her worst moments. Like maybe all men are attracted to younger women and that you have to harness yourself not to lose what's important to you . . . (*to Anne*) maybe that's how you look at your desire to have your dream condo. How do you keep from saying, "There's that rich lawyer who looks at me all of the time"? . . . (*to Dr. S*) I think that would be a pretty natural thing for her to think about.

This dialogue also reveals the unified detachment Anne and Mark are developing, when they both laugh at Anne's comment about a "trophy wife." What has previously been a very painful subject for Anne is becoming something they can joke about. The discussion then moved to exploring Anne's insecurities about Mark's relationships with other women:

DR. S: So what in your eyes is Mark's ideal "bill"? You made reference to a "bill" that is his ideal.

ANNE: Well, probably someone younger, who is able to have children, someone who plays tennis, who goes running and also cooks and cleans, makes a good living, is very good in bed . . .

DR. S: (*to Mark*) Because this is comparable to the richer man that you view with Anne. (*to Anne*) For you, it's the woman who . . .

ANNE: But that woman's out there. A lot of women are like that.

DR. S: And the way that you see and experience Mark talking to women. And at times you kind of wonder to what extent he enjoys it, and you think it's just a matter of time if you're not willing to live up to it . . .

ANNE: Right, that some other women is going to be able to step right in there without a problem.

DR. S: When the insecurities come up for both of you. For you, Mark, it's the rich man who could come along and provide what Anne longs for, and for you, Anne, it's that you don't compete physically—with the workout—so it's just a matter of time until a woman comes along and decides, "I'm going after him." Anne, can you tell me some of the things Mark does that make you feel threatened?

ANNE: When he makes comments about how attractive a woman is, like I'm one of the guys. When he tells me I'm fat, or makes comments like I have a double chin . . .

DR. S: Which then tells you that you're not cutting it.

ANNE: Yeah.

Dr. S then brought back the subject of condominium buying, and used this as a metaphor for Anne and Mark's concerns about "settling" for less than what they want in making a major commitment:

DR. S: When you make a commitment, whether it's committing to a condo, committing to a relationship—it's settling, you're settling— you're saying "This is it."

ANNE: That's a good way of looking at it. I hadn't thought of that. That's what we're having trouble with . . . the reality that we're not going to get everything that we want. The insecurity, the scariness of making the purchase, is knowing that we're never going to get what we want.

MARK: Part of it is our concern that the next condominium we see is going to be the one we want.

ANNE: Right, it's the condo over the next hill.

MARK: So you have to think about "Is 60% of what we want what we should settle for?" I'm thinking, 60? I was thinking it's more like 90. So I don't know when you're supposed to cut your losses and say we have to go for this—this is what reality dictates.

DR. S: And if we can take it a step further, that might be when you both decided to get married, you both made a settlement. You both start to wonder whether the other settled for 60 or 90%. You wonder "What did I settle for? Did I settle for 60 or 90%?"

MARK: Yeah.

ANNE: Right.

DR. S: Now let's put yourselves in a situation where you're insecure. What's gonna happen? When you're in an insecure place, that 90% might feel like . . .

ANNE: 50%.

DR. S: Exactly. When you're feeling good, you think, "She got 90% of what she wanted in me," or "I got 90%." But when you're in an insecure place, you think "I settled for 50%." Then when you look at your own insecurity, you think, "My God, she settled for 35 or 40%." You both made a settlement when you married each other. You decided, "This is it, we're gonna get married," and you settled.

MARK: But "settled" has such negative connotations.

DR. S: I think there's some feelings associated with that. And a parallel to the word "settlement" is "acceptance."

MARK: Oh, I see.

DR. S: When you go through the settlement, you think "This is who this person is." Whether it's 90, 80, 60, or 35%, you've settled—you've basically said, "I accept this."

By using condominium buying as a metaphor, Dr. S has underscored how Anne and Mark's theme of insecurity feeds itself, and how it leads them both to question whether each has "settled" for less than he or she wanted in the relationship. Adding the additional component of "insecurity about settlement" to their theme helped Anne and Mark understand the things each of them do that "threaten" the other (e.g., when Mark talks about his attraction to younger women), and also build a bridge toward working on acceptance.

Session 17

In this session, Dr. S continues to process the theme of insecurity with Anne and Mark. In this particular part of the dialogue, when Anne and Mark are discussing a familiar polarization process, Mark suggests to Anne that she work out more. Anne interprets Mark's suggestion as a criticism about her appearance, which makes her feel insecure and threatened. Anne then "fights back" against Mark's suggestions by becoming depressed and "doing nothing," which in turn makes Mark more critical of her.

Here Dr. S uses two IBCT acceptance-building techniques. The first technique is empathic joining. As Dr. S tries to "get to the bottom of" Mark's suggestions/criticisms of Anne's appearance, Mark makes the following soft disclosure about his own insecurities:

DR. S: This is a real, central question. There are some basic limits that you have, where you say, "Up to here, I accept you, but beyond that, you'd better change." On the other hand, this is who you are. *This is who you are.* But the irony of it is, that once we accept, change can come about. But there's that push to determine within ourselves not only other person's limits but also our own. I get the sense that you're both exploring yourselves and your own limits.

ANNE: Perhaps, yes.

DR. S: You're both looking at your own limits. With you, Anne, it's about your looks, your appearance. And for you, Mark, it's about you as a financial provider. And the temptation is, when that gets uncomfortable, that's where your partner comes in kind of, to redirect your focus from that versus being able to talk about how you're feeling.

ANNE: Yeah.

MARK: Yeah, I think I've noticed, since we've started therapy, that's what I do. When I get insecure about myself, I start looking outwards, saying, "You should do this," and that makes me feel better.

DR. S: Right, it's active, it can be advice giving—it can be a real male thing, "Do this, do that."

MARK: Right, I do that with her kids, too. I know I do.

Instead of focusing on the critical nature of Mark's suggestions, Dr. S has placed an emphasis on *why* Mark becomes critical. Mark is encouraged to consider the *reasons* for his behavior, and as a result he discloses that he becomes critical when he himself is feeling insecure. Mark recognizes that this happens not only with regard to his attempts to direct Anne's behavior but also in his interactions with Anne's children.

The second acceptance-building technique Dr. S uses in this portion of the session is a tolerance intervention: emphasizing the positive aspects of a partner's negative behavior. Dr. S continues:

DR. S: In some situations it might work really well [to give advice]. People might like that—like in your work as a counselor, Mark. You feel really productive.

MARK: Yeah, I change people's lives. I know I do.

DR. S: On the other hand, there might be some circumstances where it's experienced as being critical, and I think of this in terms of the two of you. It feeds in to Anne's feeling criticized.

ANNE: Yes.

DR. S: And then it feels threatening, like "If you don't do something about it, then . . . "

Here Dr. S has positively reemphasized Mark's suggestions to Anne as his attempts to give her guidance or advice. Mark, an employment counselor, is used to giving such suggestions to others as way of being constructive or helpful. Dr. S underscores this aspect of Mark's behavior—that this same "counselor" quality makes Mark very good at what he does in his career. However, Dr. S does not try to reframe

Mark's behavior as *completely* positive. Dr. S also underscores how Mark's "advice" is experienced by Anne as critical and threatening.

At the end of the session, Dr. S recharacterizes Anne and Mark's polarization process in terms of the information that has emerged from these two interventions:

DR. S: I think you put it really well, Mark. When you start to feel uncomfortable, this is your process, this is what you do. You start to look outside yourself. From your end, it might be like you're being a counselor when you start with Anne. You want to advise. But from her end, it might be like you're being authoritarian, the drill sergeant, rather than the counselor. And you, Anne, start to feel you're being berated. You start to feel worse about yourself.

ANNE: Yeah.

DR. S: So you feel like you've gotta either take it, or you've gotta fight back.

MARK: I think I can . . . the fighting back is . . . well, I can understand that. I really can.

Session 25

In their final session, Anne described a recent insight she had had about feeling "undeserving" of happiness, and her belief that happiness comes at a cost of some kind. She said that happiness made her feel guilty, because she felt that someone else must be suffering for her happiness, or that somehow she would suffer negative repercussions for being happy. Anne connected some of these feelings to her bout with an eating disorder as a teenager, and to the depressive episodes she sometimes experienced as an adult.

In the dialogue below, Dr. S uses several IBCT techniques to discuss Anne's insights and the way that her feelings contribute to the couple's polarization process. First, Dr. S uses empathic joining to help Mark understand the experience Anne is having when she gets depressed (a time when Mark regularly makes suggestions about how Anne "should" think, feel, or behave). Then Dr. S detaches Anne and Mark from their problem—that Anne feels criticized whenever Mark makes these suggestions. Rather than engaging Anne and Mark in their emotional responses to each other's behavior, Dr. S framed this problem as a consequence of basic communication problems. By describing their problem in terms of their methods of communication, Dr. S detaches Anne and Mark from the problem itself, and provides each with a new way of reacting to an old problem (without doing any formal communication training):

DR. S: I think the idea around the conflict over happiness—having the happiness—is like savoring a good meal, and that it will cost you: "OK, so it has some high fat, but I'm going to enjoy it because I deserve this, I deserve this moment—the same way that I deserve this moment of happiness, even if so-and-so doesn't have it together. I deserve this happiness." And that's going to be the struggle, to be able to react to Mark in a way that expresses, "God, I'm really feeling guilty."

ANNE: When I'm on the couch, and I'm totally immobile in my depression, that's a lot of what's going on. I'm beating myself up.

DR. S: And so Mark needs to listen, to just *listen* and say, "Gee, that must be really hard." Now there may be a pull, Mark, to problem-solve, to say, "Well, you shouldn't feel that way," or "So-and-so is that way because . . . ," but that will only bring out Anne's self-criticism and could become argumentative. When you sense the pain, Mark, and what it's costing Anne, the reaction that you have is "Let me show you what to do." But that is only going to bring out in Anne the feeling of "You see, you idiot, you're not doing it right," which will then feed into the self-criticism. So it's going to help to just listen, and simply to paraphrase, and she will hear that it's not reasonable. If, rather than criticizing, you just say, "Gee, you really don't feel worthy of these things," if you just paraphrase those themes of her insecurity, her self-criticalness, that is kind of maintaining a connection.

Finally, Dr. S uses tolerance interventions to allow Anne and Mark to see their problem as a difference in their communication styles. As he continues to describe their problem in terms of communication difficulties, Dr. S describes Anne as responding to situations based on how she *feels*, while Mark is more likely to use logic or *reason* to determine his responses to situations. Dr. S also points out how Anne and Mark's problem is often a result of this differ-

ence, and that these differences actually compliment one another:

DR. S: (*to Mark*) And that's what I want to encourage, maybe a new way of responding rather than using *reason* when you start to feel like Anne's feelings don't make sense. Rather than saying, "This doesn't make sense," say instead, "What I'm hearing you say is that you don't deserve this"—whatever it is. And what I'm expecting, Anne, is that to hear Mark express that he understands you would make you feel close to him.

ANNE: Yeah, and it would definitely not be the wedge of "you should." (*Mark laughs.*)

DR. S: Anne, you talk about things from the emotional experience, and Mark, you talk about things from the rational experience—and both are needed, both are important.

This section of the dialogue also reveals how Anne and Mark have developed unified detachment from their problem. Anne uses the phrase "the wedge of 'you should' " to describe what had previously been the "hot topic" of feeling criticized by Mark, and Mark is able to laugh about his own behavior.

CONCLUSION

Although a single case study is useful for illustrative purposes, it obviously does not establish generalizable conclusions about treatment outcome. However, the studies we have described give some promising results for the efficacy of IBCT. The major clinical trial we described earlier, in which Anne and Mark participated, is still ongoing in its 5-year follow-up. This study will provide more definitive information about the long-term impact of IBCT in the treatment of serious and chronic couple distress.

IBCT is part of what Hayes (2004) has called the "third wave" of behavior therapy. The "first wave" encompassed traditional classical and operant conditioning approaches. The "second wave" incorporated cognitive strategies. The third wave emphasizes "contextual and experiential change strategies in addition to more direct and didactic ones" (quoted in Hayes, 2004, p. 6). Acceptance and mindfulness are key aspects of these third-wave therapies. Although these therapies have generated considerable enthusiasm and confirming data, only additional outcome research will establish whether these therapies in general or IBCT in particular will work to alleviate human suffering, including the substantial suffering that occurs in couple relationships, in more powerful ways than the first two waves of behavior therapy.

NOTES

1. We use the more inclusive term "couple therapy" rather than the more limited term "marital therapy," because the term "couple therapy" can refer to unmarried couples, gay and lesbian couples, and married couples.
2. Identifying information has been changed to protect confidentiality, but clinical dynamics are accurately portrayed and quotations are taken directly from tapes of the therapy sessions but altered slightly to increase readability.
3. Not included here are case examples of the application of TBCT interventions, which can be found elsewhere (e.g., Cordova & Jacobson, 1993; Jacobson & Margolin, 1979).
4. In our project we assessed for violence using the CTS and excluded any couple in which the wife reported moderate to severe violence from the husband. We excluded the couple prior to their seeing one of our project therapists and we referred the couple to appropriate individual treatment for violence. Dr. S could proceed with the knowledge that the wife had not endorsed this kind of violence from her husband on the CTS (although she could still do so in the individual session). In a clinical setting, we recommend that practitioners give the CTS to all clients and follow up with individual sessions, where they focus specifically on violent items that the individual has endorsed as committing or receiving on the CTS. Based on these interviews, the practitioner should refer clients when appropriate (Jacobson & Gottman, 1998).

REFERENCES

Atkins, D. C., Berns, S. B., George, W., Doss, B., Gattis, K., & Christensen, A. (2005). Prediction of response to treatment in a randomized clinical trial of marital therapy. *Journal of Consulting and Clinical Psychology*, 73, 893–903.

Baucom, D. H., & Epstein, N. (1990). *Cognitive behavioral marital therapy*. New York: Brunner/Mazel.

Baucom, D. H., Epstein, N., & Rankin, L. A. (1995). Cognitive aspects of cognitive behavioral marital therapy. In N. S. Jacobson & A. S. Gurman (Eds.),

Clinical handbook of couple therapy (pp. 65–90). New York: Guilford Press.

Baucom, D. H., & Hoffman, J. A. (1986). The effectiveness of marital therapy: Current status and application to the clinical setting. In N. S. Jacobson & A. S. Gurman (Eds.), *Clinical handbook of marital therapy* (pp. 597–620). New York: Guilford Press.

Baucom, D. H., Shoham, V. M., Kim, T., Daiuto, A. D., & Stickle, T. R. (1998). Empirically supported couple and family interventions for marital distress and adult mental health problems. *Journal of Consulting and Clinical Psychology*, 66(1), 53–88.

Beach, S. R. H., Wamboldt, M. Z., Kaslow, N. J., Heyman, R. E., First, M. B., Underwood, L. G., et al. (2006). *Relational processes and DSM-V: Neuroscience, assessment, prevention, and treatment*. Washington, DC: American Psychiatric Publishing.

Buehler, C., Anthony, C., Krishnakumar, A., Stone, G., Gerard, J., & Pemberton, S. (1997). Interparental conflict and youth problems behaviors: A meta-analysis. *Journal of Child and Family Studies*, 6, 233–247.

Burman, B., & Margolin, G. (1992). Analysis of the association between marital relationships and health problems: An interactional perspective. *Psychological Bulletin*, 112, 39–63.

Christensen, A., Atkins, D. C., Berns, S., Wheeler, J., Baucom, D. H., & Simpson, L. E. (2004). Traditional versus integrative behavioral couple therapy for significantly and chronically distressed married couples. *Journal of Consulting and Clinical Psychology*, 72, 176–191.

Christensen, A., Atkins, D. C., Yi, J., Baucom, D. H., & George, W. H. (2006). Couple and individual adjustment for two years following a randomized clinical trial comparing traditional versus integrative behavioral couple therapy. *Journal of Consulting and Clinical Psychology*, 74, 1180–1191.

Christensen, A., & Heavey, C. L. (1999). Interventions for couples. *Annual Review of Psychology*, 50, 65–102.

Christensen, A., & Jacobson, N. S. (1997). *Frequency and Acceptability of Partner Behavior Inventory: Unpublished measures*. University of California, Los Angeles.

Christensen, A., & Jacobson, N. S. (2000). *Reconcilable differences*. New York: Guilford Press.

Christensen, A., Jacobson, N. S., & Babcock, J. C. (1995). Integrative behavioral couple therapy. In N. S. Jacobson & A. S. Gurman (Eds.), *Clinical handbook of couple therapy* (pp. 31–64). New York: Guilford Press.

Cordova, J., & Jacobson, N. S. (1993). Couple distress. In D. H. Barlow (Ed.), *Clinical handbook of psychological disorders* (2nd ed.). New York: Guilford Press.

Crane, D. R., & Mead, D. E. (1980). The Marital Status Inventory: Some preliminary data on an instrument to measure marital dissolution potential. *American Journal of Family Therapy*, 8(3), 31–35.

Doss, B. D., & Christensen, A. (2006). Acceptance in romantic relationships: The Frequency and Acceptability of Partner Behavior Inventory. *Psychological Assessment*, *18*, 289–302.

Doss, B. D., Thum, Y. M., Sevier, M., Atkins, D. C., & Christensen, A. (2005). Improving relationships: Mechanisms of change in couple therapy. *Journal of Consulting and Clinical Psychology*, *73*, 624–633.

Epstein, N., & Baucom, D. H. (2002). *Enhanced cognitive-behavioral therapy for couples: A contextual approach*. Washington, DC: American Psychological Association.

Floyd, F. J., & Markman, H. J. (1983). Observational biases in spouse observation: Toward a cognitive/behavioral model of marriage. *Journal of Consulting and Clinical Psychology*, *51*, 450–457.

Floyd, F. J., Markman, H. J., Kelly, S., Blumberg, S. L., & Stanley, S. M. (1995). Preventive intervention and relationship enhancement. In N. S. Jacobson & A. S. Gurman (Eds.), *Clinical handbook of couple therapy* (pp. 212–230). New York: Guilford Press.

Gottman, J., Notarius, C., Gonso, J., & Markman, H. (1976). *A couple's guide to communication*. Champaign, IL: Research Press.

Gurman, A. S., Knickerson, D. P., & Pinsoff, W. M. (1986). Research on the process and outcome of marital and family therapy. In S. L. Garfield & A. E. Bergin (Eds.), *Handbook of psychotherapy and behavior change* (3rd ed., pp. 565–624). New York: Wiley.

Hahlweg, K., Schindler, L., Revenstorf, D., & Brengelmann, J. C. (1984). The Munich Marital Therapy Study. In K. Hahlweg & N. S. Jacobson (Eds.), *Marital interaction: Analysis and modification* (pp. 3–26). New York: Guilford Press.

Halford, W. K. (2001). *Brief therapy for couples: Helping partners help themselves*. New York: Guilford Press.

Hayes, S. C. (2004). Acceptance and commitment therapy and the new behavior therapies. In S. C. Hayes, V. M. Follette, & M. M. Linehan (Eds.), *Mindfulness and acceptance: Expanding the cognitive-behavioral tradition* (pp. 1–29). New York: Guilford Press.

Holtzworth-Munroe, A., & Jacobson, N. S. (1991). Behavioral marital therapy. In A. S. Gurman & D. P. Knickerson (Eds.), *Handbook of family therapy* (2nd ed., pp. 96–133). New York: Brunner/Mazel.

Jacobson, N. S. (1977). Problem solving and contingency contracting in the treatment of marital discord. *Journal of Consulting and Clinical Psychology*, *45*, 92–100.

Jacobson, N. S. (1978a). A review of the research on the effectiveness of marital therapy. In T. J. Paolino & B. S. McGrady (Eds.), *Marriage and marital therapy: Psychoanalytic, behavioral, and systems theory perspectives* (pp. 395–444). New York: Brunner/Mazel.

Jacobson, N. S. (1978b). Specific and nonspecific factors in the effectiveness of a behavioral approach to the treatment of marital discord. *Journal of Consulting and Clinical Psychology*, *46*, 442–452.

Jacobson, N. S. (1984). A component analysis of behavioral marital therapy: The relative effectiveness of behavior exchange and problem solving training. *Journal of Consulting and Clinical Psychology*, *52*, 295–305.

Jacobson, N. S., & Addis, M. E. (1993). Research on couple therapy: What do we know? Where are we going? *Journal of Consulting and Clinical Psychology*, *61*, 85–93.

Jacobson, N. S., & Christensen, A. (1998). *Acceptance and change in couple therapy: A therapist's guide to transforming relationships*. New York: Norton.

Jacobson, N. S., Christensen, A., Prince, S. E., Cordova, J., & Eldridge, K. (2000). Integrative behavioral couple therapy: An acceptance-based, promising new treatment for couple discord. *Journal of Consulting and Clinical Psychology*, *68*(2), 351–355.

Jacobson, N. S., Follette, W. C., & Pagel, M. (1986). Predicting who will benefit from behavioral marital therapy. *Journal of Consulting and Clinical Psychology*, *54*, 518–522.

Jacobson, N. S., Follette, W. S., Revenstorf, D., Baucom, D. H., Hahlweg, K., & Margolin, G. (1984). Variability in outcome and clinical significance of behavior marital therapy: A reanalysis of outcome data. *Journal of Consulting and Clinical Psychology*, *52*, 497–564.

Jacobson, N. S., & Gottman, J. (1998). *When men batter women: New insights into ending abusive relationships*. New York: Simon & Schuster.

Jacobson, N. S., & Holtzworth-Munroe, A. (1986). Marital therapy: A social learning/cognitive perspective. In N. S. Jacobson & A. S. Gurman (Eds.), *Clinical handbook of marital therapy* (pp. 29–70). New York: Guilford Press.

Jacobson, N. S., & Margolin, G. (1979). *Marital therapy: Strategies based on social learning and behavior exchange principles*. New York: Brunner/Mazel.

Jacobson, N. S., Schmaling, K. B., & Holtzworth-Munroe, A. (1987). Component analysis of behavioral marital therapy: Two-year follow-up and prediction of relapse. *Journal of Marital and Family Therapy*, *13*, 187–195.

Knox, D. (1971). *Marital happiness: A behavioral approach to counseling*. Champaign, IL: Research Press.

Liberman, R. P. (1970). Behavioral approaches to family and couple therapy. *American Journal of Orthopsychiatry*, *40*, 106–118.

Liberman, R. P., Wheeler, E. G., deVisser, L. A., Kuehnel, J., & Kuehnel, T. (1981). *Handbook of marital therapy: A positive approach to helping troubled relationships*. New York: Plenum Press.

Simpson, L. E., Doss, B. D., Wheeler, J., & Christensen, A. (2007). Relationship violence among couples seeking therapy: Common couple violence or battering? *Journal of Marital and Family Therapy, 33,* 270–283.

Skinner, B. F. (1966). *The behavior of organisms: An experimental analysis.* Englewood Cliffs, NJ: Prentice Hall.

Snyder, D. K., Castellani, A. M., & Whisman, M. A. (2006). Current status and future directions for couple therapy. *Annual Review of Psychology, 57,* 317–344.

Snyder, D. K., Wills, R. M., & Grady-Fletcher, A. (1991). Long-term effectiveness of behavioral versus insight-oriented marital therapy: A 4-year follow-up study. *Journal of Consulting and Clinical Psychology, 59,* 138–141.

Spanier, G. B. (1976). Measuring dyadic adjustment: New scales for assessing the quality of marriage and similar dyads. *Journal of Marriage and the Family, 38,* 15–28.

Straus, M. A., Hamby, S. L., Boney-McCoy, S., & Sugarman, D. B. (1996). The Revised conflict tactics scales (CTS2): Development and preliminary psychometric data. *Journal of Family Issues, 17*(3), 283–316.

Stuart, R. B. (1969). Operant interpersonal treatment for marital discord. *Journal of Consulting and Clinical Psychology, 33,* 675–682.

Stuart, R. B. (1980). *Helping couples change: A social learning approach to marital therapy.* New York: Guilford Press.

Weiss, R. L., & Cerreto, M. C. (1980). The Marital Status Inventory: Development of a measure of dissolution potential. *American Journal of Family Therapy, 8*(2), 80–85.

Weiss, R. L., Hops, H., & Patterson, G. R. (1973). A framework for conceptualizing marital conflict, technology for altering it, some data for evaluating it. In L. A. Hamerlynck, L. C. Handy, & E. J. Mash (Eds.), *Behavior change: Methodology, concepts, and practice* (pp. 309–342). Champaign, IL: Research Press.

Whisman, M. A. (1999). Marital dissatisfaction and psychiatric disorders: Results from the national comorbidity survey. *Journal of Abnormal Psychology, 108,* 701–706.

Whisman, M. S., & Bruce, M. L. (1999). Marital dissatisfaction and incidence of major depressive episode in a community sample. *Journal of Abnormal Psychology, 108,* 674–678.

Wimberly, J. D. (1998). An outcome study of integrative couples therapy delivered in a group format. (Doctoral dissertation, University of Montana, 1997). *Dissertation Abstracts International: Section B: The Sciences and Engineering, 58*(12-B), 6832.

Author Index

Subject Index

Page numbers followed by *f* indicate figure, *t* indicate table.